Clinically Oriented ANATOMY

Seventh Edition

MOORE

Clinically Oriented
ANATOMY

Seventh Edition

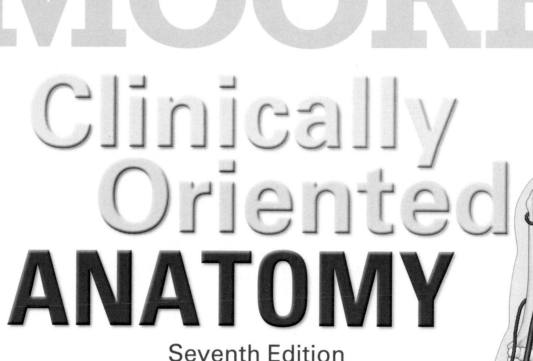

Keith L. Moore, M.Sc., Ph.D., D.Sc. (Hon), F.I.A.C., F.R.S.M., F.A.A.A.

Professor Emeritus in Division of Anatomy, Department of Surgery
Former Chair of Anatomy and Associate
Dean for Basic Medical Sciences
Faculty of Medicine, University of Toronto
Toronto, Ontario, Canada

Arthur F. Dalley II, Ph.D.

Professor, Department of Cell and Developmental Biology
Adjunct Professor, Department of Orthopaedics and Rehabilitation
Director, Programs in Medical Gross Anatomy and Anatomical Donations Program
Vanderbilt University School of Medicine
Adjunct Professor for Anatomy
Belmont University School of Physical Therapy
Nashville, Tennessee, U.S.A.

Anne M. R. Agur, B.Sc. (OT), M.Sc., Ph.D.

Professor, Division of Anatomy, Department of Surgery, Faculty of Medicine
Department of Physical Therapy
Department of Occupational Science & Occupational Therapy
Division of Physiatry, Department of Medicine
Division of Biomedical Communications
Institute of Medical Science
Graduate Department of Rehabilitation Science
Graduate Department of Dentistry
University of Toronto
Toronto, Ontario, Canada

. Wolters Kluwer | Lippincott Williams & Wilkins
Health

Philadelphia · Baltimore · New York · London
Buenos Aires · Hong Kong · Sydney · Tokyo

Acquisitions Editor: Crystal Taylor
Product Manager: Julie Montalbano
Marketing Manager: Joy Fisher Williams
Art Director, Digital Content: Jennifer Clements
Artists: Imagineeringart.com, lead artist Natalie Intven, MSc, BMC
Designer: Terry Mallon
Compositor: SPi Global

7th Edition

Copyright © 2014, 2010, 2006, 1999, 1992, 1985, 1980 Lippincott Williams & Wilkins, a Wolters Kluwer business.

351 West Camden Street   **Two Commerce Square**
Baltimore, MD 21201   **2001 Market Street**
                                 Philadelphia, PA 19103

Printed in China

All rights reserved. This book is protected by copyright. No part of this book may be reproduced or transmitted in any form or by any means, including as photocopies or scanned-in or other electronic copies, or utilized by any information storage and retrieval system without written permission from the copyright owner, except for brief quotations embodied in critical articles and reviews. Materials appearing in this book prepared by individuals as part of their official duties as U.S. government employees are not covered by the above-mentioned copyright. To request permission, please contact Lippincott Williams & Wilkins at Two Commerce Square, 2001 Market Street, Philadelphia, PA 19103, via email at permissions@lww.com, or via website at lww.com (products and services).

9 8 7 6 5 4 3 2 1

5th edition:
Italian Translation, 2008, published by Casa Editrice Ambrosiana
Portuguese Translation, 2007, published by Editora Guanabara Koogan
French Translation, 2007, published by DeBoeck Universite
Spanish Translation, 2007, published by Editorial Medica Panamericana, S.A.
Japanese Translation, 2008, published by MEDSI
Indonesian Translation, 2009, published by Penerbit Erlangga
Serbian Translation, 2009, published by Romanov Publishing Group
Korean Translation, 2009, published by Shin Heung
Complex Chinese Translation, 2009, published by The Leader Book Company
Macedonian Translation, 2010, published by Tabernakul Publishing
Albanian Translation, 2010, published by Tabernakul Publishing

6th edition:
Portuguese Translation, 2011, published by Editora Guanabara Koogan
French Translation, 2011, published by Deboeck Universite
Spanish Translation, 2010, published by Wolters Kluwer Spanish Language Program

Library of Congress Cataloging-in-Publication Data
Moore, Keith L.
   Clinically oriented anatomy / Keith L. Moore, Arthur F. Dalley, Anne M.R. Agur. — 7th ed.
   p. ; cm.
   Includes bibliographical references and index.
   ISBN 978-1-4511-1945-9 (pbk. : alk. paper)
 I. Dalley, Arthur F. II. Agur, A. M. R. III. Title.
 [DNLM: 1. Anatomy.   QS 4]

 612—dc23

 2012041233

DISCLAIMER

Care has been taken to confirm the accuracy of the information presented and to describe generally accepted practices. However, the authors, editors, and publisher are not responsible for errors or omissions or for any consequences from application of the information in this book and make no warranty, expressed or implied, with respect to the currency, completeness, or accuracy of the contents of the publication. Application of this information in a particular situation remains the professional responsibility of the practitioner; the clinical treatments described and recommended may not be considered absolute and universal recommendations.

The authors, editors, and publisher have exerted every effort to ensure that drug selection and dosage set forth in this text are in accordance with the current recommendations and practice at the time of publication. However, in view of ongoing research, changes in government regulations, and the constant flow of information relating to drug therapy and drug reactions, the reader is urged to check the package insert for each drug for any change in indications and dosage and for added warnings and precautions. This is particularly important when the recommended agent is a new or infrequently employed drug.

Some drugs and medical devices presented in this publication have Food and Drug Administration (FDA) clearance for limited use in restricted research settings. It is the responsibility of the healthcare provider to ascertain the FDA status of each drug or device planned for use in their clinical practice.

To purchase additional copies of this book, call our customer service department at **(800) 638-3030** or fax orders to **(301) 223-2320**. International customers should call **(301) 223-2300**.

Visit Lippincott Williams & Wilkins on the Internet: http://www.lww.com. Lippincott Williams & Wilkins customer service representatives are available from 8:30 am to 6:00 pm, EST.

The publishers have made every effort to trace the copyright holders for borrowed material. If they have inadvertently overlooked any, they will be pleased to make the necessary arrangements at the first opportunity.

CCS0113

In Loving Memory of Marion

My best friend, wife, colleague, mother of our five children and grandmother of our nine grandchildren for her love, unconditional support, and understanding. Wonderful memories keep you in our hearts and minds. • (KLM)

To Pam and Ron

I am grateful to my eldest daughter Pam, who assumed the office duties her mother previously carried out. She is also helpful in many other ways. I am also grateful to my son-in-law Ron Crowe whose technical skills have helped me prepare the manuscript for this book. • (KLM)

To My Grandchildren

Melissa, Kristin, Alecia, Lauren, Mitchel, Caitin, Jayme, Courtney and Brooke. With best wishes for your future endeavours. Love, Grandpa • (KLM)

To Muriel

My bride, best friend, counselor, and mother of our sons; and to our family—Tristan, Lana, Elijah, Finley and Sawyer; Denver, and Skyler—with love and great appreciation for their support, understanding, good humor, and—most of all—patience. • (AFD)

To my husband, Enno, and my children, Erik and Kristina, for their support and encouragement. • (AMRA)

To Our Students

You will remember some of what you hear, much of what you read, more of what you see, and almost all of what you experience and understand fully.

To Anatomical Donors

With sincere appreciation to all those who donate their bodies for anatomical study and research, without whom anatomical textbooks and atlases, and anatomical study in general would not be possible.

**Keith L. Moore, Ph.D.,
D.Sc. (Hon)., F.I.A.C.,
F.R.S.M., F.A.A.A.**

Dr. Moore has been the recipient of many prestigious awards and recognitions. He has received the highest awards for excellence in human anatomy education at the medical, dental, graduate, and undergraduate levels—and for his remarkable record of textbook publications in clinically oriented anatomy and embryology—from both the American Association of Anatomists (AAA: Distinguished Educator Award, 2007) and the American Association of Clinical Anatomists (AACA: Honored Member Award, 1994). In 2008 Dr. Moore was inducted as a Fellow of the American Association of Anatomists. The rank of Fellow honors distinguished members who have demonstrated excellence in science and their overall contributions to the medical sciences. In 2012, Dr. Moore received an honorary Doctor of Science degree from The Ohio State University, the Queen Elizabeth II Diamond Jubilee Medal honoring significant contributions and achievements by Canadians, and the R. Benton Adkins, Jr. Distinguished Service Award for his outstanding record of service to the American Association of Clinical Anatomists.

Arthur F. Dalley II

Arthur F. Dalley II, Ph.D.

**Anne M. R. Agur, B.Sc.
(OT), M.Sc., Ph.D.**

Preface

A third of a century has passed since the first edition of *Clinically Oriented Anatomy* appeared on bookstore shelves. Although the factual basis of anatomy is remarkable among basic sciences for its longevity and consistency, this book has evolved markedly since its inception. This is a reflection of changes in the clinical application of anatomy, new imaging technologies that reveal living anatomy in new ways, and improvements in graphic and publication technology that enable superior demonstration of this information. Efforts continue to make this book even more student friendly and authoritative. The seventh edition has been thoroughly reviewed by students, anatomists, and clinicians for accuracy and relevance and revised with significant new changes and updates.

KEY FEATURES

Clinically Oriented Anatomy has been widely acclaimed for the relevance of its clinical correlations. As in previous editions, the seventh edition places clinical emphasis on anatomy that is important in physical diagnosis for primary care, interpretation of diagnostic imaging, and understanding the anatomical basis of emergency medicine and general surgery. Special attention has been directed toward assisting students in learning the anatomy they will need to know in the twenty-first century, and to this end new features have been added and existing features updated.

Extensive art program. The seventh edition is distinguished by an extensive revision of the art program. Working with a team of artists from Imagineering, every illustration has been revised, improving accuracy and consistency and giving classical art derived from *Grant's Atlas of Anatomy* a fresh, vital, new appearance. An effort has been made to ensure that all the anatomy presented and covered in the text is also illustrated. The text and illustrations have been developed to work together for optimum pedagogical effect, aiding the learning process and markedly reducing the amount of searching required to find structures. The great majority of the clinical conditions are supported by photographs and/or color illustrations; multipart illustrations often combine dissections, line art, and medical images; tables are accompanied by illustrations to aid the student's understanding of the structures described.

Clinical correlations. Popularly known as "blue boxes," the clinical information sections have grown, and many of them are supported by photographs and/or dynamic color illustrations to help with understanding the practical value of anatomy. In response to our readers' suggestions, the blue boxes have been grouped together within chapters, enabling presentation of topics with less interruption of the running text.

Bottom line summaries. Frequent "bottom line" boxes summarize the preceding information, ensuring that primary concepts do not become lost in the many details necessary for thorough understanding. These summaries provide a convenient means of ongoing review and underscore the big picture point of view.

Anatomy described in a practical, functional context. A more realistic approach to the musculoskeletal system emphasizes the action and use of muscles and muscle groups in daily activities, emphasizing gait and grip. The eccentric contraction of muscles, which accounts for much of their activity, is now discussed along with the concentric contraction that is typically the sole focus in anatomy texts. This perspective is important to most health professionals, including the growing number of physical and occupational therapy students using this book.

Surface anatomy and medical imaging. Surface anatomy and medical imaging, formerly presented separately, are now integrated into the chapter, presented at the time each region is being discussed, clearly demonstrating anatomy's relationship to physical examination and diagnosis. Both natural views of unobstructed surface anatomy and illustrations superimposing anatomical structures on surface anatomy photographs are components of each regional chapter. Medical images, focusing on normal anatomy, include plain and contrast radiographic, MRI, CT, and ultrasonography studies, often with correlative line art as well as explanatory text, to help prepare future professionals who need to be familiar with diagnostic images.

Case studies, accompanied by clinico-anatomical problems and board review-style multiple-choice questions. Interactive case studies and multiple-choice questions are available to our readers online at http://thePoint.lww.com, providing a convenient and comprehensive means of self-testing and review.

Terminology. The terminology fully adheres to *Terminologia Anatomica* (1998), approved by the International Federation of Associations of Anatomists (IFAA). Although the official English-equivalent terms are used throughout the book, when new terms are introduced, the Latin form, used in Europe, Asia, and other parts of the world, is also provided.

The roots and derivations of terms are provided to help students understand meaning and increase retention. Eponyms, although not endorsed by the IFAA, appear in parentheses in this edition—for example, sternal angle (angle of Louis)—to assist students who will hear eponymous terms during their clinical studies. The terminology is now available online at http://www.unifr.ch/ifaa.

RETAINED AND IMPROVED FEATURES

Students and faculty have told us what they want and expect from *Clinically Oriented Anatomy,* and we listened:

- A *comprehensive text* enabling students to fill in the blanks, as time allotted for lectures continues to decrease, laboratory guides become exclusively instructional, and multiauthored lecture notes develop inconsistencies in comprehension, fact, and format.
- A *resource capable of supporting areas of special interest and emphasis* within specific anatomy courses that *serves the anatomy needs of students during both the basic science and the clinical phases of their studies.*
- A *thorough Introduction* that covers important systemic information and concepts basic to the understanding of the anatomy presented in the subsequent regional chapters. Students from many countries and backgrounds have written to express their views of this book—gratifyingly, most are congratulatory. Health professional students have more diverse backgrounds and experiences than ever before. Curricular constraints often result in unjustified assumptions concerning the prerequisite information necessary for many students to understand the presented material. The Introduction includes efficient summaries of functional systemic anatomy. Students' comments specifically emphasized the need for a systemic description of the nervous system and the peripheral autonomic nervous system (ANS) in particular.
- Routine facts (such as muscle attachments, innervations, and actions) presented in *tables organized to demonstrate shared qualities and illustrated to demonstrate the provided information. Clinically Oriented Anatomy* provides more tables than any other anatomy textbook.
- *Illustrated clinical correlations* that not only describe but also *show anatomy as it is applied clinically.*
- *Illustrations that facilitate orientation.* Many orientation figures have been added, along with arrows to indicate the locations of the inset figures (areas shown in close-up views) and viewing sequences. Labels have been placed to minimize the distance between label and object, with leader lines running the most direct course possible.

- Blue boxes are classified by the following icons to indicate the type of clinical information covered:

Anatomical variations. These blue boxes feature anatomical variations that may be encountered in the dissection lab or in practice, emphasizing the clinical importance of awareness of such variations.

Life cycle. These blue boxes emphasize prenatal developmental factors that affect postnatal anatomy and anatomical phenomena specifically associated with stages of life—childhood, adolescence, adult, and advanced age.

Trauma. The effect of traumatic events—such as fractures of bones or dislocations of joints—on normal anatomy and the clinical manifestations and dysfunction resulting from such injuries are featured in these blue boxes.

Diagnostic procedures. Anatomical features and observations that play a role in physical diagnosis are targeted in these blue boxes.

Surgical procedures. These blue boxes address such topics as the anatomical basis of surgical procedures, such as the planning of incisions, and the anatomical basis of regional anesthesia.

Pathology. The effect of disease on normal anatomy, such as cancer of the breast, and anatomical structures or principles involved in the confinement or dissemination of disease within the body are the types of topics covered in these blue boxes.

- **Boldface type** indicates the main entries of anatomical terms, when they are introduced and defined. In the index, the page numbers of these main entries also appear in boldface type, so that the main entries can be easily located. Boldface type is also used to introduce clinical terms in the clinical correlation (blue) boxes.
- *Italic type* indicates anatomical terms important to the topic and region of study or labeled in an illustration that is being referenced.
- Useful content outlines appear at the beginning of every chapter.
- Instructor's resources and supplemental materials are available at http://thePoint.lww.com.

Anne M. R. Agur, Ph.D., joined Keith Moore and Arthur Dalley as a co-author for the sixth edition. From the outset, *Clinically Oriented Anatomy* has utilized materials from *Grant's Atlas,* for which Anne has had responsibility since 1991. Anne made significant contributions to previous editions of *Clinically Oriented Anatomy* beyond the sharing of materials from *Grant's Atlas*, and has been involved in—and been an asset to—every stage of the development of this and the previous editions.

COMMITMENT TO EDUCATING STUDENTS

This book is written for health science students, keeping in mind those who may not have had a previous acquaintance with anatomy. We have tried to present the material in an interesting way so that it can be easily integrated with what will be taught in more detail in other disciplines such as physical diagnosis, medical rehabilitation, and surgery. We hope this text will serve two purposes: to educate and to excite. If students develop enthusiasm for clinical anatomy, the goals of this book will have been fulfilled.

Keith L. Moore
University of Toronto
Faculty of Medicine

Arthur F. Dalley II
Vanderbilt University
School of Medicine

Anne M. R. Agur
University of Toronto
Faculty of Medicine

ABBREVIATIONS

a., aa.	artery, arteries	lev.	levator
ant.	anterior	lit.	literally
B.C.E.	before the Common (Christian) era	M	male
C	cervical	m., mm.	muscle, muscles
C.E.	Common (Christian) era	Mediev.	medieval
Co	coccygeal	Mod.	modern
dim.	diminutive	post.	posterior
e.g.	for example	S	sacral
et al.	and others	sup.	superior, superioris
F	female	supf.	superficial
Fr.	French	T	thoracic
G.	Greek	TA	*Terminologia Anatomica*
i.e.	that is	TE	Terminologia Embryologica
inf.	inferior	TH	Terminologia Histologica
L	liter, lumbar	v., vv.	vein, veins
L.	Latin	vs.	versus

Acknowledgments

We wish to thank the following colleagues who were invited by the publisher to assist with the development of the seventh edition through their critical analysis.

- Ernest Adeghate, PhD, Chair, Department of Anatomy, United Arab Emirates University
- Christopher Bise, PT, MS, DPT, OCS, Assistant Professor, University of Pittsburgh; Physical Therapist at UPMC Children's Hospital of Pittsburgh
- Christopher Briggs, PhD, Assistant Professor, Department of Anatomy and Neuroscience, University of Melbourne, Australia
- Anjanette Clifford, BS, MS, DC, Assistant Professor of Master of Science Degree in Sports Science and Rehabilitation, Logan College of Chiropractic University
- James Culberson, PhD, Professor, Department of Neurobiology and Anatomy, West Virginia University
- Terry Dean, MD, PhD, Post-Doctoral Fellow, Department of Cell and Molecular Biology, University of Pennsylvania
- Robert Frysztak, PhD, Professor, Department of Physiology, National University Health Sciences
- Tom Gillingwater, MD, Professor, Department of Biological and Clinical Lab Sciences, University of Edinburgh, United Kingdom
- Daniel Graney, PhD, Professor, Department of Anatomy and Embryology, University of Washington School of Medicine
- Robert Hage, MD, PhD, DLO, MBA, Professor, Department of Anatomy, St.George's University, West Indies
- Beth Jones, PT, DPT, MS, OCS, Assistant Professor, Physical Therapy Program, Department of Orthopaedics and Rehabilitation, School of Medicine, University of New Mexico; Assistant Professor, Department of Cell Biology and Physiology, School of Medicine, University of New Mexico
- Randy Kulesza, PhD, Associate Professor, Department of Anatomy, Assistant Dean- Post Baccalaureate and MS in Biomedical Sciences Programs, Lake Erie College of Osteopathic Medicine
- Octavian Lucaciu, MD, PhD, Associate Professor, Department of Anatomy, Canadian Memorial Chiropractic College
- Linda McLoon, PhD, Professor, Department of Ophthalmology and Visual Neuroscience, University of Minnesota
- Gary Nieder, PhD, Professor, Department of Neuroscience, Cell Biology & Physiology, Wright State University
- El Sayed Nosair, PhD, Assistant Professor, Sharjah University, United Arab Emirates
- James Walker, PhD, Associate Professor, Department of Basic Medical Sciences, Purdue University; Associate Director, Department of Human Anatomy, Indiana University School of Medicine-Lafayette

Several students were also invited by the publisher to review the textbook:

- Shloka Ananthanarayana, Mount Sinai School of Medicine
- Jennifer Gulas, Universidad Autonoma de Guadalajara, Mexico
- Paul Johnson, Michigan State University
- Liying Low, University of Glasgow, Scotland
- Kristina Medhus, University of Texas Medical School-Houston
- Vanessa Scott, Albert Einstein College of Medicine
- Sara Thorp, Ohio University College of Osteopathic Medicine
- Ryckie Wade, University of East Anglia, United Kingdom

In addition to reviewers, many people—some of them unknowingly—helped us by perusing, discussing, or contributing to parts of the manuscript and/or providing constructive criticism of the text and illustrations in this and previous editions:

- Dr. Peter Abrahams, Prof. of Clinical Anatomy, Medical Teaching Centre, Institute of Clinical Education, Warwick Medical School, University of Warwick, Coventry, UK
- Dr. Robert D. Acland, Professor of Surgery/Microsurgery, Division of Plastic and Reconstructive Surgery, University of Louisville, Louisville, Kentucky
- Dr. Edna Becker, Associate Professor of Medical Imaging, University of Toronto Faculty of Medicine, Toronto
- Dr. Donald R. Cahill, Professor of Anatomy (retired; former Chair), Mayo Medical School; former Editor-in-Chief of Clinical Anatomy, Rochester, Minnesota
- Dr. Joan Campbell, Assistant Professor of Medical Imaging, University of Toronto Faculty of Medicine, Toronto
- Dr. Stephen W. Carmichael, Professor Emeritus, Mayo Medical School, Editor-in-Chief of Clinical Anatomy, Rochester, Minnesota
- Dr. Carmine D. Clemente, Professor of Anatomy and Orthopedic Surgery, University of California, Los Angeles School of Medicine, Los Angeles
- Dr. James D. Collins, Professor of Radiological Sciences, University of California, Los Angeles School of Medicine/Center for Health Sciences, Los Angeles

- Dr. Raymond F. Gasser, Emeritus Professor of Anatomy, Louisiana State University School of Medicine, New Orleans
- Dr. Ralph Ger (Deceased), Professor of Anatomy and Structural Biology, Albert Einstein College of Medicine, Bronx, New York
- Dr. Paul Gobee, Assistant Professor, Developer Anatomical E-Learning, Department of Anatomy & Embryology, Leiden University Medical Center, Leiden, Netherlands
- Dr. Douglas J. Gould, Professor of Biomedical Sciences, Oakland University William Beaumont School of Medicine, Detroit, Michigan
- Dr. Daniel O. Graney, Professor of Biological Structure, University of Washington School of Medicine, Seattle
- Dr. David G. Greathouse, former Professor and Chair, Belmont University School of Physical Therapy, Nashville, Tennessee
- Scott L. Hagan, 4th year Medical Student, Vanderbilt University School of Medicine, Nashville, TN
- Dr. Masoom Haider, Assistant Professor of Medical Imaging, University of Toronto Faculty of Medicine, Toronto
- Dr. John S. Halle, Professor and Chair, Belmont University School of Physical Therapy, Nashville, Tennessee
- Dr. Jennifer L. Halpern, Assistant Professor, Orthopedic Surgery—Oncology, Vanderbilt University School of Medicine, Nashville, Tennessee
- Dr. Nicole Herring, Assistant Professor, Anatomical Sciences and Neurobiology, University of Louisville School of Medicine, Louisville, Kentucky
- Dr. Walter Kuchareczyk, Professor and Neuroradiologist Senior Scientist, Department of Medical Resonance Imaging, University Health Network, Toronto, Ontario, Canada.
- Dr. Nirusha Lachman, Professor of Anatomy, Mayo Medical School, Rochester, Minnesota
- Dr. H. Wayne Lambert, Professor, Neurobiology and Anatomy Department, West Virginia University School of Medicine, Morgantown, West Virginia
- Dr. Michael von Lüdinghausen, University Professor, Anatomy Institute, University of Würzburg, Würzburg, Germany (retired)
- Dr. Shirley McCarthy, Director of MRI, Department of Diagnostic Radiology, Yale University School of Medicine, New Haven, Connecticut
- Dr. Lillian Nanney, Professor of Plastic Surgery and Cell and Developmental Biology, Vanderbilt University School of Medicine, Nashville, Tennessee
- Dr. Todd R. Olson, Professor of Anatomy and Structural Biology, Albert Einstein College of Medicine, Bronx, New York
- Dr. Wojciech Pawlina, Professor and Chair of Anatomy, Mayo Medical School, Rochester, Minnesota
- Dr. T. V. N. Persaud, Professor Emeritus of Human Anatomy and Cell Science, Faculties of Medicine and Dentistry, University of Manitoba, Winnipeg, Manitoba, Canada. Professor of Anatomy and Embryology, St. George's University, Granada, West Indies
- Dr. Cathleen C. Pettepher, Professor of Cancer Biology, Vanderbilt University School of Medicine, Nashville, Tennessee
- Dr. Thomas H. Quinn, Professor of Biomedical Sciences, Creighton University School of Medicine, Omaha, Nebraska
- Dr. Christopher Ramnanan, Assistant Professor, Department of Cellular and Functional Anatomy, Division of Clinical and Functional Anatomy, University of Ottawa Faculty of Medicine, Ottawa, Ontario, Canada
- Dr. David Resuehr, Assistant Professor, Department of Cellular, Developmental and Integrative Biology, University of Alabama at Birmingham School of Medicine, Birmingham, Alabama
- Dr. George E. Salter, Professor of Anatomy (retired), Department of Cell Biology, University of Alabama, Birmingham
- Dr. Ryan Splittgerber, Assistant Professor, Department of Genetics, Cell Biology and Anatomy, University of Nebraska Medical Center, College of Medicine, Omaha, Nebraska
- Dr. Tatsuo Sato, Professor and Head (retired), Second Department of Anatomy, Tokyo Medical and Dental University Faculty of Medicine, Tokyo
- Professor Colin P. Wendell-Smith, Department of Anatomy and Physiology, University of Tasmania, Hobart, Tasmania, Australia (retired)
- Dr. Andreas H. Weiglein, Professor, Institut fur Anatomie, Medical University Graz, Graz, Austria
- Dr. David G. Whitlock, Professor of Anatomy, University of Colorado Medical School, Denver

Art plays a major role in facilitating learning. We extend our sincere gratitude and appreciation for the skills, talents, and timely work of our medical illustrators for this edition. Wynne Auyeung and Natalie Intven from Imagineering did a superb job of managing a team of talented artists to revise all of the illustrations for a more consistent, vibrant art program. Photographs taken during a major surface anatomy photography project for the fifth edition continue to be a tremendous asset. E. Anne Rayner, Senior Photographer, Vanderbilt Medical Art Group did an excellent job photographing the surface anatomy models, working in association with authors Arthur Dalley and Anne Agur. We greatly appreciate the contribution the models made to the quality of both the previous and the current edition. Although the number of illustrations from *Grant's Atlas of Anatomy* continues to be reduced and replaced by new art, we gratefully acknowledge the excellence of Professor J. C. B. Grant's dissections and the excellent art done by the following: Dorothy Foster Chubb,

Elizabeth Blackstock, Nancy Joy, Nina Kilpatrick, David Mazierski, Stephen Mader, Bart Vallecoccia, Sari O'Sullivan, Kam Yu, Caitlin Duckwall, and Valerie Oxorn.

Many thanks also to those at Lippincott Williams & Wilkins who participated in the development of this edition: Crystal Taylor, Acquisitions Editor; Jennifer Clements, Art Director; and Julie Montalbano, Product Manager. Finally, thanks are due to the sales and marketing division at LWW, which has played a key role in the continued success of this book.

Keith L. Moore
Arthur F. Dalley II
Anne M. R. Agur

Contents

3   Pelvis and Perineum / 326

4   Back / 439

5   Lower Limb / 508

8   Neck / 981

9   Summary of Cranial Nerves / 1053

List of Clinical Blue Boxes

3   Pelvis and Perineum

7   Head

8   Neck

9 Summary of Cranial Nerves

Figure Credits

INTRODUCTION

Fig. I.20 Based on Hamill JH, Knutzan K: Biochemical Basis of Human Movement. 2nd ed. Baltimore: Williams & Wilkins, 2003.

Fig. I.22C Based on Silverthorn. Human Physiology. 4th ed. Tappan, NJ: Pearson Education, 2007. P. 459.

Fig. I.50 Daffner RH: Clinical Radiology: The Essentials. 2nd ed. Baltimore: Williams & Wilkins, 1998.

Fig. I.53 Wicke L: Atlas of Radiologic Anatomy. 6th English ed. Ed and trans: Taylor AN. Baltimore: Williams & Wilkins, 1998. [Wicke L: Roentgen-Anatomie Normalbefunde. 5th ed. Munich: Urban and Schwarzenberg, 1995.]

Fig. I.54 Atlas of Radiologic Anatomy. 6th English ed.

Fig. I.55 Atlas of Radiologic Anatomy. 6th English ed.

Fig. I.56 Atlas of Radiologic Anatomy. 6th English ed.

Fig. BI.1 Reprinted with permission from van de Graaff K: Human Anatomy. 4th ed. Dubuque, IA: WC Brown, 1995.

Fig. BI.2 Rassner G: Atlas of Dermatology. 3rd ed. Trans: Burgdorf WHC. Philadelphia: Lea & Febiger, 1994 (photo); Stedman's Medical Dictionary. 27th ed. Baltimore: Lippincott Williams & Wilkins, 2000. (artist: Neil O. Hardy, Westport, CT).

Fig. BI.4 Based on Stedman's Medical Dictionary. 27th ed. (artist: Neil O. Hardy, Westport, CT).

Fig. BI.5 Based on Stedman's Medical Dictionary. 27th ed. (artist: Neil O. Hardy, Westport, CT).

Fig. BI.8 Based on Willis MC: Medical Terminology: The Language of Health Care. Baltimore: Lippincott Williams & Wilkins, 1995.

Fig. BI.9 Reprinted with permission from Roche Lexikon Medizin. 4th ed. Munich: Urban & Schwarzenberg, 1998.

CHAPTER 1

Fig. 1.20. B&C. Based on Clay JH, Pounds DM: Basic Clinical Massage Therapy: Integrating Anatomy and Treatment. 2nd ed. Baltimore: Lippincott Williams & Wilkins, 2002.

Fig. 1.24C Based on Stedman's Medical Dictionary. 27th ed. (artist: Michael Schenk, Jackson, MS).

Fig. 1.30A Dean D, Herbener TE: Cross-Sectional Anatomy. Baltimore: Lippincott Williams & Wilkins, 2000.

Fig. 1.48 Adapted with permission from Moore KL, Persaud TVN. The Developing Human: Clinically Oriented Embryology. 7th ed. Philadelphia: Saunders, 2003. Fig. 8.5A, B, & D, p. 150.

Fig. 1.50 Adapted with permission from Torrent-Guasp F, Buckberg GD, Clemente C, et al.: The structure and function of the helical heart and its buttress wrapping. The normal macroscopic structure of the heart. Semin Thoracic Cardiovasc Surg 2001;13:30.

Fig. B1.6A Based on Bickley LS, Szilagyi PG: Bates' Guide to Physical Examination. 8th ed. Baltimore: Lippincott Williams & Wilkins, 2002.

Fig. B1.6B Brant WE, Helms CA: Fundamentals of Diagnostic Radiology. 2nd ed. Baltimore: Williams & Wilkins, 1999.

Fig. B1.7 Based on Hall-Craggs ECB: Anatomy as the Basis of Clinical Medicine. 3rd ed. Baltimore: Williams & Wilkins, 1995

Fig. B1.9 Based on Stedman's Medical Dictionary. 27th ed. (artist: Neil O. Hardy, Westport, CT).

Fig. B1.11A Based on Stedman's Medical Dictionary. 27th ed. Baltimore: Lippincott Williams & Wilkins, 2000. (artist: Mikki Senkarik, San Antonio, TX).

Fig. B1.11B Olympus America, Inc., Melville, NY.

Fig. B1.12A Based on Stedman's Medical Dictionary. 27th ed. (artist: Neil O. Hardy, Westport, CT).

Fig. B1.12B Bates' Guide to Physical Examination, 10th ed., p. 300.

Fig. B1.13 Stedman's Medical Dictionary. 27th ed. (artist: Neil O. Hardy, Westport, CT); photographs of bronchus, carina, and trachea—Feinsilver SH, Fein A: Textbook of Bronchoscopy. Baltimore: Williams & Wilkins, 1995; photograph of bronchoscopy procedure—courtesy of Temple University Hospital, Philadelphia.

Fig. B1.14 Clinical Radiology: The Essentials. 2nd ed.

Fig. B1.18 Based on Stedman's Medical Dictionary. 27th ed. (artist: Neil O. Hardy, Westport, CT).

Fig. B1.19 With permission from The Developing Human: Clinically Oriented Embryology. 7th ed. Figs. 14.15 and 14.14, p. 345–346.

Fig. B1.23 Siemens Medical Solutions USA, Inc.

Fig. B1.26 Based on figure provided by the Anatomical Chart Company.

Fig. B1.28 Based on Stedman's Medical Dictionary. 27th ed. (artist: Neil O. Hardy, Westport, CT).

Fig. B1.29 Based on Stedman's Medical Dictionary. 27th ed. (artist: Neil O. Hardy, Westport, CT); photograph—courtesy of Quinton Cardiology, Inc.

Fig. B1.34 Based on Clinical Radiology: The Essentials. 2nd ed.

Fig. B1.37 Cross-Sectional Anatomy. P. 25.

Fig. B1.38B-E Madden ME. Introduction to Sectional Anatomy. Baltimore: Lippincott Williams & Wilkins, 2000.

CHAPTER 2

Fig. 2.5 Basic Clinical Massage Therapy: Integrating Anatomy and Treatment. 2nd ed.

Fig. 2.6B Based on Bates' Guide to Physical Examination. 10th ed., p 415; Fig. 2.6B(slices) Based on Grants' Atlas of Anatomy 12th ed. fig 2.6DE

Fig. 2.18 Based on Sauerland EK: Grant's Dissector. 12th ed. Baltimore: Lippincott Williams & Wilkins, 1999.

Fig. 2.33B Cormack DH, Clinically Integrated Histology, Baltimore: Lippincott Williams and Wilkins, 1998. (Fig. 8.8 p. 191)

Fig. 2.36B Based on Agur AMR: Grant's Method of Anatomy. 9th ed. Baltimore: Williams & Wilkins, 1975.

Fig. 2.43C Based on Stedman's Medical Dictionary. 27th ed. (artist: Neil O. Hardy, Westport, CT).

Fig. 2.47 Based on McConnell TH, Hull K: Human Form, Human Function: Essentials of Anatomy and Physiology. 1st ed. Baltimore: Lippincott Williams & Wilkins, 2011. fig. 14.16a, p. 565.

Fig. 2.48B Based on Grant's Dissector. 12th ed.

Fig. 2.57A Based on Grant's Method of Anatomy. 9th ed.

Fig. 2.57B Based on Grant's Method of Anatomy. 9th ed.

Fig. 2.58C Based on Stedman's Medical Dictionary. 27th ed. (artist: Neil O. Hardy, Westport, CT)

Fig. 2.59D Gartner LP, Hiatt JL: Color Atlas of Histology. 3rd ed. Baltimore: Lippincott Williams & Wilkins, 2001.

Fig. 2.62 Based on Bates' Guide to Physical Examination. 8th ed.

Fig. 2.64E Based on Grant's Dissector. 12th ed.

Fig. 2.67B–E Reprinted with permission from Karaliotas C. et al: Liver and Biliary Tract Surgery: Embryological Anatomy to 3D-Imaging and Transplant Innovations. Vienna: Springer, 2007.

Fig. 2.90 Based on Rosse C, Gaddum-Rosse P: Hollinshead's Textbook of Anatomy. 5th ed. Philadelphia, Lippincott-Raven, 1997.

Fig. 2.91A Based on Basic Clinical Massage Therapy: Integrating Anatomy and Treatment. 2nd ed.

Fig. 2.102B & C Cross-Sectional Anatomy.

Fig. B2.2 Lockhart RD, Hamilton GF, Fyfe FW: Anatomy of the Human Body. Philadelphia: Lippincott, 1959

Fig. B2.3 ACD Based on Tank W, Gest TR: LWW Atlas of Anatomy. Baltimore: Lippincott Williams & Wilkins, 2008. Plate 5.11A

Fig. B2.7 Based on Stedman's Medical Dictionary. 27th ed.; photograph—courtesy of Mission Hospital, Mission Viejo, CA.

Fig. B2.8 Fundamentals of Diagnostic Radiology. 2nd ed

Fig. B2.9 Based on Stedman's Medical Dictionary. 27th ed. (artist: Neil O. Hardy, Westport, CT).

Fig. B2.10 Based on Stedman's Medical Dictionary. 28th ed. Baltimore: Lippincott Williams & Wilkins, 2006 (artist: Mikki Senkarik, San Antonio, TX).

Fig. B2.11 Based on Stedman's Medical Dictionary. 27th ed. (artist: Neil O. Hardy, Westport, CT).

Fig. B2.12 Based on Bates, 10th ed., p. 429

Fig. B2.15B Based on Stedman's Medical Dictionary. 27th ed. (artist: Neil O. Hardy)

Fig. B2.16 Based on Stedman's Medical Dictionary. 27th ed. (artist: Neil O. Hardy, Westport, CT).

Fig. B2.17 Photograph of colonoscope—Olympus America, Inc; photograph of diverticulosis—Schiller, KFR et al. Colour Atlas of Endoscopy. Chapman and Hall, London, 1986, Springer Science and Business Media; drawings—Stedman's Medical Dictionary. 27th ed. (diverticulosis—artist: Neil O. Hardy, Westport, CT; colonoscopy—artist: Mikki Senkarik, San Antonio, TX).

Fig. B2.18 Based on Cohen BS. Medical Terminology. 4th ed. Baltimore: Lippincott Williams & Wilkins, 2003. Fig. 12.8.

Fig. B2.19A Bates 10th ed., p. 444.

Fig. B2.22 Based on Bates' Guide to Physical Examination and History Taking. 8th ed. Baltimore: Lippincott Williams and Wilkins, 2003.

Fig. B2.27 Rubin et al., Rubin's Pathology: Clinicopathologic Foundations of Medicine. 4th ed. Baltimore: Lippincott Williams & Wilkins: 2004.

Fig. B2.29 Based on Stedman's Medical Dictionary. 27th ed. (artist: Neil O. Hardy, Westport, CT).

Fig. B2.30 (inset) Based on Stedman's Medical Dictionary. 28th ed.

Fig. B2.33 Stedman's Dictionary for Health Professionals and Nursing. 5th ed. Baltimore: Lippincott Williams & Wilkins, 2005. P. 987.

Fig. B2.34A Reprinted with permission from Moore KL, Persaud TVN: Before We Are Born. 7th ed., Saunders (Elsevier), Philadelphia, 2008. Fig. 9.10; courtesy of Dr. Nathan E. Wiseman, Professor of Surgery, Children's Hospital, University of Manitoba, Winnipeg, Manitoba, Canada.

Fig. B2.34B Reprinted with permission from Moore KL, Persaud TVN: The Developing Human. 8th ed., Saunders (Elsevier), Philadelphia 2008. Fig. 8.12C; courtesy of Dr. Prem S. Sahni, formerly of Department of Radiology, Children's Hospital, Winnipeg, Manitoba, Canada.

Fig. B2.35 Reprinted with permission from Medscape Gastroenterology 6 (1), 2004. http://www.medscape.com/viewarticle/474658 ©2004, Medscape.

Fig. 2.36 Based on Hardin, DMJr: Acute Appendicitis: Review and Update. American Family Physician. 60(7):2027-34 (1999) Fig. 1B©Floyd E. Hosmer

Fig. B 2.37B Based on Eckert, P et al.: Fibrinklebung, Indikation und Anwendung. München: Urban & Schwarzenberg, 1986.

Fig. TB 2.1 Based on LWW Atlas of Anatomy Plates 5.10B, 5.11B, and 5.11C.

CHAPTER 3

Fig. 3.14B Based on DeLancey JO. Structure support of the urethra as it relates to stress urinary incontinence: The hammock hypothesis. Am J Obstet Gynecol 1994;170:1713–1720

Fig. 3.38A Left—Based on Dauber W: Pocket Atlas of Human Anatomy. Rev. 5th ed. New York: Thieme: 2007. P. 195.

Fig. 3.51B Based on Clemente, CD: Anatomy: A Regional Atlas of the Human Body. 5th ed. Baltimore: Lippincott Williams & Wilkins, 2006. Fig. 272.1.

Fig. 3.61E Based on Das Lexicon der Gesundheit. Munich: Urban & Schwarzenberg Verlag, 1996 (artist: Jonathan Dimes), p. 3.

Fig. 3.72D Lee JKT, Sagel SS, Stanley RJ, et al.: Computed Body Tomography with MRI Correlation. 3rd ed. Baltimore: Lippincott Williams & Wilkins, 1998.

Fig. B3.2B Based on Anatomy as the Basis of Clinical Medicine. 3rd ed.

Fig. B3.7A & B Reprinted with permission from LearningRadiology. com.

Fig. B3.9 Based on Stedman's Medical Dictionary. 27th ed.

Fig. B3.10 Based on Hartwig W: Fundamental Anatomy. Baltimore: Lippincott Williams & Wilkins; 2007. P. 176.

Fig. B3.11 Based on Stedman's Medical Dictionary. 27th ed.

Fig. B3.14A & B Based on Beckmann CR. Obstetrics and Gynecology. 4th ed. Baltimore: Lippincott Williams and Wilkins, 2002.

Fig. B3.16 Reprinted with permission from Stuart GCE, Reid DF. Diagnostic studies. In: Copeland LJ, ed. Textbook of Gynecology. Philadelphia: Saunders, 1993.

Fig. B3.17A–D Based on Stedman's Medical Dictionary. 27th ed.

Fig. B3.18A & B Based on Fuller J, Schaller-Ayers J: A Nursing Approach. 2nd ed. Philadelphia: Lippincott, 1994. Fig. B3.11 (artist: Larry Ward, Salt Lake City, UT).

Fig. B3.20A & C–E Based on Stedman's Medical Dictionary. 27th ed.

Fig. B3.22 Based on Obstetrics and Gynecology. 4th ed.

Fig. B3.23 Based on A Nursing Approach. 2nd ed.

Fig. B3.24 Based on Stedman's Medical Dictionary. 27th ed.

Fig. B3.26A Based on Stedman's Medical Dictionary. 28th ed.

Fig. B3.26B With permission from Bristow RE, Johns Hopkins School of Medicine, Baltimore, MD.

Fig. 3.27A-C Based on LWW Atlas Plate 6.19A, p. 276

Fig. B3.28 Based on Obstetrics and Gynecology. 4th ed.

Fig. B3.29A and B Based on Stedman's Medical Dictionary. 27th ed.

Fig. B3.32 Based on Stedman's Medical Dictionary. 27th ed.

Fig. B3.33A Based on Stedman's Medical Dictionary. 27th ed. (artist: Neil O. Hardy, Westport, CT) and Clinically Oriented Anatomy, 7th ed., fig. B3.30B

Fig. B3.33B Edwards L, ed: Atlas of Genital Dermatology. Baltimore: Lippincott Williams & Wilkins, 2004.

CHAPTER 4

Fig. 4.1C Based on Olson TR: Student Atlas of Anatomy. Baltimore: Williams & Wilkins, 1996.

Fig. 4.4 Based on Pocket Atlas of Human Anatomy. Rev. 5th ed. Fig. B, p. 49.

Fig. 4.7D Becker RF, Wilson JW, Gehweiler JA: Anatomical Basic of Medical Practice. Baltimore: Williams & Wilkins, 1974.

Fig. 4.30 Based on Student Atlas of Anatomy.

Fig. 4.31 Based on Student Atlas of Anatomy.

Fig. B4.3A–E Based on Clark CR: The Cervical Spine. 3rd ed. Philadelphia: Lippincott Williams & Wilkins, 1998.

Fig. B4.3F & G Computed Body Tomography with MRI Correlation. 3rd ed.

Fig. B4.10 Van de Graff. Human Anatomy. 4th ed. Dubuque: WC Brown. P. 163.

Fig. B4.11 Median MRI ©LUHS2008. Loyola University Health System, Maywood, IL. transverse MRI—Choi S-J et al. The use of MRI to predict the clinical outcome of non-surgical treatment for lumbar I-V disc herniation. Korean J Radiol 2007;8:156–163:5a.

Fig. B4.13B GE Healthcare, www.medcyclo.com.

Fig. B4.13C Cross-sectional Human Anatomy.

Fig. B4.13D LearningRadiology.com.

Fig. B4.13E LearningRadiology.com.

Fig. B4.15C Based on The Cervical Spine. 3rd ed.

Fig. B4.16B Based on eMedicine.com, 2008/ http://www.emedicine.com/sports/TOPIC71.HTM.

Fig. B4.16C Based on Drake R et al.: Gray's Atlas of Anatomy. New York: Churchill Livingstone, 2004. P. 30.

Fig. B4.17F Science Photo Library/Custom Medical Stock Photo, Inc.

Fig. B4.17G Princess Margaret Rose Orthopaedic Hospital/Science Photo Library/Photo Researchers, Inc.; right—Anatomical Basic of Medical Practice.

CHAPTER 5

Fig. 5.5A Atlas of Radiologic Anatomy. 6th English ed.

Fig. 5.21E Based on Rose J, Gamble JG. Human Walking. 2nd ed. Baltimore: Williams & Wilkins, 1994.

Fig. 5.21G Based on Basic Clinical Massage Therapy: Integrating Anatomy and Treatment. 2nd ed.

Fig. 5.22C Based on Melloni, JL: Melloni's Illustrated Review of Human Anatomy: By Structures—Arteries, Bones, Muscles, Nerves, Veins. Lippincott Williams & Wilkins, 1988.

Fig. 5.34A & B Based on Basic Clinical Massage Therapy: Integrating Anatomy and Treatment. 2nd ed.

Fig. 5.40A Based on Basic Clinical Massage Therapy: Integrating Anatomy and Treatment. 2nd ed.

Fig. 5.40F Based on Basic Clinical Massage Therapy: Integrating Anatomy and Treatment. 2nd ed. Fig. 9.12, p. 342.

Fig. 5.40H Based on Basic Clinical Massage Therapy, 2nd. Ed. Fig. 9.14, p. 344.

Fig. 5.42(left) Based on Basic Clinical Massage Therapy: Integrating Anatomy and Treatment. 2nd ed.

Fig. 5.42(right) Based on Melloni's Illustrated Review of Human Anatomy: By Structures—Arteries, Bones, Muscles, Nerves, Veins. P. 173.

Fig. 5.55C–F Based on Basic Clinical Massage Therapy: Integrating Anatomy and Treatment. 2nd ed.

Fig. 5.60F–K Based on Basic Clinical Massage Therapy: Integrating Anatomy and Treatment. 2nd ed.

Fig. 5.68A & H Based on Basic Clinical Massage Therapy: Integrating Anatomy and Treatment. 2nd ed.

Fig. 5.68C Based on Basic Clinical Massage Therapy and Grant's Atlas of Anatomy, 13th ed., Fig. 78, p. 453

Fig. 5.69A,C Based on Grant's Atlas of Anatomy. 13th ed.

Fig. 5.69B Based on Grant's Atlas of Anatomy, 13th ed., Fig. 6.78C

Fig. 5.69D Based in part on Grant's Atlas of Anatomy, 13th ed., Fig. 5.80C, p. 455

Fig. 5.73 Based on Basmajian JV, Slonecker CE: Grant's Method of Anatomy: A Clinical Problem-Solving Approach. 11 ed. Baltimore: Williams & Wilkins, 1989.

Fig. 5.76A Based on Basic Clinical Massage Therapy: Integrating Anatomy and Treatment. 2nd ed.

Fig. 5.79A & B Based on Kapandji, IA. The Physiology of the Joints. Vol. 2: Lower Limb. 5th ed. Edinburgh, UK, Churchill Livingstone, 1987.

Fig. 5.79C Based on Basic Clinical Massage Therapy: Integrating Anatomy and Treatment. 2nd ed.

Fig. 5.80B Atlas of Radiologic Anatomy. 6th English ed.

Fig. 5.85B Atlas of Radiologic Anatomy. 6th English ed.

Fig. 5.92B Based on Student Atlas of Anatomy.

Fig. 5.95A Atlas of Radiologic Anatomy. 6th English ed.

Fig. B5.1A Yochum TR, Rowe LJ. Essentials of Skeletal Radiology, Vol. 1, 2nd ed., Baltimore: Lippincott Williams & Wilkins, 1996. Fig. 9.85, p. 707.

Fig. B5.1B Brunner, LC, Kuo TY: Hip fractures in adults. Am Fam Phys 2003;67(3):Fig. 2.

Fig. B5.1D Rossi F, Dragoni S. Acute avulsion fractures of the pelvis in adolescent competitive athletes. Skel Radiol 2001;30(3):Fig. 7.

Fig. B5.3D Yochum TR, Rowe LJ. Essentials of Skeletal Radiology, 3rd Ed. Baltimore: Lippincott Williams & Wilkins, 2005.

Fig. B5.4 Essentials of Skeletal Radiology, 3rd ed.

Fig. B5.5 ©eMedicine.com, 2008.

Fig. B5.8D Hatch RL et al.: Diagnosis and management of metatarsal fractures. Am Fam Phys 2007;76(6):217.

Fig. B5.8E Essentials of Skeletal Radiology, Vol. 1, 2nd edition, Fig. 9.104A, p. 737.

Fig. B5.9 Davies M. The os trigonum syndrome. Foot 2004;14(3):Fig. 2.

Fig. B5.10 Doda P, Peh W: Woman with possible right toe fracture. Asia Pacific J Fam Med 2006;5(3):50.

Fig. B5.11A Reprinted with permission from Roche Lexikon Medizin. 4th ed.

Fig. B5.11B–D Stedman's Medical Dictionary. 28th ed. (artist: Neil O. Hardy, Westport, CT), p. 2090.

Fig. B5.12 LearningRadiology.com.

Fig. B5.13B Kavanagh EC et al.: MRI findings in bipartite patella. Skel Radiol 2007;36(3):Fig. 1a.

Fig. B5.14 Bates 10e, p. 699 upper fig.

Fig. B5.22 Bates 10e, p. 700, upper fig.

Fig. B5.25 Bates 10e, p. 485, posterior tibial pulse

Fig. B5.26(top) www.xray200.co.uk

Fig. B5.27 Bates 10e, p. 485, dorsalis pedis pulse.

Fig. B5.28 Essentials of Skeletal Radiology. 2nd ed.

Fig. B5.30 Drawings—Willis MC: Medical Terminology: A Programmed Learning Approach to the Language of Health Care. Baltimore: Lippincott Williams & Wilkins, 2002; radiograph—Clinical Radiology—The Essentials.

Fig. B5.32A–C Modified from Palastanga NP, Field DG, Soames R: Anatomy and Human Movement. 4th ed. Oxford, UK: Butterworth-Heinemann, 2002.

Fig. B5.32D Clinical Radiology—The Essentials.

Fig. B5.34 Based on Roche Lexikon Medizin. 4th ed.

Fig. B5.35C Stedman's Medical Dictionary. 28th ed, p. 1184.

CHAPTER 6

Fig. 6.17 LWW Atlas of Anatomy. Baltimore: Pl. 2.53, p. 82.

Fig. 6.32 Basic Clinical Massage Therapy: Integrating Anatomy and Treatment, 2nd ed. Fig. 4.28, p. 147.

Fig. 6.49B–D, F, & G Basic Clinical Massage Therapy: Integrating Anatomy and Treatment. 2nd ed. Figs. 5.1, 5.12, 5.3, 5.6, and 5.10, pgs. 193, 201, 195, 197, and 199.

Fig. 6.53 Based on Hoppenfeld, S, de Boer P. Surgical Exposures in Orthopaedics, 3rd ed. Baltimore: Lippincott Williams & Wilkins, 2003. Fig. 2.27, p. 89.

Fig. 6.60B & C Basic Clinical Massage Therapy, 2nd ed. Fig. 5.5, p. 186.

Fig. 6.92 Modified from Biomechanical Basis of Human Motion. Fig. 5.8, p. 153.

Fig. 6.93 Platzer W. Color Atlas of Human Anatomy. Vol. 1: Locomotor System. 4th ed. New York: Thieme, 1992, p. 147 and 149.

Fig. 6.102 Based on LWW Atlas of Anatomy Plate 2.43

Fig. 6.103 B and C Based on from Anatomy as the Basis of Clinical Medicine. 3rd ed.

Fig. 6.109B Grant's Method of Anatomy: A Clinical Problem-Solving Approach. 11th ed.

Fig. B6.5 Rowland LP: Merritt's Textbook of Neurology. 9th ed. Baltimore: Williams & Wilkins, 1995.

Fig. B6.9 Left—Meschan I. An Atlas of Anatomy Basic to Radiology. Philadelphia: Saunders, 1975; right—Salter RB. Textbook of Disorders and Injuries of the Musculoskeletal System. 3rd ed. Baltimore: Williams & Wilkins, 1998.

Fig. B6.13 Bates, 10th ed, p. 697 bottom left.

Fig. B6.14 Based on Anderson MK, Hall SJ, Martin M: Foundations of Athletic Training. 3rd ed. Baltimore: Lippincott Williams & Wilkins, 1995.

Fig. B6.31 www.xray200.co.uk.

Fig. B6.37A John Sleezer/MCT/Landov.

Fig. B6.37B Basic Clinical Massage Therapy: Integrating Anatomy and Treatment, second edition. Fig. 5-35, p. 223.

Fig. B6.38 Textbook of Disorders and Injuries of the Musculoskeletal System. 3rd ed.

CHAPTER 7

Fig. 7.16 LWW Atlas of Anatomy. Plate 7.29, p. 324

Fig. 7.25 Based on LWW Atlas of Anatomy Plate 7.73, p. 368

Fig. 7.26 Based on LWW Atlas of Anatomy Plate 7.74, p. 369

Fig. 7.28A Based on LWW Atlas of Anatomy Plate 7.50B, p. 345.

Fig. 7.31C Based on LWW Atlas of Anatomy Plate 760B, p. 365.

Fig. 7.44A Based on Anatomy as the Basis of Clinical Medicine. 3rd ed.

Fig. 7.46A Based on LWW Atlas of Anatomy. Plate 7.58B, p. 353.

Fig. 7.51A Based on Melloni's Illustrated Review of Human Anatomy: By Structures—Arteries, Bones, Muscles, Nerves, Veins, p. 149.

Fig. 7.51B Based on Human Anatomy. 4th ed. Fig. 15.18, p. 419.

Fig. 7.52 Welch Allyn, Inc., Skaneateles Falls, NY.

Fig. 7.53 Based on Human Anatomy. 4th ed. Fig. 15.17.

Fig. 7.54B Melloni's Illustrated Review of Human Anatomy: By Structures—Arteries, Bones, Muscles, Nerves, Veins. P. 141.

Fig. 7.54C Based on Melloni's Illustrated Review of Human Anatomy: By Structures—Arteries, Bones, Muscles, Nerves, Veins. P. 143.

Fig. 7.56A–D Based on Girard, Louis: Anatomy of the Human Eye. II. The Extra-ocular Muscles. Teaching Films, Inc. Houston, TX.

Fig. 7.57 Based on Melloni's Illustrated Review of Human Anatomy: By Structures—Arteries, Bones, Muscles, Nerves, Veins. P. 189.

Fig. 7.65 Based in part on Clemente C. Atlas of Anatomy 6th ed., Baltimore: Lippincott Williams and Wilkins, 2011. figs. 529-531.

Fig. 7.71 Based on Paff, GH: Anatomy of the Head & Neck. Philadelphia: WB Saunders Co., 1973. Fig. 122.3, p. 62-63.

Fig. 7.72 Based on Basic Clinical Massage Therapy: Integrating Anatomy and Treatment, 2nd ed. Figs. 3.15, 3.16, and 3.19, p. 82, 84, and 86.

Fig. 7.88 Based on LWW Atlas of Anatomy Plate 7.39A

Fig. 7.90A Based on LWW Atlas of Anatomy Plate 7-40A, p. 335

Fig. 7.90C Based on LWW Atlas of Anatomy Plate 7-38C., p. 333

Fig. 7.98 Based on Anatomy of the Head & Neck. Figs. 238–240, p. 142–143 and Grant's Atlas of Anatomy, 13th ed., Fig. 7.78B, p. 705.

Fig. 7.100B & C Based on Hall-Craggs ECB: Anatomy as the Basis of Clinical Medicine. 2nd ed. Baltimore: Williams & Wilkins, 1990. Fig. 9.100, p. 536.

Fig. 7.112 Based on LWW Atlas of Anatomy. Pl. 7.66B& C.

Fig. 7.120 Seeley RR, Stephens TR, and Tate P: Anatomy & Physiology. 6th ed. New York: McGraw-Hill 2003. Fig. 15.28, p. 532.

Fig. B7.12 Ger R, Abrahams P, Olson T: Essentials of Clinical Anatomy. 3rd ed. New York: Parthenon, 1996. Fig. B7.12.

Fig. B7.14 ©LUHS2008. Loyola University Health System, Maywood, IL.

Fig. B7.15 Skin Cancer Foundation.

Fig. B7.20A Visuals Unlimited.

Fig. B7.20B Courtesy of Dr. Gerald S. Smyser, Altru Health System, Grand Forks, ND.

Fig. B7.23 Stedman's Medical Dictionary. 28th ed. (artist: Neil O. Hardy, Westport, CT).

Fig. B7.24 Mann IC: The Development of the Human Eye. New York: Grune & Stratton. 1974.

Fig. B7.25 Welch Allyn, Inc., Skaneateles Falls, NY.

Fig. B7.26 Medical Terminology. 4th ed.

Fig. B7.27 Digital Reference of Ophthalmology, Edward S. Harkness Eye Institute, Department of Ophthalmology of Columbia University.

Fig. B7.28 Stedman's Medical Dictionary. 28th ed. (artist: Neil O. Hardy, Westport, CT).

Fig. B7.29 Mehrle G, Augenheikunde fur Krankenpfegeberufe S aufl. Munchen: Urban & Fischer, 1991.

Fig. B7.32 The Developing Human: Clinically Oriented Embryology. 7th ed.

Fig. B7.33A – D Stedman's Medical Dictionary, 28th ed. (artist: Neil O. Hardy, Westport, CT).

Fig. B7.39 Courtesy of Eugene Kowaluk Photography.

Fig. B7.41 Turner, JS: An overview of head and neck. In Walker HK, Hall WD, Hurst JW, eds: Clinical Methods—The History, Physical and Laboratory Examinations. Butterworths, 1990. Figs. 119.1 and 119.2.

Fig. B7.42 Anatomy as the Basis of Clinical Medicine. 3rd ed.

Fig. B7.43 Bechara Y. Ghorayeb MD, Houston, TX.

Fig. B7.44 Welch Allyn, Inc., Skaneateles Falls, NY.

Fig. B7.45 Stedman's Medical Dictionary. 28th ed. (artist: Neil O. Hardy, Westport, CT).

CHAPTER 8

Fig. 8.1 Based on LWW Atlas of Anatomy Plate 7.13, p. 308 and Tank, PW, Grant's Dissector, 15th ed., Baltimore: Lippincott Williams and Wilkins, 2012, Fig 7.6, p. 209 and 7.10, p. 214

Fig. 8.4A Based on LWW Atlas of Anatomy Plate 7.10A&B, p. 305

Fig. 8.7A Based on Basic Clinical Massage Therapy: Integrating Anatomy and Treatment. 2nd ed., Fig. 3.28

Fig. 8.7B&F Based on Basic Clinical Massage Therapy: Integrating Anatomy and Treatment. 2nd ed., Fig. 6.24

Fig. 8.7CDE Based on Basic Clinical Massage Therapy: Integrating Anatomy and Treatment. 2nd ed. Fig. 8.7 CDE

Fig. 8.12 Based on Grant's Dissector, 15e, Fig. 7-5, p. 208

Fig. 8.20 Based on LWW Atlas of Anatomy Plate 7.73, p 368.

Fig. 8.24A Based on Grant's Dissector. 15th ed., Fig. 7.11

Fig. 8.32C Based on Pocket Atlas of Human Anatomy. 5th ed. P. 169, Fig. C, p. 169.

Fig. 8.43 Based on LWW Atlas of Anatomy Plate 7.10

Fig. 8.44A Abrahams P: The Atlas of the Human Body. San Diego, CA: Thunder Bay Press, 2002. P. 66.

Fig. 8.46B Based on LWW Atlas of Anatomy Plate 7-21, p. 316

Fig. B8.1 Based on Merritt's Textbook of Neurology. 9th ed.

Fig. B8.3 Based on Siemens Medical Solutions USA, Inc.

Fig. B8.6 Based on Sadler TW. Langman's Medical Embryology. 7th ed. Baltimore: Williams & Wilkins, 1995.

Fig. B8.7 Leung AKC, Wong Al, Robson WLLM: Ectopic thyroid gland simulating a thyroglossal duct cyst. Can J Surg 1995;38:87. ©1995 Canadian Medical Association.

Fig. B8.9 Klima: Schilddrüsen-Sonographie. München: Urban & Schwarzenberg Verlag, 1989.

Fig. B8.11 Based on Rohen JW et al.: Color Atlas of Anatomy: A Photographic Study of the Human Body. 5th ed. Baltimore: Lippincott Williams & Wilkins, 2002.

Fig. B8.12 Based on Stedman's Medical Dictionary. 27th ed.

CHAPTER 9

No credits

***Note**: Credits for figures based on* Grant's Atlas of Anatomy *and* Essential Clinical Anatomy *illustrations are available at* thePoint.lww.com.

Introduction to Clinically Oriented Anatomy

APPROACHES TO STUDYING ANATOMY

Anatomy is the setting (structure) in which the events (functions) of life occur. This book deals mainly with functional *human gross anatomy*—the examination of structures of the human that can be seen without a microscope. The three main approaches to studying anatomy are regional, systemic, and clinical (or applied), reflecting the body's organization and the priorities and purposes for studying it.

Regional Anatomy

Regional anatomy (topographical anatomy) considers the organization of the human body as major parts or segments (Fig. I.1): a main body, consisting of the head, neck, and trunk (subdivided into thorax, abdomen, back, and pelvis/perineum), and paired upper limbs and lower limbs. All the major parts may be further subdivided into areas and regions. Regional anatomy is the method of studying the body's structure by focusing attention on a specific part (e.g., the head), area (the face), or region (the orbital or eye region); examining the arrangement and relationships of the various systemic structures (muscles, nerves, arteries, etc.) within it; and then usually continuing to study adjacent regions in an ordered sequence. Outside of this Introduction, the regional approach is followed in this book, with each chapter addressing the anatomy of a major part of the body. This is the approach usually followed in anatomy courses that have a laboratory component involving dissection. When studying anatomy by this approach, it is important to routinely put the regional anatomy into the context of that of adjacent regions, parts, and of the body as a whole.

Regional anatomy also recognizes the body's organization by layers: skin, subcutaneous tissue, and deep fascia covering the deeper structures of muscles, skeleton, and cavities, which contain *viscera* (internal organs). Many of these deeper structures are partially evident beneath the body's outer covering and may be studied and examined in living individuals via surface anatomy.

Surface anatomy is an essential part of the study of regional anatomy. It is specifically addressed in this book in "surface anatomy sections" (orange background) that provide knowledge of what lies under the skin and what structures are perceptible to touch (palpable) in the living body at rest and in action. We can learn much by observing the external form and surface of the body and by observing or feeling the superficial aspects of structures beneath its surface. The aim of this method is to *visualize* (recall distinct mental images of) structures that confer contour to the surface or are palpable beneath it and, in clinical practice, to distinguish any unusual or abnormal findings. In short, surface anatomy requires a thorough understanding of the anatomy of the structures beneath the surface. In people with stab wounds, for example, a physician must be able to visualize the deep structures that may be injured. Knowledge of surface anatomy can also decrease the need to memorize facts because the body is always available to observe and palpate.

Physical examination is the clinical application of surface anatomy. **Palpation** is a clinical technique, used with **observation** and **listening** for examining the body. *Palpation of arterial pulses*, for instance, is part of a physical examination. Students of many of the health sciences will learn to use instruments to facilitate examination of the body (such as an *ophthalmoscope* for observation of features of the eyeballs) and to listen to functioning parts of the body (a *stethoscope* to auscultate the heart and lungs).

Regional study of deep structures and abnormalities in a living person is now also possible by means of radiographic and sectional imaging and endoscopy. *Radiographic and sectional imaging (radiographic anatomy)* provides useful information about normal structures in living individuals, demonstrating the effect of muscle tone, body fluids and pressures, and gravity that cadaveric study does not. *Diagnostic radiology* reveals the effects of trauma, pathology, and aging on normal structures. In this book, most radiographic and many sectional

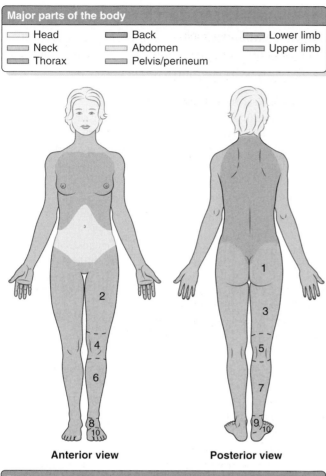

Major parts of the body

☐ Head	☐ Back	☐ Lower limb
☐ Neck	☐ Abdomen	☐ Upper limb
☐ Thorax	☐ Pelvis/perineum	

Anterior view   **Posterior view**

Regions of lower limb

1 = Gluteal region	6 = Anterior leg region
2 = Anterior thigh region	7 = Posterior leg region
3 = Posterior thigh region	8 = Anterior talocrural (ankle) region
4 = Anterior knee region	9 = Posterior talocrural region
5 = Posterior knee region	10 = Foot region

FIGURE I.1. Major parts of the body and regions of the lower limb.
Anatomy is described relative to the anatomical position illustrated here.

models. **Prosections,** carefully prepared dissections for the demonstration of anatomical structures, are also useful. However, learning is most efficient and retention is highest when didactic study is combined with the experience of first-hand **dissection**—that is, learning by doing. During dissection you observe, palpate, move, and sequentially reveal parts of the body. In 1770, Dr. *William Hunter*, a distinguished Scottish anatomist and obstetrician, stated: "Dissection alone teaches us where we may cut or inspect the living body with freedom and dispatch."

Systemic Anatomy

Systemic anatomy is the study of the body's organ systems that work together to carry out complex functions. The basic systems and the field of study or treatment of each (in parentheses) are:

- The **integumentary system** (*dermatology*) consists of the skin (L. *integumentum*, a covering) and its appendages—hairs, nails, and sweat glands, for example—and the subcutaneous tissue just beneath it. The skin, an extensive sensory organ, forms the body's outer, protective covering and container.
- The **skeletal system** (*osteology*) consists of bones and cartilage; it provides our basic shape and support for the body and is what the muscular system acts on to produce movement. It also protects vital organs such as the heart, lungs, and pelvic organs.
- The **articular system** (*arthrology*) consists of joints and their associated ligaments, connecting the bony parts of the skeletal system and providing the sites at which movements occur.
- The **muscular system** (*myology*) consists of skeletal muscles that act (contract) to move or position parts of the body (e.g., the bones that articulate at joints), or smooth and cardiac muscle that propels, expels, or controls the flow of fluids and contained substance.
- The **nervous system** (*neurology*) consists of the *central nervous system* (brain and spinal cord) and the *peripheral nervous system* (nerves and ganglia, together with their motor and sensory endings). The nervous system controls and coordinates the functions of the organ systems, enabling the body's responses to and activities within its environment. The sense organs, including the olfactory organ (sense of smell), eye or visual system (*ophthalmology*), ear (sense of hearing and balance—*otology*), and gustatory organ (sense of taste), are often considered with the nervous system in systemic anatomy.
- The **circulatory system** (*angiology*) consists of the cardiovascular and lymphatic systems, which function in parallel to transport the body's fluids.
  - The **cardiovascular system** (*cardiology*) consists of the heart and blood vessels that propel and conduct blood through the body, delivering oxygen, nutrients, and hormones to cells and removing their waste products.

images are integrated into the chapters where appropriate. The medical imaging sections at the end of each chapter provide an introduction to the techniques of radiographic and sectional imaging and include series of sectional images that apply to the chapter. *Endoscopic techniques* (using a insertable flexible fiber optic device to examine internal structures, such as the interior of the stomach) also demonstrate living anatomy. The detailed and thorough learning of the three-dimensional anatomy of deep structures and their relationships is best accomplished initially by dissection. In clinical practice, surface anatomy, radiographic and sectional images, endoscopy, and your experience from studying anatomy will combine to provide you with knowledge of your patient's anatomy.

The computer is a useful adjunct in teaching regional anatomy because it facilitates learning by allowing interactivity and manipulation of two- and three-dimensional graphic

- The **lymphatic system** is a network of lymphatic vessels that withdraws excess tissue fluid (lymph) from the body's interstitial (intercellular) fluid compartment, filters it through lymph nodes, and returns it to the bloodstream.
- The **alimentary** or **digestive system** (*gastroenterology*) consists of the digestive tract from the mouth to the anus, with all its associated organs and glands that function in ingestion, mastication (chewing), deglutition (swallowing), digestion, and absorption of food and the elimination of the solid waste (feces) remaining after the nutrients have been absorbed.
- The **respiratory system** (*pulmonology*) consists of the air passages and lungs that supply oxygen to the blood for cellular respiration and eliminate carbon dioxide from it. The diaphragm and larynx control the flow of air through the system, which may also produce tone in the larynx that is further modified by the tongue, teeth, and lips into speech.
- The **urinary system** (*urology*) consists of the kidneys, ureters, urinary bladder, and urethra, which filter blood and subsequently produce, transport, store, and intermittently excrete urine (liquid waste).
- The **genital (reproductive) system** (*gynecology* for females; *andrology* for males) consists of the gonads (ovaries and testes) that produce oocytes (eggs) and sperms, the ducts that transport them, and the genitalia that enable their union. After conception, the female reproductive tract nourishes and delivers the fetus.
- The **endocrine system** (*endocrinology*) consists of specialized structures that secrete hormones, including discrete ductless endocrine glands (such as the thyroid gland), isolated and clustered cells of the gut and blood vessel walls, and specialized nerve endings. **Hormones** are organic molecules that are carried by the circulatory system to distant effector cells in all parts of the body. The influence of the endocrine system is thus as broadly distributed as that of the nervous system. Hormones influence metabolism and other processes, such as the menstrual cycle, pregnancy, and parturition (childbirth).

None of the systems functions in isolation. The passive skeletal and articular systems and the active muscular system collectively constitute a *supersystem*, the **locomotor system** or **apparatus** (*orthopedics*), because they must work together to produce locomotion of the body. Although the structures directly responsible for locomotion are the muscles, bones, joints, and ligaments of the limbs, other systems are indirectly involved as well. The brain and nerves of the nervous system stimulate them to act; the arteries and veins of the circulatory system supply oxygen and nutrients to and remove waste from these structures; and the sensory organs (especially vision and equilibrium) play important roles in directing their activities in a gravitational environment.

In this Introduction, an overview of several systems significant to all parts and regions of the body will be provided before Chapters 1 through 8 cover regional anatomy in detail. Chapter 9 also presents systemic anatomy in reviewing the cranial nerves.

Clinical Anatomy

Clinical anatomy (applied anatomy) emphasizes aspects of bodily structure and function important in the practice of medicine, dentistry, and the allied health sciences. It incorporates the regional and systemic approaches to studying anatomy and stresses clinical application.

Clinical anatomy often involves inverting or reversing the thought process typically followed when studying regional or systemic anatomy. For example, instead of thinking, "The action of this muscle is to . . . ," clinical anatomy asks, "How would the absence of this muscle's activity be manifest?" Instead of noting, "The . . . nerve provides innervation to this area of skin," clinical anatomy asks, "Numbness in this area indicates a lesion of which nerve?"

Clinical anatomy is exciting to learn because of its role in solving clinical problems. The clinical correlation boxes (popularly called "blue boxes," appearing on a blue background) throughout this book describe practical applications of anatomy. "Case studies," such as those on the Clinically Oriented Anatomy website (http://thePoint.lww.com/COA7e), are integral parts of the clinical approach to studying anatomy.

The Bottom Line

STUDYING ANATOMY

Anatomy is the study of the structure of the human body. ♦ Regional anatomy considers the body as organized into segments or parts. ♦ Systemic anatomy sees the body as organized into organ systems. ♦ Surface anatomy provides information about structures that may be observed or palpated beneath the skin. ♦ Radiographic, sectional, and endoscopic anatomy allows appreciation of structures in living people, as they are affected by muscle tone, body fluids and pressures, and gravity. ♦ Clinical anatomy emphasizes application of anatomical knowledge to the practice of medicine.

ANATOMICOMEDICAL TERMINOLOGY

Anatomical terminology introduces and makes up a large part of medical terminology. To be understood, you must express yourself clearly, using the proper terms in the correct way. Although you are familiar with common, colloquial terms for parts and regions of the body, you must learn the *international anatomical terminology* (e.g., axillary fossa instead of armpit and clavicle instead of collarbone) that enables precise communication among healthcare professionals and scientists worldwide. Health professionals must also know the common and colloquial terms people are likely to use when they describe their complaints. Furthermore, you must be able to use terms people will understand when explaining their medical problems to them.

The terminology in this book conforms to the new *International Anatomical Terminology. Terminologia Anatomica* (TA) and *Terminologia Embryologica (TE)* list terms both in Latin and as English equivalents (e.g., the common shoulder muscle is *musculus deltoideus* in Latin and *deltoid* in English). Most terms in this book are English equivalents. Official terms are available at www.unifr.ch/ifaa. Unfortunately, the terminology commonly used in the clinical arena may differ from the official terminology. Because this discrepancy may be a source of confusion, this text clarifies commonly confused terms by placing the unofficial designations in parentheses when the terms are first used—for example, *pharyngotympanic tube* (auditory tube, eustachian tube) and *internal thoracic artery* (internal mammary artery). *Eponyms*, terms incorporating the names of people, are not used in the new terminology because they give no clue about the type or location of the structures involved. Further, many eponyms are historically inaccurate in terms of identifying the original person to describe a structure or assign its function, and do not conform to an international standard. Notwithstanding, commonly used eponyms appear in parentheses throughout the book when these terms are first used—such as *sternal angle* (angle of Louis)—since you will surely encounter them in your clinical years. Note that eponymous terms do not help to locate the structure in the body. The Clinically Oriented Anatomy website (http://thePoint.lww.com/COA7e) provides a list of eponymous terms.

Structure of terms. Anatomy is a descriptive science and requires names for the many structures and processes of the body. Because most terms are derived from Latin and Greek, medical language may seem difficult at first; however, as you learn the origin of terms, the words make sense. For example, the term *gaster* is Latin for stomach or belly. Consequently, the esophagogastric junction is the site where the esophagus connects with the stomach, gastric acid is the digestive juice secreted by the stomach, and a digastric muscle is a muscle divided into two bellies.

Many terms provide information about a structure's shape, size, location, or function or about the resemblance of one structure to another. For example, some muscles have descriptive names to indicate their main characteristics. The *deltoid muscle,* which covers the point of the shoulder, is triangular, like the symbol for *delta,* the fourth letter of the Greek alphabet. The suffix *-oid* means "like"; therefore, *deltoid* means like delta. *Biceps* means two-headed and *triceps* means three-headed. Some muscles are named according to their shape—the *piriformis muscle,* for example, is pear shaped (L. *pirum,* pear + L. *forma,* shape or form). Other muscles are named according to their location. The *temporal muscle* is in the temporal region (temple) of the cranium (skull). In some cases, actions are used to describe muscles—for example, the *levator scapulae* elevates the scapula (L. shoulder blade). Anatomical terminology applies logical reasons for the names of muscles and other parts of the body,

and if you learn their meanings and think about them as you read and dissect, it will be easier to remember their names.

Abbreviations. Abbreviations of terms are used for brevity in medical histories and in this and other books, such as in tables of muscles, arteries, and nerves. Clinical abbreviations are used in discussions and descriptions of signs and symptoms. Learning to use these abbreviations also speeds note taking. Common anatomical and clinical abbreviations are provided in this text when the corresponding term is introduced—for example, temporomandibular joint (TMJ). The Clinically Oriented Anatomy website (http://thePoint.lww.com/COA7e) provides a list of commonly used anatomical abbreviations. More extensive lists of common medical abbreviations may be found in the appendices of comprehensive medical dictionaries (e.g., *Stedman's Medical Dictionary,* 28th ed.).

Anatomical Position

All anatomical descriptions are expressed in relation to one consistent position, ensuring that descriptions are not ambiguous (Figs. I.1 and I.2). One must visualize this position in the mind when describing patients (or cadavers), whether they are lying on their sides, supine (recumbent, lying on the back, face upward), or prone (lying on the abdomen, face downward). The **anatomical position** refers to the body position as if the person were standing upright with the:

- head, gaze (eyes), and toes directed anteriorly (forward),
- arms adjacent to the sides with the palms facing anteriorly, and
- lower limbs close together with the feet parallel.

This position is adopted globally for anatomicomedical descriptions. By using this position and appropriate terminology, you can relate any part of the body precisely to any other part. It should also be kept in mind, however, that gravity causes a downward shift of internal organs (viscera) when the upright position is assumed. Since people are typically examined in the supine position, it is often necessary to describe the position of the affected organs when supine, making specific note of this exception to the anatomical position.

Anatomical Planes

Anatomical descriptions are based on four imaginary planes (median, sagittal, frontal, and transverse) that intersect the body in the anatomical position (Fig. I.2):

- The **median plane** (median sagittal plane), the vertical plane passing longitudinally through the body, divides the body into right and left halves. The plane defines the midline of the head, neck, and trunk where it intersects the surface of the body. *Midline* is often erroneously used as a synonym for the median plane.
- **Sagittal planes** are vertical planes passing through the body *parallel to the median plane. Parasagittal* is commonly used but is unnecessary because any plane parallel to and on either side of the median plane is sagittal

FIGURE I.2. **Anatomical planes.** The main planes of the body are illustrated.

by definition. However, a plane parallel and near to the median plane may be referred to as a *paramedian plane.*

- **Frontal (coronal) planes** are vertical planes passing through the body *at right angles to the median plane,* dividing the body into anterior (front) and posterior (back) parts.
- **Transverse planes** are horizontal planes passing through the body *at right angles to the median and frontal planes,* dividing the body into superior (upper) and inferior (lower) parts. Radiologists refer to transverse planes as *transaxial,* which is commonly shortened to *axial planes.*

Since the number of sagittal, frontal, and transverse planes is unlimited, a reference point (usually a visible or palpable landmark or vertebral level) is necessary to identify the location or level of the plane, such as a "transverse plane through the umbilicus" (Fig. I.2C). Sections of the head, neck, and trunk in precise frontal and transverse planes are symmetrical, passing through both the right and left members of paired structures, allowing some comparison.

The main use of anatomical planes is to describe *sections* (Fig. I.3):

- **Longitudinal sections** run lengthwise or parallel to the long axis of the body or of any of its parts, and the term applies regardless of the position of the body. Although median, sagittal, and frontal planes are the standard (most commonly used) longitudinal sections, there is a 180° range of possible longitudinal sections.
- **Transverse sections,** or cross sections, are slices of the body or its parts that are cut at right angles to the longitudinal axis of the body or of any of its parts. Because

the long axis of the foot runs horizontally, a transverse section of the foot lies in the frontal plane (Fig. I.2C).

- **Oblique sections** are slices of the body or any of its parts that are not cut along the previously listed anatomical planes. In practice, many radiographic images and anatomical sections do not lie precisely in sagittal, frontal, or transverse planes; often they are slightly oblique.

Anatomists create sections of the body and its parts anatomically, and clinicians create them by planar imaging technologies, such as computerized tomography (CT), to describe and display internal structures.

Terms of Relationship and Comparison

Various adjectives, arranged as pairs of opposites, describe the relationship of parts of the body or compare the position of two structures relative to each other (Fig. I.4). Some of these terms are specific for comparisons made in the anatomical position, or with reference to the anatomical planes:

Superior refers to a structure that is nearer the **vertex,** the topmost point of the cranium (Mediev. L., skull). **Cranial** relates to the cranium and is a useful directional term, meaning toward the head or cranium. **Inferior** refers to a structure that is situated nearer the sole of the foot. **Caudal** (L. *cauda,* tail) is a useful directional term that means toward the feet or tail region, represented in humans by the coccyx (tail bone), the small bone at the inferior (caudal) end of the vertebral column.

(A) Longitudinal section

(B) Transverse section

(C) Oblique section

FIGURE I.3. **Sections of the limbs.** Sections may be obtained by anatomical sectioning or medical imaging techniques.

Posterior (dorsal) denotes the back surface of the body or nearer to the back. **Anterior** (ventral) denotes the front surface of the body. **Rostral** is often used instead of anterior when describing parts of the brain; it means toward the rostrum (L. for beak); however, in humans it denotes nearer the anterior part of the head (e.g., the frontal lobe of the brain is rostral to the cerebellum).

Medial is used to indicate that a structure is nearer to the median plane of the body. For example, the 5th digit of the hand (little finger) is medial to the other digits. Conversely, **lateral** stipulates that a structure is farther away from the median plane. The 1st digit of the hand (thumb) is lateral to the other digits.

Dorsum usually refers to the superior aspect of any part that protrudes anteriorly from the body, such as the dorsum of the tongue, nose, penis, or foot. It is also used to describe the posterior surface of the hand, opposite the **palm.** Because the term dorsum may refer to both superior and posterior surfaces in humans, the term is easier to understand if one thinks of a quadripedal plantigrade animal that walks on its palms and soles, such as a bear. The **sole** is the inferior aspect or bottom of the foot, opposite the dorsum, much of which is in contact with the ground when standing barefoot. The surface of the hands, the feet, and the digits of both corresponding to the dorsum is the **dorsal surface,** the surface of the hand and fingers corresponding to the palm is the **palmar surface,** and the surface of the foot and toes corresponding to the sole is the **plantar surface.**

Combined terms describe intermediate positional arrangements: **inferomedial** means nearer to the feet and median plane—for example, the anterior parts of the ribs run inferomedially; **superolateral** means nearer to the head and farther from the median plane.

Other terms of relationship and comparisons are independent of the anatomical position or the anatomical planes, relating primarily to the body's surface or its central core:

Superficial, intermediate, and **deep** describe the position of structures relative to the surface of the body or the relationship of one structure to another underlying or overlying structure.

External means outside of or farther from the center of an organ or cavity, while **internal** means inside or closer to the center, independent of direction.

Proximal and **distal** are used when contrasting positions nearer to or farther from the attachment of a limb or the central aspect of a linear structure, respectively.

Terms of Laterality

Paired structures having right and left members (e.g., the kidneys) are **bilateral,** whereas those occurring on one side only (e.g., the spleen) are **unilateral.** Designating whether you are referring specifically to the right or left member of bilateral structures can be critical, and is a good habit to begin at the outset of one's training to become a health professional. Something occurring on the same side of the body as another structure is **ipsilateral;** the right thumb and right great (big) toe are ipsilateral, for example. **Contralateral** means occurring on the opposite side of the body relative to another structure; the right hand is contralateral to the left hand.

Terms of Movement

Various terms describe movements of the limbs and other parts of the body (Fig. I.5). Most movements are defined in relationship to the anatomical position, with movements occurring within, and around axes aligned with, specific anatomical planes. While most movements occur at joints where two or more bones or cartilages articulate with one another, several non-skeletal structures exhibit movement (e.g., tongue, lips, eyelids). Terms of movement may also be considered in pairs of opposing movements:

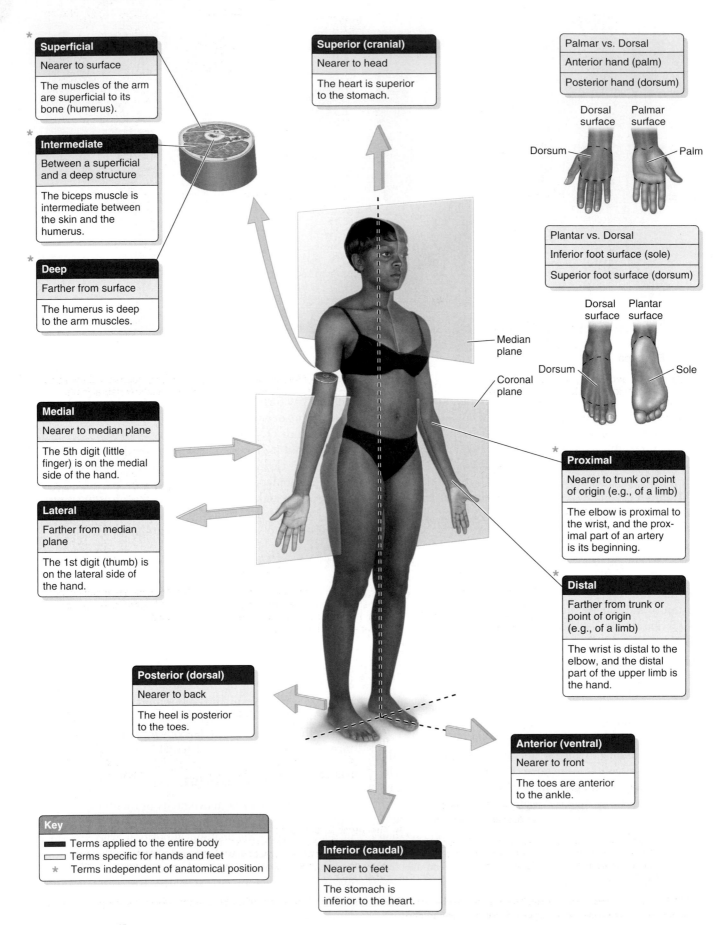

Superficial

Nearer to surface

The muscles of the arm are superficial to its bone (humerus).

Intermediate

Between a superficial and a deep structure

The biceps muscle is intermediate between the skin and the humerus.

Deep

Farther from surface

The humerus is deep to the arm muscles.

Medial

Nearer to median plane

The 5th digit (little finger) is on the medial side of the hand.

Lateral

Farther from median plane

The 1st digit (thumb) is on the lateral side of the hand.

Superior (cranial)

Nearer to head

The heart is superior to the stomach.

Median plane

Coronal plane

Palmar vs. Dorsal

Anterior hand (palm)

Posterior hand (dorsum)

Dorsal surface   Palmar surface

Dorsum   Palm

Plantar vs. Dorsal

Inferior foot surface (sole)

Superior foot surface (dorsum)

Dorsal surface   Plantar surface

Dorsum   Sole

Proximal

Nearer to trunk or point of origin (e.g., of a limb)

The elbow is proximal to the wrist, and the proximal part of an artery is its beginning.

Distal

Farther from trunk or point of origin (e.g., of a limb)

The wrist is distal to the elbow, and the distal part of the upper limb is the hand.

Posterior (dorsal)

Nearer to back

The heel is posterior to the toes.

Anterior (ventral)

Nearer to front

The toes are anterior to the ankle.

Key

▬ Terms applied to the entire body
▭ Terms specific for hands and feet
* Terms independent of anatomical position

Inferior (caudal)

Nearer to feet

The stomach is inferior to the heart.

FIGURE I.4. Terms of relationship and comparison. These terms describe the position of one structure relative to another.

(A) Flexion and extension of upper limb at shoulder joint and lower limb at hip joint

Flexion and extension of forearm at elbow joint and of leg at knee joint

Flexion and extension of vertebral column at intervertebral joints

(B) Flexion and extension of hand at wrist joint

Flexion and extension of digits (fingers) at metacarpophalangeal and interphalangeal joints

(C) Opposition and reposition of thumb and little finger at carpometacarpal joint of thumb combined with flexion at metacarpophalangeal joints

(D) Pronation and supination of forearm at radio-lnar joints

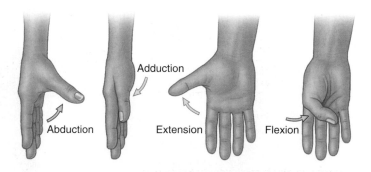

(E) Abduction and adduction of 2nd, 4th, and 5th digits at metacarpophalangeal joints

Abduction of 3rd digit at metacarpophalangeal joint

(F) The thumb is rotated 90° relative to other structures. Abduction and adduction at metacarpophalangeal joint occurs in a sagittal plane; flexion and extension at metacarpophalangeal and interphalangeal joints occurs in frontal planes, opposite to these movements at all other joints.

FIGURE I.5. Terms of movement. These terms describe movements of the limbs and other parts of the body; most movements take place at joints, where two or more bones or cartilages articulate with one another.

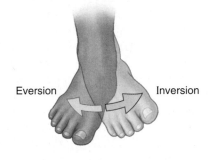

(G) Abduction and adduction of right limbs and rotation of left limbs at glenohumeral and hip joints, respectively

(H) Circumduction (circular movement) of lower limb at hip joint

(I) Inversion and eversion of foot at subtalar and transverse tarsal joints

(K) Elevation and depression of shoulders

(J) Lateral bending (lateral flexion) of trunk and rotation of upper trunk, neck, and head

(L) Protrusion and retrusion of jaw at temporomandibular joints

(M) Protraction and retraction of scapula on thoracic wall

FIGURE I.5. (Continued)

Flexion and extension movements generally occur in sagittal planes around a transverse axis (Fig. I.5A & B). **Flexion** indicates bending or decreasing the angle between the bones or parts of the body. For most joints (e.g., elbow), flexion involves movement in an anterior direction. **Extension** indicates straightening or increasing the angle between the bones or parts of the body. Extension usually occurs in a posterior direction. The knee joint, rotated 180° to other joints, is exceptional in that flexion of the knee involves posterior movement and extension involves anterior movement. **Dorsiflexion** describes flexion at the ankle joint, as occurs when walking uphill or lifting the front of the foot and toes off the ground (Fig. I.5I). **Plantarflexion** bends the foot and toes toward the ground, as when standing on your toes. Extension of a limb or part beyond the normal limit—**hyperextension** (overextension)—can cause injury, such as "whiplash" (i.e., hyperextension of the neck during a rear-end automobile collision).

Abduction and adduction movements generally occur in a frontal plane around an anteroposterior axis (Fig. I.5E & G). Except for the digits, **abduction** means moving away from the median plane (e.g., when moving an upper limb laterally away from the side of the body) and **adduction** means moving toward it. In *abduction of the digits* (fingers or toes), the term means spreading them apart—moving the other fingers away from the neutrally positioned 3rd (middle) finger or moving the other toes away from the neutrally positioned 2nd toe. The 3rd finger and 2nd toe *medially* or *laterally abduct* away from the neutral position. *Adduction of the digits* is the opposite—bringing the spread fingers or toes together, toward the neutrally positioned 3rd finger or 2nd toe. Right and left lateral flexion (lateral bending) are special forms of abduction for only the neck and trunk (Fig. I.5J). The face and upper trunk are directed anteriorly as the head and/or shoulders tilt to the right or left side, causing the midline of the body itself to become bent sideways. This is a compound movement occurring between many adjacent vertebrae.

As you can see by noticing the way the thumbnail faces (laterally instead of posteriorly in the anatomical position), the thumb is rotated 90° relative to the other digits (Fig. I.5F). Therefore, the thumb flexes and extends in the frontal plane and abducts and adducts in the sagittal plane.

Circumduction is a circular movement that involves sequential flexion, abduction, extension, and adduction (or in the opposite order) in such a way that the distal end of the part moves in a circle (Fig. I.5H). Circumduction can occur at any joint at which all the above-mentioned movements are possible (e.g., the shoulder and hip joints).

Rotation involves turning or revolving a part of the body around its longitudinal axis, such as turning one's head to face sideways (Fig. I.5G). *Medial rotation* (internal rotation) brings the anterior surface of a limb closer to the median plane, whereas *lateral rotation* (external rotation) takes the anterior surface away from the median plane.

Pronation and supination are the rotational movements of the forearm and hand that swing the distal end of the radius (the lateral long bone of the forearm) medially and laterally around and across the anterior aspect of the ulna (the other long bone of the forearm) while the proximal end of the radius rotates in place (Fig. I.5D). **Pronation** rotates the radius medially so that the palm of the hand faces posteriorly and its dorsum faces anteriorly. When the elbow joint is flexed, pronation moves the hand so that the palm faces inferiorly (e.g., placing the palms flat on a table). **Supination** is the opposite rotational movement, rotating the radius laterally and uncrossing it from the ulna, returning the pronated forearm to the anatomical position. When the elbow joint is flexed, supination moves the hand so that the palm faces superiorly. (*Memory device:* You can hold *soup* in the palm of your hand when the flexed forearm is *sup*inated but are *prone* [likely] to spill it if the forearm is then *pron*ated!)

Eversion moves the sole of the foot away from the median plane, turning the sole laterally (Fig. I.5I). When the foot is fully everted it is also dorsiflexed. **Inversion** moves the sole of the foot toward the median plane (facing the sole medially). When the foot is fully inverted it is also plantarflexed. *Pronation of the foot* actually refers to a combination of eversion and abduction that results in lowering of the medial margin of the foot (the feet of an individual with flat feet are pronated), and *supination of the foot* generally implies movements resulting in raising the medial margin of the foot, a combination of inversion and adduction.

Opposition is the movement by which the pad of the 1st digit (thumb) is brought to another digit pad (Fig. I.5C). This movement is used to pinch, button a shirt, and lift a teacup by the handle. **Reposition** describes the movement of the 1st digit from the position of opposition back to its anatomical position.

Protrusion is a movement anteriorly (forward) as in protruding the mandible (chin), lips, or tongue (Fig. I.5L). **Retrusion** is a movement posteriorly (backward), as in retruding the mandible, lips, or tongue. The similar terms **protraction** and **retraction** are used most commonly for anterolateral and posteromedial movements of the scapula on the thoracic wall, causing the shoulder region to move anteriorly and posteriorly (Fig. I.5M).

Elevation raises or moves a part superiorly, as in elevating the shoulders when shrugging, the upper eyelid when opening the eye, or the tongue when pushing it up against the palate (roof of mouth) (Fig. I.5K). **Depression** lowers or moves a part inferiorly, as in depressing the shoulders when standing at ease, the upper eyelid when closing the eye, or pulling the tongue away from the palate.

The Bottom Line

ANATOMICOMEDICAL TERMINOLOGY

Anatomical terms are descriptive terms standardized in an international reference guide, *Terminologia Anatomica* (TA). These terms, in English or Latin, are used worldwide. ♦ Colloquial terminology is used by—and to communicate with—lay people. ♦ Eponyms are often used in clinical settings but are not recommended because they do not provide anatomical context and are not standardized. ♦ Anatomical directional terms are based on the body in the anatomical position. ♦ Four anatomical planes divide the body, and sections divide the planes into visually useful and descriptive parts. ♦ Other anatomical terms describe relationships of parts of the body, compare the positions of structures, and describe laterality and movement.

ANATOMICAL VARIATIONS

Anatomy books describe (initially, at least) the structure of the body as it is usually observed in people—that is, the most common pattern. However, occasionally a particular structure demonstrates so much variation within the normal range that the most common pattern is found less than half the time! Beginning students are frequently frustrated because the bodies they are examining or dissecting do not conform to the atlas or text they are using (Bergman et al., 1988). Often students ignore the variations or inadvertently damage them by attempting to produce conformity. Therefore, you should *expect anatomical variations* when you dissect or inspect prosected specimens.

In a random group of people, individuals differ from each other in physical appearance. The bones of the skeleton vary not only in their basic shape but also in lesser details of surface structure. A wide variation is found in the size, shape, and form of the attachments of muscles. Similarly, considerable variation exists in the patterns of branching of veins, arteries, and nerves. *Veins vary the most and nerves the least.* Individual variation must be considered in physical examination, diagnosis, and treatment.

Most descriptions in this text assume a normal range of variation. However, the frequency of variation often differs among human groups, and variations collected in one population may not apply to members of another population. Some variations, such as those occurring in the origin and course of the cystic artery to the gallbladder, are clinically important (see Chapter 2), and any surgeon operating without knowledge of them is certain to have problems. Clinically significant variations are described in clinical correlation (blue) boxes identified with an Anatomical Variation icon (at left).

Apart from racial and sexual differences, humans exhibit considerable genetic variation, such as polydactyly (extra digits). Approximately 3% of newborns show one or more significant birth defects (Moore et al, 2012). Other defects (e.g., atresia or blockage of the intestine) are not detected until symptoms occur. Discovering variations and congenital anomalies in cadavers is actually one of the many benefits of firsthand dissection, because it enables students to develop an awareness of the occurrence of variations and a sense of their frequency.

The Bottom Line

ANATOMICAL VARIATIONS

Anatomical variations are common and students should expect to encounter them during dissection. It is important to know how such variations may influence physical examinations, diagnosis, and treatment.

INTEGUMENTARY SYSTEM

Because the skin (L. *integumentum,* a covering) is readily accessible and is one of the best indicators of general health, careful observation of it is important in physical examinations. It is considered in the differential diagnosis of almost every disease. The skin provides:

- *Protection* of the body from environmental effects, such as abrasions, fluid loss, harmful substances, ultraviolet radiation, and invading microorganisms.
- *Containment* for the body's structures (e.g., tissues and organs) and vital substances (especially extracellular fluids), preventing dehydration, which may be severe when extensive skin injuries (e.g., burns) are experienced.
- *Heat regulation* through the evaporation of sweat and/or the dilation or constriction of superficial blood vessels.
- *Sensation* (e.g., pain) by way of superficial nerves and their sensory endings.
- *Synthesis and storage* of vitamin D.

The **skin,** the body's largest organ, consists of the epidermis, a superficial cellular layer, and the dermis, a deep connective tissue layer (Fig. I.6).

The **epidermis** is a *keratinized epithelium*—that is, it has a tough, horny *superficial layer* that provides a protective outer surface overlying its regenerative and pigmented deep or *basal layer.* The epidermis has no blood vessels or lymphatics. The *avascular epidermis* is nourished by the underlying *vascularized dermis.* The dermis is supplied by arteries that enter its deep surface to form a cutaneous plexus of anastomosing arteries. The skin is also supplied with afferent nerve endings that are sensitive to touch, irritation (pain), and temperature. Most nerve terminals are in the dermis, but a few penetrate the epidermis.

The **dermis** is a dense layer of interlacing *collagen* and *elastic fibers.* These fibers provide skin tone and account for the strength and toughness of skin. The dermis of animals is removed and tanned to produce leather. Although the bundles of collagen fibers in the dermis run in all directions to produce a tough felt-like tissue, in any specific location most fibers run in the same direction. The predominant pattern of collagen fibers determines the characteristic tension and wrinkle lines in the skin.

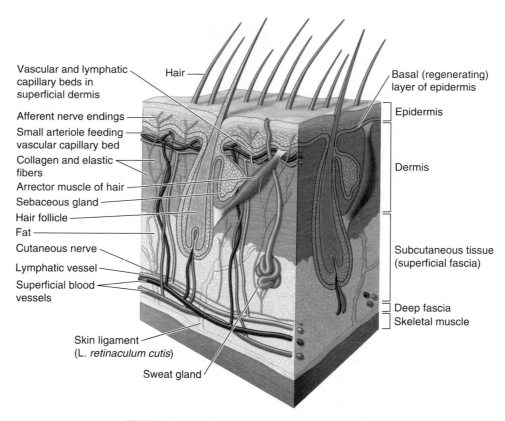

Vascular and lymphatic
capillary beds in
superficial dermis

Hair

Basal (regenerating)
layer of epidermis

Epidermis

Afferent nerve endings

Small arteriole feeding
vascular capillary bed

Dermis

Collagen and elastic
fibers

Arrector muscle of hair

Sebaceous gland

Hair follicle

Fat

Cutaneous nerve

Subcutaneous tissue
(superficial fascia)

Lymphatic vessel

Superficial blood
vessels

Deep fascia
Skeletal muscle

Skin ligament
(L. *retinaculum cutis*)

Sweat gland

FIGURE I.6. Skin and some of its specialized structures.

The **tension lines** (also called cleavage lines or Langer lines) tend to spiral longitudinally in the limbs and run transversely in the neck and trunk (Fig. I.7). Tension lines at the elbows, knees, ankles, and wrists are parallel to the transverse creases that appear when the limbs are flexed. The elastic fibers of the dermis deteriorate with age and are not replaced; consequently, in older people, the skin wrinkles and sags as it loses its elasticity.

The skin also contains many specialized structures (Fig. I.6). The deep layer of the dermis contains *hair follicles,* with associated smooth arrector muscles and sebaceous glands. Contraction of the **arrector muscles of hairs** (L. *musculi arrector pili*) erects the hairs, causing goose bumps. Hair follicles are generally slanted to one side, and several *sebaceous glands* lie on the side the hair is directed toward ("points to") as it emerges from the skin. Thus, contraction of the arrector muscles causes the hairs to stand up straighter, thereby compressing the sebaceous glands and helping them secrete their oily product onto the skin surface. The evaporation of the watery secretion (sweat) of the *sweat glands* from the skin provides a *thermoregulatory mechanism* for heat loss (cooling). Also involved in the loss or retention of body heat are the small arteries (arterioles) within the dermis. They dilate to fill *superficial capillary beds* to radiate heat (skin appears red) or constrict to minimize surface heat loss (skin, especially of the lips and fingertips, appears blue). Other skin structures or derivatives include the nails (fingernails, toenails), the mammary glands, and the enamel of teeth.

Located between the overlying skin (dermis) and underlying deep fascia, the **subcutaneous tissue** (superficial fascia) is composed mostly of *loose connective tissue* and *stored fat* and contains sweat glands, *superficial blood vessels, lymphatic vessels,* and *cutaneous nerves* (Fig. I.6). The neurovascular structures course in the subcutaneous tissue, distributing only their terminal branches to the skin.

The subcutaneous tissue provides for most of the body's fat storage, so its thickness varies greatly, depending on the person's nutritional state. In addition, the distribution of subcutaneous tissue varies considerably in different sites in the same individual. Compare, for example, the relative abundance of subcutaneous tissue evident by the thickness of the fold of skin that can be pinched at the waist or thighs with the anteromedial part of the leg (the shin, the anterior border of the tibia) or the back of the hand, the latter two being nearly devoid of subcutaneous tissue. Also consider the distribution of subcutaneous tissue and fat between the sexes: In mature females, it tends to accumulate in the breasts and thighs, whereas in males, subcutaneous fat accumulates in the lower abdominal wall.

Subcutaneous tissue participates in thermoregulation, functioning as insulation, retaining heat in the body's core. It also provides padding that protects the skin from compression by bony prominences, such as those in the buttocks.

Skin ligaments (L. *retinacula cutis*), numerous small fibrous bands, extend through the subcutaneous tissue and attach the deep surface of the dermis to the underlying

An incision made across the cleavage lines is more likely to gape, increasing healing time, and result in increased scar tissue.

An incision made parallel to the cleavage lines results in less gaping, faster healing, and less scar tissue.

FIGURE I.7. Tension lines in the skin. The *dashed lines* indicate the predominant direction of the collagen fibers in the dermis.

Anterior view   Posterior view

deep fascia (Fig. I.6). The length and density of these ligaments determines the mobility of the skin over deep structures. Where skin ligaments are longer and sparse, the skin is more mobile, such as on the back of the hand (Fig. I.8A & B). Where ligaments are short and abundant, the skin is firmly attached to the underlying deep fascia, such as in the palms and soles (Fig. I.8C). In dissection, removal of skin where the skin ligaments are short and abundant requires use of a sharp scalpel. The skin ligaments are long but particularly well developed in the breasts, where they form weight-bearing *suspensory ligaments* (see Chapter 1).

INTEGUMENTARY SYSTEM

Skin Color Signs in Physical Diagnosis

Blood flow through the superficial capillary beds of the dermis affects the color of skin and can provide important clues for diagnosing certain clinical conditions. When the blood is not carrying enough oxygen from the lungs, such as in a person who has stopped breathing or in a person having a defective circulation that is sending an inadequate amount of blood through the lungs, the skin can appear bluish (*cyanotic*). This occurs because the oxygen-carrying hemoglobin of blood is bright red when carrying oxygen (as it does in arteries and usually does in capillaries), and appears deep, purplish blue when depleted of oxygen, as it does in veins. Cyanosis is especially evident where skin is thin, such as the lips, eyelids, and deep to the transparent nails. Skin injury, exposure to excess heat, infection, inflammation, or allergic reactions may cause the superficial capillary beds to become engorged, making the skin look abnormally red, a sign called *erythema*. In certain liver disorders, a yellow pigment called bilirubin builds up in the blood, giving a yellow appearance to the whites of the eyes and skin, a condition called *jaundice*. Skin color changes are most readily observed in people with light-colored skin and may be difficult to discern in people with dark skin.

Skin Incisions and Scarring

The skin is always under tension. In general, lacerations or incisions that parallel the tension lines usually heal well with little scarring because there is minimal disruption of fibers. The uninterrupted fibers tend to retain the cut edges in place. However, a laceration or incision across the tension lines disrupts more collagen fibers. The disrupted lines of force cause the wound to gape and it may heal with excessive (keloid) scarring. When other considerations, such as adequate exposure and access or avoidance of nerves, are not of greater importance, surgeons attempting to minimize scarring for cosmetic reasons may use surgical incisions that parallel the tension lines.

Stretch Marks in Skin

The collagen and elastic fibers in the dermis form a tough, flexible meshwork of tissue. Because the skin can distend considerably, a relatively small incision can be made during surgery compared with the much larger incision required to attempt the same procedure in an embalmed cadaver, which no longer exhibits elasticity. The skin can stretch and grow to accommodate gradual increases in size. However, marked and relatively fast size increases, such as the abdominal enlargement and weight gain accompanying pregnancy, can stretch the skin too much, damaging the collagen fibers in the dermis (Fig. BI.1). Bands of thin wrinkled skin, initially red but later becoming purple, and white stretch marks (L. *striae gravidarum*) appear on the abdomen, buttocks, thighs, and breasts during pregnancy. *Stretch marks* (L. *striae cutis distensae*) also form in obese individuals and in certain diseases (e.g., hypercortisolism or Cushing syndrome); they occur along with distension and loosening of the deep fascia due to protein breakdown leading to reduced cohesion between the collagen fibers. Stretch marks generally fade after pregnancy and weight loss, but they never disappear completely.

Skin Injuries and Wounds

Lacerations. Accidental cuts and skin tears are superficial or deep. Superficial lacerations violate the epidermis and perhaps the superficial layer of the dermis; they bleed but do not interrupt the continuity of the dermis. Deep lacerations penetrate the deep layer of the dermis, extending into the subcutaneous tissue or beyond; they gape and require approximation of the cut edges of the dermis (by suturing, or stitches) to minimize scarring.

Burns are caused by thermal trauma, ultraviolet or ionizing radiation, or chemical agents. Burns are classified, in increasing order of severity, based on the depth of skin injury (Fig. BI.2):

- *1st-degree (superficial) burn* (e.g., sunburn): damage is limited to the epidermis; symptoms are *erythema* (hot red skin), pain, and *edema* (swelling); *desquamation* (peeling) of the superficial layer usually occurs several days later, but the layer is quickly replaced from the basal layer of the epidermis without significant scarring.

Inflamed

1st-degree (superficial) burn - early stage; may "peel" at later stage

Superficial

Deep

2nd-degree (partial-thickness) burn

3rd-degree (full thickness) burn

Umbilicus

Stretch mark

FIGURE BI.1.

2nd-degree (partial-thickness) burn

FIGURE BI.2.

- *2nd-degree (partial-thickness) burn:* epidermis and superficial dermis are damaged with blistering (superficial 2nd degree) or loss (deep 2nd degree); nerve endings are damaged, making this variety the most painful; except for their most superficial parts, the sweat glands and hair follicles are not damaged and can provide the source of replacement cells for the basal layer of the epidermis along with cells from the edges of the wound; healing will occur slowly (3 weeks to several months), leaving scarring and some contracture, but it is usually complete.
- *3rd-degree (full-thickness) burn:* the entire thickness of the skin is damaged and perhaps underlying muscle. There is marked edema and the burned area is numb since sensory endings are destroyed. A minor degree of healing may occur at the edges, but the open, ulcerated portions require skin grafting: dead material (*eschar*) is removed and replaced (*grafted*) over the burned area with skin *harvested* (taken) from a non-burned location (*autograft*) or using skin from human cadavers or pigs, or cultured or artificial skin.

The extent of a burn (percent of total body surface affected) is generally more significant than the degree (severity in terms of depth) in estimating the effect on the well-being of the victim. According to the American Burn Association's classification of burn injury, a major burn includes 3rd-degree burns over 10% of body surface area; 2nd-degree burns over 25% of body surface area; or any 3rd-degree burns on the face, hands, feet, or perineum (area including anal and urogenital regions). When the burn area exceeds 70% of body surface area, the mortality rate exceeds 50%. The surface area affected by a burn in an adult can be estimated by applying the "Rule of Nines" in which the body is divided into areas that are approximately 9% or multiples of 9% of the total body surface (Fig. BI.3).

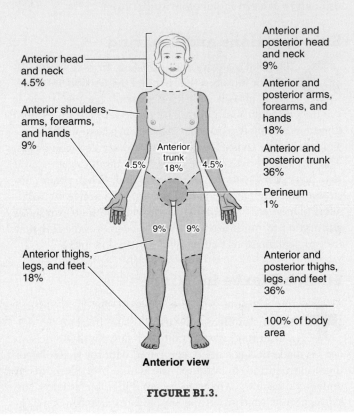

Anterior view

FIGURE BI.3.

The Bottom Line

INTEGUMENTARY SYSTEM

The integumentary system (the skin) consists of the epidermis, dermis, and specialized structures (hair follicles, sebaceous glands, and sweat glands). The skin: ♦ plays important roles in protection, containment, heat regulation, and sensation; ♦ synthesizes and stores vitamin D; ♦ features tension lines, relating to the predominant direction of collagen fibers in the skin, that have implications for surgery and wound healing. Subcutaneous tissue, located beneath the dermis, contains most of the body's fat stores.

FASCIAS, FASCIAL COMPARTMENTS, BURSAE, AND POTENTIAL SPACES

Fascias (L. *fasciae*) constitute the wrapping, packing, and insulating materials of the deep structures of the body. Underlying the *subcutaneous tissue* (superficial fascia) almost everywhere is the deep fascia (Fig. I.9). The **deep fascia** is a dense, organized connective tissue layer, devoid of fat, that covers most of the body parallel to (deep to) the skin and subcutaneous tissue. Extensions from its internal surface invest deeper structures, such as individual muscles and neurovascular bundles, as **investing fascia.** Its thickness varies widely. For example, in the face, distinct layers of deep fascia are absent.

In the limbs, groups of muscles with similar functions sharing the same nerve supply are located in **fascial compartments,** separated by thick sheets of deep fascia, called **intermuscular septa,** that extend centrally from the surrounding fascial sleeve to attach to bones. These compartments may contain or direct the spread of an infection or a tumor.

In a few places, the deep fascia gives attachment (origin) to the underlying muscles (although it is not usually included in lists or tables of origins and insertions); but in most places, the muscles are free to contract and glide deep to it. However, the deep fascia itself never passes freely over bone; where deep fascia contacts bone, it blends firmly with the *periosteum* (bone covering). The relatively unyielding deep fascia investing muscles, and especially that surrounding the fascial compartments in the limbs, limits the outward expansion of the bellies of contracting skeletal muscles. Blood is thus pushed out as the veins of the muscles and compartments are compressed. *Valves*

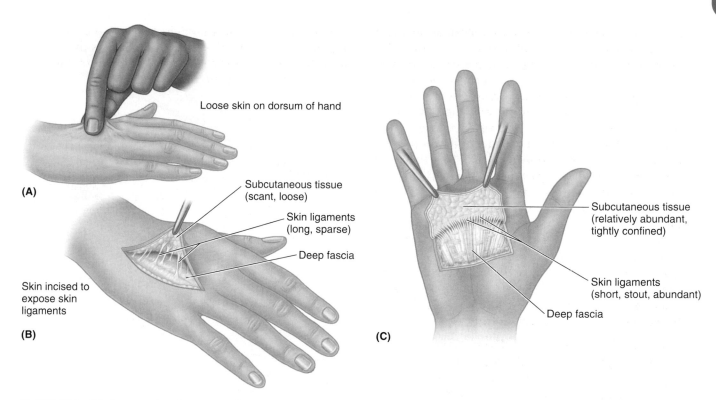

FIGURE I.8. Skin ligaments in subcutaneous tissue. A. The thickness of subcutaneous tissue can be estimated as being approximately half that of a pinched fold of skin (i.e., a fold of skin includes a double thickness of subcutaneous tissue). The dorsum of the hand has relatively little subcutaneous tissue. **B.** Long, relatively sparse skin ligaments allow the mobility of the skin demonstrated in part **A. C.** The skin of the palm (like that of the sole) is firmly attached to the underlying deep fascia.

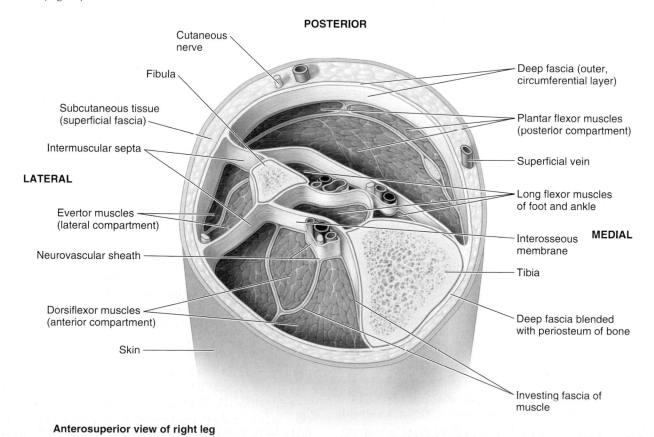

FIGURE I.9. Excavated section of the leg demonstrating the deep fascia and fascial formations.

within the veins allow the blood to flow only in one direction (toward the heart), preventing the backflow that might occur as the muscles relax. Thus deep fascia, contracting muscles, and venous valves work together as a *musculovenous pump* to return blood to the heart, especially in the lower limbs where blood must move against the pull of gravity (Fig. I.26).

Near certain joints (e.g., wrist and ankle), the deep fascia becomes markedly thickened, forming a **retinaculum** (plural = retinacula) to hold tendons in place where they cross the joint during flexion and extension, preventing them from taking a shortcut, or *bow stringing,* across the angle created (Fig. I.19).

Subserous fascia, with varying amounts of fatty tissue, lies between the internal surfaces of the musculoskeletal walls and the serous membranes lining the body cavities. These are the *endothoracic, endoabdominal,* and *endopelvic fascias;* the latter two may be referred to collectively as *extraperitoneal fascia.*

Bursae (singular = bursa; Mediev. L., a purse) are closed sacs or envelopes of **serous membrane** (a delicate connective tissue membrane capable of secreting fluid to lubricate a smooth internal surface). Bursae are normally collapsed. Unlike three-dimensional realized or actual spaces, these potential spaces have no depth; their walls are apposed with only a thin film of lubricating fluid between them that is secreted by the enclosing membranes. When the wall is interrupted at any point, or when a fluid is secreted or formed within them in excess, they become realized spaces; however, this condition is abnormal or pathological.

Usually occurring in locations subject to friction, bursae enable one structure to move more freely over another. **Subcutaneous bursae** occur in the subcutaneous tissue between the skin and bony prominences, such as at the elbow or knee; **subfascial bursae** lie beneath deep fascia; and **subtendinous bursae** facilitate the movement of tendons over bone. **Synovial tendon sheaths** are a specialized type of elongated bursae that wrap around tendons, usually enclosing them as they traverse osseofibrous tunnels that anchor the tendons in place (Fig. I.10A).

Bursae occasionally communicate with the synovial cavities of joints. Because they are formed by delicate, transparent serous membranes and are collapsed, bursae are not easily noticed or dissected in the laboratory. It is possible to display bursae by injecting and distending them with colored fluid.

Collapsed bursal sacs surround many important organs (e.g., the heart, lungs, and abdominal viscera) and structures (e.g., portions of tendons). This configuration is much like wrapping a large but empty balloon around a structure, such as a fist (Fig. I.10B). The object is surrounded by the two layers of the empty balloon but is not inside the balloon; the balloon itself remains empty. For an even more exact comparison, the balloon should first be filled with water and then emptied, leaving the empty balloon wet inside. In exactly this way, the heart is surrounded by—but is not inside—the pericardial sac. Each lung is surrounded by—but is not inside—a *pleural sac,* and the abdominal viscera are surrounded by—

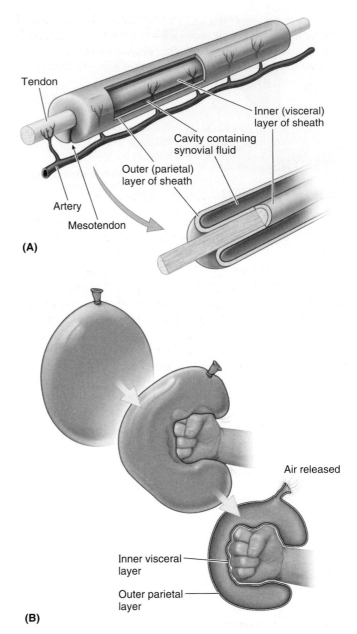

FIGURE I.10. Synovial tendon sheaths and bursal sacs. A. Synovial tendon sheaths are longitudinal bursae that surround tendons as they pass deep to retinacula or through fibrous digital sheaths. **B.** Bursal sacs enclose several structures, such as the heart, lungs, abdominal viscera, and tendons, much like this collapsed balloon encloses the fist. A thin film of lubricating fluid between the parietal and visceral layers confers mobility to the structure surrounded by the bursa within a confined compartment. The transitional folds of synovial membrane between the continuous parietal and visceral layers surrounding the connecting stalks (the wrist in this example) and/or neurovascular structures serving the surrounded mass are called mesenteries. In the case of a synovial tendon sheath, the mesentery is called a mesotendon.

but are not inside—the *peritoneal sac.* In such cases, the inner layer of the balloon or serous sac (the one adjacent to the fist, viscus, or viscera) is called the **visceral layer;** the outer layer of the balloon (or the one in contact with the body wall) is called the **parietal layer.** Such a surrounding double layer of membranes, moistened on their apposed surfaces, confers freedom of movement on the surrounded structure when it is contained within a confined space, such as the heart within its surrounding fibrous sac (*pericardium*) or flexor tendons within the fibrous tunnels that hold the tendons against the bones of the fingers.

FASCIAS

Fascial Planes and Surgery

In living people, fascial planes (*interfascial* and *intrafascial*) are potential spaces between adjacent fascias or fascia-lined structures, or within loose areolar fascias, such as the *subserous fascias*. Surgeons take advantage of these interfascial planes, separating structures to create spaces that allow movement and access to deeply placed structures. In some procedures, surgeons use extrapleural or extraperitoneal fascial planes, which allow them to operate outside the membranes lining the body cavities, minimizing the potential for contamination, the spread of infection, and consequent formation of adhesions (adherences) within the cavities. Unfortunately, these planes are often fused and difficult to establish or appreciate in embalmed cadavers.

The Bottom Line

FASCIAS AND BURSAE

Deep fascia is an organized connective tissue layer that completely envelops the body beneath the subcutaneous tissue underlying the skin. Extensions and modifications of the deep fascia: ♦ divide muscles into groups (intermuscular septa), ♦ invest individual muscles and neurovascular bundles (investing fascia), ♦ lie between musculoskeletal walls and the serous membranes lining body cavities (subserous fascia), and ♦ hold tendons in place during joint movements (retinacula). Bursae are closed sacs formed of serous membrane that occur in locations subject to friction; they enable one structure to move freely over another.

SKELETAL SYSTEM

The skeletal system may be divided into two functional parts (Fig. I.11):

- The **axial skeleton** consists of the bones of the head (*cranium* or *skull*), neck (*hyoid bone* and *cervical vertebrae*), and trunk (*ribs, sternum, vertebrae,* and *sacrum*).

- The **appendicular skeleton** consists of the *bones of the limbs,* including those forming the pectoral (shoulder) and pelvic girdles.

Cartilage and Bones

The skeleton is composed of cartilages and bones. **Cartilage** is a resilient, semirigid form of connective tissue that forms parts of the skeleton where more flexibility is required—for example, where the *costal cartilages* attach the ribs to the sternum. Also, the **articulating surfaces** (bearing surfaces) of bones participating in a synovial joint are capped with **articular cartilage** that provides smooth, low-friction, gliding surfaces for free movement (Fig. I.16A). Blood vessels do not enter cartilage (i.e., it is *avascular*); consequently, its cells obtain oxygen and nutrients by diffusion. The proportion of bone and cartilage in the skeleton changes as the body grows; the younger a person is, the more cartilage he or she has. The bones of a newborn are soft and flexible because they are mostly composed of cartilage.

Bone, a living tissue, is a highly specialized, hard form of connective tissue that makes up most of the skeleton. Bones of the adult skeleton provide:

- support for the body and its vital cavities; it is the chief supporting tissue of the body.
- protection for vital structures (e.g., the heart).
- the mechanical basis for movement (leverage).
- storage for salts (e.g., calcium).
- a continuous supply of new blood cells (produced by the marrow in the medullary cavity of many bones).

A fibrous connective tissue covering surrounds each skeletal element like a sleeve, except where articular cartilage occurs; that surrounding bones is **periosteum** (Fig. I.15), whereas that around cartilage is **perichondrium.** The periosteum and perichondrium nourish the external aspects of the skeletal tissue. They are capable of laying down more cartilage or bone (particularly during fracture healing) and provide the interface for attachment of *tendons* and *ligaments*.

The two types of bone are **compact bone** and **spongy** (trabecular) **bone.** They are distinguished by the relative amount of solid matter and by the number and size of the spaces they contain (Fig. I.12). All bones have a superficial thin layer of compact bone around a central mass of spongy bone, except where the latter is replaced by a *medullary (marrow) cavity*. Within the medullary cavity of adult bones, and between the **spicules** (trabeculae) of spongy bone, *yellow* (fatty) or *red* (blood cell and platelet forming) *bone marrow*—or a combination of both—is found.

The architecture and proportion of compact and spongy bone vary according to function. Compact bone provides strength for weight bearing. In *long bones* designed for rigidity and attachment of muscles and ligaments, the amount of compact bone is greatest near the middle of the *shaft* where the bones are liable to buckle. In addition, long bones have elevations (e.g., *ridges, crests,* and *tubercles*) that serve as *buttresses*

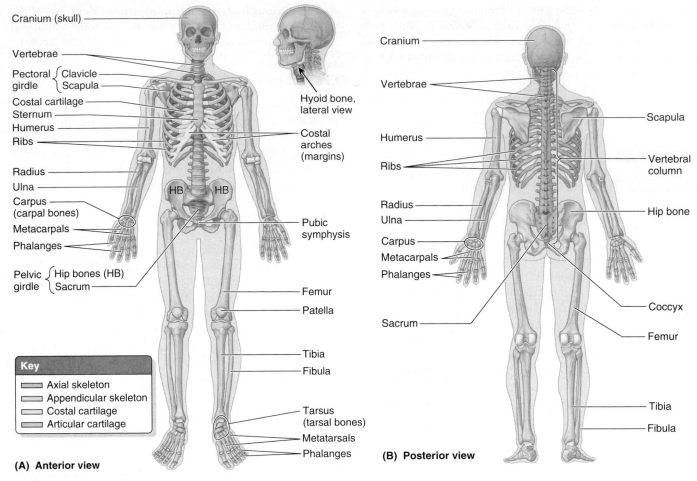

(A) Anterior view

(B) Posterior view

FIGURE I.11. Skeletal system.

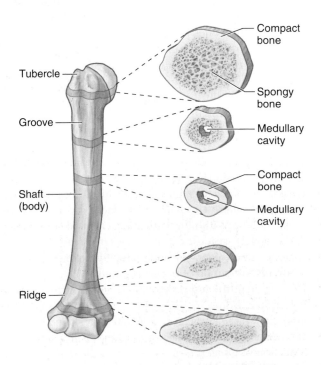

FIGURE I.12. Transverse sections of the humerus. The shaft of a living bone is a tube of compact bone that surrounds a medullary cavity.

(supports) where large muscles attach. Living bones have some *elasticity* (flexibility) and great *rigidity* (hardness).

CLASSIFICATION OF BONES

Bones are classified according to their shape.

- *Long bones* are tubular (e.g., the humerus in the arm).
- *Short bones* are cuboidal and are found only in the tarsus (ankle) and carpus (wrist).
- *Flat bones* usually serve protective functions (e.g., the flat bones of the cranium protect the brain).
- *Irregular bones* have various shapes other than long, short, or flat (e.g., bones of the face).
- *Sesamoid bones* (e.g., the patella or knee cap) develop in certain tendons and are found where tendons cross the ends of long bones in the limbs; they protect the tendons from excessive wear and often change the angle of the tendons as they pass to their attachments.

Bone Markings and Formations

Bone markings appear wherever tendons, ligaments, and fascias are attached or where arteries lie adjacent to or enter

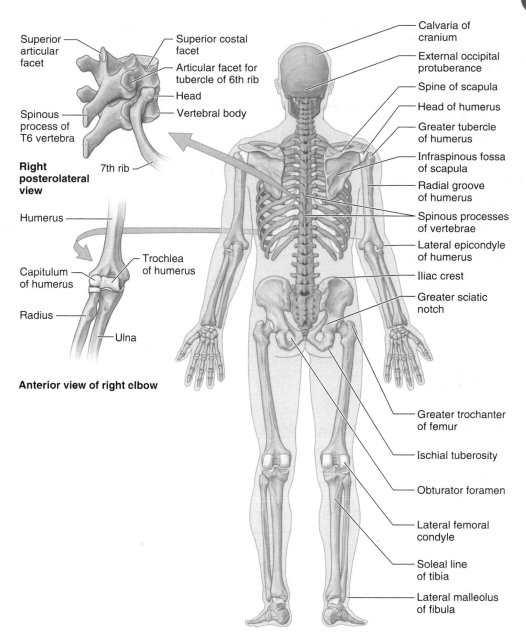

Superior articular facet

Superior costal facet

Articular facet for tubercle of 6th rib

Head

Vertebral body

Spinous process of T6 vertebra

Right posterolateral view

7th rib

Humerus

Capitulum of humerus

Trochlea of humerus

Radius

Ulna

Anterior view of right elbow

Calvaria of cranium

External occipital protuberance

Spine of scapula

Head of humerus

Greater tubercle of humerus

Infraspinous fossa of scapula

Radial groove of humerus

Spinous processes of vertebrae

Lateral epicondyle of humerus

Iliac crest

Greater sciatic notch

Greater trochanter of femur

Ischial tuberosity

Obturator foramen

Lateral femoral condyle

Soleal line of tibia

Lateral malleolus of fibula

Posterior view

FIGURE I.13. Bone markings and formations. Markings appear on bones wherever tendons, ligaments, and fascia attach. Other formations relate to joints, the passage of tendons, and the provision of increased leverage.

bones. Other formations occur in relation to the passage of a tendon (often to direct the tendon or improve its leverage) or to control the type of movement occurring at a joint. Some of the various markings and features of bones are (Fig. I.13):

- *Capitulum:* small, round, articular head (e.g., capitulum of the humerus).
- *Condyle:* rounded, knuckle-like articular area, often occurring in pairs (e.g., the lateral and medial femoral condyles).
- *Crest:* ridge of bone (e.g., the iliac crest).
- *Epicondyle:* eminence superior or adjacent to a condyle (e.g., lateral epicondyle of the humerus).
- *Facet:* smooth flat area, usually covered with cartilage, where a bone articulates with another bone (e.g., superior

costal facet on the body of a vertebra for articulation with a rib).
- *Foramen:* passage through a bone (e.g., obturator foramen).
- *Fossa:* hollow or depressed area (e.g., infraspinous fossa of the scapula).
- *Groove:* elongated depression or furrow (e.g., radial groove of the humerus).
- *Head* (L. *caput*): large, round articular end (e.g., head of the humerus).
- *Line:* linear elevation (e.g., soleal line of the tibia).
- *Malleolus:* rounded process (e.g., lateral malleolus of the fibula).
- *Notch:* indentation at the edge of a bone (e.g., greater sciatic notch).

- *Protuberance:* projection of bone (e.g., external occipital protuberance).
- *Spine:* thorn-like process (e.g., the spine of the scapula).
- *Spinous process:* projecting spine-like part (e.g., spinous process of a vertebra).
- *Trochanter:* large blunt elevation (e.g., greater trochanter of the femur).
- *Trochlea:* spool-like articular process or process that acts as a pulley (e.g., trochlea of the humerus).
- *Tubercle:* small raised eminence (e.g., greater tubercle of the humerus—Fig. I.13).
- *Tuberosity:* large rounded elevation (e.g., ischial tuberosity).

BONE DEVELOPMENT

Most bones take many years to grow and mature. The humerus (arm bone), for example, begins to ossify at the end of the embryonic period (8 weeks); however, ossification is not complete until age 20. All bones derive from *mesenchyme* (embryonic connective tissue) by two different processes: intramembranous ossification (directly from mesenchyme) and endochondral ossification (from cartilage derived from mesenchyme). The histology (microscopic structure) of a bone is the same by either process (Ross et al., 2011).

- In **intramembranous ossification** (membranous bone formation), mesenchymal models of bones form during the embryonic period, and direct ossification of the mesenchyme begins in the fetal period.
- In **endochondral ossification** (cartilaginous bone formation), cartilage models of the bones form from mesenchyme during the fetal period, and bone subsequently replaces most of the cartilage.

A brief description of endochondral ossification helps explain how long bones grow (Fig. I.14). The mesenchymal cells condense and differentiate into *chondroblasts*, dividing cells in growing cartilage tissue, thereby forming a *cartilaginous bone model.* In the midregion of the model, the cartilage *calcifies* (becomes impregnated with calcium salts), and *periosteal capillaries* (capillaries from the fibrous sheath surrounding the model) grow into the calcified cartilage of the bone model and supply its interior. These blood vessels, together with associated *osteogenic (bone-forming) cells,* form a *periosteal bud* (Fig. I.14A). The capillaries initiate the **primary ossification center,** so named because the bone tissue it forms replaces most of the cartilage in the main body of the bone model. The shaft of a bone ossified from the primary ossification center is the **diaphysis,** which grows as the bone develops.

Most **secondary ossification centers** appear in other parts of the developing bone after birth; the parts of a bone ossified from these centers are **epiphyses.** The chondrocytes in the middle of the epiphysis hypertrophy, and the *bone matrix* (extracellular substance) between them

(A)

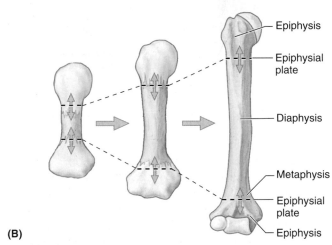

(B)

FIGURE I.14. Development and growth of a long bone. A. The formation of primary and secondary ossification centers is shown. **B.** Growth in length occurs on both sides of the cartilaginous epiphysial plates (*double-headed arrows*). The bone formed from the primary center in the diaphysis does not fuse with that formed from the secondary centers in the epiphyses until the bone reaches its adult size. When growth ceases, the depleted epiphysial plate is replaced by a synostosis (bone-to-bone fusion), observed as an epiphysial line in radiographs and sectioned bone.

calcifies. *Epiphysial arteries* grow into the developing cavities with associated osteogenic cells. The flared part of the diaphysis nearest the epiphysis is the **metaphysis.** For growth to continue, the bone formed from the primary center in the diaphysis does not fuse with that formed from the secondary centers in the epiphyses until the bone reaches its adult size. Thus, during growth of a long bone, cartilaginous **epiphysial plates** intervene between the diaphysis and epiphyses (Fig. I.14B). These growth plates are eventually replaced by bone at each of its two sides, diaphysial and epiphysial. When this occurs, bone growth ceases and the diaphysis fuses with the epiphyses.

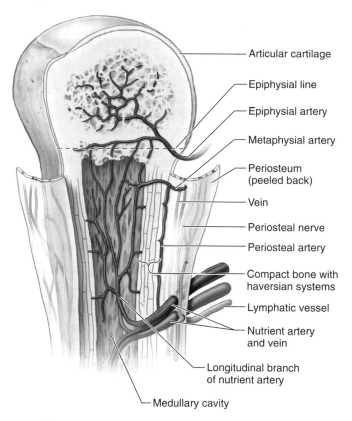

FIGURE I.15. Vasculature and innervation of a long bone.

Labels:
- Articular cartilage
- Epiphysial line
- Epiphysial artery
- Metaphysial artery
- Periosteum (peeled back)
- Vein
- Periosteal nerve
- Periosteal artery
- Compact bone with haversian systems
- Lymphatic vessel
- Nutrient artery and vein
- Longitudinal branch of nutrient artery
- Medullary cavity

The seam formed during this fusion process (*synostosis*) is particularly dense and is recognizable in sectioned bone or radiographs as an **epiphysial line** (Fig. I.15). The epiphysial fusion of bones occurs progressively from puberty to maturity. *Ossification of short bones* is similar to that of the primary ossification center of long bones, and only one short bone, the calcaneus (heel bone), develops a secondary ossification center.

VASCULATURE AND INNERVATION OF BONES

Bones are richly supplied with blood vessels. Most apparent are the **nutrient arteries** (one or more per bone) that arise as independent branches of adjacent arteries outside the periosteum and pass obliquely through the compact bone of the shaft of a long bone via **nutrient foramina.** The nutrient artery divides in the medullary cavity into longitudinal branches that proceed toward each end, supplying the bone marrow, spongy bone, and deeper portions of the compact bone (Fig. I.15). However, many small branches from the periosteal arteries of the periosteum are responsible for nourishment of most of the compact bone. Consequently, a bone from which the periosteum has been removed dies.

Blood reaches the *osteocytes* (bone cells) in the compact bone by means of **haversian systems** or *osteons* (microscopic canal systems) that house small blood vessels. The ends of the bones are supplied by metaphysial and epiphysial arteries that arise mainly from the arteries that supply the joints. In the limbs, these arteries are typically part of a *periarticular arterial plexus*, which surrounds the joint, ensuring blood flow distal to the joint regardless of the position assumed by the joint.

Veins accompany arteries through the nutrient foramina. Many large veins also leave through foramina near the articular ends of the bones. Bones containing red bone marrow have numerous large veins. *Lymphatic vessels* are also abundant in the periosteum.

Nerves accompany blood vessels supplying bones. The periosteum is richly supplied with sensory nerves—**periosteal nerves**—that carry pain fibers. The periosteum is especially sensitive to tearing or tension, which explains the acute pain from bone fractures. Bone itself is relatively sparsely supplied with sensory endings. Within bones, **vasomotor nerves** cause constriction or dilation of blood vessels, regulating blood flow through the bone marrow.

BONES

Accessory (Supernumerary) Bones

Accessory (supernumerary) bones develop when additional ossification centers appear and form extra bones. Many bones develop from several centers of ossification, and the separate parts normally fuse. Sometimes one of these centers fails to fuse with the main bone, giving the appearance of an extra bone. Careful study shows that the apparent extra bone is a missing part of the main bone. Circumscribed areas of bone are often seen along the sutures of the cranium where the flat bones abut, particularly those related to the parietal bone (see Chapter 7). These small, irregular, worm-like bones are **sutural bones** (wormian bones). It is important to know that accessory bones are common in the foot, to avoid mistaking them for bone fragments in radiographs and other medical images.

Heterotopic Bones

Bones sometimes form in soft tissues where they are not normally present (e.g., in scars). Horse riders often develop *heterotopic bones* in their thighs (*rider's bones*), probably because of chronic muscle strain resulting in small hemorrhagic (bloody) areas that undergo calcification and eventual ossification.

Trauma to Bone and Bone Changes

Bones are living organs that cause pain when injured, bleed when fractured, remodel in relationship to stresses placed on them, and change

FIGURE I.16. **Three classes of joint.** Examples of each class are shown. **A.** Two models demonstrating basic features of a synovial joint.

joint is partially movable. The interosseous membrane in the forearm is a sheet of fibrous tissue that joins the radius and ulna in a syndesmosis. A **dento-alveolar syndesmosis** (gomphosis or socket) is a fibrous joint in which a peg-like process fits into a socket articulation between the root of the tooth and the alveolar process of the jaw. Mobility of this joint (a loose tooth) indicates a pathological state affecting the supporting tissues of the tooth. However, microscopic movements here give us information (via the sense of proprioception) about how hard we are biting or clenching our teeth and whether we have a particle stuck between our teeth.

3. The articulating structures of **cartilaginous joints** are united by hyaline cartilage or fibrocartilage. In **primary cartilaginous joints,** or synchondroses, the bones are united by hyaline cartilage, which permits slight bending during early life. Primary cartilaginous joints are usually temporary unions, such as those present during the development of a long bone (Figs. I.14 and I.16C), where the bony epiphysis and the shaft are joined by an epiphysial plate. Primary cartilaginous joints permit growth in the length of a bone. When full growth is achieved, the epiphysial plate converts to bone and the epiphyses fuse with the diaphysis. **Secondary cartilaginous joints,** or symphyses, are strong, slightly movable joints united by fibrocartilage. The fibrocartilaginous *intervertebral discs* (Fig. I.16C) between the vertebrae consist of binding connective tissue that joins the vertebrae together. Cumulatively, these joints provide strength and shock absorption as well as considerable flexibility to the vertebral column (spine).

Synovial joints, the most common type of joint, provide free movement between the bones they join; they are joints of locomotion, typical of nearly all limb joints. Synovial joints are usually reinforced by **accessory ligaments** that are either separate (*extrinsic*) or are a thickening of a portion of the joint capsule (*intrinsic*). Some synovial joints have other distinguishing features, such as a fibrocartilaginous *articular disc* or meniscus, which are present when the articulating surfaces of the bones are incongruous (Fig. I.16A).

The six major types of synovial joints are classified according to the shape of the articulating surfaces and/or the type of movement they permit (Fig. I.17):

1. **Plane joints** permit gliding or sliding movements in the plane of the articular surfaces. The opposed surfaces of the bones are flat or almost flat, with movement limited by their tight joint capsules. Plane joints are numerous and are nearly always small. An example is the *acromioclavicular joint* between the acromion of the scapula and the clavicle.

2. **Hinge joints** permit flexion and extension only, movements that occur in one plane (sagittal) around a single axis that runs transversely; thus hinge joints are *uniaxial joints.* The joint capsule of these joints is thin and lax anteriorly and posteriorly where movement occurs; however, the bones are joined by strong, laterally placed collateral ligaments. The *elbow joint* is a hinge joint.

FIGURE I.17. The six types of synovial joints. Synovial joints are classified according to the shape of their articulating surfaces and/or the type of movement they permit.

3. **Saddle joints** permit abduction and adduction as well as flexion and extension, movements occurring around two axes at right angles to each other; thus saddle joints are *biaxial joints* that allow movement in two planes, sagittal and frontal. The performance of these movements in a circular sequence (circumduction) is also possible. The opposing articular surfaces are shaped like a saddle (i.e., they are reciprocally concave and convex). The *carpometacarpal joint* at the base of the 1st digit (thumb) is a saddle joint (Fig. I.17).

4. **Condyloid joints** permit flexion and extension as well as abduction and adduction; thus condyloid joints are also biaxial. However, movement in one plane (sagittal) is usually greater (freer) than in the other. Circumduction, more restricted than that of saddle joints, is also possible. The *metacarpophalangeal joints* (knuckle joints) are condyloid joints.

5. **Ball and socket joints** allow movement in multiple axes and planes: flexion and extension, abduction and adduction, medial and lateral rotation, and circumduction; thus ball and socket joints are *multiaxial joints.* In these highly mobile joints, the spheroidal surface of one bone moves within the socket of another. The *hip joint* is a ball and socket joint in which the spherical *head of the femur* rotates within the socket formed by the *acetabulum* of the hip bone.

6. **Pivot joints** permit rotation around a central axis; thus they are uniaxial. In these joints, a rounded process of bone rotates within a sleeve or ring. The *median atlantoaxial joint* is a pivot joint in which the atlas (C1 vertebra) rotates around a finger-like process, the dens of the axis (C2 vertebra), during rotation of the head.

JOINT VASCULATURE AND INNERVATION

Joints receive blood from **articular arteries** that arise from the vessels around the joint. The arteries often *anastomose* (communicate) to form networks (*peri-articular arterial anastomoses*) to ensure a blood supply to and across the joint in the various positions assumed by the joint. **Articular veins** are communicating veins that accompany arteries (L. *venae comitantes*) and, like the arteries, are located in the joint capsule, mostly in the synovial membrane.

Joints have a rich nerve supply provided by **articular nerves** with sensory nerve endings in the joint capsule. In the distal parts of the limbs (hands and feet), the articular nerves are branches of the cutaneous nerves supplying the overlying skin. However, most articular nerves are branches of nerves that supply the muscles that cross and therefore move the joint. The **Hilton law** states that the nerves supplying a joint also supply the muscles moving the joint and the skin covering their distal attachments.

Articular nerves transmit sensory impulses from the joint that contribute to the sense of **proprioception,** which provides an awareness of movement and position of the parts of the body. The synovial membrane is relatively insensitive. Pain fibers are numerous in the fibrous layer of the joint capsule and the accessory ligaments, causing considerable pain when the joint is injured. The sensory nerve endings respond to the twisting and stretching that occurs during sports activities.

JOINTS

Joints of Newborn Cranium

The bones of the *calvaria* (skullcap) of a newborn infant's cranium do not make full contact with each other (Fig. BI.6). At these sites, the sutures form wide areas of fibrous tissue called **fontanelles.** The *anterior fontanelle* is the most prominent; laypeople call it the "soft spot." The fontanelles in a newborn are often felt as ridges because of the overlapping of the cranial bones by molding of the calvaria as it passes through the birth canal. Normally, the anterior fontanelle is flat. A bulging fontanelle may indicate increased intracranial pressure; however, the fontanelle normally bulges during crying. Pulsations of the fontanelle reflect the pulse of cerebral arteries. A depressed fontanelle may be observed when the baby is dehydrated (Swartz, 2001).

FIGURE BI.6.

Labels: Anterior fontanelle; Frontal suture; Internasal suture; Intermaxillary suture; Mandibular symphysis (intermandibular suture)

Degenerative Joint Disease

Synovial joints are well designed to withstand wear, but heavy use over several years can cause degenerative changes. Some destruction is inevitable during such activities as jogging, which wears away the articular cartilages and sometimes erodes the underlying articulating surfaces of the bones. The normal aging of articular cartilage begins early in adult life and progresses slowly thereafter, occurring on the ends of the articulating bones, particularly those of the hip, knee, vertebral column, and hands (Salter, 1998). These irreversible degenerative changes in joints result in the articular cartilage becoming a less effective shock absorber and lubricated surface. As a result, the articulation becomes increasingly vulnerable to the repeated friction that occurs during joint movements. In some people, these changes do not produce significant symptoms; in others, they cause considerable pain.

Degenerative joint disease or *osteoarthritis* is often accompanied by stiffness, discomfort, and pain. Osteoarthritis is common in older people and usually affects joints that support the weight of their bodies (e.g., the hips and knees). Most substances in the bloodstream, normal or pathological, easily enter the joint cavity. Similarly, traumatic infection of a joint may be followed by *arthritis,* inflammation of a joint, and *septicemia,* blood poisoning.

Arthroscopy

The cavity of a synovial joint can be examined by inserting a cannula and an arthroscope (a small telescope) into it. This surgical procedure— *arthroscopy*—enables orthopedic surgeons to examine joints for abnormalities, such as torn menisci (partial articular discs of the knee joint). Some surgical procedures can also be performed during arthroscopy (e.g., by inserting instruments through small puncture incisions). Because the opening in the joint capsule for inserting the arthroscope is small, healing is more rapid after this procedure than after traditional joint surgery.

The Bottom Line

JOINTS

A joint is a union between two or more bones or rigid parts of the skeleton. Three general types of joints are recognized: fibrous, cartilaginous, and synovial. Freely moveable synovial joints: ♦ are the most common type; ♦ can be classified into plane, hinge, saddle, condyloid, ball and socket, and pivot; ♦ receive their blood supply from articular arteries that often form networks; ♦ are drained by articular veins originating in the synovial membrane; ♦ are richly innervated by articular nerves that transmit the sensation of proprioception, an awareness of movement and position of parts of the body.

MUSCLE TISSUE AND MUSCULAR SYSTEM

The muscular system consists of all the muscles of the body. Voluntary skeletal muscles constitute the great majority of the named muscles. All skeletal muscles are composed of one specific type of muscle tissue. However, other types of muscle tissue constitute a few named muscles (e.g., the ciliary and detrusor muscles, and the arrector muscles of hairs) and form important components of the organs of other systems, including the cardiovascular, alimentary, genitourinary, integumentary, and visual systems.

Types of Muscle (Muscle Tissue)

Muscle cells, often called *muscle fibers* because they are long and narrow when relaxed, are specialized contractile cells. They are organized into tissues that move body parts or temporarily alter the shape (reduce the circumference of all or part) of internal organs. Associated connective tissue conveys nerve fibers and capillaries to the muscle cells as it binds them into bundles or fascicles. Three types of muscle are described based on distinct characteristics relating to:

- Whether it is normally willfully controlled (*voluntary* vs. *involuntary*).
- Whether it appears striped or unstriped when viewed under a microscope (*striated* vs. *smooth* or *unstriated*).
- Whether it is located in the body wall (*soma*) and limbs or makes up the hollow organs (*viscera,* e.g., the heart) of the body cavities or blood vessels (*somatic* vs. *visceral*).

There are three muscle types (Table I.1):

1. **Skeletal striated muscle** is voluntary somatic muscle that makes up the gross *skeletal muscles* that compose the muscular system, moving or stabilizing bones and other structures (e.g., the eyeballs).
2. **Cardiac striated muscle** is involuntary visceral muscle that forms most of the walls of the heart and adjacent parts of the great vessels, such as the aorta, and pumps blood.
3. **Smooth muscle** (unstriated muscle) is involuntary visceral muscle that forms part of the walls of most vessels and hollow organs (viscera), moving substances through them by coordinated sequential contractions (pulsations or peristaltic contractions).

Skeletal Muscles

FORM, FEATURES, AND NAMING OF MUSCLES

All skeletal muscles, commonly referred to simply as "muscles," have fleshy, reddish, contractile portions (one or more heads or bellies) composed of skeletal striated muscle. Some muscles are fleshy throughout, but most also have white non-contractile portions (tendons), composed mainly of organized collagen bundles, that provide a means of attachment (Fig. I.18).

When referring to the length of a muscle, both the belly and the tendons are included. In other words, a muscle's length is the distance between its attachments. Most skeletal muscles are attached directly or indirectly to bones, cartilages, ligaments, or fascias or to some combination of these structures. Some muscles are attached to organs (the eyeball, for example), skin (such as facial muscles), and mucous

TABLE I.1. TYPES OF MUSCLE (MUSCLE TISSUE)

Muscle Type	Location	Appearance of Cells	Type of Activity	Stimulation
Skeletal striated muscle Striation Muscle fiber Nucleus Satellite cell	Composes gross, named muscles (e.g., biceps of arm) attached to skeleton and fascia of limbs, body wall, and head/neck	Large, very long, unbranched, cylindrical fibers with transverse striations (stripes) arranged in parallel bundles; multiple, peripherally located nuclei	Intermittent (phasic) contraction above a baseline tonus; acts primarily to produce movement (isotonic contraction) through shortening (concentric contraction) or controlled relaxation (eccentric contraction), or to maintain position against gravity or other resisting force without movement (isometric contraction)	Voluntary (or reflexive) by somatic nervous system
Cardiac striated muscle Nucleus Intercalated disc Striation Muscle fiber	Muscle of heart (myocardium) and adjacent portions of great vessels (aorta, vena cava)	Branching and anastomosing shorter fibers with transverse striations (stripes) running parallel and connected end to end by complex junctions (intercalated discs); single, central nucleus	Strong, quick, continuous rhythmic contraction; acts to pump blood from heart	Involuntary; intrinsically (myogenically) stimulated and propagated; rate and strength of contraction modified by autonomic nervous system
Smooth (unstriated or unstriped) muscle Smooth muscle fiber Nucleus	Walls of hollow viscera and blood vessels, iris, and ciliary body of eye; attached to hair follicles of skin (arrector muscle of hair)	Single or agglomerated small, spindle-shaped fibers without striations; single central nucleus	Weak, slow, rhythmic, or sustained tonic contraction; acts mainly to propel substances (peristalsis) and to restrict flow (vasoconstriction and sphincteric activity)	Involuntary by autonomic nervous system

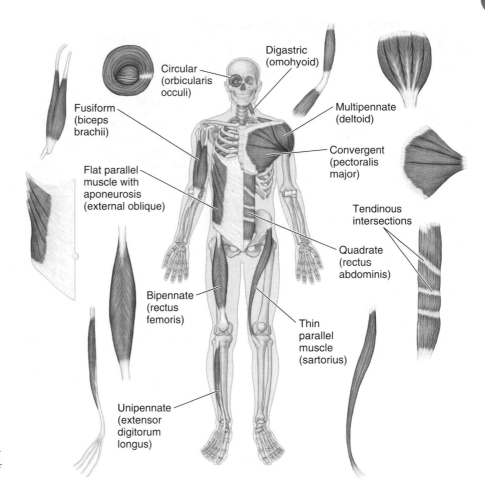

FIGURE I.18. Architecture and shape of skeletal muscles. The architecture and shape of a skeletal muscle depend on the arrangement of its fibers.

membranes (intrinsic tongue muscles). Muscles are organs of locomotion (movement), but they also provide static support, give form to the body, and provide heat. Figure I.19 identifies the skeletal muscles that lie most superficially. The deep muscles are identified when each region is studied.

The architecture and shape of muscles vary (Fig. I.18). The tendons of some muscles form flat sheets, or **aponeuroses,** that anchor the muscle to the skeleton (usually a ridge or a series of spinous processes) and/or to deep fascia (such as the latissimus dorsi muscle of the back), or to the aponeurosis of another muscle (such as the oblique muscles of the anterolateral abdominal wall). Most muscles are named on the basis of their function or the bones to which they are attached. The abductor digiti minimi muscle, for example, abducts the little finger. The sternocleidomastoid muscle (G. *kleidos,* bolt or bar, clavicle) attaches inferiorly to the sternum and clavicle and superiorly to the mastoid process of the temporal bone of the cranium. Other muscles are named on the basis of their position (medial, lateral, anterior, posterior) or length (brevis, short; longus, long). Muscles may be described or classified according to their shape, for which a muscle may also be named:

- **Flat muscles** have parallel fibers often with an aponeurosis—for example, the external oblique (broad

flat muscle). The sartorius is a narrow flat muscle with parallel fibers.
- **Pennate muscles** are feather-like (L. *pennatus,* feather) in the arrangement of their fascicles, and may be *unipennate, bipennate,* or *multipennate*—for example, extensor digitorum longus (unipennate), rectus femoris (bipennate), and deltoid (multipennate).
- **Fusiform muscles** are spindle shaped with a round, thick belly (or bellies) and tapered ends—for example, biceps brachii.
- **Convergent muscles** arise from a broad area and converge to form a single tendon—for example, pectoralis major.
- **Quadrate muscles** have four equal sides (L. *quadratus,* square)—for example, the rectus abdominis, between its tendinous intersections.
- **Circular** or **sphincteral muscles** surround a body opening or orifice, constricting it when contracted—for example, orbicularis oculi (closes the eyelids).
- **Multiheaded** or **multibellied muscles** have more than one head of attachment or more than one contractile belly, respectively. *Biceps muscles* have two heads of attachment (e.g., biceps brachii), *triceps muscles* have three heads (e.g., triceps brachii), and the digastric and gastrocnemius muscles have two bellies. (Those of the former are arranged in tandem; those of the latter lie parallel.)

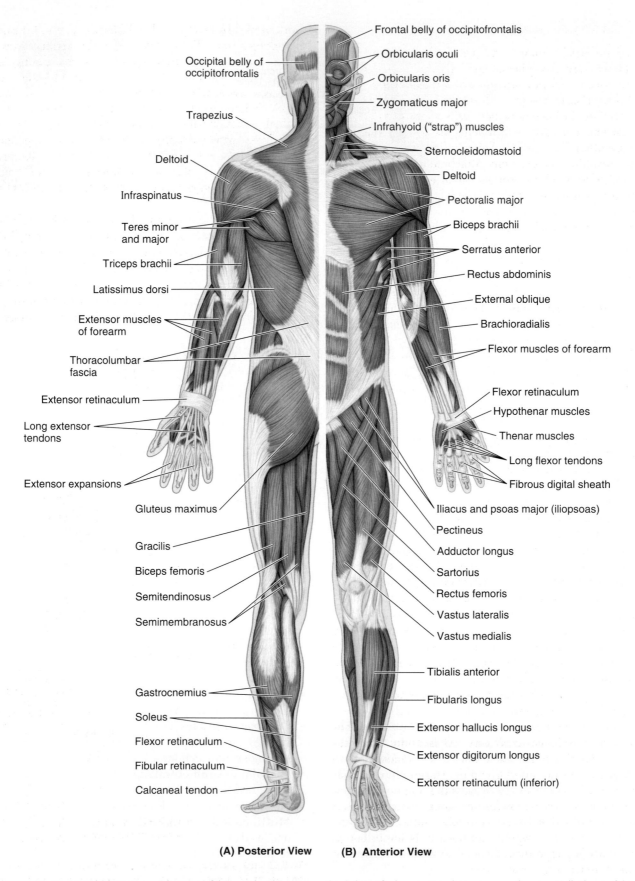

(A) Posterior View   (B) Anterior View

FIGURE I.19. Superficial skeletal muscles. Most of the muscles shown move the skeleton for locomotion, but some muscles—especially those of the head—move other structures (e.g., the eyeballs, scalp, eyelids, skin of face, and tongue). The sheath of the left rectus abdominis, formed by aponeuroses of the flat abdominal muscles, has been removed to reveal the muscle. Retinculae are deep fascial thickenings that tether tendons to underlying bones as they cross joints.

CONTRACTION OF MUSCLES

Skeletal muscles function by contracting; they pull and never push. However, certain phenomena—such as "popping of the ears" to equalize air pressure and the *musculovenous pump* (pp. 41–42, Fig. I.26)—take advantage of the expansion of muscle bellies during contraction. When a muscle contracts and shortens, one of its attachments usually remains fixed while the other (more mobile) attachment is pulled toward it, often resulting in movement. Attachments of muscles are commonly described as the origin and insertion; the *origin* is usually the proximal end of the muscle, which remains fixed during muscular contraction, and the *insertion* is usually the distal end of the muscle, which is movable. However, this is not always the case. Some muscles can act in both directions under different circumstances. For example, when doing push-ups, the distal end of the upper limb (the hand) is fixed (on the floor) and the proximal end of the limb and the trunk (of the body) are being moved. Therefore, this book usually uses the terms *proximal* and *distal* or *medial* and *lateral* when describing most muscle attachments. Note that if the attachments of a muscle are known, the action of the muscle can usually be deduced (rather than memorized). When studying muscle attachments, act out the action; you are more likely to learn things you have experienced.

Reflexive Contraction. Although skeletal muscles are also referred to as voluntary muscles, certain aspects of their activity are automatic (**reflexive**) and therefore not voluntarily controlled. Examples are the respiratory movements of the diaphragm, controlled most of the time by reflexes stimulated by the levels of oxygen and carbon dioxide in the blood (although we can willfully control it within limits), and the myotatic reflex, which results in movement after a muscle stretch produced by tapping a tendon with a reflex hammer.

Tonic Contraction. Even when "relaxed," the muscles of a conscious individual are almost always slightly contracted. This slight contraction, called **muscle tone** (tonus), does not produce movement or active resistance (as phasic contraction does) but gives the muscle a certain firmness, assisting the stability of joints and the maintenance of posture, while keeping the muscle ready to respond to appropriate stimuli. Muscle tone is usually absent only when unconscious (as during deep sleep or under general anesthesia) or after a nerve lesion resulting in paralysis.

Phasic Contraction. There are two main types of **phasic** (active) **muscle contractions**: (1) **isotonic contractions,** in which the muscle changes length in relationship to the production of movement, and (2) **isometric contractions,** in which muscle length remains the same—no movement occurs, but the force (muscle tension) is increased above tonic levels to resist gravity or other antagonistic force (Fig. I.20). The latter type of contraction is important in maintaining upright posture and when muscles act as fixators or shunt muscles as described below.

There are two types of isotonic contractions. The type we most commonly think of is **concentric contraction,** in which movement occurs as a result of the muscle

shortening—for example, when lifting a cup, pushing a door, or striking a blow. The ability to apply exceptional force by means of concentric contraction often is what distinguishes an athlete from an amateur. The other type of isotonic contraction is **eccentric contraction,** in which a contracting muscle lengthens—that is, it undergoes a controlled and gradual relaxation while continually exerting a (diminishing) force, like playing out a rope. Although people are generally not as aware of them, eccentric contractions are as important as concentric contractions for coordinated, functional movements such as walking, running, and setting objects (or one's self) down.

Often, when the main muscle of a particular movement (the *prime mover*) is undergoing a concentric contraction, its antagonist is undergoing a coordinated eccentric contraction. In walking, we contract concentrically to pull our center of gravity forward and then, as it passes ahead of the limb, we contract eccentrically to prevent a lurching during the transfer of weight to the other limb. Eccentric contractions

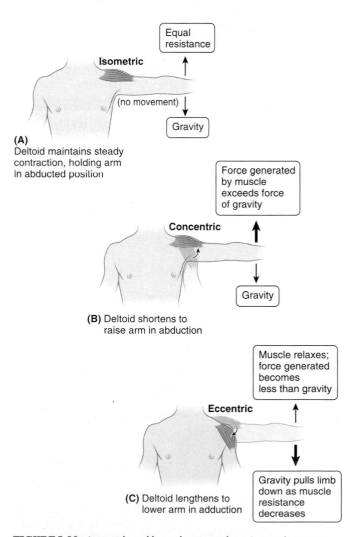

FIGURE I.20. Isometric and isotonic contractions. Isometric contraction sustains the position of a joint without producing movement. Concentric and eccentric contractions are isotonic contractions in which the muscle changes length: concentric contractions by shortening and eccentric contractions by actively controlled lengthening (relaxation).

require less metabolic energy at the same load but, with a maximal contraction, are capable of generating much higher tension levels than concentric contractions—as much as 50% higher (Marieb, 2004).

Whereas the **structural unit** of a muscle is a skeletal striated muscle fiber, the **functional unit** of a muscle is a **motor unit,** consisting of a motor neuron and the muscle fibers it controls (Fig. I.21). When a *motor neuron* in the spinal cord is stimulated, it initiates an impulse that causes all the muscle fibers supplied by that motor unit to contract simultaneously. The number of muscle fibers in a motor unit varies from one to several hundred. The number of fibers varies according to the size and function of the muscle. Large motor units, in which one neuron supplies several hundred muscle fibers, are in the large trunk and thigh muscles. In smaller eye and hand muscles, where precision movements are required, the motor units include only a few muscle fibers. Movement (phasic contraction) results from the activation of an increasing number of motor units, above the level required to maintain muscle tone.

FUNCTIONS OF MUSCLES

Muscles serve specific functions in moving and positioning the body.

- A **prime mover** (agonist) is the main muscle responsible for producing a specific movement of the body. It contracts concentrically to produce the desired movement, doing most of the work (expending most of the energy) required. In most movements, there is a single prime mover, but some movements involve two prime movers working in equal measure.
- A **fixator** steadies the proximal parts of a limb through isometric contraction while movements are occurring in distal parts.

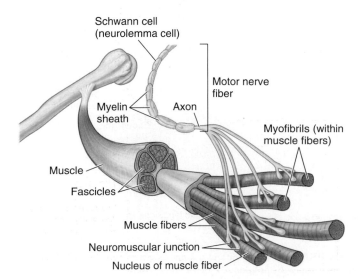

Schwann cell
(neurolemma cell)

Motor nerve
fiber

Myelin
sheath

Axon

Myofibrils (within
muscle fibers)

Muscle

Fascicles

Muscle fibers

Neuromuscular junction

Nucleus of muscle fiber

FIGURE I.21. Motor unit. A motor unit consists of a single motor neuron and the muscle fibers innervated by it.

- A **synergist** complements the action of a prime mover. It may directly assist a prime mover, providing a weaker or less mechanically advantaged component of the same movement, or it may assist indirectly, by serving as a fixator of an intervening joint when a prime mover passes over more than one joint, for example. It is not unusual to have several synergists assisting a prime mover in a particular movement.
- An **antagonist** is a muscle that opposes the action of another muscle. A primary antagonist directly opposes the prime mover, but synergists may also be opposed by secondary antagonists. As the active movers concentrically contract to produce a movement, antagonists eccentrically contract, relaxing progressively in coordination to produce a smooth movement.

The same muscle may act as a prime mover, antagonist, synergist, or fixator under different conditions. Note also that the actual prime mover in a given position may be gravity. In such cases, a paradoxical situation may exist in which the prime mover usually described as being responsible for the movement is inactive (passive), while the controlled relaxation (eccentric contraction) of the antigravity antagonist(s) is the active (energy requiring) component in the movement. An example is lowering (adducting) the upper limbs from the abducted position (stretched out laterally at 90° to the trunk) when standing erect (Fig. I.20C). The prime mover (adductor) is gravity; the muscles described as the prime movers for this movement (pectoralis major and latissimus dorsi) are inactive or passive; and the muscle being actively innervated (contracting eccentrically) is the deltoid (an abductor, typically described as the antagonist for this movement).

When a muscle's pull is exerted along a line that parallels the axis of the bones to which it is attached, it is at a disadvantage for producing movement. Instead it acts to maintain contact between the articular surfaces of the joint it crosses (i.e., it resists dislocating forces); this type of muscle is a **shunt muscle.** For example, when the arms are at one's sides, the deltoid functions as a shunt muscle. The more oblique a muscle's line of pull is oriented to the bone it moves (i.e., the *less* parallel the line of pull is to the long axis of the bone, e.g., the biceps brachii when the elbow is flexed), the more capable it is of rapid and effective movement; this type of muscle is a **spurt muscle.** The deltoid becomes increasingly effective as a spurt muscle after other muscles have initiated abduction of the arm.

NERVES AND ARTERIES TO MUSCLES

Variation in the nerve supply of muscles is rare; it is a nearly constant relationship. In the limb, muscles of similar actions are generally contained within a *common fascial compartment* and share innervation by the same nerves (Fig. I.9); therefore, you should learn the innervation of limb muscles in terms of the functional groups, making it necessary to memorize only the exceptions. Nerves supplying skeletal muscles (**motor nerves**) usually enter the fleshy portion of the muscle (vs. the tendon), almost always from the deep aspect (so the nerve is protected by the muscle it supplies). The few exceptions will be pointed out later in the text. When a nerve pierces a muscle, by passing through its fleshy portion or between its two heads of attachment, it usually supplies that muscle. Exceptions are the sensory branches that innervate the skin of the back after penetrating the superficial muscles of the back.

The blood supply of muscles is not as constant as the nerve supply and is usually multiple. Arteries generally supply the structures they contact. Thus you should learn the course of the arteries and deduce that a muscle is supplied by all the arteries in its vicinity.

SKELETAL MUSCLES

Muscle Dysfunction and Paralysis

 From the clinical perspective, it is important not only to think in terms of the action normally produced by a given muscle but also to consider what loss of function would occur if the muscle failed to function (paralysis). How would the dysfunction of a given muscle or muscle group be manifest (i.e., what are the visible signs)?

Absence of Muscle Tone

Although a gentle force, muscle tone can have important effects: the tonus of muscles in the lips helps keep the teeth aligned, for instance. When this gentle but constant pressure is absent (due to paralysis or a short lip that leaves the teeth exposed), teeth migrate, becoming everted ("buck teeth").

The absence of muscle tone in an unconscious patient (e.g., under a general anesthetic) may allow joints to be dislocated as he or she is being lifted or positioned. When a muscle is denervated (loses its nerve supply), it becomes *paralyzed* (flaccid, lacking both its tonus and its ability to contract phasically on demand or reflexively). In the absence of a muscle's normal tonus, that of opposing (*antagonist*) muscle(s) may cause a limb to assume an abnormal resting position. In addition, the denervated muscle will become fibrotic and lose its elasticity, also contributing to the abnormal position at rest.

Muscle Soreness and "Pulled" Muscles

Eccentric contractions that are either excessive or associated with a novel task are often the cause of delayed-onset *muscle soreness*. Thus walking down many flights of stairs would actually result in more soreness, owing to the eccentric contractions, than walking up the same flights of stairs. The muscle stretching that occurs during the lengthening type of eccentric contraction appears to be more likely to produce microtears in the muscles and/or periosteal irritation than that associated with concentric contraction (shortening of the muscle belly).

Skeletal muscles are limited in their ability to lengthen. Usually muscles cannot elongate beyond one third of their resting length without sustaining damage. This is reflected in their attachments to the skeleton, which usually do not permit excessive lengthening. An exception is the hamstring muscles of the posterior thigh. When the knee is extended, the hamstrings typically reach their maximum length before the hip is fully flexed (i.e., flexion at the hip is limited by the hamstring's ability to elongate). Undoubtedly this, as well as forces related to their eccentric contraction, explains why hamstring muscles are "pulled" (sustain tears) more commonly than other muscles (Fig. BI.7).

Growth and Regeneration of Skeletal Muscle

Skeletal striated muscle fibers cannot divide, but they can be replaced individually by new muscle fibers derived from **satellite cells of skeletal muscle**

FIGURE BI.7.

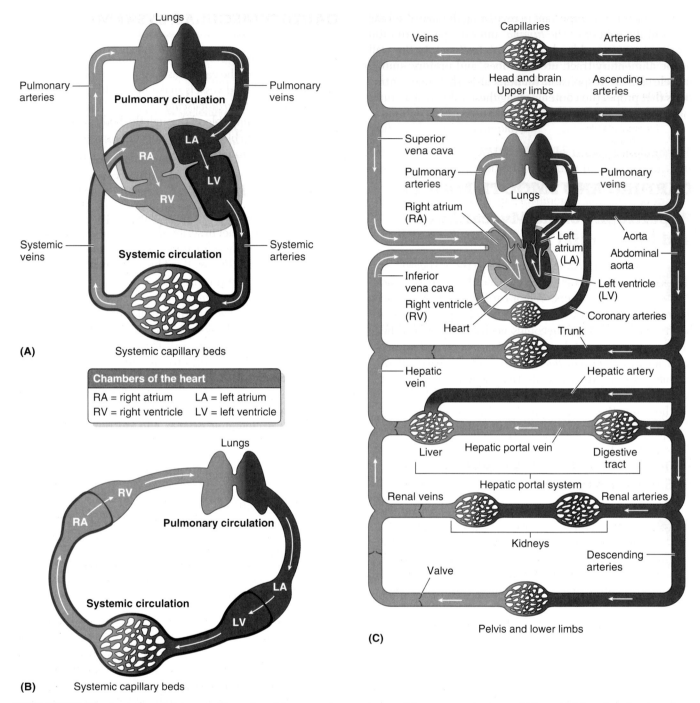

FIGURE I.22. The circulation. A. Schematic illustration of the anatomic arrangement of the two muscular pumps (right and left heart) serving the pulmonary and systemic circulations. **B.** Schematic illustration of the body's circulation, with the right and left heart depicted as two pumps in series. The pulmonary and systemic circulations are actually serial components of one continuous loop. **C.** A more detailed schematic illustration demonstrating that the systemic circulation actually consists of many parallel circuits serving the various organs and regions of the body.

- **Tunica media,** a middle layer consisting primarily of smooth muscle.
- **Tunica adventitia,** an outer connective tissue layer or sheath.

The tunica media is the most variable coat. Arteries, veins, and lymphatic ducts are distinguished by the thickness of this layer relative to the size of the lumen, its organization, and,

in the case of arteries, the presence of variable amounts of elastic fibers.

ARTERIES

Arteries are blood vessels that carry blood under relatively high pressure (compared to the corresponding veins) from the heart and distribute it to the body (Fig. I.24A). The blood

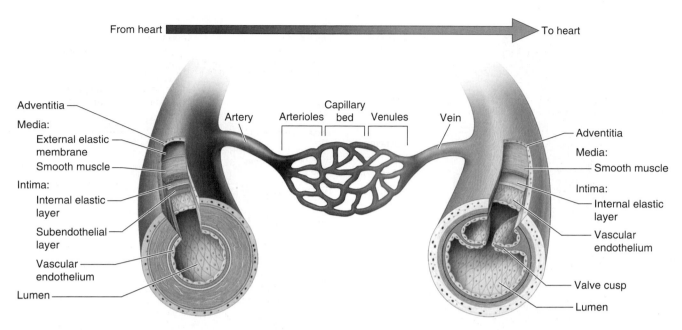

From heart   To heart

Adventitia
Media:
  External elastic membrane
  Smooth muscle
Intima:
  Internal elastic layer
  Subendothelial layer
  Vascular endothelium
Lumen

Artery   Arterioles   Capillary bed   Venules   Vein

Adventitia
Media:
  Smooth muscle
Intima:
  Internal elastic layer
  Vascular endothelium
Valve cusp
Lumen

FIGURE I.23. Blood vessel structure. The walls of most blood vessels have three concentric layers of tissue, called tunics (L. *tunicae,* coats). With less muscle, veins are thinner walled than their companion arteries and have wide lumens (L. *luminae*) that usually appear flattened in tissue sections.

passes through arteries of decreasing caliber. The different types of arteries are distinguished from each other on the basis of overall size, relative amounts of elastic tissue or muscle in the tunica media (Fig. I.23), the thickness of the wall relative to the lumen, and function. Artery size and type is a continuum—that is, there is a gradual change in morphological characteristics from one type to another. There are three types of arteries:

- **Large elastic arteries** (conducting arteries) have many elastic layers (sheets of elastic fibers) in their walls. These large arteries initially receive the cardiac output. Their elasticity enables them to expand when they receive the cardiac output from the ventricles, minimizing the pressure change, and return to normal size between ventricular contractions, as they continue to push the blood into the medium arteries downstream. This maintains the blood pressure in the arterial system between cardiac contractions (at a time when ventricular pressure falls to zero). Overall, this minimizes the ebb in blood pressure as the heart contracts and relaxes. Examples of large elastic arteries are the aorta, the arteries that originate from the arch of the aorta (brachiocephalic trunk, subclavian and carotid arteries), and the pulmonary trunk and arteries (Fig. I.24A).
- **Medium muscular arteries** (distributing arteries) have walls that consist chiefly of circularly disposed smooth muscle fibers. Their ability to decrease their diameter (*vasoconstrict*) regulates the flow of blood to different parts of the body as required by circumstance (e.g., activity, thermoregulation). Pulsatile contractions of their muscular walls (regardless of lumen caliber) temporarily and rhythmically constrict their lumina in progressive

sequence, propelling and distributing blood to various parts of the body. Most of the named arteries, including those observed in the body wall and limbs during dissection such as the brachial or femoral arteries, are medium muscular arteries.

- **Small arteries** and **arterioles** have relatively narrow lumina and thick muscular walls. The degree of filling of the capillary beds and level of arterial pressure within the vascular system are regulated mainly by the degree of tonus (firmness) in the smooth muscle of the arteriolar walls. If the tonus is above normal, *hypertension* (high blood pressure) results. Small arteries are usually not named or specifically identified during dissection, and arterioles can be observed only under magnification.

Anastomoses (communications) between multiple branches of an artery provide numerous potential detours for blood flow in case the usual pathway is obstructed by compression due to the position of a joint, pathology, or surgical ligation. If a main channel is occluded, the smaller alternate channels can usually increase in size over a period of time, providing a **collateral circulation** that ensures the blood supply to structures distal to the blockage. However, collateral pathways require time to open adequately; they are usually insufficient to compensate for sudden occlusion or ligation.

There are areas, however, where collateral circulation does not exist, or is inadequate to replace the main channel. Arteries that do not anastomose with adjacent arteries are **true** (anatomic) **terminal arteries** (end arteries). Occlusion of an end artery interrupts the blood supply to the structure or segment of an organ it supplies. True terminal arteries supply the retina, for example, where occlusion will result in blindness. While not true terminal arteries, *functional*

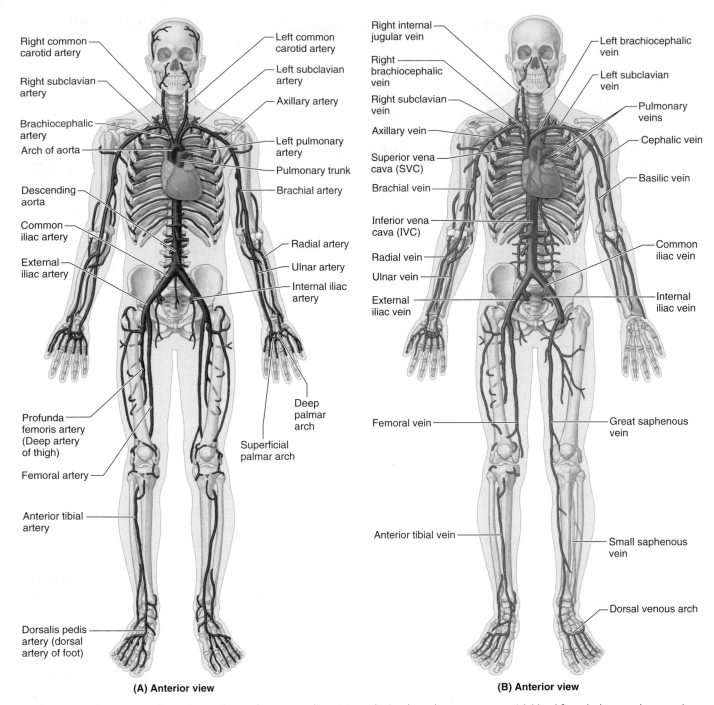

Right common carotid artery

Right subclavian artery

Brachiocephalic artery

Arch of aorta

Descending aorta

Common iliac artery

External iliac artery

Profunda femoris artery (Deep artery of thigh)

Femoral artery

Anterior tibial artery

Dorsalis pedis artery (dorsal artery of foot)

Left common carotid artery

Left subclavian artery

Axillary artery

Left pulmonary artery

Pulmonary trunk

Brachial artery

Radial artery

Ulnar artery

Internal iliac artery

Deep palmar arch

Superficial palmar arch

(A) Anterior view

Right internal jugular vein

Right brachiocephalic vein

Right subclavian vein

Axillary vein

Superior vena cava (SVC)

Brachial vein

Inferior vena cava (IVC)

Radial vein

Ulnar vein

External iliac vein

Femoral vein

Anterior tibial vein

Left brachiocephalic vein

Left subclavian vein

Pulmonary veins

Cephalic vein

Basilic vein

Common iliac vein

Internal iliac vein

Great saphenous vein

Small saphenous vein

Dorsal venous arch

(B) Anterior view

FIGURE I.24. Systemic portion of the cardiovascular system. The arteries and veins shown here carry oxygen-rich blood from the heart to the systemic capillary beds and return low-oxygen blood from the capillary beds to the heart, respectively, constituting the systemic circulation. Although commonly depicted and considered as single vessels, as shown here, the deep veins of the limbs usually occur as pairs of accompanying veins.

terminal arteries (arteries with ineffectual anastomoses) supply segments of the brain, liver, kidneys, spleen, and intestines; they may also exist in the heart.

VEINS

Veins generally return low-oxygen blood from the capillary beds to the heart, which gives the veins a dark blue appearance (Fig. I.24B). The large pulmonary veins are atypical in

that they carry oxygen-rich blood from the lungs to the heart. Because of the lower blood pressure in the venous system, the walls (specifically, the tunica media) of veins are thinner than those of their companion arteries (Fig. I.23). Normally, veins do not pulsate and do not squirt or spurt blood when severed. There are three sizes of veins:

- **Venules** are the smallest veins. Venules drain capillary beds and join similar vessels to form small veins.

Magnification is required to observe venules. Small veins are the tributaries of larger veins that unite to form **venous plexuses,** such as the dorsal venous arch of the foot (Fig. I.24B). Small veins are unnamed.

- **Medium veins** drain venous plexuses and accompany medium arteries. In the limbs, and in some other locations where the flow of blood is opposed by the pull of gravity, the medium veins have **venous valves,** passive flap valves that permit blood to flow toward the heart but not in the reverse direction (Fig. I-26). Examples of medium veins include the named superficial veins (cephalic and basilic veins of the upper limbs and great and small saphenous veins of the lower limbs) and the accompanying veins that are named according to the artery they accompany (Fig. I-24B).
- **Large veins** are characterized by wide bundles of longitudinal smooth muscle and a well-developed tunica adventitia. An example is the superior vena cava.

Veins are more abundant than arteries. Although their walls are thinner, their diameters are usually larger than those of the corresponding artery. The thin walls allow veins to have a large capacity for expansion, and do so when blood return to the heart is impeded by compression or internal pressures (e.g., after taking a large breath and holding it; this is the *Valsalva maneuver*).

Since the arteries and veins make up a circuit, it might be expected that half the blood volume would be in the arteries and half in the veins. Because of the veins' larger diameter and ability to expand, typically only 20% of the blood occupies arteries, whereas 80% is in the veins.

Although often depicted as single vessels in illustrations for simplicity, veins tend to be double or multiple. Those that accompany deep arteries—**accompanying veins** (L. *venae comitantes*)—surround them in an irregular branching network (Fig. I.25). This arrangement serves as a *countercurrent heat exchanger*, the warm arterial blood warming the cooler venous blood as it returns to the heart from a cold limb. The accompanying veins occupy a relatively unyielding fascial **vascular sheath** with the artery they accompany. As a

FIGURE I.26. Musculovenous pump. Muscular contractions in the limbs function with the venous valves to move blood toward the heart. The outward expansion of the bellies of contracting muscles is limited by deep fascia and becomes a compressive force, propelling the blood against gravity.

result, they are stretched and flattened as the artery expands during contraction of the heart, which aids in driving venous blood toward the heart—an *arteriovenous pump.*

Systemic veins are more variable than arteries, and *venous anastomoses*—natural communications, direct or indirect, between two veins—occur more often between them. The outward expansion of the bellies of contracting skeletal muscles in the limbs, limited by the deep fascia, compresses the veins, "milking" the blood superiorly toward the heart; another (musculovenous) type of venous pump (Fig. I.26). The valves of the veins break up the columns of blood, thus relieving the more dependent parts of excessive pressure, allowing venous blood to flow only toward the heart. The venous congestion that hot and tired feet experience at the end of a busy day is relieved by resting the feet on a footstool that is higher than the trunk (of the body). This position of the feet also helps the veins return blood to the heart.

BLOOD CAPILLARIES

For the oxygen and nutrients carried by the arteries to benefit the cells that make up the tissues of the body, they must leave the transporting vessels and enter the *extravascular space* between the cells, the extracellular (intercellular) space in which the cells live. **Capillaries** are simple

FIGURE I.25. Accompanying veins. Although most veins of the trunk occur as large single vessels, veins in the limbs occur as two or more smaller vessels that accompany an artery in a common vascular sheath.

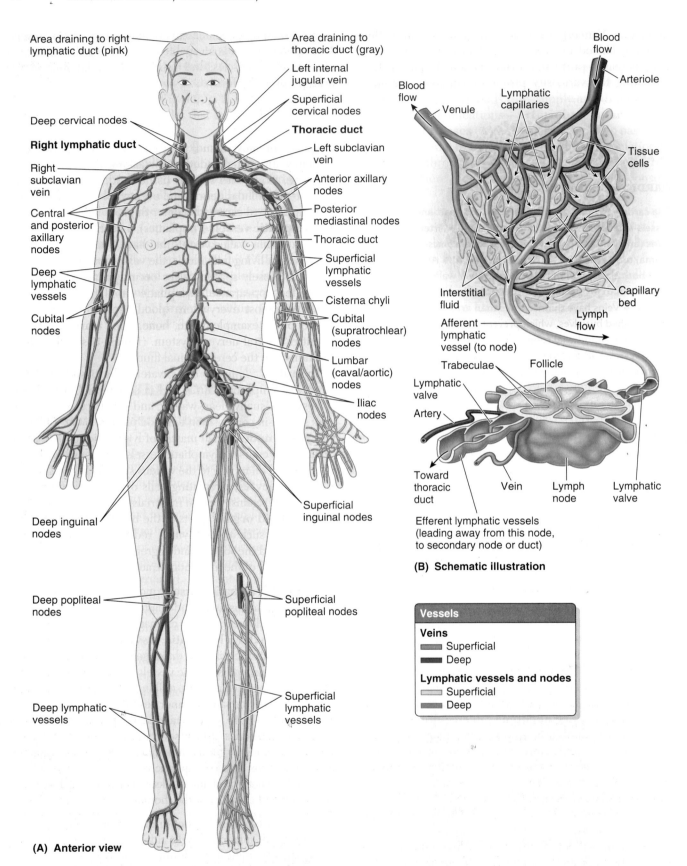

Area draining to right lymphatic duct (pink)

Area draining to thoracic duct (gray)

Left internal jugular vein

Superficial cervical nodes

Deep cervical nodes

Right lymphatic duct

Thoracic duct

Right subclavian vein

Left subclavian vein

Central and posterior axillary nodes

Anterior axillary nodes

Posterior mediastinal nodes

Thoracic duct

Deep lymphatic vessels

Superficial lymphatic vessels

Cisterna chyli

Cubital nodes

Cubital (supratrochlear) nodes

Lumbar (caval/aortic) nodes

Iliac nodes

Deep inguinal nodes

Superficial inguinal nodes

Deep popliteal nodes

Superficial popliteal nodes

Deep lymphatic vessels

Superficial lymphatic vessels

(A) Anterior view

Blood flow

Arteriole

Blood flow

Venule

Lymphatic capillaries

Tissue cells

Interstitial fluid

Capillary bed

Lymph flow

Afferent lymphatic vessel (to node)

Trabeculae

Follicle

Lymphatic valve

Artery

Toward thoracic duct

Vein

Lymph node

Lymphatic valve

Efferent lymphatic vessels (leading away from this node, to secondary node or duct)

(B) Schematic illustration

Vessels

Veins
- Superficial
- Deep

Lymphatic vessels and nodes
- Superficial
- Deep

FIGURE I.27. Lymphoid system. A. Pattern of lymphatic drainage. Except for the right superior quadrant of the body (pink), lymph ultimately drains into the left venous angle via the thoracic duct. The right superior quadrant drains to the right venous angle, usually via a right lymphatic duct. Lymph typically passes through several sets of lymph nodes, in a generally predictable order, before it enters the venous system. **B.** Schematic illustration of lymph flow from extracellular spaces through a lymph node. *Small black arrows* indicate the flow (leaking) of interstitial fluid out of blood capillaries and (absorption) into the lymphatic capillaries.

of the body merge in the abdomen, sometimes forming a dilated collecting sac, the cisterna chyli. From this sac (if present), or from the merger of the trunks, the thoracic duct ascends into and then through the thorax to enter the **left venous angle** (junction of left internal jugular and left subclavian veins).

Although this is the typical drainage pattern of most lymph, lymphatic vessels communicate with veins freely in many parts of the body. Consequently, ligation of a lymphatic trunk or even the thoracic duct itself may have only a transient effect as a new pattern of drainage is established through more peripheral lymphaticovenous—and later interlymphatic—anastomoses.

Additional functions of the lymphoid system include:

- *Absorption and transport of dietary fat.* Special lymphatic capillaries, called *lacteals* (L. *lacteus*, milk), receive all lipid and lipid-soluble vitamins absorbed by the intestine. Visceral lymphatics then convey the milky fluid, *chyle* (G. *chylos*, juice), to the thoracic duct and into the venous system.
- *Formation of a defense mechanism for the body.* When foreign protein drains from an infected area, antibodies specific to the protein are produced by immunologically competent cells and/or lymphocytes and dispatched to the infected area.

LYMPHOID SYSTEM

Spread of Cancer

Cancer invades the body by *contiguity* (growing into adjacent tissue) or by *metastasis* (the dissemination of tumor cells to sites distant from the original or primary tumor). Metastasis occurs three ways:

1. *Direct seeding* of serous membranes of body cavities.
2. *Lymphogenous spread* (via lymphatic vessels).
3. *Hematogenous spread* (via blood vessels).

It is surprising that often even a thin fascial sheet or serous membrane deflects tumor invasion. However, once a malignancy penetrates into a potential space, the direct seeding of cavities—that is, of its serous membranes—is likely.

Lymphogenous spread of cancer is the most common route for the initial dissemination of *carcinomas* (epithelial tumors), the most common type of cancer. Cells loosened from the primary cancer site enter and travel via lymphatics. The lymph-borne cells are filtered through and trapped by lymph nodes, which thus become secondary (metastatic) cancer sites.

The pattern of cancerous lymph node involvement follows the natural routes of lymph drainage. Thus when removing a potentially metastatic tumor, surgeons *stage the metastasis* (determine the degree to which cancer has spread) by removing and examining lymph nodes that receive lymph from the organ or region in the order the lymph normally passes through them. Therefore, it is important for physicians to literally know the lymphatic drainage "backward and forward"—that is, (1) to know what nodes are likely to be affected when a tumor is identified in a certain site or organ (and the order in which they receive lymph) and (2) to be able to determine likely sites of primary cancer sites (sources of metastasis) when an enlarged node is detected. *Cancerous nodes* enlarge as the tumor cells within them increase; however, unlike swollen infected nodes, cancerous nodes are not usually painful when compressed.

Hematogenous spread of cancer is the most common route for the metastasis of the less common (but more malignant) *sarcomas* (connective tissue cancers). Because veins are more abundant and have thinner walls that offer less resistance, metastasis occurs more often by venous than arterial routes. Since the blood-borne cells follow venous flow, the liver and lungs are the most common sites of secondary sarcomas. Typically, the treatment or removal of a primary tumor is not difficult, but the treatment or removal of all the affected lymph nodes or other secondary (metastatic) tumors may be impossible (Cotran et al., 1999).

Lymphangitis, Lymphadenitis, and Lymphedema

Lymphangitis and *lymphadenitis* are secondary inflammations of lymphatic vessels and lymph nodes, respectively. These conditions may occur when the lymphoid system is involved in chemical or bacterial transport after severe injury or infection. The lymphatic vessels, not normally evident, may become apparent as red streaks in the skin, and the nodes become painfully enlarged. This condition is potentially dangerous because the uncontained infection may lead to *septicemia* (blood poisoning). *Lymphedema*, a localized type of edema, occurs when lymph does not drain from an area of the body. For instance, if cancerous lymph nodes are surgically removed from the axilla (compartment superior to the armpit), lymphedema of the limb may occur. Solid cell growths may permeate lymphatic vessels and form minute *cellular emboli* (plugs), which may break free and pass to regional lymph nodes. In this way, further lymphogenous spread to other tissues and organs may occur.

The Bottom Line

LYMPHOID SYSTEM

The lymphoid system drains surplus fluid from the extracellular spaces to the bloodstream. ♦ The lymphoid system also constitutes a major part of the body's defense system. ♦ Important components of the lymphoid system are networks of lymphatic capillaries, the lymphatic plexuses; lymphatic vessels; lymph; lymph nodes; lymphocytes; and the lymphoid organs. ♦ The lymphoid system provides a (relatively) predictable route for the spread of certain types of cancerous cells throughout the body. ♦ Inflammation of lymphatic vessels and/or enlargement of lymph nodes is an important indicator of possible injury, infection, or disease (e.g., cancer).

NERVOUS SYSTEM

The nervous system enables the body to react to continuous changes in its internal and external environments. It also controls and integrates the various activities of the body, such as circulation and respiration. For descriptive purposes, the nervous system is divided:

- Structurally into the *central nervous system* (CNS), consisting of the brain and spinal cord, and the *peripheral nervous system* (PNS), the remainder of the nervous system outside of the CNS.
- Functionally into the *somatic nervous system* (SNS) and the *autonomic nervous system* (ANS).

Nervous tissue consists of two main cell types: neurons (*nerve cells*) and neuroglia (*glial cells*), which support the neurons.

- **Neurons** are the structural and functional units of the nervous system specialized for rapid communication (Figs. I.28 and I.29). A neuron is composed of a **cell body** with processes (extensions) called **dendrites** and an **axon,** which carry impulses to and away from the cell body, respectively. *Myelin,* layers of lipid, and protein substances form a **myelin sheath** around some axons, greatly increasing the velocity of impulse conduction. Two types of neurons constitute the majority of neurons comprising the nervous system (and the peripheral nervous system in particular) (Fig. I.28):
  1. **Multipolar motor neurons** have two or more dendrites and a single axon that may have one or more collateral branches. They are the most common type of neuron in the nervous system (CNS and PNS). All of the motor neurons that control skeletal muscle and those comprising the ANS are multipolar neurons.
  2. **Pseudounipolar sensory neurons** have a short, apparently single (but actually double) process

extending from the cell body. This common process separates into a peripheral process, conducting impulses from the receptor organ (touch, pain, or temperature sensors in the skin, for example) toward the cell body, and a central process that continues from the cell body into the CNS. The cell bodies of pseudounipolar neurons are located outside the CNS in sensory ganglia and are thus part of the PNS.

Neurons communicate with each other at **synapses,** points of contact between neurons (Fig. I.29). The communication occurs by means of *neurotransmitters,* chemical agents released or secreted by one neuron, which may excite or inhibit another neuron, continuing or terminating the relay of impulses or the response to them.

- **Neuroglia** (glial cells or glia), approximately five times as abundant as neurons, are non-neuronal, non-excitable cells that form a major component of nervous tissue, supporting, insulating, and nourishing the neurons. In the CNS, neuroglia include *oligodendroglia, astrocytes, ependymal cells,* and *microglia* (small glial cells). In the

FIGURE I.28. Neurons. The most common types of neurons are shown. **A.** Multipolar motor neurons. All of the motor neurons that control skeletal muscle and those comprising the ANS are multipolar neurons. **B.** Except for some of the special senses (for example, olfaction and vision), all sensory neurons of the PNS are pseudounipolar neurons with cell bodies located in sensory ganglia.

FIGURE I.29. Multipolar motor neurons synapsing. A neuron influences other neurons at synapses. *Inset:* Detailed structure of an axodendritic synapse. Neurotransmitters diffuse across the synaptic cleft between the two cells and become bound to receptors.

PNS, neuroglia include *satellite cells* around the neurons in the spinal (posterior root) and autonomic ganglia and Schwann (*neurolemma*) cells (Figs. I.28 and I.29).

Central Nervous System

The **central nervous system** (CNS) consists of the brain and spinal cord (Fig. I.30). The principal roles of the CNS are to integrate and coordinate incoming and outgoing neural signals and to carry out higher mental functions, such as thinking and learning.

A **nucleus** is a collection of nerve cell bodies in the CNS. A bundle of nerve fibers (axons) within the CNS connecting neighboring or distant nuclei of the cerebral cortex is a **tract.** The brain and spinal cord are composed of gray matter and white matter. The nerve cell bodies lie within and constitute the **gray matter;** the interconnecting fiber tract systems form the **white matter** (Fig. I.31). In transverse sections of the spinal cord, the gray matter appears roughly as an H-shaped area embedded in a matrix of white matter. The struts (supports) of the H are **horns;** hence there are right and left posterior (dorsal) and anterior (ventral) gray horns.

Three membranous layers—pia mater, arachnoid mater, and dura mater—collectively constitute the **meninges.** The meninges and the **cerebrospinal fluid** (CSF) surround and protect the CNS. The brain and spinal cord are intimately

covered on their outer surface by the innermost meningeal layer, a delicate, transparent covering, the **pia mater.** The CSF is located between the pia mater and the **arachnoid mater.** External to the pia mater and arachnoid mater is the thick, tough **dura mater**. The *dura mater of the brain is* intimately related to the internal aspect of the bone of the surrounding *neurocranium* (braincase); *the dura mater of the spinal cord* is separated from the surrounding bone of the vertebral column by a fat-filled *epidural space.*

Peripheral Nervous System

The **peripheral nervous system** (PNS) consists of nerve fibers and cell bodies outside the CNS that conduct impulses to or away from the CNS (Fig. I.30). The PNS is organized into nerves that connect the CNS with peripheral structures.

A **nerve fiber** consists of an axon, its neurolemma (G. *neuron,* nerve + G. *lemma,* husk), and surrounding endoneurial connective tissue (Figs. I.32). The **neurolemma** consists of the cell membranes of Schwann cells that immediately surround the axon, separating it from other axons. In the PNS, the neurolemma may take two forms, creating two classes of nerve fibers:

1. The neurolemma of myelinated nerve fibers consists of Schwann cells specific to an individual axon, organized into a continuous series of enwrapping cells that form myelin.
2. The neurolemma of unmyelinated nerve fibers is composed of Schwann cells that do not make up such an apparent series; multiple axons are separately embedded within the cytoplasm of each cell. These Schwann cells do not produce myelin. Most fibers in cutaneous nerves (nerves supplying sensation to the skin) are unmyelinated.

A **nerve** consists of:

- a bundle of nerve fibers outside the CNS (or a "bundle of bundled fibers," or *fascicles,* in the case of a larger nerve),
- the connective tissue coverings that surround and bind the nerve fibers and fascicles together, and
- the blood vessels (*vasa nervorum*) that nourish the nerve fibers and their coverings (Fig. I.33).

Nerves are fairly strong and resilient because the nerve fibers are supported and protected by three connective tissue coverings:

1. **Endoneurium,** delicate connective tissue immediately surrounding the neurilemma cells and axons.
2. **Perineurium,** a layer of dense connective tissue that encloses a fascicle of nerve fibers, providing an effective barrier against penetration of the nerve fibers by foreign substances.
3. **Epineurium,** a thick connective tissue sheath that surrounds and encloses a bundle of fascicles, forming the outermost covering of the nerve; it includes fatty tissue, blood vessels, and lymphatics.

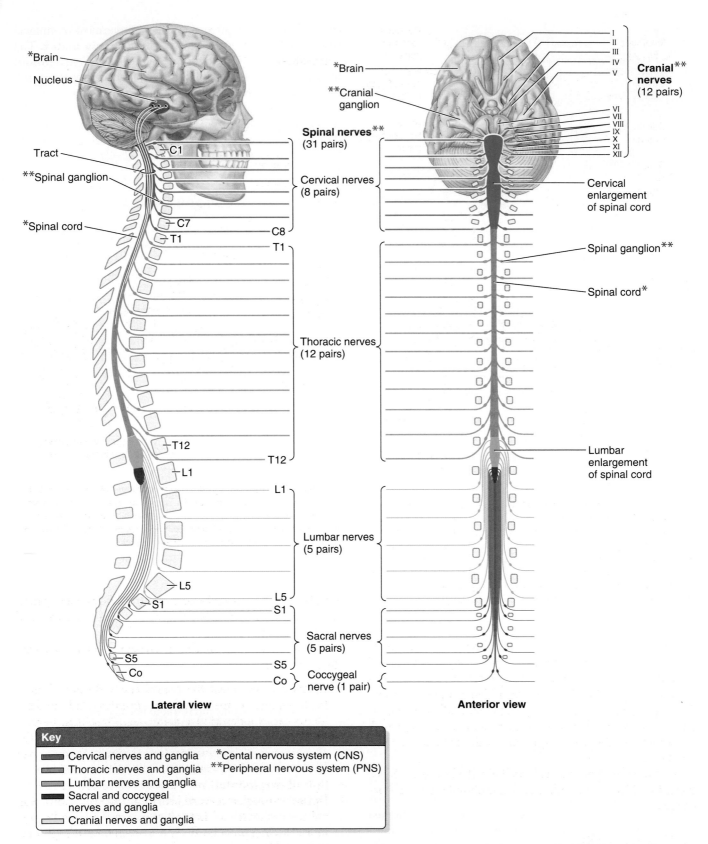

Lateral view

Anterior view

Key

- Cervical nerves and ganglia
- Thoracic nerves and ganglia
- Lumbar nerves and ganglia
- Sacral and coccygeal nerves and ganglia
- Cranial nerves and ganglia

*Cental nervous system (CNS)
**Peripheral nervous system (PNS)

FIGURE I.30. Basic organization of the nervous system. The CNS consists of the brain and spinal cord. The PNS consists of nerves and ganglia. Nerves are either cranial nerves or spinal (segmental) nerves, or derivatives of them. Except in the cervical region, each spinal nerve bears the same letter–numeral designation as the vertebra forming the superior boundary of its exit from the vertebral column. In the cervical region, each spinal nerve bears the same letter–numeral designation as the vertebra forming its inferior boundary. Spinal nerve C8 exits between vertebrae C7 and T1. The cervical and lumbar enlargements of the spinal cord occur in relationship to the innervation of the limbs.

FIGURE I.31. **Spinal cord and spinal meninges.** The dura mater and arachnoid mater are incised and reflected to show the posterior and anterior roots and the denticulate ligament (a bilateral, longitudinal, toothed thickening of the pia mater that anchors the cord in the center of the vertebral canal). The spinal cord is sectioned to show its horns of gray matter. The meninges extend along the nerve roots then blend with the epineurium at the point where the posterior and anterior roots join, forming the dural root sleeves that enclose the sensory (posterior root) ganglia.

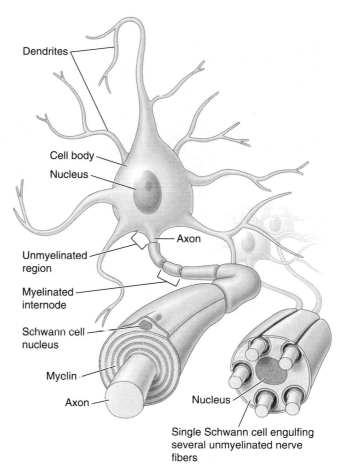

FIGURE I.32. **Myelinated and unmyelinated nerve fibers.** Myelinated nerve fibers have a sheath composed of a continuous series of neurilemma (Schwann) cells that surround the axon and form a series of myelin segments. Multiple unmyelinated nerve fibers are individually engulfed within a single neurilemma cell that does not produce myelin.

Nerves are organized much like a telephone cable: The axons are like individual wires insulated by the neurolemma and endoneurium; the insulated wires are bundled by the perineurium, and the bundles are surrounded by the epineurium forming the cable's outer wrapping (Fig. I.33). It is important to distinguish between *nerve fibers* and *nerves*, which are sometimes depicted diagrammatically as being one and the same.

A collection of neuron cell bodies outside the CNS is a **ganglion.** There are both motor (autonomic) and sensory ganglia.

TYPES OF NERVES

The PNS is anatomically and operationally continuous with the CNS (Fig. I.30). Its **afferent (sensory) fibers** convey neural impulses to the CNS from the sense organs (e.g., the eyes) and from sensory receptors in various parts of the body (e.g., in the skin). Its **efferent (motor) fibers** convey neural impulses from the CNS to *effector organs* (muscles and glands).

Nerves are either cranial nerves or spinal nerves, or derivatives of them.

- **Cranial nerves** exit the cranial cavity through foramina (openings) in the cranium (G. *kranion,* skull) and are identified by a descriptive name (e.g., "trochlear nerve") or a Roman numeral (e.g., "CN IV"). Only 11 of the 12 pairs of cranial nerves arise from the brain; the other pair (CN XI) arises from the superior part of the spinal cord.
- **Spinal (segmental) nerves** exit the vertebral column (spine) through intervertebral foramina (Fig. I.30). Spinal nerves arise in bilateral pairs from a specific segment of the spinal cord. The 31 spinal cord segments and the 31 pairs of nerves arising from them are identified by a letter and number (e.g., "T4") designating the region of the spinal cord and their superior-to-inferior order (*C*, cervical; *T*, thoracic; *L*, lumbar; *S*, sacral; *Co*, coccygeal).

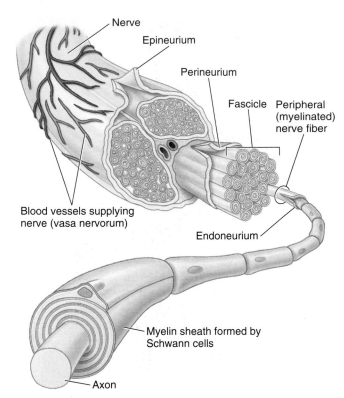

FIGURE I.33. Arrangement and ensheathment of myelinated nerve fibers. Nerves consist of the bundles of nerve fibers, the layers of connective tissue binding them together, and the blood vessels (vasa nervorum) that serve them. All but the smallest nerves are arranged in bundles called fascicles.

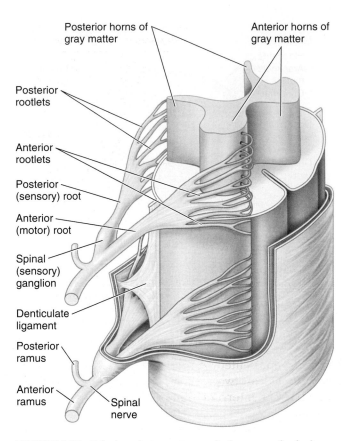

FIGURE I.34. Spinal cord gray matter, spinal roots, and spinal nerves. The meninges are incised and reflected to show the H-shaped gray matter in the spinal cord and the posterior and anterior rootlets and roots of two spinal nerves. The posterior and anterior rootlets enter and leave the posterior and anterior gray horns, respectively. The posterior and anterior nerve roots unite distal to the spinal ganglion to form a mixed spinal nerve, which immediately divides into posterior and anterior rami.

Spinal Nerves. Spinal nerves initially arise from the spinal cord as *rootlets* (a detail commonly omitted from diagrams for the sake of simplicity); the rootlets converge to form two *nerve roots* (Fig. I.34):

1. An **anterior (ventral) nerve root,** consisting of motor (efferent) fibers passing from nerve cell bodies in the anterior horn of spinal cord gray matter to effector organs located peripherally.
2. A **posterior (dorsal) nerve root,** consisting of sensory (afferent) fibers from cell bodies in the spinal (sensory) or posterior (dorsal) root ganglion (commonly abbreviated in clinical use as "DRG") that extend peripherally to sensory endings and centrally to the posterior horn of spinal cord gray matter.

The posterior and anterior nerve roots unite, within or just proximal to the intervertebral foramen, to form a *mixed* (both motor and sensory) *spinal nerve,* which immediately divides into two *rami* (L., branches): a *posterior (dorsal) ramus* and an *anterior (ventral) ramus.* As branches of the mixed spinal nerve, the posterior and anterior rami carry both motor and sensory fibers, as do all their subsequent branches. The terms *motor nerve* and *sensory nerve* are almost always relative terms, referring to the *majority* of fiber types conveyed

by that nerve. Nerves supplying muscles of the trunk or limbs (motor nerves) also contain about 40% sensory fibers, which convey pain and proprioceptive information. Conversely, cutaneous (sensory) nerves contain motor fibers, which serve sweat glands and the smooth muscle of blood vessels and hair follicles.

The unilateral area of skin innervated by the sensory fibers of a single spinal nerve is called a **dermatome;** the unilateral muscle mass receiving innervation from the fibers conveyed by a single spinal nerve is a **myotome** (Fig. I.35). From clinical studies of lesions of the posterior roots or spinal nerves, dermatome maps have been devised to indicate the typical pattern of innervation of the skin by specific spinal nerves (Fig. I.36). However, a lesion of a single posterior root or spinal nerve would rarely result in numbness over the area demarcated for that nerve in these maps because the fibers conveyed by adjacent spinal nerves overlap almost completely as they are distributed to the skin, providing a type of double coverage. The lines indicating dermatomes on dermatome maps would thus

FIGURE I.35. Dermatomes and myotomes. Schematic representation of a dermatome (the unilateral area of skin) and myotome (the unilateral portion of skeletal muscle) receiving innervation from a single spinal nerve.

be better represented by smudges or gradations of color. Generally, at least two adjacent spinal nerves (or posterior roots) must be interrupted to produce a discernible area of numbness.

As they emerge from the intervertebral foramina, spinal nerves are divided into two rami (Fig. I.37):

1. **Posterior (primary) rami of spinal nerves** supply nerve fibers to the synovial joints of the vertebral column, deep muscles of the back, and the overlying skin in a segmental pattern. As a general rule, the posterior rami remain separate from each other (do not merge to form major somatic nerve plexuses).
2. **Anterior (primary) rami of spinal nerves** supply nerve fibers to the much larger remaining area, consisting of the anterior and lateral regions of the trunk and the upper and lower limbs. The anterior rami that are distributed exclusively to the trunk generally remain separate from each other, also innervating muscles and skin in a segmental pattern (Figs. I.38 and I.39). However, primarily in relationship to the innervation of the limbs, the majority of anterior rami merge with one or more adjacent anterior rami, forming the major *somatic nerve plexuses* (networks) in which their fibers intermingle and from which a new set of *multisegmental peripheral nerves* emerges (Figs. I.39 and I.40A & B). The anterior rami of spinal nerves participating in plexus formation contribute fibers to multiple peripheral nerves arising from the plexus (Fig. I.40A); conversely, most peripheral nerves arising from the plexus contain fibers from multiple spinal nerves (Fig. I.40B).

Although the spinal nerves lose their identity as they split and merge in the plexus, the fibers arising from a specific

Anterior view   Posterior view

FIGURE I.36. Dermatomes (segmental cutaneous innervation). Dermatome maps of the body are based on an accumulation of clinical findings following spinal nerve injuries. This map is based on the studies of Foerster (1933) and reflects both anatomical (actual) distribution or segmental innervation and clinical experience. Another popular but more schematic map is that of Keegan and Garrett (1948), which is appealing for its regular, more easily extrapolated pattern. Spinal nerve C1 lacks a significant afferent component and does not supply the skin; therefore, no C1 dermatome is depicted. Note that in the Foerster map, C5–T1 and L3–S1 are distributed almost entirely in the limbs (i.e., have little or no representation on the trunk).

spinal cord segment and conveyed from it by a single spinal nerve are ultimately distributed to one segmental dermatome, although they may reach it by means of a multisegmental peripheral nerve arising from the plexus that also conveys fibers to all or parts of other adjacent dermatomes (Fig. I.40C).

It is therefore important to distinguish between the distribution of the fibers carried by spinal nerves (*segmental innervation* or *distribution*—i.e., dermatomes and myotomes labeled with a letter and a number, such as "T4") and of the fibers carried by branches of a plexus (*peripheral nerve innervation* or *distribution*, labeled with the names of peripheral nerves, such as "the median

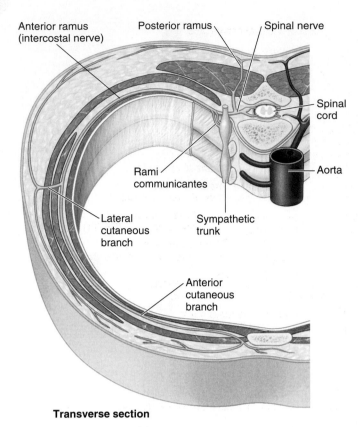

Transverse section

FIGURE I.37. Distribution of spinal nerves. Almost as soon as they are formed by the merging of posterior and anterior roots, spinal nerves divide into anterior and posterior (primary) rami. Posterior rami are distributed to the synovial joints of the vertebral column, deep muscles of the back, and the overlying skin. The remaining anterolateral body wall, including the limbs, is supplied by anterior rami. Posterior rami and the anterior rami of spinal nerves T2–T12 generally do not merge with the rami of adjacent spinal nerves to form plexuses.

nerve") (Figs. I.36 and I.38). Mapping segmental innervation (dermatomes, determined by clinical experience) and mapping the distribution of peripheral nerves (determined by dissecting the branches of a named nerve distally) produce entirely different maps, except for most of the trunk where, in the absence of plexus formation, segmental and peripheral distributions are the same. The overlapping in the cutaneous distribution of nerve fibers conveyed by adjacent spinal nerves also occurs in the cutaneous distribution of nerve fibers conveyed by adjacent peripheral nerves.

Cranial Nerves. As they arise from the CNS, some cranial nerves convey only sensory fibers, some only motor fibers, and some carry a mixture of both types of fibers (Fig. I.41). Communication occurs between cranial nerves, and between cranial nerves and upper cervical (spinal) nerves; thus a nerve that initially conveys only motor fibers may receive sensory fibers distally in its course, and vice

versa. Except for the first two (those involved in the senses of smell and sight), cranial nerves that convey sensory fibers into the brain bear sensory ganglia (similar to spinal or posterior root ganglia), where the cell bodies of the pseudounipolar fibers are located. Although, by definition, the term *dermatome* applies only to spinal nerves, similar areas of skin supplied by single cranial nerves can be identified and mapped. Unlike dermatomes, however, there is little overlap in the innervation of zones of skin supplied by cranial nerves.

SOMATIC AND VISCERAL FIBERS

The types of fibers conveyed by cranial or spinal nerves are as follows (Fig. I.41):

- Somatic fibers
  - **General sensory fibers** (*general somatic afferent* [*GSA*] *fibers*) transmit sensations from the body to the CNS; they may be *exteroceptive sensations* from the skin (pain, temperature, touch, and pressure) or pain and *proprioceptive sensations* from muscles, tendons, and joints. Proprioceptive sensations are usually subconscious, providing information regarding joint position and the tension of tendons and muscles. This information is combined with input from the vestibular apparatus of the internal ear, resulting in awareness of the orientation of the body and limbs in space, independent of visual input.
  - **Somatic motor fibers** (*general somatic efferent* [*GSE*] *fibers*) transmit impulses to skeletal (voluntary) muscles.
- Visceral fibers
  - **Visceral sensory fibers** (*general visceral afferent* [*GVA*] *fibers*) transmit pain or subconscious visceral *reflex sensations* (information concerning distension, blood gas, and blood pressure levels, for example) from hollow organs and blood vessels to the CNS.
  - **Visceral motor fibers** (*general visceral efferent* [*GVE*] *fibers*) transmit impulses to smooth (involuntary) muscle and glandular tissues. Two varieties of fibers, *presynaptic* and *postsynaptic*, work together to conduct impulses from the CNS to smooth muscle or glands.

Both types of sensory fibers—visceral sensory and general sensory—are processes of pseudounipolar neurons with cell bodies located outside of the CNS in spinal or cranial sensory ganglia (Figs. I.41 and I.42). The motor fibers of nerves are axons of multipolar neurons. The cell bodies of somatic motor and presynaptic visceral motor neurons are located in the gray matter of the spinal cord. Cell bodies of postsynaptic motor neurons are located outside the CNS in autonomic ganglia.

Trigeminal nerve (CN V)
Great auricular nerve (C2,3)
Transverse cervical nerve (C2,3)
Supraclavicular nerves (C3,4)
Superior lateral cutaneous nerve of arm (C5,6)
Medial cutaneous nerve of arm (C5,6)
Inferior lateral cutaneous nerve of arm (C5,6)
Lateral cutaneous nerve of forearm (C5,6)
Medial cutaneous nerve of forearm (C8, T1)
Radial nerve (C6–8)
Median nerve (C6–8)
Ulnar nerve (C8, T1)
Lateral cutaneous nerve of thigh (L2,3)
Obturator nerve (L2–4)
Femoral nerve (L2–4)
Lateral sural cutaneous nerve (L4–S1)
Superficial fibular nerve (L5, S1)
Sural nerve (L5–S2)
Deep fibular nerve (L5)

Lesser occipital nerve (C2,3)
Supraclavicular nerves (C3,4)
Superior lateral cutaneous nerve of arm (C5,6)
Inferior lateral cutaneous nerve of arm (C5,6)
Posterior cutaneous nerve of arm (C7)
Medial cutaneous nerve of arm (C7)
Lateral cutaneous nerve of forearm (C5,6)
Medial cutaneous nerve of forearm (C8, T1)
Posterior cutaneous nerve of forearm (C6–8)
Ulnar nerve (C8, T1)
Radial nerve (C6–8)
Lateral cutaneous nerve of thigh (L2,3)
Posterior cutaneous nerve of thigh (S1–3)
Saphenous nerve (L3,4)
Lateral sural cutaneous nerve (L4–S1)
Medial sural cutaneous nerve (L5–S2)
Sural nerve (L5–S2)
Calcaneal branches of sural and tibial nerve (L5–S2)

Anterior view   **Posterior view**

FIGURE I.38. Distribution of peripheral cutaneous nerves. Maps of the cutaneous distribution of peripheral nerves are based on dissection and supported by clinical findings.

In addition to the fiber types listed above, some cranial nerves also convey **special sensory fibers** for the special senses (smell, sight, hearing, balance, and taste). On the basis of the embryologic/phylogenetic derivation of certain muscles of the head and neck, some motor fibers conveyed by cranial nerves to striated muscle have traditionally been classified as "special visceral"; however, since the designation is confusing and not applied clinically, that term will not be used here. These fibers are occasionally designated as *branchial motor*, referring to muscle tissue derived from the pharyngeal arches in the embryo.

CENTRAL AND PERIPHERAL NERVOUS SYSTEMS

Damage to the CNS

When the *brain or spinal cord is damaged*, the injured axons do not recover in most circumstances. Their proximal stumps begin to regenerate, sending sprouts into the area of the lesion; however, this growth is blocked by *astrocyte proliferation* at the injury site, and the axonal sprouts are soon retracted. As a result, permanent disability follows destruction of a tract in the CNS.

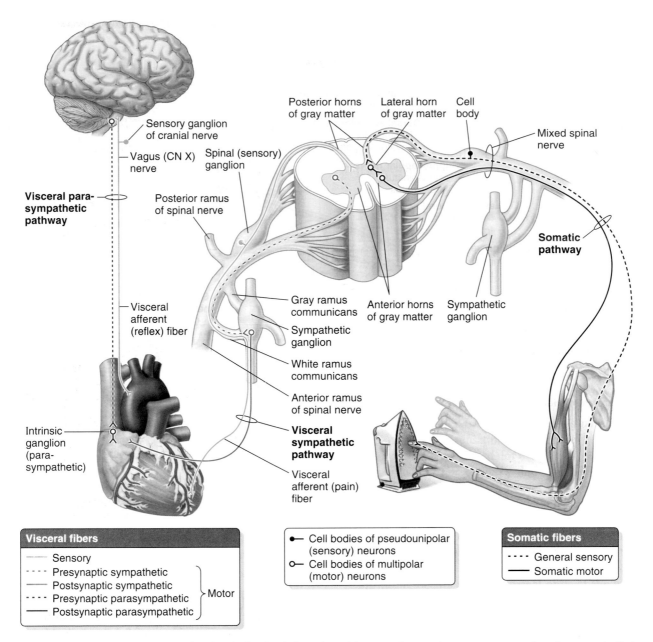

FIGURE I.41. Somatic and visceral innervation via spinal, splanchnic, and cranial nerves. The somatic motor system permits voluntary and reflexive movement caused by contraction of skeletal muscles, such as occurs when one touches a hot iron.

Labels in figure:

Posterior horns of gray matter
Lateral horn of gray matter
Cell body
Mixed spinal nerve
Sensory ganglion of cranial nerve
Vagus (CN X) nerve
Spinal (sensory) ganglion
Visceral parasympathetic pathway
Posterior ramus of spinal nerve
Somatic pathway
Visceral afferent (reflex) fiber
Gray ramus communicans
Anterior horns of gray matter
Sympathetic ganglion
Sympathetic ganglion
White ramus communicans
Anterior ramus of spinal nerve
Intrinsic ganglion (parasympathetic)
Visceral sympathetic pathway
Visceral afferent (pain) fiber

Visceral fibers
— Sensory
- - - Presynaptic sympathetic
— Postsynaptic sympathetic
- - - Presynaptic parasympathetic
— Postsynaptic parasympathetic } Motor

●— Cell bodies of pseudounipolar (sensory) neurons
○— Cell bodies of multipolar (motor) neurons

Somatic fibers
- - - General sensory
— Somatic motor

The Bottom Line

CENTRAL AND PERIPHERAL NERVOUS SYSTEMS

The nervous system can be functionally divided into the central nervous system (CNS), which consists of the brain and spinal cord, and the peripheral nervous system (PNS), which consists of the nerve fibers and their nerve cell bodies that reside outside the CNS. ♦ Neurons are the functional units of the nervous system. They are composed of a cell body, dendrites, and axons. ♦ The neuronal axons (nerve fibers) transmit impulses to other neurons or to a target organ or muscle, or in the case of sensory nerves, transmit impulses to the CNS from peripheral sensory organs. ♦ Neuroglia are non-neuronal, supporting cells of the nervous system.

♦ Within the CNS, a collection of nerve cell bodies is called a nucleus; in the PNS, nerve cell body aggregations (or even solitary nerve cell bodies) constitute a ganglion. ♦ In the CNS, a bundle of nerve fibers that connect the nuclei is called a tract; in the PNS, a bundle of nerve fibers, the connective tissue holding it together, and the blood vessels serving it (vasa nervorum) constitute a nerve. ♦ Nerves exiting the cranium are cranial nerves; those exiting the vertebral column (formerly, the spine), are spinal nerves. ♦ Although some cranial nerves convey a single type of fiber, most nerves convey a variety of visceral or somatic and sensory or motor fibers.

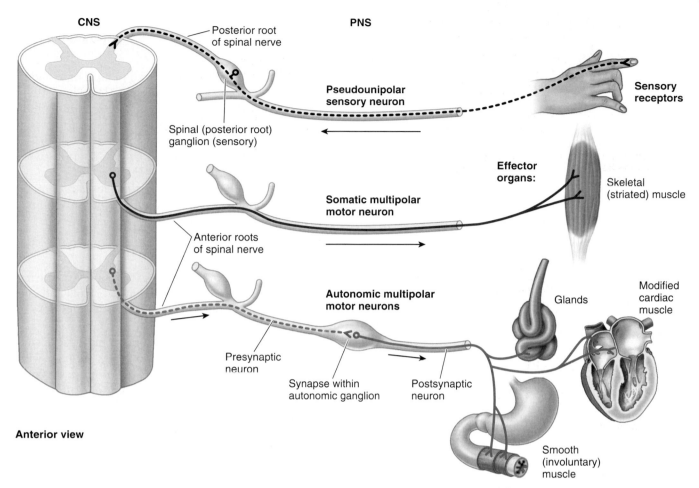

FIGURE I.42. Neurons of the PNS. Note the types of neurons involved in the somatic and visceral nervous systems, the general location of their cell bodies in relation to the CNS, and their receptors or effector organs.

Somatic Nervous System

The somatic nervous system (SNS), composed of somatic parts of the CNS and PNS, provides sensory and motor innervation to all parts of the body (G. *soma*), except the viscera in the body cavities, smooth muscle, and glands (Figs. I.41 and I.42). The **somatic sensory system** transmits sensations of touch, pain, temperature, and position from sensory receptors. Most of these sensations reach conscious levels (i.e., we are aware of them). The **somatic motor system** innervates only skeletal muscle, stimulating voluntary and reflexive movement by causing the muscle to contract, as occurs in response to touching a hot iron.

Autonomic Nervous System (ANS)

The **autonomic nervous system** (ANS), classically described as the *visceral nervous system* or *visceral motor system* (Figs. I.41 and I.42), consists of motor fibers that stimulate smooth (involuntary) muscle, modified cardiac muscle (the intrinsic stimulating and conducting tissue of the heart), and glandular (secretory) cells. However, the visceral efferent fibers of the ANS are accompanied by visceral afferent fibers. As the afferent component of autonomic reflexes and in conducting visceral pain impulses, these visceral afferent fibers also play a role in the regulation of visceral function.

The efferent nerve fibers and ganglia of the ANS are organized into two systems or divisions: the *sympathetic (thoracolumbar) division* and the *parasympathetic (craniosacral) division.* Unlike sensory and somatic motor innervation, in which the passage of impulses between the CNS and the sensory ending or effector organ involves a single neuron, in both divisions of the ANS, conduction of impulses from the CNS to the effector organ involves a series of two *multipolar neurons* (Fig. I.42). The nerve cell body of the first **presynaptic (preganglionic) neuron** is located in the gray matter of the CNS. Its fiber (axon) synapses only on the cell body of a **postsynaptic (postganglionic) neuron,** the second neuron in the series. The cell bodies of these second neurons are located outside the CNS in autonomic ganglia, with fibers terminating on the effector organ (smooth muscle, modified cardiac muscle, or glands).

The anatomical distinction between the sympathetic and parasympathetic divisions of the ANS is based primarily on:

1. The location of the presynaptic cell bodies, and
2. Which nerves conduct the presynaptic fibers from the CNS.

A functional distinction of pharmacological importance for medical practice is that the postsynaptic neurons of the two divisions generally liberate different neurotransmitter substances: *norepinephrine* by the sympathetic division (except in the case of sweat glands) and *acetylcholine* by the parasympathetic division.

SYMPATHETIC (THORACOLUMBAR) DIVISION OF ANS

The cell bodies of the presynaptic neurons of the sympathetic division of the ANS are found in only one location: the **intermediolateral cell columns** (IMLs) or nuclei of the spinal cord (Fig. I.43). The paired (right and left) IMLs are a part of the gray matter of the thoracic (T1–12) and the upper lumbar (L1–L2 or 3) segments of the spinal cord (hence the alternate name "thoracolumbar" for the division). In transverse sections of this part of the spinal cord, the IMLs appear as small lateral horns of the H-shaped gray matter, looking somewhat like an extension of the cross-bar of the H between the posterior and the anterior horns. The IMLs are organized *somatotopically* (i.e., arranged like the body, the cell bodies involved with innervation of the head located superiorly, and those involved with innervation of the pelvic viscera and lower limbs located inferiorly). Thus it is possible to deduce the location of the presynaptic sympathetic cell bodies involved in innervation of a specific part of the body.

The cell bodies of postsynaptic neurons of the sympathetic nervous system occur in two locations, the paravertebral and prevertebral ganglia (Fig. I.44):

- **Paravertebral ganglia** are linked to form right and left *sympathetic trunks* (*chains*) on each side of the vertebral column and extend essentially the length of this column. The *superior paravertebral ganglion* (the superior cervical ganglion of each sympathetic trunk) lies at the base of the cranium. The *ganglion impar* forms inferiorly where the two trunks unite at the level of the coccyx.
- **Prevertebral ganglia** are in the plexuses that surround the origins of the main branches of the abdominal aorta (for which they are named), such as the two large *celiac ganglia* that surround the origin of the *celiac trunk* (a major artery arising from the aorta).

Because they are motor fibers, the axons of presynaptic neurons leave the spinal cord through anterior roots and enter the anterior rami of spinal nerves T1–L2 or 3 (Figs. I.45 and I.46). Almost immediately after entering, all the presynaptic sympathetic fibers leave the anterior rami of these spinal nerves and pass to the sympathetic trunks through **white rami communicantes** (*communicating branches*). Within the sympathetic trunks, presynaptic fibers follow one of four possible courses:

- Ascend in the sympathetic trunk to synapse with a postsynaptic neuron of a higher paravertebral ganglion.

FIGURE I.43.   Intermediolateral cell columns. Each IML or nucleus constitutes the lateral horn of gray matter of spinal cord segments T1–L2 or 3 and consists of the cell bodies of the presynaptic neurons of the sympathetic nervous system, which are somatotopically arranged.

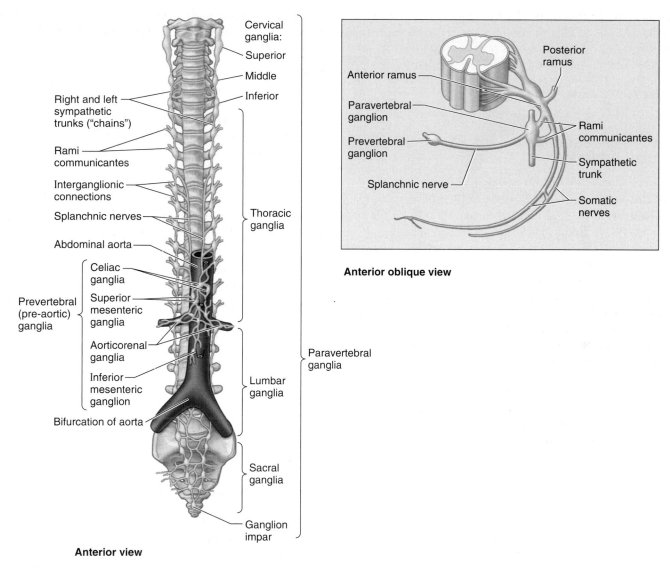

Cervical ganglia:
- Superior
- Middle
- Inferior

Right and left sympathetic trunks ("chains")

Rami communicantes

Interganglionic connections

Splanchnic nerves

Abdominal aorta

Prevertebral (pre-aortic) ganglia
- Celiac ganglia
- Superior mesenteric ganglia
- Aorticorenal ganglia
- Inferior mesenteric ganglion

Bifurcation of aorta

Thoracic ganglia

Paravertebral ganglia

Lumbar ganglia

Sacral ganglia

Ganglion impar

Anterior view

Anterior ramus

Paravertebral ganglion

Prevertebral ganglion

Splanchnic nerve

Posterior ramus

Rami communicantes

Sympathetic trunk

Somatic nerves

Anterior oblique view

FIGURE I.44. Ganglia of the sympathetic nervous system. In the sympathetic nervous system, cell bodies of postsynaptic neurons occur either in the paravertebral ganglia of the sympathetic trunks or in the prevertebral ganglia that occur mainly in relationship to the origins of the main branches of the abdominal aorta. Prevertebral ganglia are specifically involved in the innervation of abdominopelvic viscera. The cell bodies of postsynaptic neurons distributed to the remainder of the body occur in the paravertebral ganglia.

- Descend in the sympathetic trunk to synapse with a postsynaptic neuron of a lower paravertebral ganglion.
- Enter and synapse immediately with a postsynaptic neuron of the paravertebral ganglion at that level.
- Pass through the sympathetic trunk without synapsing, continuing through an abdominopelvic splanchnic nerve (a branch of the trunk involved in innervating abdominopelvic viscera) to reach the prevertebral ganglia.

Presynaptic sympathetic fibers that provide autonomic innervation within the head, neck, body wall, limbs, and thoracic cavity follow one of the first three courses, synapsing within the paravertebral ganglia. Presynaptic sympathetic fibers innervating viscera within the abdominopelvic cavity follow the fourth course.

Postsynaptic sympathetic fibers greatly outnumber the presynaptic fibers; each presynaptic sympathetic fiber synapses with 30 or more postsynaptic fibers. Those postsynaptic sympathetic fibers, destined for distribution within the neck, body wall, and limbs, pass from the paravertebral ganglia of the sympathetic trunks to adjacent anterior rami of spinal nerves through **gray rami communicantes** (Fig. I.46). By this means, they enter all branches of all 31 pairs of spinal nerves, including the posterior rami.

The postsynaptic sympathetic fibers stimulate contraction of the blood vessels (*vasomotion*) and arrector muscles associated with hairs (*pilomotion,* resulting in "goose bumps"), and to cause sweating (*sudomotion*). Postsynaptic sympathetic fibers that perform these functions in the

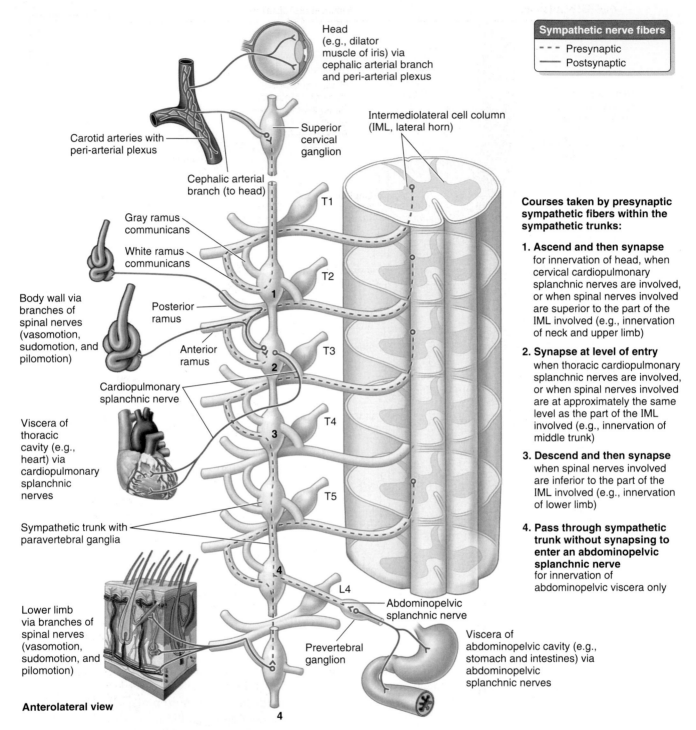

Head
(e.g., dilator
muscle of iris) via
cephalic arterial branch
and peri-arterial plexus

Sympathetic nerve fibers
- - - Presynaptic
——— Postsynaptic

Intermediolateral cell column
(IML, lateral horn)

Carotid arteries with
peri-arterial plexus

Superior
cervical
ganglion

Cephalic arterial
branch (to head)

T1

Gray ramus
communicans

White ramus
communicans

T2

Body wall via
branches of
spinal nerves
(vasomotion,
sudomotion, and
pilomotion)

Posterior
ramus

Anterior
ramus

T3

Cardiopulmonary
splanchnic nerve

T4

Viscera of
thoracic
cavity (e.g.,
heart) via
cardiopulmonary
splanchnic
nerves

T5

Sympathetic trunk with
paravertebral ganglia

L4

Lower limb
via branches of
spinal nerves
(vasomotion,
sudomotion, and
pilomotion)

Abdominopelvic
splanchnic nerve

Prevertebral
ganglion

Viscera of
abdominopelvic cavity (e.g.,
stomach and intestines) via
abdominopelvic
splanchnic nerves

Anterolateral view

**Courses taken by presynaptic
sympathetic fibers within the
sympathetic trunks:**

1. **Ascend and then synapse**
   for innervation of head, when
   cervical cardiopulmonary
   splanchnic nerves are involved,
   or when spinal nerves involved
   are superior to the part of the
   IML involved (e.g., innervation
   of neck and upper limb)

2. **Synapse at level of entry**
   when thoracic cardiopulmonary
   splanchnic nerves are involved,
   or when spinal nerves involved
   are at approximately the same
   level as the part of the IML
   involved (e.g., innervation of
   middle trunk)

3. **Descend and then synapse**
   when spinal nerves involved
   are inferior to the part of the
   IML involved (e.g., innervation
   of lower limb)

4. **Pass through sympathetic
   trunk without synapsing to
   enter an abdominopelvic
   splanchnic nerve**
   for innervation of
   abdominopelvic viscera only

FIGURE I.45. Courses taken by sympathetic motor fibers. All presynaptic fibers follow the same course until they reach the sympathetic trunks. In the trunks, they follow one of four possible courses. Fibers involved in providing sympathetic innervation to the body wall and limbs or viscera above the level of the diaphragm follow paths 1–3 to synapse in the paravertebral ganglia of the sympathetic trunks. Fibers involved in innervating abdominopelvic viscera follow path 4 to prevertebral ganglion via abdominopelvic splanchnic nerves.

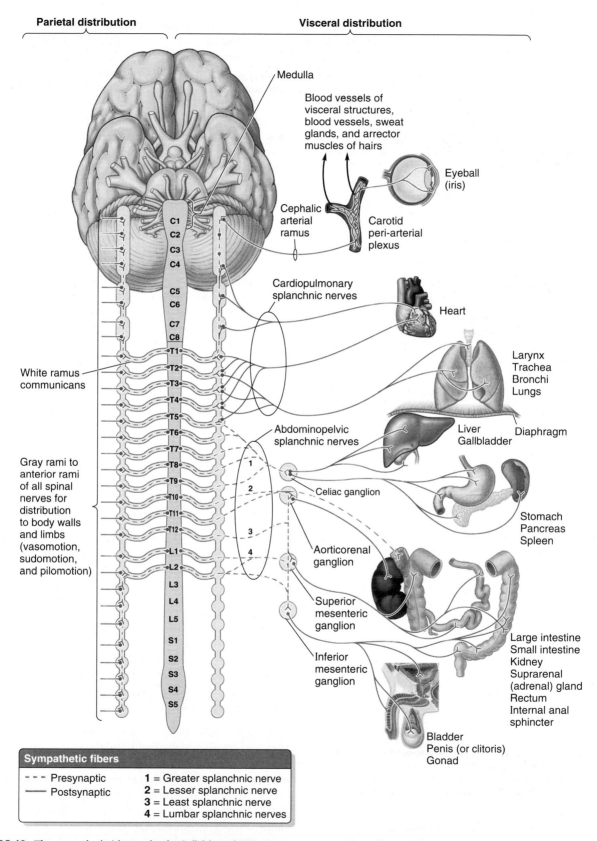

Parietal distribution

Visceral distribution

Medulla

Blood vessels of visceral structures, blood vessels, sweat glands, and arrector muscles of hairs

Eyeball (iris)

Cephalic arterial ramus

Carotid peri-arterial plexus

Cardiopulmonary splanchnic nerves

Heart

White ramus communicans

Larynx
Trachea
Bronchi
Lungs

Diaphragm

Liver
Gallbladder

Abdominopelvic splanchnic nerves

Celiac ganglion

Gray rami to anterior rami of all spinal nerves for distribution to body walls and limbs (vasomotion, sudomotion, and pilomotion)

Stomach
Pancreas
Spleen

Aorticorenal ganglion

Superior mesenteric ganglion

Large intestine
Small intestine
Kidney
Suprarenal (adrenal) gland
Rectum
Internal anal sphincter

Inferior mesenteric ganglion

Bladder
Penis (or clitoris)
Gonad

Sympathetic fibers	
- - - Presynaptic	**1** = Greater splanchnic nerve
——— Postsynaptic	**2** = Lesser splanchnic nerve
	3 = Least splanchnic nerve
	4 = Lumbar splanchnic nerves

FIGURE I.46. The sympathetic (thoracolumbar) division of ANS. Postsynaptic sympathetic fibers exit from the sympathetic trunks by different means, depending on their destination: Those destined for parietal distribution within the neck, body wall, and limbs pass from the sympathetic trunks to adjacent anterior rami of all spinal nerves through gray communicating branches (L. rami communicantes); those destined for the head pass from cervical ganglia by means of cephalic arterial rami to form a carotid peri-arterial plexus; and those destined for viscera of the thoracic cavity (e.g., the heart) pass through cardiopulmonary splanchnic nerves. Presynaptic sympathetic fibers involved in the innervation of viscera of the abdominopelvic cavity (e.g., the stomach) pass through the sympathetic trunks to the prevertebral ganglia by means of abdominopelvic splanchnic nerves. Postsynaptic fibers from the prevertebral ganglia form peri-arterial plexuses, which follow branches of the abdominal aorta to reach their destination.

head (plus innervation of the dilator muscle of the iris—dilator pupillae) all have their cell bodies in the *superior cervical ganglion* at the superior end of the sympathetic trunk. They pass from the ganglion by means of a **cephalic arterial branch** to form *peri-arterial plexuses of nerves*, which follow the branches of the carotid arteries, or they may pass directly to nearby cranial nerves, to reach their destination in the head (Maklad et al., 2001).

Splanchnic nerves convey visceral efferent (autonomic) and afferent fibers to and from the viscera of the body cavities. Postsynaptic sympathetic fibers destined for the viscera of the thoracic cavity (e.g., the heart, lungs, and esophagus) pass through **cardiopulmonary splanchnic nerves** to enter the cardiac, pulmonary, and esophageal plexuses (Figs. I.45 and I.46). The presynaptic sympathetic fibers involved in the innervation of viscera of the abdominopelvic cavity (e.g., the stomach and intestines) pass to the prevertebral ganglia through **abdominopelvic splanchnic nerves** (including the greater, lesser, least thoracic, and lumbar splanchnic nerves) (Figs. I.45–I.47). All presynaptic sympathetic fibers of the abdominopelvic splanchnic nerves, except those involved in innervating the suprarenal (adrenal) glands, synapse in prevertebral ganglia. The postsynaptic fibers from the prevertebral ganglia form peri-arterial plexuses, which follow branches of the abdominal aorta to reach their destination.

Some presynaptic sympathetic fibers pass through the celiac prevertebral ganglia without synapsing, continuing to terminate directly on cells of the medulla of the suprarenal gland (Fig. I.47). The suprarenal medullary cells function as a special type of postsynaptic neuron that, instead of releasing their neurotransmitter substance onto the cells of a specific effector organ, release it into the bloodstream to circulate throughout the body, producing a widespread sympathetic response. Thus the sympathetic innervation of this gland is exceptional.

As described earlier, postsynaptic sympathetic fibers are components of virtually all branches of all spinal nerves. By this means and via peri-arterial plexuses, they extend to and innervate all the body's blood vessels (the sympathetic system's primary function) as well as sweat glands, arrector muscles of hairs, and visceral structures. Thus the sympathetic nervous system reaches virtually all parts of the body, with the rare exception of such avascular tissues as cartilage and nails. Because the two sets of sympathetic ganglia (para- and prevertebral) are centrally placed in the body and are close to the midline (hence relatively close to the spinal cord), in this division the presynaptic fibers are relatively short, whereas the postsynaptic fibers are relatively long, having to extend to all parts of the body.

PARASYMPATHETIC (CRANIOSACRAL) DIVISION OF ANS

Presynaptic parasympathetic nerve cell bodies are located in two sites within the CNS, and their fibers exit by two routes. This arrangement accounts for the alternate name "craniosacral" for the parasympathetic division of the ANS (Fig. I.48):

- In the gray matter of the brainstem, the fibers exit the CNS within cranial nerves III, VII, IX, and X; these fibers constitute the **cranial parasympathetic outflow**.
- In the gray matter of the sacral segments of the spinal cord (S2–4), the fibers exit the CNS through the anterior roots of sacral spinal nerves S2–4 and the pelvic splanchnic nerves that arise from their anterior rami; these fibers constitute the **sacral parasympathetic outflow.**

Not surprisingly, the cranial outflow provides parasympathetic innervation of the head, and the sacral outflow provides the parasympathetic innervation of the pelvic viscera. However, in terms of the innervation of thoracic and abdominal viscera, the cranial outflow through the vagus nerve (CN X) is dominant. It provides innervation to all thoracic viscera and most of the gastrointestinal (GI) tract from the esophagus through most of the large intestine (to its left colic flexure).

The sacral outflow to the GI tract supplies only the descending and sigmoid colon and rectum.

Regardless of the extensive influence of its cranial outflow, the parasympathetic system is much more restricted

Abdominopelvic splanchnic nerves

Prevertebral (pre-aortic) ganglion

Paravertebral ganglion

Via peri-arterial plexus

Cells of suprarenal medulla

Cortex of suprarenal gland

Abdominopelvic viscera

Sympathetic motor fibers

\- \- \- Presynaptic

——— Postsynaptic

FIGURE I.47. Sympathetic supply to medulla of suprarenal (adrenal) gland. The sympathetic supply to the suprarenal gland is exceptional. The secretory cells of the medulla are postsynaptic sympathetic neurons that lack axons or dendrites. Consequently, the suprarenal medulla is supplied directly by presynaptic sympathetic neurons. The neurotransmitters produced by medullary cells are released into the bloodstream to produce a widespread sympathetic response.

FIGURE I.48. Parasympathetic (craniosacral) division of ANS. Presynaptic parasympathetic nerve cell bodies are located in opposite ends of the CNS and their fibers exit by two different routes: (1) in the gray matter of the brainstem, with fibers exiting the CNS within cranial nerves III, VII, IX, and X (these fibers constitute the cranial parasympathetic outflow), and (2) in the gray matter of the sacral (S2–4) segments of the spinal cord, with fibers exiting the CNS via the anterior roots of spinal nerves S2–4 and the pelvic splanchnic nerves that arise from their anterior rami. (These fibers constitute the sacral parasympathetic outflow.) The cranial outflow provides parasympathetic innervation of the head, neck, and most of the trunk; the sacral outflow provides the parasympathetic innervation of the pelvic viscera.

than the sympathetic system in its distribution. The parasympathetic system distributes only to the head, visceral cavities of the trunk, and erectile tissues of the external genitalia. With the exception of the latter, it does not reach the body wall or limbs, and except for the initial parts of the anterior rami of spinal nerves S2–4, its fibers are not components of spinal nerves or their branches.

Four discrete pairs of parasympathetic ganglia occur in the head. Elsewhere, presynaptic parasympathetic fibers synapse with postsynaptic cell bodies, which occur singly in or on the wall of the target organ (**intrinsic** or **enteric ganglia**). Consequently, in this division, most presynpatic fibers are very long, extending from the CNS to the effector organ, whereas the postsynaptic fibers are very short, running from a ganglion located near or embedded in the effector organ.

FUNCTIONS OF DIVISIONS OF ANS

Although both sympathetic and parasympathetic systems innervate involuntary (and often affect the same) structures, they have different, usually contrasting yet coordinated, effects (Figs. I.46 and I.48). In general, the *sympathetic system* is a **catabolic** (energy-expending) **system** that enables the body to deal with stresses, such as when preparing the body for the fight-or-flight response. The *parasympathetic system* is primarily a **homeostatic** or **anabolic** (energy-conserving) **system,** promoting the quiet and orderly processes of the body, such as those that allow the body to feed and assimilate. Table I.2 summarizes the specific functions of the ANS and its divisions.

The primary function of the sympathetic system is to regulate blood vessels. This is accomplished by several means having different effects. Blood vessels throughout the body are tonically innervated by sympathetic nerves, maintaining a resting state of moderate vasoconstriction. In most vascular beds, an increase in sympathetic signals causes increased vasoconstriction, and a decrease in the rate of sympathetic signals allows vasodilation. However, in certain regions of the body, sympathetic signals are vasodilatory (i.e., sympathetic transmitter substances inhibit active vasoconstriction, allowing the blood vessels to be passively dilated by the blood pressure). In the coronary vessels, the vessels of skeletal muscles, and the external genitalia, sympathetic stimulation results in vasodilation (Wilson-Pauwels et al., 2010).

VISCERAL SENSATION

Visceral afferent fibers have important relationships to the ANS, both anatomically and functionally. We are usually unaware of the sensory input of these fibers, which provides information about the condition of the body's internal environment. This information is integrated in the CNS, often triggering visceral or somatic reflexes or both. Visceral reflexes regulate blood pressure and chemistry by altering such functions as heart and respiratory rates and vascular resistance.

Visceral sensation that reaches a conscious level is generally perceived as pain that is either poorly localized or felt as cramps or that may convey a feeling of hunger, fullness, or nausea. Surgeons operating on patients who are under local anesthesia may handle, cut, clamp, or even burn (cauterize) visceral organs without evoking conscious sensation. However, adequate stimulation, such as the following, may elicit visceral pain:

- Sudden distension.
- Spasms or strong contractions.
- Chemical irritants.
- Mechanical stimulation, especially when the organ is active.
- Pathological conditions (especially ischemia) that lower the normal thresholds of stimulation.

Normal activity usually produces no sensation, but it may do so when the blood supply is inadequate (ischemia). Most visceral reflex (unconscious) sensation and some pain travel in visceral afferent fibers that accompany the parasympathetic fibers retrograde (backward). Most visceral pain impulses (from the heart and most organs of the peritoneal cavity) travel centrally along visceral afferent fibers accompanying sympathetic fibers.

The Bottom Line

AUTONOMIC NERVOUS SYSTEM (ANS)

The autonomic nervous system is a subdivision of the motor nervous system that controls functions of the body not under conscious control. ♦ Two neurons, a presynaptic and a postsynaptic fiber, connect the CNS with an end organ, consisting of smooth muscle, gland, or modified cardiac muscle. ♦ Based on the location of the cell body of the presynaptic fibers, the ANS can be subdivided into two divisions: the sympathetic and parasympathetic. ♦ Presynaptic cell bodies of the sympathetic division are found only in the intermediolateral cell columns of gray matter in the thoracolumbar spinal cord, which are organized somatotopically. ♦ The presynaptic sympathetic nerve fibers terminate in sympathetic ganglia formed of the cell bodies of postsynaptic sympathetic neurons. ♦ Sympathetic ganglia are in the sympathetic trunks (paravertebral ganglia) or around the roots of the major branches of the abdominal aorta (prevertebral ganglia). ♦ Cell bodies of the presynaptic neurons of the parasympathetic division are in the gray matter of the brainstem and sacral segments of the spinal cord. ♦ Cell bodies of postsynaptic parasympathetic neurons of the trunk are located in or on the structure being innervated, whereas those in the head are organized into discrete ganglia. ♦ The sympathetic and parasympathetic divisions usually have opposite but coordinated effects.
♦ The sympathetic system primarily regulates blood vessels and facilitates emergency (flight-or-fight) responses.

TABLE I.2. FUNCTIONS OF AUTONOMIC NERVOUS SYSTEM (ANS)

Organ, Tract, or System		Effect of Sympathetic Stimulation[a]	Effect of Parasympathetic Stimulation[b]
Eyes	Pupil	Dilates pupil (admits more light for increased acuity at a distance)	Constricts pupil (protects pupil from excessively bright light)
	Ciliary body		Contracts ciliary muscle, allowing lens to thicken for near vision (accommodation)
Skin	Arrector muscles of hair	Causes hairs to stand on end ("goose-flesh" or "goose bumps")	No effect (does not reach)[c]
	Peripheral blood vessels	Vasoconstricts (blanching of skin, lips, and turning fingertips blue)	No effect (does not reach)[c]
	Sweat glands	Promotes sweating[d]	No effect (does not reach)[c]
Other glands	Lacrimal glands	Slightly decreases secretion[e]	Promotes secretion
	Salivary glands	Secretion decreases, becomes thicker, more viscous[e]	Promotes abundant, watery secretion
Heart		Increases the rate and strength of contraction; inhibits the effect of parasympathetic system on coronary vessels, allowing them to dilate[e]	Decreases the rate and strength of contraction (conserving energy); constricts coronary vessels in relation to reduced demand
Lungs		Inhibits effect of parasympathetic system, resulting in bronchodilation and reduced secretion, allowing for maximum air exchange	Constricts bronchi (conserving energy) and promotes bronchial secretion
Digestive tract		Inhibits peristalsis, and constricts blood vessels to digestive tract so that blood is available to skeletal muscle; contracts internal anal sphincter to aid fecal continence	Stimulates peristalsis and secretion of digestive juices Contracts rectum, inhibits internal anal sphincter to cause defecation
Liver and gallbladder		Promotes breakdown of glycogen to glucose (for increased energy)	Promotes building/conservation of glycogen; increases secretion of bile
Urinary tract		Vasoconstriction of renal vessels slows urine formation; internal sphincter of bladder contracted to maintain urinary continence	Inhibits contraction of internal sphincter of bladder, contracts detrusor muscle of the bladder wall causing urination
Genital system		Causes ejaculation and vasoconstriction resulting in remission of erection	Produces engorgement (erection) of erectile tissues of the external genitals
Suprarenal medulla		Release of adrenaline into blood	No effect (does not innervate)

[a]In general, the effects of sympathetic stimulation are catabolic, preparing body for the fight-or-flight response.

[b]In general, the effects of parasympathetic stimulation are anabolic, promoting normal function and conserving energy.

[c]The parasympathetic system is restricted in its distribution to the head, neck, and body cavities (except for erectile tissues of genitalia); otherwise, parasympathetic fibers are never found in the body wall and limbs. Sympathetic fibers, by comparison, are distributed to all vascularized portions of the body.

[d]With the exception of the sweat glands, glandular secretion is parasympathetically stimulated.

[e]With the exception of the coronary arteries, vasoconstriction is sympathetically stimulated; the effects of sympathetic stimulation on glands (other than sweat glands) are the indirect effects of vasoconstriction.

♦ The parasympathetic system—distributed only to the viscera of the head, neck, and cavities of the trunk and the erectile tissues of the genitalia—is primarily concerned with body conservation, often reversing the effects of sympathetic stimulation. ♦ Some nerves distributing autonomic nerve fibers to the body cavities also convey visceral sensory nerve fibers from the viscera that conduct impulses for pain or reflexes.

MEDICAL IMAGING TECHNIQUES

Radiologic anatomy is the study of the structure and function of the body using medical imaging techniques. It is an important part of clinical anatomy and is the anatomic basis of radiology, the branch of medical science dealing with the use of radiant energy in the diagnosis and treatment of disease. Being able to identify normal structures on radiographs (X-rays) makes it easier to recognize the changes caused by disease and injury. Familiarity with medical imaging techniques commonly used in clinical settings enables one to recognize congenital anomalies, tumors, and fractures. The most commonly used medical imaging techniques are

- Conventional radiography (X-ray images).
- Computerized tomography (CT).
- Ultrasonography (US).
- Magnetic resonance imaging (MRI).
- Nuclear medicine imaging.

Although the techniques differ, each is based on the receipt of attenuated beams of energy that have been passed through, reflected off of, or generated by the body's tissues. Medical imaging techniques permit the observation of anatomical structures in living people and the study of their movements in normal and abnormal activities (e.g., the heart and stomach).

Conventional Radiography

Conventional radiographic studies, in which special techniques such as contrast media have not been used, is referred to clinically as *plain film studies* (Fig. I.49), although today most images are produced and viewed digitally on monitors instead of film. In a radiologic examination, a highly penetrating beam of X-rays transilluminates the patient, showing tissues of differing densities of mass within the body as images of differing intensities (areas of relative light and dark) on the film or monitor (Fig. I.50). A tissue or organ that is relatively dense in mass (e.g., compact bone) absorbs or reflects more X-rays than does a less dense tissue (e.g., spongy bone). Consequently, a dense tissue or organ produces a somewhat transparent area on the X-ray film or bright area on a monitor because fewer X-rays reach the film or detector. A dense substance is *radiopaque*, whereas a substance of less density is *radiolucent*.

Many of the same principles that apply to making a shadow apply to conventional radiography. When making a shadow of your hand on a wall, the closer your hand is to the wall, the sharper the shadow produced. The farther your hand is from the wall (and therefore the closer to the light source), the more the shadow is magnified. Radiographs are made with the part of the patient's body being studied close to the X-ray film or detector to maximize the clarity of the image and minimize magnification artifacts. In basic radiologic nomenclature, *postero-anterior (PA) projection* refers to a radiograph in which the X-rays traversed the patient from posterior (P) to anterior (A); the X-ray tube was posterior to the patient and the X-ray film or detector was anterior (Fig. I.51A). A radiograph using *anteroposterior (AP) projection* radiography is the opposite. Both PA and AP projection radiographs are viewed as if you and the patient were facing each other (the patient's right side is opposite your left); this is referred to as an *anteroposterior (AP) view*. (Thus the standard chest X-ray, taken to examine the heart and lungs, is an AP view of

Trachea

1st rib

Superior vena cava

Rib

Right atrium

Right dome of diaphragm

Clavicle

Coracoid process of scapula

Arch of aorta

Pulmonary artery

Left auricle

Left ventricle

Apex of heart

FIGURE I.49. Radiograph of thorax (chest). AP view of a PA projection radiograph demonstrates the arch of the aorta, parts of the heart, and domes of the diaphragm. Note that the dome of the diaphragm is higher on the right side. (Courtesy of Dr. E. L. Lansdown, Professor of Medical Imaging, University of Toronto, Toronto, ON, Canada.)

(A)   **(B)**

FIGURE I.51. Orientation of patient's thorax during radiography.
A. When taking a PA projection, the X-rays from the X-ray tube pass through the thorax from the back to reach the X-ray film or detector anterior to the person. **B.** When taking a lateral projection, the X-rays pass through the thorax from the side to reach the X-ray film adjacent to the person's other side.

FIGURE I.50. Principles of X-ray image formation. Portions of the beam of X-rays traversing the body become attenuated to varying degrees based on tissue thickness and density. The beam is diminished by structures that absorb or reflect it, causing less reaction on the film or by the detector compared with areas that allow the beam to pass relatively uninterrupted.

a PA projection.) For lateral radiographs, radiopaque letters (R or L) are used to indicate the side placed closest to the film or detector, and the image is viewed from the same direction that the beam was projected (Fig. I.51B).

The introduction of contrast media (radiopaque fluids such as iodine compounds or barium) allows the study of various luminal or vascular organs and potential or actual spaces—such as the digestive tract, blood vessels, kidneys, synovial cavities, and the subarachnoid space—that are not visible in plain films (Fig. I.52). Most radiologic examinations are performed in at least two projections at right angles to each other. Because each radiograph presents a two-dimensional representation of a three-dimensional structure, structures sequentially penetrated by the X-ray beam overlap each other. Thus more than one view is usually necessary to detect and localize an abnormality accurately.

Computed Tomography

In computed tomography (CT), the scans show radiographic images of the body that resemble transverse anatomical sections (Fig. I.53). In this technique, a beam of X-rays passes through the body as the X-ray tube and detector rotate around the axis of the body. Multiple overlapping radial energy absorptions are measured, recorded, and compared by a computer to determine the radiodensity of each volumetric pixel (*voxel*) of the chosen body plane. The radiodensity of

(amount of radiation absorbed by) each voxel is determined by factors that include the amount of air, water, fat, or bone in that element. The computer maps the voxels into a planar image (slice) that is displayed on a monitor or printout. CT images relate well to conventional radiographs, in that areas of great absorption (e.g., bone) are relatively transparent (white) and those with little absorption are black (Fig. I.53). CT scans are always displayed as if the viewer were standing at a supine patient's feet—i.e., from an inferior view.

Ultrasonography

Ultrasonography (US) is a technique that visualizes superficial or deep structures in the body by recording pulses of ultrasonic waves reflecting off the tissues (Fig. I.54). US has the advantage of a lower cost than CT and MRI, and the machine is portable. The technique can be performed virtually anywhere, including the clinic examination room, bedside, or on the operating table. A transducer in contact with the skin generates high-frequency soundwaves that pass through the body and reflect off tissue interfaces between tissues of differing characteristics, such as soft tissue and bone. Echoes from the body reflect into the transducer and convert to electrical energy. The electrical signals are recorded and displayed on a monitor as a cross-sectional image, which can be viewed in real time and recorded as a single image or on videotape.

A major advantage of US is its ability to produce real-time images, demonstrating motion of structures and flow within blood vessels. In *Doppler ultrasonography*, the shifts in frequency between emitted ultrasonic waves and their echoes are used to measure the velocities of moving objects. This technique is based on the principle of the *Doppler effect*. Blood flow through vessels is displayed in color, superimposed on the two-dimensional cross-sectional image.

Gallbladder

Duodenal cap

Pylorus of stomach

Pyloric antrum of
stomach

Jejunum

Fundus of stomach

Peristaltic wave

Rugae

Greater curvature

FIGURE I.52. Radiograph of stomach, small intestine, and gallbladder. Observe the gastric folds, or rugae (longitudinal folds of the mucous membrane). Also note the peristaltic wave that is moving the gastric contents toward the duodenum, which is closely related to the gallbladder. (Courtesy of Dr. J. Heslin, Toronto, ON, Canada.)

Scanning of the pelvic viscera from the surface of the abdomen requires a fully distended bladder. The urine serves as an "acoustical window," transmitting soundwaves to and from the posteriorly placed pelvic viscera with minimal attenuation. The distended bladder also displaces gas-filled intestinal loops out of the pelvis. *Transvaginal sonography* permits the positioning of the transducer closer to the organ of interest (e.g., the ovary) and avoids fat and gas, which absorb or reflect soundwaves. Bone reflects nearly all ultrasound waves, whereas air conducts them poorly. Consequently, US is not generally used for examining the CNS and aerated lungs of adults.

The appeal of ultrasonography in obstetrics is that it is a non-invasive procedure that does not use radiation; it can yield useful information about the pregnancy, such as determining whether it is intra-uterine or extra-uterine (ectopic) and whether the embryo or fetus is living. It has also become a standard method of evaluating the growth and development of the embryo and fetus.

Magnetic Resonance Imaging

Magnetic resonance imaging (MRI) provides images of the body similar to those of CT scans, but MRI is better for tissue differentiation. MRI studies closely resemble ana-tomical sections, especially of the brain (Fig. I.55). The person is placed in a scanner with a strong magnetic field, and the body is pulsed with radiowaves. Signals subsequently emitted from the patient's tissues are stored in a computer and reconstructed into various images of the body. The appearance of tissues on the generated images can be varied by controlling how radiofrequency pulses are sent and received.

Free protons in the tissues that become aligned by the surrounding magnetic field are excited (flipped) with a radiowave pulse. As the protons flip back, minute but measurable energy signals are emitted. Tissues that are high in proton density, such as fat and water, emit more signals than tissues that are low in proton density. The tissue signal is based primarily on three properties of protons in a particular region of the body. These are referred to as T1 and T2 relaxation (producing T1- and T2-weighted images), and proton density. Although liquids have a high density of free protons, the excited free protons in moving fluids such as blood tend to move out of the field before they flip and give off their signal and are replaced by unexcited protons. Consequently, moving fluids appear black in T1-weighted images.

Computers associated with MRI scanners have the capacity to reconstruct tissues in any plane from the data acquired: transverse, median, sagittal, frontal, and even arbitrary oblique planes. The data may also be used to generate

CT image of the upper abdomen

FIGURE I.53. Technique for producing a CT scan. The X-ray tube rotates around the person in the CT scanner and sends a fan-shaped beam of X-rays through the upper abdomen from a variety of angles. X-ray detectors on the opposite side of the body measure the amount of radiation that passes through a horizontal section. A computer reconstructs the images from several scans, and a CT scan is produced. The scan is oriented so it appears the way an examiner would view it when standing at the foot of the bed and looking toward a supine person's head.

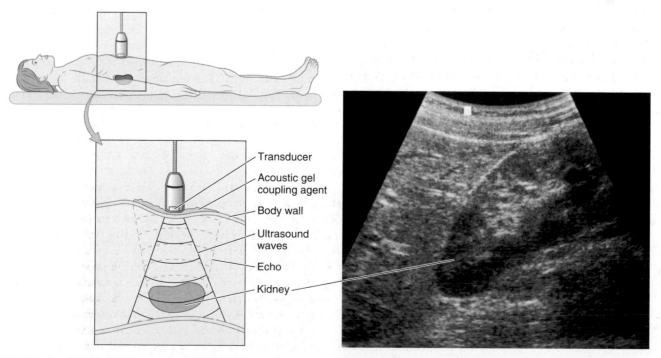

FIGURE I.54. Technique for producing an ultrasound image of the upper abdomen. The image results from the echo of ultrasound waves from abdominal structures of different densities. The image of the right kidney is displayed on a monitor.

Compact bone (black lines)

Air-filled sinuses

Nasal cavity

Tooth

Tongue

Brain (cerebrum)

Venous sinus (fluid-filled)

Cerebellum

Fluid-filled subarachnoid space

Spinal cord

C2 vertebra

Pharynx   Subcutaneous tissue (fat) and connective tissue

FIGURE I.55. Median MRI of head. Many details of the CNS and structures in the nasal and oral cavities and upper neck are seen in this study. The black low-signal areas superior to the anterior and posterior aspects of the nasal cavity are the air-filled frontal and sphenoidal sinuses.

three-dimensional reconstructions. MRI scanners produce good images of soft tissues without the use of ionizing radiation. Motion made by the patient during long scanning sessions created problems for early-generation scanners, but fast scanners now in use can be gated or paced to visualize moving structures, such as the heart and blood flow, in real time.

Nuclear Medicine Imaging

Nuclear medicine imaging techniques provide information about the distribution or concentration of trace amounts of radioactive substances introduced into the body. Nuclear medicine scans show images of specific organs after intravenous (IV) injection of a small dose of radioactive material. The radionuclide is tagged to a compound that is selectively taken up by an organ, such as technetium-99m methylene diphosphonate (^{99m}Tc-MDP) for bone scanning (Fig. I.56).

Positron emission tomography (PET) scanning uses cyclotron-produced isotopes of extremely short half-life that emit positrons. PET scanning is used to evaluate the physiologic

FIGURE I.56. Bone scans of head and neck, thorax, and pelvis. These nuclear medicine images can be viewed as a whole or in cross section.

function of organs, such as the brain, on a dynamic basis. Areas of increased brain activity will show selective uptake of the injected isotope. Images can be viewed as the whole organ or in cross sections. Single-photon emission computed tomography (SPECT) scans are similar but use longer lasting tracers. They are less costly, but require more time and have lower resolution.

The Bottom Line

MEDICAL IMAGING TECHNIQUES

Medical imaging techniques enable the visualization of anatomy in living people. These techniques enable structures to be examined with their normal tonus, fluid volumes, internal pressures, etc., which are not present in the cadaver. The primary goal of medical imaging is, of course, to detect pathology. However, a sound knowledge of radiologic anatomy is required to distinguish pathologies and abnormalities from normal anatomy.

Thorax

OVERVIEW OF THORAX

The **thorax** is the part of the body between the neck and abdomen. Commonly the term *chest* is used as a synonym for thorax, but the chest is much more extensive than the thoracic wall and cavity contained within it. The **chest** is generally conceived as the superior part of the trunk that is broadest superiorly owing to the presence of the *pectoral (shoulder) girdle* (clavicles and scapulae), with much of its girth accounted for by the pectoral and scapular musculature and, in adult females, the breasts.

The **thoracic cavity** and its wall have the shape of a truncated cone, being narrowest superiorly, with the circumference increasing inferiorly, and reaching its maximum size at the junction with the abdominal portion of the trunk. The *wall of the thoracic cavity* is relatively thin, essentially as thick as its skeleton. The thoracic skeleton takes the form of a domed birdcage. The **thoracic cage** (rib cage), with the horizontal bars formed by ribs and costal cartilages, is also supported by the vertical sternum (breastbone) and thoracic vertebrae (Fig. 1.1). Furthermore, the floor of the thoracic cavity (thoracic diaphragm) is deeply invaginated inferiorly (i.e., is pushed upward) by viscera of the abdominal cavity. Consequently, nearly the lower half of the thoracic wall surrounds and protects abdominal rather than thoracic viscera (e.g., liver). Thus the thorax and its cavity are much smaller than one might expect based on external appearances of the chest.

The thorax includes the primary organs of the respiratory and cardiovascular systems. The thoracic cavity is divided into three major spaces: the central compartment or *mediastinum* that houses the thoracic viscera except for the lungs and, on each side, the *right* and *left pulmonary cavities* housing the lungs.

The majority of the thoracic cavity is occupied by the lungs, which provide for the exchange of oxygen and carbon dioxide between the air and blood. Most of the remainder of the thoracic cavity is occupied by the heart and structures involved in conducting the air and blood to and from the lungs. Additionally, nutrients (food) traverse the thoracic cavity via the esophagus, passing from the site of entry in the head to the site of digestion and absorption in the abdomen.

Although in terms of function and development the mammary glands are most related to the reproductive system, the breasts are located on and are typically dissected with the thoracic wall; thus they are included in this chapter.

THORACIC WALL

The true thoracic wall includes the thoracic cage and the muscles that extend between the ribs as well as the skin, subcutaneous tissue, muscles, and fascia covering its anterolateral aspect. The same structures covering its posterior aspect are considered to belong to the back. The mammary glands of the breasts lie within the subcutaneous tissue of the thoracic wall. The anterolateral axio-appendicular muscles (see Chapter 6) that overlie the thoracic cage and form the bed of the breast are encountered in the thoracic wall and may be

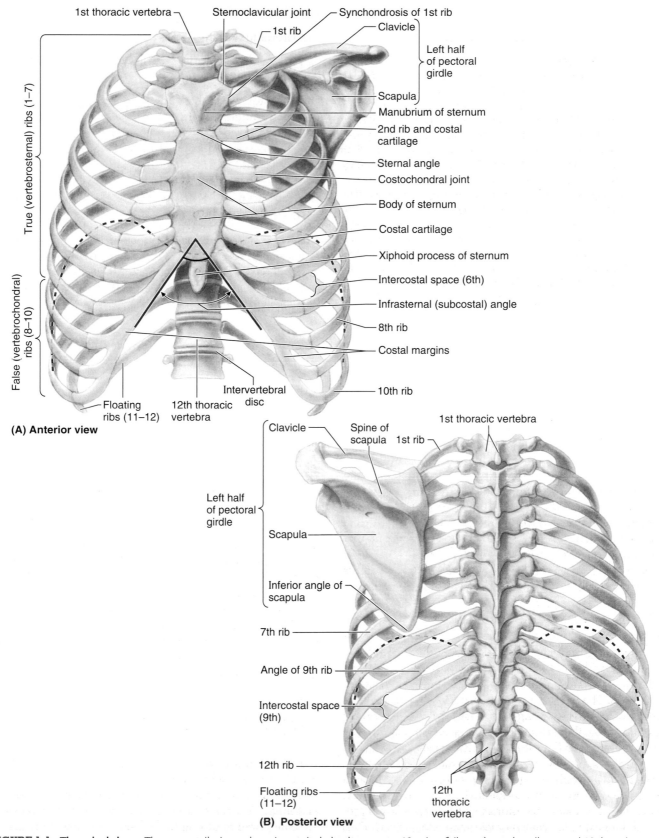

FIGURE 1.1. Thoracic skeleton. The osteocartilaginous thoracic cage includes the sternum, 12 pairs of ribs and costal cartilages, and 12 thoracic vertebrae and intervertebral discs. The clavicles and scapulae form the pectoral (shoulder) girdle, one side of which is included here to demonstrate the relationship between the thoracic (axial) and upper limb (appendicular) skeletons. The red dotted line indicates the position of the diaphragm, which separates the thoracic and abdominal cavities.

considered part of it, but are distinctly upper limb muscles based on function and innervation. They will be mentioned only briefly here.

The domed shape of the thoracic cage provides remarkable rigidity, given the light weight of its components, enabling it to:

- Protect vital thoracic and abdominal organs (most air or fluid filled) from external forces.
- Resist the negative (sub-atmospheric) internal pressures generated by the elastic recoil of the lungs and inspiratory movements.
- Provide attachment for and support the weight of the upper limbs.
- Provide the anchoring attachment (origin) of many of the muscles that move and maintain the position of the upper limbs relative to the trunk, as well as provide the attachments for muscles of the abdomen, neck, back, and respiration.

Although the shape of the thoracic cage provides rigidity, its joints and the thinness and flexibility of the ribs allow it to absorb many external blows and compressions without fracture and to change its shape for respiration. Because the most important structures within the thorax (heart, great vessels, lungs, and trachea), as well as its floor and walls, are constantly in motion, the thorax is one of the most dynamic regions of the body. With each breath, the muscles of the thoracic wall—working in concert with the diaphragm and muscles of the abdominal wall—vary the volume of the thoracic cavity, first by expanding the capacity of the cavity, thereby causing the lungs to expand and draw air in and then, due to lung elasticity and muscle relaxation, decreasing the volume of the cavity and causing them to expel air.

The Bottom Line

OVERVIEW OF THORAX

The thorax, consisting of the thoracic cavity, its contents, and the wall that surrounds it, is the part of the trunk between the neck and abdomen. ◆ The shape and size of the thoracic cavity and thoracic wall are different from that of the chest (upper trunk or torso) because the latter includes some upper limb bones and muscles and, in adult females, the breasts. ◆ The thorax includes the primary organs of the respiratory and cardiovascular systems. ◆ The thoracic cavity is divided into three compartments: the central mediastinum, occupied by the heart and structures transporting air, blood, and food; and the right and left pulmonary cavities, occupied by the lungs.

Skeleton of Thoracic Wall

The **thoracic skeleton** forms the osteocartilaginous *thoracic cage* (Fig. 1.1), which protects the thoracic viscera and some abdominal organs. The thoracic skeleton includes 12 pairs of ribs and associated costal cartilages, 12 thoracic vertebrae and the intervertebral (IV) discs interposed between them, and the sternum. The ribs and costal cartilages form the largest part of the thoracic cage; both are identified numerically, from the most superior (1st rib or costal cartilage) to the most inferior (12th).

RIBS, COSTAL CARTILAGES, AND INTERCOSTAL SPACES

Ribs (L. *costae*) are curved, flat bones that form most of the thoracic cage (Figs. 1.1 and 1.2). They are remarkably light in weight yet highly resilient. Each rib has a spongy interior containing *bone marrow* (hematopoietic tissue), which forms blood cells. There are *three types of ribs* that can be classified as typical or atypical:

1. **True (vertebrosternal) ribs** (1st–7th ribs): They attach directly to the sternum through their own costal cartilages.
2. **False (vertebrochondral) ribs** (8th, 9th, and usually 10th ribs): Their cartilages are connected to the cartilage of the rib above them; thus their connection with the sternum is indirect.
3. **Floating (vertebral, free) ribs** (11th, 12th, and sometimes 10th ribs): The rudimentary cartilages of these ribs do not connect even indirectly with the sternum; instead they end in the posterior abdominal musculature.

Typical ribs (3rd–9th) have the following components:

- **Head:** wedge-shaped and has two facets, separated by the **crest of the head** (Figs. 1.2 and 1.3); one facet for articulation with the numerically corresponding vertebra and one facet for the vertebra superior to it.
- **Neck:** connects the head of the rib with the body at the level of the tubercle.
- **Tubercle:** located at the junction of the neck and body; a smooth *articular part* articulates with the corresponding transverse process of the vertebra, and a rough *non-articular part* provides attachment for the costotransverse ligament (see Fig. 1.8B).
- **Body** (shaft): thin, flat, and curved, most markedly at the **costal angle** where the rib turns anterolaterally. The angle also demarcates the lateral limit of attachment of the deep back muscles to the ribs (see Table 4.6 in Chapter 4). The concave internal surface of the body has a **costal groove** paralleling the inferior border of the rib, which provides some protection for the intercostal nerve and vessels.

Atypical ribs (1st, 2nd, and 10th–12th) are dissimilar (Fig. 1.3):

- The **1st rib** is the broadest (i.e., its body is widest and nearly horizontal), shortest, and most sharply curved of

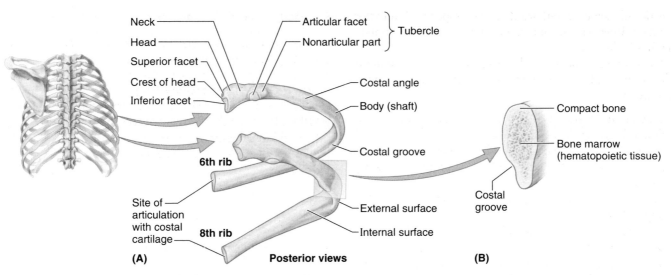

FIGURE 1.2. Typical ribs. A. The 3rd–9th ribs have common characteristics. Each rib has a head, neck, tubercle, and body (shaft). **B.** Cross section of the midbody of a rib.

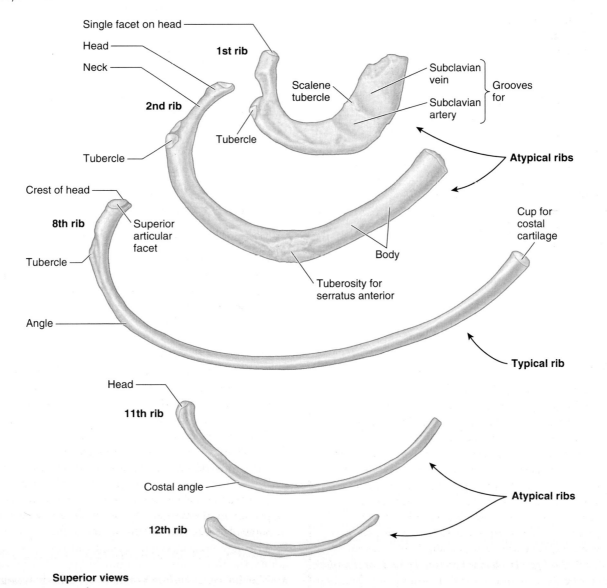

FIGURE 1.3. Atypical ribs. The atypical 1st, 2nd, 11th, and 12th ribs differ from typical ribs (e.g., the 8th rib, shown in center).

the seven true ribs. It has a single facet on its head for articulation with the T1 vertebra only and two transversely directed grooves crossing its superior surface for the subclavian vessels; the grooves are separated by a **scalene tubercle** and ridge, to which the anterior scalene muscle is attached.

- The **2nd rib** is has a thinner, less curved body and is substantially longer than the 1st rib. Its head has two facets for articulation with the bodies of the T1 and T2 vertebrae; its main atypical feature is a rough area on its upper surface, the **tuberosity for serratus anterior,** from which part of that muscle originates.
- The *10th–12th ribs*, like the 1st rib, have only one facet on their heads and articulate with a single vertebra.
- The *11th and 12th ribs* are short and have no neck or tubercle.

Costal cartilages prolong the ribs anteriorly and contribute to the elasticity of the thoracic wall, providing a flexible attachment for their anterior ends (tips). The cartilages increase in length through the first 7 and then gradually decrease. The first 7 costal cartilages attach directly and independently to the sternum; the 8th, 9th, and 10th articulate with the costal cartilages just superior to them, forming a continuous, articulated, cartilaginous **costal margin** (Fig. 1.1A; see also Fig. 1.13). The 11th and 12th costal cartilages form caps on the anterior ends of the corresponding ribs and do not reach or attach to any other bone or cartilage. The costal cartilages of ribs 1–10 clearly anchor the anterior end of the rib to the sternum, limiting its overall movement as the posterior end rotates around the transverse axis of the rib (Fig. 1.5).

Intercostal spaces separate the ribs and their costal cartilages from one another (Fig. 1.1A). The spaces are named according to the rib forming the superior border of the space—for example, the 4th intercostal space lies between ribs 4 and 5. There are 11 intercostal spaces and 11 intercostal nerves. Intercostal spaces are occupied by intercostal muscles and membranes, and two sets (main and collateral) of intercostal blood vessels and nerves, identified by the same number assigned to the space. The space below the 12th rib does not lie between ribs and thus is referred to as the **subcostal space,** and the anterior ramus (branch) of spinal nerve T12 is the subcostal nerve. The intercostal spaces are widest anterolaterally, and they widen further with inspiration. They can also be further widened by extension and/or lateral flexion of the thoracic vertebral column to the contralateral side.

THORACIC VERTEBRAE

Most **thoracic vertebrae** are typical in that they are independent, have bodies, vertebral arches, and seven processes for muscular and articular connections (Figs. 1.4 and 1.5). Characteristic features of thoracic vertebrae include:

- Bilateral *costal facets (demifacets) on the vertebral bodies,* usually occurring in inferior and superior pairs, for articulation with the heads of ribs.

- *Costal facets on the transverse processes* for articulation with the tubercles of ribs, except for the inferior two or three thoracic vertebrae.
- Long, inferiorly slanting *spinous processes.*

Superior and **inferior costal facets,** most of which are small *demifacets,* occur as bilaterally paired, planar surfaces on the superior and inferior posterolateral margins of the bodies of typical thoracic vertebrae (T2–T9). Functionally, the facets are arranged in pairs on adjacent vertebrae, flanking an interposed IV disc: an inferior (demi)facet of the superior vertebra and a superior (demi)facet of the inferior vertebra. Typically, two demifacets paired in this manner and the posterolateral margin of the IV disc between them form a single socket to receive the head of the rib of the same identifying number as the inferior vertebra (e.g., head of rib 6 with the superior costal facet of vertebra T6). Atypical thoracic vertebrae bear whole costal facets in place of demifacets:

- The superior costal facets of vertebra T1 are not demifacets because there are no demifacets on the C7 vertebra above, and rib 1 articulates only with vertebra T1. T1 has a typical inferior costal (demi)facet.
- T10 has only one bilateral pair of (whole) costal facets, located partly on its body and partly on its pedicle.
- T11 and T12 also have only a single pair of (whole) costal facets, located on their pedicles.

The *spinous processes* projecting from the vertebral arches of typical thoracic vertebrae (e.g., vertebrae T6 or T7) are long and slope inferiorly, usually overlapping the vertebra below (Figs. 1.4D and 1.5). They cover the intervals between the *laminae* of adjacent vertebrae, thereby preventing sharp objects such as a knife from entering the *vertebral canal* and injuring the spinal cord. The convex superior articular facets of the *superior articular processes* face mainly posteriorly and slightly laterally, whereas the concave inferior articular facets of the *inferior articular processes* face mainly anteriorly and slightly medially. The bilateral joint planes between the respective articular facets of adjacent thoracic vertebrae define an arc, centering on an axis of rotation within the vertebral body (Fig. 1.4A–C). Thus small rotatory movements are permitted between adjacent vertebrae, limited by the attached rib cage.

THE STERNUM

The **sternum** (G. *sternon,* chest) is the flat, elongated bone that forms the middle of the anterior part of the thoracic cage (Fig. 1.6). It directly overlies and affords protection for mediastinal viscera in general and much of the heart in particular. The sternum consists of three parts: manubrium, body, and xiphoid process. In adolescents and young adults, the three parts are connected together by cartilaginous joints (*synchondroses*) that ossify during middle to late adulthood.

FIGURE 1.4. Thoracic vertebrae. A. T1 has a vertebral foramen and body similar in size and shape to a cervical vertebra. **B.** T5–T9 vertebrae have typical characteristics of thoracic vertebrae. **C.** T12 has bony processes and a body size similar to a lumbar vertebra. The planes of the articular facets of thoracic vertebrae define an arc (*red arrows*) that centers on an axis traversing the vertebral bodies vertically. **D.** Superior and inferior costal facets (demifacets) on the vertebral body and costal facets on the transverse processes. Long sloping spinous processes are characteristic of thoracic vertebrae.

FIGURE 1.5. Costovertebral articulations of a typical rib. The costovertebral joints include the joint of head of rib, in which the head articulates with two adjacent vertebral bodies and the intervertebral disc between them, and the costotransverse joint, in which the tubercle of the rib articulates with the transverse process of a vertebra. The rib moves (elevates and depresses) around an axis that traverses the head and neck of the rib (*arrows*).

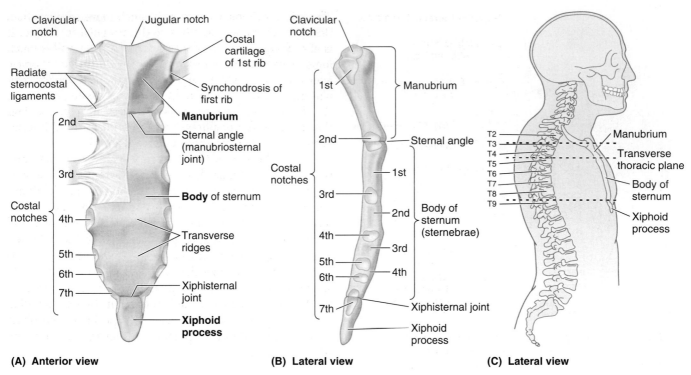

FIGURE 1.6. Sternum. A. The thin, broad membranous bands of the radiate sternocostal ligaments pass from the costal cartilages to the anterior and posterior surfaces of the sternum—is shown on the upper right side. **B.** Observe the thickness of the superior third of the manubrium between the clavicular notches. **C.** The relationship of the sternum to the vertebral column is shown.

The **manubrium** (L. handle, as in the handle of a sword, with the sternal body forming the blade) is a roughly trapezoidal bone. The manubrium is the widest and thickest of the three parts of the sternum. The easily palpated concave center of the superior border of the manubrium is the **jugular notch (suprasternal notch).** The notch is deepened by the medial (sternal) ends of the clavicles, which are much larger than the relatively small **clavicular notches** in the manubrium that receive them, forming the *sternoclavicular (SC) joints* (Fig. 1.1A). Inferolateral to the clavicular notch, the costal cartilage of the 1st rib is tightly attached to the lateral border of the manubrium—the **synchondrosis of the first rib** (Figs. 1.1A and 1.6A). The manubrium and body of the sternum lie in slightly different planes superior and inferior to their junction, the **manubriosternal joint** (Fig. 1.6A & B); hence, their junction forms a projecting **sternal angle** (of Louis).

The **body of the sternum,** is longer, narrower, and thinner than the manubrium, and is located at the level of the T5–T9 vertebrae (Fig. 1.6A–C). Its width varies because of the scalloping of its lateral borders by the **costal notches.** In young people, four *sternebrae* (primordial segments of the sternum) are obvious. The sternebrae articulate with each other at primary cartilaginous joints (*sternal synchondroses*). These joints begin to fuse from the inferior end between puberty (sexual maturity) and age 25. The nearly flat anterior surface of the body of the sternum is marked in adults by three variable **transverse ridges** (Fig. 1.6A), which represent the lines of fusion (*synostosis*) of its four originally separate sternebrae.

The **xiphoid process,** the smallest and most variable part of the sternum, is thin and elongated. Its inferior end lies at the level of T10 vertebra. Although often pointed, the process may be blunt, bifid, curved, or deflected to one side or anteriorly. It is cartilaginous in young people but more or less ossified in adults older than age 40. In elderly people, the xiphoid process may fuse with the sternal body.

The xiphoid process is an important landmark in the median plane because

- Its junction with the sternal body at the **xiphisternal joint** indicates the inferior limit of the central part of the thoracic cavity projected onto the anterior body wall; this joint is also the site of the **infrasternal angle** (subcostal angle) formed by the right and left costal margins (Fig. 1.1A).
- It is a midline marker for the superior limit of the liver, the central tendon of the diaphragm, and the inferior border of the heart.

Thoracic Apertures

While the thoracic cage provides a complete wall peripherally, it is open superiorly and inferiorly. The much smaller superior opening (aperture) is a passageway that allows communication with the neck and upper limbs. The larger inferior opening provides the ring-like origin of the diaphragm, which completely occludes the opening. Excursions of the diaphragm primarily control the volume/internal pressure of the thoracic cavity, providing the basis for tidal respiration (air exchange).

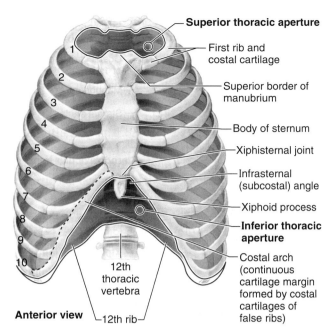

Superior thoracic aperture

First rib and costal cartilage

Superior border of manubrium

Body of sternum

Xiphisternal joint

Infrasternal (subcostal) angle

Xiphoid process

Inferior thoracic aperture

Costal arch (continuous cartilage margin formed by costal cartilages of false ribs)

12th thoracic vertebra

12th rib

Anterior view

FIGURE 1.7. Thoracic apertures. The superior thoracic aperture is the "doorway" between the thoracic cavity and the neck and upper limb. The inferior thoracic aperture provides attachment for the diaphragm, which protrudes upward so that upper abdominal viscera (e.g., liver) receive protection from the thoracic cage. The continuous cartilaginous bar formed by the articulated cartilages of the 7th–10th (false) ribs forms the costal margin.

SUPERIOR THORACIC APERTURE

The **superior thoracic aperture** is bounded (Fig. 1.7):

- Posteriorly, by vertebra T1, the body of which protrudes anteriorly into the opening.
- Laterally, by the 1st pair of ribs and their costal cartilages.
- Anteriorly, by the superior border of the manubrium.

Structures that pass between the thoracic cavity and the neck through the oblique, kidney-shaped superior thoracic aperture include the trachea, esophagus, nerves, and vessels that supply and drain the head, neck, and upper limbs.

The adult superior thoracic aperture measures approximately 6.5 cm anteroposteriorly and 11 cm transversely. To visualize the size of this opening, note that this is slightly larger than necessary to allow the passage of a 2-inch × 4-inch piece of lumber. Because of the obliquity of the 1st pair of ribs, the aperture slopes antero-inferiorly.

INFERIOR THORACIC APERTURE

The **inferior thoracic aperture,** the anatomical *thoracic outlet*, is bounded as follows:

- Posteriorly, by the 12th thoracic vertebra, the body of which protrudes anteriorly into the opening.
- Posterolaterally, by the 11th and 12th pairs of ribs.
- Anterolaterally, by the joined costal cartilages of ribs 7–10, forming the costal margins.
- Anteriorly, by the xiphisternal joint.

The inferior thoracic aperture is much more spacious than the superior thoracic aperture and is irregular in outline. It is also oblique because the posterior thoracic wall is much longer than the anterior wall. By closing the inferior thoracic aperture, the diaphragm separates the thoracic and abdominal cavities almost completely. Structures passing from or to the thorax to or from the abdomen pass through openings that traverse the diaphragm (e.g., esophagus and inferior vena cava), or pass posterior to it (e.g., aorta).

Just as the size of the thoracic cavity (or its contents) is often overestimated, its inferior extent (corresponding to the boundary between the thoracic and abdominal cavities) is often incorrectly estimated because of the discrepancy between the inferior thoracic aperture and the location of the diaphragm (floor of the thoracic cavity) in living persons. Although the diaphragm takes origin from the structures that make up the inferior thoracic aperture, the domes of the diaphragm rise to the level of the 4th intercostal space, and abdominal viscera, including the liver, spleen, and stomach, lie superior to the plane of the inferior thoracic aperture, within the thoracic wall (Fig. 1.1A & B).

Joints of Thoracic Wall

Although movements of the joints of the thoracic wall are frequent—for example, in association with normal respiration—the range of movement at the individual joints is relatively small. Nonetheless, any disturbance that reduces the mobility of these joints interferes with respiration. During deep breathing, the excursions of the thoracic cage (anteriorly, superiorly, or laterally) are considerable. Extending the vertebral column further increases the anteroposterior (AP) diameter of the thorax. The joints of the thoracic wall are illustrated in Figure 1.8. The type, participating articular surfaces, and ligaments of the joints of the thoracic wall are provided in Table 1.1.

The *intervertebral joints* between the bodies of adjacent vertebrae are joined by longitudinal ligaments and *intervertebral discs*. These joints are discussed with the back in Chapter 4; the sternoclavicular joints are discussed in Chapter 6.

COSTOVERTEBRAL JOINTS

A typical rib articulates posteriorly with the vertebral column at two joints, the joints of heads of ribs and costotransverse joints (Fig. 1.5).

Joints of Heads of Ribs. The *head of the rib* articulates with the *superior costal facet* of the corresponding (same-numbered) vertebra, the *inferior costal facet* of the vertebra superior to it, and the adjacent intervertebral (IV) disc uniting the two vertebrae (Figs. 1.4 and 1.8A). For example, the head of the 6th rib articulates with the superior costal facet of the body of the T6 vertebra, the inferior costal facet of T5, and the IV disc between these vertebrae.

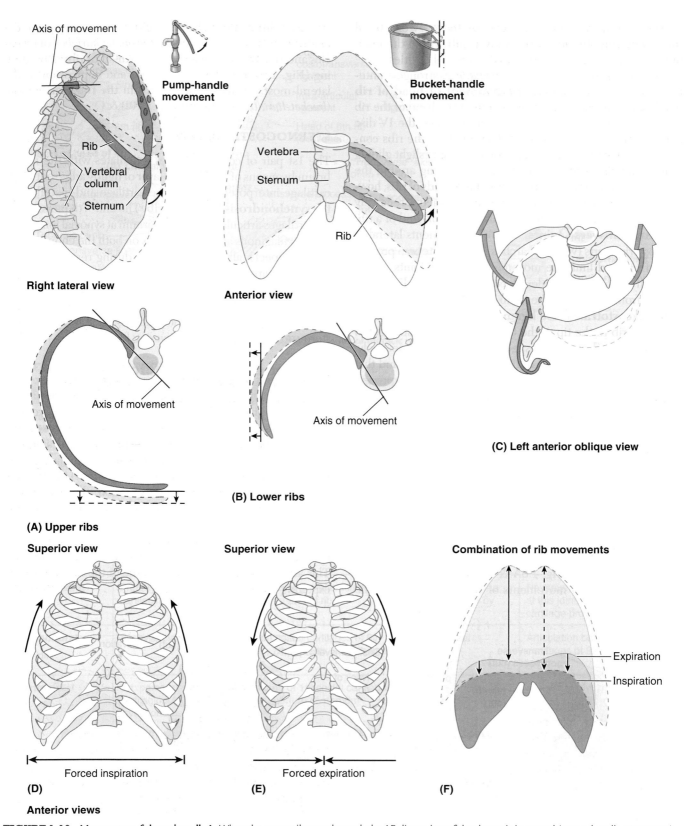

FIGURE 1.10. Movements of thoracic wall. A. When the upper ribs are elevated, the AP dimension of the thorax is increased (pump-handle movement), with a greater excursion (increase) occurring inferiorly, at the end of the pump handle. **B.** The middle parts of the lower ribs move laterally when they are elevated, increasing the transverse dimension (bucket-handle movement). **C.** The combination of rib movements (*arrows*) that occur during forced inspiration increase the AP and transverse dimensions of the thoracic cage. **D.** The thorax widens during forced inspiration as the ribs are elevated (*arrows*). **E.** The thorax narrows during expiration as the ribs are depressed (*arrows*). **F.** The primary movement of inspiration (resting or forced) is contraction of the diaphragm, which increases the vertical dimension of the thoracic cavity (*arrows*). When the diaphragm relaxes, decompression of the abdominal viscera pushes the diaphragm upward, reducing the vertical dimension for expiration.

The *vertical dimension* (height) of the central part of the thoracic cavity increases during inspiration as contraction of the diaphragm causes it to descend, compressing the abdominal viscera (Fig. 1.10F). During expiration, the vertical dimension returns to the neutral position as the elastic recoil of the lungs produces sub-atmospheric pressure in the pleural cavities, between the lungs and the thoracic wall. As a result of this and the absence of resistance to the previously compressed viscera, the domes of the diaphragm ascend, diminishing the vertical dimension.

The *AP dimension* of the thorax increases considerably when the intercostal muscles contract. Movement of the ribs (primarily 2nd–6th) at the costovertebral joints around an axis passing through the necks of the ribs causes the anterior ends of the ribs to rise—*the pump-handle movement* (Fig. 1.10A & C). Because the ribs slope inferiorly, their elevation also results in anterior–posterior movement of the sternum, especially its inferior end, with slight movement occurring at the manubriosternal joint in young people, in whom this joint has not yet synostosed (united).

The *transverse dimension* of the thorax also increases slightly when the intercostal muscles contract, raising the middle (lateral-most parts) of the ribs (especially the lower ones)—*the bucket-handle movement* (Fig. 1.10B & C). The combination of all these movements moves the thoracic cage anteriorly, superiorly, and laterally (Fig. 1.10C & F).

THORACIC WALL

Chest Pain

Although *chest pain* can result from pulmonary disease, it is probably the most important symptom of cardiac disease (Swartz, 2009). However, chest pain may also occur in intestinal, gallbladder, and musculoskeletal disorders. When evaluating a patient with chest pain, the examination is largely concerned with discriminating between serious conditions and the many minor causes of pain. People who have had a *heart attack* usually describe the associated pain as a "crushing" sub-sternal pain (deep to the sternum) that does not disappear with rest.

Rib Fractures

The short, broad 1st rib, posteroinferior to the clavicle, is rarely fractured because of its protected position (it cannot be palpated). When it is broken, however, structures crossing its superior aspect may be injured, including the brachial plexus of nerves and subclavian vessels that serve the upper limb. The middle ribs are most commonly fractured. *Rib fractures* usually result from blows or crushing injuries. The weakest part of a rib is just anterior to its angle; however, direct violence may fracture a rib anywhere, and its broken end may injure internal organs such as a lung and/or the spleen. Fractures of the lower ribs may tear the diaphragm and result in a *diaphragmatic hernia* (see Chapter 2). Rib fractures are painful because the broken parts move during respiration, coughing, laughing, and sneezing.

Flail Chest

Multiple rib fractures may allow a sizable segment of the anterior and/or lateral thoracic wall to move freely. The loose segment of the wall moves paradoxically (inward on inspiration and outward on expiration). *Flail chest* is an extremely painful injury and impairs ventilation, thereby affecting oxygenation of the blood. During treatment, the loose segment may be fixed by hooks and/or wires so that it cannot move.

Thoracotomy, Intercostal Space Incisions, and Rib Excision

The surgical creation of an opening through the thoracic wall to enter a pleural cavity is a *thoracotomy* (Fig. B1.1). An anterior thoracotomy may involve making H-shaped cuts through the perichondrium of one or more costal cartilages and then shelling out segments of costal cartilage to gain entrance to the thoracic cavity (see Fig 1.13, right side).

The posterolateral aspects of the 5th–7th intercostal spaces are important sites for *posterior thoracotomy incisions*. In general, a lateral approach is most satisfactory for entry through the thoracic cage (Fig. B1.1). With the patient lying on the contralateral side, the upper limb is fully abducted, placing the forearm beside the patient's head. This elevates and laterally rotates the inferior angle of scapula, allowing access as high as the 4th intercostal space.

Surgeons use an H-shaped incision to incise the superficial aspect of the periosteum that ensheaths the rib, strip the periosteum from the rib, and then *excise a wide segment of the rib* to gain better access, as might be required to enter the thoracic cavity and remove a lung (*pneumonectomy*), for example. In the rib's absence, entry into the thoracic cavity can be made through the deep aspect of the periosteal sheath, sparing the adjacent intercostal muscles. After the operation, the missing pieces of ribs regenerate from the intact periosteum, although imperfectly.

Supernumerary Ribs

People usually have 12 ribs on each side, but the number is increased by the presence of *cervical* and/or *lumbar ribs*, or decreased by failure of

The Bottom Line

Skeleton of thoracic wall: The thoracic wall (1) protects the contents of the thoracic cavity; (2) provides the mechanics for breathing; and (3) provides for attachment of neck, back, upper limb, and abdominal musculature. ◆ The domed shape of the thoracic cage gives it strength, and its osteocartilaginous elements and joints give it flexibility. ◆ Posteriorly the thoracic cage consists of a column of 12 thoracic vertebrae and interposed IV discs. ◆ Laterally and anteriorly the cage consists of 12 ribs that are continued anteriorly by costal cartilages. Anteriorly, the 3-part sternum protects the central thoracic viscera.

Apertures of thoracic wall: Although the thoracic cage is complete peripherally, it is open superiorly and inferiorly. ◆ The superior thoracic aperture is a small passageway for the transmittal of structures to and from the neck and upper limbs. ◆ The large inferior thoracic aperture provides a rim to which the diaphragm is attached. Structures passing between the thorax and abdomen traverse openings in the diaphragm (e.g., esophagus) or pass posterior to it (e.g., aorta).

Joints of thoracic wall: The joints enable and determine movements of the thoracic wall. ◆ Posteriorly, ribs articulate with the semiflexible thoracic vertebral column via costovertebral joints. These include joints of heads of ribs and costotransverse joints, both strongly supported by multiple ligaments. ◆ Anteriorly, ribs articulate with costal cartilages via costochondral joints. ◆ Costal cartilages 1–7 articulate directly and costal cartilages 8–10 articulate indirectly with the sternum via the synchondrosis of the 1st rib, synovial sternocostal joints, and interchondral joints.

Movements of thoracic wall: The movements of most ribs occur around a generally transverse axis that passes through the head, neck, and tubercle of the rib. ◆ This axis, plus the slope and curvature of the ribs, results in pump-handle-type movements of the upper ribs that alter the AP diameter of the thorax and bucket-handle-type movements of lower ribs that alter its transverse diameter. ◆ Contraction and relaxation of the superiorly convex diaphragm alters its vertical dimensions. ◆ Increasing dimensions produce inhalation, and decreasing dimensions produce exhalation.

Muscles of Thoracic Wall

Some muscles attached to and/or covering the thoracic cage are primarily involved in serving other regions. **Axio-appendicular muscles** extend from the thoracic cage (axial skeleton) to bones of the upper limb (appendicular skeleton). Similarly, some muscles of the anterolateral abdominal wall, back, and neck muscles have attachments to the thoracic cage (Fig. 1.11). The axio-appendicular muscles act primarily on the upper limbs (see Chapter 6). But several of them, including the *pectoralis major* and *pectoralis minor* and the inferior part of the *serratus anterior,* may also function as accessory muscles of respiration, helping elevate the ribs to expand the thoracic cavity when inspiration is deep and forceful (e.g., after a 100-m dash). The *scalene muscles* of the neck, which descend from vertebrae of the neck to the 1st and 2nd ribs, act primarily on the vertebral column. However, they also serve as *accessory respiratory muscles* by fixing these ribs and enabling the muscles connecting the ribs below to be more effective in elevating the lower ribs during forced inspiration.

The true **muscles of the thoracic wall** are the serratus posterior, levatores costarum, intercostal, subcostal, and transversus thoracis. They are demonstrated in Figure 1.12A & B, and their attachments, innervations, and functions are listed in Table 1.2.

The *serratus posterior muscles* have traditionally been described as inspiratory muscles, but this function is not supported by electromyography or other evidence. On the basis of its attachments and disposition, the **serratus posterior superior** was said to elevate the superior four ribs, thus increasing the AP diameter of the thorax and raising the sternum. On the basis of its attachments and disposition, the **serratus posterior inferior** was said to depress the inferior ribs, preventing them from being pulled superiorly by the diaphragm. However, recent studies (Vilensky et al., 2001) suggest that these muscles, which span the superior and inferior thoracic apertures as well as the transitions from the relatively inflexible thoracic vertebral column to the much more flexible cervical and lumbar segments of the column, may not be primarily motor in function. Rather, they may have a proprioceptive function. These muscles, particularly the serratus posterior superior, have been implicated as a source of chronic pain in myofascial pain syndromes.

The **levatores costarum muscles** (L. *levator,* a lifter) are 12 fan-shaped muscles that elevate the ribs (Fig. 1.17), but their role, if any, in normal inspiration is uncertain. They may play a role in vertebral movement and/or proprioception.

The *intercostal muscles* occupy the intercostal spaces (Figs. 1.11–1.14; Table 1.2). The superficial layer is formed by the external intercostals, the inner layer by the internal intercostals. The deepest fibers of the latter, lying internal to the intercostal vessels, are somewhat artificially designated as a separate muscle, the *innermost intercostals.*

• The **external intercostal muscles** (11 pairs) occupy the intercostal spaces from the tubercles of the ribs posteriorly to the costochondral junctions anteriorly (Figs. 1.11–1.13, and 1.15). Anteriorly, the muscle fibers are replaced

Scaleni

Pectoralis major

Serratus
anterior

Anterolateral
abdominal
muscles
{
External
oblique

Rectus
abdominis
}

Cut end of clavicular head
of pectoralis major

Subclavius

Cut ends (proximal and
distal attachments) of
sternocostal head of
pectoralis major

Pectoralis minor

External
intercostal

Humerus

Serratus
anterior

Internal intercostal

Anterior view

FIGURE 1.11. **Axio-appendicular, neck, and anterolateral abdominal muscles overlying thoracic wall.** The pectoralis major has been removed on the left side to expose the pectoralis minor, subclavius, and external intercostal muscles. When the upper limb muscles are removed, the superiorly tapering domed shape of the thoracic cage is revealed.

by the **external intercostal membranes** (Fig. 1.15A). These muscles run infero-anteriorly from the rib above to the rib below. Each muscle attaches superiorly to the inferior border of the rib above and inferiorly to the superior border of the rib below (Fig. 1.15C). These muscles are continuous inferiorly with the *external oblique muscles* in the anterolateral abdominal wall. The external intercostals are most active during inspiration.

- The **internal intercostal muscles** (11 pairs) run deep to and at right angles to the external intercostals (Figs. 1.12B, 1.14, and 1.15C). Their fibers run inferoposteriorly from the floors of the costal grooves to the superior borders of the ribs inferior to them. The internal intercostals attach to the bodies of the ribs and their costal cartilages as far anteriorly as the sternum and as far posteriorly as the angles of the ribs (Fig. 1.16). Between the ribs posteriorly, medial to the angles, the internal intercostals are replaced by the **internal intercostal membranes** (Fig. 1.15A). The inferior internal intercostal muscles are continuous with the *internal oblique muscles* in the anterolateral abdominal wall. The internal intercostals—weaker than the external intercostal muscles—are most active during expiration—especially their interosseous (vs. interchondral) portions.

- The **innermost intercostal muscles** are similar to the internal intercostals and are essentially their deeper parts. The innermost intercostals are separated from the internal intercostals by intercostal nerves and vessels (Figs. 1.15A & B and 1.16). These muscles pass between the internal

surfaces of adjacent ribs and occupy the lateral-most parts of the intercostal spaces. It is likely (but undetermined) that their actions are the same as those of the internal intercostal muscles.

The **subcostal muscles** are variable in size and shape, usually being well developed only in the lower thoracic wall. These thin muscular slips extend from the internal surface of the angle of one rib to the internal surface of the second or third rib inferior to it. Crossing one or two intercostal spaces, the subcostals run in the same direction as the internal intercostals and blend with them (Fig. 1.15B).

The **transversus thoracis muscles** consist of four or five slips that radiate superolaterally from the posterior aspect of the inferior sternum (Figs. 1.13–1.15A). The transversus thoracis muscles are continuous inferiorly with the *transversus abdominis muscles* in the anterolateral body wall. These muscles appear to have a weak expiratory function and may also provide proprioceptive information.

Although the external and internal intercostals are active during inspiration and expiration, respectively, most activity is isometric (increases tonus without producing movement); the role of these muscles in producing movement of the ribs appears to be related mainly to *forced respiration.* The diaphragm is the primary muscle of inspiration. Expiration is passive unless one is exhaling against resistance (e.g., inflating a balloon) or trying to expel air more rapidly than usual (e.g., coughing, sneezing, blowing one's nose, or shouting). The elastic recoil of the lungs and decompression of

FIGURE 1.12. Muscles of thoracic wall.

TABLE 1.2. MUSCLES OF THORACIC WALL

Muscle	Superior Attachment	Interior Attachment	Innervation	Main Action	
Serratus posterior superior	Nuchal ligament, spinous processes of C7 to T3 vertebrae	Superior borders of 2nd to 4th ribs	2nd to 5th intercostal nerves	Proprioception (elevate ribs)[b]	
Serratus posterior inferior	Spinous processes of T11 to L2 vertebrae	Inferior borders of 8th to 12th ribs near their angles	Anterior rami to T9 to T12 thoracic spinal nerves	Proprioception (depress ribs)[b]	
Levator costarum	Transverse processes of T7–11	Subjacent ribs between tubercle and angle	Posterior primary rami of C8–T11 nerves	Elevate ribs	
External intercostal	Inferior border of ribs	Superior border of ribs below	Intercostal nerve	Elevate ribs during forced inspiration[a]	
Internal intercostal				Interosseous part: depresses ribs	During active (forced) respiration[a]
Innermost intercostal				Interchondral part: elevates ribs	
Subcostal	Internal surface of lower ribs near their angles	Superior borders of 2nd or 3rd ribs below		Probably act in same manner as internal intercostal muscles	
Transversus thoracis	Posterior surface of lower sternum	Internal surface of costal cartilages 2–6		Weakly depress ribs[b] Proprioception?	

[a]All intercostal muscles keep intercostal spaces rigid, thereby preventing them from bulging out during expiration and from being drawn in during inspiration. The role of individual intercostal muscles and accessory muscles of respiration in moving the ribs is difficult to interpret despite many electromyographic studies.

[b]Action traditionally assigned based on attachments; appear to be largely proprioceptive in function.

abdominal viscera expel previously inhaled air. The primary role of the intercostal muscles in respiration is to support (increase the tonus or rigidity of) the intercostal space, resisting paradoxical movement especially during inspiration when internal thoracic pressures are lowest (most negative). This is most apparent following a high spinal cord injury, when there is an initial flaccid paralysis of the entire trunk but the diaphragm remains active. In these circumstances, the vital capacity is markedly compromised by the paradoxical incursion of the thoracic wall during inspiration. Several weeks later, the paralysis becomes spastic; the thoracic wall stiffens and vital capacity rises (Standring, 2008).

The mechanical action of the intercostal muscles in rib movement, especially during forced respiration, can be

Anterior view

Labels (clockwise from top left):
Scaleni { Posterior, Medius, Anterior }
Sternocleidomastoid
Brachial plexus / Axillary artery / Axillary vein
Subclavian vein
Pectoralis minor
Sternothyroid / Sternohyoid
Pectoralis major (cut)
1st intercostal nerve
2nd intercostal nerve
Internal thoracic vein and artery
3rd
4th
External intercostal muscle
Internal intercostal muscle deep to **external intercostal membrane**
Parasternal lymph node
Transversus thoracis
Pectoralis major (cut)
Serratus anterior
Rectus abdominis
External oblique
Costal margin

FIGURE 1.13. Dissection of anterior aspect of anterior thoracic wall. The external intercostal muscles are replaced by membranes between costal cartilages. The H-shaped cuts through the perichondrium of the 3rd and 4th costal cartilages are used to shell out pieces of cartilage, as was done with the 4th costal cartilage. It is not uncommon for the 8th rib to attach to the sternum, as in this specimen. The internal thoracic vessels and parasternal lymph nodes (*green*) lie inside the thoracic cage lateral to the sternum.

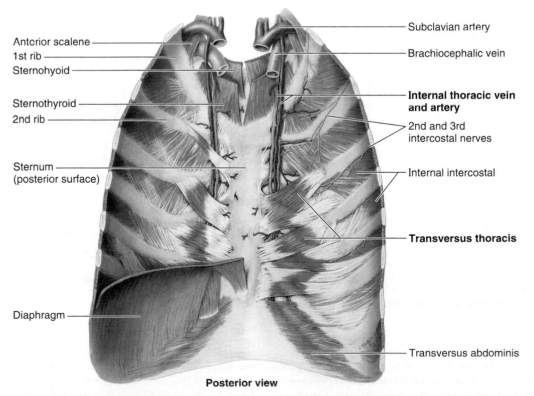

Posterior view

Labels:
Anterior scalene
Subclavian artery
1st rib
Brachiocephalic vein
Sternohyoid
Sternothyroid
Internal thoracic vein and artery
2nd rib
2nd and 3rd intercostal nerves
Internal intercostal
Sternum (posterior surface)
Transversus thoracis
Diaphragm
Transversus abdominis

FIGURE 1.14. Posterior aspect of anterior thoracic wall. The internal thoracic arteries arise from the subclavian arteries and have paired accompanying veins (L. *venae comitantes*) inferiorly. Superior to the 2nd costal cartilage, there is only a single internal thoracic vein on each side, which drains into the brachiocephalic vein. The continuity of the transversus thoracis muscle with the transversus abdominis muscle becomes apparent when the diaphragm is removed, as has been done here on the right side.

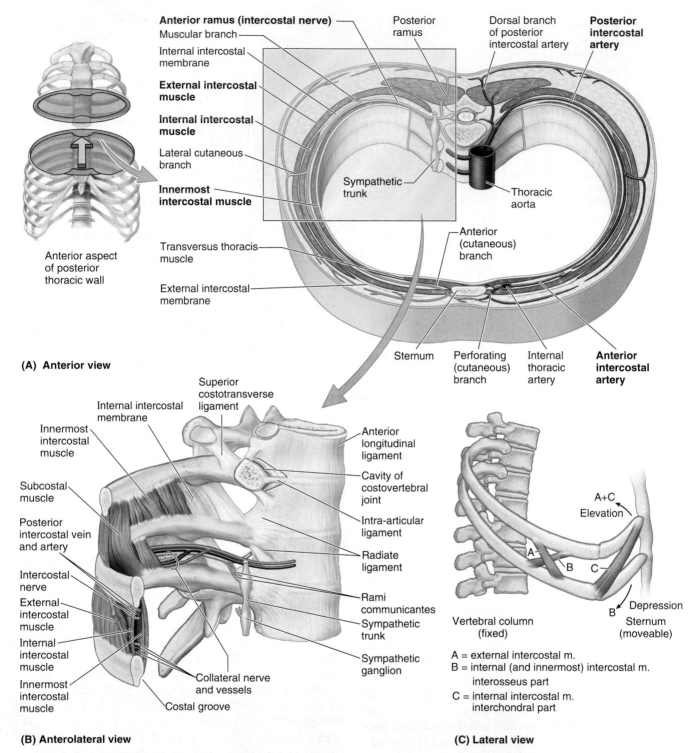

(A) Anterior view

(B) Anterolateral view

(C) Lateral view

A = external intercostal m.
B = internal (and innermost) intercostal m.
    interosseus part
C = internal intercostal m.
    interchondral part

FIGURE 1.15. Contents of an intercostal space. A. This transverse section shows nerves (*right side*) and arteries (*left side*) in relation to the intercostal muscles. **B.** The posterior part of an intercostal space is shown. The joint capsule (radiate ligament) of one costovertebral joint has been removed. Innermost intercostal muscles bridge one intercostal space; subcostal muscles bridge two. The mnemonic for the order of the neurovascular structures in the intercostal space from superior to inferior is VAN—vein, artery, and nerve. Communicating branches (L. *rami communicantes*) extend between the intercostal nerves and the sympathetic trunk. **C.** A simple model of the action of the intercostal muscles is shown. Contraction of the muscle fibers that most closely parallel the slope of the ribs at a given point (fibers *A* and *C*) will elevate the ribs and sternum; contraction of muscle fibers that are approximately perpendicular to the slope of the ribs (fibers *B*) will depress the ribs.

Supraclavicular nerves (C3 and C4)

Deltoid

Deltopectoral triangle

Cephalic vien

Platysma

Skin

Pectoralis major

Subcutaneous tissue

Intercostobrachial nerve (T2)

Anterior branches of **lateral cutaneous nerves** (derived from intercostal nerves)

Anterior and posterior branches of **lateral cutaneous nerves** (derived from intercostal nerves)

Pectoral fascia covering pectoralis major

Serratus anterior

Anterior cutaneous nerves

External oblique and nerve supply

6th cartilage

Anterior view (slightly oblique)

FIGURE 1.16. Superficial dissection of male pectoral region. The platysma is cut short on the right side and is reflected on the left side, together with the underlying supraclavicular nerves. Filmy pectoral fascia covers the right pectoralis major. The fascia has been removed on the left side. The cutaneous branches of the intercostal nerves that supply the breast are shown.

appreciated by means of a simple model (Fig. 1.15C). A pair of curved levers, representing the ribs bordering an intercostal space, are hinged posteriorly to a fixed vertebral column and anteriorly to a moveable sternum. The ribs (and intervening intercostal space) descend as they run anteriorly, reaching their low point approximately at the costochondral junction, and then ascend to the sternum. Muscles with fibers that most closely approximate the slope of the ribs at their attachments (external intercostal and interchondral portion of the internal intercostal muscles) rotate the ribs superiorly at their posterior axes, elevating the ribs and sternum. Muscle with fibers that are approximately perpendicular to the slope of the ribs at their attachment (interosseous part of internal intercostal muscles) rotate the ribs inferiorly at their posterior axes, depressing the ribs and sternum (Slaby et al., 1994).

The (thoracic) *diaphragm* is a shared wall (actually floor/ceiling) separating the thorax and abdomen. Although it has functions related to both compartments of the trunk, its most important (vital) function is serving as the *primary muscle of inspiration*. The detailed description of the diaphragm appears in Chapter 2 because the attachments of its crura occur at abdominal levels (i.e., to lumbar vertebrae) and all of its attachments are best observed from its inferior (abdominal) aspect.

Fascia of Thoracic Wall

Each part of the deep fascia is named for the muscle it invests or for the structure(s) to which it is attached. Consequently, a large portion of the deep fascia overlying the anterior thoracic wall is called **pectoral fascia** for its association with the pectoralis major muscles (Fig. 1.16). In turn, much of the pectoral fascia forms a major part of the *bed of the breast* (structures against which the posterior surface of the breast lies). Deep to the pectoralis major and its fascia is another layer of deep fascia suspended from the clavicle and investing the pectoralis minor muscle, the *clavipectoral fascia*.

The thoracic cage is lined internally with **endothoracic fascia** (see Fig. 1.30C). This thin fibro-areolar layer attaches the adjacent portion of the lining of the lung cavities (costal parietal pleura) to the thoracic wall. It becomes more fibrous over the apices of the lungs (*suprapleural membrane*).

Nerves of Thoracic Wall

The 12 pairs of *thoracic spinal nerves* supply the thoracic wall. As soon as they leave the IV foramina in which they are formed, the mixed thoracic spinal nerves divide into anterior and posterior (primary) rami or branches (Fig. 1.15A and 1.17). The *anterior rami of nerves T1–T11* form the **intercostal nerves** that run along the extent of the intercostal

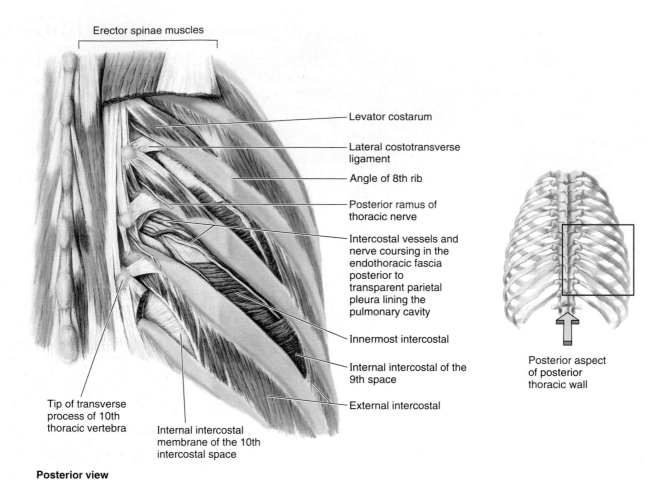

Erector spinae muscles

Levator costarum

Lateral costotransverse
ligament

Angle of 8th rib

Posterior ramus of
thoracic nerve

Intercostal vessels and
nerve coursing in the
endothoracic fascia
posterior to
transparent parietal
pleura lining the
pulmonary cavity

Innermost intercostal

Internal intercostal of the
9th space

External intercostal

Tip of transverse
process of 10th
thoracic vertebra

Internal intercostal
membrane of the 10th
intercostal space

Posterior view

Posterior aspect
of posterior
thoracic wall

FIGURE 1.17. Dissection of posterior aspect of thoracic wall. Most of the deep muscles of the back have been removed to expose the levatores costarum muscles. In the 8th and 10th intercostal spaces, varying parts of the external intercostal muscle have been removed to expose the underlying internal intercostal membrane, which is continuous with the internal intercostal muscle. In the 9th intercostal space, the levator costorum has been removed to expose the intercostal vessels and nerve.

spaces. The *anterior ramus of nerve T12,* coursing inferior to the 12th rib, is the **subcostal nerve.** The *posterior rami of thoracic spinal nerves* pass posteriorly, immediately lateral to the articular processes of the vertebrae, to supply the joints, deep back muscles, and skin of the back in the thoracic region.

TYPICAL INTERCOSTAL NERVES

The 3rd–6th intercostal nerves enter the medial-most parts of the posterior intercostal spaces, running initially within the endothoracic fascia between the parietal pleura (serous lining of pulmonary cavity) and the internal intercostal membrane nearly in the middle of the intercostal spaces (Figs. 1.15A & B and 1.17). Near the angles of the ribs, the nerves pass between the internal intercostal and the innermost intercostal muscles. At this point, the intercostal nerves pass to and then continue to course in or just inferior to the *costal grooves,* running inferior to the intercostal arteries (which, in turn, run inferior to the intercostal veins). The neurovascular bundles (especially the vessels) are thus sheltered by the inferior margins of the overlying ribs. Collateral branches of

these nerves arise near the angles of the ribs and run along the superior border of the rib below. The nerves continue anteriorly between the internal and innermost intercostal muscles, supplying these and other muscles and giving rise to lateral cutaneous branches in approximately the midaxillary line (**MAL**). Anteriorly, the nerves appear on the internal surface of the internal intercostal muscle. Near the sternum, the nerves turn anteriorly, passing between the costal cartilages to become anterior cutaneous branches.

Through its posterior ramus and the lateral and anterior cutaneous branches of its anterior ramus, most thoracic spinal nerves (T2–T12) supply a strip-like *dermatome* of the trunk extending from the posterior median line to the anterior median line (Fig. 1.18). The group of muscles supplied by the posterior ramus and anterior ramus (intercostal nerve) of each pair of thoracic spinal nerves constitutes a *myotome.* The myotomes of most thoracic spinal nerves (T2–T11) include the intercostal, subcostal, transversus thoracis, levatores costarum, and serratus posterior muscles associated with the intercostal space that includes the anterior ramus (intercostal nerve) of the specific spinal nerve, plus the overlying portion of the deep muscles of the back.

FIGURE 1.18. Segmental innervation (dermatomes) of thoracic wall (after Foerster). Dermatomes C5–T1 are located mostly in the upper limbs and are not represented significantly on the body wall. Since the anterior rami of spinal nerves T2–T12 are not involved in plexus formation, there is no difference between the dermatomes and the zones of peripheral nerve distribution here. Dermatome T4 includes the nipple; dermatome T10 includes the umbilicus.

The *branches of a typical intercostal nerve* are (Fig. 1.15A & B):

- **Rami communicantes,** or communicating branches, that connect each intercostal nerve to the ipsilateral sympathetic trunk. Presynaptic fibers leave the initial portions of the anterior ramus of each thoracic (and upper lumbar) spinal nerve by means of a white communicating ramus and pass to the *sympathetic trunk.* Postsynaptic fibers distributed to the body wall and limbs pass from the ganglia of the sympathetic trunk via gray rami to join the anterior ramus of the nearest spinal nerve, including all intercostal nerves. Sympathetic nerve fibers are distributed through all branches of all spinal nerves (anterior and posterior rami) to reach the blood vessels, sweat glands, and smooth muscle of the body wall and limbs.
- **Collateral branches** that arise near the angles of the ribs and descend to course along the superior margin of the lower rib, helping supply intercostal muscles and parietal pleura.
- **Lateral cutaneous branches** that arise near the MAL, pierce the internal and external intercostal muscles, and divide in turn into *anterior and posterior branches.* These terminal branches supply the skin of the lateral thoracic and abdominal walls.
- **Anterior cutaneous branches** pierce the muscles and membranes of the intercostal space in the parasternal line and divide into *medial and lateral branches.* These terminal branches supply the skin on the anterior aspect of the thorax and abdomen.
- **Muscular branches** that supply the intercostal, subcostal, transversus thoracis, levatores costarum, and serratus posterior muscles.

ATYPICAL INTERCOSTAL NERVES

Although the anterior ramus of most thoracic spinal nerves is simply the intercostal nerve for that level, the *anterior ramus*

of the 1st thoracic (T1) spinal nerve first divides into a large superior and a small inferior part. The superior part joins the *brachial plexus,* the nerve plexus supplying the upper limb, and the inferior part becomes the 1st intercostal nerve. Other atypical features of specific intercostal nerves include the following:

- The *1st and 2nd intercostal nerves* course on the internal surface of the 1st and 2nd ribs, instead of along the inferior margin in costal grooves (Fig. 1.14).
- The *1st intercostal nerve* has no anterior cutaneous branch and often no lateral cutaneous branch. When there is a lateral cutaneous branch, it supplies the skin of the axilla and may communicate with either the intercostobrachial nerve or the medial cutaneous nerve of the arm.
- The *2nd* (and sometimes 3rd) *intercostal nerve* gives rise to a large lateral cutaneous branch, the **intercostobrachial nerve;** it emerges from the 2nd intercostal space at the MAL, penetrates the serratus anterior, and enters the axilla and arm. The intercostobrachial nerve usually supplies the floor—skin and subcutaneous tissue—of the axilla and then communicates with the *medial cutaneous nerve of the arm* to supply the medial and posterior surfaces of the arm. The lateral cutaneous branch of the 3rd intercostal nerve frequently gives rise to a second intercostobrachial nerve.
- The *7th–11th intercostal nerves,* after giving rise to lateral cutaneous branches, cross the costal margin posteriorly and continue on to supply abdominal skin and muscles. No longer being between ribs (intercostal), they now become *thoraco-abdominal nerves* of the anterior abdominal wall (see Chapter 2). Their anterior cutaneous branches pierce the rectus sheath, becoming cutaneous close to the median plane.

Vasculature of Thoracic Wall

In general, the pattern of vascular distribution in the thoracic wall reflects the structure of the thoracic cage—that is, it runs in the intercostal spaces, parallel to the ribs.

ARTERIES OF THORACIC WALL

The arterial supply to the thoracic wall (Fig. 1.19; Table 1.3) derives from the:

- *Thoracic aorta,* through the posterior intercostal and subcostal arteries.
- *Subclavian artery,* through the internal thoracic and supreme intercostal arteries.
- *Axillary artery,* through the superior and lateral thoracic arteries.

The **intercostal arteries** course through the thoracic wall between the ribs. With the exception of the 10th and 11th intercostal spaces, each intercostal space is supplied by three arteries: a large posterior intercostal artery (and its collateral branch) and a small pair of anterior intercostal arteries.

(A) Anterosuperior view

Anterior aspect of posterior thoracic wall

Dorsal branch of posterior intercostal a.

Posterior intercostal a.

Thoracic aorta

Perforating (cutaneous) branch

Internal thoracic a.

Anterior intercostal a.

Lateral cutaneous branch

(B) Anterior view

Right common carotid a.

Brachiocephalic trunk

Left common carotid a.

Vertebral a.

Left subclavian a.

Thyrocervical trunk

Sternum

Costocervical trunk

Axillary a.

Supreme (superior) intercostal a.

Ascending aorta

Fourth posterior intercostal a.

Internal thoracic a.

Bronchial a.

Descending aorta

Esophageal branch

Anterior intercostal a.

Musculophrenic a.

11th posterior intercostal a.

Superior epigastric a.

Subcostal a.

(C) Posterior view

Manubrium of sternum

Internal thoracic a.

Anterior intercostal a. and its collateral branch

Transversus thoracis muscle

Musculophrenic a.

Diaphragm

Superior epigastric aa.

Transversus abdominis

Rectus sheath

(D) Anterior view

Supreme (superior) intercostal a.

Internal thoracic a.

Posterior intercostal a.

Anterior intercostal a.

Subcostal a.

FIGURE 1.19. Arteries of thoracic wall. The arterial supply to the thoracic wall derives from the thoracic aorta through the posterior intercostal and subcostal arteries (**A, B,** and **D**), from the axillary artery (**B**), and from the subclavian artery through the internal thoracic (**C**) and supreme intercostal arteries (**B**). Connections (anastomoses) between the arteries permit collateral circulation pathways to develop (**D**).

TABLE 1.3. ARTERIAL SUPPLY OF THORACIC WALL

Artery	Origin	Course	Distribution
Posterior intercostals	Superior intercostal artery (intercostal spaces 1 and 2) and thoracic aorta (remaining intercostal spaces)	Pass between internal and innermost intercostal muscles	Intercostal muscles, overlying skin, and parietal pleura
Anterior intercostals	Internal thoracic (intercostal spaces 1–6) and musculophrenic arteries (intercostal spaces 7–9)		
Internal thoracic	Subclavian artery	Passes inferiorly and lateral to sternum between costal cartilages and transversus thoracic muscle to divide into superior epigastric and musculophrenic arteries	By way of anterior intercostal arteries to intercostal spaces 1–6 and musculophrenic artery (lateral terminal branch)
Subcostal	Thoracic aorta	Courses along inferior border of 12th rib	Muscles of anterolateral abdominal wall

The **posterior intercostal arteries:**

- Of the 1st and 2nd intercostal spaces arise from the **supreme (superior) intercostal artery,** a branch of the costocervical trunk of the subclavian artery.
- Of the 3rd–11th intercostal spaces (and the subcostal arteries of the subcostal space) arise posteriorly from the thoracic aorta (Fig. 1.19). Because the aorta is slightly to the left of the vertebral column, the right 3rd–11th intercostal arteries cross the vertebral bodies, running a longer course than those on the left side (Fig. 1.19B).
- All give off a posterior branch that accompanies the posterior ramus of the spinal nerve to supply the spinal cord, vertebral column, back muscles, and skin.
- Give rise to a small collateral branch that crosses the intercostal space and runs along the superior border of the rib.
- Accompany the intercostal nerves through the intercostal spaces. Close to the angle of the rib, the arteries enter the costal grooves, where they lie between the intercostal vein and nerve. At first the arteries run in the endothoracic fascia between the parietal pleura and the internal intercostal membrane (Fig. 1.17); then they run between the innermost intercostal and internal intercostal muscles.
- Have terminal and collateral branches that anastomose anteriorly with anterior intercostal arteries (Fig. 1.19A).

The **internal thoracic arteries** (historically, the internal mammary arteries):

- Arise in the root of the neck from the inferior surfaces of the first parts of the *subclavian arteries.*
- Descend into the thorax posterior to the clavicle and 1st costal cartilage (Figs. 1.13, 1.14, and 1.19).
- Are crossed near their origins by the ipsilateral phrenic nerve.
- Descend on the internal surface of the thorax slightly lateral to the sternum and posterior to the upper six costal cartilages and intervening internal intercostal muscles. After descending past the 2nd costal cartilage, the internal thoracic arteries run anterior to the transversus thoracis muscle (Figs. 1.15A and 1.19C). Between slips of the transversus thoracis muscle, the arteries contact parietal pleura posteriorly.
- Terminate in the 6th intercostal space by dividing into the *superior epigastric* and the **musculophrenic arteries.**
- Directly give rise to the anterior intercostal arteries supplying the superior 6 intercostal spaces.

Ipsilateral pairs of **anterior intercostal arteries:**

- Supply the anterior parts of the upper 9 intercostal spaces.
- Pass laterally in the intercostal space, one near the inferior margin of the superior rib and the other near the superior margin of the inferior rib.
- Of the first 2 intercostal spaces lie initially in the endothoracic fascia between the parietal pleura and the internal intercostal muscles.
- Supplying the 3rd–6th intercostal spaces are separated from the pleura by slips of the transversus thoracis muscle.
- Of the 7th–9th intercostal spaces derive from the *musculophrenic arteries,* also branches of the internal thoracic arteries.
- Supply the intercostal muscles and send branches through them to supply the pectoral muscles, breasts, and skin.
- Are absent from the inferior two intercostal spaces; these spaces are supplied only by the posterior intercostal arteries and their collateral branches.

VEINS OF THORACIC WALL

The **intercostal veins** accompany the intercostal arteries and nerves and lie most superior in the costal grooves (Figs. 1.15B and 1.20). There are 11 **posterior intercostal**

Left brachiocephalic v.
Right subclavian v.
Right brachiocephalic v.
Right superior intercostal v.
Superior vena cava (SVC)
Left superior intercostal v.
Azygos v.
Posterior intercostal v.
Internal thoracic v.
Accessory hemi-azygos v.
Anterior intercostal v.
Musculophrenic v.
Hemi-azygos v.
Superior epigastric v.
Subcostal v.
Inferior vena cava (IVC)
Diaphragm

Anterior view

FIGURE 1.20. Veins of thoracic wall. Although depicted here as continuous channels, the anterior and posterior intercostal veins are separate vessels, normally draining in opposite directions, the tributaries of which communicate (anastomose) in approximately the anterior axillary line. Because these veins lack valves, however, flow can be reversed.

veins and one **subcostal vein** on each side. The posterior intercostal veins anastomose with the **anterior intercostal veins** (tributaries of internal thoracic veins). As they approach the vertebral column, the posterior intercostal veins receive a *posterior branch*, which accompanies the posterior ramus of the spinal nerve of that level, and an *intervertebral vein* draining the vertebral venous plexuses associated with the vertebral column. Most posterior intercostal veins (4–11) end in the *azygos/hemi-azygos venous system*, which conveys venous blood to the superior vena cava (SVC). The posterior intercostal veins of the 1st intercostal space usually enter directly into the right and left brachiocephalic veins. The posterior intercostal veins of the 2nd and 3rd (and occasionally 4th) intercostal spaces unite to form a trunk, the *superior intercostal vein* (Fig. 1.20).

The **right superior intercostal vein** is typically the final tributary of the *azygos vein*, before it enters the SVC. The **left superior intercostal vein,** however, usually empties into the *left brachiocephalic vein*. This requires the vein to pass anteriorly along the left side of the superior mediastinum, specifically across the arch of the aorta or the root of the great vessels arising from it, and between the vagus and phrenic nerves (see Fig. 1.70B). It usually receives the left bronchial veins and may receive the left pericardiacophrenic vein as well. Typically, it communicates inferiorly with the *accessory hemi-azygos vein*. The **internal thoracic veins** are the companion veins (L. *venae comitantes*) of the internal thoracic arteries.

MUSCLES AND NEUROVASCULATURE OF THORACIC WALL

Dyspnea: Difficult Breathing

When people with respiratory problems (e.g., *asthma*) or with *heart failure* have difficulty breathing (*dypsnia*), they use their accessory respiratory muscles to assist the expansion of their thoracic cavity. They lean on their knees or on the arms of a chair to fix their pectoral girdle, so these muscles are able to act on their rib attachments and expand the thorax.

Extrapleural Intrathoracic Surgical Access

Fixation makes it difficult to appreciate in the embalmed cadaver, but in surgery the relatively loose nature of the thin endothoracic fascia provides a natural cleavage plane, allowing the surgeon to separate the costal parietal pleura lining the lung cavity from the thoracic wall. This allows *intrathoracic access to extrapleural structures* (e.g., lymph nodes) and instrument placement without opening and perhaps contaminating the potential space (pleural cavity) that surrounds the lungs.

Herpes Zoster Infection of Spinal Ganglia

A *herpes zoster infection* causes a classic, dermatomally distributed skin lesion—*shingles*—an agonizingly painful condition (Fig. B1.3). Herpes zoster is primarily a viral disease of spinal ganglia, usually a reactivation of the varicella-zoster virus (VZV), or

FIGURE B1.3. Herpes zoster.

chickenpox virus. After invading a ganglion, the virus produces a sharp burning pain in the dermatome supplied by the involved nerve (Fig. 1.18). The affected skin area becomes red, and vesicular eruptions appear. The pain may precede or follow the skin eruptions. Although primarily a *sensory neuropathy* (pathological change in the nerve), weakness from motor involvement occurs in 0.5–5.0% of people, commonly in elderly cancer patients (Rowland, 2010). Muscular weakness usually occurs in the same myotomal distribution, as do the dermatomal pain and vesicular eruptions.

Intercostal Nerve Block

Local anesthesia of an intercostal space is produced by injecting an anesthetic agent around the intercostal nerves between the paravertebral line and the area of required anesthesia. This procedure, an *intercostal nerve block*, involves infiltration of the anesthetic around the intercostal nerve trunk and its collateral branches (Fig. B1.4). The term *block* indicates that the nerve endings in the skin and transmission of impulses through the sensory nerves carrying information about pain are interrupted (blocked)

FIGURE B1.4. Intercostal nerve block.

before the impulses reach the spinal cord and brain. Because any particular area of skin usually receives innervation from two adjacent nerves, considerable overlapping of contiguous dermatomes occurs. Therefore, complete loss of sensation usually does not occur unless two or more intercostal nerves are anesthetized.

The Bottom Line

MUSCLES AND NEUROVASCULATURE OF THORACIC WALL

Muscles of thoracic wall: The thorax is overlapped by the axio-appendicular muscles of the upper limb as well as some neck, back, and abdominal muscles. ♦ Most of these muscles can affect deep respiration when the pectoral girdle is fixed and account for many of the surface features of the thoracic region. The muscles that are truly thoracic, however, provide few if any surface features.
♦ The serratus posterior muscles are thin with small bellies that may be proprioceptive organs. ♦ The costal muscles can move the ribs during forced respiration. The costal muscles function primarily to support (provide tonus for) the intercostal spaces, resisting negative and positive intrathoracic pressures. ♦ The diaphragm is the primary muscle of respiration, responsible for most of inspiration (normally expiration is mostly passive).
♦ Deep fascia overlies and invests the muscles of the thoracic wall, as it does elsewhere. ♦ Where the fleshy portions of the intercostal muscles are absent, their fascia is continued as intercostal membranes so that the wall is complete. ♦ The endothoracic fascia is a thin, fibro-areolar layer between the internal aspect of the

thoracic cage and the lining of the pulmonary cavities, which can be opened surgically to gain access to intrathoracic structures.

Neurovasculature of thoracic wall: The pattern of distribution of neurovascular structures to the thoracic wall reflects the construction of the thoracic cage. ♦ These neurovascular structures course in the intercostal spaces, parallel to the ribs, and serve the intercostal muscles as well as the integument and parietal pleura on their superficial and deep aspects.
♦ Because plexus formation does not occur in relationship to the thoracic wall, the pattern of peripheral and segmental (dermatomal) innervation is identical in this region. ♦ The intercostal nerves run a posterior to anterior course along the length of each intercostal space, and the anterior and posterior intercostal arteries and veins converge toward and anastomose in approximately the anterior axillary line. ♦ The posterior vessels arise from the thoracic aorta and drain to the azygos venous system. ♦ The anterior vessels arise from the internal thoracic artery, branches, and tributaries and drain to the internal thoracic vein, branches, and tributaries.

Breasts

The breasts are the most prominent superficial structures in the anterior thoracic wall, especially in women. The **breasts** (L. *mammae*) consist of glandular and supporting fibrous tissue embedded within a fatty matrix, together with blood vessels, lymphatics, and nerves. Both men and women have breasts; normally they are well developed only in women (Figs. 1.21 and 1.22). The **mammary glands** are in the subcutaneous tissue overlying the pectoralis major and minor muscles. At the greatest prominence of the breast is the *nipple,* surrounded by a circular pigmented area of skin, the **areola** (L. small area).

The mammary glands within the breasts are accessory to reproduction in women. They are rudimentary and functionless in men, consisting of only a few small ducts or epithelial cords. Usually, the fat present in male breasts is not different from that of subcutaneous tissue elsewhere, and the glandular system does not normally develop.

FEMALE BREASTS

The amount of fat surrounding the glandular tissue determines the size of non-lactating breasts. The roughly circular body of the female breast rests on a **bed of the breast** that extends transversely from the lateral border of the sternum to the midaxillary line and vertically from the 2nd through 6th ribs. Two thirds of the bed are formed by the *pectoral fascia* overlying the pectoralis major; the other third, by the fascia covering the serratus anterior. Between the breast and the pectoral fascia is a loose subcutaneous tissue plane or

FIGURE 1.22. Sagittal section of female breast and anterior thoracic wall. The superior two thirds of the figure demonstrates the suspensory ligaments and alveoli of the breast with resting lobules of mammary gland; the inferior part shows lactating lobules of mammary gland.

potential space—the **retromammary space** (bursa). This plane, containing a small amount of fat, allows the breast some degree of movement on the pectoral fascia. A small part of the mammary gland may extend along the inferolateral edge of the pectoralis major toward the axillary fossa (armpit), forming an **axillary process** or tail (of Spence). Some women discover this (especially when it may enlarge during a menstrual cycle) and become concerned that it may be a lump (tumor) or enlarged lymph nodes.

The mammary glands are firmly attached to the dermis of the overlying skin, especially by substantial skin ligaments (L. *retinacula cutis*), the **suspensory ligaments** (of Cooper). These condensations of fibrous connective tissue, particularly well developed in the superior part of the gland, help support the *lobes* and *lobules of the mammary gland.*

During puberty (ages 8–15 years), the breasts normally enlarge, owing in part to glandular development but primarily from increased fat deposition. The areolae and nipples also enlarge. Breast size and shape are determined in part by genetic, ethnic, and dietary factors. The **lactiferous ducts** give rise to buds that develop into 15–20 **lobules of the mammary gland,** which constitute the **parenchyma** (functional substance) of the mammary gland. Thus each lobule is drained by a lactiferous duct, all of which converge to open independently. Each duct has a dilated portion deep to the areola, the **lactiferous sinus,** in which a small droplet of milk accumulates or remains in the nursing mother. As the neonate begins to suckle, compression of the areola (and lactiferous sinus beneath it) expresses the accumulated droplets and encourages the neonate to continue nursing as the hormonally mediated *let-down reflex* ensues. The mother's milk is secreted into—not sucked from the gland by—the baby's mouth.

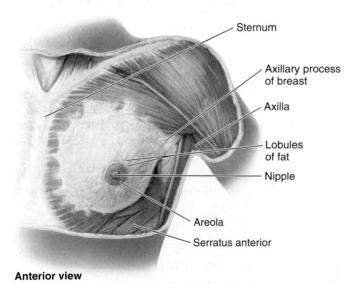

Anterior view

FIGURE 1.21. Superficial dissection of female pectoral region. The pectoral fascia has been removed, except where it lies deep to the breast. The bed of the breast extends from the 2nd through the 6th ribs. The axillary process of the breast extends toward or into the axillary fossa.

The areolae contain numerous **sebaceous glands,** which enlarge during pregnancy and secrete an oily substance that provides a protective lubricant for the areola and nipple. The areola and nipple are particularly subject to chaffing and irritation as mother and baby begin the nursing experience. The **nipples** are conical or cylindrical prominences in the centers of the areolae. The nipples have no fat, hair, or sweat glands. The tips of the nipples are fissured with the lactiferous ducts opening into them. The nipples are composed mostly of circularly arranged smooth muscle fibers that compress the lactiferous ducts during lactation and erect the nipples in response to stimulation, as when a baby begins to suckle.

The mammary glands are modified sweat glands; therefore, they have no capsule or sheath. The rounded contour and most of the volume of the breasts are produced by subcutaneous fat, except during pregnancy when the mammary glands enlarge and new glandular tissue forms. The milk-secreting **alveoli** (L. small hollow spaces) are arranged in grape-like clusters. In most women, the breasts enlarge slightly during the menstrual period from increased release of gonadotropic hormones—follicle-stimulating hormone (FSH) and luteinizing hormone (LH)—on the glandular tissue.

VASCULATURE OF BREAST

The *arterial supply of the breast* (Fig. 1.23A & B) derives from the:

- **Medial mammary branches of perforating branches** and *anterior intercostal branches of the internal thoracic artery,* originating from the subclavian artery.
- *Lateral thoracic* and *thoraco-acromial arteries,* branches of the axillary artery.
- *Posterior intercostal arteries,* branches of the thoracic aorta in the 2nd, 3rd, and 4th intercostal spaces.

The *venous drainage of the breast* is mainly to the *axillary vein,* but there is some drainage to the internal thoracic vein (Fig. 1.23C).

The *lymphatic drainage of the breast* is important because of its role in the metastasis of cancer cells. Lymph passes from the nipple, areola, and lobules of the gland to the **subareolar lymphatic plexus** (Fig. 1.24A & B). From this plexus:

- Most lymph (>75%), especially from the lateral breast quadrants, drains to the *axillary lymph nodes,* initially to the *anterior* or *pectoral nodes* for the most part. However, some lymph may drain directly to other axillary nodes or even to interpectoral, deltopectoral, supraclavicular, or inferior deep cervical nodes. (The axillary lymph nodes are covered in detail in Chapter 6.)
- Most of the remaining lymph, particularly from the medial breast quadrants, drains to the *parasternal lymph nodes* or to the opposite breast, whereas lymph from the inferior quadrants may pass deeply to abdominal lymph nodes (subdiaphragmatic *inferior phrenic lymph nodes*).

Lymph from the skin of the breast, except the nipple and areola, drains into the ipsilateral axillary, inferior deep cervical, and infraclavicular lymph nodes and into the parasternal lymph nodes of both sides.

Lymph from the axillary nodes drains into *clavicular* (*infraclavicular* and *supraclavicular*) *lymph nodes* and from them into the *subclavian lymphatic trunk,* which also drains lymph from the upper limb. Lymph from the parasternal nodes enters the *bronchomediastinal lymphatic trunks,* which also drain lymph from the thoracic viscera. The termination of the lymphatic trunks varies; traditionally, these trunks are described as merging with each other and with the *jugular lymphatic trunk,* draining the head and neck to form a short *right lymphatic duct* on the right side or entering the termination at the *thoracic duct* on the left side. However, in many (perhaps most) cases, the trunks open independently into the junction of the internal jugular and subclavian veins, the *right or left venous angles,* that form the *right* and *left brachiocephalic veins* (Fig. 1.24C). In some cases, they open into both contributing veins immediately prior to the angle.

NERVES OF BREAST

The *nerves of the breast* derive from *anterior and lateral cutaneous branches of the 4th–6th intercostal nerves* (Fig. 1.15). The branches of the intercostal nerves pass through the pectoral fascia covering the pectoralis major to reach overlying subcutaneous tissue and skin of the breast. The branches of the intercostal nerves convey sensory fibers from the skin of the breast and sympathetic fibers to the blood vessels in the breasts and smooth muscle in the overlying skin and nipple.

Surface Anatomy of Thoracic Wall

The *clavicles* (collar bones) lie subcutaneously, forming bony ridges at the junction of the thorax and neck (Fig. 1.25). They can be palpated easily throughout their length, especially where their medial ends articulate with the manubrium of the sternum. The clavicles demarcate the superior division between zones of lymphatic drainage: above the clavicles, lymph flows ultimately to inferior jugular lymph nodes; below them, parietal lymph (that from the body wall and upper limbs) flows to the axillary lymph nodes.

The *sternum* (breastbone) lies subcutaneously in the anterior median line and is palpable throughout its length. Between the prominences of the medial ends of the clavicles at the sternoclavicular joints, the *jugular notch* in the manubrium can be palpated between the prominent medial ends of the clavicles. The notch lies at the level of the inferior border of the body of T2 vertebra and the space between the 1st and 2nd thoracic spinous processes.

The *manubrium,* approximately 4 cm long, lies at the level of the bodies of T3 and T4 vertebrae (Fig. 1.26). The *sternal angle* is palpable and often visible in young people because of the slight movement that occurs at the manubriosternal joint during forced respiration. The sternal angle lies at the level

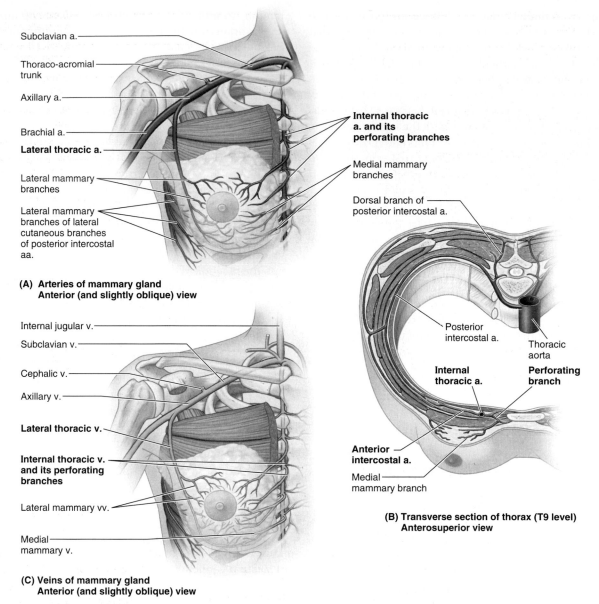

Subclavian a.

Thoraco-acromial trunk

Axillary a.

Brachial a.

Lateral thoracic a.

Lateral mammary branches

Lateral mammary branches of lateral cutaneous branches of posterior intercostal aa.

Internal thoracic a. and its perforating branches

Medial mammary branches

(A) Arteries of mammary gland Anterior (and slightly oblique) view

Dorsal branch of posterior intercostal a.

Posterior intercostal a.

Thoracic aorta

Internal thoracic a.

Perforating branch

Anterior intercostal a.

Medial mammary branch

(B) Transverse section of thorax (T9 level) Anterosuperior view

Internal jugular v.

Subclavian v.

Cephalic v.

Axillary v.

Lateral thoracic v.

Internal thoracic v. and its perforating branches

Lateral mammary vv.

Medial mammary v.

(C) Veins of mammary gland Anterior (and slightly oblique) view

FIGURE 1.23. Vasculature of breast. A. The mammary gland is supplied from its medial aspect mainly by perforating branches of the internal thoracic artery and by several branches of the axillary artery (principally the lateral thoracic artery) superiorly and laterally. **B.** The breast is supplied deeply by branches arising from the intercostal arteries. **C.** Venous drainage is to the axillary vein (mainly) and the internal thoracic veins. [a., artery; v., vein; vv. veins]

of the T4–T5 IV disc and the space between the 3rd and 4th thoracic spinous processes. The sternal angle marks the level of the 2nd pair of costal cartilages. The left side of the manubrium is anterior to the arch of the aorta, and its right side directly overlies the merging of the brachiocephalic veins to form the *superior vena cava* (SVC) (Fig. 1.24C). Because it is common clinical practice to insert catheters into the SVC for intravenous feeding of extremely ill patients and for other purposes, it is essential to know the surface anatomy of this large vein. The SVC passes inferiorly deep to the manubrium and manubriosternal junction but projects as much as a fingerbreadth to the right of the margin of the manubrium. The SVC enters the right atrium of the heart opposite the right 3rd costal cartilage.

The *body of the sternum,* approximately 10 cm long, lies anterior to the right border of the heart and vertebrae T5–T9 (Fig. 1.26). The **intermammary cleft** (midline depression or cleavage between the mature female breasts) overlies the sternal body (Figs. 1.25 & 1.29). The *xiphoid process* lies in a slight depression, the **epigastric fossa.** This fossa is used as a guide in cardiopulmonary resuscitation (CPR) to properly position the hand on the inferior part of the sternum. The *xiphisternal joint* is palpable and is often seen as a ridge, at the level of the inferior border of T9 vertebra.

The *costal margins,* formed by the joined costal cartilages of the 7th–10th ribs, are easily palpable because they extend inferolaterally from the xiphisternal joint. The converging right and left costal margins form the *infrasternal angle.*

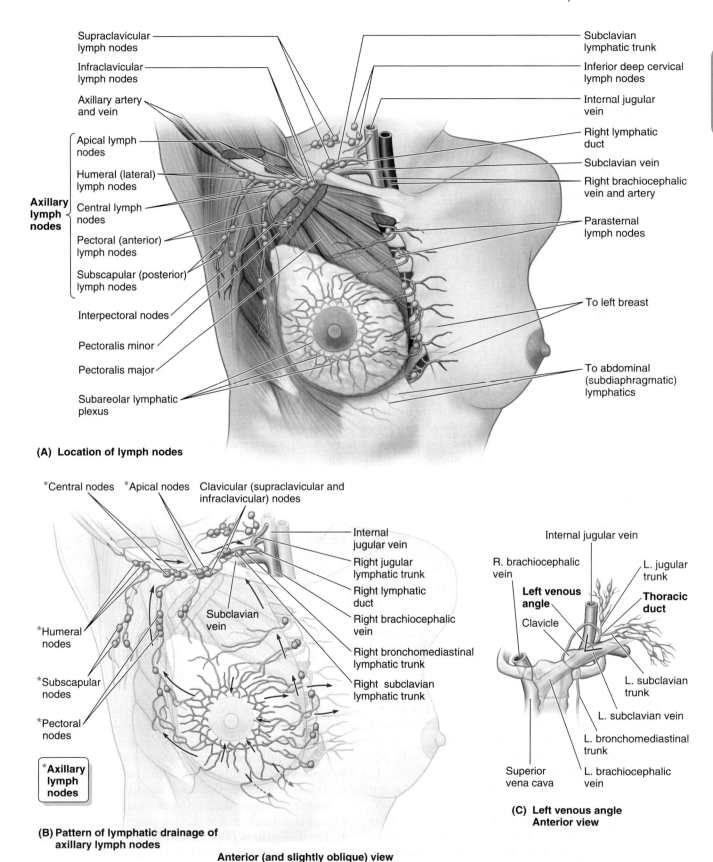

(A) Location of lymph nodes

Supraclavicular lymph nodes

Infraclavicular lymph nodes

Axillary artery and vein

Axillary lymph nodes

Apical lymph nodes

Humeral (lateral) lymph nodes

Central lymph nodes

Pectoral (anterior) lymph nodes

Subscapular (posterior) lymph nodes

Interpectoral nodes

Pectoralis minor

Pectoralis major

Subareolar lymphatic plexus

Subclavian lymphatic trunk

Inferior deep cervical lymph nodes

Internal jugular vein

Right lymphatic duct

Subclavian vein

Right brachiocephalic vein and artery

Parasternal lymph nodes

To left breast

To abdominal (subdiaphragmatic) lymphatics

(B) Pattern of lymphatic drainage of axillary lymph nodes

*Central nodes   *Apical nodes   Clavicular (supraclavicular and infraclavicular) nodes

*Humeral nodes

*Subscapular nodes

*Pectoral nodes

*Axillary lymph nodes

Subclavian vein

Internal jugular vein

Right jugular lymphatic trunk

Right lymphatic duct

Right brachiocephalic vein

Right bronchomediastinal lymphatic trunk

Right subclavian lymphatic trunk

(C) Left venous angle Anterior view

Internal jugular vein

R. brachiocephalic vein

Left venous angle

Clavicle

L. jugular trunk

Thoracic duct

L. subclavian trunk

L. subclavian vein

L. bronchomediastinal trunk

Superior vena cava

L. brachiocephalic vein

Anterior (and slightly oblique) view

FIGURE 1.24. Lymphatic drainage of breast. A. The lymph nodes receiving drainage from the breast. **B.** The *red arrows* indicate lymph flow from the right breast. Most lymph, especially that from the superior lateral quadrant and center of the breast, drains to the axillary lymph nodes, which, in turn, are drained by the subclavian lymphatic trunk. On the right side, it enters the venous system via the right lymphatic duct. **C.** Most lymph from the left breast returns to the venous system via the thoracic duct.

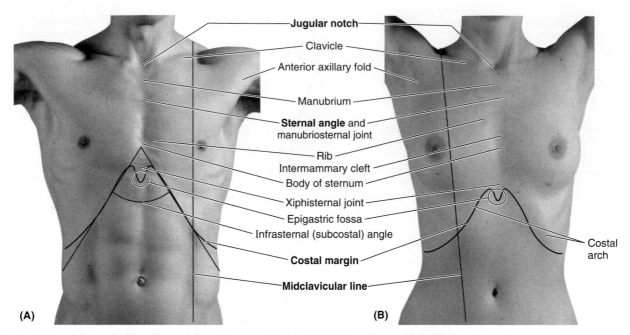

FIGURE 1.25. Surface features of anterior thoracic wall.

The *ribs* and *intercostal spaces* provide a basis for locating or describing the position of structures or sites of trauma or pathology on or deep to the thoracic wall. Because the 1st rib is not palpable, rib counting in physical examinations starts with the 2nd rib adjacent to the subcutaneous and easily palpated sternal angle. To count the ribs and intercostal spaces anteriorly, slide the fingers (digits) laterally from the sternal angle onto the 2nd costal cartilage and begin counting the ribs and spaces by moving the fingers from here. The 1st intercostal space is that superior to the 2nd costal cartilage—that is, intercostal spaces are numbered according to the rib forming their superior boundary. Generally, it is more reliable to count intercostal spaces, since the fingertip tends to rest in (slip into) the gaps between the ribs. One finger should remain in place while another is used to locate the next space. Using all the fingers, it is possible to locate four spaces at a time. The spaces are widest anterolaterally (approximately in the midclavicular line). If the fingers are removed from the thoracic wall while counting spaces, the finger may easily be returned to the same space, mistaking it for the one below. Posteriorly, the medial end of the spine of the scapula overlies the 4th rib.

While the ribs and/or intercostal spaces provide the "latitude" for navigation and localization on the thoracic wall, several imaginary lines facilitate anatomical and clinical descriptions by providing "longitude." The following lines are extrapolated over the thoracic wall based on visible or palpable superficial features:

- The **anterior median (midsternal) line** (AML) indicates the intersection of the median plane with the anterior thoracic wall (Fig. 1.27A).
- The **midclavicular line** (MCL) passes through the midpoint of the clavicle, parallel to the AML.
- The **anterior axillary line** (AAL) runs vertically along the anterior axillary fold that is formed by the inferolateral border of the pectoralis major as it spans from the thoracic cage to the humerus in the arm (Figs. 1.27B).
- The **midaxillary line** (MAL) runs from the apex (deepest part) of the axillary fossa (armpit), parallel to the AAL.
- The **posterior axillary line** (PAL), also parallel to the AAL, is drawn vertically along the posterior axillary fold formed by the latissimus dorsi and teres major muscles as they span from the back to the humerus.

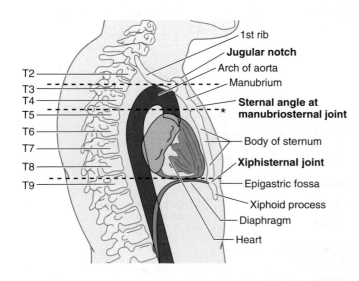

*** Transverse thoracic plane**

FIGURE 1.26. Vertebral levels of sternum and transverse thoracic plane.

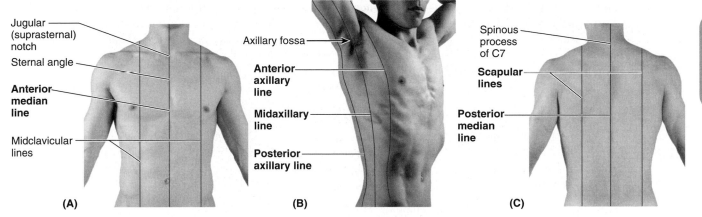

FIGURE 1.27. Vertical lines of thoracic wall.

- The **posterior median (midvertebral) line** (PML) is a vertical line along the tips of the spinous processes of the vertebrae (Fig. 1.27C).
- The **scapular lines** (SLs) are parallel to the posterior median line and intersect the inferior angles of the scapula.

Additional lines (not illustrated) are extrapolated along the borders of palpable bony formations such as the sternum and vertebral column, such as the parasternal and paravertebral lines (G. *para,* alongside of, adjacent to).

Breasts are the most prominent surface features of the anterior thoracic wall, especially in women. Except when there is an overabundance of subcutaneous tissue, the breasts in men are mostly an accentuation of the contour of the *pectoralis major muscles,* highlighted by the presence of the nipple in the 4th intercostal space, lateral to the MCL (Fig. 1.28). In moderately athletic individuals, the contour of the pectoralis major muscles is apparent, separated in the midline by the intermammary cleft overlying the sternum, with the lateral border forming the *anterior axillary fold* (Fig. 1.25). Inferolaterally, finger-like slips, or **digitations of the serratus anterior,** have a serrated (sawtooth) appearance as they attach to the ribs and interdigitate with the *external oblique* (Fig. 1.28).

The *inferior ribs* and *costal margins* are often apparent, especially when the abdominal muscles are contracted to "pull the belly in." The intercostal musculature is not normally evident; however, in (rare) cases in which there is an absence or atrophy of the intercostal musculature, the intercostal spaces become apparent with respiration: during inspiration, they are concave; during expiration, they protrude.

The female breasts vary in the size, shape, and symmetry—even in the same person. Their flattened superior surfaces show no sharp demarcation from the anterior surface of the thoracic wall, but laterally and inferiorly, their borders are well defined (Fig. 1.29). A venous pattern over the breasts is often visible, especially during pregnancy.

The *nipple* is surrounded by the slightly raised and circular pigmented *areola,* the color of which depends on the woman's complexion. The areola usually darkens during pregnancy and retains the darkened pigmentation thereafter. The areola is normally dotted with the papular (small elevated) openings of the *areolar glands* (sebaceous glands in the skin of the areola). On occasion, one or both nipples are inverted (retracted); this minor congenital anomaly may make breast feeding difficult.

FIGURE 1.28. Surface anatomy of thoracic wall musculature.

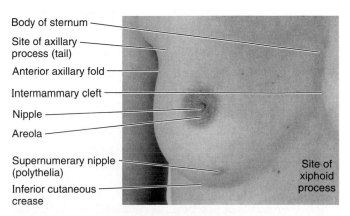

FIGURE 1.29. Surface anatomy of female breast.

In men and young *nulliparous women*—those who have never borne a viable child—with moderate breast size, the nipple lies anterior to the 4th intercostal space, approximately 10 cm from the AML. Usually, however, the position of nipples varies considerably with breast size, especially in *multiparous women*—those who have given birth to two or more children. Consequently, because of variations in size and shape, the nipples are not a reliable guide to the 4th intercostal spaces in adult females.

BREASTS

Changes in Breasts

Changes in breast tissue, such as branching of the lactiferous ducts, occur during menstrual periods and pregnancy. Although mammary glands are prepared for secretion by midpregnancy, they do not produce milk until shortly after the baby is born. *Colostrum,* a creamy white to yellowish premilk fluid, may secrete from the nipples during the last trimester of pregnancy and during initial episodes of nursing. Colostrum is believed to be especially rich in protein, immune agents, and a growth factor affecting the infant's intestines. In multiparous women (those who have given birth two or more times), the breasts often become large and pendulous. The breasts in elderly women are usually small because of the decrease in fat and the atrophy of glandular tissue.

Breast Quadrants

For the anatomical location and description of tumors and cysts, the surface of the breast is divided into *four quadrants* (Fig. B1.5). For example, a physician's record might state: "A hard irregular mass was felt in the superior medial quadrant of the breast at the 2 o'clock position, approximately 2.5 cm from the margin of the areola."

Right breast

FIGURE B1.5. Breast quadrants.

Carcinoma of the Breast

Understanding the lymphatic drainage of the breasts is of practical importance in predicting the metastases (dispersal) of cancer cells from a *carci-noma of the breast* (breast cancer). Carcinomas of the breast are malignant tumors, usually *adenocarcinomas* (glandular cancer) arising from the epithelial cells of the lactiferous ducts in the mammary gland lobules (Fig. B1.6A). Metastatic cancer cells that enter a lymphatic vessel usually pass through two or three groups of lymph nodes before entering the venous system.

Interference with the lymphatic drainage by cancer may cause *lymphedema* (*edema,* excess fluid in the subcutaneous tissue), which in turn may result in deviation of the nipple and a thickened, leather-like appearance of the skin. Prominent "puffy" skin between dimpled pores give it an orange-peel appearance (*peau d'orange sign*). Larger dimples (fingertip size or bigger) result from cancerous invasion of the glandular tissue and fibrosis (fibrous degeneration), which causes shortening or places traction on the suspensory ligaments. *Subareolar breast cancer* may cause retraction of the nipple by a similar mechanism involving the lactiferous ducts.

Breast cancer typically spreads by means of lymphatic vessels (*lymphogenic metastasis*), which carry cancer cells from the breast to the lymph nodes, chiefly those in the axilla. The cells lodge in the nodes, producing nests of tumor cells (*metastases*). Abundant communications among lymphatic pathways and among axillary, cervical, and parasternal nodes may also cause metastases from the breast to develop in the supraclavicular lymph nodes, the opposite breast, or the abdomen (Fig. 1.24A & B). Because most of lymphatic drainage of the breast is to the *axillary lymph nodes*, they are the most common site of metastasis from a breast cancer. Enlargement of these palpable nodes suggests the possibility of breast cancer and may be key to early detection. However, the absence of enlarged axillary lymph nodes is no guarantee that metastasis from a breast cancer has not occurred; the malignant cells may have passed to other nodes, such as the infraclavicular and supraclavicular lymph nodes.

The posterior intercostal veins drain into the *azygos/hemi-azygos system of veins* alongside the bodies of the vertebrae (see Fig. 1.38B) and communicate with the internal vertebral venous plexus surrounding the spinal cord. Cancer cells can also spread from the breast by these venous routes to the vertebrae, and from there to the cranium and brain. Cancer also spreads by contiguity (invasion of adjacent tissue). When breast cancer cells invade the *retromammary space* (Fig. 1.22), attach to or invade the pectoral fascia overlying the pectoralis major, or metastasize to the interpectoral nodes, the breast elevates when the muscle contracts. This movement is a clinical sign of advanced cancer of the breast.

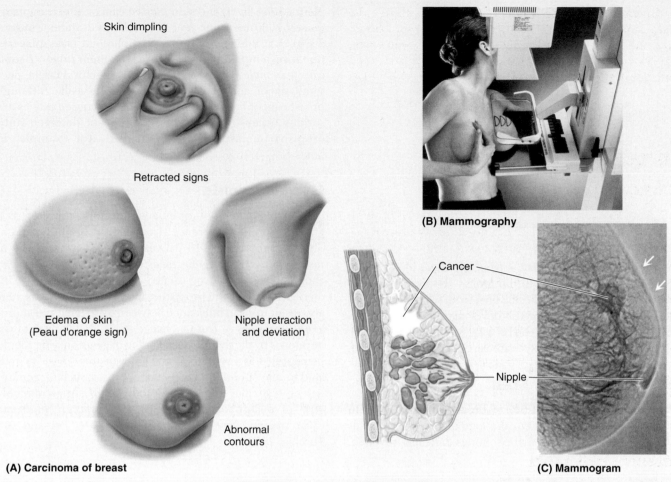

Skin dimpling

Retracted signs

Edema of skin
(Peau d'orange sign)

Nipple retraction
and deviation

Abnormal
contours

(A) Carcinoma of breast

(B) Mammography

Cancer

Nipple

(C) Mammogram

FIGURE B1.6. Detection of breast cancer.

To observe this upward movement, the physician has the patient place her hands on her hips and press while pulling her elbows forward to tense her pectoral muscles.

Mammography

Radiographic examination of the breasts, *mammography,* is one of the techniques used to detect breast masses (Fig. B1.6B). A carcinoma appears as a large, jagged density in the *mammogram.* The skin is thickened over the tumor (*upper two arrows* in Fig. B1.6C) and the nipple is depressed. Surgeons use mammography as a guide when removing breast tumors, cysts, and abscesses.

Surgical Incisions of Breast

Surgical incisions are made in the inferior breast quadrants when possible because these quadrants are less vascular than the superior ones. The transition between the thoracic wall and breast is most abrupt inferiorly, producing a line, crease, or deep skin fold—the *inferior cutaneous crease* (Fig. 1.29). Incisions made along this crease will be least evident and may be hidden by overlap of the breast. Incisions that must be made near the areola, or on the breast itself, are usually directed

radially to either side of the nipple (Langer tension lines run transversely here) or circumferentially (Fig. I.7 in Introduction).

Mastectomy (breast excision) is not as common as it once was as a treatment for breast cancer. In *simple mastectomy,* the breast is removed down to the retromammary space. *Radical mastectomy,* a more extensive surgical procedure, involves removal of the breast, pectoral muscles, fat, fascia, and as many lymph nodes as possible in the axilla and pectoral region. In current practice, often only the tumor and surrounding tissues are removed—a *lumpectomy* or *quadrantectomy* (known as *breast-conserving surgery,* a wide local excision)—followed by radiation therapy (Goroll, 2009).

Polymastia, Polythelia, and Amastia

Polymastia (supernumerary breasts) or *polythelia* (accessory nipples) may occur superior or inferior to the normal pair, occasionally developing in the axillary fossa or anterior abdominal wall (Figs. 1.29 and B1.7). Supernumerary breasts usually consist of only a rudimentary nipple and areola, which may be mistaken for a mole (nevus) until they change pigmentation with the normal nipples during pregnancy. However, glandular tissue may also be present and further develop with lactation. These small

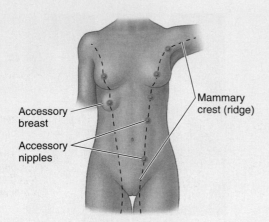

FIGURE B1.7. Polymastia and polythelia.

supernumerary breasts may appear anywhere along a line extending from the axilla to the groin—the location of the *embryonic mammary crest* (milk line) from which the breasts develop, and along which breasts develop in animals with multiple breasts. There may be no breast development (*amastia*), or there may be a nipple and/or areola, but no glandular tissue.

Breast Cancer in Men

 Approximately 1.5% of breast cancers occur in men. As in women, the cancer usually metastasizes to axillary lymph nodes but also to bone,

pleura, lung, liver, and skin. Breast cancer affects approximately 1000 men per year in the United States (Swartz, 2009). A visible and/or palpable subareolar mass or secretion from a nipple may indicate a *malignant tumor. Breast cancer in males* tends to infiltrate the pectoral fascia, pectoralis major, and apical lymph nodes in the axilla. Although breast cancer is uncommon in men, the consequences are serious because they are frequently not detected until extensive metastases have occurred—for example, in bone.

Gynecomastia

 Slight temporary enlargement of the breasts is a normal occurrence (frequency = 70%) in males at puberty (age 10–12 years). Breast hypertrophy in males after puberty (*gynecomastia*) is relatively rare (<1%) and may be age or drug related (e.g., after treatment with diethylstilbestrol for prostate cancer). Gynecomastia may also result from an imbalance between estrogenic and androgenic hormones or from a change in the metabolism of sex hormones by the liver. Thus a finding of gynecomastia should be regarded as a symptom, and an evaluation must be initiated to rule out important potential causes, such as suprarenal or testicular cancers (Goroll, 2009). Approximately 40% of postpubertal males with *Klinefelter syndrome* (XXY trisomy) have gynecomastia (Moore, Persaud and Torchia, 2012).

The Bottom Line

BREASTS AND SURFACE ANATOMY OF THORACIC WALL

Breasts: The mammary glands are in the subcutaneous tissue of the breast, overlying the pectoralis major and serratus anterior muscles and associated deep fascia (bed of the breast). ♦ Lobules of glandular tissue converge toward the nipple, each having its own lactiferous duct, which opens there. ♦ The superior lateral quadrant of the breast has the most glandular tissue, largely owing to an extension toward or into the axilla (axillary process) and, therefore, is the site of most tumors. ♦ The breast is served by the internal thoracic and lateral thoracic vessels and the 2nd–6th intercostal vessels and nerves. Most lymph from the breast drains to the axillary lymph nodes; this is significant when treating breast cancer.

♦ Because the mammary glands and axillary lymph nodes are superficial, the ability to palpate primary and metastatic tumors during routine breast examination enables early detection and treatment.

Surface anatomy of thoracic wall: The thoracic wall is especially well provided with visible and/or palpable features useful in examining the wall and underlying visceral features. ♦ Ribs and intercostal spaces, counted from the 2nd rib at the level of the sternal angle, provide latitude. ♦ Clavicles, nipples, axillary folds, scapulae, and the vertebral column provide longitude. ♦ The breasts are prominent features and, in males, the nipples demarcate the 4th intercostal space.

VISCERA OF THORACIC CAVITY

When sectioned transversely, it is apparent that the *thoracic cavity* is kidney shaped: a transversely ovoid space deeply indented posteriorly by the thoracic vertebral column and the heads and necks of the ribs that articulate with it

(Fig. 1.30A). The thoracic cavity is divided into three compartments (Figs. 1.30A & C):

• Right and left **pulmonary cavities,** bilateral compartments that contain the lungs and *pleurae* (lining membranes) and occupy the majority of the thoracic cavity.

Transverse CT scan

1 Sternum	7 Right pulmonary cavity
2 Vertebral body	8 Left pulmonary cavity
3-6 Ribs	9 Mediastinum

(A) Inferior views

Cervical pleura
Bronchial tree (representing root of lung)
Costal pleura
Pleural cavity
Visceral pleura

Trachea
Cervical pleura
*Costal part
Costal surface of left lung covered with visceral pleura
Cardiac notch
*Mediastinal part
Lingula
*Diaphragmatic part
Costodiaphragmatic recesses

(B) Anterior view

Collapsed lung

Pleural cavity
Collapsed lung
Visceral pleura
Parietal pleura
Thoracic wall lined with endothoracic fascia
Phrenico-pleural fascia (part of endothoracic fascia)

Hilum of lung (site of entry of root of lung)   **Inflated lung**
Suprapleural membrane
Cervical pleura
Mediastinal part
Costal part
Diaphragmatic part   } Parts of parietal pleura
Endothoracic fascia
Visceral pleura
Mediastinum (contains heart)
Diaphragm

Layers

▬	Visceral pleura
▬	Parietal pleura
▬	Costal pleura
▬	Diaphragmatic pleura
▬	Mediastinal pleura
▬	Cervical pleura
—	Fascial membranes (Suprapleural and mediastinal fascia, fibrous pericardium)
- - -	Endothoracic fascia
*	Parts of parietal pleura

The right and left pulmonary cavities, separated by the mediastinum, are lined with parietal pleura that reflects onto the lungs as visceral pleura.

(C) Anterior view

FIGURE 1.30. Divisions of thoracic cavity and lining of pulmonary cavities. A. The CT scan and interpretive diagram above it are transverse cross-sectional views of the thoracic cavity demonstrating its kidney-like shape, resulting from the protruding vertebral bodies, and division into three compartments. The dimensional (**B**) and coronal cross-sectional (**C**) diagrams demonstrate the linings of the pleural cavities and lungs (pleurae). Each lung is invested by the inner layer of a closed sac that has been invaginated by the lung. **Inset:** A fist invaginating an underinflated balloon demonstrates the relationship of the lung (represented by the fist) to walls of the pleural sac (parietal and visceral layers of pleura).

- A central **mediastinum,** a compartment intervening between and completely separating the two pulmonary cavities, which contains essentially all other thoracic structures—the heart, thoracic parts of the great vessels, thoracic part of the trachea, esophagus, thymus, and other structures (e.g., lymph nodes). It extends vertically from the superior thoracic aperture to the diaphragm and anteroposteriorly from the sternum to the thoracic vertebral bodies.

Pleurae, Lungs, and Tracheobronchial Tree

Each *pulmonary cavity* (right and left) is lined by a *pleural membrane* (**pleura**) that also reflects onto and covers the external surface of the lungs occupying the cavities (Fig. 1.30B & C). To visualize the relationship of the pleurae and lungs, push your fist into an underinflated balloon (Fig. 1.30C). The inner part of the balloon wall (adjacent to your fist, which represents the lung), is comparable to the *visceral pleura;* the remaining outer wall of the balloon represents the *parietal pleura.* The cavity between the layers of the balloon, here filled with air, is analogous to the pleural cavity, although the pleural cavity contains only a thin film of fluid. At your wrist (representing the root of the lung), the inner and outer walls of the balloon are continuous, as are the visceral and parietal layers of pleura, together forming a *pleural sac.* Note that the lung is outside of but surrounded by the pleural sac, just as your fist is surrounded by but outside of the balloon.

The inset in Figure 1.30C is also helpful in understanding the development of the lungs and pleurae. During the embryonic period, the developing lungs invaginate (grow into) the **pericardioperitoneal canals,** the precursors of the pleural cavities. The invaginated *coelomic epithelium* covers the primordia of the lungs and becomes the visceral pleura in the same way that the balloon covers your fist. The epithelium lining the walls of the pericardioperitoneal canals forms the parietal pleura. During embryogenesis, the pleural cavities become separated from the pericardial and peritoneal cavities.

PLEURAE

Each lung is invested by and enclosed in a serous **pleural sac** that consists of two continuous membranes: the *visceral pleura,* which invests all surfaces of the lungs forming their shiny outer surface, and the *parietal pleura,* which lines the pulmonary cavities (Fig. 1.30B & C).

The **pleural cavity**—the potential space between the layers of pleura—contains a capillary layer of **serous pleural fluid,** which lubricates the pleural surfaces and allows the layers of pleura to slide smoothly over each other during respiration. The surface tension of the pleural fluid provides the cohesion that keeps the lung surface in contact with the thoracic wall; consequently, the lung expands and fills with air

when the thorax expands while still allowing sliding to occur, much like a film of water between two glass plates.

The **visceral pleura** (pulmonary pleura) closely covers the lung and adheres to all its surfaces, including those within the horizontal and oblique fissures (Figs. 1.30B & C and 1.31A). In cadaver dissection, the visceral pleura cannot usually be dissected from the surface of the lung. It provides the lung with a smooth slippery surface, enabling it to move freely on the parietal pleura. The visceral pleura is continuous with the parietal pleura at the **hilum of the lung,** where structures making up the *root of the lung* (e.g., bronchus and pulmonary vessels) enter and leave the lung (Fig. 1.30C).

The **parietal pleura** lines the pulmonary cavities, thereby adhering to the thoracic wall, mediastinum, and diaphragm. It is thicker than the visceral pleura, and during surgery and cadaver dissections, it may be separated from the surfaces it covers. The parietal pleura consists of three *parts—costal, mediastinal,* and *diaphragmatic—*and the *cervical pleura.*

The **costal part of the parietal pleura** (costovertebral or costal pleura) covers the internal surfaces of the thoracic wall (Figs. 1.30B & C and 1.32). It is separated from the internal surface of the thoracic wall (sternum, ribs and costal cartilages, intercostal muscles and membranes, and sides of thoracic vertebrae) by *endothoracic fascia.* This thin, extrapleural layer of loose connective tissue forms a natural cleavage plane for surgical separation of the costal pleura from the thoracic wall (see the blue box "Extrapleural Intrathoracic Surgical Access," p. 96).

The **mediastinal part of the parietal pleura** (mediastinal pleura) covers the lateral aspects of the mediastinum, the partition of tissues and organs separating the pulmonary cavities and their pleural sacs. It continues superiorly into the root of the neck as cervical pleura. It is continuous with costal pleura anteriorly and posteriorly, and with the diaphragmatic pleura inferiorly. Superior to the root of the lung, the mediastinal pleura is a continuous sheet passing anteroposteriorly between the sternum and the vertebral column. At the *hilum of the lung,* it is the mediastinal pleura that reflects laterally onto the root of the lung to become continuous with the visceral pleura.

The **diaphragmatic part of the parietal pleura** (diaphragmatic pleura) covers the superior (thoracic) surface of the diaphragm on each side of the mediastinum, except along its costal attachments (origins) and where the diaphragm is fused to the *pericardium,* the fibroserous membrane surrounding the heart (Figs. 1.30B & C and 1.32). A thin, more elastic layer of endothoracic fascia, the **phrenicopleural fascia,** connects the diaphragmatic pleura with the muscular fibers of the diaphragm (Fig. 1.30C).

The **cervical pleura** covers the apex of the lung (the part of the lung extending superiorly through the superior thoracic aperture into the root of the neck—Figs. 1.30B & C and 1.31A). It is a superior continuation of the costal and mediastinal parts of the parietal pleura. The cervical pleura forms a cup-like dome (**pleural cupula**) over the apex that reaches its summit 2–3 cm superior to the level of the

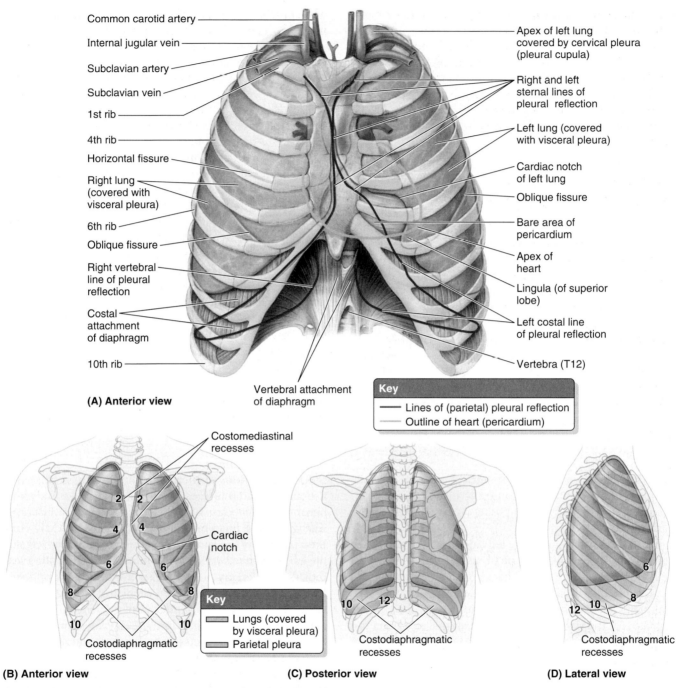

(A) Anterior view

Common carotid artery

Internal jugular vein

Subclavian artery

Subclavian vein

1st rib

4th rib

Horizontal fissure

Right lung (covered with visceral pleura)

6th rib

Oblique fissure

Right vertebral line of pleural reflection

Costal attachment of diaphragm

10th rib

Vertebral attachment of diaphragm

Apex of left lung covered by cervical pleura (pleural cupula)

Right and left sternal lines of pleural reflection

Left lung (covered with visceral pleura)

Cardiac notch of left lung

Oblique fissure

Bare area of pericardium

Apex of heart

Lingula (of superior lobe)

Left costal line of pleural reflection

Vertebra (T12)

Key
— Lines of (parietal) pleural reflection
— Outline of heart (pericardium)

Costomediastinal recesses

2 2

4 4

6 6

8 8

10 10

Cardiac notch

Key
▭ Lungs (covered by visceral pleura)
▭ Parietal pleura

Costodiaphragmatic recesses

(B) Anterior view

10 12

Costodiaphragmatic recesses

(C) Posterior view

6

8

12 10

Costodiaphragmatic recesses

(D) Lateral view

FIGURE 1.31. Relationship of thoracic contents and linings of thoracic cage. A. The apices of the lungs and cervical pleura extend into the neck. The left sternal reflection of parietal pleura and anterior border of the left lung deviate from the median plane, circumventing the area where the heart is, lies adjacent to the anterior thoracic wall. In this "bare area" the pericardial sac is accessible for needle puncture with less risk of puncturing the pleural cavity or lung. **B–D.** The shapes of the lungs and the larger pleural sacs that surround them during quiet respiration are demonstrated. The costodiaphragmatic recesses, not occupied by lung, are where pleural exudate accumulates when the body is erect. The outline of the horizontal fissure of the right lung clearly parallels the 4th rib. The ribs are identified by number.

medial third of the clavicle at the level of the neck of the 1st rib. The cervical pleura is reinforced by a fibrous extension of the endothoracic fascia, the **suprapleural membrane** (Sibson fascia). The membrane attaches to the internal border of the 1st rib and the transverse process of C7 vertebra (Fig. 1.30C).

The relatively abrupt lines along which the parietal pleura changes direction as it passes (reflects) from one wall of the pleural cavity to another are the *lines of pleural reflection* (Figs. 1.31 and 1.32). Three lines of pleural reflection outline the extent of the pulmonary cavities on each side: *sternal, costal,* and *diaphragmatic.* The outlines of the right and

Bare area of pericardium
Costomediastinal recess
Sternal reflection of left pleura
Fat pad
Left phrenic nerve
Pericardial sac fused with central tendon
Esophagus
Central tendon of diaphragm
Aorta
Diaphragmatic part*
Costodiaphragmatic recess
Costal part*

Superior view

Sternal reflection of right pleura
Internal thoracic vessels
Transversus thoracis muscle
External oblique
Diaphragmatic part*
Right phrenic nerve
Inferior vena cava
Central tendon
Thoracic duct
Azygos vein
Splanchnic nerve
Sympathetic trunk
Latissimus dorsi m.
Serratus posterior inferior m.

* of parietal pleura

FIGURE 1.32. Diaphragm, base of pulmonary cavities and mediastinum, and costodiaphragmatic recesses. Most of the diaphragmatic pleura has been removed. At this level, the mediastinum consists of the pericardial sac (middle mediastinum) and the posterior mediastinum, mainly containing the esophagus and aorta. The deep groove surrounding the convexity of the diaphragm is the costodiaphragmatic recess, lined with parietal pleura. Anteriorly at this level, the pericardium and costomediastinal recesses and, between the sternal reflections of pleura, an area of pericardium only (the bare area) lie between the heart and the thoracic wall.

left pulmonary cavities are asymmetrical (i.e., are not mirror images of each other) because the heart is turned and extends toward the left side, imposing on the left cavity more markedly than on the right.

Deviation of the heart to the left side primarily affects the **right** and **left sternal lines of pleural reflection,** which are asymmetrical. The sternal lines are sharp or abrupt and occur where the costal pleura is continuous with the mediastinal pleura anteriorly. Starting superiorly from the cupulae (Fig. 1.31A), the right and left lines of sternal reflection run inferomedially, passing posterior to the sternoclavicular joints to meet at the anterior median line (AML), posterior to the sternum at the level of its sternal angle. Between the levels of costal cartilages 2–4, the right and left lines descend in contact. The pleural sacs may even slightly overlap each other.

The *sternal line of pleural reflection on the right side* continues to pass inferiorly in the AML to the posterior aspect of the xiphoid process (level of the 6th costal cartilage), where it turns laterally (Fig. 1.31). The *sternal line of reflection on the left side*, however, descends in the AML only to the level of the 4th costal cartilage. Here it passes to the left margin of the sternum and continues inferiorly to the 6th costal cartilage, creating a shallow notch as it runs lateral to an area of direct contact between the pericardium (heart sac) and the anterior thoracic wall. This shallow notch in the pleural sac, and the "bare area" of pericardial contact with the anterior wall, are important for *pericardiocentesis* (see blue box, "Pericardiocentesis," later in this chapter).

The **costal lines of pleural reflection** are sharp continuations of the sternal lines, occurring where the costal pleura becomes continuous with diaphragmatic pleura inferiorly. The right costal line proceeds laterally from the AML. However, because of the bare area of pericardium on the left side, the left costal line begins at the midclavicular line; otherwise, the right and left costal lines are symmetrical as they proceed laterally, posteriorly, and then medially, passing obliquely across the 8th rib in the midclavicular line (MCL) and the 10th rib in the midaxillary line (MAL), becoming continuous posteriorly with the vertebral lines at the necks of the 12th ribs inferior to them.

The **vertebral lines of pleural reflection** are much rounder, gradual reflections and occur where the costal pleura becomes continuous with the mediastinal pleura posteriorly. The vertebral lines of pleural reflection parallel the vertebral column, running in the paravertebral planes from vertebral level T1 through T12, where they become continuous with the costal lines.

The lungs do not fully occupy the pulmonary cavities during expiration; thus the peripheral diaphragmatic pleura is in contact with the lowermost parts of the costal pleura. The potential pleural spaces here are the **costodiaphragmatic recesses,** pleura-lined "gutters," which surround the upward convexity of the diaphragm inside the thoracic wall (Figs. 1.30B, 1.32, and 1.33C). Similar but smaller pleural recesses are located posterior to the sternum where the costal pleura is in contact with the mediastinal pleura. The potential pleural spaces here are the **costomediastinal recesses.** The left recess is larger (less occupied) because the *cardiac notch* in the left lung is more pronounced than the corresponding notch in the pleural sac. The *inferior borders of the lungs* move farther into the pleural recesses during deep inspiration and retreat from them during expiration (Fig. 1.33B & C).

LUNGS

The **lungs** are the vital organs of respiration. Their main function is to oxygenate the blood by bringing inspired air

into close relation with the venous blood in the pulmonary capillaries. Although cadaveric lungs may be shrunken, firm or hard, and discolored, healthy lungs in living people are normally light, soft, and spongy, and fully occupy the pulmonary cavities. They are also elastic and recoil to approximately one third their size when the thoracic cavity is opened (Fig. 1.30C). The lungs are separated from each other by the mediastinum. Each lung has (Figs. 1.33 and 1.34):

- An **apex,** the blunt superior end of the lung ascending above the level of the 1st rib into the root of the neck; the apex is covered by cervical pleura.

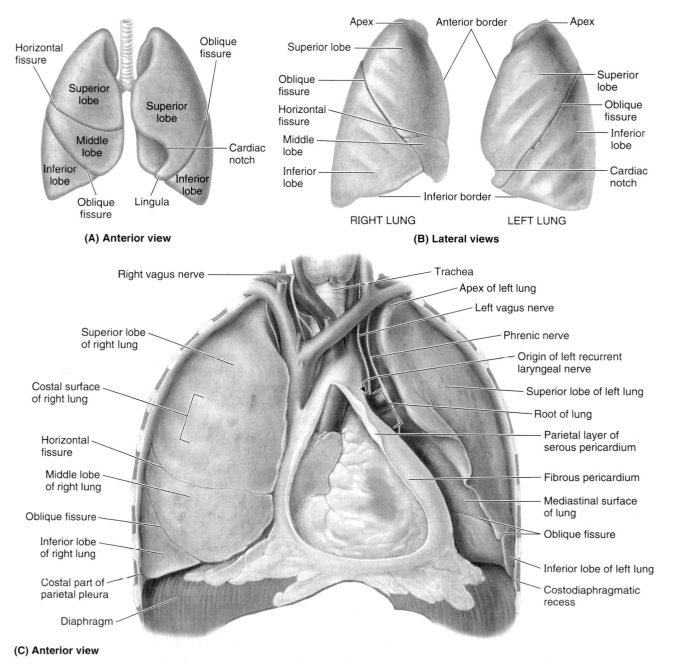

FIGURE 1.33. Costal surfaces of lungs. The lungs are shown in isolation in anterior (**A**) and lateral views (**B**), demonstrating lobes and fissures. **C.** The heart and lungs are shown in situ. The left lung is retracted from the heart (covered by fibrous pericardium) revealing the phrenic nerve as it passes anterior to the root of the lung, while the vagus nerve (CN X) passes posterior to the root. The superior lobe of the left lung in **C** is a variation that has neither a marked cardiac notch nor a lingula.

- Usually 18–20 in number (10 in the right lung; 8–10 in the left lung, depending on the combining of segments).
- Surgically resectable.

Beyond the tertiary segmental bronchi (Fig. 1.35B), there are 20 to 25 generations of branching *conducting bronchioles* that eventually end as **terminal bronchioles,** the smallest conducting bronchioles (Fig. 1.36). **Bronchioles** lack cartilage in their walls. **Conducting bronchioles** transport air but lack glands or alveoli. Each terminal bronchiole gives rise to several generations of **respiratory bronchioles,** characterized by scattered, thin-walled outpocketings (alveoli) that extend from their lumens. The **pulmonary alveolus** is the basic structural unit of gas exchange in the lung. Due to the presence of the alveoli, the respiratory bronchioles are involved both in air transportation and gas exchange. Each respiratory bronchiole gives rise to 2–11 *alveolar ducts,* each of which gives rise to 5–6 *alveolar sacs.* **Alveolar ducts** are elongated airways densely lined with alveoli, leading to common spaces, the **alveolar sacs,** into which clusters of alveoli open. New alveoli continue to develop until about age 8 years, by which time there are approximately 300 million alveoli.

VASCULATURE OF LUNGS AND PLEURAE

Each lung has a pulmonary artery supplying blood to it and two pulmonary veins draining blood from it (Fig. 1.37). The **right** and **left pulmonary arteries** arise from the *pulmonary trunk* at the level of the *sternal angle;* they carry low-oxygen ("venous") blood to the lungs for oxygenation. (They are usually colored blue, like veins, or bluish-purple in anatomical illustrations.) Each pulmonary artery becomes part of the root of the corresponding lung and divides secondary **lobar arteries.** The *right* and *left superior lobar arteries* to the superior lobes arise first, before entering the hilum. Continuing into the lung, the artery descends posterolateral to the main bronchus as the *inferior lobar artery of the left lung* and as an intermediate artery that will divide into *middle* and *inferior lobar arteries of the right lung.* Lobar arteries divide into tertiary **segmental arteries.** The arteries and bronchi are paired in the lung, branching simultaneously and running parallel courses. Consequently, a paired secondary lobar artery and bronchus serves each lobe. Likewise, a paired tertiary segmental artery and bronchus supply each bronchopulmonary segment of the lung. Usually, the artery is located on the anterior aspect of the corresponding bronchus.

Two *pulmonary veins,* a **superior** and an **inferior pulmonary vein** on each side, carry oxygen-rich ("arterial") blood from corresponding lobes of each lung to the left atrium of the heart. The **middle lobe vein** is a tributary of the right superior pulmonary vein. (Pulmonary veins are commonly colored red, like arteries, or reddish-purple in anatomical illustrations.) The pulmonary veins run independently of the arteries and bronchi in the lung, coursing between and receiving blood from adjacent bronchopulmonary segments

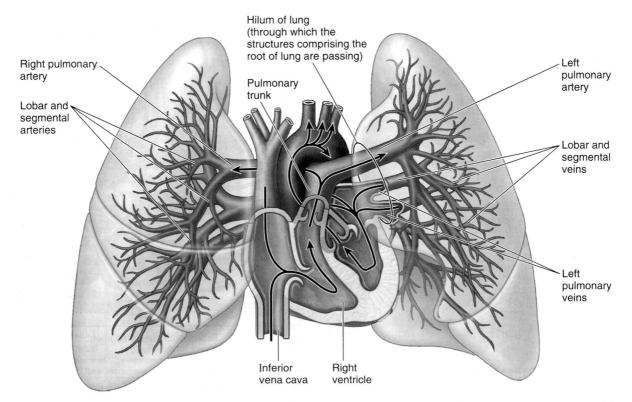

FIGURE 1.37. Pulmonary circulation. Although the intrapulmonary relationships are accurately demonstrated, the separation of the vessels of the root of the lung has been exaggerated in the hilar region to show them as they enter and leave the lung. Note that the right pulmonary artery passes under the arch of the aorta to reach the right lung and that the left pulmonary artery lies completely to the left of the arch.

as they run toward the hilum. Except in the central, perihilar region of the lung, the veins from the visceral pleura and the bronchial venous circulation drain into the pulmonary veins, the relatively small volume of low-oxygen blood entering the large volume of oxygen-rich blood returning to the heart. Veins from the parietal pleura join systemic veins in adjacent parts of the thoracic wall.

Bronchial arteries supply blood for nutrition of the structures making up the root of the lungs, the supporting

tissues of the lungs, and the visceral pleura (Fig. 1.38A). The two **left bronchial arteries** usually arise directly from the thoracic aorta. The single **right bronchial artery** may also arise directly from the aorta; however it commonly arises indirectly, either by way of the proximal part of one of the upper posterior intercostal arteries (usually the right 3rd posterior intercostal artery), or from a common trunk with the left superior bronchial artery.

The small bronchial arteries provide branches to the upper esophagus. Then they typically pass along the posterior aspects of the main bronchi, supplying them and their branches as far distally as the respiratory bronchioles. (However, see the variation shown in Figs. 1.63 and 1.69, drawn from a cadaver dissection.) The most distal branches of the bronchial arteries anastomose with branches of the pulmonary arteries in the walls of the bronchioles and in the visceral pleura. The parietal pleura is supplied by the arteries that supply the thoracic wall.

The **bronchial veins** (Fig. 1.38B) drain only part of the blood supplied to the lungs by the bronchial arteries, primarily that distributed to or near the more proximal part of the roots of the lungs. The remainder of the blood is drained by the pulmonary veins, specifically the blood returning from the visceral pleura, the more peripheral regions of the lung, and the distal components of the root of the lung. The *right bronchial vein* drains into the *azygos vein,* and the *left bronchial vein* drains into the *accessory hemi-azygos vein* or the *left superior intercostal vein.* Bronchial veins also receive some blood from esophageal veins.

The **pulmonary lymphatic plexuses** communicate freely (Fig. 1.39). The superficial **subpleural\lymphatic plexus** lies deep to the visceral pleura and drains the lung parenchyma (tissue) and visceral pleura. Lymphatic vessels from this superficial plexus drain into the **bronchopulmonary lymph nodes** (hilar lymph nodes) in the region of the lung hilum.

The deep **bronchopulmonary lymphatic plexus** is located in the submucosa of the bronchi and in the peribronchial connective tissue. It is largely concerned with draining the structures that form the root of the lung. Lymphatic vessels from this deep plexus drain initially into the intrinsic **pulmonary lymph nodes,** located along the lobar bronchi. Lymphatic vessels from these nodes continue to follow the bronchi and pulmonary vessels to the hilum of the lung, where they also drain into the bronchopulmonary lymph nodes. From them, lymph from both the superficial and deep lymphatic plexuses drains to the **superior** and **inferior tracheobronchial lymph nodes,** superior and inferior to the bifurcation of the trachea and main bronchi, respectively. The right lung drains primarily through the consecutive sets of nodes on the right side, and the superior lobe of the left lung drains primarily through corresponding nodes of the left side. Many, but not all, of the lymphatics from the lower lobe of the left lung, however, drain to the right superior tracheobronchial nodes; the lymph then continues to follow the right-side pathway.

Right superior posterior intercostal artery

Right 3rd intercostal artery

Arch of aorta

Left superior intercostal artery

Bronchial arteries

Esophageal artery

Thoracic aorta

(A) Bronchial arteries

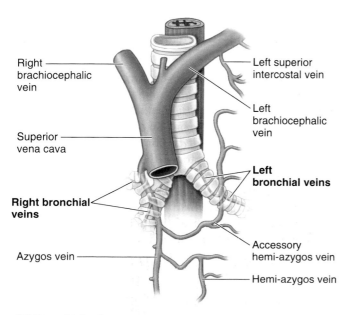

Right brachiocephalic vein

Superior vena cava

Right bronchial veins

Azygos vein

Left superior intercostal vein

Left brachiocephalic vein

Left bronchial veins

Accessory hemi-azygos vein

Hemi-azygos vein

(B) Bronchial veins

FIGURE 1.38. Bronchial arteries and veins. A. The bronchial arteries supply the supporting tissues of the lungs and visceral pleura. **B.** The bronchial veins drain the more proximal capillary beds supplied by the bronchial arteries; the rest is drained by the pulmonary veins.

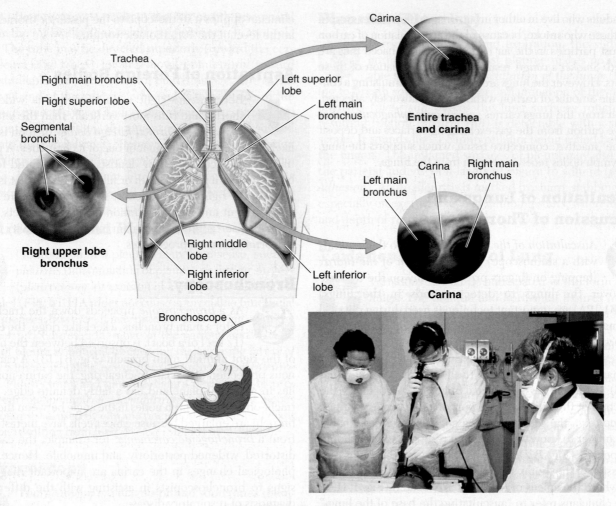

FIGURE B1.13. Bronchoscopy.

aspirates a peanut, they choke and cough. Once the peanut passes the carina, coughing usually stops. If the choking victim is inverted to make use of gravity to expel the foreign body (postural drainage of the lungs), lung secretions passing the carina also cause coughing, which assists the expellation.

Lung Resections

Knowledge of the anatomy of the bronchopulmonary segments (Fig. 1.35) is essential for precise interpretation of radiographs and other medical images of the lungs. Awareness of these segments is also essential for surgical resection of diseased segments. Bronchial and pulmonary disorders such as tumors or abscesses (collections of pus) often localize in a bronchopulmonary segment, which may be surgically resected. During treatment of *lung cancer*, the surgeon may remove a whole lung (*pneumonectomy*), a lobe (*lobectomy*), or a bronchopulmonary segment (*segmentectomy*).

Segmental Atelectasis

Blockage of a segmental bronchus (Fig. 1.35E, e.g., by an aspirated object) will prevent air from reaching the bronchopulmonary segment it supplies. The air

in the blocked segment will gradually be absorbed into the blood, and the segment will collapse. A segmental collapse does not require compensating space in the pleural cavity to be realized because adjacent segments will expand to compensate for the reduced volume of the collapsed segment.

Pulmonary Embolism

Obstruction of a pulmonary artery by a blood clot (*embolus*) is a common cause of morbidity (sickness) and mortality (death). An embolus in a pulmonary artery forms when a blood clot, fat globule, or air bubble travels in the blood to the lungs from a leg vein, for example, after a compound fracture. The embolus passes through the right side of the heart to a lung through a pulmonary artery. It may block a pulmonary artery—*pulmonary embolism (PE)*—or one of its branches. The pulmonary arteries carry all the blood that has returned to the right heart via the vena caval system. Consequently, the immediate result of PE is partial or complete obstruction of blood flow to the lung. The blockage results in a lung or a sector of a lung that is ventilated with air but not perfused with blood.

When a large embolus occludes a pulmonary artery, the patient suffers *acute respiratory distress* because of a major decrease in the oxygenation of blood, owing to blockage of blood flow through the lung. Conversely, the right side of the heart may become acutely dilated because the volume of blood arriving from the systemic circuit cannot be pushed through the pulmonary circuit (*acute cor pulmonale*). In either case, death may occur in a few minutes. A medium-size embolus may block an artery supplying a bronchopulmonary segment, producing a *pulmonary infarct,* an area of necrotic (dead) lung tissue.

In physically active people, a collateral circulation—an indirect, accessory blood supply—often exists and develops further when there is a PE so that infarction is not as likely to occur, or at least not be as devastating. Anastomoses with branches of the bronchial arteries abound in the region of the terminal bronchioles. In ill people with impaired circulation in the lung, such as *chronic congestion,* PE commonly results in lung infarction. When an area of visceral pleura is also deprived of blood, it becomes inflamed (*pleuritis*) and irritates or becomes fused to the sensitive parietal pleura, resulting in pain. Pain from the parietal pleura is referred to the cutaneous distribution of the intercostal nerves to the thoracic wall, or, in the case of inferior nerves, to the anterior abdominal wall.

Lymphatic Drainage and Pleural Adhesion

If the parietal and visceral layers of pleura adhere (*pleural adhesion*), the lymphatic vessels in the lung and visceral pleura may *anastomose* (join) with parietal lymphatic vessels that drain into the axillary lymph nodes. The presence of carbon particles in these nodes is presumptive evidence of pleural adhesion.

Hemoptysis

Spitting of blood or blood-stained sputum derived from the lungs and/or bronchial tree is due to bronchial or pulmonary hemorrhage. In about 95% of cases, the bleeding is from branches of the bronchial arteries. The most common causes include *bronchitis* (inflammation of the bronchi), *lung cancer, pneumonia, bronchiectasis, pulmonary embolism,* and *tuberculosis.*

Bronchogenic Carcinoma

The term *bronchogenic carcinoma* was once a specific designation for cancer arising in a bronchus—usually squamous- (oat) or small-cell carcinoma (cancer)—but now the term refers to any lung cancer. *Lung cancer* (carcinoma—CA) is mainly caused by cigarette smoking; most cancers arise in the mucosa of the large bronchi and produce a persistent, productive cough or *hemoptysis* (spitting of blood). Malignant (cancer) cells can be detected in the sputum (saliva-borne matter). The primary tumor, observed radiologically as an enlarging lung mass (Fig. B1.14), metastasizes early to the bronchopulmonary lymph nodes and subsequently to other thoracic lymph

Lung carcinoma: CT scan shows a mass in anterior segment of right upper lobe (arrow) adjacent to pleura.

FIGURE B1.14. Lung cancer.

nodes. Common sites of *hematogenous metastases* (spreading through the blood) of cancer cells from a bronchogenic carcinoma are the brain, bones, lungs, and suprarenal glands. The tumor cells probably enter the systemic circulation by invading the wall of a sinusoid or venule in a lung. It is then transported through the pulmonary veins, left heart, and aorta to these structures. Often the lymph nodes superior to the clavicle—the *supraclavicular lymph nodes*—are enlarged when bronchogenic carcinoma develops owing to metastases of cancer cells from the tumor. Consequently, the supraclavicular lymph nodes were once referred to as *sentinel lymph nodes* because their enlargement alerted the physician to the possibility of malignant disease in the thoracic and/or abdominal organs. More recently, the term sentinel lymph node has been applied to a node or nodes that first receive lymph draining from a cancer-containing area, regardless of location, following injection of blue dye containing radioactive tracer (technetium-99).

Lung Cancer and Mediastinal Nerves

Lung cancer involving a phrenic nerve may result in paralysis of one half of the diaphragm (hemidiaphragm). Because of the intimate relationship of the *recurrent laryngeal nerve* to the apex of the lung (Fig. 1.33C), this nerve may be involved in *apical lung cancers.* This involvement usually results in hoarseness owing to paralysis of a vocal fold (cord) because the recurrent laryngeal nerve supplies all but one of the laryngeal muscles.

Pleural Pain

The visceral pleura is insensitive to pain because it receives no nerves of general sensation. The parietal pleura (particularly the costal part) is extremely sensitive to pain. The parietal pleura is richly supplied by branches of the intercostal and phrenic nerves. Irritation of the parietal pleura may produce local pain or referred pain projected to dermatomes supplied by the same spinal (posterior root) ganglia and segments of the spinal cord. Irritation of the costal and peripheral parts of the diaphragmatic pleura results in local pain and referred pain to the dermatomes of

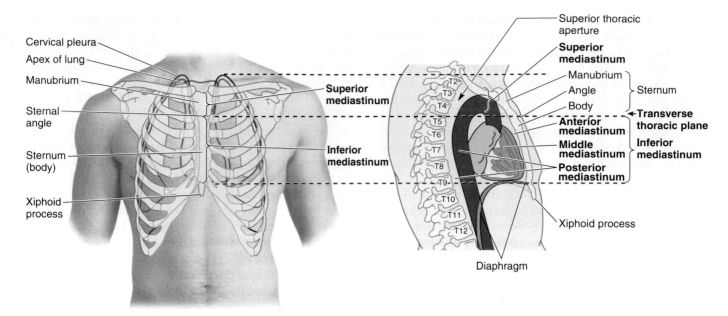

FIGURE 1.42. Subdivisions and levels of mediastinum. The subdivisions of the mediastinum are demonstrated as if the person were in the supine position. The level of the viscera relative to the subdivisions as defined by thoracic cage landmarks depends on the individual's position because the soft tissue of the mediastinum sags with the pull of gravity.

Overview of Mediastinum

The **mediastinum** (Mod. L. middle septum), occupied by the mass of tissue between the two pulmonary cavities, is the central compartment of the thoracic cavity (Fig. 1.42). It is covered on each side by *mediastinal pleura* and contains all the thoracic viscera and structures except the lungs. The mediastinum extends from the superior thoracic aperture to the diaphragm inferiorly, and from the sternum and costal cartilages anteriorly to the bodies of the thoracic vertebrae posteriorly. Unlike the rigid structure observed in the embalmed cadaver, the mediastinum in living people is a highly mobile region because it consists primarily of hollow (liquid- or air-filled) visceral structures united only by loose connective tissue, often infiltrated with fat. The major structures in the mediastinum are also surrounded by blood and lymphatic vessels, lymph nodes, nerves, and fat.

The looseness of the connective tissue and the elasticity of the lungs and parietal pleura on each side of the mediastinum enable it to accommodate movement as well as volume and pressure changes in the thoracic cavity; for example, those resulting from movements of the diaphragm, thoracic wall, and tracheobronchial tree during respiration, contraction (beating) of the heart and pulsations of the great arteries, and passage of ingested substances through the esophagus. The connective tissue becomes more fibrous and rigid with age; hence the mediastinal structures become less mobile. The mediastinum is divided into superior and inferior parts for purposes of description (Fig. 1.42).

The **superior mediastinum** extends inferiorly from the superior thoracic aperture to the horizontal plane that includes the *sternal angle* anteriorly and passes approximately through the *junction (IV disc) of T4 and T5 vertebrae* posteriorly, often referred to as the **transverse thoracic plane.** The **inferior mediastinum**—between the transverse thoracic plane and the diaphragm—is further subdivided by the pericardium into anterior, middle, and posterior parts. The pericardium and its contents (heart and roots of its great vessels) constitute the **middle mediastinum.** Some structures, such as the esophagus, pass vertically through the mediastinum and therefore lie in more than one mediastinal compartment.

Pericardium

The middle mediastinum includes the pericardium, heart, and roots of its great vessels (Fig. 1.34)—ascending aorta, pulmonary trunk, and SVC—passing to and from the heart.

The **pericardium** is a fibroserous membrane that covers the heart and the beginning of its great vessels (Figs. 1.33B and 1.43). The pericardium is a closed sac composed of two layers. The tough external layer, the **fibrous pericardium,** is continuous with the central tendon of the diaphragm (Fig. 1.32). The internal surface of the fibrous pericardium is lined with a glistening serous membrane, the **parietal layer of serous pericardium.** This layer is reflected onto the heart at the great vessels (aorta, pulmonary trunk and veins, and superior and inferior venae cavae) as the **visceral layer of serous pericardium.** The **serous pericardium** is composed mainly of mesothelium, a single layer of flattened cells forming an epithelium that lines both the internal surface of the fibrous pericardium and the external surface of the heart. The fibrous pericardium is:

- Continuous superiorly with the *tunica adventitia* (perivascular connective tissue) of the great vessels entering and leaving the heart and with the pretracheal layer of deep cervical fascia.
- Attached anteriorly to the posterior surface of the sternum by the **sternopericardial ligaments,** which are highly variable in their development.

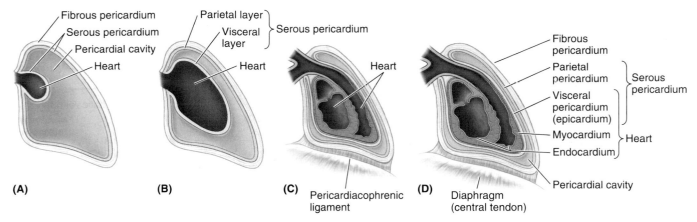

Diagrammatic right lateral views

FIGURE 1.43. Pericardium and heart. A. The heart occupies the middle mediastinum and is enclosed by pericardium, composed of two parts. The tough, outer fibrous pericardium stabilizes the heart and helps prevent it from overdilating. Between the fibrous pericardium and the heart is a "collapsed" sac, the serous pericardium. The embryonic heart invaginates the wall of the serous sac (**B**) and soon practically obliterates the pericardial cavity (**C**), leaving only a potential space between the layers of serous pericardium. **C.** and **D.** The pericardiacophrenic ligament is the continuity of the fibrous pericardium with the central tendon of the diaphragm.

- Bound posteriorly by loose connective tissue to structures in the posterior mediastinum.
- Continuous inferiorly with the central tendon of the diaphragm (Fig. 1.43C & D).

The inferior wall (floor) of the fibrous pericardial sac is firmly attached and confluent (partially blended) centrally with the central tendon of the diaphragm. The site of continuity has been referred to as the **pericardiacophrenic ligament;** however, the fibrous pericardium and central tendon are not separate structures that fused together secondarily, nor are they separable by dissection. As a result of the attachments just described, the heart is relatively well tethered in place inside this fibrous sac. The pericardium is influenced by movements of the heart and great vessels, the sternum, and the diaphragm.

The heart and roots of the great vessels within the pericardial sac lie posterior to the sternum, costal cartilages, and anterior ends of the 3rd–5th ribs on the left side (Fig. 1.44). The heart and pericardial sac are situated obliquely, approximately two thirds to the left and one third to the right of the median plane. If you turn your face to the left about 45° without rotating your shoulders, the rotation of your head approximates that of the heart relative to the trunk.

The fibrous pericardium protects the heart against sudden overfilling because it is so unyielding and closely related to the great vessels that pierce it superiorly. The ascending aorta carries the pericardium superiorly beyond the heart to the level of the sternal angle.

The **pericardial cavity** is the potential space between opposing layers of the parietal and visceral layers of serous pericardium. It normally contains a thin film of fluid that enables the heart to move and beat in a frictionless environment.

The *visceral layer of serous pericardium* forms the *epicardium,* the outermost of three layers of the heart wall. It extends onto the beginning of the great vessels, becoming continuous with the parietal layer of serous pericardium (1) where the aorta and pulmonary trunk leave the heart and (2) where the SVC,

inferior vena cava (IVC), and pulmonary veins enter the heart. The **transverse pericardial sinus** is a transversely running passage within the pericardial cavity between these two groups of vessels and the reflections of serous pericardium around them. The reflection of the serous pericardium around the second group of vessels defines the *oblique pericardial sinus.* The pericardial sinuses form during development of the heart as a consequence of the folding of the primordial heart tube. As the heart tube folds, its venous end moves posterosuperiorly (Fig. 1.45) so that the venous end of the tube lies adjacent to the arterial end, separated only by the transverse pericardial sinus (Fig. 1.46). Thus the transverse sinus is posterior to the intrapericardial parts of the pulmonary trunk and ascending aorta, anterior to the SVC, and superior to the atria of the heart.

As the veins of the heart develop and expand, a pericardial reflection surrounding them forms the **oblique pericardial sinus,** a wide pocket-like recess in the pericardial cavity posterior to the base (posterior aspect) of the heart, formed by the left atrium (Figs. 1.45 and 1.46). The oblique sinus is bounded laterally by the pericardial reflections surrounding the pulmonary veins and IVC and posteriorly by the pericardium overlying the anterior aspect of the esophagus. The oblique sinus can be entered inferiorly and will admit several fingers; however, they cannot pass around any of these structures because the sinus is a blind sac (cul-de-sac).

The **arterial supply of the pericardium** (Fig. 1.47) is mainly from a slender branch of the internal thoracic artery, the **pericardiacophrenic artery,** that often accompanies or at least parallels the phrenic nerve to the diaphragm. Smaller contributions of blood come from the:

- *Musculophrenic artery,* a terminal branch of the internal thoracic artery.
- *Bronchial, esophageal,* and *superior phrenic arteries,* branches of the thoracic aorta.
- *Coronary arteries* (visceral layer of serous pericardium only), the first branches of the aorta.

from perforation of a weakened area of heart muscle owing to a previous *myocardial infarction (MI)* or heart attack, from bleeding into the pericardial cavity after cardiac operations, or from stab wounds. This situation is especially lethal because of the high pressure involved and the rapidity with which the fluid accumulates. The heart is increasingly compressed and circulation fails. The veins of the face and neck become engorged because of the backup of blood, beginning where the SVC enters the pericardium.

In patients with *pneumothorax*—air or gas in the pleural cavity—the air may dissect along connective tissue planes and enter the pericardial sac, producing a *pneumopericardium*.

Pericardiocentesis

Drainage of fluid from the pericardial cavity, *pericardiocentesis,* is usually necessary to relieve cardiac tamponade. To remove the excess fluid, a wide-bore needle may be inserted through the left 5th or 6th intercostal space near the sternum. This approach to the pericardial sac is possible because the cardiac notch in the left lung and the shallower notch in the left pleural sac leaves part of the pericardial sac exposed—the bare area of the pericardium (Figs. 1.31A and 1.32). The pericardial sac may also be reached via the infrasternal angle by passing the needle superoposteriorly (Fig. B1.18). At this site, the needle avoids the lung and pleurae and enters the pericardial cavity; however, care must be taken not to puncture the internal thoracic artery or its terminal branches. In acute cardiac tamponade from hemopericardium, an emergency thoracotomy may be performed (the thorax is rapidly opened) so that the pericardial sac may be incised to immediately relieve the tamponade and establish *stasis of the hemorrhage* (stop the escape of blood) from the heart (see blue box "Thoracotomy, Intercostal Space Incisions, and Rib Excision," earlier in this chapter).

FIGURE B1.18. Pericardiocentesis.

Positional Abnormalities of the Heart

Abnormal folding of the embryonic heart may cause the position of the heart to be completely reversed so that the apex is misplaced to the right instead of the left—*dextrocardia.* This congenital anomaly is the most common positional abnormality of the heart, but it is still relatively uncommon. Dextrocardia is associated with mirror image positioning of the great vessels and arch of the aorta. This anomaly may be part of a general transposition of the thoracic and abdominal viscera (*situs inversus*), or the transposition may affect only the heart (*isolated dextrocardia*). In dextrocardia with situs inversus, the incidence of accompanying cardiac defects is low, and the heart usually functions normally. In isolated dextrocardia, however, the congenital anomaly is complicated by severe cardiac anomalies, such as *transposition of the great arteries.*

The Bottom Line

MEDIASTINUM OVERVIEW AND PERICARDIUM

Mediastinum overview: The mediastinum is the central compartment of the thoracic cavity and contains all thoracic viscera except the lungs. ♦ Occupying structures are hollow (fluid or air filled), and although contained between bony formations anteriorly and posteriorly, lie between "pneumatic packing," inflated to constantly changing volumes on each side. ♦ The mediastinum is a pliable, dynamic structure that is moved by structures contained within it (e.g., heart) and surrounding it (the diaphragm and other movements of respiration), as well as by the effect of gravity and body position. ♦ The superior mediastinum (above the transverse thoracic plane) is occupied by the trachea and upper parts of the great vessels. ♦ The middle part (most) of the inferior mediastinum is occupied by the heart. ♦ Most of the posterior mediastinum is occupied by structures vertically traversing all or much of the thorax.

Pericardium: The pericardium is a fibroserous sac, invaginated by the heart and roots of the great vessels, that encloses the serous cavity surrounding the heart. ♦ The fibrous pericardium is inelastic, attached anteriorly and inferiorly to the sternum and diaphragm, and blends with the adventitia of the great vessels as they enter or leave the sac. Thus it holds the heart in its middle mediastinal position and limits expansion (filling) of the heart. ♦ If fluid or a tumor occupies the pericardial space, the capacity of the heart is compromised. ♦ The serous pericardium lines the fibrous pericardium and the exterior of the heart. This glistening lubricated surface allows the heart (attached only by its afferent and efferent vessels and related reflections of serous membrane) the free movement required for its "wringing-out" motions during contraction. ♦ The parietal layer of the serous pericardium is sensitive. Pain impulses conducted from it by the somatic phrenic nerves result in referred pain sensations.

Heart

The **heart,** slightly larger than one's loosely clenched fist, is a double, self-adjusting suction and pressure pump, the parts of which work in unison to propel blood to all parts of the body. The right side of the heart (*right heart*) receives poorly oxygenated (venous) blood from the body through the SVC and IVC and pumps it through the pulmonary trunk and arteries to the lungs for oxygenation (Fig. 1.49A). The left side of the heart (*left heart*) receives well-oxygenated (arterial) blood from the lungs through the pulmonary veins and pumps it into the aorta for distribution to the body.

The heart has four chambers: **right** and **left atria** and **right** and **left ventricles.** The atria are receiving chambers that pump blood into the ventricles (the discharging chambers). The synchronous pumping actions of the heart's

FIGURE 1.49. Cardiac cycle. The cardiac cycle describes the complete movement of the heart or heartbeat and includes the period from the beginning of one heartbeat to the beginning of the next one. The cycle consists of diastole (ventricular relaxation and filling) and systole (ventricular contraction and emptying). The right heart (blue side) is the pump for the pulmonary circuit; the left heart (red side) is the pump for the systemic circuit.

two atrioventricular (AV) pumps (right and left chambers) constitute the **cardiac cycle** (Fig. 1.49B–F). The cycle begins with a period of ventricular elongation and filling (**diastole**) and ends with a period of ventricular shortening and emptying (**systole**).

Two **heart sounds** are heard with a stethoscope: a *lub* (1st) sound as the blood is transferred from the atria into the ventricles, and a *dub* (2nd) sound as the ventricles expel blood from the heart. The heart sounds are produced by the snapping shut of the oneway valves that normally keep blood from flowing backward during contractions of the heart.

The wall of each heart chamber consists of three layers, from superficial to deep (Fig. 1.43):

1. **Endocardium,** a thin internal layer (endothelium and subendothelial connective tissue) or lining membrane of the heart that also covers its valves.
2. **Myocardium,** a thick, helical middle layer composed of cardiac muscle.
3. **Epicardium,** a thin external layer (mesothelium) formed by the visceral layer of serous pericardium.

The walls of the heart consist mostly of myocardium, especially in the ventricles. When the ventricles contract, they produce a wringing motion because of the double helical orientation of the cardiac muscle fibers (Torrent-Guasp et al., 2001) (Fig. 1.50). This motion initially ejects the blood from the ventricles as the outer (basal) spiral contracts, first narrowing and then shortening the heart, reducing the volume of the ventricular chambers. Continued sequential contraction of the inner (apical) spiral elongates the heart, followed by widening as the myocardium briefly relaxes, increasing the volume of the chambers to draw blood from the atria.

The cardiac muscle fibers are anchored to the **fibrous skeleton of the heart** (Fig. 1.51). This is a complex framework of dense collagen forming four **fibrous rings** (L. *anuli fibrosi*) that surround the orifices of the valves, a right and left **fibrous trigone** (formed by connections between rings), and the membranous parts of the interatrial and interventricular septa. The fibrous skeleton of the heart:

• Keeps the orifices of the AV and semilunar valves patent and prevents them from being overly distended by an increased volume of blood pumping through them.
• Provides attachments for the leaflets and cusps of the valves.
• Provides attachment for the myocardium, which, when uncoiled, forms a continuous **ventricular myocardial band** that originates primarily from the fibrous ring of the pulmonary valve and inserts primarily into the fibrous ring of the aortic valve (Fig. 1.50).
• Forms an electrical "insulator," by separating the myenterically conducted impulses of the atria and ventricles so that they contract independently and by surrounding and providing passage for the initial part of the AV bundle of the conducting system of the heart (discussed later in this chapter).

Externally, the atria are demarcated from the ventricles by the **coronary sulcus** (**atrioventricular groove**), and

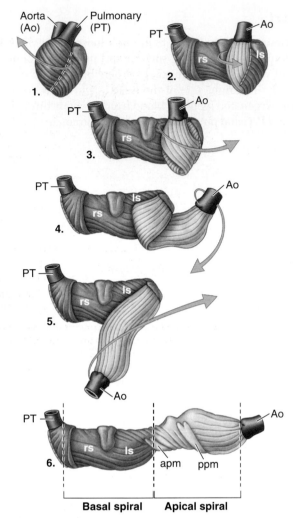

FIGURE 1.50. Arrangement of the myocardium and the fibrous skeleton of heart. The helical (double spiral) arrangement of the myocardium (modified from Torrent-Guasp et al., 2001). When the superficial myocardium is incised along the anterior interventricular groove (*dashed red line*) and peeled back starting at its origin from the fibrous ring of the pulmonary trunk (*PT*), the thick double spirals of the ventricular myocardial band are revealed. The ventricular myocardial band is progressively unwrapped. A band of nearly horizontal fibers forms an outer basal spiral (*dark brown*) that comprises the outer wall of the right ventricle (right segment; *rs*) and external layer of the outer wall of the left ventricle (left segment; *ls*). The deeper apical spiral (*light brown*), comprises the internal layer of the outer wall of the left ventricle. Its criss crossing fibers make up the interventricular septum. Thus the septum, like the outer wall of the left ventricle, is also double layered. The sequential contraction of the myocardial band enables the ventricles to function as parallel, sucking and propelling pumps; on contraction, the ventricles do not merely collapse inward but rather wring themselves out. *apm,* anterior papillary muscles; *ppm,* posterior papillary muscles.

the right and left ventricles are demarcated from each other by **anterior** and **posterior interventricular (IV) sulci** (grooves) (Fig. 1.52B & D). The heart appears trapezoidal from an anterior or posterior view (Fig. 1.52A), but in three dimensions it is shaped like a tipped-over pyramid with its apex (directed anteriorly and to the left), a base (opposite the apex, facing mostly posteriorly), and four sides.

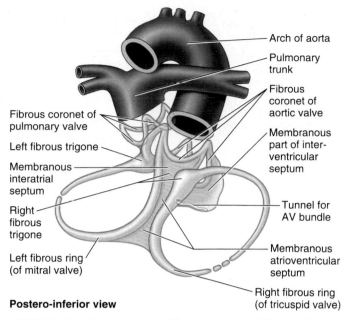

Fibrous coronet of pulmonary valve

Left fibrous trigone

Membranous interatrial septum

Right fibrous trigone

Left fibrous ring (of mitral valve)

Arch of aorta

Pulmonary trunk

Fibrous coronet of aortic valve

Membranous part of interventricular septum

Tunnel for AV bundle

Membranous atrioventricular septum

Right fibrous ring (of tricuspid valve)

Postero-inferior view

FIGURE 1.51. Fibrous skeleton of heart. The isolated fibrous skeleton is composed of four fibrous rings (or two rings and two "coronets"), each encircling a valve; two trigones; and the membranous portions of the interatrial, interventricular, and atrioventricular septa.

The **apex of the heart** (Fig. 1.52B):

- Is formed by the inferolateral part of the left ventricle.
- Lies posterior to the left 5th intercostal space in adults, usually approximately 9 cm (a hand's breadth) from the median plane.
- Remains motionless throughout the cardiac cycle.
- Is where the sounds of mitral valve closure are maximal (**apex beat**); the apex underlies the site where the heartbeat may be auscultated on the thoracic wall.

The **base of the heart** (Fig. 1.52C & D):

- Is the heart's posterior aspect (opposite the apex).
- Is formed mainly by the left atrium, with a lesser contribution by the right atrium.
- Faces posteriorly toward the bodies of vertebrae T6–T9 and is separated from them by the pericardium, oblique pericardial sinus, esophagus, and aorta.
- Extends superiorly to the bifurcation of the pulmonary trunk and inferiorly to the coronary sulcus.
- Receives the pulmonary veins on the right and left sides of its left atrial portion, and the superior and inferior venae cavae at the superior and inferior ends of its right atrial portion.

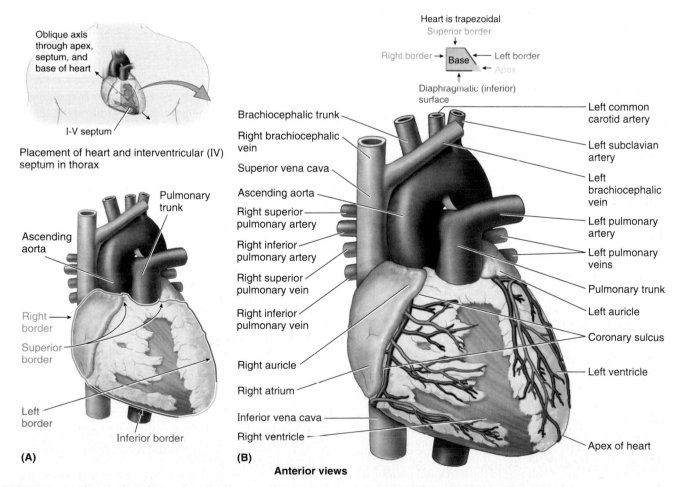

Oblique axis through apex, septum, and base of heart

I-V septum

Placement of heart and interventricular (IV) septum in thorax

Ascending aorta

Pulmonary trunk

Right border

Superior border

Left border

Inferior border

(A)

Heart is trapezoidal

Superior border

Right border → Base ← Left border

← Apex

Diaphragmatic (inferior) surface

Brachiocephalic trunk

Right brachiocephalic vein

Superior vena cava

Ascending aorta

Right superior pulmonary artery

Right inferior pulmonary artery

Right superior pulmonary vein

Right inferior pulmonary vein

Right auricle

Right atrium

Inferior vena cava

Right ventricle

Left common carotid artery

Left subclavian artery

Left brachiocephalic vein

Left pulmonary artery

Left pulmonary veins

Pulmonary trunk

Left auricle

Coronary sulcus

Left ventricle

Apex of heart

(B)

Anterior views

FIGURE 1.52. Shape, orientation, surfaces, and borders of heart. A, B. The sternocostal surface of the heart and the relationship of the great vessels are shown. The ventricles dominate this surface (two thirds right ventricle, one third left ventricle).

(C)

Base of heart
Pulmonary (left) surface
Left border
Sulcus terminalis
Right border
Diaphragmatic surface
Inferior border
Line separating base and pulmonary surface of heart from diaphragmatic surface

(D)

Left common carotid artery
Left subclavian artery
Left pulmonary artery
Left superior pulmonary vein
Left inferior pulmonary vein
Left atrium
Coronary sulcus
Left ventricle

Brachiocephalic trunk
Right brachiocephalic vein
Arch of azygos vein
Arch of aorta
Superior vena cava
Right pulmonary artery
Right superior pulmonary vein
Right inferior pulmonary vein
Right atrium
Inferior vena cava
Coronary sinus

Right ventricle

Postero-inferior views

FIGURE 1.52. *(Continued)* **C, D.** The pulmonary (left) and diaphragmatic (inferior) surfaces and the base of the heart are shown as well as the relationship of the great vessels.

The four *surfaces of the heart* (Fig. 1.52A–D) are the:

1. **Anterior (sternocostal) surface,** formed mainly by the right ventricle.
2. **Diaphragmatic (inferior) surface,** formed mainly by the left ventricle and partly by the right ventricle; it is related mainly to the central tendon of the diaphragm.
3. **Right pulmonary surface,** formed mainly by the right atrium.
4. **Left pulmonary surface,** formed mainly by the left ventricle; it forms the cardiac impression in the left lung.

The heart appears trapezoidal in both anterior (Fig. 1.52A & B) and posterior views (Fig. 1.52C & D). The four *borders of the heart* are the:

1. **Right border** (slightly convex), formed by the right atrium and extending between the SVC and the IVC.
2. **Inferior border** (nearly horizontal), formed mainly by the right ventricle and slightly by the left ventricle.
3. **Left border** (oblique, nearly vertical), formed mainly by the left ventricle and slightly by the left auricle.
4. **Superior border,** formed by the right and left atria and auricles in an anterior view; the ascending aorta and pulmonary trunk emerge from this border and the SVC enters its right side. Posterior to the aorta and pulmonary trunk and anterior to the SVC, this border forms the inferior boundary of the transverse pericardial sinus.

The **pulmonary trunk,** approximately 5 cm long and 3 cm wide, is the arterial continuation of the right ventricle and divides into *right* and *left pulmonary arteries*. The pulmonary trunk and arteries conduct low-oxygen blood to the lungs for oxygenation (Figs. 1.49A and 1.52B).

RIGHT ATRIUM

The right atrium forms the right border of the heart and receives venous blood from the SVC, IVC, and coronary sinus (Fig. 1.52B & D). The ear-like **right auricle** is a conical muscular pouch that projects from this chamber like an add-on room, increasing the capacity of the atrium as it overlaps the ascending aorta.

The *interior of the right atrium* (Fig. 1.53A & B) has a:

- Smooth, thin-walled, posterior part (the **sinus venarum**) on which the venae cavae (SVC and IVC) and coronary sinus open, bringing poorly oxygenated blood into the heart.
- Rough, muscular anterior wall composed of pectinate muscles (L. *musculi pectinati*).
- Right AV orifice through which the right atrium discharges the poorly oxygenated blood it has received into the right ventricle.

The smooth and rough parts of the atrial wall are separated externally by a shallow vertical groove, the **sulcus terminalis**

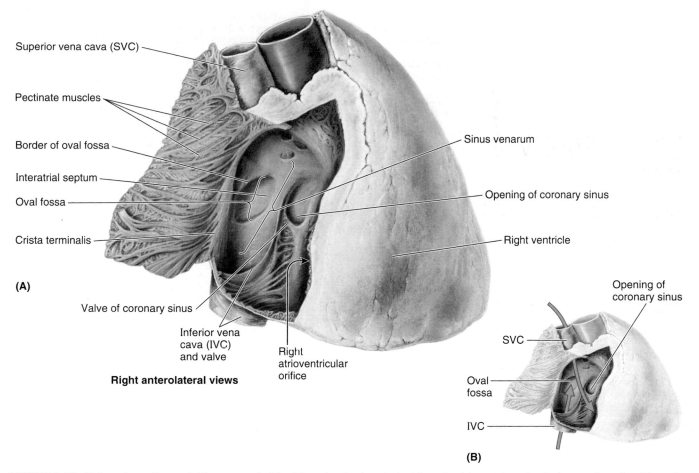

Superior vena cava (SVC)

Pectinate muscles

Border of oval fossa

Interatrial septum

Oval fossa

Crista terminalis

Sinus venarum

Opening of coronary sinus

Right ventricle

(A)

Valve of coronary sinus

Inferior vena cava (IVC) and valve

Right atrioventricular orifice

Right anterolateral views

Opening of coronary sinus

SVC

Oval fossa

IVC

(B)

FIGURE 1.53. Right atrium of heart. A. The outer wall of the right atrium has been incised from the right auricle to the diaphragmatic surface. The wall has been retracted to reveal the smooth-walled part of the atrium, the sinus venarum, derived from absorption of the venous sinus of the embryonic heart. All of the venous structures entering the right atrium (superior and inferior vena cavae and coronary sinus) open into the sinus venarum. The shallow oval fossa is the site of fusion of the embryonic valve of the oval foramen with the interatrial septum. **B.** The inflow from the superior vena cava (*SVC*) is directed toward the right atrioventricular orifice, whereas blood from the inferior vena cava (*IVC*) is directed toward the oval fossa, as it was before birth.

or terminal groove (Fig. 1.52C), and internally by a vertical ridge, the **crista terminalis** or terminal crest (Fig. 1.53A). The SVC opens into the superior part of the right atrium at the level of the right 3rd costal cartilage. The IVC opens into the inferior part of the right atrium almost in line with the SVC at approximately the level of the 5th costal cartilage.

The **opening of the coronary sinus,** a short venous trunk receiving most of the cardiac veins, is between the right AV orifice and the IVC orifice. The **interatrial septum** separating the atria has an oval, thumbprint-size depression, the **oval fossa** (L. *fossa ovalis*), which is a remnant of the **oval foramen** (L. *foramen ovale*) and its valve in the fetus. Full understanding of the features of the right atrium requires an awareness of the development of the heart; see the blue box "Embryology of the Right Atrium," p. 151.

RIGHT VENTRICLE

The right ventricle forms the largest part of the anterior surface of the heart, a small part of the diaphragmatic surface, and almost the entire inferior border of the heart (Fig. 1.52B).

Superiorly it tapers into an arterial cone, the **conus arteriosus** (infundibulum), which leads into the pulmonary trunk (Fig. 1.54). The interior of the right ventricle has irregular muscular elevations (**trabeculae carneae**). A thick muscular ridge, the **supraventricular crest,** separates the ridged muscular wall of the inflow part of the chamber from the smooth wall of the conus arteriosus, or outflow part. The inflow part of the ventricle receives blood from the right atrium through the **right AV (tricuspid) orifice** (Fig. 1.55A), located posterior to the body of the sternum at the level of the 4th and 5th intercostal spaces. The right AV orifice is surrounded by one of the fibrous rings of the *fibrous skeleton of the heart* (Fig. 1.51). The fibrous ring keeps the caliber of the orifice constant (large enough to admit the tips of three fingers), resisting the dilation that might otherwise result from blood being forced through it at varying pressures.

The **tricuspid valve** (Figs. 1.54 and 1.55) guards the right AV orifice. The bases of the valve cusps are attached to the fibrous ring around the orifice. Because the fibrous ring maintains the caliber of the orifice, the attached valve cusps contact each other in the same way with each heartbeat. **Tendinous**

Pulmonary trunk

Aorta

Superior vena cava

Right atrium

Anterior cusp

Septal cusp

Posterior papillary muscle

Tendinous cords (L. *chordae tendineae*)

Posterior cusp of tricuspid valve

Anterior papillary muscle

(A) Anterior view

Septomarginal trabecula (moderator band)

Right (R), left (L) and anterior (A) cusps of the pulmonary trunk (closing pulmonary orifice)

Conus arteriosus (infundibulum)

Supraventricular crest

Septal papillary muscles

Trabeculae carneae

Opened chamber is right ventricle

Muscular part

Membranous part

Interventricular septum

Cusp

Tendinous cords

Papillary muscles

Direction of blood flow

Cusp

Open valve   Closed valve

(C)

Pulmonary trunk

Pulmonary valve

Conus arteriosus (outflow part of right ventricle)

Supraventricular crest

Anterior cusp of tricuspid valve

Inflow part of right ventricle

SVC

Right atrium

IVC

(B) Anterior view

FIGURE 1.54. Interior of right ventricle of heart. The sternocostal wall of the right ventricle has been excised. **A.** The tricuspid valve at the entrance to the ventricle (right atrioventricular [AV] orifice) is open and the pulmonic valve at the exit to the pulmonary trunk is closed, as they would be during ventricular filling (diastole). The smooth funnel-shaped conus arteriosus is the outflow tract of the chamber. **B.** The inflow of blood enters the chamber from its posterior and inferior aspect, flowing anteriorly and to the left (toward the apex); the outflow of blood to the pulmonary trunk leaves superiorly and posteriorly. *IVC,* inferior vena cava; *SVC,* superior vena cava.

cords (L. *chordae tendineae*) attach to the free edges and ventricular surfaces of the anterior, posterior, and septal cusps, much like the cords attaching to a parachute (Fig. 1.54A). The tendinous cords arise from the apices of **papillary muscles,** which are conical muscular projections with bases attached to the ventricular wall. The papillary muscles begin to contract before contraction of the right ventricle, tightening the tendinous cords and drawing the cusps together. Because the cords are attached to adjacent sides of two cusps, they prevent separation of the cusps and their inversion when tension is applied to the tendinous cords and maintained throughout ventricular contraction (*systole*)—that is, the cusps of the tricuspid valve are prevented from prolapsing (being driven into the right atrium) as ventricular pressure rises. Thus, regurgitation of

blood (backward flow of blood) from the right ventricle back into the right atrium is blocked during ventricular systole by the valve cusps (Fig. 1.55C).

Three papillary muscles in the right ventricle correspond to the cusps of the tricuspid valve (Fig. 1.54A):

1. The **anterior papillary muscle,** the largest and most prominent of the three, arises from the anterior wall of the right ventricle; its tendinous cords attach to the anterior and posterior cusps of the tricuspid valve.
2. The **posterior papillary muscle,** smaller than the anterior muscle, may consist of several parts; it arises from the inferior wall of the right ventricle, and its tendinous cords attach to the posterior and septal cusps of the tricuspid valve.

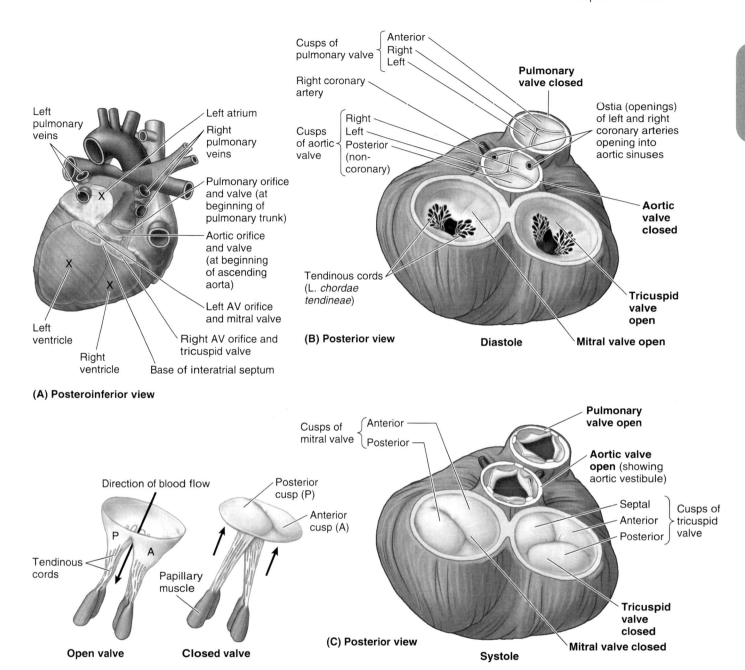

FIGURE 1.55. Valves of heart and great vessels. A. The coronary valves are shown in situ. *AV*, atrioventricular. **B.** At the beginning of diastole (ventricular relaxation and filling), the aortic and pulmonary valves are closed; shortly thereafter, the tricuspid and mitral valves open (also shown in Fig. 1.49). **C.** Shortly after systole (ventricular contraction and emptying) begins, the tricuspid and mitral valves close and the aortic and pulmonary valves open.

3. The **septal papillary muscle** arises from the interventricular septum, and its tendinous cords attach to the anterior and septal cusps of the tricuspid valve.

The **interventricular septum (IVS),** composed of muscular and membranous parts, is a strong, obliquely placed partition between the right and left ventricles (Fig. 1.54A and 1.57), forming part of the walls of each. Because of the much higher blood pressure in the left ventricle, the **muscular part of the IVS,** which forms the majority of the septum, has the thickness of the remainder of the wall of the left ventricle (two to three times as thick as the wall of the right ventricle)

and bulges into the cavity of the right ventricle. Superiorly and posteriorly, a thin membrane, part of the fibrous skeleton of the heart (Fig. 1.51), forms the much smaller **membranous part of the IVS.** On the right side, the septal cusp of the tricuspid valve (Fig. 1.54) is attached to the middle of this membranous part of the fibrous skeleton. This means that inferior to the cusp, the membrane is an interventricular septum, but superior to the cusp it is an *atrioventricular septum,* separating the right atrium from the left ventricle.

The **septomarginal trabecula (moderator band)** is a curved muscular bundle that traverses the right ventricular

Right vagus nerve (CN X)
Recurrent laryngeal nerve
Anterior scalene muscle
Right phrenic nerve
Right subclavian artery
Brachiocephalic trunk
Right brachiocephalic vein
Superior vena cava
Pulmonary trunk

Left phrenic nerve
Left common carotid artery
Recurrent laryngeal nerve
Left internal jugular vein
Left brachiocephalic vein
Left subclavian artery
Left phrenic nerve
Left vagus nerve (CN X)
Arch of aorta
Ligamentum arteriosum
Descending (thoracic) aorta

(A) Anterior view

Trachea

Left pulmonary artery

Azygos vein

Right pulmonary artery

Right and left main bronchi

Esophagus

(1)   (2)   (3)   (4)

(B) Anterior views

Right vagus nerve
Right recurrent laryngeal nerve
Right pulmonary plexus

Left vagus nerve
Left recurrent laryngeal nerve
Cardiac plexus
Left pulmonary plexus
Esophageal (nerve) plexus

(C) Anterior view

FIGURE 1.68. Great vessels and nerves. A. The relationships of the vessels and nerves in the superior mediastinum are shown. The ligamentum arteriosum is the remnant of the fetal shunt (ductus arteriosus) that bypasses the prefunctional lungs. **B.** The relationships at the bifurcation of the trachea from superficial to deep are shown. (1) Most anterior. The left brachiocephalic vein passes across the roots of the three major branches of the arch of the aorta. (2) The ascending aorta and arch pass anterior and superior, respectively, to the right pulmonary artery. (3) The bifurcation of the pulmonary trunk and right pulmonary artery lie directly anterior to the bifurcation of the trachea. (4) The cardiac plexus remains on the anterior aspect of the tracheal bifurcation after removal of the pulmonary trunk and arteries, the ascending aorta, and the arch of the aorta, to which the plexus is primarily related. **C.** The nerves in the superior and posterior mediastina are seen after the viscera that lie anterior to the trachea and esophagus have been removed.

The **left vagus nerve** (LVN) descends in the neck posterior to the left common carotid artery (Fig. 1.68A). It enters the mediastinum between the left common carotid artery and left subclavian artery. When the LVN reaches the left side of the arch of the aorta, it diverges posteriorly from the left phrenic nerve. The LVN is separated laterally from the phrenic nerve by the left superior intercostal vein. As the LVN curves medially at the inferior border of the arch of the aorta, it gives off the **left recurrent laryngeal nerve.** The left recurrent laryngeal nerve passes inferior to the arch of the aorta, immediately lateral to the ligamentum arteriosum, and ascends to the larynx in the groove between the trachea and the esophagus (Figs. 1.63, 1.66B, 1.68A–C, and 1.69). The LVN passes posterior to the root of the left lung, where it breaks up into many branches that contribute to the **left pulmonary plexus.** The LVN leaves this plexus as a single trunk and passes to the esophagus, where it joins fibers from the right vagus in the *esophageal (nerve) plexus* (Fig. 1.68B & C).

The *phrenic nerves* (Fig. 1.68A) supply the diaphragm with motor and sensory fibers, the latter accounting for approximately one third of the nerve's fibers. The phrenic nerves also supply sensory fibers to the pericardium and mediastinal pleura. Each phrenic nerve enters the superior mediastinum between the subclavian artery and the origin

of the brachiocephalic vein (see Table 1.6). The fact that the phrenic nerves pass anterior to the roots of the lungs provides an important means of distinguishing them from the vagus nerves, which pass posterior to the roots.

The **right phrenic nerve** passes along the right side of the right brachiocephalic vein, SVC, and the pericardium over the right atrium. It also passes anterior to the root of the right lung and descends on the right side of the IVC to the diaphragm, which it pierces near the caval opening (Fig. 1.70A).

The **left phrenic nerve** descends between the left subclavian and left common carotid arteries. It crosses the left surface of the arch of the aorta anterior to the left vagus nerve and passes over the left superior intercostal vein. The left phrenic nerve then descends anterior to the root of the left lung and runs along the fibrous pericardium, superficial to the left atrium and ventricle of the heart, where it pierces the diaphragm to the left of the pericardium (Fig. 1.70B). Most branching of the phrenic nerves for distribution to the diaphragm occurs on the diaphragm's inferior (abdominal) surface.

TRACHEA

The **trachea** descends anterior to the esophagus and enters the superior mediastinum, inclining a little to the right of

Vertebral column

Cervical parietal pleura

Arch of azygos vein

Right main bronchus

Left main bronchus

Esophagus

Left vagus nerve (CN X)

Esophagus

Left recurrent laryngeal nerve

Thoracic duct

Trachea

1st rib

Arch of aorta

Bronchial arteries

Root of lung (entering lung at hilum)

Intrapulmonary bronchi

Descending (thoracic) aorta

Anterior view

FIGURE 1.69. Deep dissection of superior mediastinum. Four structures run parallel as they traverse the superior thoracic aperture: trachea, esophagus, left recurrent laryngeal nerve, and thoracic duct. The right main bronchus is more vertical, shorter, and wider than the left main bronchus. The course of the right bronchial artery shown here is aberrant; usually it passes posterior to the bronchus.

the median plane (Figs. 1.68B & C and 1.69). The posterior surface of the trachea is flat where it is applied to the esophagus (Fig. 1.65B). The trachea ends at the level of the sternal angle by dividing into the right and left main bronchi (Figs. 1.65A and 1.69). The trachea terminates superior to the level of the heart and is not a component of the posterior mediastinum.

ESOPHAGUS

The **esophagus** is a fibromuscular tube that extends from the pharynx to the stomach (Figs. 1.65A & B, 1.68B & C, 1.69, 1.70A, and 1.71). The esophagus enters the superior mediastinum between the trachea and vertebral column, where it lies anterior to the bodies of the T1–T4 vertebrae. The esophagus is usually flattened anteroposteriorly. Initially, it inclines to the left but is pushed back to the median plane by the arch of the aorta. It is then compressed anteriorly by the root of the left lung. In the superior mediastinum, the *thoracic duct* usually lies on the left side of the esophagus,

deep (medial) to the arch of the aorta (Figs. 1.69 and 1.70B). Inferior to the arch, the esophagus again inclines to the left as it approaches and passes through the **esophageal hiatus** in the diaphragm (Fig. 1.71).

Posterior Mediastinum

The **posterior mediastinum** (the posterior part of the inferior mediastinum) is located inferior to the transverse thoracic plane, anterior to the T5–T12 vertebrae, posterior to the pericardium and diaphragm, and between the parietal pleura of the two lungs (Figs. 1.65A and 1.68C). The posterior mediastinum contains the thoracic aorta, thoracic duct and lymphatic trunks, posterior mediastinal lymph nodes, azygos and hemi-azygos veins, and esophagus and esophageal nerve plexus. Some authors also include the thoracic sympathetic trunks and thoracic splanchnic nerves; however, these structures lie lateral to the vertebral bodies and are not within the posterior mediastinal compartment or space per se.

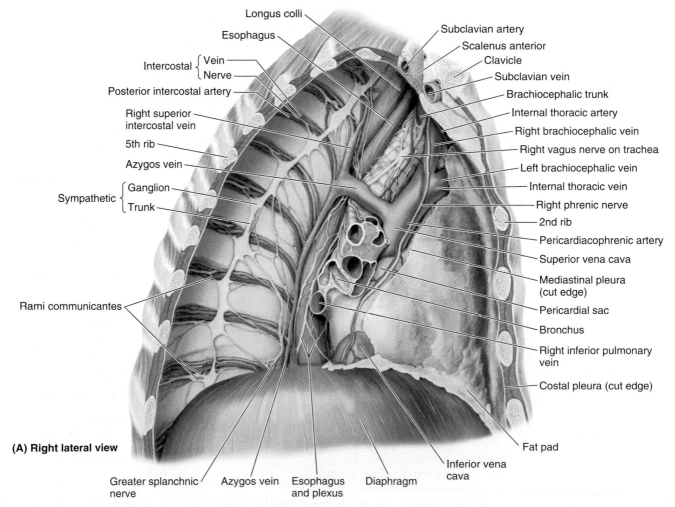

FIGURE 1.70. Lateral exposures of mediastinum. A. In this right side view, most of the costal and mediastinal pleura has been removed to expose the underlying structures. This side of the mediastinum, the "blue side," is dominated by venous structures: the azygos vein and arch, superior vena cava, right atrium, and inferior vena cava.

THORACIC AORTA

The **thoracic aorta** is the continuation of the arch of the aorta). (Figs. 1.69, 1.71, and 1.72; Table 1.5). It begins on the left side of the inferior border of the body of the T4 vertebra and descends in the posterior mediastinum on the left sides of the T5–T12 vertebrae. As it descends, the thoracic aorta approaches the median plane and displaces the esophagus to the right. The **thoracic aortic plexus** (Fig. 1.70B), an autonomic nerve network, surrounds it. The thoracic aorta lies posterior to the root of the left lung (Figs. 1.69 and 1.70B), pericardium, and esophagus. It terminates (with a name change to *abdominal aorta*) anterior to the inferior border of the T12 vertebra and enters the abdomen through the **aortic hiatus** in the diaphragm (Fig. 1.71). The thoracic duct and azygos vein ascend on its right side and accompany it through this hiatus.

In a pattern that will be more evident in the abdomen, the *branches of the descending aorta* arise and course within three "vascular planes" (Fig. 1.72):

- An *anterior, midline plane* of *unpaired visceral branches* to the gut (embryonic digestive tube) and its derivatives (A in Fig. 1.72 inset).
- *Lateral planes* of *paired visceral branches* serving viscera other than the gut and its derivatives (B).
- *Posterolateral planes* of *paired (segmental) parietal branches* to the body wall (C).

In the thorax, the *unpaired visceral branches* of the anterior vascular plane are the **esophageal arteries**—usually two, but there may be as many as five (Fig. 1.72; Table 1.5). The *paired visceral branches* of the lateral plane are represented in the thorax by the *bronchial arteries* (Fig. 1.69). Although the right and left bronchial arteries may arise directly from the aorta, most commonly only the paired left bronchial arteries do so; the right bronchial arteries arise indirectly as branches of a right posterior intercostal artery (usually the 3rd). The *paired parietal branches* of the thoracic aorta that arise posterolaterally are the nine *posterior intercostal arteries* that supply all but the upper two intercostal spaces and

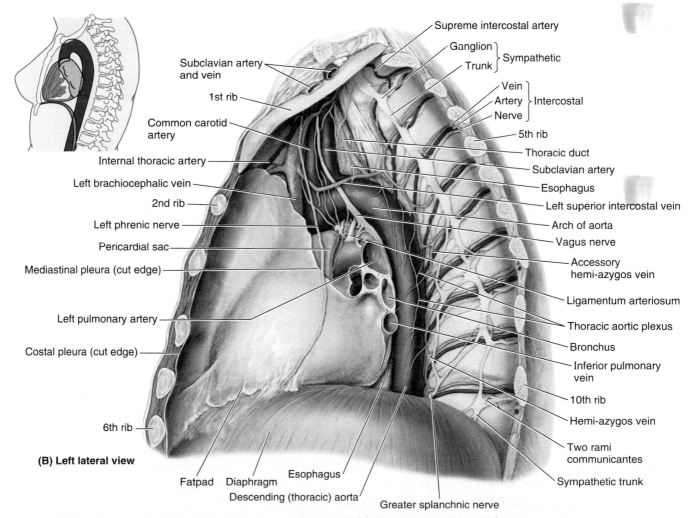

FIGURE 1.70. *(Continued)* **B.** The left side of the mediastinum, the "red side," is dominated by arterial structures: the arch of aorta and thoracic aorta, left common carotid and subclavian arteries, and left ventricle (plus the pulmonary trunk and left pulmonary artery). At the thoracic and superior lumbar levels, the sympathetic trunk is attached to intercostal nerves by paired (white and gray) rami communicantes. The left superior intercostal vein, draining the upper two to three intercostal spaces, passes anteriorly to enter the left brachiocephalic vein.

Anterior view

FIGURE 1.71. Anterior view of esophagus, trachea, bronchi, and aorta. The arch of aorta curves posteriorly on the left side of the trachea and esophagus. Enlargement of the inferior tracheobronchial (carinal) nodes may widen the angle between the main bronchi. In this specimen, the thoracic duct enters the left subclavian vein.

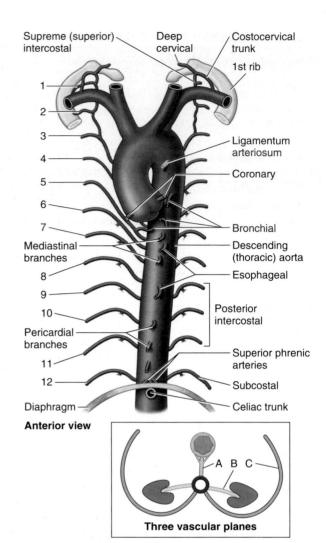

Anterior view

Three vascular planes

Superior view

FIGURE 1.72. Branches of thoracic aorta. Branches of the thoracic aorta tend to arise within three vascular planes (*inset*). Esophageal and pericardial branches represent unpaired visceral branches (*A* in inset) arising anteriorly; the bronchial arteries represent paired lateral visceral branches (*B* in inset); posterior intercostal and subcostal arteries (*1–12*) represent paired, segmental parietal branches that mostly arise posterolaterally (*C* in inset). The paired superior phrenic arteries arising from the inferior part of the thoracic aorta that supply the diaphragm are exceptions to the pattern; they are paired parietal branches that have migrated anteriorly.

the *subcostal arteries* (Fig. 1.72). The latter vessels arise from the thoracic aorta but course below the diaphragm. They are in series with the posterior intercostal arteries.

Exceptions to this pattern include the:

- **Superior phrenic arteries,** paired parietal branches that pass anterolaterally to the superior surface of the diaphragm (which is actually facing posteriorly at this level owing to the convexity of the diaphragm), where they anastomose with the musculophrenic and pericardiacophrenic branches of the internal thoracic artery.
- **Pericardial branches,** unpaired branches that arise anteriorly but, instead of passing to the gut, send twigs to the pericardium. The same is true for the small **mediastinal arteries** that supply the lymph nodes and other tissues of the posterior mediastinum.

ESOPHAGUS

The **esophagus** descends into the posterior mediastinum from the superior mediastinum, passing posterior to and to the right of the arch of the aorta (Figs. 1.68C, 1.69, and 1.71) and posterior to the pericardium and left atrium. The esophagus constitutes the primary posterior relationship of the base of the heart. It then deviates to the left and passes through the *esophageal hiatus* in the diaphragm at the level of the T10 vertebra, anterior to the aorta.

The esophagus may have three impressions, or "constrictions," in its thoracic part. These may be observed as narrowings of the lumen in oblique chest radiographs that are taken as barium is swallowed. The esophagus is compressed by three structures: (1) the arch of the aorta, (2) the left main bronchus, and (3) the diaphragm. The first two impressions occur in close proximity. The aortic arch compression is most evident in a postero-anterior (PA) radiograph after a barium swallow, and the bronchial impression is more evident in lateral views. No constrictions are visible in the empty esophagus; however, as it expands during filling, the structures noted above compress its walls.

TABLE 1.5. AORTA AND ITS BRANCHES IN THORAX

Artery	Origin	Course	Branches
Ascending aorta	Aortic orifice of left ventricle	Ascends approximately 5 cm to sternal angle where it becomes arch of aorta	Right and left coronary arteries
Arch of aorta	Continuation of ascending aorta	Arches posteriorly on left side of trachea and esophagus and superior to left main bronchus	Brachiocephalic, left common carotid, left subclavian
Thoracic (descending) aorta	Continuation of arch of aorta	Descends in posterior mediastinum to left of vertebral column; gradually shifts to right to lie in median plane at aortic hiatus	Posterior intercostal arteries, subcostal, some phrenic arteries and visceral branches (e.g., esophageal)
Posterior intercostal	Posterior aspect of thoracic aorta	Pass laterally and then anteriorly parallel to ribs	Lateral and anterior cutaneous branches
Bronchial (1–2 branches)	Anterior aspect of aorta or posterior intercostal artery	Run with the tracheobronchial tree	Bronchial and peribronchial tissue, visceral pleura
Esophageal (4–5 branches)	Anterior aspect of thoracic aorta	Run anteriorly to esophagus	To esophagus
Superior phrenic (vary in number)	Anterior aspects of thoracic aorta	Arise at aortic hiatus and pass to superior aspect of diaphragm	To diaphragm

THORACIC DUCT AND LYMPHATIC TRUNKS

The **thoracic duct** is the largest lymphatic channel in the body. In the posterior mediastinum, it lies on the anterior aspect of the bodies of the inferior 7 thoracic vertebrae (Fig. 1.73). The thoracic duct conveys most lymph of the body to the venous system: that from the lower limbs; pelvic cavity; abdominal cavity; left upper limb; and left side of the thorax, head, and neck—that is, all lymph except that from the right superior quadrant (see the overview of the lymphatic system in the Introduction chapter).

The thoracic duct originates from the **cisterna chyli** (chyle cistern) in the abdomen and ascends through the aortic hiatus in the diaphragm (Fig. 1.71). The duct is usually thin walled and dull white. Often it is beaded because of its numerous valves. It ascends in the posterior mediastinum among the thoracic aorta on its left, the azygos vein on its right, the esophagus anteriorly, and the vertebral bodies posteriorly. At the level of the T4, T5, or T6 vertebra, the thoracic duct crosses to the left, posterior to the esophagus, and ascends into the superior mediastinum.

The thoracic duct receives branches from the middle and superior intercostal spaces of both sides through several collecting trunks. It also receives branches from posterior mediastinal structures. Near its termination, the thoracic duct often receives the *jugular, subclavian,* and *bronchomediastinal lymphatic trunks* (although any or all these vessels may terminate independently). The thoracic duct usually empties into the venous system near the union of the left internal jugular and subclavian veins—the left *venous angle* or origin of the left brachiocephalic vein (Figs. 1.72 and 1.73A)—but it may open into the left subclavian vein as shown in Figure 1.71.

VESSELS AND LYMPH NODES OF POSTERIOR MEDIASTINUM

The thoracic aorta and its branches have been discussed earlier. **Posterior mediastinal lymph nodes** (Fig. 1.73A & B) lie posterior to the pericardium, where they are related to the esophagus and thoracic aorta. There are several nodes posterior to the inferior part of the esophagus and more (up to eight) anterior and lateral to it. The posterior mediastinal lymph nodes receive lymph from the esophagus, the posterior aspect of the pericardium and diaphragm, and the middle posterior intercostal spaces. Lymph from the nodes drains to the right or left venous angles via the right lymphatic duct or the thoracic duct.

The **azygos system of veins,** on each side of the vertebral column, drains the back and thoracoabdominal walls (Figs. 1.73A and 1.74A & B) and mediastinal viscera. The azygos system exhibits much variation in its origin, course, tributaries, and anastomoses. The *azygos vein* (G., *azygos,* unpaired) and its main tributary, the *hemi-azygos vein,* usually arise from "roots" arising from the posterior aspect of the IVC and/or renal vein, respectively, which merge with the ascending *lumbar veins.*

The **azygos vein** forms a collateral pathway between the SVC and IVC and drains blood from the posterior walls of the thorax and abdomen. It ascends in the posterior mediastinum, passing close to the right sides of the bodies of the inferior 8 thoracic vertebrae. It arches over the superior aspect of the root of the right lung to join the SVC, similar to the way the arch of the aorta passes over the root of the left lung. In addition to the *posterior intercostal veins,* the azygos vein communicates with the vertebral venous plexuses that drain the back, vertebrae, and structures in the vertebral canal.

(A) Anterior view

(B) Right anterolateral view

FIGURE 1.73. Thoracic duct and bronchomediastinal trunks. A. The thoracic aorta has been pulled slightly to the left and the azygos vein slightly to the right to expose the thoracic duct. At approximately the transverse thoracic plane (sternal angle, T4–T5 intervertebral disc level), the thoracic duct passes to the left and continues its ascent to the neck where it arches laterally to enter the left venous angle. The right lymphatic duct is formed by the union of the contralateral partners of the ducts that join the termination of the thoracic duct. **B.** Lymph nodes and pathways that provide lymphatic drainage of the thoracic cavity.

The azygos vein also receives the mediastinal, esophageal, and bronchial veins (Fig. 1.74).

The **hemi-azygos vein** arises on the left side by the junction of the left subcostal and ascending lumbar veins. It ascends on the left side of the vertebral column, posterior to the thoracic aorta as far as the T9 vertebra. Here it crosses to the right, posterior to the aorta, thoracic duct, and esophagus, and joins the azygos vein. The hemi-azygos vein receives the inferior three posterior intercostal veins, the inferior esophageal veins, and several small mediastinal veins. The **accessory hemi-azygos vein** begins at the medial end of the 4th or 5th intercostal space and descends on the left side of the vertebral column from T5 through T8. It receives tributaries from veins in the 4th–8th intercostal spaces and sometimes from the left bronchial veins. It crosses over the T7 or T8 vertebra, posterior to the thoracic aorta and thoracic duct, where it joins the azygos vein. Sometimes the accessory hemi-azygos vein joins the hemi-azygos vein and opens with it into the azygos vein. The accessory hemi-azygos

is frequently connected to the left superior intercostal vein, as shown in Figure 1.74. The left superior intercostal vein, which drains the 1st–3rd intercostal spaces, may communicate with the accessory hemi-azygos vein; however, it drains primarily into the left brachiocephalic vein.

NERVES OF POSTERIOR MEDIASTINUM

The sympathetic trunks and their associated ganglia form a major portion of the autonomic nervous system (Fig. 1.75; Table 1.6). The **thoracic sympathetic trunks** are in continuity with the cervical and lumbar sympathetic trunks. The thoracic trunks lie against the heads of the ribs in the superior part of the thorax, the costovertebral joints in the midthoracic level, and the sides of the vertebral bodies in the inferior part of the thorax. The **lower thoracic splanchnic nerves**—also known as greater, lesser, and least splanchnic nerves—are part of the *abdominopelvic splanchnic nerves* because they supply viscera inferior to the diaphragm. They consist of presynaptic

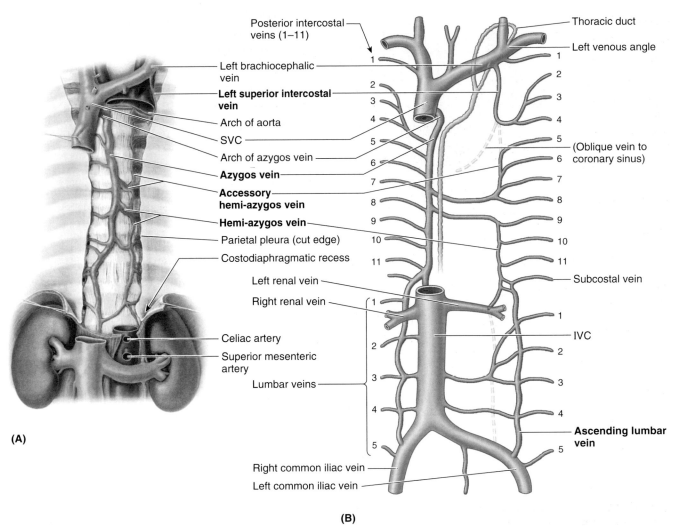

Posterior intercostal veins (1–11)
Thoracic duct
Left brachiocephalic vein
Left venous angle
Left superior intercostal vein
Arch of aorta
SVC
Arch of azygos vein
(Oblique vein to coronary sinus)
Azygos vein
Accessory hemi-azygos vein
Hemi-azygos vein
Parietal pleura (cut edge)
Costodiaphragmatic recess
Left renal vein
Subcostal vein
Right renal vein
Celiac artery
Superior mesenteric artery
Lumbar veins
IVC
Ascending lumbar vein
Right common iliac vein
Left common iliac vein

(A)

(B)

FIGURE 1.74. Azygos system of veins. The azygos vein forms a direct connection between the inferior vena cava (*IVC*) and the superior vena cava (*SVC*). The azygos and hemi-azygos veins are also continuous inferiorly (below diaphragm) with the ascending lumbar veins.

fibers from the 5th through the 12th sympathetic ganglia, which pass through the diaphragm and synapse in prevertebral ganglia in the abdomen. They supply sympathetic innervation for most of the abdominal viscera. These splanchnic nerves are discussed further in Chapter 2.

Anterior Mediastinum

The **anterior mediastinum,** the smallest subdivision of the mediastinum (Fig. 1.42), lies between the body of the sternum and the transversus thoracis muscles anteriorly and the pericardium posteriorly. It is continuous with the superior mediastinum at the sternal angle and is limited inferiorly by the diaphragm. The anterior mediastinum consists of loose connective tissue (**sternopericardial ligaments**), fat, lymphatic vessels, a few lymph nodes, and branches of the internal thoracic vessels. In infants and children, the anterior mediastinum contains the inferior part of the thymus. In unusual cases, this lymphoid organ may extend to the level of the 4th costal cartilages.

Surface Anatomy of Heart and Mediastinal Viscera

The heart and great vessels are approximately in the middle of the thorax, surrounded laterally and posteriorly by the lungs and anteriorly by the sternum and the central part of the thoracic cage (Fig. 1.76). The borders of the heart are variable and depend on the position of the diaphragm and the build and physical condition of the person. The outline of the heart can be traced on the anterior surface of the thorax by using the following guidelines (Fig. 1.76C):

• The *superior border* corresponds to a line connecting the inferior border of the 2nd left costal cartilage to the superior border of the 3rd right costal cartilage.
• The *right border* corresponds to a line drawn from the 3rd right costal cartilage to the 6th right costal cartilage; this border is slightly convex to the right.
• The *inferior border* corresponds to a line drawn from the inferior end of the right border to a point in the 5th

Middle cervical ganglion

Cervicothoracic (stellate) ganglion (fusion of inferior cervical and first thoracic ganglion)

T2 sympathetic ganglion

Trachea

Cardiac plexus

Left pulmonary plexus

Aorta

Esophagus

T8 sympathetic ganglion

Esophageal (nerve) plexus

Splanchnic nerve

Thoracic sympathetic trunk

FIGURE 1.75. Autonomic nerves of superior and posterior mediastina.

TABLE 1.6. NERVES OF THORAX

Nerve	Origin	Course	Distribution
Vagus (CN X)	8–10 rootlets from medulla of brainstem	Enters superior mediastinum posterior to sternoclavicular joint and brachiocephalic vein; gives rise to recurrent laryngeal nerve; continues into abdomen	Pulmonary plexus, esophageal plexus, and cardiac plexus
Phrenic	Anterior rami of C3–C5 nerves	Passes through superior thoracic aperture and runs between mediastinal pleura and pericardium	Central portion of diaphragm
Intercostals (1–11)	Anterior rami of T1–T11 nerves	Run in intercostal spaces between internal and innermost layers of intercostal muscles	Muscles in and skin over intercostal space; lower nerves supply muscles and skin of anterolateral abdominal wall
Subcostal	Anterior ramus of T12 nerve	Follows inferior border of 12th rib and passes into abdominal wall	Abdominal wall and skin of gluteal region
Recurrent laryngeal	Vagus nerve	Loops around subclavian artery on right; on left runs around arch of aorta and ascends in tracheo-esophageal groove	Intrinsic muscles of larynx (except cricothyroid); sensory inferior to level of vocal folds
Cardiac plexus	Cervical and cardiac branches of vagus nerve and sympathetic trunk	From arch of aorta and posterior surface of heart, fibers extend along coronary arteries and to sinu-atrial node	Impulses pass to sinu-atrial node; parasympathetic fibers slow rate, reduce force of heartbeat, and constrict coronary arteries; sympathetic fibers have the opposite effect
Pulmonary plexus	Vagus nerve and sympathetic trunk	Forms on root of lung and extends along bronchial subdivisions	Parasympathetic fibers constrict bronchioles; sympathetic fibers dilate them; afferents convey reflexes
Esophageal plexus	Vagus nerve, sympathetic ganglia, greater splanchnic nerve	Distal to tracheal bifurcation; vagus and sympathetic nerves form a plexus around esophagus	Vagal and sympathetic fibers to smooth muscle and glands of inferior two thirds of esophagus

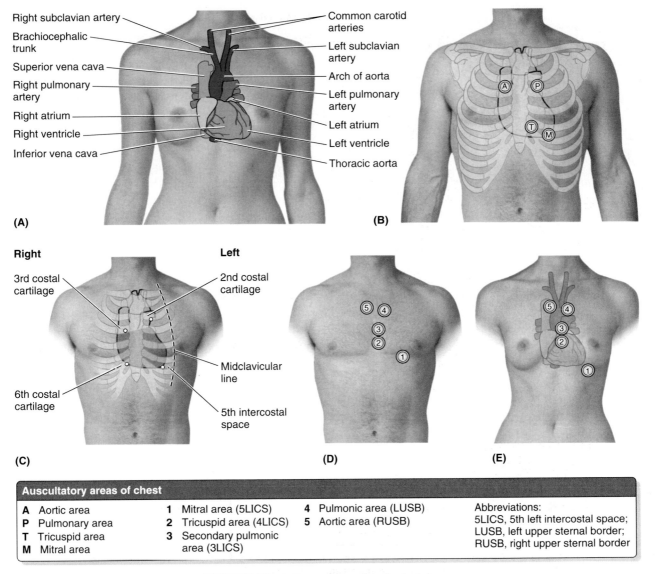

FIGURE 1.76. Surface anatomy of mediastinal viscera.

intercostal space close to the left MCL; the left end of this line corresponds to the location of the apex of the heart and the apex beat.

- The *left border* corresponds to a line connecting the left ends of the lines representing the superior and inferior borders.

- The valves are located posterior to the sternum; however, the sounds produced by them are projected to the areas shown in Figure 1.76—pulmonary (*P*), aortic (*A*), mitral (*M*), and tricuspid (*T*)—where the stethoscope may be placed to avoid intervening bone.

The **apex beat** is the impulse that results from the apex of the heart being forced against the anterior thoracic wall when the left ventricle contracts. The location of the apex beat (mitral area, M) varies in position and may be located in the 4th or 5th intercostal spaces, 6–10 cm from the AML (anterior median line).

Auscultatory Areas

Clinicians' interest in the surface anatomy of the heart and cardiac valves results from their need to listen to valve sounds. The five areas (two areas are for the pulmonary valve) are as wide apart as possible so that the sounds produced at any given valve may be clearly distinguished from those produced at other valves (Fig. 1.76D & E). Blood tends to carry the sound in the direction of its flow; consequently, each area is situated superficial to the chamber or vessel into which the blood has passed and in a direct line with the valve orifice.

SUPERIOR, POSTERIOR, AND ANTERIOR MEDIASTINUM

Variations of Great Arteries

BRANCHES OF ARCH OF AORTA

The usual pattern of branches of the arch of the aorta is present in approximately 65% of people (Fig. 1.64). *Variations in the origin of the branches of the arch* are fairly common (Fig. B1.32A). In approximately 27% of people, the left common carotid artery originates from the brachiocephalic trunk. A brachiocephalic trunk fails to form in approximately 2.5% of people; in these cases each of the four arteries (right and left common carotid and subclavian arteries) originate independently from the arch of the aorta. The left vertebral artery originates from the arch of the aorta in approximately 5% of people. Both right and left brachiocephalic trunks originate from the arch in approximately 1.2% of people (Bergman et al., 1988).

A *retro-esophageal right subclavian artery* sometimes arises as the last (most-left-sided) branch of the arch of the aorta (Fig. B1.32B). The artery crosses posterior to the esophagus to reach the right upper limb and may compress the esophagus, causing difficulty in swallowing (*dysphagia*). An accessory artery to the thyroid gland, the **thyroid ima artery** (L. *arteria thyroidea ima*), may arise from the arch of the aorta or the brachiocephalic artery.

ANOMALIES OF ARCH OF AORTA

The most superior part of the arch of the aorta is usually approximately 2.5 cm inferior to the superior border of the manubrium, but it may be more superior or inferior. Sometimes the arch curves over the root of the right lung and passes inferiorly on the right side, forming a **right arch of the aorta.** In some cases, the abnormal arch, after passing over the root of the right lung, passes posterior to the esophagus to reach its usual position on the left side. Less frequently, a **double arch of the aorta** forms a vascular ring around the esophagus and trachea (Fig. B1.32C). A trachea that is compressed enough to affect breathing may require surgical division of the vascular ring.

(A) Variations in the origins of the branches of the arch of the aorta

(B) Retro-esophageal right subclavian artery

(C) Double aortic arch

FIGURE B1.32. **Variations and anomalies of branches of aortic arch.**

Aneurysm of the aortic arch: MR angiogram in a sagittal oblique plane; injected contrast medium shows vascular structures as bright; (5) superior vena cava, (6) aortic arch, (a) left common carotid artery, (b) brachiocephalic artery, (c) left subclavian artery, (d) ascending aorta, (e) right pulmonary vein, (f) left pulmonary vein, (g) left pulmonary artery (h) pulmonary trunk, (i) left atrium, (j) left ventricle, (k) diaphragm, (l) liver, (m) large saccular aneurysm arising from the ascending aorta.

FIGURE B1.33. Aneurysm of the aortic arch (magnetic resonance [*MR*] angiogram).

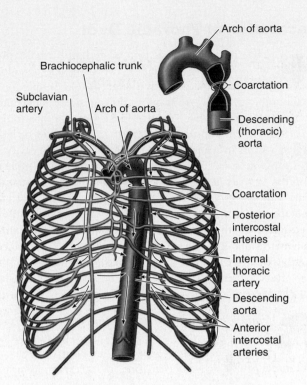

FIGURE B1.34. Coarctation of aorta.

Aneurysm of Ascending Aorta

The distal part of the ascending aorta receives a strong thrust of blood when the left ventricle contracts. Because its wall is not yet reinforced by fibrous pericardium (the fibrous pericardium blends with the aortic adventitia at the beginning of the arch; Fig. 1.66B), an *aneurysm* (localized dilation) may develop. An aortic aneurysm is evident on a chest film (radiograph of the thorax) or an MR angiogram (Fig. B1.33) as an enlarged area of the ascending aorta silhouette. Individuals with an aneurysm usually complain of chest pain that radiates to the back. The aneurysm may exert pressure on the trachea, esophagus, and recurrent laryngeal nerve, causing difficulty in breathing and swallowing.

Coarctation of Aorta

In *coarctation of the aorta*, the arch of the aorta or thoracic aorta has an abnormal narrowing (stenosis) that diminishes the caliber of the aortic lumen, producing an obstruction to blood flow to the inferior part of the body (Fig. B1.34). The most common site for a coarctation is near the ligamentum arteriosum (Fig. 1.63). When the coarctation is inferior to this site (*postductal coarctation*), a good collateral circulation usually develops between the proximal and distal parts of the aorta through the intercostal and inter-

nal thoracic arteries. This type of coarctation is compatible with many years of life because the collateral circulation carries blood to the thoracic aorta inferior to the stenosis. The collateral vessels may become so large that they cause notable pulsation in the intercostal spaces and erode the adjacent surfaces of the ribs, which is visible in radiographs of the thorax.

Injury to Recurrent Laryngeal Nerves

The recurrent laryngeal nerves supply all intrinsic muscles of the larynx, except one. Consequently, any investigative (diagnostic) procedure (e.g., *mediastinotomy*) or disease process in the superior mediastinum may injure these nerves and affect the voice. Because the left recurrent laryngeal nerve winds around the arch of the aorta and ascends between the trachea and esophagus, it may be involved in a bronchogenic or esophageal carcinoma, enlargement of mediastinal lymph nodes, or an *aneurysm of the arch of the aorta*. In the latter condition, the nerve may be stretched by the dilated arch.

Blockage of Esophagus

The impressions produced in the esophagus by adjacent structures are of clinical interest because of the slower passage of substances at these sites. The impressions indicate where swallowed foreign objects are most likely to lodge and where a stricture may develop, e.g., after the accidental drinking of a caustic liquid such as lye.

Laceration of Thoracic Duct

 The thoracic duct is thin walled and usually dull white in living persons. However it may be colorless, making it difficult to identify. Consequently, it is vulnerable to inadvertent injury during investigative and/or surgical procedures in the posterior mediastinum. *Laceration of the thoracic duct* during an accident or lung surgery results in lymph escaping into the thoracic cavity at rates ranging from 75 to 200 mL per hour. Lymph or chyle from the lacteals of the intestine may also enter the pleural cavity, producing *chylothorax*. This fluid may be removed by a needle tap or by thoracentesis; in some cases it may be necessary to ligate (tie off) the thoracic duct. The lymph then returns to the venous system by other lymphatic channels that join the thoracic duct superior to the ligature.

Variations of Thoracic Duct

Variations of the thoracic duct are common because the superior part of the duct represents the original left member of a pair of lymphatic vessels in the embryo. Sometimes two thoracic ducts are present for a short distance.

Alternate Venous Routes to Heart

 The azygos, hemi-azygos, and accessory hemi-azygos veins offer alternate means of venous drainage from the thoracic, abdominal, and back regions when *obstruction of the IVC* occurs. In some people, an accessory azygos vein parallels the azygos vein on the right side. Other people have no hemi-azygos system of veins. A clinically important variation, although uncommon, is when the azygos system receives all the blood from the IVC except that from the liver. In these people, the azygos system drains nearly all the blood inferior to the diaphragm, except from the digestive tract. If *obstruction of the SVC* occurs superior to the entrance of the azygos vein, blood can drain inferiorly into the veins of the abdominal wall and return to the right atrium through the azygos venous system and the IVC.

Age Changes in Thymus

The thymus is a prominent feature of the superior mediastinum during infancy and childhood. In some infants, the thymus may compress the trachea. The thymus plays an important role in the development and maintenance of the immune system. As puberty is reached, the thymus begins to diminish in relative size. By adulthood, it is usually replaced by adipose tissue and is often scarcely recognizable; however, it continues to produce T-lymphocytes.

Aortic Angiography

To radiographically visualize the arch of the aorta and the branches arising from it, a long, narrow catheter is passed into the ascending

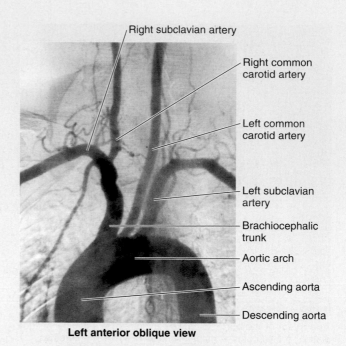

Left anterior oblique view

FIGURE B1.35. Aortic angiogram (aortogram).

aorta via the femoral or brachial artery in the inguinal or elbow region, respectively. Under fluoroscopic control, the tip of the catheter is placed just inside the opening of a coronary artery; an **aortic angiogram** can be made by injecting radiopaque contrast material into the aorta and into openings of the arteries arising from the arch of the aorta (Fig. B1.35).

Radiography of Mediastinum

 The heart casts most of the central radiopaque shadow in PA projections (Fig. B1.36), but the separate chambers of the heart are not distinguishable. Knowledge of the structures forming the **cardiovascular shadow** or silhouette is important because changes in the shadow may indicate anomalies or functional disease (Fig. B1.36A). In PA radiographs (AP views), the borders of the cardiovascular shadow are as follows:

- *Right border,* right brachiocephalic vein, SVC, right atrium, and IVC.
- *Left border,* terminal part of the arch of aorta, pulmonary trunk, left auricle, and left ventricle.

The left inferior part of the cardiovascular shadow presents the region of the apex. The typical anatomical apex, if present, is often inferior to the shadow of the diaphragm. Three main types of cardiovascular shadows occur, depending primarily on body type or habitus (Fig. B1.36B):

- *Transverse type,* observed in obese persons, pregnant women, and infants.
- *Oblique type,* characteristic of most people.
- *Vertical type,* present in people with narrow chests.

Anterior views

(B)   Transverse   Oblique   Vertical

FIGURE B1.36. Cardiovascular shadows (mediastinal silhouettes). A. Composition of the margins of the cardiovascular shadow. **B.** Common types of cardiovascular shadow.

CT and MRI of Mediastinum

CT and MRI are commonly used to examine the thorax. CT is sometimes combined with mammography to examine the breasts (Fig. B1.37). Before CT scans are taken, an iodide contrast material is given intravenously. Because breast cancer cells have an unusual affinity for iodide, they become recognizable. MRI is usually better for detecting and delineating soft tissue lesions. It is especially useful for examining the viscera and lymph nodes of the mediastinum and roots of the lungs, by means of both planar (Fig. B1.38) and reconstructed (Fig. B1.39) images. Transverse (axial) CT and MR scans are always oriented to show how a horizontal section of a patient's body lying on an examination table would appear to the physician who is at the patient's feet. Therefore, the top of the image is anterior, and the left lateral edge of the image represents the right lateral surface of the patient's body. Data from CT and MR scans can be graphically reconstructed by the computer as transverse, sagittal, oblique, or coronal sections of the body.

CT examination of breasts

Circled numbers = corresponding ribs

1. Nipple	7. Left lung
2. Lactiferous ducts	8. Liver
3. Suspensory ligaments	9. Inferior vena cava
4. Left ventricle	10. Esophagus
5. Right atrium	11. Descending aorta
6. Right lung	12. T9 vertebra

FIGURE B1.37. CT examination of breasts.

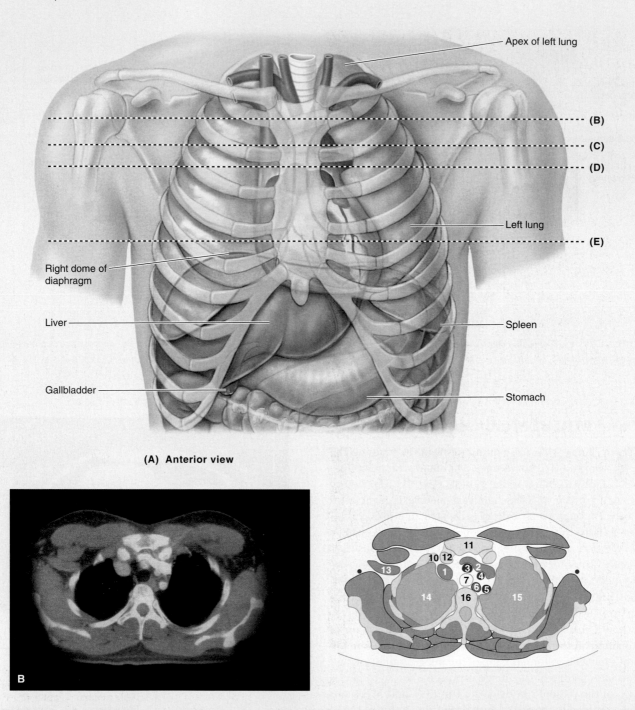

Apex of left lung

(B)

(C)

(D)

Left lung

(E)

Right dome of diaphragm

Liver

Spleen

Gallbladder

Stomach

(A) Anterior view

B

FIGURE B1.38. Serial transverse CT scans of thorax. A. The level of each scan is indicated (broken lines). **B.** At the level of the sternoclavicular joints, the left brachiocephalic vein (*2*) *crosses the midline anterior to the three branches of the arch of the aorta* (*3, 4,* and *5*) to join the right brachiocephalic vein (*1*), forming the superior vena cava [SVC] (*22*) at a more inferior level.

FIGURE B1.38. *(Continued)* **C.** The arch of the aorta (*20*) is obliquely placed (more sagittal than transverse), with the ascending end anteriorly in the mid-line, and the descending end posteriorly and to the left of the vertebral bodies (*17*). The SVC (*22*) on the right side receives the arch of the azygos vein (*23*) from its posterior aspect. **D.** The pulmonary trunk (*27*) forms the stem of an inverted Y, with the arms formed by the right (*28*) and left (*29*) pulmonary arteries. The right pulmonary artery (*28*) passes beneath the arch of the aorta [between ascending (*24*) and descending (*25*) aortae]. **E.** A scan at the level of the maximum diameter of the heart demonstrates all four chambers (*32–35*) and the diagonal slant of the interventricular septum (between *33* and *35*).

Key to Structures in Transverse CT Scans of Thorax

1 Right brachiocephalic vein	**14** Right lung	**26** Conus arteriosus
2 Left brachiocephalic vein	**15** Left lung	**27** Pulmonary trunk
3 Brachiocephalic artery	**16** T4 vertebral body	**28** Right pulmonary artery
4 Left common carotid artery	**17** T5 vertebral body	**29** Left pulmonary artery
5 Left subclavian artery	**18** T6 vertebral body	**30** Hemi-azygos vein
6 Esophagus	**19** T8 vertebral body	**31** Internal thoracic vessels
7 Trachea	**20** Arch of aorta	**32** Right atrium
8 Right main bronchus	**21** Anterior mediastinum	**33** Right ventricle
9 Left main bronchus	(region of thymic remnant)	**34** Left atrium
10 Costal cartilage	**22** Superior vena cava	**35** Left ventricle
11 Sternum	**23** Arch of azygos vein	**36** Inferior right pulmonary vein
12 Clavicle	**24** Ascending aorta	**37** Inferior left pulmonary vein
13 Axillary vein	**25** Descending aorta	

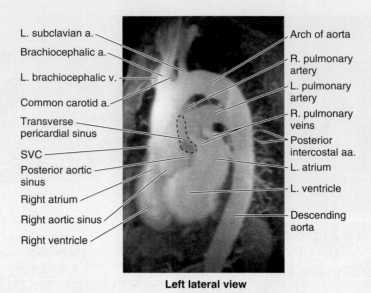

L. subclavian a.

Brachiocephalic a.

L. brachiocephalic v.

Common carotid a.

Transverse
pericardial sinus

SVC

Posterior aortic
sinus

Right atrium

Right aortic sinus

Right ventricle

Arch of aorta

R. pulmonary
artery

L. pulmonary
artery

R. pulmonary
veins

Posterior
intercostal aa.

L. atrium

L. ventricle

Descending
aorta

Left lateral view

FIGURE B1.39. **Magnetic resonance reconstructed angiogram of heart and great vessels.** Lateral view (from left and slightly anterior). Reconstructed from data generated and accumulated by spiral magnetic resonance imaging. All chambers of the heart and great vessels are clearly visible. *SVC*, superior vena cava.

The Bottom Line

SUPERIOR, POSTERIOR, AND ANTERIOR MEDIASTINUM; SURFACE ANATOMY OF THORACIC VISCERA

Superior mediastinum: The superior mediastinum extends between the superior thoracic aperture and the transverse thoracic plane. The only organ that belongs exclusively to this region is the adult thymus. ♦ The remainder of the structures in the superior mediastinum pass through the superior thoracic aperture to the root of the neck, or pass between the neck and abdomen. ♦ Within the superior mediastinum, structures occur in systemic layers, proceeding from anterior to posterior: (1) lymphoid system (thymus), (2) blood vascular system (veins first, then arteries), (3) respiratory system (trachea), (4) alimentary system (esophagus), and (5) lymph vascular system. ♦ The nervous system does not have its own layer in the superior mediastinum, but it is integrated with layer 2 (phrenic and vagus nerves) and lies between layers 3 and 4 (recurrent laryngeal nerves). ♦ The pattern of the branches of the arch of the aorta is atypical in approximately 35% of people.

Posterior mediastinum: The posterior mediastinum is the narrow passageway that lies posterior to the heart and diaphragm and between the lungs. It contains structures passing from thorax to abdomen or vice versa. ♦ Contents include the esophagus and esophageal nerve plexus, thoracic aorta, thoracic duct and lymphatic trunks, posterior mediastinal lymph nodes, and azygos and hemi-azygos veins. ♦ Branches of the thoracic aorta occur primarily within three vascular planes. ♦ The azygos/hemi-azygos venous system constitutes the venous counterpart to the thoracic aorta and its posterior mediastinal branches.

♦ The thoracic portion of the sympathetic trunks and thoracic splanchnic nerves may or may not be considered components of the posterior mediastinum.

Anterior mediastinum: The smallest subdivision of the mediastinum, between sternum and transversus thoracis muscles, significant primarily as a surgical plane, contains primarily loose connective tissue and, in infants and children, the inferior extend of the thymus.

Surface anatomy of thoracic viscera: The heart and great vessels are in the central thorax, surrounded laterally and posteriorly by the lungs, and are overlapped anteriorly by the lines of pleural reflection and anterior borders of the lungs, sternum and the central part of the thoracic cage.

♦ The position of the mediastinal viscera depends on position relative to gravity, phase of respiration, and the build and physical condition of the person. ♦ Apical portions of pleurae and lungs lie posterior to the supraclavicular fossa.

♦ The transverse thoracic plane intersects the sternal angle and demarcates the great vessels superiorly from the pericardium/heart. ♦ The xiphisternal junction provides an indication of the central tendon of the diaphragm.

Abdomen

The **abdomen** is the part of the trunk between the thorax and the pelvis (Fig. 2.1). It is a flexible, dynamic container, housing most of the organs of the alimentary system and part of the urogenital system. Containment of the abdominal organs and their contents is provided by *musculo-aponeurotic walls* anterolaterally, the diaphragm superiorly, and the muscles of the pelvis inferiorly. The anterolateral musculo-aponeurotic

walls are suspended between and supported by two bony rings (the inferior margin of the thoracic skeleton superiorly and the pelvic girdle inferiorly) linked by a semirigid lumbar vertebral column in the posterior abdominal wall. Interposed between the more rigid thorax and pelvis, this arrangement enables the abdomen to enclose and protect its contents while providing the flexibility required by respiration, posture, and locomotion.

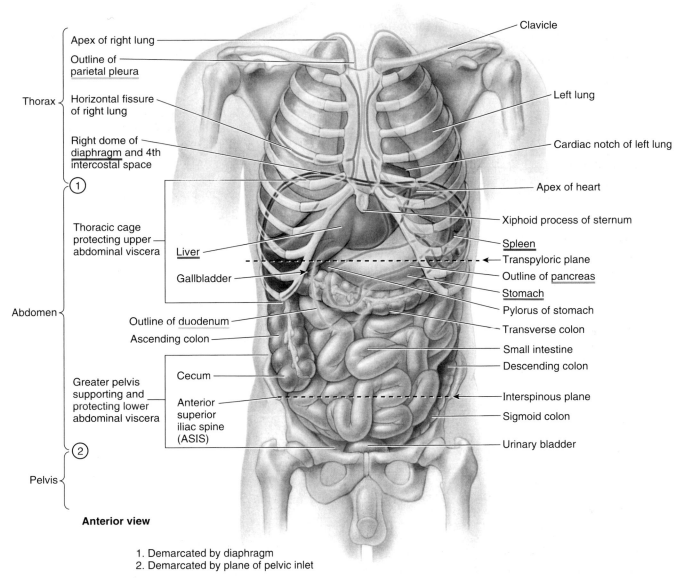

Anterior view

1. Demarcated by diaphragm
2. Demarcated by plane of pelvic inlet

FIGURE 2.1. Overview of viscera of thorax and abdomen *in situ*.

Through voluntary or reflexive contraction, its muscular roof, anterolateral walls, and floor can raise internal (intra-abdominal) pressure to aid expulsion of air from the thoracic cavity (lungs and bronchi) or of fluid (e.g., urine or vomitus), flatus, feces, or fetuses from the abdominopelvic cavity.

OVERVIEW: WALLS, CAVITIES, REGIONS, AND PLANES

The dynamic, multi-layered, musculo-aponeurotic **abdominal walls** not only contract to increase intra-abdominal pressure, but also distend considerably, accommodating expansions caused by ingestion, pregnancy, fat deposition, or pathology.

The *anterolateral abdominal wall* and several organs lying against the *posterior wall* are covered on their internal aspects with a serous membrane or *peritoneum* (serosa) that *reflects* (turns sharply and continues) onto the **abdominal viscera** (L., soft parts, internal organs), such as the stomach, intestine, liver, and spleen. Thus, a bursal sac or lined potential space (*peritoneal cavity*) is formed between the walls and the viscera that normally contains only enough extracellular (parietal) fluid to lubricate the membrane covering most of the surfaces of the structures forming or occupying the abdominal cavity. Visceral movement associated with digestion occurs freely, and the double-layered reflections of peritoneum passing between the walls and the viscera provide passage for the blood vessels, lymphatics, and nerves. Variable amounts of fat may also occur between the walls and viscera and the peritoneum lining them.

The **abdominal cavity:**

- forms the superior and major part of the **abdominopelvic cavity** (Fig. 2.2), the continuous cavity that extends between the *thoracic diaphragm* and *pelvic diaphragm.*
- has no floor of its own because it is continuous with the *pelvic cavity.* The plane of the *pelvic inlet* (superior pelvic aperture) arbitrarily, but not physically, separates the abdominal and the pelvic cavities.
- extends superiorly into the osseocartilaginous *thoracic cage* to the 4th intercostal space (Fig. 2.1). Consequently, the more superiorly placed abdominal organs (spleen, liver, part of the kidneys, and stomach) are protected by the thoracic cage. The *greater pelvis* (expanded part of the pelvis superior to the pelvic inlet) supports and partly protects the lower abdominal viscera (part of the ileum, cecum, appendix, and sigmoid colon).
- is the location of most digestive organs, parts of the urogenital system (kidneys and most of the ureters), and the spleen.

Nine regions of the abdominal cavity are used to describe the location of abdominal organs, pains, or pathologies (Table 2.1A & B). The regions are delineated by four planes: two sagittal (vertical) and two transverse (horizontal) planes. The two sagittal planes are usually the *midclavicular planes* that pass from the midpoint of the clavicles (approximately 9 cm

from the midline) to the **midinguinal points,** midpoints of the lines joining the *anterior superior iliac spine* (ASIS) and the *pubic tubercles* on each side.

Most commonly, the transverse planes are the **subcostal plane,** passing through the inferior border of the 10th costal cartilage on each side, and the **transtubercular plane,** passing through the iliac tubercles (approximately 5 cm posterior to the ASIS on each side) and the body of the L5 vertebra. Both of these planes have the advantage of intersecting palpable structures.

Some clinicians use the transpyloric and interspinous planes to establish the nine regions. The **transpyloric plane,** extrapolated midway between the superior borders of the manubrium of the sternum and the pubic symphysis (typically the L1 vertebral level), commonly transects the *pylorus* (the distal, more tubular part of the stomach) when the patient is recumbent (supine or prone) (Fig. 2.1). Because the viscera sag with the pull of gravity, the pylorus usually lies at a lower level when the individual is standing erect. The transpyloric plane is a useful landmark because it also transects many other important structures: the fundus of the gallbladder, neck of the pancreas, origins of the superior mesenteric artery (SMA) and hepatic portal vein, root of the transverse mesocolon, duodenojejunal junction, and hila of the kidneys. The **interspinous plane** passes through the easily palpated ASIS on each side (Table 2.1B).

For more general clinical descriptions, four quadrants of the abdominal cavity (right and left upper and lower quadrants) are defined by two readily defined planes: (1) the transverse **transumbilical plane,** passing through the umbilicus (and the intervertebral [IV] disc between the L3 and L4 vertebrae), dividing it into upper and lower halves, and (2) the vertical *median plane,* passing longitudinally through the body, dividing it into right and left halves (Table 2.1C).

It is important to know what organs are located in each abdominal region or quadrant so that one knows where to auscultate, percuss, and palpate them (Table 2.1), and to record the locations of findings during a physical examination.

ANTEROLATERAL ABDOMINAL WALL

Although the abdominal wall is continuous, it is subdivided into the *anterior wall, right and left lateral walls,* and *posterior wall* for descriptive purposes (Fig. 2.3). The wall is musculo-aponeurotic, except for the posterior wall, which includes the lumbar region of the vertebral column. The boundary between the anterior and lateral walls is indefinite, therefore the term **anterolateral abdominal wall** is often used. Some structures, such as muscles and cutaneous nerves, are in both the anterior and lateral walls. The anterolateral abdominal wall extends from the thoracic cage to the pelvis.

The anterolateral abdominal wall is bounded superiorly by the cartilages of the 7th–10th ribs and the xiphoid process of the sternum, and inferiorly by the inguinal ligament and the

Body cavities
- Thoracic cavity
- Abdominal cavity
- Pelvic cavity

Plane of superior thoracic aperture (thoracic inlet)

Thoracic cage

Thoracic diaphragm

Plane of superior pelvic aperture (pelvic inlet)

Abdominopelvic cavity

Pubic symphysis

Pelvic diaphragm

Medial view

FIGURE 2.2. Abdominopelvic cavity. The body has been sectioned in the median plane to show the abdominal and pelvic cavities as subdivisions of the continuous abdominopelvic cavity.

TABLE 2.1. ABDOMINAL REGIONS (A), REFERENCE PLANES (B), AND QUADRANTS (C)

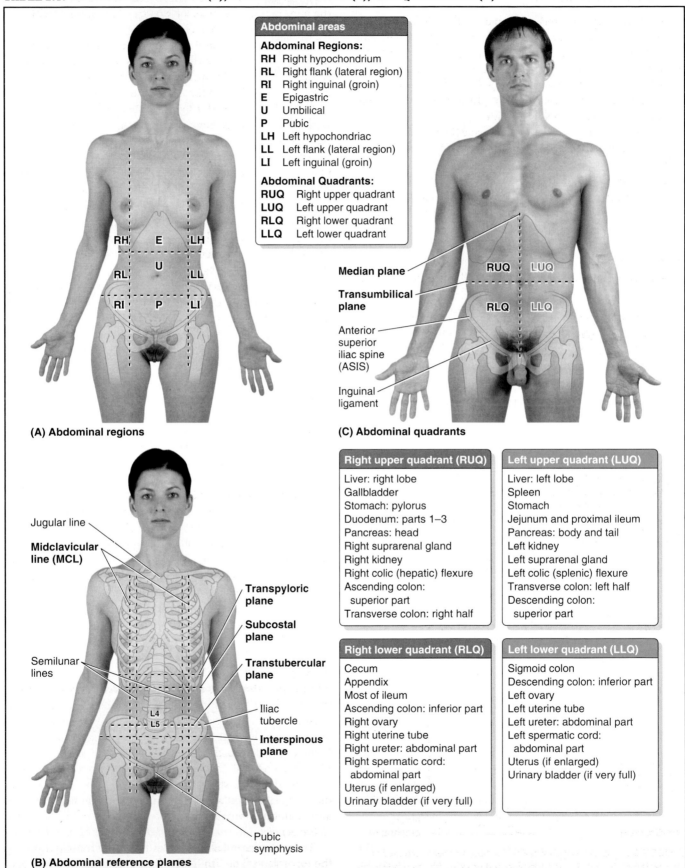

Abdominal areas

Abdominal Regions:
- **RH** Right hypochondrium
- **RL** Right flank (lateral region)
- **RI** Right inguinal (groin)
- **E** Epigastric
- **U** Umbilical
- **P** Pubic
- **LH** Left hypochondriac
- **LL** Left flank (lateral region)
- **LI** Left inguinal (groin)

Abdominal Quadrants:
- **RUQ** Right upper quadrant
- **LUQ** Left upper quadrant
- **RLQ** Right lower quadrant
- **LLQ** Left lower quadrant

(A) Abdominal regions

(C) Abdominal quadrants

Median plane
Transumbilical plane
Anterior superior iliac spine (ASIS)
Inguinal ligament

(B) Abdominal reference planes

Jugular line
Midclavicular line (MCL)
Semilunar lines
Transpyloric plane
Subcostal plane
Transtubercular plane
Iliac tubercle
Interspinous plane
Pubic symphysis
L4
L5

Right upper quadrant (RUQ)	Left upper quadrant (LUQ)
Liver: right lobe	Liver: left lobe
Gallbladder	Spleen
Stomach: pylorus	Stomach
Duodenum: parts 1–3	Jejunum and proximal ileum
Pancreas: head	Pancreas: body and tail
Right suprarenal gland	Left kidney
Right kidney	Left suprarenal gland
Right colic (hepatic) flexure	Left colic (splenic) flexure
Ascending colon: superior part	Transverse colon: left half
Transverse colon: right half	Descending colon: superior part

Right lower quadrant (RLQ)	Left lower quadrant (LLQ)
Cecum	Sigmoid colon
Appendix	Descending colon: inferior part
Most of ileum	Left ovary
Ascending colon: inferior part	Left uterine tube
Right ovary	Left ureter: abdominal part
Right uterine tube	Left spermatic cord: abdominal part
Right ureter: abdominal part	Uterus (if enlarged)
Right spermatic cord: abdominal part	Urinary bladder (if very full)
Uterus (if enlarged)	
Urinary bladder (if very full)	

Vertical anterior abdominal muscles

Linea alba

Flat anterolateral abdominal muscles

Anterior

Anterolateral

Left lateral (flank)

of abdomen

of back

Vertical posterior muscles

Posterior

Axio-appendicular muscles*

Lumbar vertebra

Inferior view

* Boundary indefinite and overlapping

FIGURE 2.3. Subdivisions of abdominal wall. A transverse section of the abdomen demonstrates various aspects of the wall and its components. [*The relatively superficial latissimus dorsi and deeper psoas major muscles are axioappendicular muscles that attach distally in the upper and lower limbs, respectively.]

superior margins of the anterolateral aspects of the pelvic girdle (iliac crests, pubic crests, and pubic symphysis) (Fig. 2.4A).

The anterolateral abdominal wall consists of skin and subcutaneous tissue (superficial fascia) composed mainly of fat, muscles and their aponeuroses and deep fascia, extraperitoneal fat, and parietal peritoneum (Fig. 2.4B). The skin attaches loosely to the subcutaneous tissue, except at the umbilicus, where it adheres firmly. Most of the anterolateral wall includes three musculotendinous layers; the fiber bundles of each layer run in different directions. This three-ply structure is similar to that of the intercostal spaces in the thorax.

Fascia of the Anterolateral Abdominal Wall

The subcutaneous tissue over most of the wall includes a variable amount of fat. It is a major site of fat storage. Males are especially susceptible to subcutaneous accumulation of fat in the lower anterior abdominal wall. In *morbid obesity*, the fat is many inches thick, often forming one or more sagging folds (L. *panniculi;* singular = *panniculus*, apron).

Superior to the umbilicus, the subcutaneous tissue is consistent with that found in most regions. Inferior to the umbilicus, the deepest part of the subcutaneous tissue is reinforced by many elastic and collagen fibers, so it has two layers: the **superficial fatty layer** (Camper fascia) and the **deep membranous layer** (Scarpa fascia) **of subcutaneous tissue.** The membranous layer continues inferiorly into

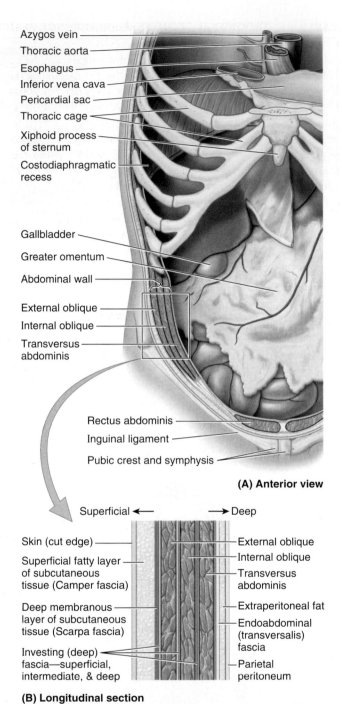

Azygos vein

Thoracic aorta

Esophagus

Inferior vena cava

Pericardial sac

Thoracic cage

Xiphoid process of sternum

Costodiaphragmatic recess

Gallbladder

Greater omentum

Abdominal wall

External oblique

Internal oblique

Transversus abdominis

Rectus abdominis

Inguinal ligament

Pubic crest and symphysis

(A) Anterior view

Superficial ← → Deep

Skin (cut edge)

Superficial fatty layer of subcutaneous tissue (Camper fascia)

Deep membranous layer of subcutaneous tissue (Scarpa fascia)

Investing (deep) fascia—superficial, intermediate, & deep

External oblique

Internal oblique

Transversus abdominis

Extraperitoneal fat

Endoabdominal (transversalis) fascia

Parietal peritoneum

(B) Longitudinal section

FIGURE 2.4. Abdominal contents, undisturbed, and layers of antero-lateral abdominal wall. A. The anterior abdominal wall and soft tissues of the anterior thoracic wall have been removed. Most of the intestine is covered by the apron-like greater omentum, a peritoneal fold hanging from the stomach. B. Layers of the anterolateral abdominal wall, including the trilaminar flat muscles, are shown.

the perineal region as the superficial perineal fascia (Colles fascia), but not into the thighs.

Superficial, intermediate, and deep layers of investing fascia cover the external aspects of the three muscle layers of the anterolateral abdominal wall and their *aponeuroses* (flat expanded tendons) and cannot be easily separated from them.

The investing fascias here are extremely thin, being represented mostly by the *epimysium* (outer fibrous connective tissue layer surrounding all muscles—see Introduction) superficial to or between muscles. The internal aspect of the abdominal wall is lined with membranous and areolar sheets of varying thickness constituting **endoabdominal fascia.** Although continuous, different parts of this fascia are named according to the muscle or aponeurosis it is lining. The portion lining the deep surface of the transversus abdominis muscle and its aponeurosis is the **transversalis fascia.** The glistening lining of the abdominal cavity, the *parietal peritoneum,* is formed by a single layer of epithelial cells and supporting connective tissue. The parietal peritoneum is internal to the transversalis fascia and is separated from it by a variable amount of **extraperitoneal fat.**

Muscles of Anterolateral Abdominal Wall

There are five (bilaterally paired) muscles in the anterolateral abdominal wall (Fig. 2.3): three flat muscles and two vertical muscles. Their attachments are demonstrated in Figure 2.5 and listed, along with their nerve supply and main actions, in Table 2.2.

The *three flat muscles* are the *external oblique, internal oblique,* and *transversus abdominis.* The muscle fibers of these three concentric muscle layers have varying orientations, with the fibers of the outer two layers running diagonally and perpendicular to each other for the main part, and the fibers of the deep layer running transversely. All three flat muscles are continued anteriorly and medially as strong,

(A) Layer 1

Free posterior border of external oblique
Internal oblique
External oblique
Rectus sheath (anterior layer)
Anterior superior iliac spine (ASIS)
Inguinal ligament
Attachment of external oblique to iliac crest

(B) Layer 2

External oblique (cut)
Thoracolumbar fascia
Internal oblique
Inguinal ligament

(C) Layer 3

Cut attachments of internal oblique
Transversus abdominis
12th rib
Quadratus lumborum (posterior abdominal wall)

(D) Anterior & posterior wall muscles

Costal cartilages
Rectus abdominis
Tendinous intersections
Pubic crest

Lateral views

(A) - (C) = Three layers of muscles of anterolateral abdominal wall

(E) Inferior view of transverse section of posterolateral abdominal wall

Psoas muscle
Quadratus lumborum
Thoracolumbar fascia:
Anterior layer
Middle layer
Posterior layer

Origin of (2) & (3) from lateral part of thoracolumbar fascia

Layers of anterolateral abdominal wall muscle:
(1) External oblique
(2) Internal oblique
(3) Transversus abdominis
Free posterior border of external oblique (1)
Latissimus dorsi
Deep muscles of back

FIGURE 2.5. Muscles of anterolateral abdominal wall.

TABLE 2.2. MUSCLES OF ANTEROLATERAL ABDOMINAL WALL

Muscle	Origin	Insertion	Innervation	Main Action[a]
External oblique (A)	External surfaces of 5th–12th ribs	Linea alba, pubic tubercle, and anterior half of iliac crest	Thoraco-abdominal nerves (T7–T11 spinal nerves) and subcostal nerve	Compresses and supports abdominal viscera,[b] flexes and rotates trunk
Internal oblique (B)	Thoracolumbar fascia, anterior two thirds of iliac crest, and connective tissue deep to lateral third of inguinal ligament	Inferior borders of 10th–12th ribs, linea alba, and pecten pubis via conjoint tendon	Thoraco-abdominal nerves (anterior rami of T6–T12 spinal nerves) and first lumbar nerves	
Transversus abdominis (C)	Internal surfaces of 7th–12th costal cartilages, thoracolumbar fascia, iliac crest, and connective tissue deep to lateral third of inguinal ligament	Linea alba with aponeurosis of internal oblique, pubic crest, and pecten pubis via conjoint tendon		Compresses and supports abdominal viscera[b]
Rectus abdominis (D)	Pubic symphysis and pubic crest	Xiphoid process and 5th–7th costal cartilages	Thoraco-abdominal nerves (anterior rami of T6–T12 spinal nerves)	Flexes trunk (lumbar vertebrae) and compresses abdominal viscera;[b] stabilizes and controls tilt of pelvis (antilordosis)

[a]Approximately 80% of people have an insignificant muscle, the *pyramidalis*, which is located in the rectus sheath anterior to the most inferior part of the rectus abdominis. It extends from the pubic crest of the hip bone to the linea alba. This small muscle draws down on the linea alba.

[b]In so doing, these muscles act as antagonists of the diaphragm to produce expiration.

sheet-like aponeuroses (Fig. 2.6A). Between the midclavicular line (MCL) and the midline, the aponeuroses form the tough, aponeurotic, tendinous *rectus sheath* enclosing the rectus abdominis muscle (Fig. 2.6B). The aponeuroses then interweave with their fellows of the opposite side, forming a midline raphe (G. *rhaphe,* suture, seam), the **linea alba** (L. white line), which extends from the xiphoid process to the pubic symphysis. The decussation and interweaving of the aponeurotic fibers here is not only between right and left sides but also between superficial and intermediate and intermediate and deep layers.

The *two vertical muscles* of the anterolateral abdominal wall, contained within the rectus sheath, are the large *rectus abdominis* and the small *pyramidalis.*

EXTERNAL OBLIQUE MUSCLE

The **external oblique muscle** is the largest and most superficial of the three flat anterolateral abdominal muscles (Fig. 2.7). The attachments of the external oblique are demonstrated in Figure 2.5A, and listed, along with the nerve supply, and main actions, in Table 2.2. In contrast to the two deeper layers, the external oblique does not originate posteriorly from the thoracolumbar fascia; its posteriormost fibers (the thickest part of the muscle) have a free edge where they span between its costal origin and the iliac crest (Fig 2.5D & E). The fleshy part of the muscle contributes primarily to the lateral part of the abdominal wall. Its aponeurosis contributes to the anterior part of the wall.

Although the posteriormost fibers from rib 12 are nearly vertical as they run to the iliac crest, more anterior fibers fan out, taking an increasingly medial direction so that most of the fleshy fibers run inferomedially—in the same direction as the fingers do when the hands are in one's side pockets—with the most anterior and superior fibers approaching a horizontal course. The muscle fibers become aponeurotic approximately at the MCL medially and at the **spino-umbilical line** (line running from the umbilicus to the ASIS) inferiorly, forming a sheet of tendinous fibers that decussate at the linea alba, most becoming continuous with tendinous fibers of the contralateral internal oblique (see Fig. 2.6A). Thus, the contralateral external and internal oblique muscles together form a "digastric muscle," a two-bellied muscle sharing a common central tendon that works as a unit (see Introduction chapter). For example, the right external oblique and left internal oblique work together when flexing and rotating to bring the right shoulder toward the left hip (torsional movement of trunk).

Inferiorly, the external oblique aponeurosis attaches to the *pubic crest* medial to the *pubic tubercle.* The inferior margin of the external oblique aponeurosis is thickened as an undercurving fibrous band with a free posterior edge that spans between the ASIS and the pubic tubercle as the *inguinal ligament* (Poupart ligament) (Figs. 2.7B and 2.8).

Palpate your inguinal ligament by pressing deeply into the center of the crease between the thigh and trunk and moving the fingertips up and down. Inferiorly the

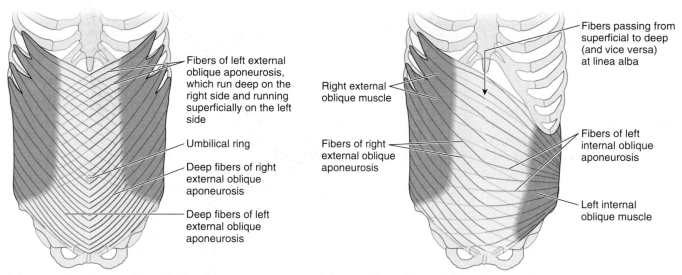

Fibers of left external oblique aponeurosis, which run deep on the right side and running superficially on the left side

Umbilical ring

Deep fibers of right external oblique aponeurosis

Deep fibers of left external oblique aponeurosis

Fibers passing from superficial to deep (and vice versa) at linea alba

Right external oblique muscle

Fibers of right external oblique aponeurosis

Fibers of left internal oblique aponeurosis

Left internal oblique muscle

Intramuscular exchange of superficial and deep fibers within aponeuroses of contralateral external oblique muscles.

Intermuscular exchange of fibers between aponeuroses of contralateral external and internal oblique muscles.

(A) Anterior views

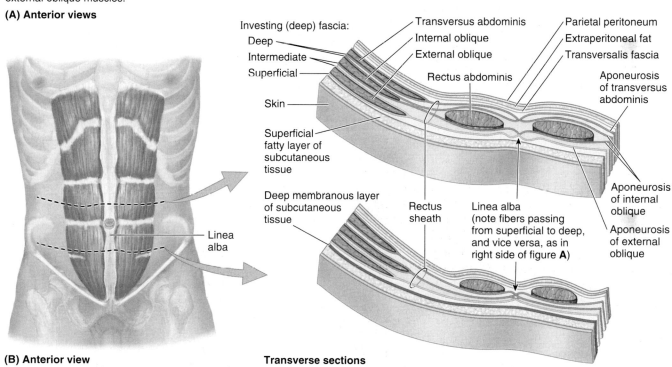

Linea alba

Investing (deep) fascia:
Deep
Intermediate
Superficial

Skin

Superficial fatty layer of subcutaneous tissue

Deep membranous layer of subcutaneous tissue

Rectus sheath

Transversus abdominis
Internal oblique
External oblique

Rectus abdominis

Linea alba (note fibers passing from superficial to deep, and vice versa, as in right side of figure **A**)

Parietal peritoneum
Extraperitoneal fat
Transversalis fascia

Aponeurosis of transversus abdominis

Aponeurosis of internal oblique

Aponeurosis of external oblique

(B) Anterior view   **Transverse sections**

FIGURE 2.6. Structure of anterolateral abdominal wall. A. Intramuscular and intermuscular fiber exchanges within the bilaminar aponeuroses of the external and internal oblique muscles are shown. **B.** Transverse sections of the wall superior and inferior to the umbilicus show the makeup of the rectus sheath.

inguinal ligament is continuous with the deep fascia of the thigh. The inguinal ligament is therefore not a free-standing structure, although—as a useful landmark—it is frequently depicted as such. It serves as a *retinaculum* (retaining band) for the muscular and neurovascular structures passing deep to it to enter the thigh. The inferior parts of the two deeper anterolateral abdominal muscles arise in relationship to the lateral portion of the inguinal ligament. The complex modifications and attachments of the inguinal ligament, and of the inferomedial portions

of the aponeuroses of the anterolateral abdominal wall muscles, are discussed in detail with the inguinal region (later in this chapter).

INTERNAL OBLIQUE MUSCLE

The intermediate of the three flat abdominal muscles, the **internal oblique** is a thin muscular sheet that fans out anteromedially (Figs. 2.5B, 2.8, and 2.9A). Except for its lowermost fibers, which arise from the lateral half of the

Serratus anterior

5th costal cartilage

Anterior layer of rectus sheath

Anterior layer of
rectus sheath

Rectus abdominis

Linea alba

External oblique

External oblique

Lateral abdominal
cutaneous branches

Tendinous intersection

Anterior abdominal
cutaneous branches

Anterior superior iliac spine

External oblique aponeurosis

Superficial circumflex iliac
artery and vein

Deep membranous layer
of subcutaneous tissue

Superficial epigastric
artery and vein

Intercrural fibers

Superficial inguinal ring

External pudendal
artery and vein

Ilio-inguinal nerve
Spermatic cord

Great saphenous vein

(A) Anterior view

Internal oblique

External oblique

Transversus abdominis

Anterior superior iliac spine

External oblique aponeurosis

Musculo-aponeurotic arcade of
transversus abdominis

Deep inguinal ring
(transversalis fascia)

Spermatic cord

Incurved lower margin
(gutter) of aponeurosis
forming inguinal ligament
(floor of inguinal canal)

Inguinal ligament (passing
anterior to pecten pubis)

Nerve
Femoral Artery
Vein

Pubic tubercle

Pubic crest

(B) Anterior view

Testis

FIGURE 2.7. Anterolateral abdominal wall. A. In this superficial dissection, the anterior layer of the rectus sheath is reflected on the left side. Observe the anterior cutaneous nerves (T7–T12) piercing the rectus abdominis and the anterior layer of the rectus sheath. **B.** The three flat abdominal muscles and the formation of the inguinal ligament are demonstrated.

FIGURE 2.8. Inferior abdominal wall and inguinal region of a male. The aponeurosis of the external oblique is partly cut away, and the spermatic cord has been cut and removed from the inguinal canal.

inguinal ligament, its fleshy fibers run perpendicular to those of the external oblique, running superomedially (like your fingers when the hand is placed over your chest). Its fibers also become aponeurotic at the MCL and participate in the formation of the rectus sheath. The attachments of the internal oblique are demonstrated in Figure 2.5B, and listed, along with the nerve supply and main actions, in Table 2.2.

TRANSVERSUS ABDOMINIS MUSCLE

The fibers of the **transversus abdominis,** the innermost of the three flat abdominal muscles (see Figs. 2.5C and 2.7B), run more or less transversally, except for the inferior ones, which run parallel to those of the internal oblique. This transverse, circumferential orientation is ideal for compressing the abdominal contents, increasing intra-abdominal pressure. The fibers of the transversus abdominis muscle also end in an aponeurosis, which contributes to the formation of the rectus sheath (Fig. 2.9). The attachments of the transversus abdominis are demonstrated in Figure 2.5C, and listed, along with the nerve supply and main actions, in Table 2.2.

Between the internal oblique and the transversus abdominis muscles is a *neurovascular plane,* which corresponds with a similar plane in the intercostal spaces. In both regions, the

plane lies between the middle and deepest layers of muscle (Fig. 2.9A). The **neurovascular plane of the anterolateral abdominal wall** contains the nerves and arteries supplying the anterolateral abdominal wall. In the anterior part of the abdominal wall, the nerves and vessels leave the neurovascular plane and lie mostly in the subcutaneous tissue.

RECTUS ABDOMINIS MUSCLE

A long, broad, strap-like muscle, the **rectus abdominis** (L. *rectus,* straight) is the principal vertical muscle of the anterior abdominal wall (Figs. 2.5D, 2.6A, and 2.8B). The attachments of the rectus abdominis are demonstrated in Figure 2.5D, and listed, along with the nerve supply and main actions, in Table 2.2. The paired rectus muscles, separated by the linea alba, lie close together inferiorly. The rectus abdominis is three times as wide superiorly as inferiorly; it is broad and thin superiorly and narrow and thick inferiorly. Most of the rectus abdominis is enclosed in the rectus sheath. The rectus muscle is anchored transversely by attachment to the anterior layer of the rectus sheath at three or more **tendinous intersections** (see Figs. 2.5D and 2.7A). When tensed in muscular people, the areas of muscle between the tendinous intersections bulge outward. The intersections,

(A) Anterior view   **(B) Schematic sagittal section**

FIGURE 2.9. Formation of rectus sheath and neurovascular structures of anterolateral abdominal wall. A. In this deep dissection, the fleshy portion of the external oblique is excised on the right side, but its aponeurosis and the anterior wall of the rectus sheath are intact. The anterior wall of the sheath and the rectus abdominis are removed on the left side so that the posterior wall of the sheath may be seen. Lateral to the left rectus sheath, the fleshy part of the internal oblique has been cut longitudinally; the edges of the cut are retracted to reveal the thoraco-abdominal nerves coursing in the neurovascular plane between the internal oblique and the transversus abdominis. **B.** Sagittal section through the rectus sheath of the anterior abdominal wall.

indicated by grooves in the skin between the muscular bulges, usually occur at the level of the xiphoid process, umbilicus, and halfway between these structures.

PYRAMIDALIS

The **pyramidalis** is a small, insignificant triangular muscle that is absent in approximately 20% of people. It lies anterior to the inferior part of the rectus abdominis and attaches to the anterior surface of the pubis and the anterior pubic ligament. It ends in the linea alba, which is especially thickened for a variable distance superior to the pubic symphysis. The pyramidalis tenses the linea alba. When present, surgeons use the attachment of the pyramidalis to the linea alba as a landmark for median abdominal incision (Skandalakis et al., 2009).

RECTUS SHEATH, LINEA ALBA, AND UMBILICAL RING

The **rectus sheath** is the strong, incomplete fibrous compartment of the rectus abdominis and pyramidalis muscles (Figs. 2.7–2.9). Also found in the rectus sheath are the superior and inferior epigastric arteries and veins, lymphatic vessels, and distal portions of the thoraco-abdominal nerves (abdominal portions of the anterior rami of spinal nerves T7–T12).

The rectus sheath is formed by the decussation and interweaving of the aponeuroses of the flat abdominal muscles (Fig. 2.6B). The external oblique aponeurosis contributes to the anterior wall of the sheath throughout its length. The superior two thirds of the internal oblique aponeurosis splits into two layers (laminae) at the lateral border of the rectus abdominis; one lamina passing anterior to the muscle and the other passing posterior to it. The anterior lamina joins the aponeurosis of the external oblique to form the anterior layer of the rectus sheath. The posterior lamina joins the aponeurosis of the transversus abdominis to form the posterior layer of the rectus sheath.

Beginning approximately one third of the distance from the umbilicus to the pubic crest, the aponeuroses of the three flat muscles pass anterior to the rectus abdominis to form the anterior layer of the rectus sheath, leaving only the relatively thin transversalis fascia to cover the rectus abdominis posteriorly. A crescentic **arcuate line** (Fig. 2.9) demarcates the transition between the aponeurotic posterior wall of the sheath covering the superior three quarters of the rectus and the transversalis fascia covering the inferior quarter. Throughout the length of the sheath, the fibers of the anterior and posterior layers of the sheath interlace in the anterior median line to form the complex *linea alba*.

The posterior layer of the rectus sheath is also deficient superior to the costal margin because the transversus abdominis is continued superiorly as the transversus thoracis, which lies internal to the costal cartilages (see Fig. 1.14, p. 89), and the internal oblique attaches to the costal margin. Hence, superior to the costal margin, the rectus abdominis lies directly on the thoracic wall (Fig. 2.9B).

The linea alba, running vertically the length of the anterior abdominal wall and separating the bilateral rectus sheaths (Fig. 2.7A), narrows inferior to the umbilicus to the width of the pubic symphysis and widens superiorly to the width of the xiphoid process. The linea alba transmits small vessels and nerves to the skin. In thin muscular people, a groove is visible in the skin overlying the linea alba. At its middle, underlying the umbilicus, the linea alba contains the **umbilical ring,** a defect in the linea alba through which the fetal umbilical vessels passed to and from the umbilical cord and placenta. All layers of the anterolateral abdominal wall fuse at the umbilicus. As fat accumulates in the subcutaneous tissue postnatally, the skin becomes raised around the umbilical ring and the umbilicus becomes depressed. This occurs 7–14 days after birth, when the atrophic umbilical cord "falls off."

FUNCTIONS AND ACTIONS OF ANTEROLATERAL ABDOMINAL MUSCLES

The muscles of the anterolateral abdominal wall:

- Form a strong expandable support for the anterolateral abdominal wall.
- Support the abdominal viscera and protect them from most injuries.
- Compress the abdominal contents to maintain or increase the intra-abdominal pressure and, in so doing, oppose the diaphragm (increased intra-abdominal pressure facilitates expulsion).
- Move the trunk and help to maintain posture.

The oblique and transverse muscles, acting together bilaterally, form a muscular girdle that exerts firm pressure on the abdominal viscera. The rectus abdominis participates little, if at all, in this action. Compressing the abdominal viscera and increasing intra-abdominal pressure elevates the relaxed diaphragm to expel air during respiration, and more forcibly for coughing, sneezing, nose blowing, voluntary eructation (burping), and yelling or screaming. When the diaphragm contracts during inspiration, the anterolateral abdominal wall expands as its muscles relax to make room for the organs, such as the liver, that are pushed inferiorly. The combined actions of the anterolateral muscles also produce the force required for defecation (discharge of feces), micturition (urination), vomiting, and parturition (childbirth). Increased intra-abdominal (and intrathoracic) pressure is also involved in heavy lifting, the resulting force sometimes producing a hernia.

The anterolateral abdominal muscles are also involved in movements of the trunk at the lumbar vertebrae and in controlling the tilt of the pelvis when standing for maintenance of posture (resisting lumbar lordosis). Consequently, strengthening the anterolateral abdominal wall musculature improves standing and sitting posture. The rectus abdominis is a powerful flexor of the thoracic and especially lumbar regions of the vertebral column, pulling the anterior costal margin and pubic crest toward each other. The oblique abdominal muscles also assist in movements of the trunk, especially lateral flexion and rotation of the lumbar and lower thoracic vertebral column. The transversus abdominis probably has no appreciable effect on the vertebral column (Standring, 2008).

Neurovasculature of Anterolateral Abdominal Wall

DERMATOMES OF ANTEROLATERAL ABDOMINAL WALL

The map of dermatomes of the anterolateral abdominal wall is almost identical to the map of peripheral nerve distribution (Fig. 2.10). This is because the anterior rami of spinal nerves T7–T12, which supply most of the abdominal wall, do not participate in plexus formation. The exception occurs at the L1 level, where the L1 anterior ramus bifurcates into two named peripheral nerves. Each dermatome begins posteriorly overlying the intervertebral foramen by which the spinal nerve exits the vertebral column and follows the slope of the ribs around the trunk. Dermatome T10 includes the umbilicus, whereas dermatome L1 includes the inguinal fold.

NERVES OF ANTEROLATERAL ABDOMINAL WALL

The skin and muscles of the anterolateral abdominal wall are supplied mainly by the following nerves (Fig. 2.9A and 2.10; Table 2.3):

- **Thoraco-abdominal nerves:** these are the distal, abdominal parts of the anterior rami of the inferior six thoracic spinal nerves (T7–T11); they are the former inferior intercostal nerves distal to the costal margin.

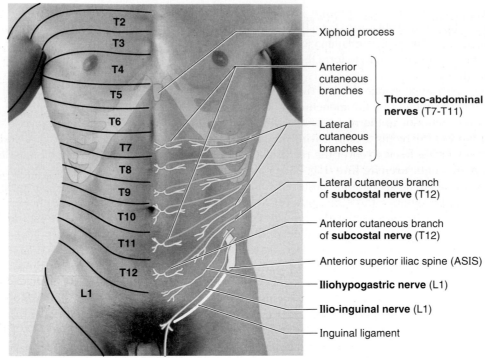

FIGURE 2.10. Dermatomes and nerves of anterolateral abdominal wall.

TABLE 2.3. NERVES OF ANTEROLATERAL ABDOMINAL WALL

Nerves	Origin	Course	Distribution
Thoraco-abdominal (T7–T11)	Continuation of lower (7th–11th) intercostal nerves distal to costal margin	Run between second and third layers of abdominal muscles; branches enter subcutaneous tissue as lateral cutaneous branches of T10–T11 (in anterior axillary line) and anterior cutaneous branches of T7–T11 (parasternal line)	Muscles of anterolateral abdominal wall and overlying skin
7th–9th lateral cutaneous branches	7th–9th intercostal nerves (anterior rami of spinal nerves T7–T9)	Anterior divisions continue across costal margin in subcutaneous tissue	Skin of right and left hypochondriac regions
Subcostal (anterior ramus of T12)	Spinal nerve T12	Runs along inferior border of 12th rib; then passes onto subumbilical abdominal wall between second and third layers of abdominal muscles	Muscles of anterolateral abdominal wall (including most inferior slip of external oblique) and overlying skin, superior to iliac crest and inferior to umbilicus
Iliohypogastric (L1)	As superior terminal branch of anterior ramus of spinal nerve L1	Pierces transversus abdominis muscle to course between second and third layers of abdominal muscles; branches pierce external oblique aponeuroses of most inferior abdominal wall	Skin overlying iliac crest, upper inguinal, and hypogastric regions; internal oblique and transversus abdominis muscles
Ilio-inguinal (L1)	As inferior terminal branch of anterior ramus of spinal nerve L1	Passes between second and third layers of abdominal muscles; then traverses inguinal canal	Skin of lower inguinal region, mons pubis, anterior scrotum or labium majus, and adjacent medial thigh; inferiormost internal oblique and transversus abdominis

- **Lateral (thoracic) cutaneous branches:** of the thoracic spinal nerves T7–T9 or T10.
- **Subcostal nerve:** the large anterior ramus of spinal nerve T12.
- **Iliohypogastric** and **ilio-inguinal nerves:** terminal branches of the anterior ramus of spinal nerve L1.

The *thoraco-abdominal nerves* pass inferoanteriorly from the intercostal spaces and run in the neurovascular plane between the internal oblique and the transversus abdominis muscles to supply the abdominal skin and muscles. The *lateral cutaneous branches* emerge from the musculature of the anterolateral wall to enter the subcutaneous tissue along the anterior axillary line (as anterior and posterior divisions), whereas the anterior abdominal cutaneous branches pierce the rectus sheath to enter the subcutaneous tissue a short distance from the median plane. *Anterior abdominal cutaneous branches of thoraco-abdominal nerves* (Fig. 2.10; Table 2.3):

- *T7–T9* supply the skin superior to the umbilicus.
- *T10* supplies the skin around the umbilicus.
- *T11*, plus the cutaneous branches of the subcostal (T12), iliohypogastric, and ilio-inguinal (L1), supply the skin inferior to the umbilicus.

During their course through the anterolateral abdominal wall, the thoraco-abdominal, subcostal, and iliohypogastric nerves communicate with each other.

VESSELS OF ANTEROLATERAL ABDOMINAL WALL

The skin and subcutaneous tissue of the abdominal wall are served by an intricate subcutaneous venous plexus, draining superiorly to the internal thoracic vein medially and the lateral thoracic vein laterally and inferiorly to the superficial and inferior epigastric veins, tributaries of the femoral and external iliac veins, respectively (Fig. 2.11). Cutaneous veins surrounding the umbilicus anastomose with *para-umbilical veins*, small tributaries of the *hepatic portal vein* that parallel the *obliterated umbilical vein* (round ligament of the liver). A relatively direct lateral superficial anastomotic channel, the **thoraco-epigastric vein,** may exist or develop (as a result of

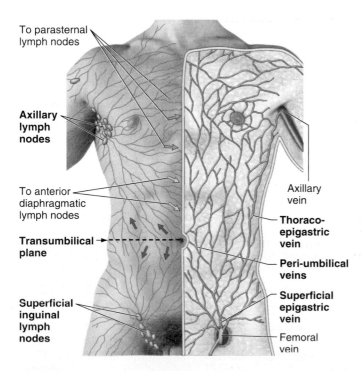

Anterior view

FIGURE 2.11. Lymphatics and superficial veins of anterolateral abdominal wall.

altered venous flow) between the *superficial epigastric vein* (a femoral vein tributary) and the *lateral thoracic vein* (an axillary vein tributary). The deeper veins of the anterolateral abdominal wall accompany the arteries, bearing the same name. A deeper, medial venous anastomosis may exist or develop between the *inferior epigastric vein* (an external iliac vein tributary) and the *superior epigastric/internal thoracic veins* (subclavian vein tributaries). The superficial and deep anastomoses may afford collateral circulation during blockage of either vena cava.

The primary blood vessels (arteries and veins) of the anterolateral abdominal wall are the

- *Superior epigastric vessels* and branches of the *musculophrenic vessels* from the internal thoracic vessels.
- *Inferior epigastric* and *deep circumflex iliac vessels* from the external iliac vessels.
- *Superficial circumflex iliac* and *superficial epigastric vessels* from the femoral artery and greater saphenous vein, respectively.
- *Posterior intercostal vessels* of the 11th intercostal space and the anterior branches of *subcostal vessels.*

The *arterial supply to the anterolateral abdominal wall* is demonstrated in Figure 2.12 and summarized in Table 2.4. The distribution of the deep abdominal blood vessels reflects the arrangement of the muscles: The vessels of the anterolateral abdominal wall have an oblique, circumferential pattern (similar to the intercostal vessels; Fig. 2.11), whereas the vessels of the central anterior abdominal wall are oriented more vertically.

The **superior epigastric artery** is the direct continuation of the *internal thoracic artery*. It enters the rectus sheath superiorly through its posterior layer and supplies the superior part of the rectus abdominis and anastomoses with the inferior epigastric artery approximately in the umbilical region (see Fig. 2.9, Table 2.4)

The **inferior epigastric artery** arises from the *external iliac artery* just superior to the inguinal ligament. It runs superiorly in the transversalis fascia to enter the rectus sheath below the arcuate line. It enters the lower rectus abdominis and anastomoses with the superior epigastric artery (Fig. 2.9).

Lymphatic drainage of the anterolateral abdominal wall follows the following patterns (Fig. 2.11):

- *Superficial lymphatic vessels* accompany the subcutaneous veins; those superior to the transumbilical plane drain mainly to the **axillary lymph nodes;** however, a few drain to the **parasternal lymph nodes.** Superficial lymphatic vessels inferior to the transumbilical plane drain to the **superficial inguinal lymph nodes.**
- *Deep lymphatic vessels* accompany the deep veins of the abdominal wall and drain to the *external iliac, common iliac,* and *right* and *left lumbar* (*caval* and *aortic*) *lymph nodes.*

For an overview of superficial and deep lymphatic drainage, see the Introduction to Clinically Oriented Anatomy.

Internal thoracic a.

Musculophrenic a.

Superior epigastric a.

10th posterior intercostal a.

External oblique

11th posterior intercostal a.

Internal oblique

Subcostal a.

Transversus abdominis

Inferior epigastric a.

Deep circumflex iliac a.

Superficial epigastric a.

Superficial circumflex iliac a.

External iliac a.

Femoral a.

Transversalis fascia

FIGURE 2.12. Arteries of anterolateral abdominal wall.

TABLE 2.4. ARTERIES OF ANTEROLATERAL ABDOMINAL WALL

Artery	Origin	Course	Distribution
Musculophrenic	Internal thoracic artery	Descends along costal margin	Superficial and deep abdominal wall of hypochondriac region; anterolateral diaphragm
Superior epigastric		Descends in rectus sheath deep to rectus abdominis	Rectus abdominis muscle; superficial and deep abdominal wall of epigastric and upper umbilical regions
10th and 11th posterior intercostal arteries	Aorta	Arteries continue beyond ribs to descend in abdominal wall between internal oblique and transversus abdominis muscles	Superficial and deep abdominal wall of lateral (lumbar or flank) region
Subcostal artery			
Inferior epigastric	External iliac artery	Runs superiorly and enters rectus sheath; runs deep to rectus abdominis	Rectus abdominis muscle; deep abdominal wall of pubic and inferior umbilical regions
Deep circumflex iliac		Runs on deep aspect of anterior abdominal wall, parallel to inguinal ligament	Iliacus muscle and deep abdominal wall of inguinal region; iliac fossa
Superficial circumflex iliac	Femoral artery	Runs in subcutaneous tissue along inguinal ligament	Superficial abdominal wall of inguinal region and adjacent anterior thigh
Superficial epigastric		Runs in subcutaneous tissue toward umbilicus	Superficial abdominal wall of pubic and inferior umbilic regions

FASCIA AND MUSCLES OF ANTEROLATERAL ABDOMINAL WALL

Clinical Significance of Fascia and Fascial Spaces of Abdominal Wall

 Liposuction is a surgical method for removing unwanted subcutaneous fat using a percutaneously placed suction tube and high vacuum pressure. The tubes are inserted subdermally through small skin incisions.

When closing abdominal skin incisions inferior to the umbilicus, surgeons include the membranous layer of subcutaneous tissue when suturing because of its strength. Between this layer and the deep fascia covering the rectus abdominis and external oblique muscles is a potential space where fluid may accumulate (e.g., urine from a ruptured urethra). Although there are no barriers (other than gravity) to prevent fluid from spreading superiorly from this space, it cannot spread inferiorly into the thigh because the deep membranous layer of subcutaneous tissue fuses with the deep fascia of the thigh (*fascia lata*) along a line approximately 2.5 cm inferior and parallel to the inguinal ligament.

The endoabdominal fascia is of special importance in surgery. It provides a plane that can be opened, enabling the surgeon to approach structures on or in the anterior aspect of the posterior abdominal wall, such as the kidneys or bodies of lumbar vertebrae, without entering the membranous peritoneal sac containing the abdominal viscera. Thus, the risk of contamination is minimized. An anterolateral part of this potential space between the transversalis fascia and the parietal peritoneum (*space of Bogros*) is used for placing prostheses (Gore-Tex mesh, for example) when repairing inguinal hernias (Skandalakis et al., 1996) (see Fig. 2.15A & B).

Protuberance of Abdomen

 A prominent abdomen is normal in infants and young children because their gastrointestinal tracts contain considerable amounts of air. In addition, their anterolateral abdominal cavities are enlarging and their abdominal muscles are gaining strength. An infant's and young child's relatively large liver also accounts for some bulging.

Abdominal muscles protect and support the viscera most effectively when they are well toned; thus the well-conditioned adult of normal weight has a flat or scaphoid (lit. boat shaped; i.e., hollowed or concave) abdomen when in the supine position.

The six common causes of *abdominal protrusion* begin with the letter *F*: food, fluid, fat, feces, flatus, and fetus. Eversion of the umbilicus may be a sign of increased intra-abdominal pressure, usually resulting from ascites (abnormal accumulation of serous fluid in the peritoneal cavity), or a large mass (e.g., a tumor, a fetus, or an enlarged organ such as the liver).

Excess fat accumulation owing to overnourishment most commonly involves the subcutaneous fatty layer; however, there may also be excessive depositions of extraperitoneal fat in some types of obesity.

Tumors and organomegaly (organ enlargement such as splenomegaly—enlargement of the spleen) also produce abdominal enlargement. When the anterior abdominal muscles are underdeveloped or become atrophic, as a result of old age or insufficient exercise, they provide insufficient tonus to resist the increased weight of a protuberant abdomen on the anterior pelvis. The pelvis tilts anteriorly at the hip joints when standing (the pubis descends and the sacrum ascends) producing excessive *lordosis* (sway back) of the lumbar region.

Abdominal Hernias

 The anterolateral abdominal wall may be the site of *abdominal hernias*. Most hernias occur in the inguinal, umbilical, and epigastric regions (see the blue box "Inguinal Hernias," p. 212). *Umbilical hernias* are common in neonates because the anterior abdominal wall is relatively weak in the umbilical ring, especially in low-birth-weight infants. Umbilical hernias are usually small and result from increased intra-abdominal pressure in the presence of weakness and incomplete closure of the anterior abdominal wall after ligation of the umbilical cord at birth. Herniation occurs through the umbilical ring. *Acquired umbilical hernias* occur most commonly in women and obese people. Extraperitoneal fat and/or peritoneum protrude into the hernial sac. The lines along which the fibers of the abdominal aponeuroses interlace are also potential sites of herniation (see Fig. 2.6B). Occasionally, gaps exist where these fiber exchanges occur—for example, in the midline or in the transition from aponeurosis to rectus sheath. These gaps may be congenital, the result of the stresses of obesity and aging, or the consequence of surgical or traumatic wounds.

An *epigastric hernia*, a hernia in the epigastric region through the linea alba, occurs in the midline between the xiphoid process and the umbilicus. *Spigelian hernias* are those occurring along the semilunar lines (see Table 2.1B). These types of hernia tend to occur in people older than 40 years and are usually associated with obesity. The hernial sac, composed of peritoneum, is covered with only skin and fatty subcutaneous tissue.

NEUROVASCULATURE OF ANTEROLATERAL ABDOMINAL WALL

Palpation of Anterolateral Abdominal Wall

 Warm hands are important when palpating the abdominal wall because cold hands make the anterolateral abdominal muscles tense, producing involuntary spasms of the muscles, known as *guarding*. Intense guarding, board-like reflexive muscular rigidity that cannot be willfully suppressed, occurs during palpation when an organ (such as the appendix) is inflamed and in itself constitutes a clinically significant sign of *acute abdomen*. The involuntary muscular spasms attempt to protect the viscera from pressure, which is painful when an abdominal infection is present. The common nerve supply of the skin and muscles of the wall explains why these spasms occur.

Palpation of abdominal viscera is performed with the patient in the supine position with thighs and knees semiflexed to enable adequate relaxation of the anterolateral abdominal wall. Otherwise, the deep fascia of the thighs pulls on the membranous layer of abdominal subcutaneous tissue, tensing the abdominal wall. Some people tend to place their hands behind their heads when lying supine, which also tightens the muscles and makes the examination difficult. Placing the upper limbs at the sides and putting a pillow under the person's knees tends to relax the anterolateral abdominal muscles.

Superficial Abdominal Reflexes

The abdominal wall is the only protection most of the abdominal organs have. Consequently, the wall will react if an organ is diseased or injured. With the person supine and the muscles relaxed, the *superficial abdominal reflex* is elicited by quickly stroking horizontally, lateral to medial, toward the umbilicus. Usually, contraction of the abdominal muscles is felt; this reflex may not be observed in obese people. Similarly, any injury to the abdominal skin results in a rapid reflex contraction of the abdominal muscles.

Injury to Nerves of Anterolateral Abdominal Wall

The inferior thoracic spinal nerves (T7–T12) and the iliohypogastric and ilio-inguinal nerves (L1) approach the abdominal musculature separately to provide the multi-segmental innervation of the abdominal muscles. Thus, they are distributed across the anterolateral abdominal wall, where they run oblique but mostly horizontal courses. They are susceptible to injury in surgical incisions or from trauma at any level of the abdominal wall. *Injury to nerves of the anterolateral abdominal wall* may result in weakening of the muscles. In the inguinal region, such a weakness may predispose an individual to development of an inguinal hernia (see the blue box "Inguinal Hernias" on p. 212).

Abdominal Surgical Incisions

Surgeons use various *abdominal surgical incisions* to gain access to the abdominal cavity. When possible, the incisions follow the *cleavage lines* (Langer lines)

in the skin (see Introduction for discussion of these lines). The incision that allows adequate exposure, and secondarily, the best possible cosmetic effect, is chosen. The location of the incision also depends on the type of operation, the location of the organ(s) the surgeon wants to reach, bony or cartilaginous boundaries, avoidance of (especially motor) nerves, maintenance of blood supply, and minimizing injury to muscles and fascia of the abdominal wall while aiming for favorable healing. Thus, before making an incision, the surgeon considers the direction of the muscle fibers and the location of the aponeuroses and nerves. Consequently, a variety of incisions are routinely used, each having specific advantages and limitations.

Instead of transecting muscles, causing irreversible necrosis (death) of muscle fibers, the surgeon splits them in the direction of (and between) their fibers. The rectus abdominis is an exception; it can be transected because its muscle fibers run short distances between tendinous intersections, and the segmental nerves supplying it enter the lateral part of the rectus sheath where they can be located and preserved. Generally, incisions are made in the part of the anterolateral abdominal wall that gives the freest access to the targeted organ with the least disturbance to the nerve supply to the muscles. Muscles and viscera are retracted toward, not away from, their neurovascular supply.

Cutting a motor nerve paralyzes the muscle fibers supplied by it, thereby weakening the anterolateral abdominal wall. However, because of overlapping areas of innervation between nerves, one or two small branches of nerves may usually be cut without a noticeable loss of motor supply to the muscles or loss of sensation to the skin.

LONGITUDINAL INCISIONS

Longitudinal incisions, such as median and paramedian incisions (Fig. B2.1), are preferred for exploratory operations because they offer good exposure of and access to the viscera, and can be extended as necessary with minimal complication.

Median or *midline incisions* can be made rapidly without cutting muscle, major blood vessels, or nerves. Median incisions can be made along any part or the length of the linea alba from the xiphoid process to pubic symphysis. Because the linea alba transmits only small vessels and nerves to the skin, a midline incision is relatively bloodless, and avoids major nerves; however, incisions in some people may reveal abundant and well-vascularized fat. Conversely, because of its relatively poor blood supply, the linea alba may undergo necrosis and subsequent degeneration after incision if its edges are not aligned properly during closure.

Paramedian incisions (lateral to the median plane) are made in a sagittal plane and may extend from the costal margin to the pubic hairline. After the incision passes through the anterior layer of the rectus sheath, the muscle is freed and retracted laterally to prevent tension and injury to the vessels and nerves. The posterior layer of the rectus sheath and the peritoneum are then incised to enter the peritoneal cavity.

McBurney
point

Key

— Median or midline incision
— Left paramedian incision
— Gridiron (muscle-splitting) incision
   (traditional McBurney incision)
— Transverse (abdominal) incision
— Suprapubic (Pfannenstiel) incision
— Subcostal incision

FIGURE B2.1.

OBLIQUE AND TRANSVERSE INCISIONS

The direction of *oblique* and *transverse incisions* is related to muscle fiber orientation, nearby hard tissue (costal margin or iliac or pubic crest), or minimizing potential nerve damage. *Gridiron (muscle-splitting) incisions* are often used for an appendectomy. The oblique *McBurney incision* is made at the *McBurney point,* approximately 2.5 cm superomedial to the ASIS on the *spino-umbilical line.* The external oblique aponeurosis is incised inferomedially in the direction of its fibers and retracted. The musculoaponeurotic fibers of the internal oblique and transversus abdominis are then split in the line of their fibers and retracted. The iliohypogastric nerve, running deep to the internal oblique, is identified and preserved. Carefully made, the entire exposure cuts no musculo-aponeurotic fibers; therefore, when the incision is closed, the muscle fibers move together and the abdominal wall is as strong after the operation as it was before.

Suprapubic (Pfannenstiel) incisions ("bikini" incisions) are made at the pubic hairline. These incisions—horizontal with a slight convexity—are used for most gynecological and obstetrical operations (e.g., for cesarean section). The linea alba and anterior layers of the rectus sheaths are transected and resected superiorly, and the rectus muscles are retracted laterally or divided through their tendinous parts allowing reattachment without muscle fiber injury.

The iliohypogastric and ilio-inguinal nerves are identified and preserved.

Transverse incisions through the anterior layer of the rectus sheath and rectus abdominis provide good access and cause the least possible damage to the nerve supply of the rectus abdominis. This muscle may be divided transversely without serious damage because a new transverse band forms when the muscle segments are rejoined. Transverse incisions are not made through the tendinous intersections because cutaneous nerves and branches of the superior epigastric vessels pierce these fibrous regions of the muscle. Transverse incisions can be increased laterally as needed to increase exposure but are not utilized for exploratory procedures because superior and inferior extension is difficult.

Subcostal incisions provide access to the gallbladder and biliary ducts on the right side and the spleen on the left. The incision is made parallel but at least 2.5 cm inferior to the costal margin to avoid the 7th and 8th thoracic spinal nerves (Table 2.3).

HIGH-RISK INCISIONS

High-risk incisions include pararectus and inguinal incisions. *Pararectus incisions* along the lateral border of the rectus sheath are undesirable because they may cut the nerve supply to the rectus abdominis. *Inguinal incisions* for repairing hernias may injure the ilio-inguinal nerve.

INCISIONAL HERNIA

An *incisional hernia* is a protrusion of *omentum* (a fold of peritoneum) or an organ through a surgical incision. If the muscular and aponeurotic layers of the abdomen do not heal properly, an incisional hernia can result.

MINIMALLY INVASIVE (ENDOSCOPIC) SURGERY

Many abdominopelvic surgical procedures (e.g., removal of the gallbladder) are now performed using an *endoscope,* in which tiny perforations of the abdominal wall allow the entry of remotely operated instruments, replacing the larger conventional incisions. Thus, the potential for nerve injury, incisional hernia, or contamination through the open wound and the time required for healing are minimized.

Reversal of Venous Flow and Collateral Pathways of Superficial Abdominal Veins

 When flow in the superior or inferior vena cava is obstructed, anastomoses between the tributaries of these systemic veins, such as the thoraco-epigastric vein, may provide collateral pathways by which the obstruction may be bypassed, allowing blood to return to the heart (Fig. B2.2).

Thoraco-epigastric vein

Superficial epigastric vein

FIGURE B2.2.

The Bottom Line

FASCIA, MUSCLES, AND NEUROVASCULATURE OF ANTEROLATERAL ABDOMINAL WALL

Fascia: The fascia of the anterolateral abdominal wall consists of subcutaneous (superficial), investing (deep), and endoabdominal portions. ♦ The subcutaneous layer is modified inferior to the umbilicus to include a superficial fatty layer and a deep membranous layer. ♦ The superficial fatty layer is specialized here, particularly in males, for lipid storage, whereas the deep membranous layer is sufficiently complete to compartmentalize extravasated fluids (blood or urine) and allow placement of sutures during surgery. ♦ The investing layer is typical of deep fascias ensheathing voluntary muscles, and here reflects the trilaminar arrangement of the flat abdominal muscles and their aponeuroses. ♦ The endoabdominal fascia is of particular importance in surgery, enabling the establishment of an extraperitoneal space that allows anterior access to retroperitoneal structures (e.g., kidneys, ureters, and bodies of lumbar vertebra) without entering the peritoneal cavity.

Muscles: The anterolateral abdominal muscles consist of concentric, flat muscles located anterolaterally and vertical muscles placed anteriorly adjacent to the midline. ♦ A trilaminar arrangement of the flat muscles, like that in the thorax, also occurs here; however, other than their innervation by multiple but separate segmental nerves, the metamerism (segmentation) characteristic of the thoracic intercostal musculature is not apparent in the abdomen. ♦ The fleshy portions of the flat muscles become aponeurotic anteriorly. The fibers of the aponeuroses interlace in the midline, forming the linea alba, and continue into the aponeuroses of the contralateral muscles. ♦ The aponeurotic fibers of the external obliques are also continuous across the midline with those of the contralateral internal oblique muscles. ♦ Three layers of flat, bilateral digastric muscles encircle the trunk, forming oblique and transverse girdles that enclose the abdominal cavity. ♦ In the upper two thirds of the abdominal wall, the aponeurotic layers separate on each side of the linea alba to form longitudinal sheaths that contain the rectus muscles. This brings them into a functional relationship with the flat muscles in which the vertical muscles brace the girdles anteriorly. ♦ In the lower third of the anterior abdominal wall, the aponeuroses of all three layers of flat muscles pass anterior to the rectus muscles (recti). ♦ As flexors of the trunk, the recti are the antagonistic partners of the deep (extensor) muscles of the back. Balance in the development and tonus of these partners affects posture (and thus weakness of the abdominal muscles may result in excessive lumbar lordosis—an abnormally convex curvature of the lower vertebral column). ♦ The special arrangements of the anterolateral abdominal muscles enable them to provide flexible containing walls for the abdominal contents, to increase intra-abdominal pressure or decrease abdominal volume for expulsion, and to produce anterior and lateral flexion and torsional (rotatory) movements of the trunk.

Nerves: The anterolateral abdominal muscles receive multi-segmental innervation via the anterior rami of lower thoracic (T7–T12) and the L1 spinal nerves. ♦ The rami pass separately to the muscles as five thoraco-abdominal nerves (T7–T11), a subcostal nerve (T12), and iliohypogastric and ilio-inguinal nerves (L1) that course in a plane between the second and third layers. ♦ Lateral cutaneous branches supply the overlying abdominal skin lateral to the MCL. ♦ Anterior cutaneous branches supply skin medial to the MCL. ♦ Except for L1, the maps of the abdominal dermatomes and of the peripheral nerves are thus identical. ♦ Landmark dermatomes are dermatome T10, which includes the umbilicus, and dermatome L1, which includes the inguinal fold.

Vessels: ♦ The skin and subcutaneous tissue of the abdominal wall drain superiorly (ultimately to the superior vena caval system) via the internal thoracic vein medially and the lateral thoracic vein laterally, and inferiorly (ultimately to the inferior vena caval system) via the superficial and inferior epigastric veins. ♦ Cutaneous veins surrounding the umbilicus anastomose with small tributaries of the hepatic portal vein. ♦ The distribution of the deeper abdominal blood vessels reflects the arrangement of the muscles: an oblique, circumferential pattern (similar to the intercostal vessels above)

over the anterolateral abdominal wall and a vertical pattern anteriorly. ♦ The circumferential vessels of the anterolateral wall are continuations of the 7th–11th posterior intercostal vessels, subcostal vessels, and deep circumflex iliac vessels. ♦ Vertical vessels include an anastomosis between the superior and the inferior epigastric vessels within the rectus sheath. ♦ A superficial anastomotic channel, the thoraco-epigastric vein, and the deeper medial pathway between the inferior and the superior epigastric veins afford collateral circulation during blockage of superior or inferior vena cava. ♦ Superficial abdominal lymphatic vessels superior to the transumbilical plane drain primarily to the axillary lymph nodes; those inferior to the plane drain to the superficial inguinal lymph nodes. ♦ Deep lymphatic vessels accompany deep veins of the abdominal wall to the iliac and right and left lumbar (caval and aortic) lymph nodes.

Internal Surface of Anterolateral Abdominal Wall

The internal (posterior) surface of the anterolateral abdominal wall is covered with transversalis fascia, a variable amount of extraperitoneal fat, and parietal peritoneum (Fig. 2.13).

The infraumbilical part of this surface exhibits five *umbilical peritoneal folds* passing toward the umbilicus, one in the median plane and two on each side:

- The **median umbilical fold** extends from the apex of the urinary bladder to the umbilicus and covers the **median**

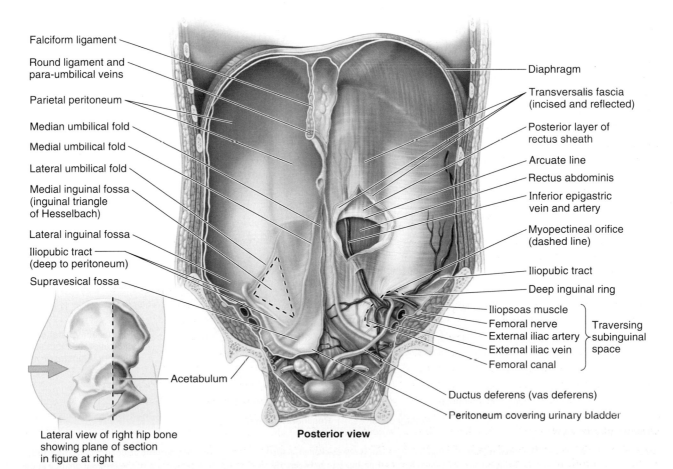

Falciform ligament
Round ligament and para-umbilical veins
Parietal peritoneum
Median umbilical fold
Medial umbilical fold
Lateral umbilical fold
Medial inguinal fossa (inguinal triangle of Hesselbach)
Lateral inguinal fossa
Iliopubic tract (deep to peritoneum)
Supravesical fossa
Acetabulum

Diaphragm
Transversalis fascia (incised and reflected)
Posterior layer of rectus sheath
Arcuate line
Rectus abdominis
Inferior epigastric vein and artery
Myopectineal orifice (dashed line)
Iliopubic tract
Deep inguinal ring
Iliopsoas muscle
Femoral nerve
External iliac artery
External iliac vein
Femoral canal
⎱ Traversing subinguinal space
Ductus deferens (vas deferens)
Peritoneum covering urinary bladder

Lateral view of right hip bone showing plane of section in figure at right

Posterior view

FIGURE 2.13. Posterior aspect of anterolateral abdominal wall of a male. The peritoneal ligaments, folds, and fossae are the main features of this aspect.

umbilical ligament, a fibrous remnant of the *urachus* that joined the apex of the fetal bladder to the umbilicus.

- Two **medial umbilical folds,** lateral to the median umbilical fold, cover the **medial umbilical ligaments,** formed by *occluded parts of the umbilical arteries.*
- Two **lateral umbilical folds,** lateral to the medial umbilical folds, cover the *inferior epigastric vessels* and therefore bleed if cut.

The depressions lateral to the umbilical folds are the *peritoneal fossae,* each of which is a potential site for a hernia. The location of a hernia in one of these fossae determines how the hernia is classified. The shallow fossae between the umbilical folds are the:

- **Supravesical fossae** between the median and the medial umbilical folds, formed as the peritoneum reflects from the anterior abdominal wall onto the bladder. The level of the supravesical fossae rises and falls with filling and emptying of the bladder.
- **Medial inguinal fossae** between the medial and the lateral umbilical folds, areas also commonly called **inguinal triangles** (Hesselbach triangles), which are potential sites for the less common direct inguinal hernias.
- **Lateral inguinal fossae,** lateral to the lateral umbilical folds, include the *deep inguinal rings* and are potential sites for the most common type of hernia in the lower abdominal wall, the *indirect inguinal hernia* (see clinical correlation [blue] box "Inguinal Hernias," on p. 212).

The supra-umbilical part of the internal surface of the anterior abdominal wall has a sagittally oriented peritoneal reflection, the **falciform ligament,** that extends between the superior anterior abdominal wall and the liver. It encloses the *round ligament of the liver* (L. *ligamentum teres hepatis*) and *para-umbilical veins* in its inferior free edge. The round ligament is a fibrous remnant of the *umbilical vein,* which passed from the umbilicus to the liver prenatally (Fig. 2.13).

Inguinal Region

The **inguinal region** (groin) extends between the ASIS and pubic tubercle. It is an important area anatomically and clinically: anatomically because it is a region where structures exit and enter the abdominal cavity, and clinically because the pathways of exit and entrance are potential sites of herniation.

Although the testis is located in the perineum postnatally, the male gonad originally forms in the abdomen. Its relocation out of the abdomen into the perineum through the inguinal canal accounts for many of the structural features of the region. Traditionally, the testis and scrotum are dissected and studied in relation to the anterior abdominal wall and the inguinal region. For this reason, male anatomy receives greater emphasis in this section.

INGUINAL LIGAMENT AND ILIOPUBIC TRACT

Thickened fibrous bands, or *retinacula,* occur in relationship to many joints that have a wide range of movement to retain structures against the skeleton during the various positions of the joint (see Introduction). The *inguinal ligament* and *iliopubic tract,* extending from the ASIS to the *pubic tubercle,* constitute a bilaminar anterior (flexor) retinaculum of the hip joint (Figs. 2.13 and 2.14). The retinaculum spans the **subinguinal**

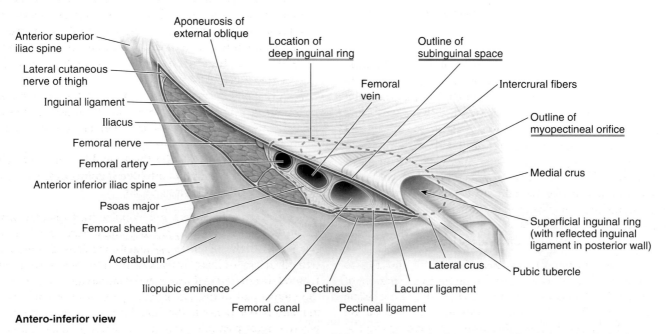

Anterior superior iliac spine
Lateral cutaneous nerve of thigh
Inguinal ligament
Iliacus
Femoral nerve
Femoral artery
Anterior inferior iliac spine
Psoas major
Femoral sheath
Acetabulum
Iliopubic eminence
Femoral canal
Pectineus
Pectineal ligament
Lacunar ligament
Lateral crus
Pubic tubercle
Superficial inguinal ring (with reflected inguinal ligament in posterior wall)
Medial crus
Outline of myopectineal orifice
Intercrural fibers
Outline of subinguinal space
Femoral vein
Location of deep inguinal ring
Aponeurosis of external oblique

Antero-inferior view

FIGURE 2.14. Formations of inguinal region. The inguinal ligament is the thickened, underturned, inferior margin of the aponeurosis of the external oblique, forming a retinaculum that bridges the subinguinal space. A slit-like gap between the medial and the lateral crura of the external oblique aponeurosis, bridged by intercrural fibers, forms the superficial inguinal ring.

space, through which pass the flexors of the hip and neurovascular structures serving much of the lower limb. These fibrous bands are the thickened inferolateral-most portions of the external oblique and aponeurosis and the inferior margin of the transversalis fascia. They are major landmarks of the region.

The **inguinal ligament** is a dense band constituting the inferiormost part of the external oblique aponeurosis. Although most fibers of the ligament's medial end insert into the pubic tubercle, some follow other courses (Fig. 2.14):

- Some of the deeper fibers pass posteriorly to attach to the *superior pubic ramus* lateral to the tubercle, forming the arching **lacunar ligament** (of Gimbernat), which forms the medial boundary of the subinguinal space. The most lateral of these fibers continue to run along the *pecten pubis* as the **pectineal ligament** (of Cooper).
- Some of the more superior fibers fan upward, bypassing the *pubic tubercle* and crossing the linea alba to blend with the lower fibers of the contralateral external oblique aponeurosis. These fibers form the **reflected inguinal ligament** (Figs. 2.8, 2.14, and 2.15A).

The **iliopubic tract** is the thickened inferior margin of the transversalis fascia, which appears as a fibrous band running parallel and posterior (deep) to the inguinal ligament (Figs. 2.13 and 2.15B). The iliopubic tract, seen in the place of the inguinal ligament when the inguinal region is viewed from its internal (posterior) aspect (e.g., during laparoscopy), reinforces the posterior wall and floor of the inguinal canal as it bridges the structures traversing the subinguinal space.

The inguinal ligament and iliopubic tract span an area of innate weakness in the body wall in the inguinal region called the **myopectineal orifice** (Fruchaud, 1956). This weak area, occurring in relation to structures traversing the body wall, is the site of direct and indirect inguinal and femoral hernias.

INGUINAL CANAL

The **inguinal canal** is formed in relation to the relocation of the testis during fetal development. The inguinal canal in adults is an oblique passage, approximately 4 cm long, directed inferomedially through the inferior part of the anterolateral abdominal wall. It lies parallel and superior to the medial half of the inguinal ligament (see Figs. 2.14 and 2.15). The main occupant of the inguinal canal is the spermatic cord in males and the round ligament of the uterus in females. These are functionally and developmentally distinct structures that occur in the same location. The inguinal canal also contains blood and lymphatic vessels and the ilio-inguinal nerve in both sexes. The inguinal canal has an opening at each end:

- The **deep (internal) inguinal ring** is the entrance to the inguinal canal. It is located superior to the middle of the inguinal ligament and lateral to the inferior epigastric artery (Fig. 2.14). It is the beginning of an evagination in the transversalis fascia that forms an opening like the entrance to a cave (Figs. 2.7B, 2.13, and 2.15). Through this opening, the extraperitoneal ductus deferens (vas deferens) and testicular vessels in males (or round ligament

of the uterus in females) pass to enter the inguinal canal. The transversalis fascia itself continues into the canal, forming the innermost covering (internal fascia) of the structures traversing the canal.

- The **superficial (external) inguinal ring** is the exit by which the spermatic cord in males, or the round ligament in females, emerges from the inguinal canal (Figs. 2.7A, 2.14, and 2.15). The superficial ring is a split that occurs in the diagonal, otherwise parallel fibers of the external oblique aponeurosis just superolateral to the pubic tubercle. The parts of the aponeurosis that lie lateral and medial to, and form the margins of, the superficial ring are *crura* (L. leg-like parts). The **lateral crus** attaches to the pubic tubercle, and the **medial crus** attaches to the pubic crest. Fibers of the superficial layer of investing (deep) fascia overlying the external oblique muscle and aponeurosis, running perpendicular to the fibers of the aponeurosis, pass from one crus to the other across the superolateral part of the ring. These **intercrural fibers** help prevent the crura from spreading apart (i.e., they keep the "split" in the aponeurosis from expanding).

The *inguinal canal* is normally collapsed anteroposteriorly against the structures it conveys. Between its two openings (rings), the inguinal canal has two walls (anterior and posterior), as well as a roof and floor (Figs. 2.14 and 2.15A & B). The structures forming these boundaries are listed in Table 2.5.

The inguinal canal has two walls (anterior and posterior), a roof, and a floor (Figs. 2.8 and 2.15A & B):

- *Anterior wall:* formed by the external oblique aponeurosis throughout the length of the canal; its lateral part is reinforced by muscle fibers of the internal oblique.
- *Posterior wall:* formed by the transversalis fascia; its medial part is reinforced by pubic attachments of the internal oblique and transversus abdominis aponeuroses that frequently merge to variable extents into a common tendon—the **inguinal falx** (conjoint tendon)—and the reflected inguinal ligament.
- *Roof:* formed laterally by the transversalis fascia, centrally by musculo-aponeurotic arches of the internal oblique and transversus abdominis, and medially by the medial crus of the external oblique aponeurosis.
- *Floor:* formed laterally by the iliopubic tract, centrally by gutter formed by the infolded inguinal ligament, and medially by the lacunar ligament.

As the inguinal ligament and iliopubic tract span the *myopectineal orifice* (Fig. 2.13), they demarcate the inferior boundaries of the inguinal canal and its openings. The inguinal triangle separates these formations from the structures of the femoral sheath (femoral vessels and femoral canal) that traverse the medial part of the subinguinal space. Most groin hernias in males pass superior to the iliopubic tract (inguinal hernias), whereas most pass inferior to it in females (femoral hernias). Because of its relative weakness, the myopectineal orifice is overlaid with prosthetic mesh placed in the extraperitoneal retro-inguinal space ("space of Bogros") in many hernia repairs.

Peritoneum
Transversalis fascia
Transversus abdominis muscle
Internal oblique muscle
External oblique muscle
Testicular artery and veins
External oblique aponeurosis
Ductus deferens
Ilio-inguinal nerve
Inferior epigastric vessels
Retro-inguinal space (of Bogros)
Deep inguinal ring
Plane of section for (B)
Intercrural fibers

Internal
spermatic fascia
*
Inguinal
ligament
Origin of
cremasteric muscle
Inguinal falx
(conjoint tendon)
Femoral vessels
Superficial inguinal ring
External spermatic fascia
Reflected inguinal ligament
Cremasteric muscle and fascia
Internal spermatic
fascia
Spermatic cord
External spermatic fascia
Testis

* Musculo-aponeurotic arcades of
internal oblique & transversus abdominis

(A) Anterior view

Aponeuroses of:
external ⎫
           ⎬ oblique
internal ⎭
Skin
Fatty layer
Inguinal canal
Spermatic cord
Membranous
layer of sub-
cutaneous
tissue
Anterior wall
of inguinal canal
(intercrural
fibers)
Ductus
deferens
Transversus
abdominis
Transversalis fascia
Retro-inguinal space
(of Bogros)
Peritoneum
Inguinal falx (conjoint
tendon) forming
posterior wall of canal
Iliopubic tract
Inguinal ligament
forming "gutter" (floor
of inguinal canal)
Superior ramus
of pubis
Fascia lata
of thigh

(B) Schematic sagittal section of inguinal canal

FIGURE 2.15. Inguinal canal and spermatic cord. A. The layers of the abdominal wall and the coverings of the spermatic cord and testis derived from them are shown. **B.** Sagittal section of the anterior abdominal wall and inguinal canal at the plane shown in part **A.**

TABLE 2.5. BOUNDARIES OF INGUINAL CANAL

Boundary	Lateral Third/Deep Ring	Middle Third	Medial Third/Superficial Ring
Posterior wall	Transversalis fascia	Transversalis fascia	Inguinal falx (conjoint tendon) plus reflected inguinal ligament
Anterior wall	Internal oblique plus lateral crus of aponeurosis of external oblique	Aponeurosis of external oblique (lateral crus and intercrural fibers)	Aponeurosis of external oblique (intercrural fibers), with fascia of external oblique continuing onto cord as external spermatic fascia
Roof	Transversalis fascia	Musculo-aponeurotic arches of internal oblique and transverse abdominal	Medial crus of aponeurosis of external oblique
Floor	Iliopubic tract	Inguinal ligament	Lacunar ligament

Development of Inguinal Canal. The testes develop in the extraperitoneal connective tissue in the superior lumbar region of the posterior abdominal wall (Fig. 2.16A). The **male gubernaculum** is a fibrous tract connecting the **primordial testis** to the anterolateral abdominal wall at the site of the future deep ring of the inguinal canal. A peritoneal diverticulum, the **processus vaginalis,** traverses the developing inguinal canal, carrying muscular and fascial layers of the anterolateral abdominal wall before it as it enters the **primordial scrotum.** By the 12th week, the testis is in the pelvis, and by 28 weeks (7th month), it lies close to the developing deep inguinal ring (Fig. 2.16B). The testis begins to pass through the inguinal canal during the 28th week and takes approximately 3 days to traverse it. Approximately 4 weeks later, the testis enters the scrotum (Fig. 2.16C). As the testis, its duct (*ductus deferens*), and its vessels and nerves relocate, they are ensheathed by musculofascial extensions of the anterolateral abdominal wall, which account for the presence of their derivatives in the adult scrotum: the internal and external *spermatic fasciae* and cremaster muscle (Fig. 2.15). The stalk of the processus vaginalis normally degenerates; however, its distal saccular part forms the *tunica vaginalis,* the serous sheath of the testis and epididymis (Moore et al., 2012).

The *ovaries* also develop in the superior lumbar region of the posterior abdominal wall and relocate to the lateral wall of the pelvis (Fig. 2.17). The processus vaginalis of the peritoneum traverses the transversalis fascia at the site of the deep inguinal ring, forming the inguinal canal as in the male, and protrudes into the developing labium majus.

The **female gubernaculum,** a fibrous cord connecting the ovary and primordial uterus to the developing labium majus, is represented postnatally by the **ovarian ligament,** between the ovary and uterus, and the **round ligament of the uterus** (L. *ligamentum teres uteri*), between the uterus and labium majus. Because of the attachment of the ovarian ligaments to the uterus, the ovaries do not relocate to the inguinal region; however, the round ligament passes through the inguinal canal and attaches to the subcutaneous tissue of the labium majus (Fig. 2.17B & C).

Except for its most inferior part, which becomes a serous sac engulfing the testis, the *tunica vaginalis,* the processus vaginalis obliterates by the 6th month of fetal development. The inguinal canals in females are narrower than those in males, and the canals in infants of both sexes are shorter and much less oblique than in adults. The superficial inguinal rings in infants lie almost directly anterior to the deep inguinal rings.

Inguinal Canal and Increased Intra-Abdominal Pressure. The deep and superficial inguinal rings in the adult do not overlap because of the oblique path of the inguinal canal. Consequently, increases in intra-abdominal pressure act on the inguinal canal, forcing the posterior wall of the canal against the anterior wall and strengthening this wall, thereby decreasing the likelihood of herniation until the pressures overcome the resistant effect of this mechanism.

Diagrammatic oblique sagittal section to right of midline

(A) Seventh week

Diagrammatic oblique sagittal section to right of midline

(B) Seventh month

Diagrammatic oblique sagittal section to right of midline

(C) Ninth month

FIGURE 2.16. Formation of inguinal canals and relocation of testes. A. In a 7-week embryo, the testis is attached to the posterior abdominal wall. **B.** A fetus at 28 weeks (seventh month) shows the processus vaginalis and testis passing through the inguinal canal. The testis passes posterior to the processus vaginalis, not through it. **C.** In a newborn infant, obliteration of the stalk of the processus vaginalis has occurred. The remains of the processus vaginalis have formed the tunica vaginalis of the testis. The remnant of the gubernaculum has disappeared.

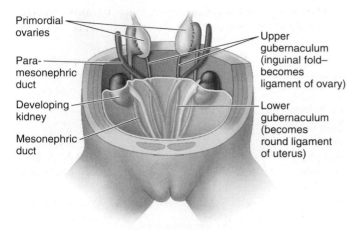

(A) 2 months

Primordial ovaries

Para-mesonephric duct

Developing kidney

Mesonephric duct

Upper gubernaculum (inguinal fold– becomes ligament of ovary)

Lower gubernaculum (becomes round ligament of uterus)

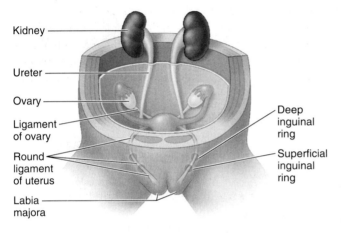

(B) 15 weeks

Kidney

Ureter

Ovary

Ligament of ovary

Round ligament of uterus

Labia majora

Deep inguinal ring

Superficial inguinal ring

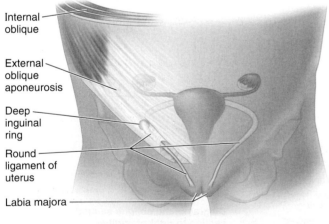

(C) Mature

Internal oblique

External oblique aponeurosis

Deep inguinal ring

Round ligament of uterus

Labia majora

Anterior view

FIGURE 2.17. Formation of inguinal canals in females. A. At 2 months the undifferentiated gonads (primordial ovaries) are located on the dorsal abdominal wall. **B.** At 15 weeks the ovaries have descended into the greater pelvis. The processus vaginalis (not shown) passes through the abdominal wall, forming the inguinal canal on each side as in the male fetus. The round ligament passes through the canal and attaches to the subcutaneous tissue of the labium majus. **C.** In the mature female, the processus vaginalis has degenerated but the round ligament persists and passes through the inguinal canal.

Musculo-aponeurotic arcades of

Internal oblique   Superficial inguinal ring

Transversus abdominis

Relaxed   Contracted

Anterior view

FIGURE 2.18. Arcades of inguinal canal. The inguinal canal consists of a series of three musculo-aponeurotic arcades traversed by the spermatic cord or round ligament of the uterus (*arrow*). The muscular contraction that increases intra-abdominal pressure also causes the roof of the canal to descend, narrowing the canal as it is simultaneously collapsed anteroposteriorly by the increased internal pressure.

Simultaneously, contraction of the external oblique approximates the anterior wall of the canal to the posterior wall. It also increases tension on the medial and lateral crura, resisting enlargement (dilation) of the superficial inguinal ring. Contraction of the musculature that forms the lateral part of the arcades of the internal oblique and transversus abdominis muscles makes the roof of the canal descend, constricting the canal (Fig. 2.18).

Spermatic Cord, Scrotum, and Testes

SPERMATIC CORD

The **spermatic cord** contains structures running to and from the testis and suspends the testis in the scrotum (see Fig. 2.19; Table 2.6). The spermatic cord begins at the deep inguinal ring lateral to the inferior epigastric vessels, passes through the inguinal canal, exits at the superficial inguinal ring, and ends in the scrotum at the posterior border of the testis. Fascial coverings derived from the anterolateral abdominal wall during prenatal development surround the spermatic cord. The *coverings of the spermatic cord* include the following:

- **Internal spermatic fascia:** derived from the transversalis fascia.
- **Cremasteric fascia:** derived from the investing fascia of both the superficial and deep surfaces of the internal oblique muscle.
- **External spermatic fascia:** derived from the external oblique aponeurosis and its investing fascia.

The cremasteric fascia contains loops of **cremaster muscle,** which is formed by the lowermost fascicles of the internal oblique muscle arising from the inguinal ligament (Figs. 2.8 and 2.15A). The cremaster muscle reflexively draws the testis superiorly in the scrotum, particularly in response to cold. In a warm environment, such as a hot bath, the cremaster relaxes and the testis descends deeply in the scrotum. Both responses occur in an attempt to regulate the temperature of the testis for **spermatogenesis** (formation of sperms), which requires a constant temperature approximately one degree cooler than core temperature, or during sexual activity as a protective response. The cremaster typically acts coincidentally with the **dartos muscle,** smooth muscle of the fat-free subcutaneous tissue of the scrotum (*dartos fascia*), which inserts into the skin, assisting testicular elevation as it produces contraction of the skin of the scrotum in response to the same stimuli. The cremaster muscle is innervated by the *genital branch of the genitofemoral nerve* (L1, L2), a derivative of the *lumbar plexus* (Fig. 2.19). The cremaster is striated muscle receiving somatic innervation, whereas the dartos is smooth muscle receiving autonomic innervation. Although less well developed and usually indistinct, the round ligament of the female receives similar contributions from the layers of the abdominal wall as it traverses the inguinal canal. The constituents of the spermatic cord are the following (Figs. 2.19 and 2.21; Table 2.6):

- *Ductus deferens* (vas deferens): a muscular tube approximately 45 cm long that conveys sperms from the epididymis to the ejaculatory duct.
- *Testicular artery:* arising from the aorta and supplying the testis and epididymis.
- *Artery of ductus deferens:* arising from the inferior vesical artery.
- *Cremasteric artery:* arising from the inferior epigastric artery.
- *Pampiniform venous plexus:* a network formed by up to 12 veins that converge superiorly as right or left testicular veins.
- Sympathetic *nerve fibers* on arteries and sympathetic and parasympathetic nerve fibers on the ductus deferens.
- *Genital branch of the genitofemoral nerve:* supplying the cremaster muscle.
- *Lymphatic vessels:* draining the testis and closely associated structures and passing to the lumbar lymph nodes.
- **Vestige of processus vaginalis:** may be seen as a fibrous thread in the anterior part of the spermatic cord extending between the abdominal peritoneum and the tunica vaginalis; it may not be detectable.

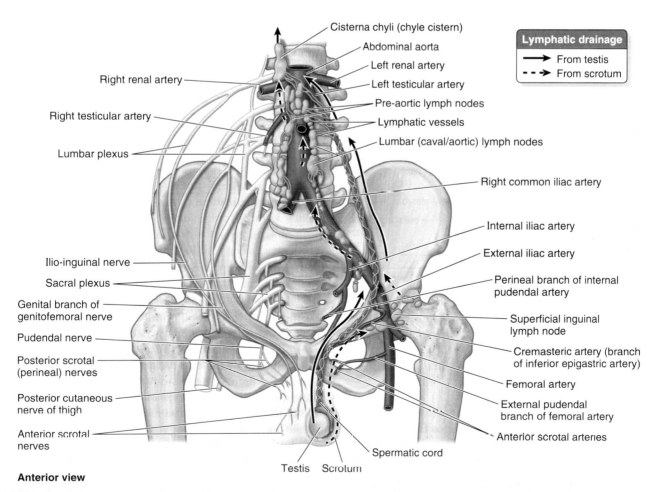

FIGURE 2.19. Arterial supply and lymphatic drainage of testis and scrotum; innervation of scrotum. Lymph draining from the testis and scrotum follows different courses. The lumbar plexus provides innervation to the anterolateral aspect of the scrotum; the sacral plexus provides innervation to the postero-inferior aspect.

The long **testicular arteries** arise from the anterolateral aspect of the *abdominal aorta* just inferior to the *renal arteries* (Fig. 2.19). They pass retroperitoneally (posterior to the peritoneum) in an oblique direction, crossing over the ureters and the inferior parts of the external iliac arteries to reach the deep inguinal rings. They enter the inguinal canals through the deep rings, pass through the canals, exit them through the superficial inguinal rings, and enter the spermatic cords to supply the testes. The testicular artery or one of its branches anastomoses with the *artery of the ductus deferens*.

The veins emerging from the testis and epididymis form the **pampiniform venous plexus,** a network of 8–12 veins lying anterior to the ductus deferens and surrounding the testicular artery in the spermatic cord (Fig. 2.21). The pampiniform plexus is part of the thermoregulatory system of the testis (along with the cremasteric and dartos muscles) helping to keep this gland at a constant temperature. The veins of each pampiniform plexus converge superiorly, forming a **right testicular vein,** which enters the inferior vena cava (IVC), and a **left testicular vein,** which enters the left renal vein.

The lymphatic drainage of the testis follows the testicular artery and vein to the *right* and *left lumbar (caval/aortic)* and *pre-aortic lymph nodes* (see Fig. 2.19). The autonomic nerves of the testis arise as the **testicular plexus of nerves** on the testicular artery, which contains vagal parasympathetic and visceral afferent fibers and sympathetic fibers from the T10(–T11) segment of the spinal cord.

EPIDIDYMIS

The **epididymis** is an elongated structure on the posterior surface of the testis (Fig. 2.20). **Efferent ductules** of the testis transport newly developed sperms to the epididymis from the rete testis. The epididymis is formed by minute convolutions

of the **duct of the epididymis,** so tightly compacted that they appear solid (Fig. 2.21). The duct becomes progressively smaller as it passes from the head of the epididymis on the superior part of the testis to its tail. At the **tail of the epididymis,** the ductus deferens begins as the continuation of the epididymal duct. In the lengthy course of this duct, the sperms are stored and continue to mature. The epididymis consists of the:

- **Head of the epididymis:** the superior expanded part that is composed of lobules formed by the coiled ends of 12–14 *efferent ductules.*
- **Body of the epididymis:** major part consisting of the tightly convoluted duct of the epididymis.
- **Tail of the epididymis:** tapering continuation with the ductus deferens, the duct that transports the sperms from the epididymis to the ejaculatory duct for expulsion via the urethra during ejaculation (see Chapter 3).

Surface Anatomy of Anterolateral Abdominal Wall

The **umbilicus** is an obvious feature of the anterolateral abdominal wall and is the reference point for the *transumbilical plane* (Fig. 2.22). This puckered indentation of skin in the center of the anterior abdominal wall is typically at the level of the IV disc between the L3 and L4 vertebrae. However, its position varies with the amount of subcutaneous fat present. The umbilicus indicates the level of the T10 dermatome. The **epigastric fossa** (pit of the stomach) is a slight depression in the epigastric region, just inferior to the *xiphoid process*. This fossa is particularly noticeable when a person is in the supine position because the abdominal organs spread out, drawing the anterolateral abdominal wall posteriorly in this region. The pain caused by pyrosis ("heartburn," result-

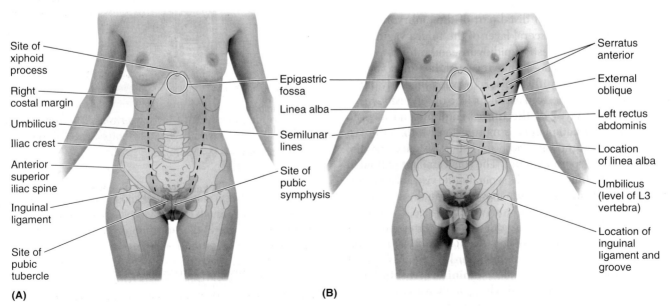

(A)

Site of xiphoid process
Right costal margin
Umbilicus
Iliac crest
Anterior superior iliac spine
Inguinal ligament
Site of pubic tubercle

Epigastric fossa
Linea alba
Semilunar lines
Site of pubic symphysis

(B)

Serratus anterior
External oblique
Left rectus abdominis
Location of linea alba
Umbilicus (level of L3 vertebra)
Location of inguinal ligament and groove

FIGURE 2.22. Surface anatomy of the anterolateral abdominal wall.

ing from reflux of gastric acid into the esophagus) is often felt at this site. The 7th–10th costal cartilages unite on each side of the epigastric fossa, their medial borders forming the *costal margin.* Although the abdominal cavity extends higher, the costal margin is the demarcation between the thoracic and abdominal portions of the body wall. When a person is in the supine position, observe the rise and fall of the abdominal wall with respiration: superiorly with inspiration and inferiorly with expiration. The rectus abdominis muscles can be palpated and observed when a supine person is asked to raise their head and shoulders against resistance.

The location of the *linea alba* is visible in lean individuals because of the vertical skin groove superficial to this raphe. The groove is usually obvious because the linea alba is approximately 1 cm wide between the two parts of the rectus abdominis superior to the umbilicus. Inferior to the umbilicus, the linea alba is not indicated by a groove. Some pregnant women, especially those with dark hair and a dark complexion, have a heavily pigmented line, the **linea nigra,** in the midline skin external to the linea alba. After pregnancy, the color of this line fades.

The upper margins of the pubic bones (*pubic crest*) and the cartilaginous joint that unite them (*pubic symphysis*) can be felt at the inferior end of the linea alba. The inguinal fold is a shallow oblique groove overlying the inguinal ligament as it extends between the *anterior superior iliac spine* (ASIS) and the *pubic tubercle.* The bony *iliac crest* at the level of L4 vertebra can be easily palpated as it extends posteriorly from the ASIS. The pubic crest, inguinal folds, and iliac crests demarcate the inferior limit of the anterior abdominal wall, distinguishing it from the perineum centrally and the lower limbs (thighs) laterally.

The **semilunar lines** (L. *lineae semilunares*) are slightly curved, linear impressions in the skin that extend from the inferior costal margin near the 9th costal cartilages to the pubic tubercles. These semilunar skin grooves (5–8 cm from the midline) are clinically important because they are parallel with the lateral edges of the rectus sheath.

Skin grooves also overlie the *tendinous intersections* of the rectus abdominis, which are clearly visible in persons with well-developed rectus muscles. The interdigitating bellies of the *serratus anterior* and *external oblique* muscles are also visible.

The site of the inguinal ligament is indicated by the **inguinal groove,** a skin crease that is parallel and just inferior to the inguinal ligament. This groove is readily visualized by having the person drop one leg to the floor while lying supine on an examining table. The inguinal groove marks the division between the anterolateral abdominal wall and the thigh.

INTERNAL SURFACE OF ANTEROLATERAL ABDOMINAL WALL AND INGUINAL REGION

Undescended (Cryptorchid) Testis

 The testes are undescended in approximately 3% of full-term and 30% of premature infants (Moore, Persaud, and Torchia, 2012). About 95% of undescended testes occur unilaterally. If a testis has not descended or is not retractable (capable of being drawn down), the condition is *cryptorchidism* (G. *orchis,* testis + L. from G. *kryptos,* hidden). The *undescended testis* usually lies somewhere along the normal path of its prenatal descent, commonly in the inguinal canal. The importance of cryptorchidism is a greatly increased risk for developing malignancy in the undescended testis, particularly problematic because it is not palpable and is not usually detected until cancer has progressed.

External Supravesical Hernia

 An *external supravesical hernia* leaves the peritoneal cavity through the supravesical fossa (Fig. 2.13). The site of the hernia is medial to that of a direct inguinal hernia (see the blue box "Inguinal Hernias," on p. 212). The iliohypogastric nerve is in danger of injury during the repair of this rare type of hernia.

Postnatal Patency of Umbilical Vein

Before the birth of a fetus, the umbilical vein carries well-oxygenated, nutrient-rich blood from the placenta to the fetus. Although reference is often made to the "occluded" umbilical vein forming the *round ligament of the liver,* this vein is patent for some time after birth, and is used for *umbilical vein catheterization* for exchange transfusion during early infancy—for example, in infants with *erythroblastosis fetalis* or *hemolytic disease* of the newborn (Kliegman et al., 2011).

Metastasis of Uterine Cancer to Labium Majus

Lymphogenous metastasis of cancer most commonly occurs along lymphatic pathways that parallel the venous drainage of the organ that is the site of the primary tumor. This is also true of the uterus, the veins and lymph vessels of which mostly drain via deep routes. However, some lymphatic vessels follow the course of the round ligament through the inguinal canal. Thus, while occurring less often, metastatic uterine cancer cells (especially from tumors adjacent to the proximal attachment of the round ligament) can spread from the uterus to the labium majus (the developmental homolog of the scrotum and site of distal attachment of the round ligament), and from there to the superficial inguinal nodes, which receive lymph from the skin of the perineum (including the labia).

SPERMATIC CORD, SCROTUM, AND TESTES

Inguinal Hernias

The majority of abdominal hernias occur in the inguinal region. Inguinal hernias account for 75% of abdominal hernias. These herniations occur in both sexes, but most inguinal hernias (approximately 86%) occur in males because of the passage of the spermatic cord through the *inguinal canal.*

An *inguinal hernia* is a protrusion of parietal peritoneum and viscera, such as the small intestine, through a normal or abnormal opening from the cavity in which they belong. Most hernias are reducible, meaning they can be returned to their normal place in the peritoneal cavity by appropriate manipulation. The two types of inguinal hernia are *direct* and *indirect inguinal hernias.* More than two thirds are indirect hernias. Characteristics of direct and indirect inguinal hernias are listed and illustrated in Table B2.1, with related anatomy illustrated in Figure B2.3A–C.

Normally, most of the processus vaginalis obliterates before birth, except for the distal part that forms the tunica vaginalis of the testis (Table 2.6). The peritoneal part of the hernial sac of an indirect inguinal hernia is formed by the persisting processus vaginalis. If the entire stalk of the processus vaginalis persists, the hernia extends into the scrotum superior to the testis, forming a complete indirect inguinal hernia (Table B2.1).

The *superficial inguinal ring* is palpable superolateral to the pubic tubercle by invaginating the skin of the upper scrotum with the index finger (Fig. B2.3D). The examiner's finger follows the spermatic cord superolaterally to the superficial inguinal ring. If the ring is dilated, it may admit the finger without causing pain. Should a hernia be present, a sudden impulse is felt against either the tip or pad of the examining finger when the patient is asked to cough (Swartz, 2009). However, because both inguinal hernia types exit the superficial ring, palpation of an impulse at this site does not discriminate type.

With the palmar surface of the finger against the anterior abdominal wall, the *deep inguinal ring* may be felt as a skin depression superior to the inguinal ligament, 2–4 cm superolateral to the pubic tubercle. Detection of an impulse at the superficial ring and a mass at the site of the deep ring suggests an indirect hernia.

Palpation of a direct inguinal hernia is performed by placing the palmar surface of the index and/or middle finger over the inguinal triangle and asking the person to cough or bear down (strain). If a hernia is present, a forceful impulse is felt against the pad of the finger. The finger can also be placed in the superficial inguinal ring; if a direct hernia is present, a sudden impulse is felt medial to the finger when the person coughs or bears down.

Cremasteric Reflex

Contraction of the cremaster muscle is elicited by lightly stroking the skin on the medial aspect of the superior part of the thigh with an applicator stick or tongue depressor. The *ilio-inguinal nerve* supplies this area of skin. The rapid elevation of the testis on the same side is the *cremasteric reflex.* This reflex is extremely active in children; consequently, hyperactive cremasteric reflexes may simulate undescended testes. A hyperactive reflex can be abolished by having the child sit in a cross-legged, squatting position; if the testes are descended, they can then be palpated in the scrotum.

Cysts and Hernias of Canal of Nuck

Indirect inguinal hernias can occur in women; however, they are approximately 20 times more common in men. If the processus vaginalis persists in females, it forms a small peritoneal pouch, the *canal of Nuck,* in the inguinal canal that may extend to the labium majus. In female infants, such remnants can enlarge and form cysts in the inguinal canal. The cysts may produce a bulge in the anterior part of the labium majus and have the potential to develop into an indirect inguinal hernia.

Hydrocele of Spermatic Cord and/or Testis

A *hydrocele* is the presence of excess fluid in a *persistent processus vaginalis.* This congenital anomaly may be associated with an indirect inguinal hernia. The fluid accumulation results from secretion of an abnormal amount of serous fluid from the visceral layer of the tunica vaginalis. The size of the hydrocele depends on how much of the processus vaginalis persists.

A *hydrocele of the testis* is confined to the scrotum and distends the tunica vaginalis (Fig. B2.4A). A *hydrocele of the spermatic cord* is confined to the spermatic cord and distends the persistent part of the stalk of the processus vaginalis (Fig. B2.4B). A congenital hydrocele of the cord and testis may communicate with the peritoneal cavity.

Detection of a hydrocele requires *transillumination,* a procedure during which a bright light is applied to the side of the scrotal enlargement in a darkened room. The transmission of light as a red glow indicates excess serous fluid in the scrotum. Newborn male infants often have residual peritoneal fluid in their tunica vaginalis; however, this fluid is usually absorbed during the 1st year of life. Certain pathological conditions, such as injury and/or inflammation of the epididymis, may also produce a hydrocele in adults.

Hematocele of Testis

A *hematocele of the testis* is a collection of blood in the tunica vaginalis that results, for example, from rupture of branches of the testicular artery by trauma to the testis (Fig. B2.4C). Trauma may produce a scrotal and/or testicular *hematoma* (accumulation of blood, usually clotted, in any extravascular location). Blood does not transilluminate; therefore, transillumination can differentiate a hematocele or hematoma from a hydrocele. A hematocele of the testis may be associated with a *scrotal hematocele,* resulting from effusion of blood into the scrotal tissues.

TABLE B2.1. CHARACTERISTICS OF INGUINAL HERNIAS

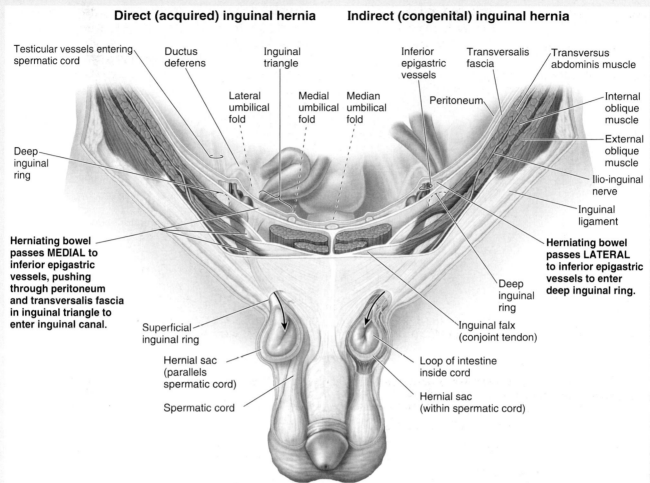

Characteristic	Direct (Acquired)	Indirect (Congenital)
Predisposing factors	Weakness of anterior abdominal wall in inguinal triangle (e.g., owing to distended superficial ring, narrow inguinal falx, or attenuation of aponeurosis in males >40 years of age)	Patency of processus vaginalis (complete or at least superior part) in younger persons, the great majority of which are males
Frequency	Less common (one third to one quarter of inguinal hernias)	More common (two thirds to three quarters) of inguinal hernias
Exit from abdominal cavity (Fig. B2.3A & B)	Peritoneum plus transversalis fascia (lies outside inner one or two fascial coverings of cord)	Peritoneum of persistent processus vaginalis plus all three fascial coverings of cord/round ligament
Course (Fig. B2.3C)	Passes through or around inguinal canal, usually traversing only medial third of canal, external and parallel to vestige of processus vaginalis	Traverses inguinal canal (entire canal if it is of sufficient size) within processus vaginalis
Exit from anterior abdominal wall	Via superficial ring, lateral to cord; rarely enters scrotum	Via superficial ring inside cord, commonly passing into scrotum/labium majus

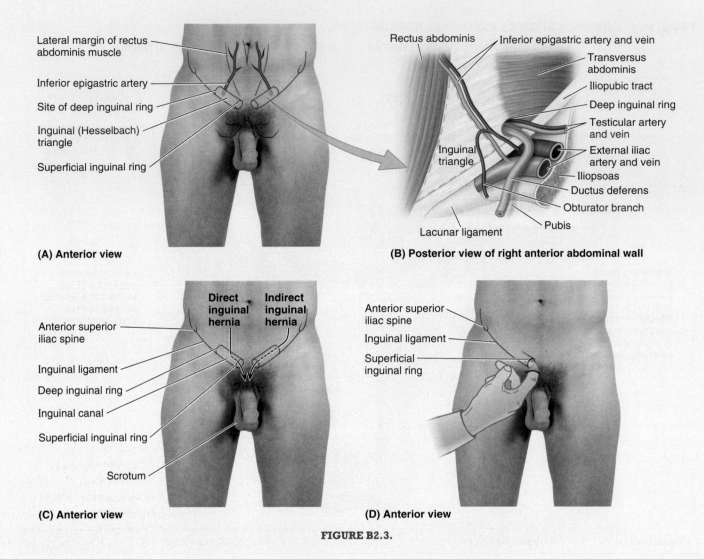

(A) Anterior view

Lateral margin of rectus abdominis muscle
Inferior epigastric artery
Site of deep inguinal ring
Inguinal (Hesselbach) triangle
Superficial inguinal ring

(B) Posterior view of right anterior abdominal wall

Rectus abdominis
Inferior epigastric artery and vein
Transversus abdominis
Iliopubic tract
Deep inguinal ring
Testicular artery and vein
External iliac artery and vein
Iliopsoas
Ductus deferens
Obturator branch
Pubis
Inguinal triangle
Lacunar ligament

(C) Anterior view

Direct inguinal hernia
Indirect inguinal hernia
Anterior superior iliac spine
Inguinal ligament
Deep inguinal ring
Inguinal canal
Superficial inguinal ring
Scrotum

(D) Anterior view

Anterior superior iliac spine
Inguinal ligament
Superficial inguinal ring

FIGURE B2.3.

Torsion of Spermatic Cord

Torsion of the spermatic cord is a surgical emergency because necrosis (pathologic death) of the testis may occur. The torsion (twisting) obstructs the venous drainage, with resultant edema and hemorrhage, and subsequent arterial obstruction. The twisting usually occurs just above the upper pole of the testis (Fig. B2.4D). To prevent recurrence or occurrence on the contralateral side, which is likely, both testes are surgically fixed to the scrotal septum.

Ductus deferens and spermatic cord
Head of epididymis
Tunica vaginalis
Testis
Fluid in tunica vaginalis

(A) Hydrocele (H) of testis

(B) Hydrocele (H) of cord

Hemorrhage into the tunica vaginalis due to injury to the spermatic vessels

(C) Hematocele (H) of testis

Spermatic cord
Upper pole of testis
Testis

(D) Torsion of spermatic cord

FIGURE B2.4.

Anesthetizing Scrotum

Since the anterolateral surface of the scrotum is supplied by the lumbar plexus (primarily L1 fibers via the ilio-inguinal nerve) and the postero-inferior aspect is supplied by the sacral plexus (primarily S3 fibers via the pudendal nerve), a spinal anesthetic agent must be injected more superiorly to anesthetize the anterolateral surface of the scrotum than is necessary to anesthetize its postero-inferior surface.

Spermatocele and Epididymal Cyst

A *spermatocele* is a retention cyst (collection of fluid) in the epididymis (Fig. B2.5A), usually near its head. Spermatoceles contain a milky fluid and are generally asymptomatic. An *epididymal cyst* is a collection of fluid anywhere in the epididymis (Fig. B2.5B).

Vestigial Remnants of Embryonic Genital Ducts

When the tunica vaginalis is opened, rudimentary structures may be observed at the superior aspects of the testes and epididymis (Fig. B2.6). These structures are small remnants of genital ducts in the embryo. They are rarely observed unless pathological changes occur. The **appendix of the testis** is a vesicular remnant of the cranial end of the *paramesonephric (müllerian) duct,* the embryonic genital duct that in the female forms half of the uterus. It is attached to the upper pole of the testis. The **appendices of the epididymis** are remnants of the cranial end of the *mesonephric (wolffian) duct,* the embryonic genital duct that in the male forms part of the ductus deferens. The appendices are attached to the head of the epididymis.

Varicocele

The vine-like *pampiniform plexus of veins* may become dilated (varicose) and tortuous, producing a *varicocele,* which is usually visible only when the man is standing or straining. The enlargement usually disappears when the person lies down, particularly if the scrotum is ele-

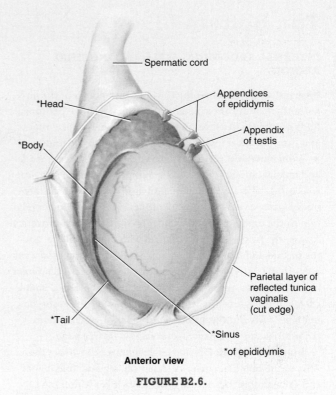

Anterior view

FIGURE B2.6.

vated while supine, allowing gravity to empty the veins. Palpating a varicocele can be likened to feeling a bag of worms. Varicoceles may result from defective valves in the testicular vein, but kidney or renal vein problems can also result in distension of the pampiniform veins. Varicocele occurs predominantly on the left side, probably because the acute angle at which the right vein enters the IVC is more favorable to flow than the nearly 90° angle at which the left testicular vein enters the left renal vein, making it more susceptible to obstruction or reversal of flow.

Cancer of Testis and Scrotum

Lymphogenous metastasis is common to all testicular tumors, so a knowledge of lymphatic drainage is helpful in treatment (Kumar et al., 2009). Because the testes relocate from the posterior abdominal wall to the scrotum during fetal development, their lymphatic drainage differs from that of the scrotum, which is an outpouching of anterolateral abdominal skin (see Fig. 2.15). Consequently:

- *Cancer of the testis:* metastasizes initially to the retroperitoneal *lumbar lymph nodes,* which lie just inferior to the renal veins. Subsequent spread may be to mediastinal and supraclavicular nodes.
- *Cancer of the scrotum:* metastasizes to the *superficial inguinal lymph nodes,* which lie in the subcutaneous tissue inferior to the inguinal ligament and along the terminal part of the great saphenous vein.

Metastasis of testicular cancer may also occur by hematogenous spread of cancer cells (via the blood) to the lungs, liver, brain, and bone.

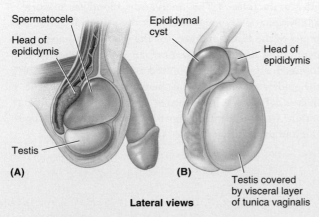

FIGURE B2.5. A. Spermatocele. **B.** Epididymal cyst.

The Bottom Line

INTERNAL ABDOMINAL WALL AND INGUINAL REGION

Internal abdominal wall: The primary features of the internal surface of the anterolateral abdominal wall are peritoneal folds overlying structures radiating from the umbilical ring and the peritoneal fossae formed in relation to the folds. ♦ Of the umbilical peritoneal folds, the central three (median and medial umbilical folds) cover remnants of embryological structures, whereas the lateral umbilical folds cover the inferior epigastric vessels. ♦ The peritoneal fossae formed in relation to the umbilical folds include the transitional supravesical fossae, the height of which changes with bladder filling, and the medial and lateral inguinal fossa, overlying potential weak areas in the anterior abdominal wall where direct and indirect inguinal hernias, respectively, may occur. ♦ The supra-umbilical falciform ligament encloses the remnant of the embryonic umbilical vein and the accompanying para-umbilical veins (tributaries of the hepatic portal vein) in its free edge.

Inguinal region: The inguinal region extends from the ASIS to the pubic tubercle; its superficial inguinal fold demarcates the abdomen from the lower limb. It lies within the L1 dermatome. ♦ Most structures and formations in the inguinal region relate to a double (bilaminar) retinaculum formed by the inguinal ligament and iliopubic tract as they extend between the two bony points. These two bands are thickenings of the inferior margins of the external oblique aponeurosis and transversalis fascia of the abdominal wall, respectively.

To allow the testis to descend prenatally to a subcutaneous location that will be cooler postnatally (a requirement for the development of sperms), the inguinal canal traverses the abdominal wall superior and parallel to the medial half of the inguinal ligament. ♦ In females, only the inferior portion of the gubernaculum traverses the canal, becoming the round ligament of the uterus. ♦ The inguinal canal itself consists of a deep ring internally, a superficial ring externally, and two musculo-aponeurotic arches in between. ♦ The oblique passageway through the offset rings and arches collapses when intra-abdominal pressure increases. ♦ Collapse of the canal, combined with the prenatal occlusion of the peritoneal evagination (processus vaginalis) and the contraction of the arches, normally resists the tendency for abdominal contents to herniate (protrude through) the canal. ♦ Failure of the processus vaginalis to occlude, or defective anatomy, or degeneration of tissues, may result in the development of inguinal hernias.

SPERMATIC CORD, SCROTUM, AND TESTES

Spermatic cord: In their passage through the inguinal canal, the processus vaginalis, testis, ductus deferens, and neurovascular structures of the testis (or processus vaginalis and lower ovarian gubernaculum of the female) become engulfed by fascial extensions derived from most (three of four) of the layers traversed. This results in a trilaminar covering. ♦ The transversalis fascia, internal oblique, and external oblique layers contribute the internal spermatic fascia, cremasteric muscle and fascia, and external spermatic fascia, respectively, to the spermatic cord. ♦ Although the portion of the processus vaginalis within the spermatic cord occludes, that adjacent to the testis remains patent as the tunica vaginalis testis. ♦ The contents of the spermatic cord are the ductus deferens and neurovascular structures, which trailed the testis as it relocated from the posterior abdominal wall during development.

Scrotum: The scrotum is the integumentary sac formed from the labioscrotal swellings of the male to house the testes after their relocation. The fatty layer of subcutaneous tissue of the abdominal wall is replaced in the scrotum by the smooth dartos muscle, whereas the membranous layer is continued as the dartos fascia and scrotal septum. ♦ The scrotum receives anterior scrotal arteries from the thigh (via the external pudendal artery), posterior scrotal arteries from the perineum (internal pudendal artery), and internally cremasteric arteries from the abdomen (inferior epigastric artery). ♦ Anterior scrotal nerves are derived from the lumbar plexus (via the genitofemoral and ilio-inguinal nerves), and posterior scrotal nerves from the sacral plexus (via the pudendal nerve).

Testes: The testes are the male gonads, shaped and sized like large olives or small plums, that produce sperms and male hormones. ♦ Each testis is engulfed, except posteriorly and superiorly, by a double-layered serous sac, the tunica vaginalis, derived from the peritoneum. ♦ The outer surface of the testis is covered with the fibrous tunica albuginea, which is thickened internally and posteriorly as the mediastinum of the testis from which septa radiate. ♦ Between the septa are loops of fine seminiferous tubules in which the sperms develop. The tubules converge and empty into the rete testis in the mediastinum, which is connected in turn to the epididymis by the efferent ductules. ♦ The innervation, blood vasculature, and lymphatic drainage all reflect the posterior abdominal origin of the testes and are, for the main part, independent of the surrounding scrotal sac. ♦ The epididymis is formed by the highly convoluted and compacted duct of the epididymis leading from the efferent ductules to the ductus deferens. It is the site of sperm storage and maturation. The epididymis clings to the more protected superior and posterior aspects of the testis.

PERITONEUM AND PERITONEAL CAVITY

The **peritoneum** is a continuous, glistening, and slippery transparent serous membrane. It lines the abdominopelvic cavity and invests the viscera (Fig. 2.23). The peritoneum consists of two continuous layers: the *parietal peritoneum*, which lines the internal surface of the abdominopelvic wall, and the *visceral peritoneum*, which invests viscera such as the stomach and intestines. Both layers of peritoneum consist of *mesothelium*, a layer of simple squamous epithelial cells.

The **parietal peritoneum** is served by the same blood and lymphatic vasculature and the same somatic nerve supply, as is the region of the wall it lines. Like the overlying skin, the peritoneum lining the interior of the body wall is sensitive to pressure, pain, heat and cold, and laceration. Pain from the parietal peritoneum is generally well localized, except for that on the inferior surface of the central part of the diaphragm, where innervation is provided by the phrenic nerves (discussed later in this chapter); irritation here is often referred to the C3–C5 dermatomes over the shoulder.

The **visceral peritoneum** and the organs it covers are served by the same blood and lymphatic vasculature and visceral nerve supply. The visceral peritoneum is insensitive to touch, heat and cold, and laceration; it is stimulated primarily by stretching and chemical irritation. The pain produced is poorly localized, being referred to the dermatomes of the spinal ganglia providing the sensory fibers, particularly to midline portions of these dermatomes. Consequently, pain

from foregut derivatives is usually experienced in the epigastric region, that from midgut derivatives in the umbilical region, and that from hindgut derivatives in the pubic region.

The peritoneum and viscera are in the abdominopelvic cavity. The relationship of the viscera to the peritoneum is as follows:

- *Intraperitoneal organs* are almost completely covered with visceral peritoneum (e.g., the stomach and spleen). *Intraperitoneal* in this case does *not* mean inside the peritoneal cavity (although the term is used clinically for substances injected into this cavity). Intraperitoneal organs have conceptually, if not literally, invaginated into the closed sac, like pressing your fist into an inflated balloon (see the discussion of potential spaces in the Introduction).
- *Extraperitoneal, retroperitoneal,* and *subperitoneal organs* are also outside the peritoneal cavity—external to the parietal peritoneum—and are only partially covered with peritoneum (usually on just one surface). Retroperitoneal organs such as the kidneys are between the parietal peritoneum and the posterior abdominal wall and have parietal peritoneum only on their anterior surfaces (often with a variable amount of intervening fat). Similarly, the subperitoneal urinary bladder has parietal peritoneum only on its superior surface.

The **peritoneal cavity** is within the abdominal cavity and continues inferiorly into the pelvic cavity. The peritoneal cavity is a potential space of capillary thinness between the parietal and visceral layers of peritoneum. It contains no organs but contains a thin film of **peritoneal fluid,** which is composed of

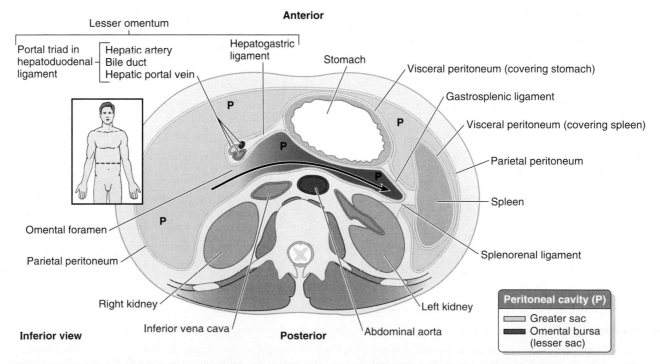

FIGURE 2.23. Transverse section of abdomen at level of omental bursa. The orientation figure (inset) indicates the level of the section superficially. The *dark arrow* passes from the greater sac of the peritoneal cavity (*P*) through the omental (epiploic) foramen and across the full extent of the omental bursa (lesser sac).

water, electrolytes, and other substances derived from interstitial fluid in adjacent tissues. Peritoneal fluid lubricates the peritoneal surfaces, enabling the viscera to move over each other without friction, and allowing the movements of digestion. In addition to lubricating the surfaces of the viscera, the peritoneal fluid contains leukocytes and antibodies that resist infection. Lymphatic vessels, particularly on the inferior surface of the constantly active diaphragm, absorb the peritoneal fluid. The peritoneal cavity is completely closed in males. However, there is a communication pathway in females to the exterior of the body through the uterine tubes, uterine cavity, and vagina. This communication constitutes a potential pathway of infection from the exterior.

Embryology of Peritoneal Cavity

When it is initially formed, the gut is the same length as the developing body. It undergoes exuberant growth, however, to provide the large absorptive surface required by nutrition. By the end of the 10th week of development, the gut is much longer than the body that contains it. For this increase in length to occur, the gut must gain freedom of movement relative to the body wall at an early stage, while still maintaining the connection with it necessary for innervation and blood supply. This growth (and later, the activity of the gut) is accommodated by the development of a serous cavity within the trunk that houses the increasingly lengthy and convoluted gut in a relatively compact space. The rate of growth of the gut initially outpaces the development of adequate space within the trunk (body), and for a time the rapidly lengthening gut extends outside the developing anterior body wall (see "Brief Review of the Embryological Rotation of the Midgut," on p. 258).

Early in its development, the embryonic body cavity (*intraembryonic coelom*) is lined with *mesoderm*, the primordium of the peritoneum. At a slightly later stage, the primordial abdominal cavity is lined with *parietal peritoneum* derived from

mesoderm, which forms a closed sac. The lumen of the peritoneal sac is the *peritoneal cavity*. As the organs develop, they invaginate (protrude) to varying degrees into the peritoneal sac, acquiring a peritoneal covering, the *visceral peritoneum*. A viscus (organ) such as the kidney protrudes only partially into the peritoneal cavity; hence, it is primarily retroperitoneal, always remaining external to the peritoneal cavity and posterior to the peritoneum lining the abdominal cavity. Other viscera, such as the stomach and spleen, protrude completely into the peritoneal sac and are almost completely invested by visceral peritoneum—that is, they are *intraperitoneal*.

These viscera are connected to the abdominal wall by a *mesentery* of variable length, which is composed of two layers of peritoneum with a thin layer of loose connective tissue between them. Generally, viscera that vary relatively little in size and shape, such as the kidneys, are retroperitoneal, whereas viscera that undergo marked changes in shape owing to filling, emptying, and peristalsis, such as the stomach, are invested with visceral peritoneum. Intraperitoneal viscera with a mesentery, such as most of the small intestine, are mobile, the degree of which varies with the length of the mesentery. Although the liver and spleen do not change shape as a result of intrinsic activity (although they may slowly change in size when engorged with blood), their need for a covering of visceral peritoneum is dictated by the need to accommodate passive changes in position imposed by the adjacent, highly active diaphragm.

As organs protrude into the peritoneal sac, their vessels, nerves, and lymphatics remain connected to their extraperitoneal (usually retroperitoneal) sources or destinations so that these connecting structures lie between the layers of the peritoneum forming their mesenteries. Initially, the entire primordial gut is suspended in the center of the peritoneal cavity by a posterior mesentery attached to the midline of the posterior body wall. As the organs grow, they gradually reduce the size of the peritoneal cavity until it is only a potential space

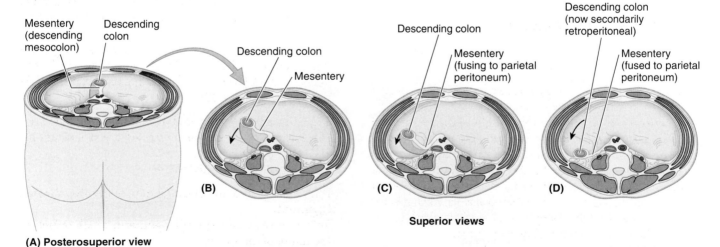

FIGURE 2.24. Migration and fusion of descending mesocolon. Starting from the primordial position, suspended from the midline of the posterior abdominal wall (**A**), the mesocolon shifts to the left (**B**) and gradually fuses with the left posterior parietal peritoneum (**C**). **D.** The descending colon has become secondarily retroperitoneal. The *arrow* indicates the left paracolic gutter, the site where an incision is made during mobilization of the colon during surgery. Sometimes the descending colon retains a short mesentery, similar to the stage shown in **C,** especially where the colon is in the iliac fossa.

between the parietal and visceral layers of peritoneum. As a consequence, several parts of the gut come to lie against the posterior abdominal wall, and their posterior mesenteries become gradually reduced because of pressure from overlying organs (Fig. 2.24). For example, during development, the growing coiled mass of small intestine pushes the part of the gut that will become the descending colon to the left side and presses its mesentery against the posterior abdominal wall. The mesentery is held there until the layer of peritoneum that formed the left side of the mesentery and the part of the visceral peritoneum of the colon lying against the body wall fuse with the parietal peritoneum of the body wall. As a result, the colon becomes fixed to the posterior abdominal wall on the left side with peritoneum covering only its anterior aspect. The descending colon (as well as the ascending colon on the right side) has thus become *secondarily retroperitoneal,* having once been intraperitoneal (Moore et al., 2012).

The layers of peritoneum that fused now form a **fusion fascia,** a connective tissue plane in which the nerves and vessels of the descending colon continue to lie. Thus, the descending colon of the adult can be freed from the posterior body wall (surgically mobilized) by incising the peritoneum along the lateral border of the descending colon and then bluntly dissecting along the plane of the fusion fascia, elevating the neurovascular structures from the posterior body wall until the midline is reached. The ascending colon can be similarly mobilized on the right side.

Several parts of the gastrointestinal tract and associated organs become secondarily retroperitoneal (e.g., most of the duodenum and pancreas as well as the ascending and descending parts of the colon). They are covered with peritoneum only on their anterior surface. Other parts of the viscera (e.g., the sigmoid colon and spleen) retain a relatively short mesentery. However, the roots of the short mesenteries do not remain attached to the midline but shift to the left or right by a fusion process like that described for the descending colon.

Peritoneal Formations

The *peritoneal cavity* has a complex shape. Some of the facts relating to this include the following:

- The peritoneal cavity houses a great length of gut, most of which is covered with peritoneum.
- Extensive continuities are required between the parietal and visceral peritoneum to convey the necessary neurovascular structures from the body wall to the viscera.
- Although the volume of the abdominal cavity is a fraction of the body's volume, the parietal and visceral peritoneum lining the peritoneal cavity within it have a much greater surface area than the body's outer surface (skin); therefore, the peritoneum is highly convoluted.

Various terms are used to describe the parts of the peritoneum that connect organs with other organs, or to the abdominal wall, and the compartments and recesses that are formed as a consequence.

A **mesentery** is a double layer of peritoneum that occurs as a result of the invagination of the peritoneum by an organ and constitutes a continuity of the visceral and parietal peritoneum. It provides a means for neurovascular communications between the organ and the body wall (Fig. 2.25A & E). A mesentery connects an intraperitoneal organ to the body wall—usually the posterior abdominal wall (e.g., mesentery of the small intestine).

The **small intestine mesentery** is usually referred to simply as "the mesentery"; however, mesenteries related to other specific parts of the alimentary tract are named accordingly—for example, the *transverse* and *sigmoid mesocolons* (Fig. 2.25B), *mesoesophagus, mesogastrium,* and *mesoappendix.* Mesenteries have a core of connective tissue containing blood and lymphatic vessels, nerves, lymph nodes, and fat (see Fig. 2.48A).

An **omentum** is a double-layered extension or fold of peritoneum that passes from the stomach and proximal part of the duodenum to adjacent organs in the abdominal cavity (Fig. 2.25).

- The **greater omentum** is a prominent, four-layered peritoneal fold that hangs down like an apron from the greater curvature of the stomach and the proximal part of the duodenum (Fig. 2.25A, C, & E). After descending, it folds back and attaches to the anterior surface of the transverse colon and its mesentery.
- The **lesser omentum** is a much smaller, double-layered peritoneal fold that connects the lesser curvature of the stomach and the proximal part of the duodenum to the liver (Fig. 2.25B & D). It also connects the stomach to a triad of structures that run between the duodenum and liver in the free edge of the lesser omentum (Fig. 2.23).

A **peritoneal ligament** consists of a double layer of peritoneum that connects an organ with another organ or to the abdominal wall.

The liver is connected to the:

- Anterior abdominal wall by the *falciform ligament* (Fig. 2.26).
- Stomach by the **hepatogastric ligament,** the membranous portion of the lesser omentum.
- Duodenum by the **hepatoduodenal ligament,** the thickened free edge of the lesser omentum, which conducts the *portal triad:* portal vein, hepatic artery, and bile duct (Figs. 2.23 and 2.26).

The hepatogastric and hepatoduodenal ligaments are continuous parts of the lesser omentum and are separated only for descriptive convenience.

The stomach is connected to the:

- Inferior surface of the diaphragm by the **gastrophrenic ligament.**
- Spleen by the **gastrosplenic ligament,** which reflects to the hilum of the spleen.
- Transverse colon by the **gastrocolic ligament,** the apron-like part of the greater omentum, which descends from the greater curvature, turns under, and then ascends to the transverse colon.

inflammation of the peritoneum—*peritonitis*. Exudation of serum, fibrin, cells, and pus into the peritoneal cavity occurs, accompanied by pain in the overlying skin and an increase in the tone of the anterolateral abdominal muscles. Given the extent of the peritoneal surfaces and the rapid absorption of material, including bacterial toxins, from the peritoneal cavity, when a peritonitis becomes *generalized* (widespread in the peritoneal cavity), the condition is dangerous and perhaps lethal. In addition to the severe abdominal pain, tenderness, nausea and/or vomiting, fever, and constipation are present.

General peritonitis also occurs when an ulcer perforates the wall of the stomach or duodenum, spilling acid content into the peritoneal cavity. Excess fluid in the peritoneal cavity is called *ascitic fluid*. The clinical condition in which one has ascitic fluid is referred to as *ascites*. Ascites may also occur as a result of mechanical injury (which may also produce internal bleeding) or other pathological conditions, such as portal hypertension (venous congestion), widespread metastasis of cancer cells to the abdominal viscera, and starvation (when plasma proteins fail to be produced, altering concentration gradients and producing a paradoxically protuberant abdomen). In all these cases, the peritoneal cavity may be distended with several liters of abnormal fluid, interfering with movements of the viscera.

Rhythmic movements of the anterolateral abdominal wall normally accompany respirations. If the abdomen is drawn in as the chest expands (*paradoxical abdominothoracic rhythm*) and muscle rigidity is present, either peritonitis or pneumonitis (inflammation of the lungs) may be present. Because the intense pain worsens with movement, people with peritonitis commonly lie with their knees flexed to relax their anterolateral abdominal muscles. They also breath shallowly (and hence more rapidly), reducing the intra-abdominal pressure and pain.

Peritoneal Adhesions and Adhesiotomy

 If the peritoneum is damaged, by a stab wound for example, or infected, the peritoneal surfaces become inflamed, making them sticky with *fibrin*. As healing occurs, the fibrin may be replaced with fibrous tissue, forming abnormal attachments between the visceral peritoneum of adjacent viscera, or between the visceral peritoneum of an organ and the parietal peritoneum of the adjacent abdominal wall. *Adhesions* (scar tissue) may also form after an abdominal operation (e.g., owing to a ruptured appendix) and limit the normal movements of the viscera. This tethering may cause chronic pain or emergency complications such as intestinal obstruction when the intestine becomes twisted around an adhesion (*volvulus*).

Adhesiotomy refers to the surgical separation of adhesions. Adhesions are often found during dissection of cadavers (see the adhesion binding the spleen to the diaphragm in Fig. 2.39B, for example).

Abdominal Paracentesis

 Treatment of generalized peritonitis includes removal of the ascitic fluid and, in the presence of infection, administration of large doses of antibiotics. Occasionally, more localized accumulations of fluid may have to be removed for analysis. Surgical puncture of the peritoneal cavity for the aspiration or drainage of fluid is called *paracentesis*. After injection of a local anesthetic agent, a needle or trocar and a cannula are inserted through the anterolateral abdominal wall into the peritoneal cavity through the linea alba, for example. The needle is inserted superior to the empty urinary bladder, in a location that avoids the inferior epigastric artery.

Intraperitoneal Injection and Peritoneal Dialysis

 The peritoneum is a semipermeable membrane with an extensive surface area, much of which (subdiaphragmatic portions in particular) overlies blood and lymphatic capillary beds. Therefore, fluid injected into the peritoneal cavity is absorbed rapidly. For this reason, anesthetic agents, such as solutions of barbiturate compounds, may be injected into the peritoneal cavity by *intraperitoneal (I.P.) injection*.

In *renal failure*, waste products such as urea accumulate in the blood and tissues and ultimately reach fatal levels. *Peritoneal dialysis* may be performed in which soluble substances and excess water are removed from the system by transfer across the peritoneum, using a dilute sterile solution that is introduced into the peritoneal cavity on one side and then drained from the other side. Diffusible solutes and water are transferred between the blood and the peritoneal cavity as a result of concentration gradients between the two fluid compartments. Peritoneal dialysis is usually employed only temporarily, however. For the long term, it is preferable to use direct blood flow through a renal dialysis machine.

Functions of Greater Omentum

 The greater omentum, large and fat laden, prevents the visceral peritoneum from adhering to the parietal peritoneum. It has considerable mobility and moves around the peritoneal cavity with peristaltic movements of the viscera. It often forms adhesions adjacent to an inflamed organ, such as the appendix, sometimes walling it off and thereby protecting other viscera from it. Thus, it is common when entering the abdominal cavity, in either dissection or surgery, to find the omentum markedly displaced from the "normal" position in which it is almost always depicted in anatomical illustrations. The greater omentum also cushions the abdominal organs against injury and forms insulation against loss of body heat.

Abscess Formation

Perforation of a duodenal ulcer, rupture of the gall-bladder, or perforation of the appendix may lead to the formation of a an *abscess* (circumscribed collection of purulent exudate, i.e., pus) in the subphrenic recess. The abscess may be walled inferiorly by adhesions (see the blue box "Subphrenic Abscesses," p. 283).

Spread of Pathological Fluids

Peritoneal recesses are of clinical importance in connection with the spread of pathological fluids such as pus, a product of inflammation. The recesses determine the extent and direction of the spread of fluids that may enter the peritoneal cavity when an organ is diseased or injured.

Flow of Ascitic Fluid and Pus

The *paracolic gutters* are of clinical importance because they provide pathways for the flow of ascitic fluid and the spread of intraperitoneal infections (Fig. 2.27B). Purulent material (consisting of or containing pus) in the abdomen can be transported along the paracolic gutters into the pelvis, especially when the person is upright. Thus, to facilitate the flow of exudate into the pelvic cavity where absorption of toxins is slow, patients with peritonitis are often placed in the sitting position (at least a 45° angle). Conversely, infections in the pelvis may extend superiorly to a subphrenic recess situated under the diaphragm (see the blue box "Subphrenic Abscesses," p. 283), especially when the person is supine. Similarly, the paracolic gutters provide pathways for the spread of cancer cells that have sloughed from the ulcerated surface of a tumor and entered the peritoneal cavity.

Fluid in Omental Bursa

Perforation of the posterior wall of the stomach results in the passage of its fluid contents into the omental bursa. An inflamed or injured pancreas can also result in the passage of pancreatic fluid into the bursa, forming a *pancreatic pseudo-cyst*.

Intestine in Omental Bursa

Although uncommon, a loop of small intestine may pass through the omental foramen into the omental bursa and be strangulated by the edges of the foramen. As none of the boundaries of the foramen can be incised because each contains blood vessels, the swollen intestine must be decompressed using a needle so it can be returned to the greater sac of the peritoneal cavity through the omental foramen.

Severance of Cystic Artery

The cystic artery must be ligated or clamped and then severed during *cholecystectomy*, removal of the gall-bladder. Sometimes, however, the artery is accidentally severed before it has been adequately ligated. The surgeon can control the hemorrhage by compressing the hepatic artery as it traverses the hepatoduodenal ligament. The index finger is placed in the omental foramen and the thumb on its anterior wall (Fig. 2.29). Alternate compression and release of pressure on the hepatic artery allows the surgeon to identify the bleeding artery and clamp it.

The Bottom Line

PERITONEUM, PERITONEAL CAVITY, AND PERITONEAL FORMATIONS

Peritoneum and peritoneal cavity: The peritoneum is a continuous, serous membrane that lines the abdominopelvic cavity (the parietal peritoneum) and the contained viscera (the visceral peritoneum). ♦ The collapsed peritoneal cavity between the parietal and visceral peritoneum normally contains only enough peritoneal fluid (about 50 mL) to lubricate the inner surface of the peritoneum. This arrangement allows the gut the freedom of movement required for alimentation (digestion). ♦ Adhesions formed as a result of infection or injury interfere with these movements. ♦ The parietal peritoneum is a sensitive, semipermeable membrane, with blood and lymphatic capillary beds especially abundant deep to its subdiaphragmatic surface.

Peritoneal formations and subdivisions of peritoneal cavity: Continuities and connections between the visceral and parietal peritoneum occur where the gut enters and exits the abdominopelvic cavity. ♦ Parts of the peritoneum also occur as double folds (mesenteries and omenta, and subdivisions called ligaments) that convey neurovascular structures and the ducts of accessory organs to and from the viscera. ♦ Peritoneal ligaments are named for the particular structures connected by them. ♦ As a result of the rotation and exuberant growth of the intestine during development, the disposition of the peritoneal cavity becomes complex. The main part of the peritoneal cavity (greater sac) is divided by the transverse mesocolon into supracolic and infracolic compartments. ♦ A smaller part of the peritoneal cavity, the omental bursa (lesser sac) lies posterior to the stomach, separating it from retroperitoneal viscera on the posterior wall. It communicates with the greater sac via the omental foramen. ♦ The complex disposition of the peritoneal cavity determines the flow and pooling of excess (ascitic) fluid occupying the peritoneal cavity during pathological conditions.

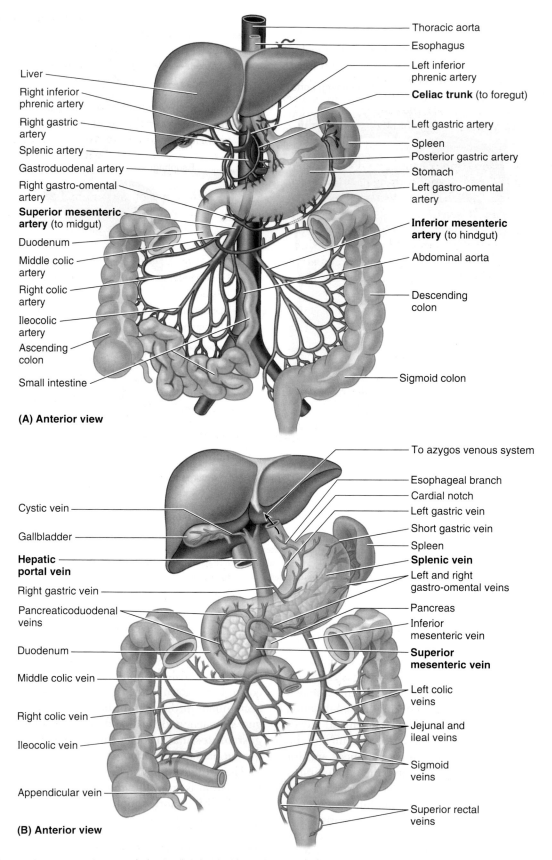

(A) Anterior view

Liver
Right inferior phrenic artery
Right gastric artery
Splenic artery
Gastroduodenal artery
Right gastro-omental artery
Superior mesenteric artery (to midgut)
Duodenum
Middle colic artery
Right colic artery
Ileocolic artery
Ascending colon
Small intestine

Thoracic aorta
Esophagus
Left inferior phrenic artery
Celiac trunk (to foregut)
Left gastric artery
Spleen
Posterior gastric artery
Stomach
Left gastro-omental artery
Inferior mesenteric artery (to hindgut)
Abdominal aorta
Descending colon
Sigmoid colon

(B) Anterior view

Cystic vein
Gallbladder
Hepatic portal vein
Right gastric vein
Pancreaticoduodenal veins
Duodenum
Middle colic vein
Right colic vein
Ileocolic vein
Appendicular vein

To azygos venous system
Esophageal branch
Cardial notch
Left gastric vein
Short gastric vein
Spleen
Splenic vein
Left and right gastro-omental veins
Pancreas
Inferior mesenteric vein
Superior mesenteric vein
Left colic veins
Jejunal and ileal veins
Sigmoid veins
Superior rectal veins

FIGURE 2.32.   Arterial supply and venous drainage of abdominal parts of alimentary system. A. The arterial supply is demonstrated. The three unpaired branches of the abdominal aorta supply, in succession, the derivatives of the foregut, midgut, and hindgut. **B.** The venous drainage is shown. The nutrient-rich blood from the gastrointestinal tract and that from the spleen, pancreas, and gallbladder all drain to the liver via the portal vein. The *black arrow* indicates the communication of the esophageal vein with the azygos (systemic) venous system.

Esophagus

The **esophagus** is a muscular tube (approximately 25 cm [10 in] long) with an average diameter of 2 cm that conveys food from the pharynx to the stomach (Fig. 2.33A). As seen during *fluoroscopy* (x-ray, using a fluoroscope) after a barium swallow (Fig. 2.34), the esophagus normally has three constrictions where adjacent structures produce impressions:

- **Cervical constriction (upper esophageal sphincter):** at its beginning at the **pharyngoesophageal junction,** approximately 15 cm from the incisor teeth; caused by the *cricopharyngeus muscle* (see Chapter 8).
- **Thoracic (broncho-aortic) constriction:** a compound constriction where it is first crossed by the arch of the aorta, 22.5 cm from the incisor teeth, and then where it is crossed by the left main bronchus, 27.5 cm from the

incisor teeth; the former is seen in anteroposterior views, the latter in lateral views.
- **Diaphragmatic constriction:** where it passes through the *esophageal hiatus* of the diaphragm, approximately 40 cm from the incisor teeth (Fig. 2.33A).

Awareness of these constrictions is important when passing instruments through the esophagus into the stomach, and when viewing radiographs of patients who are experiencing *dysphagia* (difficulty in swallowing).

The esophagus:

- Follows the curve of the vertebral column as it descends through the neck and mediastinum—the median partition of the thoracic cavity (Fig. 2.33A).
- Has internal *circular* and external *longitudinal layers of muscle* (Fig. 2.33B). In its superior third, the external layer consists of voluntary striated muscle; the inferior

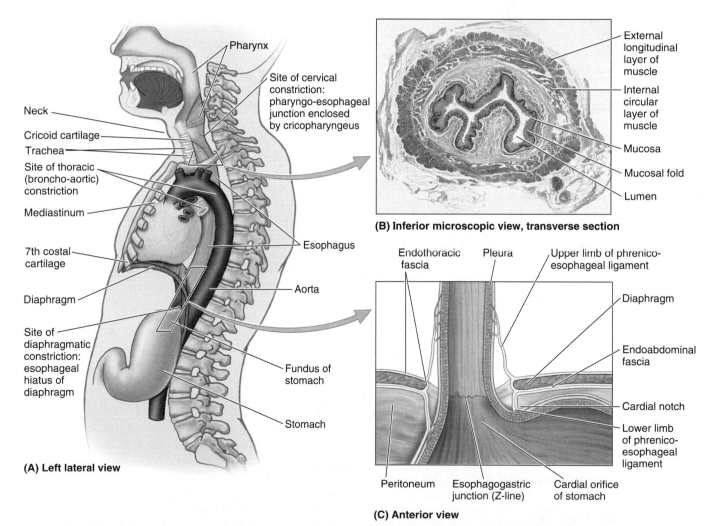

FIGURE 2.33. The esophagus and its relationships. A. This view shows the full length of the esophagus and structures related to it. The esophagus begins at the level of the cricoid cartilage and descends posterior to the trachea. It leaves the thorax through the esophageal hiatus of the diaphragm. **B.** The transverse section of the esophagus shows the double muscular and plicated mucosal layers of its wall. **C.** A coronal section of the inferior esophagus, diaphragm, and superior stomach is shown. The phrenicoesophageal ligament connects the esophagus flexibly to the diaphragm; it limits upward movement of the esophagus while permitting some movement during swallowing and respiration.

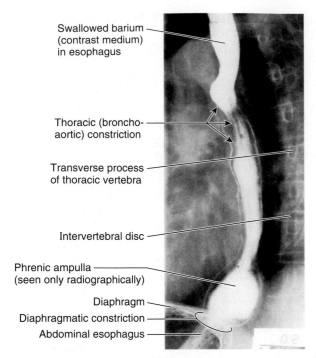

Swallowed barium (contrast medium) in esophagus

Thoracic (broncho-aortic) constriction

Transverse process of thoracic vertebra

Intervertebral disc

Phrenic ampulla (seen only radiographically)

Diaphragm

Diaphragmatic constriction

Abdominal esophagus

FIGURE 2.34. Radiograph of esophagus after swallowing barium meal. This left posterior oblique (LPO) view demonstrates two of the three normal "constrictions" (impressions) caused by the arch of the aorta and left main bronchus. The phrenic ampulla, which is seen only radiographically, is the distensible part of the esophagus superior to the diaphragm. (Courtesy of Dr. E. L. Lansdown, Professor of Medical Imaging, University of Toronto, Toronto, ON, Canada.)

third is composed of smooth muscle, and the middle third is made up of both types of muscle.

- Passes through the elliptical *esophageal hiatus* in the muscular *right crus of the diaphragm,* just to the left of the median plane at the level of the T10 vertebra.
- Terminates by entering the stomach at the *cardial orifice of the stomach* (Fig. 2.33C) to the left of the midline at the level of the 7th left costal cartilage and T11 vertebra.
- Is encircled by the esophageal (nerve) plexus distally (Fig. 2.35).

Food passes through the esophagus rapidly because of the peristaltic action of its musculature, aided by but not dependent on gravity (one can still swallow if inverted). The esophagus is attached to the margins of the esophageal hiatus in the diaphragm by the **phrenico-esophageal ligament** (Fig. 2.33C), an extension of inferior diaphragmatic fascia. This ligament permits independent movement of the diaphragm and esophagus during respiration and swallowing.

The trumpet-shaped **abdominal part of the esophagus,** only 1.25 cm long, passes from the esophageal hiatus in the right crus of the diaphragm to the *cardial orifice of the stomach,* widening as it approaches, passing anteriorly and to the left as it descends inferiorly. Its anterior surface is covered with peritoneum of the greater sac, continuous with that covering the anterior surface of the stomach. It fits into a groove on the posterior (visceral) surface of the liver.

The posterior surface of the abdominal part of the esophagus is covered with peritoneum of the omental bursa, continuous with that covering the posterior surface of the stomach. The right border of the abdominal esophagus is continuous with the lesser curvature of the stomach; however, its left border is separated from the fundus of the stomach by the *cardial notch* between the esophagus and fundus (Fig. 2.37A).

The **esophagogastric junction** lies to the left of the T11 vertebra on the horizontal plane that passes through the tip of the xiphoid process. Surgeons and endoscopists designate the **Z-line** (Fig. 2.33C), a jagged line where the mucosa abruptly changes from esophageal to gastric mucosa, as the junction. Immediately superior to this junction, the diaphragmatic musculature forming the esophageal hiatus functions as a physiological *inferior esophageal sphincter* that contracts and relaxes. Radiologic studies show that food stops here momentarily and that the sphincter mechanism is normally efficient in preventing reflux of gastric contents into the esophagus. When one is not eating, the lumen of the esophagus is normally collapsed superior to this level to prevent food or stomach juices from regurgitating into the esophagus.

Details concerning the neurovasculature of the cervical and thoracic portions of the esophagus are provided in Chapters 1 and 8. The arterial supply of the abdominal part of the esophagus is from the *left gastric artery,* a branch of the celiac trunk, and the *left inferior phrenic artery* (Fig. 2.32A). The venous drainage from the *submucosal veins* of this part of the esophagus is both to the *portal venous system* through the *left gastric vein* (Fig. 2.32B) and into the *systemic venous system* through **esophageal veins** entering the *azygos vein.*

The lymphatic drainage of the abdominal part of the esophagus is into the *left gastric lymph nodes* (Fig. 2.35); efferent lymphatic vessels from these nodes drain mainly to *celiac lymph nodes.*

The esophagus is innervated by the **esophageal plexus,** formed by the *vagal trunks* (becoming anterior and posterior gastric branches), and the *thoracic sympathetic trunks* via the *greater (abdominopelvic) splanchnic nerves* and *periarterial plexuses* around the left gastric and inferior phrenic arteries. (See also "Summary of Innervation of Abdominal Viscera," p. 300.)

Stomach

The **stomach** is the expanded part of the digestive tract between the esophagus and small intestine (Fig. 2.31B). It is specialized for the accumulation of ingested food, which it chemically and mechanically prepares for digestion and passage into the duodenum. The stomach acts as a food blender and reservoir; its chief function is enzymatic digestion. The *gastric juice* gradually converts a mass of food into a semiliquid mixture, *chyme* (G. juice), which passes fairly quickly into the duodenum. An empty stomach is only of slightly larger caliber than the large intestine; however, it is capable of considerable expansion and can hold 2–3 L of food.

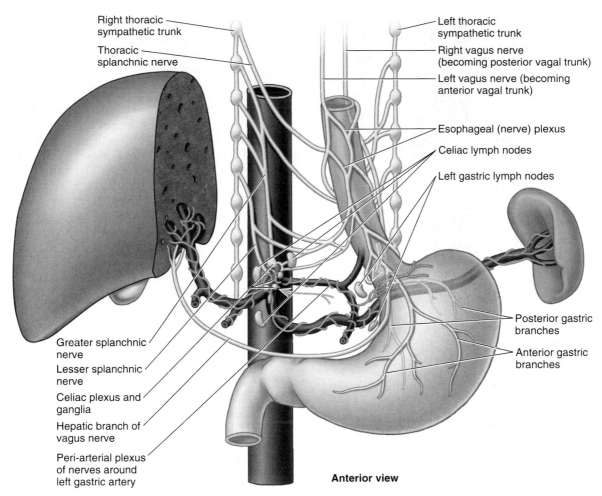

Right thoracic sympathetic trunk

Thoracic splanchnic nerve

Left thoracic sympathetic trunk

Right vagus nerve (becoming posterior vagal trunk)

Left vagus nerve (becoming anterior vagal trunk)

Esophageal (nerve) plexus

Celiac lymph nodes

Left gastric lymph nodes

Posterior gastric branches

Anterior gastric branches

Greater splanchnic nerve

Lesser splanchnic nerve

Celiac plexus and ganglia

Hepatic branch of vagus nerve

Peri-arterial plexus of nerves around left gastric artery

Anterior view

FIGURE 2.35.   Nerves and lymphatics of abdominal esophagus and stomach. The vagus nerves (CN X) divide into branches that form the esophageal (nerve) plexus around the inferior esophagus. Anterior and posterior gastric branches of the plexus accompany the esophagus through the esophageal hiatus for distribution to the anterior and posterior aspects of the stomach. The anterior branches also extend to the pylorus and liver. Postsynaptic sympathetic nerve fibers from the celiac plexus are distributed to these organs through peri-arterial plexuses. The lymphatic vessels of the stomach follow a pattern similar to that of the arteries, although the flow is in the opposite direction. Thus, lymph from the stomach and abdominal part of the esophagus drains to the gastric and then celiac lymph nodes.

POSITION, PARTS, AND SURFACE ANATOMY OF STOMACH

The size, shape, and position of the stomach can vary markedly in persons of different body types (bodily habitus) and may change even in the same individual as a result of diaphragmatic movements during respiration, the stomach's contents (empty vs. after a heavy meal), and the position of the person. In the supine position, the stomach commonly lies in the right and left upper quadrants, or epigastric, umbilical, and left hypochondrium and flank regions (Fig. 2.36A). In the erect position, the stomach moves inferiorly. In asthenic (thin, weak) individuals, the body of the stomach may extend into the pelvis (Fig. 2.36B).

The stomach has four parts (Figs. 2.36A and 2.37A–C):

- **Cardia:** the part surrounding the **cardial orifice** (opening), the superior opening or inlet of the stomach. In the supine position, the cardial orifice usually lies posterior to

the 6th left costal cartilage, 2–4 cm from the median plane at the level of the T11 vertebra.

- **Fundus:** the dilated superior part that is related to the left dome of the diaphragm, limited inferiorly by the horizontal plane of the cardial orifice. The **cardial notch** is between the esophagus and the fundus. The fundus may be dilated by gas, fluid, food, or any combination of these. In the supine position, the fundus usually lies posterior to the left 6th rib in the plane of the MCL (Fig. 2.36A).
- **Body:** the major part of the stomach between the fundus and pyloric antrum.
- **Pyloric part:** the funnel-shaped outflow region of the stomach; its wider part, the **pyloric antrum,** leads into the **pyloric canal,** its narrower part (Fig. 2.37A–E). The **pylorus** (G., gatekeeper) is the distal, sphincteric region of the pyloric part. It is a marked thickening of the circular layer of smooth muscle that controls discharge of the stomach contents through the **pyloric orifice** (infe-

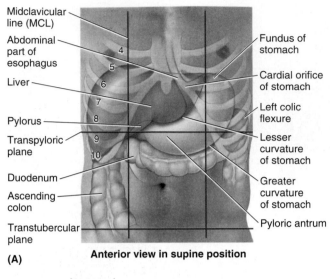

Midclavicular line (MCL)
Abdominal part of esophagus
Liver
Pylorus
Transpyloric plane
Duodenum
Ascending colon
Transtubercular plane

Fundus of stomach
Cardial orifice of stomach
Left colic flexure
Lesser curvature of stomach
Greater curvature of stomach
Pyloric antrum

(A)   **Anterior view in supine position**

(B)   **Anterior views**

FIGURE 2.36. Surface anatomy and effect of body type (bodily habitus) on disposition and shape of stomach. A. The most common position of the stomach in a person of medium build in the supine or prone position. **B.** A heavily built hyperasthenic individual with a short thorax and long abdomen is likely to have a stomach that is placed high and more transversely disposed. In people with a slender asthenic physique, the stomach is likely to be low and vertical.

rior opening or outlet of the stomach) into the duodenum (Fig. 2.37D). Intermittent emptying of the stomach occurs when intragastric pressure overcomes the resistance of the pylorus. The pylorus is normally tonically contracted so that the pyloric orifice is reduced, except when emitting *chyme* (semifluid mass). At irregular intervals, *gastric peristalsis* pushes the chyme through the pyloric canal and orifice into the small intestine for further mixing, digestion, and absorption.

In the supine position, the pyloric part of the stomach lies at the level of the **transpyloric plane,** midway between the jugular notch superiorly and the pubic crest inferiorly

(Fig. 2.36A). The plane transects the 8th costal cartilages and the L1 vertebra. When erect its location varies from the L2 through L4 vertebra. The pyloric orifice is approximately 1.25 cm right of the midline.

The stomach also features two curvatures (Fig. 2.37A–C):

- **Lesser curvature:** forms the shorter concave right border of the stomach. The **angular incisure** (notch), the most inferior part of the curvature, indicates the junction of the body and pyloric part of the stomach (Fig. 2.37A & B). The angular incisure lies just to the left of the midline.
- **Greater curvature:** forms the longer convex left border of the stomach. It passes inferiorly to the left from the junction of the 5th intercostal space and MCL, then curves to the right, passing deep to the 9th or 10th left cartilage as it continues medially to reach the pyloric antrum.

Because of the unequal lengths of the lesser curvature on the right and the greater curvature on the left, in most people the shape of the stomach resembles the letter J.

INTERIOR OF STOMACH

The smooth surface of the gastric mucosa is reddish brown during life, except in the pyloric part, where it is pink. In life, it is covered by a continuous mucous layer that protects its surface from the gastric acid the stomach's glands secrete. When contracted, the gastric mucosa is thrown into longitudinal ridges or wrinkles called **gastric folds** (gastric rugae) (Fig. 2.38A & B); they are most marked toward the pyloric part and along the greater curvature. During swallowing, a temporary groove or furrow-like **gastric canal** forms between the longitudinal gastric folds along the lesser curvature. It can be observed radiographically and endoscopically. The gastric canal forms because of the firm attachment of the gastric mucosa to the muscular layer, which does not have an oblique layer at this site. Saliva and small quantities of masticated food and other fluids drain along the gastric canal to the pyloric canal when the stomach is mostly empty. The gastric folds diminish and obliterate as the stomach is distended (fills).

RELATIONS OF STOMACH

The stomach is covered by visceral peritoneum, except where blood vessels run along its curvatures and in a small area posterior to the cardial orifice (Fig. 2.36A). The two layers of the lesser omentum extend around the stomach and leave its greater curvature as the greater omentum (Figs. 2.28, 2.31, and 2.37A). Anteriorly, the stomach is related to the diaphragm, left lobe of liver, and anterior abdominal wall. Posteriorly, the stomach is related to the omental bursa and pancreas; the posterior surface of the stomach forms most of the anterior wall of the omental bursa (Fig. 2.39A). The transverse colon is related inferiorly and laterally to the stomach as it courses along the greater curvature of the stomach to the left colic flexure.

The **bed of the stomach,** on which the stomach rests in the supine position, is formed by the structures forming the posterior wall of the omental bursa. From superior to inferior,

(A) Anterior view

Lesser curvature*
Falciform ligament
Lesser omentum
Esophagus
Cardial notch*
Fundus*
Diaphragm
Cardia*
Body*
Liver
7th rib
Porta hepatis
Omental foramen
Pylorus
Gallbladder
Pyloric canal
10th rib
Angular incisure (notch)
Pyloric antrum

Transverse colon appearing in an unusual gap in the greater omentum
Anastomosis between right and left gastro-omental arteries
Greater omentum, gastrocolic portion
Greater curvature*
*of stomach

Pyloric part of stomach
Pyloric orifice
Duodenum

(D)
Internal (lateral) view from duodenum

Ampulla
Pylorus
Pyloric antrum
Duodenum

(E) Anterior view

(B)
Esophagus
Cardial notch
Cardia
Fundus
Angular incisure
Lesser curvature
Pylorus
Pyloric canal
Body
Duodenum
Pyloric antrum
Greater curvature
Anterior views

(C)
Gallbladder
Ampulla (duodenal cap)
Pylorus
Pyloric antrum
Fundus
Gas
Peristaltic wave
Gastric folds (rugae)
Greater curvature
Jejunum

FIGURE 2.37. Abdominal part of esophagus and stomach. A. The stomach is inflated with air. The left part of the liver is cut away so that the lesser omentum and omental foramen can be seen. The extent of the intact liver is indicated by the longer *dotted lines*. **B.** Parts of the stomach. **C.** Radiograph of the stomach after a barium meal. Circular peristaltic waves begin in the body of the stomach and sweep toward the pyloric canal, as shown in **E** *(arrowheads)*, where they stop. Gas can be seen in the cardia and fundus of this supine patient. **D.** The pylorus is the significantly constricted terminal part of the stomach. The pyloric orifice is the opening of the pyloric canal into the duodenum. **E.** Radiograph demonstrating the pyloric region of the stomach and the superior part of the duodenum. (**C** and **E** courtesy of Dr. E. L. Lansdown, Professor of Medical Imaging, University of Toronto, Toronto, ON, Canada.)

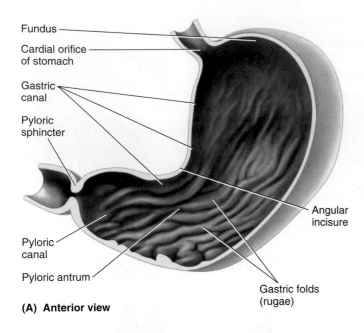

Fundus

Cardial orifice
of stomach

Gastric
canal

Pyloric
sphincter

Pyloric
canal

Pyloric antrum

Angular
incisure

Gastric folds
(rugae)

(A) Anterior view

Fundus

Ampulla
(duodenal
cap)

Pylorus

Pyloric
canal

Duodenum

Pyloric
antrum

Greater
curvature

Angular
incisure

Gastric
folds

(B) AP view

FIGURE 2.38. The internal surface of the stomach. A. The anterior wall of the stomach has been removed to demonstrate its interior. The longitudinal gastric folds disappear on distension. Along the lesser curvature, several longitudinal mucosal folds extend from the esophagus to the pylorus, making up the gastric canal along which ingested liquids pass. **B.** Radiograph of stomach after a barium meal. Observe the peristaltic wave in the stomach and the longitudinal gastric folds (rugae) of mucous membrane. (**A** courtesy of Dr. J. Helsin, Toronto, ON, Canada.)

the bed of the stomach is formed by the left dome of the diaphragm, spleen, left kidney and suprarenal gland, splenic artery, pancreas, and transverse mesocolon (Fig. 2.39B).

VESSELS AND NERVES OF STOMACH

The rich *arterial supply of the stomach* arises from the celiac trunk and its branches (Fig. 2.40; Table 2.7). Most blood is supplied by anastomoses formed along the lesser curvature by the **right** and **left gastric arteries,** and along the greater curvature by the **right** and **left gastro-omental (gastro-epiploic) arteries.** The fundus and upper body receive blood from the **short** and **posterior gastric arteries.**

The *veins of the stomach* parallel the arteries in position and course (Fig. 2.41). The **right** and **left gastric veins** drain into the *hepatic portal vein;* the **short gastric veins** and **left gastro-omental veins** drain into the *splenic vein,* which joins the superior mesenteric vein (SMV) to form the hepatic portal vein. The **right gastro-omental vein** empties in the SMV. A **prepyloric vein** ascends over the pylorus to the right gastric vein. Because this vein is obvious in living persons, surgeons use it for identifying the pylorus.

The **gastric lymphatic vessels** (Fig. 2.42A) accompany the arteries along the greater and lesser curvatures of the stomach. They drain lymph from its anterior and posterior surfaces toward its curvatures, where the **gastric** and **gastro-omental lymph nodes** are located. The efferent vessels from these nodes accompany the large arteries to the *celiac lymph nodes.* The following is a summary of the *lymphatic drainage of the stomach:*

- Lymph from the superior two thirds of the stomach drains along the right and left gastric vessels to the **gastric lymph nodes;** lymph from the fundus and superior part of the body of the stomach also drains along the short gastric arteries and left gastro-omental vessels to the *pancreaticosplenic lymph nodes.*
- Lymph from the right two thirds of the inferior third of the stomach drains along the right gastro-omental vessels to the **pyloric lymph nodes.**
- Lymph from the left one third of the greater curvature drains to the **pancreaticoduodenal lymph nodes,** which are located along the short gastric and splenic vessels.

The *parasympathetic nerve supply of the stomach* (Fig. 2.42B) is from the anterior and posterior vagal trunks and their branches, which enter the abdomen through the esophageal hiatus.

The *anterior vagal trunk,* derived mainly from the left vagus nerve (CN X), usually enters the abdomen as a single branch that lies on the anterior surface of the esophagus. It runs toward the lesser curvature of the stomach, where it gives off hepatic and duodenal branches, which leave the stomach in the hepatoduodenal ligament. The rest of the anterior vagal trunk continues along the lesser curvature, giving rise to anterior gastric branches.

The larger *posterior vagal trunk,* derived mainly from the right vagus nerve, enters the abdomen on the posterior surface of the esophagus and passes toward the lesser curvature of the stomach. The posterior vagal trunk supplies branches to the anterior and posterior surfaces of the stomach. It gives off a celiac branch, which passes to the *celiac plexus,* and then continues along the lesser curvature, giving rise to posterior gastric branches.

The *sympathetic nerve supply of the stomach,* from the T6 through T9 segments of the spinal cord, passes to the celiac plexus through the *greater splanchnic nerve* and is distributed through the plexuses around the gastric and gastroomental arteries. (See also "Summary of Innervation of Abdominal Viscera," p. 301).

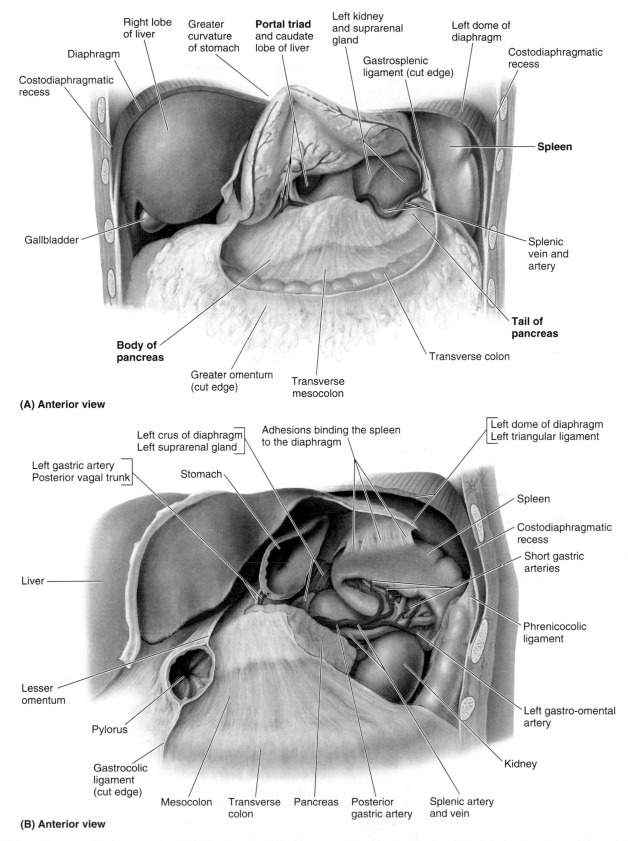

(A) Anterior view

(B) Anterior view

FIGURE 2.39. Omental bursa and stomach bed. A. The omental bursa, the greater omentum, and gastrosplenic ligament have been cut along the greater curvature of the stomach, and the stomach has been reflected superiorly to open the bursa anteriorly. At the right end of the bursa, two of the boundaries of the omental foramen can be seen: the inferior root of the hepatoduodenal ligament (containing the portal triad) and caudate lobe of the liver. **B.** The stomach and most of the lesser omentum have been excised, and the peritoneum of the posterior wall of the omental bursa covering the stomach bed is largely removed to reveal the organs in the bed. Although adhesions, such as those binding the spleen to the diaphragm here, are common postmortem findings, they are not normal anatomy.

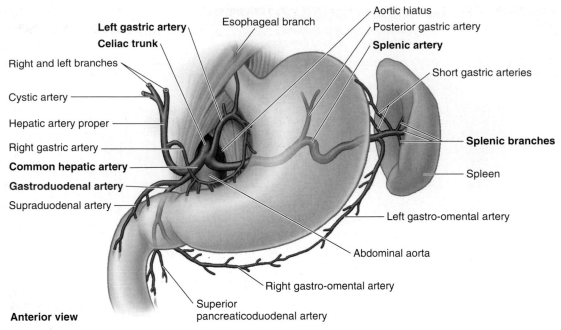

FIGURE 2.40. Arteries of stomach, duodenum, and spleen. The arterial supply of the abdominal part of the esophagus, stomach, upper (superior and upper descending parts) duodenum, and spleen is from the celiac artery. The direct branches of the celiac trunk appear in boldface.

TABLE 2.7. ARTERIAL SUPPLY TO ABDOMINAL FOREGUT DERIVATIVES: ESOPHAGUS, STOMACH, LIVER, GALLBLADDER, PANCREAS, AND SPLEEN

Artery	Origin	Course	Distribution
Celiac trunk	Abdominal aorta (at level of aortic hiatus)	After short antero-inferior course, bifurcates into splenic and common hepatic arteries	Esophagus, stomach, proximal duodenum, liver/biliary apparatus, pancreas
Left gastric	Celiac trunk	Ascends retroperitoneally to esophageal hiatus, giving rise to an esophageal branch; then descending along lesser curvature to anastomose with right gastric artery	Distal (mostly abdominal) part of esophagus and lesser curvature of stomach
Splenic		Runs retroperitoneally along superior border of pancreas; traverses splenorenal ligament to hilum of spleen	Body of pancreas, spleen, and greater curvature and posterior stomach body
Posterior gastric	Splenic artery posterior to stomach	Ascends retroperitoneally along posterior wall of lesser omental bursa to enter gastrophrenic ligament	Posterior wall and fundus of stomach
Left gastro-omental (left gastroepiploic)	Splenic artery in hilum of spleen	Passes between layers of gastrosplenic ligament to stomach, then along greater curvature in greater omentum to anastomose with right gastro-omental artery	Left portion of greater curvature of stomach
Short gastric ($n = 4$–5)		Passes between layers of gastrosplenic ligament to fundus of stomach	Fundus of stomach
Hepatic[a]	Celiac trunk	Passes retroperitoneally to reach hepatoduodenal ligament; passing between layers to porta hepatis; bifurcates into right and left hepatic arteries	Liver, gallbladder and biliary ducts, stomach, duodenum, pancreas, and respective lobes of liver

TABLE 2.7. ARTERIAL SUPPLY TO ABDOMINAL FOREGUT DERIVATIVES: ESOPHAGUS, STOMACH, LIVER, GALLBLADDER, PANCREAS, AND SPLEEN (Continued)

Artery	Origin	Course	Distribution
Cystic	Right hepatic artery	Arises within hepatoduodenal ligament (in cysto-hepatic triangle of Calot)	Gallbladder and cystic duct
Right gastric	Hepatic artery	Runs along lesser curvature of stomach to anastomose with left gastric artery	Right portion of lesser curvature of stomach
Gastroduodenal		Descends retroperitoneally, posterior to gastro-duodenal junction	Stomach, pancreas, first part of duodenum, and distal part of bile duct
Right gastro-omental (right gastroepiploic)	Gastroduodenal artery	Passes between layers of greater omentum along greater curvature of stomach to anastomose with left gastro-omental artery	Right portion of greater curvature of stomach
Superior pancreaticoduodenal		Divides into anterior and posterior arteries that descend on each side of pancreatic head, anastomosing with similar branches of inferior pancreaticoduodenal artery	Proximal portion of duodenum and superior part of head of pancreas
Inferior pancreaticoduodenal	Superior mesenteric artery	Divides into anterior and posterior arteries that ascend on each side of pancreatic head, anastomosing with similar branches of superior pancreaticoduodenal artery	Distal portion of duodenum and head of pancreas

[a]For descriptive purposes, the hepatic artery is often divided into the *common hepatic artery,* from its origin to the origin of the gastroduodenal artery, and *hepatic artery proper,* made up of the remainder of the vessel.

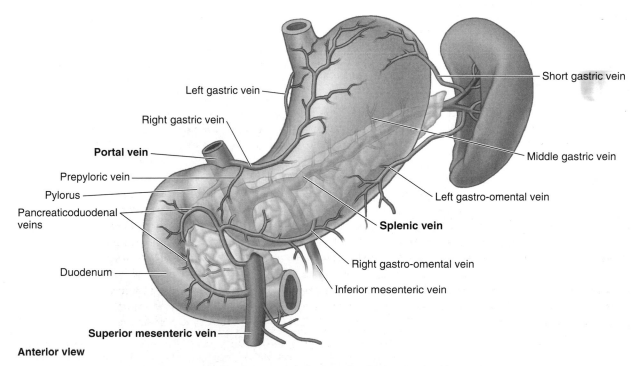

Anterior view

FIGURE 2.41.   Veins of stomach, duodenum, and spleen. Venous drainage from the abdominal part of the esophagus, stomach, upper (superior and upper descending parts) duodenum, pancreas, and spleen is into the portal vein, either directly or indirectly via the splenic or superior mesenteric vein (SMV). The gastric veins parallel the arteries in position and course.

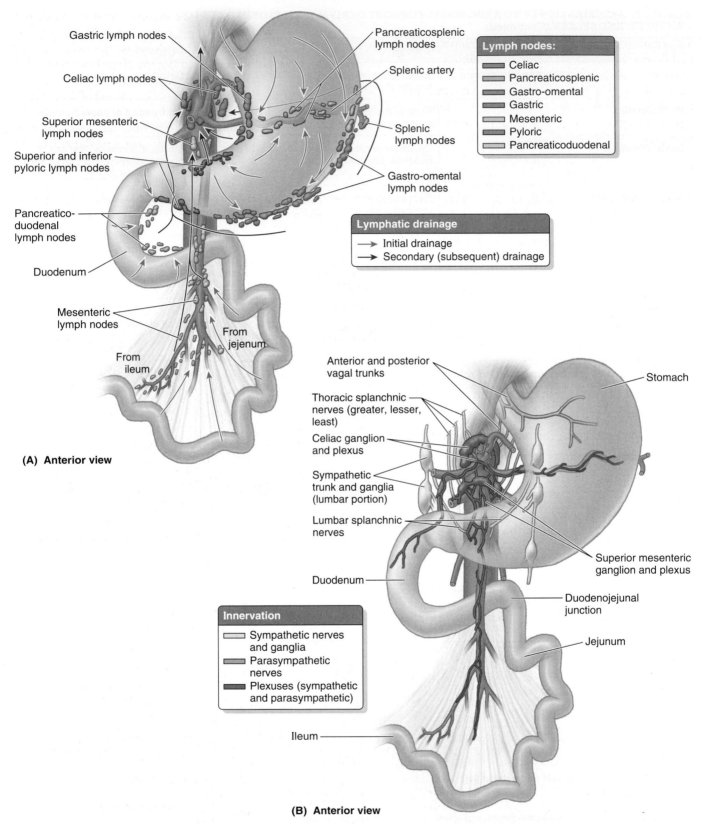

(A) Anterior view

(B) Anterior view

FIGURE 2.42. Lymphatic drainage and innervation of stomach and small intestine. A. The arrows indicate the direction of lymph flow to the lymph nodes. **B.** Innervation of the stomach is both parasympathetic, from the vagus nerves (CN X) via the esophageal plexus, and sympathetic, via the greater (abdominopelvic) splanchnic, the celiac plexus, and peri-arterial plexuses.

Small Intestine

The **small intestine,** consisting of the duodenum, jejunum, and ileum (Fig. 2.43), is the primary site for absorption of nutrients from ingested materials. It extends from the pylorus to the ileocecal junction where the ileum joins the cecum (the first part of the large intestine). The pyloric part of the stomach empties into the duodenum, duodenal admission being regulated by the pylorus.

DUODENUM

The **duodenum** (L. breadth of 12 fingers), the first and shortest (25 cm) part of the small intestine, is also the widest and most fixed part. The duodenum pursues a C-shaped course around the head of the pancreas (Figs. 2.43C and 2.44A & C). It begins at the pylorus on the right side and ends at the **duodenojejunal flexure (junction)** on the left side (Fig. 2.44B & C). This junction occurs approximately at the level of the L2 vertebra, 2–3 cm to the left of the midline. The junction usually takes the form of an acute angle, the **duodenojejunal flexure.** Most of the duodenum is fixed by peritoneum to structures on the posterior abdominal wall and is considered partially retroperitoneal. The duodenum is divisible into four parts (Figs. 2.44C and 2.45; Table 2.8):

- *Superior* (first) *part:* short (approximately 5 cm) and lies anterolateral to the body of the L1 vertebra.

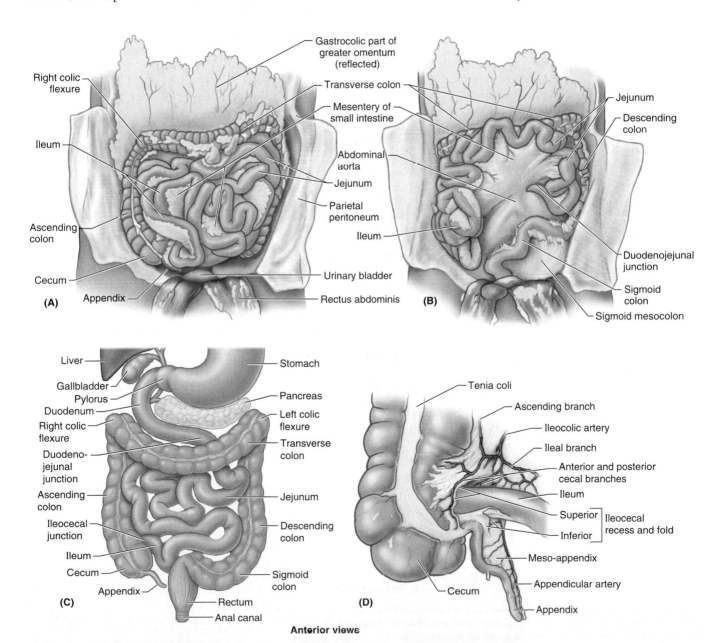

FIGURE 2.43. Small and large intestines. A. Note the convolutions of small intestine in situ, encircled on three sides by the large intestine and revealed by elevating the greater omentum. **B.** The convolutions of small intestine have been retracted superiorly to demonstrate the mesentery. **C.** This orientation drawing of the alimentary system indicates the general position and relationships of the intestines. **D.** The blood supply of the ileocecal region is shown.

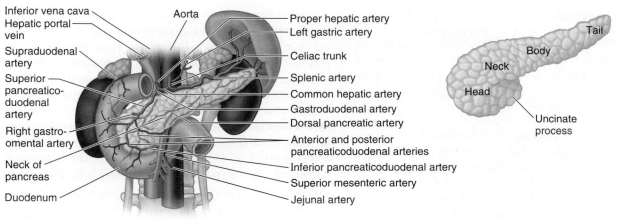

Inferior vena cava
Hepatic portal vein
Supraduodenal artery
Superior pancreatico-duodenal artery
Right gastro-omental artery
Neck of pancreas
Duodenum

Aorta

Proper hepatic artery
Left gastric artery
Celiac trunk
Splenic artery
Common hepatic artery
Gastroduodenal artery
Dorsal pancreatic artery
Anterior and posterior pancreaticoduodenal arteries
Inferior pancreaticoduodenal artery
Superior mesenteric artery
Jejunal artery

(A) Anterior view

Tail
Body
Neck
Head
Uncinate process

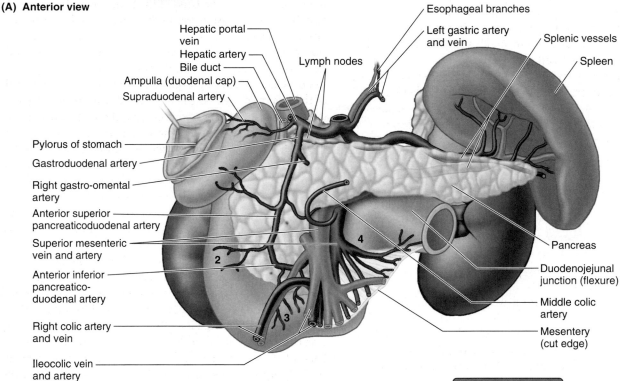

Hepatic portal vein
Hepatic artery
Bile duct
Ampulla (duodenal cap)
Supraduodenal artery

Esophageal branches
Left gastric artery and vein
Lymph nodes
Splenic vessels
Spleen

Pylorus of stomach
Gastroduodenal artery
Right gastro-omental artery
Anterior superior pancreaticoduodenal artery
Superior mesenteric vein and artery
Anterior inferior pancreatico-duodenal artery
Right colic artery and vein
Ileocolic vein and artery

Pancreas
Duodenojejunal junction (flexure)
Middle colic artery
Mesentery (cut edge)

(B) Anterior view

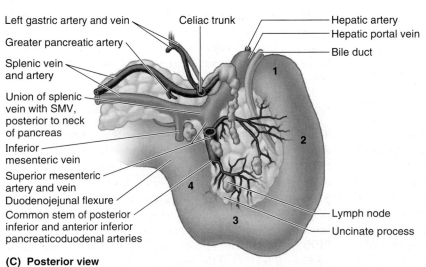

Left gastric artery and vein
Greater pancreatic artery
Splenic vein and artery
Union of splenic vein with SMV, posterior to neck of pancreas
Inferior mesenteric vein
Superior mesenteric artery and vein
Duodenojejunal flexure
Common stem of posterior inferior and anterior inferior pancreaticoduodenal arteries

Celiac trunk

Hepatic artery
Hepatic portal vein
Bile duct

Lymph node
Uncinate process

(C) Posterior view

Parts of duodenum:	
1	Superior
2	Descending
3	Horizontal
4	Ascending

FIGURE 2.44. Duodenum, pancreas, and spleen.
A. The duodenum, pancreas, and spleen and their blood supply are revealed by removal of the stomach, transverse colon, and peritoneum. **B.** The anterior aspect of the duodenum, pancreas, and related vasculature is shown. The duodenum is molded around the head of the pancreas. **C.** The posterior aspect of the duodenum and pancreas is shown. The abdominal aorta and inferior vena cava occupy the vertical concavity posterior to the head of the pancreas and third part of the duodenum. The uncinate process is the extension of the head of the pancreas that passes posterior to the superior mesenteric vessels. The bile duct is descending in a fissure (opened up) in the posterior part of the head of the pancreas. *SMV*, superior mesenteric vein.

- *Descending* (second) *part:* longer (7–10 cm) and descends along the right sides of the L1–L3 vertebrae.
- *Inferior* (third) *part:* 6–8 cm long and crosses the L3 vertebra.
- *Ascending* (fourth) *part:* short (5 cm) and begins at the left of the L3 vertebra and rises superiorly as far as the superior border of the L2 vertebra.

The first 2 cm of the superior part of the duodenum, immediately distal to the pylorus, has a mesentery and is mobile. This free part, called the **ampulla** (duodenal cap), has an appearance distinct from the remainder of the duodenum when observed radiographically using contrast medium (Fig. 2.37C & E). The distal 3 cm of the superior part and the other three parts of the duodenum have no mesentery and are immobile because they are retroperitoneal. The principal relationships of the duodenum are illustrated in Figures 2.44 and 2.45 and summarized in Table 2.8.

The **superior part of the duodenum** ascends from the pylorus and is overlapped by the liver and gallbladder. Peritoneum covers its anterior aspect, but it is bare of peritoneum posteriorly, except for the ampulla. The proximal part has the *hepatoduodenal ligament* (part of the lesser omentum) attached superiorly and the greater omentum attached inferiorly (see Fig. 2.26).

The **descending part of the duodenum** runs inferiorly, curving around the head of the pancreas (Figs. 2.44 and 2.45; Table 2.8). Initially, it lies to the right of and parallel to the IVC. The *bile* and *main pancreatic ducts* enter its posteromedial wall. These ducts usually unite to form the **hepatopancreatic ampulla,** which opens on an eminence, called the **major duodenal papilla,** located posteromedially in the descending duodenum. The descending part of the duodenum is entirely retroperitoneal. The anterior surface of its proximal and distal thirds is covered with peritoneum; however, the peritoneum reflects from its middle third to form the double-layered mesentery of the transverse colon, the transverse mesocolon.

The **inferior (horizontal) part of the duodenum** runs transversely to the left, passing over the IVC, aorta, and L3 vertebra. It is crossed by the superior mesenteric artery and vein and the root of the mesentery of the jejunum and ileum. Superior to it is the head of the pancreas and its uncinate process. The anterior surface of the inferior part is covered with peritoneum, except where it is crossed by the superior mesenteric vessels and the root of the mesentery. Posteriorly it is separated from the vertebral column by the right psoas major, IVC, aorta, and the right testicular or ovarian vessels.

The **ascending part of the duodenum** runs superiorly and along the left side of the aorta to reach the inferior border of the body of the pancreas. Here it curves anteriorly to join the jejunum at the duodenojejunal flexure, supported by the attachment of a **suspensory muscle of the duodenum** (ligament of Treitz). This muscle is composed of a slip of skeletal muscle from the diaphragm and a fibromuscular band of smooth muscle from the third and fourth parts of the duodenum. Contraction of this muscle widens the angle of the duodenojejunal flexure, facilitating movement of the intestinal contents. The suspensory muscle passes posterior to the pancreas and splenic vein and anterior to the left renal vein.

The *arteries of the duodenum* arise from the celiac trunk and the superior mesenteric artery (Fig. 2.44). The celiac trunk, via the **gastroduodenal artery** and its branch, the **superior pancreaticoduodenal artery,** supplies the duodenum proximal to the entry of the bile duct into the descending part of the duodenum. The superior mesenteric artery, through its branch, the **inferior pancreaticoduodenal artery,** supplies the duodenum distal to the entry of the bile duct. The pancreaticoduodenal arteries lie in the curve between the duodenum and the head of the pancreas and supply both structures. The anastomosis of the superior and inferior pancreaticoduodenal arteries (i.e., between the celiac and superior mesenteric arteries) occurs between the entry of the bile duct and the junction of the descending and inferior parts of the duodenum. An important transition in the blood supply of the digestive tract occurs here: proximally, extending *orad* (toward the mouth) to and including the abdominal part of the esophagus, the blood is supplied to the digestive tract by the celiac trunk; distally, extending *aborad* (away from the mouth) to the left colic flexure, the blood is supplied by the SMA. The basis of this transition in blood supply is embryological; this is the junction of the foregut and midgut.

The *veins of the duodenum* follow the arteries and drain into the *hepatic portal vein,* some directly and others indirectly, through the superior mesenteric and splenic veins (Fig. 2.41).

The *lymphatic vessels of the duodenum* follow the arteries. The *anterior lymphatic vessels* drain into the *pancreaticoduodenal lymph nodes,* located along the superior and inferior pancreaticoduodenal arteries, and into the *pyloric lymph nodes,* which lie along the gastroduodenal artery (Fig. 2.46). The *posterior lymphatic vessels* pass posterior to the head of the pancreas and drain into the **superior mesenteric lymph nodes.** Efferent lymphatic vessels from the duodenal lymph nodes drain into the *celiac lymph nodes.*

The *nerves of the duodenum* derive from the *vagus* and *greater* and *lesser (abdominopelvic) splanchnic nerves* by way of the celiac and superior mesenteric plexuses. The nerves are next conveyed to the duodenum via peri-arterial plexuses extending to the pancreaticoduodenal arteries (see also "Summary of the Innervation of the Abdominal Viscera," p. 300).

JEJUNUM AND ILEUM

The second part of the small intestine, the **jejunum,** begins at the duodenojejunal flexure where the gastrointestinal tract resumes an intraperitoneal course. The third part of the small intestine, the **ileum,** ends at the **ileocecal junction,** the union of the terminal ileum and the cecum (Figs. 2.43C and 2.47). Together, the jejunum and ileum are 6–7 m long, the jejunum constituting approximately two fifths and the ileum approximately three fifths of the intraperitoneal section of the small intestine.

FIGURE 2.45. Relationships of duodenum. The duodenum pursues a C-shaped course around the head of the pancreas.

TABLE 2.8. RELATIONSHIPS OF DUODENUM

Part of Duodenum	Anterior	Posterior	Medial	Superior	Inferior	Vertebral Level
Superior (1st part) **(A & B)**	Peritoneum Gallbladder Quadrate lobe of liver	Bile duct Gastroduodenal artery Hepatic portal vein IVC	Pylorus	Neck of gallbladder	Neck of pancreas	Anterolateral to L1 vertebra
Descending (2nd part) **(C)**	Transverse colon Transverse mesocolon Coils of small intestine	Hilum of right kidney Renal vessels Ureter Psoas major	Head of pancreas Pancreatic duct Bile duct	Superior part of duodenum	Inferior part of duodenum	Right of L2–L3 vertebrae
Inferior (horizontal) (3rd part) **(D)**	SMA SMV Coils of small intestine	Right psoas major IVC Aorta Right ureter		Head and uncinate Process of pancreas Superior mesenteric vessels	Coils of small intestine (ilium)	Anterior to L3 vertebra
Ascending (4th part) **(E)**	Beginning of root of mesentery Coils of jejunum	Left psoas major Left margin of aorta	SMA, SMV, uncinate process of pancreas	Body of pancreas	Coils of jejunum	Left of L3 vertebra

IVC, inferior vena cava; *SMA,* superior mesenteric artery; *SMV,* superior mesenteric vein.

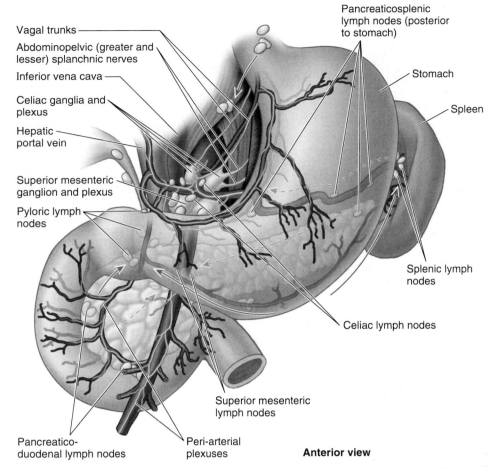

Anterior view

FIGURE 2.46. Lymphatic drainage and innervation of duodenum, pancreas, and spleen. The close positional relationship of these organs results in sharing of blood vessels, lymphatic vessels, and nerve pathways, in whole or in part.

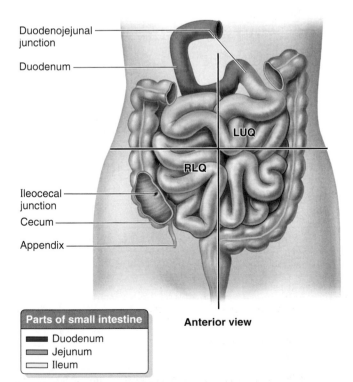

Anterior view

Parts of small intestine
- Duodenum
- Jejunum
- Ileum

FIGURE 2.47. Jejunum and ileum. The jejunum begins at the duodeno-jejunal flexure and the ileum ends at the cecum. The combined term *jejuno-ileum* is sometimes used as an expression of the fact that there is no clear external line of demarcation between the jejunum and the ileum. *LUQ,* left upper quadrant; *RLQ,* right lower quadrant.

Most of the jejunum lies in the left upper quadrant (LUQ) of the infracolic compartment, whereas most of the ileum lies in the right lower quadrant (RLQ). The terminal ileum usually lies in the pelvis from which it ascends, ending in the medial aspect of the cecum. Although no clear line of demarcation between the jejunum and ileum exists, they have distinctive characteristics that are surgically important (Fig. 2.48B–E; Table 2.9).

The **mesentery** is a fan-shaped fold of peritoneum that attaches the jejunum and ileum to the posterior abdominal wall (Fig. 2.43B and 2.48A). The origin or **root of the mesentery** (approximately 15 cm long) is directed obliquely, inferiorly, and to the right (Fig. 2.49A). It extends from the duodenojejunal junction on the left side of vertebra L2 to the ileocolic junction and the right sacro-iliac joint. The average length of the mesentery from its root to the intestinal border is 20 cm. The root of the mesentery crosses (successively) the ascending and inferior parts of the duodenum, abdominal aorta, IVC, right ureter, right psoas major, and right testicular or ovarian vessels. Between the two layers of the mesentery are the superior mesenteric vessels, lymph nodes, a variable amount of fat, and autonomic nerves.

The **superior mesenteric artery** (SMA) supplies the jejunum and ileum via **jejunal** and **ileal arteries** (Fig. 2.49B).

The SMA usually arises from the abdominal aorta at the level of the L1 vertebra, approximately 1 cm inferior to the

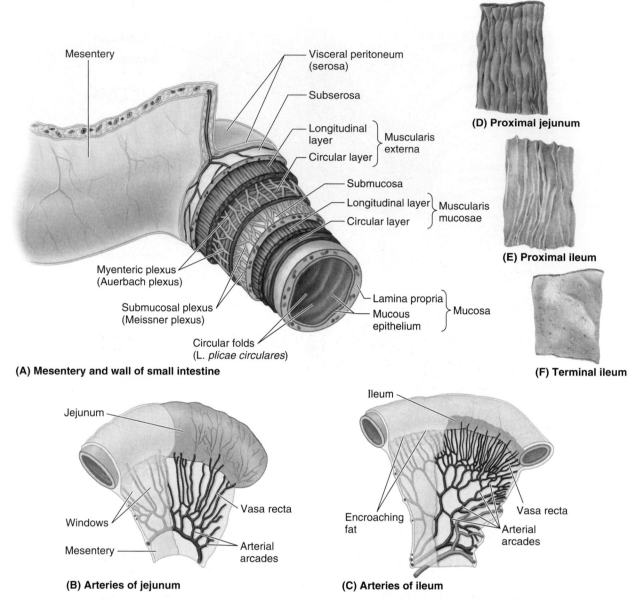

(A) Mesentery and wall of small intestine

Mesentery

Visceral peritoneum (serosa)

Subserosa

Longitudinal layer
Circular layer
} Muscularis externa

Submucosa

Longitudinal layer
Circular layer
} Muscularis mucosae

Myenteric plexus (Auerbach plexus)

Submucosal plexus (Meissner plexus)

Circular folds (L. *plicae circulares*)

Lamina propria
Mucous epithelium
} Mucosa

(D) Proximal jejunum

(E) Proximal ileum

(F) Terminal ileum

(B) Arteries of jejunum

Jejunum

Windows

Mesentery

Vasa recta

Arterial arcades

(C) Arteries of ileum

Ileum

Encroaching fat

Vasa recta

Arterial arcades

FIGURE 2.48. Structure of mesentery and small intestine: distinctive features of jejunum and ileum. A. The mesentery is a double-layered fold of visceral peritoneum that suspends the gut and conducts neurovasculature from the posterior body wall. **B–E.** Distinctive features of the jejunum and ileum, outlined in Table 2.9, are illustrated.

TABLE 2.9. DISTINGUISHING CHARACTERISTICS OF JEJUNUM AND ILEUM IN LIVING BODY (FIG. 2.48)

Characteristic	Jejunum (B & D)*		Ileum (C, E & F)*	
Color	Deeper red		Paler pink	
Caliber	2–4 cm		2–3 cm	
Wall	Thick and heavy		Thin and light	
Vascularity	Greater		Less	
Vasa recta	Long	} (B)	Short	} (C)
Arcades	A few large loops		Many short loops	
Fat in mesentery	Less		More	
Circular folds (L. *plicae circulares*)	Large, tall, and closely packed (**D**)		Low and sparse (**E**); absent in distal part (**F**)	
Lymphoid nodules (Peyer patches)	Few		Many (**F**)	

*Letters in parentheses refer to individual figures in Fig. 2.48.

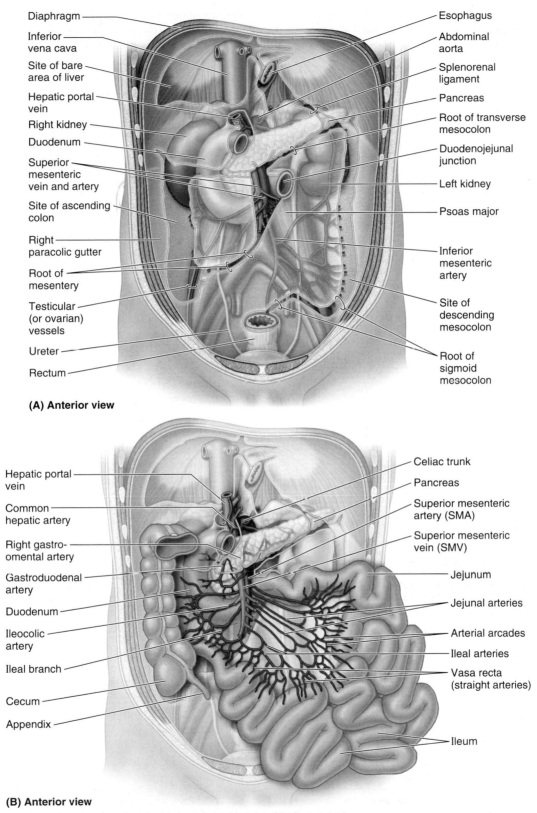

(A) Anterior view

(B) Anterior view

FIGURE 2.49. Arterial supply and mesenteries of intestines. A. Arterial supply of the large intestine. The transverse and sigmoid mesocolons and the mesentery of the jejunum and ileum have been cut at their roots. The ileocolic and right colic arteries on the right side and the left colic and sigmoid arteries on the left side originally coursed within mesenteries (ascending and descending mesocolons) that later fused to the posterior wall, they can be re-established surgically. **B.** Arterial supply and venous drainage of the small intestine. Except for the proximal duodenum, all of the intestine depicted in **B** is supplied by the SMA (as is most of the transverse colon, not shown). The SMV drains blood from the same portions of the intestine into the hepatic portal vein.

celiac trunk, and runs between the layers of the mesentery, sending 15–18 branches to the jejunum and ileum (see also Figs. 2.54 and 2.55). The arteries unite to form loops or arches, called **arterial arcades,** which give rise to straight arteries, called **vasa recta** (Figs. 2.48B and 2.49B).

The *superior mesenteric vein* drains the jejunum and ileum (Fig. 2.49B). It lies anterior and to the right of the SMA in the root of the mesentery (Fig. 2.49A). The SMV ends posterior to the neck of the pancreas, where it unites with the splenic vein to form the hepatic portal vein (Fig. 2.44C).

Specialized lymphatic vessels in the **intestinal villi** (tiny projections of the mucous membrane) that absorb fat are called **lacteals.** They empty their milk-like fluid into the lymphatic plexuses in the walls of the jejunum and ileum. The lacteals drain in turn into lymphatic vessels between the layers of the mesentery. Within the mesentery, the lymph passes sequentially through three groups of lymph nodes (Fig. 2.50):

- **Juxta-intestinal lymph nodes:** located close to the intestinal wall.
- **Mesenteric lymph nodes:** scattered among the arterial arcades.
- **Superior central nodes:** located along the proximal part of the SMA.

Efferent lymphatic vessels from the mesenteric lymph nodes drain to the *superior mesenteric lymph nodes.* Lymphatic

vessels from the terminal ileum follow the ileal branch of the ileocolic artery to the **ileocolic lymph nodes.**

The SMA and its branches are surrounded by a *peri-arterial nerve plexus* through which the nerves are conducted to the parts of the intestine supplied by this artery (Fig. 2.51). The sympathetic fibers in the nerves to the jejunum and ileum originate in the T8–T10 segments of the spinal cord and reach the **superior mesenteric nerve plexus** through the *sympathetic trunks* and *thoracic abdominopelvic* (*greater, lesser,* and *least*) *splanchnic nerves.* The presynaptic sympathetic fibers synapse on cell bodies of postsynaptic sympathetic neurons in the *celiac* and *superior mesenteric* (*prevertebral*) *ganglia.* The parasympathetic fibers in the nerves to the jejunum and ileum derive from the *posterior vagal trunks.* The presynaptic parasympathetic fibers synapse with postsynaptic parasympathetic neurons in the *myenteric* and *submucosal plexuses* in the intestinal wall (see also "Summary of Innervation of Abdominal Viscera," p. 301).

Sympathetic stimulation reduces peristaltic and secretory activity of the intestine and acts as a vasoconstrictor, reducing or stopping digestion and making blood (and energy) available for "fleeing or fighting." Parasympathetic stimulation increases peristaltic and secretory activity of the intestine, restoring the digestion process following a sympathetic reaction. The small intestine also has sensory (visceral afferent) fibers. The intestine is insensitive to most pain stimuli, including cutting and burning; however, it is sensitive to distension that is perceived as *colic* (spasmodic abdominal pains or "intestinal cramps").

Large Intestine

The **large intestine** is where water is absorbed from the indigestible residues of the liquid chyme, converting it into semisolid stool or feces that is stored temporarily and allowed to accumulate until defecation occurs. The large intestine consists of the *cecum; appendix; ascending, transverse, descending,* and *sigmoid colon; rectum;* and *anal canal* (Fig. 2.52). The large intestine can be distinguished from the small intestine by:

- **Omental appendices:** small, fatty, omentum-like projections.
- **Teniae coli:** three distinct longitudinal bands: (1) **mesocolic tenia,** to which the transverse and sigmoid mesocolons attach; (2) **omental tenia,** to which the omental appendices attach; and (3) **free tenia** (L. *t. libera*), to which neither mesocolons nor omental appendices are attached.
- **Haustra:** sacculations of the wall of the colon between the teniae
- A much greater caliber (internal diameter).

The *teniae coli* (thickened bands of smooth muscle representing most of the longitudinal coat) begin at the base of the appendix as the thick longitudinal layer of the appendix separates into three bands. The teniae run the length of the large intestine, abruptly broadening and merging with each other again at the rectosigmoid junction into a continuous

FIGURE 2.50. Mesenteric lymph nodes. The superior nodes form a system in which the central nodes, at the root of the superior mesenteric artery, receive lymph from the mesenteric, ileocolic, right colic, and middle colic nodes, which in turn receive lymph from juxta-intestinal lymph nodes. The juxta-intestinal nodes adjacent to the intestines are most abundant. Fewer occur along the arteries.

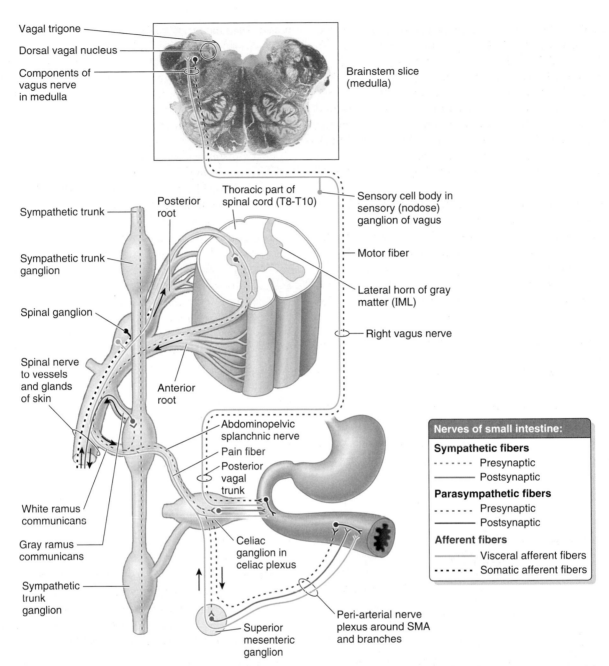

Vagal trigone

Dorsal vagal nucleus

Components of vagus nerve in medulla

Brainstem slice (medulla)

Sympathetic trunk

Posterior root

Thoracic part of spinal cord (T8-T10)

Sensory cell body in sensory (nodose) ganglion of vagus

Sympathetic trunk ganglion

Motor fiber

Lateral horn of gray matter (IML)

Spinal ganglion

Right vagus nerve

Spinal nerve to vessels and glands of skin

Anterior root

Abdominopelvic splanchnic nerve

Pain fiber

Posterior vagal trunk

White ramus communicans

Gray ramus communicans

Celiac ganglion in celiac plexus

Sympathetic trunk ganglion

Superior mesenteric ganglion

Peri-arterial nerve plexus around SMA and branches

Nerves of small intestine:

Sympathetic fibers
- - - - - Presynaptic
———— Postsynaptic

Parasympathetic fibers
- - - - - Presynaptic
———— Postsynaptic

Afferent fibers
———— Visceral afferent fibers
- - - - - Somatic afferent fibers

FIGURE 2.51. Innervation of small intestine. Presynaptic sympathetic nerve fibers originate in the T8 or T9 through T10 or T11 segments of the spinal cord and reach the celiac plexus through the sympathetic trunks and greater and lesser (abdominopelvic) splanchnic nerves. After synapsing in the celiac and superior mesenteric ganglia, postsynaptic nerve fibers accompany the arteries to the intestine. Afferent fibers are concerned with reflexes and pain. Presynaptic parasympathetic (vagus) nerves originate in the medulla (oblongata) and pass to the intestine via the posterior vagal trunk. They synapse with intrinsic postsynaptic neurons located in the intestinal wall. *SMA,* superior mesenteric artery.

longitudinal layer around the rectum. Because their tonic contraction shortens the part of the wall with which they are associated, the colon becomes sacculated or "baggy" between the teniae, forming the haustra.

CECUM AND APPENDIX

The **cecum** is the first part of the large intestine; it is continuous with the ascending colon. The cecum is a blind intestinal pouch, approximately 7.5 cm in both length and

breadth. It lies in the iliac fossa of the right lower quadrant of the abdomen, inferior to the junction of the terminal ileum and cecum (Figs. 2.52 and 2.53). If distended with feces or gas, the cecum may be palpable through the anterolateral abdominal wall.

The cecum usually lies within 2.5 cm of the inguinal ligament; it is almost entirely enveloped by peritoneum and can be lifted freely. However, the cecum has no mesentery. Because of its relative freedom, it may be displaced from the iliac fossa, but it is commonly bound to the lateral abdominal wall by one

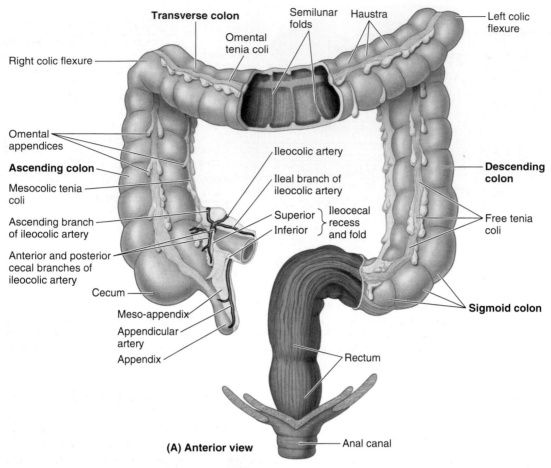

Transverse colon

Semilunar folds   Haustra

Left colic flexure

Right colic flexure

Omental tenia coli

Omental appendices

Ascending colon

Mesocolic tenia coli

Ascending branch of ileocolic artery

Anterior and posterior cecal branches of ileocolic artery

Cecum

Meso-appendix

Appendicular artery

Appendix

Ileocolic artery

Ileal branch of ileocolic artery

Superior ⎫ Ileocecal
Inferior ⎭ recess and fold

Descending colon

Free tenia coli

Sigmoid colon

Rectum

Anal canal

(A) Anterior view

(B) Anteroposterior view (with contrast medium)

(C) Anteroposterior view (double contrast study)

FIGURE 2.52. Terminal ileum and large intestine (including appendix). A. Teniae, haustra, and fatty omental appendices (characteristic of the colon) are not associated with the rectum. **B.** To examine the colon, a barium enema has been given after the bowel is cleared of fecal material by a cleansing enema. Single contrast barium studies demonstrate the semilunar folds demarcating the haustra. **C.** Following the single contrast study, the patient has evacuated the barium and the colon was distended with air for this double-contrast study. The luminal surface remains coated with a thin layer of barium. *A,* ascending colon; *C,* cecum; *D,* descending colon; *G,* sigmoid colon; *H,* hepatic or right colic flexure; *R,* rectum; *S,* splenic or left colic flexure; *T,* transverse colon; *U,* haustra. (**B** courtesy of Dr. C. S. Ho, Professor of Medical Imaging, University of Toronto, Toronto, ON, Canada; **C** courtesy of Dr. E. L. Lansdown, Professor of Medical Imaging, University of Toronto, Toronto, ON, Canada.)

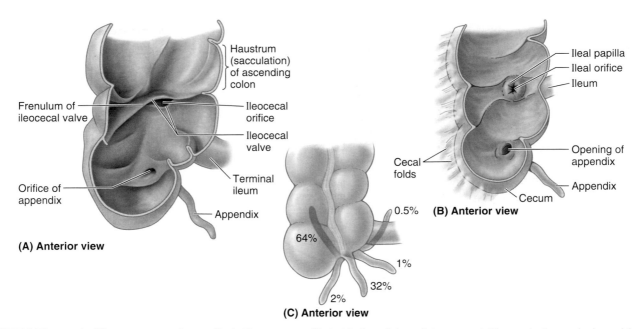

FIGURE 2.53. Terminal ileum, cecum, and appendix. A. The cecum was filled with air until dry and then opened. Observe the ileocecal valve and ileal orifice. The frenulum is a fold (more evident in cadavers) that runs from the ileocecal valve along the wall at the junction of the cecum and ascending colon. **B.** The interior of the cecum showing the endoscopic (living) appearance of the ileocecal valve. **C.** The approximate incidences of various locations of the appendix, based on an analysis of 10,000 cases, are shown.

or more **cecal folds** of peritoneum (Fig. 2.53B). The terminal ileum enters the cecum obliquely and partly invaginates into it.

In dissection, the **ileal orifice** enters the cecum between **ileocolic lips** (superior and inferior), folds that meet laterally forming ridges called the **frenula of the ileal orifice** (Fig. 2.53A). It was believed that when the cecum is distended or when it contracts, the lips and frenula actively tighten, closing the valve to prevent reflux from the cecum into the ileum. However, direct observation by endoscopy in living persons does not support this description. The circular muscle is poorly developed around the orifice; therefore, the valve is unlikely to have any sphincteric action that controls passage of the intestinal contents from the ileum into the cecum. The orifice is usually closed by tonic contraction, however, appearing as an **ileal papilla** on the cecal side (Fig. 2.53B). The papilla probably serves as a relatively passive flap valve, preventing reflux from the cecum into the ileum as contractions occur to propel contents up the ascending colon and into the transverse colon (Magee and Dalley, 1986).

The **appendix** (vermiform appendix; L. *vermis,* worm-like) is a blind intestinal diverticulum (6–10 cm in length) that contains masses of lymphoid tissue. It arises from the posteromedial aspect of the cecum inferior to the ileocecal junction. The appendix has a short triangular mesentery, the **meso-appendix,** which derives from the posterior side of the mesentery of the terminal ileum (Fig. 2.52A). The meso-appendix attaches to the cecum and the proximal part of the appendix. The position of the appendix is variable, but it is usually retrocecal (Fig. 2.53C). Clinical correlations involving the appendix are included in the blue box on pp. 259–260.

The *arterial supply of the cecum* is from the **ileocolic artery,** the terminal branch of the SMA (Figs. 2.54 and 2.55; Table 2.10). The **appendicular artery,** a branch of the ileocolic artery, supplies the appendix. *Venous drainage* from the

cecum and appendix flow through a tributary of the SMV, the **ileocolic vein** (Fig. 2.56A).

Lymphatic drainage of the cecum and appendix passes to lymph nodes in the meso-appendix and to the *ileocolic lymph nodes* that lie along the ileocolic artery (Fig. 2.56B). Efferent lymphatic vessels pass to the *superior mesenteric lymph nodes.*

The *nerve supply to the cecum and appendix* derives from the sympathetic and parasympathetic nerves from the *superior mesenteric plexus* (Fig. 2.56C). The *sympathetic nerve fibers* originate in the lower thoracic part of the spinal cord, and the *parasympathetic nerve fibers* derive from the vagus nerves. Afferent nerve fibers from the appendix accompany the sympathetic nerves to the T10 segment of the spinal cord (see also "Summary of Innervation of Abdominal Viscera," p. 300).

COLON

The **colon** has four parts—ascending, transverse, descending, and sigmoid—that succeed one another in an arch (Figs. 2.43C and 2.52). The colon encircles the small intestine, the ascending colon lying to the right of the small intestine, the transverse colon superior and/or anterior to it, the descending colon to the left if it, and the sigmoid colon inferior to it.

The **ascending colon** is the second part of the large intestine. It passes superiorly on the right side of the abdominal cavity from the cecum to the right lobe of the liver, where it turns to the left at the **right colic flexure** (*hepatic flexure*). This flexure lies deep to the 9th and 10th ribs and is overlapped by the inferior part of the liver.

The ascending colon is narrower than the cecum and is secondarily retroperitoneal along the right side of the posterior abdominal wall. The ascending colon is usually covered by peritoneum anteriorly and on its sides; however, in

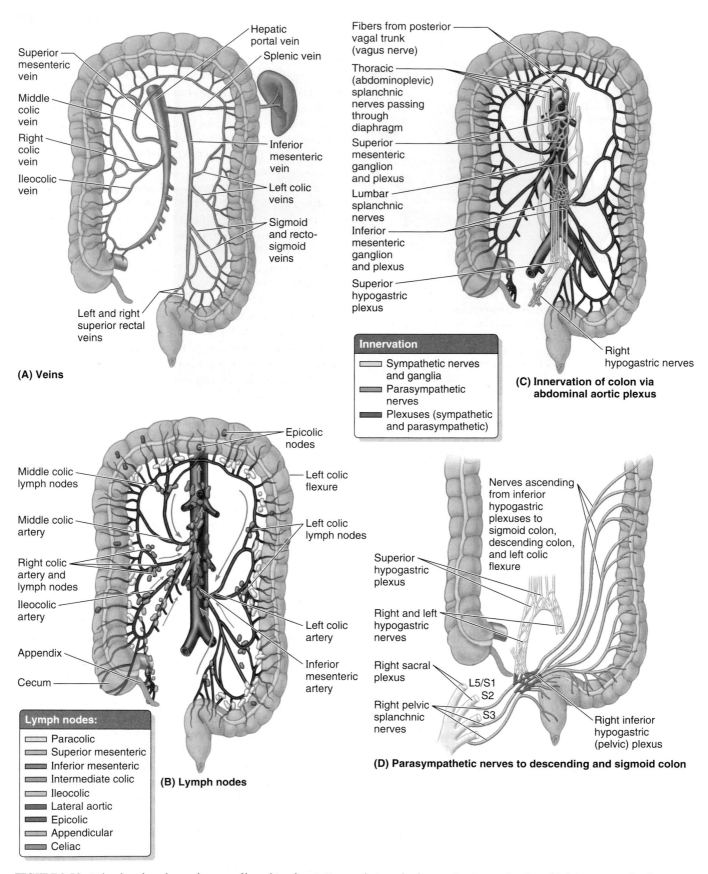

(A) Veins

Superior mesenteric vein
Middle colic vein
Right colic vein
Ileocolic vein
Hepatic portal vein
Splenic vein
Inferior mesenteric vein
Left colic veins
Sigmoid and rectosigmoid veins
Left and right superior rectal veins

(C) Innervation of colon via abdominal aortic plexus

Fibers from posterior vagal trunk (vagus nerve)
Thoracic (abdominoplevic) splanchnic nerves passing through diaphragm
Superior mesenteric ganglion and plexus
Lumbar splanchnic nerves
Inferior mesenteric ganglion and plexus
Superior hypogastric plexus
Right hypogastric nerves

Innervation
- Sympathetic nerves and ganglia
- Parasympathetic nerves
- Plexuses (sympathetic and parasympathetic)

(B) Lymph nodes

Middle colic lymph nodes
Middle colic artery
Right colic artery and lymph nodes
Ileocolic artery
Appendix
Cecum
Epicolic nodes
Left colic flexure
Left colic lymph nodes
Left colic artery
Inferior mesenteric artery

Lymph nodes:
- Paracolic
- Superior mesenteric
- Inferior mesenteric
- Intermediate colic
- Ileocolic
- Lateral aortic
- Epicolic
- Appendicular
- Celiac

(D) Parasympathetic nerves to descending and sigmoid colon

Nerves ascending from inferior hypogastric plexuses to sigmoid colon, descending colon, and left colic flexure
Superior hypogastric plexus
Right and left hypogastric nerves
Right sacral plexus
L5/S1
S2
Right pelvic splanchnic nerves
S3
Right inferior hypogastric (pelvic) plexus

FIGURE 2.56. Veins, lymph nodes, and nerves of large intestine. A. Venous drainage by the superior mesenteric vein and inferior mesenteric vein corresponds to the pattern of the superior mesenteric artery and inferior mesenteric artery. **B.** Lymph from the large intestine flows sequentially to epicolic nodes (on the gut), paracolic nodes (along mesenteric border), intermediate colic nodes (along the colic arteries), and then to the superior or inferior mesenteric nodes and the intestinal trunks. **C.** Innervation of the colon occurs by means of mixed peri-aterial plexuses extending from the superior and inferior mesenteric ganglia along the respective arteries. **D.** Parasympathetic fibers from S2–S4 spinal cord levels ascend independently from the inferior hypogastric (pelvic) plexuses to reach the sigmoid colon, descending colon, and distal transverse colon.

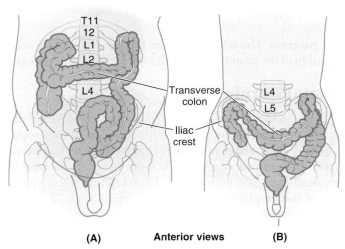

T11
12
L1
L2

L4

Transverse
colon

L4
L5

Iliac
crest

(A) Anterior views **(B)**

FIGURE 2.57. Effect of body type (body habitus) on disposition of the transverse colon. A. A heavily built hyperesthenic individual with a short thorax and a long abdomen is likely to have a transverse colon that is placed high. **B.** Individuals with a slender asthenic physique are likely to have a transverse colon that dips down toward or into the pelvis.

The **descending colon** occupies a secondarily retroperitoneal position between the left colic flexure and the left iliac fossa, where it is continuous with the sigmoid colon (Fig. 2.52). Thus, peritoneum covers the colon anteriorly and laterally and binds it to the posterior abdominal wall. Although retroperitoneal, the descending colon, especially in the iliac fossa, has a short mesentery in approximately 33% of people; however, it is usually not long enough to cause volvulus (twisting) of the colon. As it descends, the colon passes anterior to the lateral border of the left kidney. As with the ascending colon, the descending colon has a *paracolic gutter* (the left one) on its lateral aspect (see Fig. 2.49A).

The **sigmoid colon,** characterized by its S-shaped loop of variable length, links the descending colon and the rectum (Fig. 2.52). The sigmoid colon extends from the iliac fossa to the third sacral (S3) vertebra, where it joins the rectum. The termination of the teniae coli, approximately 15 cm from the anus, indicates the *rectosigmoid junction.*

The sigmoid colon usually has a long mesentery—the **sigmoid mesocolon**—and therefore has considerable freedom of movement, especially its middle part. (See the blue box "Volvulus of Sigmoid Colon," p. 261.) The **root of the sigmoid mesocolon** has an inverted V-shaped attachment, extending first medially and superiorly along the external iliac vessels and then medially and inferiorly from the bifurcation of the common iliac vessels to the anterior aspect of the sacrum. The *left ureter* and the division of the left common iliac artery lie retroperitoneally, posterior to the apex of the root of the sigmoid mesocolon. The *omental appendices of the sigmoid colon* are long (Fig. 2.52A); they disappear when the sigmoid mesentery terminates. The teniae coli also disappear as the longitudinal muscle in the wall of the colon broadens to form a complete layer in the rectum.

The *arterial supply of the descending and sigmoid colon* is from the *left colic* and **sigmoid arteries,** branches of the inferior mesenteric artery (Fig. 2.54; Table 2.10). Thus, at approximately the left colic flexure, a second transition occurs in the blood supply of the abdominal part of the alimentary canal: the SMA supplying blood to that part orad (proximal) to the flexure (derived from the embryonic midgut), and the IMA supplying blood to the part aborad (distal) to the flexure (derived from the embryonic hindgut). The sigmoid arteries descend obliquely to the left, where they divide into ascending and descending branches. The superior branch of the most superior sigmoid artery anastomoses with the descending branch of the left colic artery, thereby forming a part of the *marginal artery. Venous drainage from the descending colon and sigmoid colon* is provided by the *inferior mesenteric vein,* flowing usually into the splenic vein and then the hepatic portal vein on its way to the liver (see Figs. 2.56A and 2.75B).

Lymphatic drainage from the descending colon and sigmoid colon is conducted through vessels passing to the epicolic and paracolic nodes, and then through the **intermediate colic lymph nodes** along the left colic artery (Fig. 2.56B). Lymph from these nodes passes to the **inferior mesenteric lymph nodes** that lie around the IMA. However, lymph from the left colic flexure may also drain to the *superior mesenteric lymph nodes.*

Orad (toward the mouth, or proximal) to the left colic flexure, sympathetic and parasympathetic fibers travel together from the abdominal aortic plexus via peri-arterial plexuses to reach the abdominal part of the alimentary tract (Fig. 2.56C); however, aborad (away from the mouth, or distal) to the flexure, they follow separate routes.

The *sympathetic nerve supply of the descending and sigmoid colon* is from the lumbar part of the sympathetic trunk via lumbar (abdominopelvic) splanchnic nerves, the superior mesenteric plexus, and the peri-arterial plexuses following the inferior mesenteric artery and its branches.

The *parasympathetic nerve supply* is from the *pelvic splanchnic nerves* via the inferior hypogastric (pelvic) plexus and nerves, which ascend retroperitoneally from the plexus, independent of the arterial supply to this part of the gastrointestinal tract (Fig. 2.56D). Orad to the middle of the sigmoid colon, visceral afferents conveying pain sensation pass retrogradely with sympathetic fibers to thoracolumbar spinal sensory ganglia, whereas those carrying reflex information travel with the parasympathetic fibers to vagal sensory ganglia. Aborad to the middle of the sigmoid colon, all visceral afferents follow the parasympathetic fibers retrogradely to the sensory ganglia of spinal nerves S2–S4 (see also "Summary of Innervation of Abdominal Viscera," p. 300).

RECTUM AND ANAL CANAL

The **rectum** is the fixed (primarily retroperitoneal and subperitoneal) terminal part of the large intestine. It is continuous with the sigmoid colon at the level of S3 vertebra. The junction is at the inferior end of the mesentery of the sigmoid colon (Fig. 2.52). The rectum is continuous inferiorly with the *anal canal.* These parts of the large intestine are described with the pelvis in Chapter 3.

Gastroscope is introduced nasally or orally and led slowly down the esophagus and gastrointestinal tract until desired level is reached.

FIGURE B2.10.

Gastrectomy and Lymph Node Resection

Total gastrectomy (removal of the entire stomach) is uncommon. *Partial gastrectomy* (removal of part of the stomach) may be performed to remove a region of the stomach involved by a carcinoma, for example. Because the anastomoses of the arteries supplying the stomach provide good collateral circulation, one or more arteries may be ligated during this procedure without seriously affecting the blood supply to the part of the stomach remaining in place. When removing the pyloric antrum, for example, the greater omentum is incised parallel and inferior to the right gastro-omental artery, requiring ligation of all the omental branches of this artery. The omentum does not degenerate, however, because of anastomoses with other arteries, such as the omental branches of the left gastro-omental artery, which are still intact. Partial gastrectomy to remove a carcinoma usually also requires removal of all involved regional lymph nodes. Because cancer frequently occurs in the pyloric region, removal of the *pyloric lymph nodes* as well as the right *gastro-omental lymph nodes* also receiving lymph drainage from this region is especially important. As stomach cancer becomes more advanced, the lymphogenous dissemination of malignant cells involves the *celiac lymph nodes*, to which all gastric nodes drain.

Gastric Ulcers, Peptic Ulcers, *Helicobacter pylori,* and Vagotomy

Gastric ulcers are open lesions of the mucosa of the stomach, whereas *peptic ulcers* are lesions of the mucosa of the pyloric canal or, more often, the duodenum. Most ulcers of the stomach and duodenum are associated with an infection of a specific bacterium, *Helicobacter pylori* (*H. pylori*). People experiencing severe chronic anxiety are most prone to the development of peptic ulcers. They often have gastric acid secretion rates that are markedly higher than normal between meals. It is thought that the high acid in the stomach and duodenum overwhelms the bicarbonate normally

produced by the duodenum and reduces the effectiveness of the mucous lining, leaving it vulnerable to *H. pylori.* The bacteria erode the protective mucous lining of the stomach, inflaming the mucosa and making it vulnerable to the effects of the gastric acid and digestive enzymes (pepsin) produced by the stomach.

If the ulcer erodes into the gastric arteries, it can cause life-threatening bleeding. Because the secretion of acid by parietal cells of the stomach is largely controlled by the vagus nerves, *vagotomy* (surgical section of the vagus nerves) is performed in some people with chronic or recurring ulcers to reduce the production of acid. Vagotomy may also be performed in conjunction with resection of the ulcerated area (*antrectomy,* or resection of the pyloric antrum) to reduce acid secretion. A *truncal vagotomy* (surgical section of the vagal trunks) is rarely performed because the innervation of other abdominal structures is also sacrificed (Fig. B2.11A). In *selective gastric vagotomy,* the stomach is denervated but the vagal branches to the pylorus, liver and biliary ducts, intestines, and celiac plexus are preserved (Fig. B2.11B). A *selective proximal vagotomy* attempts to denervate even more specifically the area in which the parietal cells are located, hoping to affect the acid-producing cells while sparing other gastric function (motility) stimulated by the vagus nerve (Fig. B2.11C).

A *posterior gastric ulcer* may erode through the stomach wall into the pancreas, resulting in referred pain to the back. In such cases, *erosion of the splenic artery* results in severe hemorrhage into the peritoneal cavity. Pain impulses from the stomach are carried by visceral afferent fibers that accompany sympathetic nerves. This fact is evident because the pain of a recurrent peptic ulcer may persist after complete vagotomy, whereas patients who have had a bilateral

FIGURE B2.11. Vagotomy. Truncal (**A**), selective gastric (**B**), and selective proximal (**C**) vagotomy are shown. *Red bars* indicate site of surgical section of nerve.

sympathectomy may have a perforated peptic ulcer and experience no pain.

Visceral Referred Pain

 Pain is an unpleasant sensation associated with actual or potential tissue damage and mediated by specific nerve fibers to the brain, where its conscious appreciation may be modified. *Organic pain* arising from an organ such as the stomach varies from dull to severe; however, the pain is poorly localized. It radiates to the dermatome level, which receives visceral afferent fibers from the organ concerned. *Visceral referred pain* from a gastric ulcer, for example, is referred to the epigastric region because the stomach is supplied by pain afferents that reach the T7 and T8 spinal sensory ganglia and spinal cord segments through the greater splanchnic nerve (Fig. B2.12). The brain interprets the pain as though the irritation occurred in the skin of the epigastric region, which is also supplied by the same sensory ganglia and spinal cord segments.

Pain arising from the parietal peritoneum is of the somatic type and is usually severe. The site of its origin can be localized. The anatomical basis for this localization of pain is that the parietal peritoneum is supplied by somatic sensory fibers through thoracic nerves, whereas a viscus such as the appendix is supplied by visceral afferent fibers in the lesser splanchnic nerve. Inflamed parietal peritoneum is extremely sensitive to stretching. When digital pressure is applied to the anterolateral abdominal wall over the site of inflammation, the parietal peritoneum is stretched. When the fingers are suddenly removed, extreme localized pain is usually felt, known as *rebound tenderness*.

SMALL AND LARGE INTESTINE

Duodenal Ulcers

 Duodenal ulcers (peptic ulcers) are inflammatory erosions of the duodenal mucosa. Most (65%) duodenal ulcers occur in the posterior wall of the superior part of the duodenum within 3 cm of the pylorus. Occasionally, an ulcer perforates the duodenal wall, permitting the contents to enter the peritoneal cavity and causing *peritonitis*. Because the superior part of the duodenum closely relates to the liver, gallbladder, and pancreas, any of these structures may become adherent to the inflamed duodenum. They may also become ulcerated as the lesion continues to erode the tissue that surrounds it. Although bleeding from duodenal ulcers commonly occurs, *erosion of the gastroduodenal artery* (a posterior relation of the superior part of the duodenum) by a duodenal ulcer results in severe hemorrhage into the peritoneal cavity and subsequent peritonitis.

Developmental Changes in Mesoduodenum

 During the early fetal period, the entire duodenum has a mesentery; however, most of it fuses with the posterior abdominal wall because of pressure from the overlying transverse colon. Because the attachment of the mesoduodenum to the wall is secondary (occurred through formation of a *fusion fascia;* discussed under "Embryology of Peritoneal Cavity," p. 218), the duodenum and the closely associated pancreas can be separated (surgically mobilized) from the underlying retroperitoneal viscera during surgical operations involving the duodenum without endangering the blood supply to the kidney or the ureter.

Paraduodenal Hernias

There are two or three inconstant folds and fossae (recesses) around the duodenojejunal flexure (Fig. B2.13). The *paraduodenal fold and fossa* are large and lie to the left of the ascending part of the duodenum. If a loop of intestine enters this fossa, it may strangulate. During repair of a *paraduodenal hernia*, care must be taken not to injure the branches of the inferior mesenteric artery

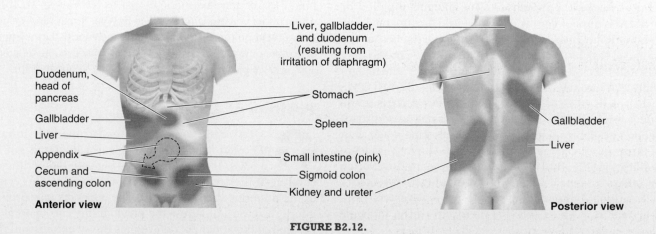

Liver, gallbladder, and duodenum (resulting from irritation of diaphragm)

Duodenum, head of pancreas

Gallbladder

Liver

Appendix

Cecum and ascending colon

Stomach

Spleen

Small intestine (pink)

Sigmoid colon

Kidney and ureter

Gallbladder

Liver

Anterior view

Posterior view

FIGURE B2.12.

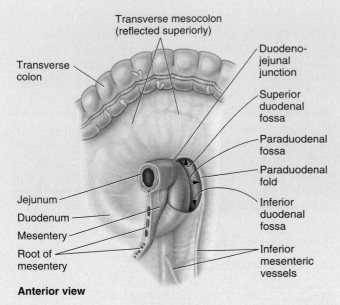

Anterior view

FIGURE B2.13.

and vein or the ascending branches of the left colic artery, which are closely related to the paraduodenal fold and fossa.

Brief Review of Embryological Rotation of Midgut

An understanding of the rotation of the midgut clarifies the adult arrangement of the intestines. The primordial gut comprises the foregut, midgut, and hindgut. Pain arising from foregut derivatives—esophagus, stomach, pancreas, duodenum, liver, and biliary ducts—localizes in the *epigastric region*. Pain arising from midgut derivatives—the small intestine distal to bile duct, cecum, appendix, ascending colon, and most of the transverse colon—localizes in the *peri-umbilical region*. Pain arising from hindgut derivatives—the distal part of the transverse colon, descending colon, sigmoid colon, and rectum—localizes in the *hypogastric region* (see Table 2.1).

For 4 weeks, the rapidly growing midgut, supplied by the SMA, is physiologically herniated into the proximal part of the umbilical cord (Fig. B2.14A). It is attached to the umbilical vesicle (yolk sac) by the omphalo-enteric duct (yolk stalk). As it returns to the abdominal cavity, the midgut rotates 270° around the axis of the SMA (Fig. B2.14B & C). As the relative size of the liver and kidneys decreases, the midgut returns to the abdominal cavity as increased space becomes available. As the parts of the intestine reach their definitive positions, their mesenteric attachments undergo modification (Fig. B2.14D & E). Some mesenteries shorten and others disappear (e.g., most of duodenal mesentery). Malrotation of the midgut results in several congenital anomalies such as volvulus (twisting) of the intestine (Moore et al., 2012).

Navigating Small Intestine

When portions of the small intestine have been delivered through a surgical wound, the proximal (orad—toward the mouth) and distal (aborad—away from the mouth) ends of a loop of intestine are not apparent. If you try to follow the intestine in a particular direction (e.g., attempting to follow the ileum to the ileocecal junction), it is important to know which end is which. Normal peristalsis may not be present to provide a clue. Place your hands on each side of the intestine and its mesentery and then follow the mesentery with your fingers to its root (its attachment to the posterior abdominal wall), untwisting the loop of intestine as necessary. Once the mesentery and intestine are straightened to match the direction of the root, the cranial end must be the orad end, and the caudal end the aborad end.

Ischemia of Intestine

Occlusion of the vasa recta (see Fig. 2.48B) by emboli (e.g., blood clots) results in *ischemia* of the part of the intestine concerned. If the ischemia is severe, *necrosis* (tissue death) of the involved segment results and *ileus* (obstruction of the intestine) of the paralytic type occurs. Ileus is accompanied by a severe colicky pain, along with abdominal distension, vomiting, and often fever and dehydration. If the condition is diagnosed early (e.g., using a *superior mesenteric arteriogram*), the obstructed part of the vessel may be cleared surgically.

Ileal Diverticulum

An *ileal diverticulum* (or Meckel diverticulum) is a congenital anomaly that occurs in 1–2% of the population. A remnant of the proximal part of the embryonic omphaloenteric duct (yolk stalk), the diverticulum usually appears as a finger-like pouch (Fig. B2.15A). It is always at the site of attachment of the omphaloenteric duct on the anti-mesenteric border (border opposite the mesenteric attachment) of the ileum. The diverticulum is usually located 30–60 cm from the ileocecal junction in infants and 50 cm in adults. It may be free (74%) or attached to the umbilicus (26%) (Fig. B2.15B). Although its mucosa is mostly ileal in type, it may also include areas of acid-producing gastric tissue, pancreatic tissue, or jejunal or colonic mucosa. An ileal diverticulum may become inflamed and produce pain mimicking that produced by appendicitis.

Position of Appendix

A *retrocecal appendix* extends superiorly toward the right colic flexure and is usually free (see Fig. 2.53C). It occasionally lies beneath the peritoneal covering of the cecum, where it is often fused to the cecum or the posterior abdominal wall. The appendix may project inferiorly toward or across the pelvic brim. The anatomical position of the appendix determines the symptoms and the

(A)

Stomach
Liver
Ventral mesentery
Midgut loop { Cranial limb
Caudal limb
Omphalo-enteric duct (yolk sac)
Vitelline artery

Dorsal aorta
Celiac artery
Elongated dorsal mesentery
Superior mesenteric artery
Plane of section A₁
Inferior mesenteric artery
Cranial limb
A_1 Superior mesenteric artery
Caudal limb
Hindgut

(B)

Falciform ligament
Small intestine
Umbilical vein
Degenerating omphalo-enteric duct
Cecal diverticulum

Duodenum
Plane of section B₁
B_1

(C)

Former site of omphalo-enteric duct
Umbilical cord

Aorta
Superior mesenteric artery
Cecal diverticulum
C_1

(D)

Superior mesenteric artery

Omental bursa
D_1

(E)

Omental foramen
Right colic flexure
Cecum
Appendix

Lesser omentum
Greater omentum
Left colic flexure
Small intestine
Large intestine

Left anterior oblique views

FIGURE B2.14.

site of muscular spasm and tenderness when the appendix is inflamed. The base of the appendix lies deep to a point that is one third of the way along the oblique line joining the right ASIS (anterior superior iliac spine) to the umbilicus (*McBurney point* on *spino-umbilical line*).

Appendicitis

Acute inflammation of the appendix, *appendicitis,* is a common cause of an *acute abdomen* (severe abdominal pain arising suddenly). Usually, digital

FIGURE B2.15.

pressure over the McBurney point registers maximum abdominal tenderness. Appendicitis in young people is usually caused by hyperplasia of lymphatic follicles in the appendix that occludes the lumen. In older people, the obstruction usually results from a *fecalith* (*coprolith*), a concretion that forms around a center of fecal matter. When secretions from the appendix cannot escape, the appendix swells, stretching the visceral peritoneum. The pain of appendicitis usually commences as a vague pain in the peri-umbilical region because afferent pain fibers enter the spinal cord at the T10 level. Later, severe pain in the right lower quadrant results from irritation of the parietal peritoneum lining the posterior abdominal wall. Extending the thigh at the hip joint elicits pain.

Acute infection of the appendix may result in *thrombosis* (clotting of blood) in the appendicular artery, which often results in ischemia, gangrene (death of tissue), and perforation of an inflamed appendix. *Rupture of the appendix* results in infection of the peritoneum (*peritonitis*), increased abdominal pain, nausea and/or vomiting, and *abdominal rigidity* (stiffness of abdominal muscles). Flexion of the right thigh ameliorates the pain because it causes relaxation of the right psoas muscle, a flexor of the thigh.

Appendectomy

Surgical removal of the appendix (**appendectomy**) may be performed through a transverse or gridiron (muscle-splitting) incision centered at the McBurney point in the right lower quadrant (see the blue box "Abdominal Surgical Incisions," p. 198). Traditionally, a gridiron incision is

made perpendicular to the spino-umbilical line, but a transverse incision is also commonly used. The choice of incision site and type is at the surgeon's discretion. While typically the inflamed appendix is deep to the McBurney point, the site of maximal pain and tenderness indicates the actual location.

Laparoscopic appendectomy has become a standard procedure selectively utilized for removing the appendix. The peritoneal cavity is first inflated with carbon dioxide gas, distending the abdominal wall, to provide viewing and working space. The laparoscope is passed through a small incision in the anterolateral abdominal wall (e.g., near or through the umbilicus). One or two other small incisions ("portals") are required for surgical (instrument) access to the appendix and related vessels.

In unusual cases of *malrotation of the intestine,* or failure of descent of the cecum, the appendix is not in the lower right quadrant (LRQ). When the cecum is high (*subhepatic cecum*), the appendix is in the right hypochondriac region (see Table 2.1) and the pain localizes there, not in the LRQ.

Mobile Ascending Colon

When the inferior part of the ascending colon has a mesentery, the cecum and proximal part of the colon are abnormally mobile. This condition, present in approximately 11% of individuals, may cause *volvulus of the colon* (L. *volvo,* to roll), an obstruction of the intestine resulting from twisting. *Cecopexy* (fixation) may avoid volvulus and possible obstruction of the colon. In this anchoring procedure, a tenia coli of the cecum and proximal ascending colon is sutured to the abdominal wall.

Colitis, Colectomy, Ileostomy, and Colostomy

  Chronic inflammation of the colon (*ulcerative* **colitis,** *Crohn disease*) is characterized by severe inflammation and ulceration of the colon and rectum. In some cases, a **colectomy** is performed, during which the terminal ileum and colon, as well as the rectum and anal canal, are removed. An **ileostomy** is then constructed to establish a *stoma,* an artificial opening of the ileum through the skin of the anterolateral abdominal wall (Fig. B2.16A). The terminating ileum is delivered through and sutured to the periphery of an opening in the anterolateral abdominal wall, allowing the egress of its contents. Following a partial colectomy, a **colostomy** or *sigmoidostomy* is performed to create an artificial cutaneous opening for the terminal part of the colon (Fig. B2.16B).

Colonoscopy

The interior of the colon can be observed and photographed in a procedure called **colonoscopy** or *coloscopy,* using a long, flexible fiberoptic endoscope (*colonoscope*) inserted into the colon through the anus and rectum (Fig. B2.17A). Small instruments can be passed through

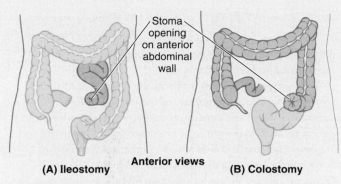

(A) Ileostomy   **Anterior views**   **(B) Colostomy**

Stoma opening on anterior abdominal wall

FIGURE B2.16. **A.** Ileostomy. **B.** Colostomy.

Descending colon

(A)   **(B)**

FIGURE B2.18. Volvulus of sigmoid colon.

the colonoscope and used to facilitate minor operative procedures, such as biopsies or removal of polyps. Most tumors of the large intestine occur in the sigmoid colon and rectum; they often appear near the rectosigmoid junction. The interior of the sigmoid colon is observed with a *sigmoidoscope*, a shorter endoscope, in a procedure called *sigmoidoscopy*.

Diverticulosis

Diverticulosis is a disorder in which multiple false *diverticula* (external evaginations or out-pocketings of the mucosa of the colon) develop along the intestine. It primarily affects middle-aged and elderly people. Diverticulosis is commonly found in the sigmoid colon (Fig. B2.17C & D). *Colonic diverticula* are not true diverticula because they are formed from protrusions of mucous membrane only, evaginated through weak points (separations) developed between muscle fibers rather than involving the whole wall of the colon. They occur most commonly on the

mesenteric side of the two nonmesenteric teniae coli, where nutrient arteries perforate the muscle coat to reach the submucosa. Diverticula are subject to infection and rupture, leading to diverticulitis, which can distort and erode the nutrient arteries, leading to hemorrhage. Diets high in fiber have proven beneficial in reducing the occurrence of diverticulosis.

Volvulus of Sigmoid Colon

Rotation and twisting of the mobile loop of the sigmoid colon and mesocolon—**volvulus of the sigmoid colon** (Fig. B2.18)—results in obstruction of the lumen of the descending colon and any part of the sigmoid colon proximal to the twisted segment. *Constipation* (inability of the stool to pass) and *ischemia* (absence of blood flow) of the looped part of the sigmoid colon result, which may progress to *fecal impaction* (an immovable collection of compressed or hardened feces) of the colon and possible *necrosis* (tissue death) of the involved segment if untreated.

Transverse colon
Decending colon
Flexible colonoscope
Ascending colon
Presence of diverticula
Sigmoid colon
Rectum

(A)

(B)

Light source

Flexible fiberoptic tube

Eyepiece

Viewing lens

(C)

Diverticula

(D) Anterior view

FIGURE B2.17. **Examination of large intestine. A.** The colonoscopic procedure. **B.** Diverticulosis of the colon, as photographed through a colonoscope. **C.** The parts of a colonoscope. Photographs can be taken by a camera attached to the colonoscope. **D.** Diverticula in the sigmoid colon are shown.

The Bottom Line

ESOPHAGUS AND STOMACH

Esophagus: The esophagus is a tubular conveyer of food, delivering it from the pharynx to the stomach. ♦ The esophagus penetrates the diaphragm at the T10 vertebral level, passing through its right crus, which decussates around it to form the physiological inferior esophageal sphincter. ♦ The trumpet-shaped abdominal part, composed entirely of smooth muscle innervated by the esophageal nerve plexus, enters the cardial part of the stomach. ♦ The abdominal part of the esophagus receives blood from esophageal branches of the left gastric artery (from the celiac trunk). ♦ Submucosal veins drain to both the systemic and portal venous systems and thus constitute portocaval anastomoses that may become varicose in the presence of portal hypertension. ♦ Internally, in living people, the esophagus is demarcated from the stomach by an abrupt mucosal transition, the Z-line.

Stomach: The stomach is the dilated portion of the alimentary tract between the esophagus and the duodenum, specialized to accumulate ingested food and prepare it chemically and mechanically for digestion. ♦ The stomach lies asymmetrically in the abdominal cavity, to the left of the midline and usually in the upper left quadrant. However, the position of the stomach can vary markedly in persons of different body types. ♦ The abdominal portion of the esophagus enters its cardial portion, and its pyloric part leads to the exit to the duodenum. ♦ Gastric emptying is controlled by the pylorus. ♦ In life, the internal surface of the stomach is covered with a protective layer of mucus, overlying gastric folds that disappear with distension. ♦ The stomach is intraperitoneal, with the lesser omentum (enclosing the anastomoses between right and left gastric vessels) attached to its lesser curvature, and the greater omentum (enclosing the anastomoses between right and left gastro-omental vessels) attached to its greater curvature. ♦ The vessels of its curvatures serve the body and pyloric antrum of the stomach. The upper body and fundus are served by short and posterior gastric vessels. ♦ The trilaminar smooth muscle of the stomach and gastric glands receive parasympathetic innervation from the vagus; sympathetic innervation to the stomach is vasoconstrictive and antiperistaltic.

SMALL AND LARGE INTESTINES

Small intestine: The duodenum is the first part of the small intestine, receiving chyme mixed with gastric acid and pepsin directly from the stomach via the pylorus. ♦ The duodenum follows a mostly secondarily retroperitoneal, C-shaped course around the head of the pancreas. ♦ The descending part of the duodenum receives both the bile and the pancreatic ducts. ♦ At or just distal to this level, a transition occurs in the blood supply of the abdominal part of the digestive tract. Proximal to this point it is supplied by branches of the celiac trunk; distal to this point, it is supplied by branches of the superior mesenteric artery.

The jejunum and ileum make up the convolutions of the small intestine occupying most of the infracolic division of the greater sac of the peritoneal cavity. ♦ The jejunum is mostly to the upper right, and the ileum to the lower left. Together they are 3–4 m in length (in the cadaver; less in living people owing to the structures' tonicity). The orad (proximal relative to the mouth) two fifths is jejunum and the aborad (distal) three fifths is ileum, although there is no clear line of transition. The diameter of the small intestine becomes increasingly smaller as the semifluid chyme progresses through it. ♦ Its blood vessels also become smaller, but the number of tiers of arcades increases while the length of the vasa recta decreases. ♦ The fat in which the vessels are embedded within the mesentery increases, making these features more difficult to see. ♦ The ileum is characterized by an abundance of lymphoid tissue, aggregated into lymphoid nodules (Peyer patches). ♦ The intraperitoneal portion of the small intestine (jejunum and ileum) is suspended by the mesentery, the root of which extends from the duodenojejunal junction to the left of the midline at the L2 level to the ileocecal junction in the right iliac fossa. ♦ An ileal diverticulum is a congenital anomaly present in 1–2% of the population. It is 3–6 cm in length and is typically located 50 cm from the ileocecal junction in adults.

Large intestine: The large intestine consists of the cecum; appendix; ascending, transverse, descending, and sigmoid colon; rectum; and anal canal. ♦ The large intestine is characterized by teniae coli, haustra, omental appendices, and a large caliber. ♦ The large intestine begins at the ileocecal valve; but its first part, the cecum, is a pocket that hangs inferior to the valve. ♦ The pouch-like cecum, the widest part of the large intestine, is completely intraperitoneal and has no mesentery, so that it is mobile within the right iliac fossa. ♦ The ileocecal valve is a combination valve and weak sphincter, actively opening periodically to allow entry of ileal contents and forming a largely passive one-way valve between the ileum and the cecum, preventing reflux. ♦ The appendix is an intestinal diverticulum, rich in lymphoid tissue, that enters the medial aspect of the cecum, usually deep to the junction of the lateral third and medial two thirds of the spino-umbilical line. Most commonly, the appendix is retrocecal in position, but 32% of the time it descends into the lesser pelvis. ♦ The cecum and appendix are supplied by branches of the ileocecal vessels.

The colon has four parts: ascending, transverse, descending, and sigmoid. ♦ The ascending colon is a superior, secondarily retroperitoneal continuation of the cecum, extending between the level of the ileocecal valve and the right colic flexure. ♦ The transverse colon, suspended by the transverse mesocolon between the right and left flex-ures, is the longest and most mobile part of the large intes-tine. The level to which it descends depends largely on body type (habitus). ♦ The descending colon occupies a second-arily retroperitoneal position between the left colic flexure and left iliac fossa, where it is continuous with the sigmoid colon. ♦ The S-shaped sigmoid colon, suspended by the sigmoid mesocolon, is highly variable in length and disposi-tion, ending at the rectosigmoid junction. The teniae, haus-tra, and omental appendices cease at the junction, located anterior to the third sacral segment.

The part of large intestine orad (proximal) to the left colic flexure (cecum, appendix, and ascending and transverse colons) is served by branches of the superior mesenteric vessels. Aborad (distal) to the flexure, most of the remainder of the large intestine (descending and sig-moid colons and superior rectum) is served by the inferior mesenteric vessels. ♦ The left colic flexure also marks the divide between cranial (vagal) and sacral (pelvic splanch-nic) parasympathetic innervation of the alimentary tract. ♦ Sympathetic fibers are conveyed to the large intestine via abdominopelvic (lesser and lumbar) splanchnic nerves via the prevertebral (superior and inferior mesenteric) ganglia and peri-arterial plexuses. ♦ The middle of the sigmoid colon marks a divide in the sensory innervation of the abdominal alimentary tract: orad, visceral affer-ents for pain travel retrogradely with sympathetic fibers to spinal sensory ganglia, whereas those conveying reflex information travel with parasympathetic fibers to vagal sensory ganglia; aborad, both types of visceral afferent fibers travel with parasympathetic fibers to spinal sensory ganglia.

Spleen

The **spleen** is an ovoid, usually purplish, pulpy mass about the size and shape of one's fist. It is relatively delicate and considered the most vulnerable abdominal organ. The spleen is located in the superolateral part of the left upper quadrant (LUQ), or hypochondrium of the abdomen, where it enjoys protection of the inferior thoracic cage (Fig. 2.58A & B). As the largest of the lymphatic organs, it participates in the body's defense system as a site of lymphocyte (white blood cell) proliferation and of immune surveillance and response.

Prenatally, the spleen is a hematopoietic (blood-forming) organ, but after birth it is involved primarily in identifying, removing, and destroying expended red blood cells (RBCs) and broken-down platelets, and in recycling iron and globin. The spleen serves as a blood reservoir, storing RBCs and plate-lets, and, to a limited degree, can provide a sort of "self-trans-fusion" as a response to the stress imposed by hemorrhage. In spite of its size and the many useful and important functions it provides, it is not a vital organ (not necessary to sustain life).

To accommodate these functions, the spleen is a soft, vas-cular (sinusoidal) mass with a relatively delicate fibroelastic capsule (Fig. 2.58E). The thin capsule is covered with a layer of visceral peritoneum that entirely surrounds the spleen except at the **splenic hilum,** where the splenic branches of the splenic artery and vein enter and leave (Fig. 2.58D). Consequently, it is capable of marked expansion and some relatively rapid contraction.

The spleen is a mobile organ although it normally does not descend inferior to the costal (rib) region; it rests on the *left colic flexure* (Fig. 2.58A & B). It is associated posteriorly with the left 9th–11th ribs (its long axis is roughly parallel to the 10th rib) and separated from them by the diaphragm and the *costodiaphragmatic recess*—the cleft-like extension of the pleural cavity between the diaphragm and the lower part of the thoracic cage. The **relations of the spleen** are:

- Anteriorly, the stomach
- Posteriorly, the left part of the diaphragm, which sepa-rates it from the pleura, lung, and ribs 9–11
- Inferiorly, the left colic flexure
- Medially, the left kidney.

The spleen varies considerably in size, weight, and shape; how-ever, it is usually approximately 12 cm long and 7 cm wide. (A nonmetric memory device exploits odd numbers: the spleen is 1 inch thick, 3 inches wide, 5 inches long, and weighs 7 ounces.)

The **diaphragmatic surface of the spleen** is convexly curved to fit the concavity of the diaphragm and curved bod-ies of the adjacent ribs (Fig. 2.58A–C). The close relation-ship of the spleen to the ribs that normally protect it can be a detrimental one in the presence of rib fractures (see the blue box "Rupture of Spleen," p. 281). The **anterior** and **superior borders of the spleen** are sharp and often notched, whereas its **posterior (medial) end** and **inferior border** are rounded (Fig. 2.58D). Normally, the spleen does not extend inferior to the left costal margin; thus it is seldom palpable through the anterolateral abdominal wall unless it is enlarged. When it is hardened and enlarged to approxi-mately three times its normal size, it moves inferior to the left costal margin, and its **superior (notched) border** lies inferomedially (see the blue box "Splenectomy and Spleno-megaly," p. 281). The notched border is helpful when palpat-ing an enlarged spleen because when the person takes a deep breath, the notches can often be palpated.

The spleen normally contains a large quantity of blood that is expelled periodically into the circulation by the action of the smooth muscle in its capsule and trabeculae. The large size of the splenic artery (or vein) indicates the volume of

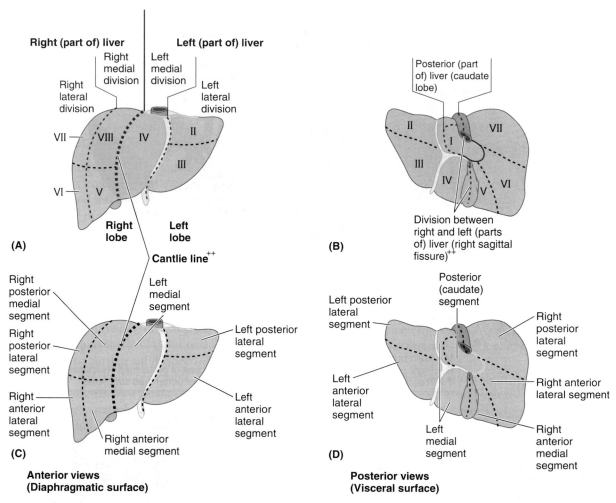

FIGURE 2.68. **Parts, divisions, and segments of liver.** Each part, division, and segment has an identifying name; segments are also identified by Roman numerals.

TABLE 2.11. TERMINOLOGY FOR SUBDIVISIONS OF LIVER

Anatomical Term	Right Lobe				Left Lobe	Caudate Lobe	
	Right (part of) liver [Right portal lobe*]		Left (part of) liver [Left portal lobe+]			Posterior (part of) liver	
	Right lateral division	Right medial division	Left medial division	Left lateral division		[Right caudate lobe*]	[Left caudate lobe+]
Functional/ Surgical Term**	Posterior lateral segment **Segment VII** [Posterior superior area]	Posterior lateral segment **Segment VIII** [Anterior superior area]	[Medial superior area] Left medial segment	Lateral segment **Segment II** [Lateral superior area]		Posterior segment **Segment I**	
	Right anterior lateral segment **Segment VI** [Posterior inferior area]	Anterior medial segment **Segment V** [Anterior inferior area]	**Segment IV** [Medial inferior area = quadrate lobe]	Left lateral anterior segment **Segment III** [Lateral inferior area]			

**The labels in the table and figures above reflect the new *Terminologia Anatomica: International Anatomical Terminology (1998)*. Previous terminology is in brackets.

Under the schema of the previous terminology, the caudate lobe was divided into right and left halves, and

*The right half of the caudate lobe was considered a subdivision of the right portal lobe.

+The left half of the caudate lobe was considered a subdivision of the left portal lobe.

++Cantlie line and the right sagittal fissure are surface markings defining the main portal fissure.

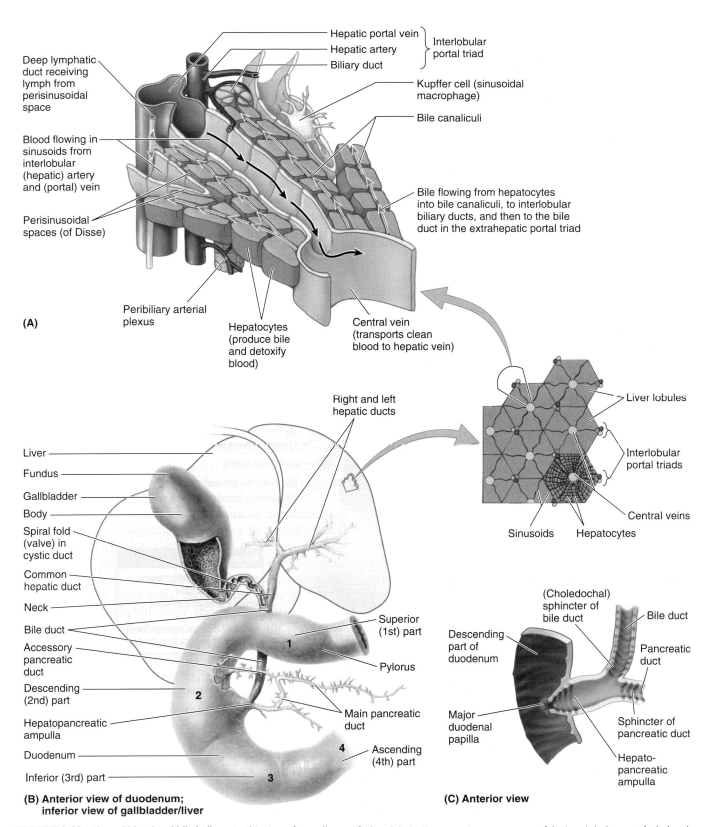

Deep lymphatic duct receiving lymph from perisinusoidal space

Blood flowing in sinusoids from interlobular (hepatic) artery and (portal) vein

Perisinusoidal spaces (of Disse)

Hepatic portal vein ⎫ Interlobular
Hepatic artery ⎬ portal triad
Biliary duct ⎭

Kupffer cell (sinusoidal macrophage)

Bile canaliculi

Bile flowing from hepatocytes into bile canaliculi, to interlobular biliary ducts, and then to the bile duct in the extrahepatic portal triad

Peribiliary arterial plexus

(A)

Hepatocytes (produce bile and detoxify blood)

Central vein (transports clean blood to hepatic vein)

Right and left hepatic ducts

Liver lobules

Interlobular portal triads

Central veins

Sinusoids   Hepatocytes

Liver

Fundus

Gallbladder

Body

Spiral fold (valve) in cystic duct

Common hepatic duct

Neck

Bile duct

Accessory pancreatic duct

Descending (2nd) part

Hepatopancreatic ampulla

Duodenum

Inferior (3rd) part

Superior (1st) part

Pylorus

Main pancreatic duct

Ascending (4th) part

1

2

3

4

(B) Anterior view of duodenum; inferior view of gallbladder/liver

(Choledochal) sphincter of bile duct

Descending part of duodenum

Major duodenal papilla

Bile duct

Pancreatic duct

Sphincter of pancreatic duct

Hepato-pancreatic ampulla

(C) Anterior view

FIGURE 2.69. Flow of blood and bile in liver. A. This view of a small part of a liver lobule illustrates the components of the interlobular portal triad and the positioning of the sinusoids and bile canaliculi. The enlarged view of the surface of a block of parenchyma removed from the liver in **B** shows the hexagonal pattern of lobes and the place of **A** within that pattern. **B.** Extrahepatic bile passages, gallbladder, and pancreatic ducts are demonstrated. **C.** The bile duct and pancreatic duct enter the hepatopancreatic ampulla, which opens into the descending part of the duodenum.

causes contractions of the gallbladder and relaxation of the sphincters at the hepatopancreatic ampulla. However, these responses are generally stimulated by the hormone *cholecystokinin* (CCK), produced by the duodenal walls (in response to the arrival of a fatty meal), and circulated through the bloodstream.

HEPATIC PORTAL VEIN AND PORTAL–SYSTEMIC ANASTOMOSES

The **hepatic portal vein** (HPV) is the main channel of the portal venous system (Fig. 2.75A & B). It is formed anterior to the IVC and posterior to the neck of the pancreas (close to the level of the L1 vertebra and the transpyloric plane) by the union of the superior mesenteric and splenic veins. In approximately one third of individuals, the IMV joins the confluence of the superior mesenteric and splenic veins; hence, all three veins form the hepatic portal vein. In most people, the IMV enters the splenic vein (60%—see Fig. 2.56A) or the SMV (40%).

Although the HPV is a large vessel, it runs a short course (7–8 cm), most of which is contained within the hepatoduodenal ligament. As it approaches the porta hepatis, the hepatic portal vein divides into right and left branches. The hepatic portal vein collects blood with reduced oxygenation but rich in nutrients from the abdominal part of the alimentary system, including the gallbladder and pancreas, as well as the spleen, and carries it to the liver. Streaming of the blood flow is said to occur in which blood from the splenic vein, carrying the products of RBC breakdown from the spleen, passes mostly to the left liver. Blood from the SMV, rich in absorbed nutrients from the intestines, passes mostly to the right liver. Within the liver, its branches are distributed in a segmental pattern (see "Blood Vessels of Liver," p. 272) and end in expanded capillaries, the *venous sinusoids of the liver* (see Fig. 2.69A).

(A) Anterior view

(B) Anteroposterior view, reconstructed MR angiogram

FIGURE 2.75. Tributaries of hepatic portal vein and portal–systemic anastomoses. A. Anastomoses provide a collateral circulation in cases of obstruction in the liver or portal vein. Here, the portal tributaries are darker blue and systemic tributaries are lighter blue. *A–D* indicate sites of anastomoses. *A* is between the submucosal esophageal veins draining into either the azygos vein (systemic) or the left gastric vein (portal); when dilated these are esophageal varices. *B* is between the inferior and middle rectal veins draining into the inferior vena cava (systemic) and the superior rectal vein, continuing as the inferior mesenteric vein (portal). The submucosal veins involved are normally dilated (varicose in appearance), even in newborns. When the mucosa containing them prolapses, they form *hemorrhoids*. (The varicose appearance of the veins and the occurrence of hemorrhoids are not typically related to portal hypertension, as is commonly stated.) *C* shows para-umbilical veins (portal) anastomosing with small epigastric veins of the anterior abdominal wall (systemic); this may produce the "caput medusae" (Fig. B2.24). *D* is on the posterior aspects (bare areas) of secondarily retroperitoneal viscera, or the liver, where twigs of visceral veins—for example, the colic vein, splenic veins, or the portal vein itself (portal system)—anastomose with retroperitoneal veins of the posterior abdominal wall or diaphragm (systemic system). **B.** Magnetic resonance (MR) angiogram (portal venogram) demonstrating the tributaries and formation of the portal vein in a living person.

Portal–systemic anastomoses, in which the portal venous system communicates with the systemic venous system, are formed in the submucosa of the inferior esophagus, in the submucosa of the anal canal, in the peri-umbilical region, and on the posterior aspects (bare areas) of secondarily retroperitoneal viscera, or the liver (Fig. 2.75; see legend for details). When portal circulation through the liver is diminished or obstructed because of liver disease or physical pressure from a tumor, for example, blood from the gastrointestinal tract can still reach the right side of the heart through the IVC by way of these collateral routes. These alternate routes are available because the hepatic portal vein and its tributaries have no valves; hence blood can flow in a reverse direction to the IVC. However, the volume of blood forced through the collateral routes may be excessive, resulting in potentially fatal *varices* (abnormally dilated veins) (see the blue box "Portal Hypertension" on p. 288) if the obstruction is not surgically bypassed (see the blue box "Portosystemic Shunts" on p. 288).

SPLEEN AND PANCREAS

Rupture of Spleen

Although well protected by the 9th–12th ribs (Fig. 2.30B), the spleen is the most frequently injured organ in the abdomen. The close relationship of the spleen to the ribs that normally protect it can be detrimental when there are rib fractures. Severe blows on the left side may fracture one or more of these ribs, resulting in sharp bone fragments that may lacerate the spleen. In addition, blunt trauma to other regions of the abdomen that cause a sudden, marked increase in intra-abdominal pressure (e.g., by impalement on the handlebars of a motorcycle) can cause the thin fibrous capsule and overlying peritoneum of the spleen to rupture, disrupting its soft pulp (*ruptured spleen*). If ruptured, there is profuse bleeding (*intraperitoneal hemorrhage*) and shock.

Splenectomy and Splenomegaly

Repair of a ruptured spleen is difficult; consequently, *splenectomy* (removal of the spleen) is often performed to prevent the person from bleeding to death. *Sub-total (partial) splenectomy*, when possible, is followed by rapid regeneration. Even *total splenectomy* usually does not produce serious effects, especially in adults, because most of its functions are assumed by other reticuloendothelial organs (e.g., liver and bone marrow), but there is a greater susceptibility to certain bacterial infections. When the spleen is diseased, resulting from, for example, granulocytic leukemia (high leukocyte and white blood cell count), it may enlarge to 10 or more times its normal size and weight (*splenomegaly*). Spleen engorgement sometimes accompanies hypertension (high blood pressure). The spleen is not usually palpable in the adult. Generally, if its lower edge can be detected when palpating below the left costal margin at the end of inspiration (Fig. B2.19A), it is enlarged about three times its "normal" size. Splenomegaly also occurs in some forms of hemolytic or granulocytic anemias, in which RBCs or white blood cells (WBCs), respectively, are destroyed at abnormally high rates (Fig. B2.19B). In such cases, a splenectomy may be life-saving.

Accessory Spleen(s)

One or more small **accessory spleens** may develop prenatally near the splenic hilum. They may be embedded partly or wholly in the tail of the pancreas, between the layers of the gastrosplenic ligament, in the infracolic compartment, in the mesentery, or in close proximity to an ovary or testis (Fig. B2.20). In most affected individuals, only one accessory spleen is present. Accessory spleens are relatively common, are usually small (approximately 1 cm in diameter, and range from 0.2 to 10 cm), and may resemble a lymph node. Awareness of the possible presence of an accessory spleen is important because if not removed during a splenectomy, the symptoms that indicated removal of the spleen (e.g., *splenic anemia*) may persist.

Splenic Needle Biopsy and Splenoportography

The relationship of the costodiaphragmatic recess of the pleural cavity to the spleen is clinically important (see Fig. 2.31A). This potential space descends to the

Thoracic (rib) cage

Splenomegaly (enlarged spleen)

Descending colon

FIGURE B2.19. Examination of spleen. A. Palpation of the spleen is demonstrated. **B.** This 4200-g spleen was seen at autopsy.

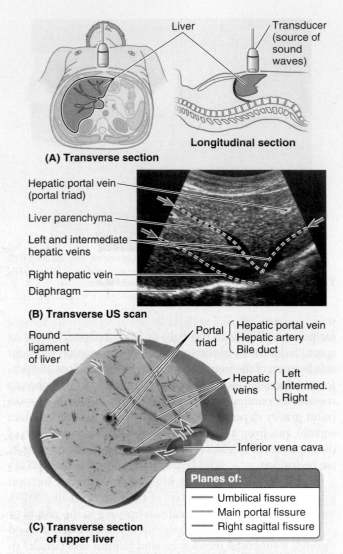

(A) Transverse section

Liver

Transducer (source of sound waves)

Longitudinal section

Hepatic portal vein (portal triad)

Liver parenchyma

Left and intermediate hepatic veins

Right hepatic vein

Diaphragm

(B) Transverse US scan

Round ligament of liver

Portal triad { Hepatic portal vein
Hepatic artery
Bile duct

Hepatic veins { Left
Intermed.
Right

Inferior vena cava

Planes of:
— Umbilical fissure
— Main portal fissure
— Right sagittal fissure

(C) Transverse section of upper liver

FIGURE B2.23. Ultrasonography (US) of hepatic veins.

pattern, the segments vary considerably in size and shape as a result of individual variation in the branching of the hepatic and portal vessels. Each hepatic resection is empirical, requiring ultrasonography, injection of dye, or balloon catheter occlusion to establish the patient's segmental pattern (Cheng et al., 1997). A more extensive injury that is likely to leave large areas of the liver devascularized may still require lobectomy.

Rupture of Liver

The liver is easily injured because it is large, fixed in position, and friable (easily crumbled). Often a fractured rib that perforates the diaphragm tears the liver. Because of the liver's great vascularity and friability, liver lacerations often cause considerable hemorrhage and right upper quadrant pain. In such cases, the surgeon must decide whether to remove foreign material and the contaminated or devitalized tissue by dissection or to perform a segmentectomy.

Aberrant Hepatic Arteries

The more common variety of right or left hepatic artery that arises as a terminal branch of the hepatic artery proper (Fig. B2.24A) may be replaced in part or entirely by an aberrant (accessory or replaced) artery arising from another source. The most common source of an *aberrant right hepatic artery* is the SMA (Fig. B2.24B). The most common source of an *aberrant left hepatic artery* is the left gastric artery (Fig. B2.24C).

Variations in Relationships of Hepatic Arteries

In most people, the right hepatic artery crosses anterior to the hepatic portal vein (Fig. B2.24D); however, in some people, the artery crosses posterior to the hepatic portal vein (Fig. B2.24E). In most people, the right hepatic artery runs posterior to the common hepatic duct (Fig. B2.24G). In some individuals, the right hepatic artery crosses anterior to the common hepatic duct (Fig. B2.24F), or the right hepatic artery arises from the SMA and so does not cross the common hepatic duct at all (Fig. B2.24H).

Hepatomegaly

The liver is a soft highly vascular organ that receives a large amount of blood immediately before it enters the heart. Both the IVC and hepatic veins lack valves. Any rise in central venous pressure is directly transmitted to the liver, which enlarges as it becomes engorged with blood. Marked temporary engorgement stretches the fibrous capsule of the liver, producing pain around the lower ribs, particularly in the right hypochondrium. This engorgement, particularly in conjunction with increased or sustained diaphragmatic activity, may be an underlying cause of "runner's stitch," perhaps explaining why it is a right-sided phenomenon.

In addition to diseases that produce hepatic engorgement such as congestive heart failure, bacterial and viral diseases such as *hepatitis* cause *hepatomegaly* (liver enlargement). When the liver is massively enlarged, its inferior edge may be readily palpated below the right costal margin and may even reach the pelvic brim in the right lower quadrant of the abdomen.

Tumors also enlarge the liver. The liver is a common site of *metastatic carcinoma* (secondary cancers spreading from organs drained by the portal system of veins, e.g., the large intestine). Cancer cells may also pass to the liver from the thorax, especially from the right breast, because of the communications between thoracic lymph nodes and the lymphatic vessels draining the bare area of the liver. Metastatic tumors form hard, rounded nodules within the hepatic parenchyma.

Cirrhosis of Liver

The liver is the primary site for detoxification of substances absorbed by the gastrointestinal tract; thus it is vulnerable to cellular damage and

(A) Typical pattern of branching of celiac trunk and hepatic arteries

Right hepatic artery
Left hepatic artery
Common hepatic artery
Cystic artery
Hepatic artery proper
Gastro-duodenal artery
Right renal artery
Abdominal aorta
Left gastric artery
Celiac trunk
Splenic artery
Left crus of diaphragm
Left renal artery
Superior mesenteric artery
Inferior mesenteric artery

(B)

Left hepatic branch
Left gastric artery
Splenic artery
Superior mesenteric artery
Gastroduodenal artery
Accessory or replaced right hepatic artery may originate from superior mesenteric artery

(C)

Left gastric artery
Accessory or replaced left hepatic artery may originate from left gastric artery

(B–C) Aberrant hepatic arteries

Right hepatic artery
Hepatic portal vein
(D) 91%

Right hepatic artery
Hepatic portal vein
(E) 9%

(D–E) Relationships of right hepatic artery to portal vein

Left hepatic artery
Right hepatic artery
Common hepatic duct
Hepatic artery
(F) 24%

Left hepatic artery
Right hepatic artery
Common hepatic duct
Hepatic artery
(G) 64%

Left hepatic artery
Right hepatic artery
Common hepatic duct
Hepatic artery
(H) 12%

(F–G) Relationships of right hepatic artery to common hepatic duct
Anterior views

FIGURE B2.24. Variations of right and left hepatic arteries.

consequent scarring, accompanied by regenerative nodules. There is progressive destruction of hepatocytes (Fig. 2.69) in *hepatic cirrhosis* and replacement of these cells by fat and fibrous tissue. Although many industrial solvents, such as carbon tetrachloride, produce cirrhosis, the condition develops most frequently in persons suffering from chronic alcoholism.

Alcoholic cirrhosis, the most common of many causes of *portal hypertension*, is characterized by hepatomegaly and a "hobnail" appearance of the liver surface (see Fig. B2.30B

the blue box "Portosystemic Shunts" on p. 288) resulting from fatty changes and fibrosis. The liver has great functional reserve; therefore the metabolic evidence of liver failure is late to appear. Fibrous tissue surrounds the intrahepatic blood vessels and biliary ducts, making the liver firm, and impeding the circulation of blood through it (*portal hypertension*). The treatment of advanced hepatic cirrhosis may include the surgical creation of a *portosystemic* or *portocaval shunt*, anastomosing the portal and systemic venous systems (see the blue box "Portosystemic Shunts," p. 288).

Liver Biopsy

Hepatic tissue may be obtained for diagnostic purposes by *liver biopsy*. Because the liver is located in the right hypochondriac region where it receives protection from the overlying thoracic cage, the needle is commonly directed through the right 10th intercostal space in the midaxillary line. Before the physician takes the biopsy, the person is asked to hold his or her breath in full expiration to reduce the costodiaphragmatic recess and to lessen the possibility of damaging the lung and contaminating the pleural cavity.

Mobile Gallbladder

In most people the gallbladder is closely attached to the fossa for the gallbladder on the visceral surface of the liver (Fig. 2.72). In approximately 4% of people, however, the gallbladder is suspended from the liver by a short mesentery, increasing its mobility. *Mobile gallbladders* are subject to vascular torsion and infarction (sudden insufficiency of arterial or venous blood supply).

Variations in the Cystic and Hepatic Ducts

Occasionally the cystic duct runs alongside the common hepatic duct and adheres closely to it. The cystic duct may be short or even absent. In some people, there is low union of the cystic and common hepatic ducts (Fig. B2.25A). As a result, the bile duct is short and lies posterior to the superior part of the duodenum, or even inferior to it. When there is low union, the two ducts may be joined by fibrous tissue, making surgical clamping of the cystic duct difficult without injuring the common hepatic duct.

Occasionally, there is high union of the cystic and common hepatic ducts near the porta hepatis (Fig. B2.25B). In other cases, the cystic duct spirals anteriorly over the common hepatic duct before joining it on the left side (Fig. B2.25C). Awareness of the variations in arteries and

bile duct formation is important for surgeons when they ligate the cystic duct during *cholecystectomy* (surgical removal of the gallbladder).

Accessory Hepatic Ducts

Accessory (aberrant) hepatic ducts are common and are in positions of danger during cholecystectomy. An accessory duct is a normal segmental duct that joins the biliary system outside the liver instead of within it (Fig. B2.26). Because it drains a normal segment of the liver, it leaks bile if inadvertently cut during surgery (Skandalakis et al., 2009). Of 95 gallbladders and biliary ducts studied, 7 had accessory ducts: 4 joined the common hepatic duct near the cystic ducts, 2 joined the cystic duct, and 1 was an anastomosing duct connecting the cystic duct with the common hepatic duct (Grant, in Agur and Dalley, 2013).

Gallstones

A *gallstone* is a concretion in the gallbladder, cystic duct, or bile duct composed chiefly of cholesterol crystals (Fig. B2.27). Gallstones (*cholelithiasis*) are much more common in females and their incidence increases with age. However, in approximately 50% of persons, gallstones are "silent" (asymptomatic). Over a 20-year period, two thirds of asymptomatic people with gallstones remain symptom free. The longer stones remain quiescent, the less likely symptoms are to develop. For gallstones to cause clinical symptoms, they must obtain a size sufficient to produce mechanical injury to the gallbladder or obstruction of the biliary tract (Townsend et al., 2012).

The distal end of the hepatopancreatic ampulla is the narrowest part of the biliary passages and is the common site for impaction of gallstones. Gallstones may also lodge in the hepatic and cystic ducts. A stone lodged in the cystic duct causes *biliary colic* (intense, spasmodic pain). When the gallbladder relaxes, the stone may move back into the gallbladder. If the stone blocks the cystic duct, *cholecystitis* (inflammation

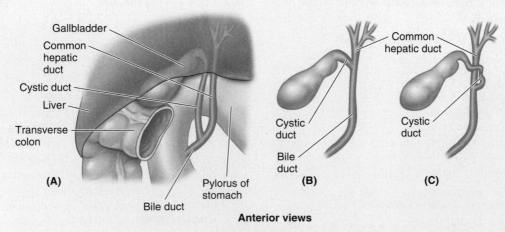

Anterior views

FIGURE B2.25. Union of cystic and common hepatic ducts. A. Low union. **B.** High union. **C.** Swerving course.

FIGURE B2.26.

of the gallbladder) occurs because of bile accumulation, causing enlargement of the gallbladder.

Another common site for impaction of gallstones is in an abnormal sacculation (Hartmann pouch), that appears in diseased states at the junction of the neck of the gallbladder and the cystic duct. When this pouch is large, the cystic duct arises from its upper left aspect, not from what appears to be the apex of the gallbladder. Gallstones commonly collect in the pouch. If a peptic duodenal ulcer ruptures, a false passage may form between the pouch and the superior part of the duodenum, allowing gallstones to enter the duodenum. (See the following blue box, "Gallstones in Duodenum.")

Pain from an *impaction of the gallbladder* develops in the epigastric region and later shifts to the right hypochondriac region at the junction of the 9th costal cartilage and the lateral border of the rectus sheath. *Inflammation of the gallbladder* may cause pain in the posterior thoracic wall, or right shoulder owing to irritation of the diaphragm. If bile cannot leave the gallbladder, it enters the blood and causes *jaundice* (see the blue box "Pancreatic Cancer," p. 283). Ultrasound and CT scans are common non-invasive techniques for locating stones.

Gallstones in Duodenum

A gallbladder that is dilated and inflamed owing to an impacted gallstone in its duct may develop adhesions with adjacent viscera. Continued inflammation may break down (ulcerate) the tissue boundaries between the gallbladder and a part of the gastrointestinal tract adherent to it, resulting in a *cholecysto-enteric fistula* (Fig. B2.28). Because of their proximity to the gallbladder, the superior part of the duodenum and the transverse colon are most likely to develop a fistula of this type. The fistula would enable a large gallstone, incapable of passing though the cystic duct, to enter the gastrointestinal tract. A large gallstone entering the small intestine in this way may become trapped at the ileocecal valve, producing a bowel obstruction (*gallstone ileus*). A cholecysto-enteric fistula also permits gas from the gastrointestinal tract to enter the gallbladder, providing a diagnostic radiographic sign.

Cholecystectomy

People with severe *biliary colic* usually have their gallbladders removed. *Laparoscopic cholecystectomy* often replaces the open-incision surgical method. The cystic artery most commonly arises from the right hepatic artery in the **cystohepatic triangle** (Calot triangle) (see Figs. 2.72 and 2.74A). In current clinical use, the cystohepatic triangle is defined inferiorly by the cystic duct,

Cholelithiasis. The gallbladder has been opened to reveal numerous yellow cholesterol gallstones.

FIGURE B2.27. Gallstones (cholelithiasis). The gallbladder has been opened to reveal numerous yellow cholesterol gallstones.

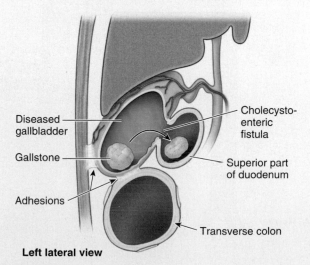

Left lateral view

FIGURE B2.28.

medially by the common hepatic duct, and superiorly by the inferior surface of the liver. Careful dissection of the cystohepatic triangle early during cholecystectomy safeguards these important structures should there be anatomical variations. Errors during gallbladder surgery commonly result from failure to appreciate the common variations in the anatomy of the biliary system, especially its blood supply. Before dividing any structure and removing the gallbladder, surgeons identify all three biliary ducts, as well as the cystic and hepatic arteries. It is usually the right hepatic artery that is in danger during surgery and must be located before ligating the cystic artery.

Portal Hypertension

When scarring and fibrosis from cirrhosis obstruct the hepatic portal vein in the liver, pressure rises in the vein and its tributaries, producing *portal hypertension*. The large volume of blood flowing from the portal system to the systemic system at the sites of portal–systemic anastomoses may produce *varicose veins*, especially in the lower esophagus. The veins may become so dilated that their walls rupture, resulting in hemorrhage (see Fig. B2.7).

Bleeding from esophageal varices (abnormally dilated veins) at the distal end of the esophagus is often severe and may be fatal. In severe cases of portal obstruction, the veins of the anterior abdominal wall (normally caval tributaries) that anastomose with the para-umbilical veins (normally portal tributaries) may become varicose and look somewhat like small snakes radiating under the skin around the umbilicus. This condition is referred to as *caput medusae* because of its resemblance to the serpents

Caput medusae in cirrhosis of liver

FIGURE B2.29.

on the head of Medusa, a character in Greek mythology (Fig. B2.29).

Portosystemic Shunts

A common method for reducing portal hypertension is to divert blood from the portal venous system to the systemic venous system by creating a communication between the hepatic portal vein and the IVC. This *portocaval anastomosis* or *portosystemic shunt* may be done where these vessels lie close to each other posterior to the liver (Fig. B2.30A–C). Another way of reducing portal pressure is to join the splenic vein to the left renal vein, after splenectomy (*splenorenal anastomosis* or *shunt*) (Fig. B2.30B–D) (Skandalakis et al., 2009).

"Hobnail" appearance of cirrhotic liver

Hepatic portal vein

Splenic vein

Inferior vena cava

Left renal vein

Superior mesenteric vein

(A) Normal

(B) Side to side

(C) End to side

(D) Central splenorenal

Portosystemic shunts *(yellow arrows)*

FIGURE B2.30. Portosystemic shunts *(red arrows)*.

The Bottom Line

SPLEEN AND PANCREAS

Spleen: The spleen is a highly vascular (sinusoidal), pulpy mass surrounded by a delicate fibroelastic capsule. ♦ The spleen is completely covered by peritoneum, except at the splenic hilum, where the splenorenal ligament (conveying splenic vessels to the spleen) and gastrosplenic ligament (conveying the short gastric and left gastro-omental vessels to the stomach) attach. ♦ The average spleen is about the size of one's fist, within a considerable range of normal variation. ♦ The spleen is the largest of the lymphoid organs, but it is not vital. ♦ As a blood reservoir, it is normally capable of considerable temporary expansion and contraction, but it may undergo much more marked, chronic enlargement when diseased. ♦ Although it receives protection from the overlying left 9th–11th ribs, the relatively delicate spleen is the abdominal organ most vulnerable to indirect trauma. ♦ Strong blows to the abdomen can cause a sudden increase in intra-abdominal pressure that may rupture the spleen, resulting in profuse intraperitoneal hemorrhage.

Pancreas: The pancreas is both an exocrine gland, producing pancreatic juice that is secreted into the duodenum for digestion, and an endocrine gland, producing insulin and glucagon that are released as hormones into the blood. ♦ The secondarily retroperitoneal pancreas consists of a head, an uncinate process, neck, body, and tail. ♦ The head, to the right of the SMA, is embraced by the C-shaped duodenum and penetrated by the termination of the bile duct, whereas its extension, the uncinate process, passes posterior to the SMA. ♦ The neck passes anterior to the SMA and SMV, the latter merging there with the splenic vein to form the hepatic portal vein. ♦ The body lies to the left of the SMA, running transversely across the posterior wall of the omental bursa and crossing anteriorly over the L2 vertebral body and abdominal aorta. ♦ The tail enters the splenorenal ligament as it approaches the splenic hilum. ♦ The splenic vein runs parallel and posterior to the tail and body of the pancreas as it runs from the spleen to the hepatic portal vein. ♦ The main pancreatic duct runs a similar course within the pancreas, continuing transversely through the head to merge with the bile duct to form the hepatopancreatic ampulla, which enters the descending part of the duodenum. ♦ As an endocrine gland, the pancreas receives an abundant blood supply from the pancreaticoduodenal and splenic arteries. ♦ Although it receives vasomotor sympathetic and secretomotor parasympathetic nerve fibers, regulation of pancreatic secretion is primarily hormonal. ♦ The pancreas is well protected by its central location in the abdomen. The exocrine pancreas is seldom the cause of clinical problems, although diabetes, involving the endocrine pancreas, has become increasingly common.

LIVER, BILIARY DUCTS, GALLBLADDER, AND PORTAL VEIN

Liver: The liver has multiple functions. ♦ It is our major metabolic organ, initially receiving all absorbed foodstuffs, except fats. ♦ It is also our largest gland, functioning as an extrinsic intestinal gland in producing bile. ♦ The liver occupies essentially all of the right dome of the diaphragm and extends to the apex of the left dome. Consequently, it enjoys protection from the lower thoracic cage and moves with respiratory excursions. ♦ The liver is divided superficially by the falciform ligament and a groove for the ligamentum venosum into a large anatomical right lobe and a much smaller left one; formations on its visceral surface demarcate caudate and quadrate lobes. ♦ The liver is covered with peritoneum except for the bare area, demarcated by peritoneal reflections comprising the coronary ligaments. ♦ Based on interdigitated branchings of the portal triad (hepatic portal vein, hepatic artery, and intrahepatic bile ducts) and hepatic veins, the continuous parenchyma of the liver can be divided into right and left livers (plus the caudate lobe). ♦ The liver can be further subdivided into four divisions and then eight surgically resectable hepatic segments. ♦ The liver, like the lungs, receives a dual blood supply, with 75–80% of the blood arriving via the hepatic portal vein, meeting the nutritional needs of the hepatic parenchyma; 20–25% arrives via the hepatic artery, delivered primarily to the non-parenchymal elements. The hepatic portal vein and hepatic artery enter the liver via the porta hepatis, where the hepatic ducts exit. ♦ Three large hepatic veins drain directly to the IVC as it is embedded in the liver's bare area. ♦ The liver is also the body's largest lymph-producing organ. The liver's visceral aspect drains via an abdominal route, and its diaphragmatic aspect drains via a thoracic route.

Biliary ducts and gallbladder: Right and left hepatic ducts drain the bile produced by the right and left livers into the common hepatic duct, which thus carries all bile from the liver. ♦ The common hepatic duct merges with the cystic duct to form the bile duct, which conveys the bile to the descending part of the duodenum. ♦ When the sphincter of the bile duct is closed, bile backs up in the bile and cystic ducts, filling the gallbladder, where bile is stored and concentrated between meals. ♦ Although parasympathetic innervation can open the sphincter of the bile duct (and the weaker sphincter of the hepatopancreatic ampulla) and contract the gallbladder, typically these are hormonally regulated responses to fat entering the duodenum, emptying the accumulated bile into the duodenum. ♦ The pear-shaped gallbladder is attached to the visceral surface of the liver, with its fundus projecting from the liver's inferior border against the anterior abdominal wall at the intersection of the transpyloric plane and the right MCL. ♦ The gallbladder, cystic duct, and uppermost bile duct are supplied by the cystic artery, a branch arising from the right hepatic artery within the cystohepatic triangle. ♦ In addition to drainage via cystic veins that accompany the cystic artery and enter the hepatic portal vein, veins from the fundus and body make up a mini-portal system that drains directly into the hepatic sinusoids deep to the visceral surface of the liver.

Hepatic portal vein: The large but short hepatic portal vein, formed posterior to the neck of the pancreas by the merger of the SMV and splenic vein, conveys all venous blood and bloodborne nutrients from the gastrointestinal tract to the liver. ♦ The hepatic portal vein terminates at the porta hepatis, bifurcating into the right and left portal veins, distributed in a segmental pattern to the right and left livers. ♦ The hepatic portal vein traverses the hepatoduodenal ligament (free edge of lesser omentum and anterior boundary of omental foramen) as part of an extrahepatic portal triad (hepatic portal vein, hepatic artery, bile duct). ♦ Portal–systemic anastomoses provide a potential collateral pathway by which blood can return to the heart when there is an obstruction of the hepatic portal vein or disease of the liver. However, when the collateral pathways must convey large volumes, potentially lethal esophageal varices may develop.

Kidneys, Ureters, and Suprarenal Glands

The *kidneys* produce urine that is conveyed by the *ureters* to the *urinary bladder* in the pelvis. The superomedial aspect of each kidney normally contacts a *suprarenal gland*. A weak fascial septum separates the glands from the kidneys; thus they are not actually attached to each other (Fig. 2.76). The suprarenal glands function as part of the endocrine system, completely separate in function from the kidneys. The superior urinary organs (kidneys and ureters), their vessels, and the suprarenal glands are primary retroperitoneal structures

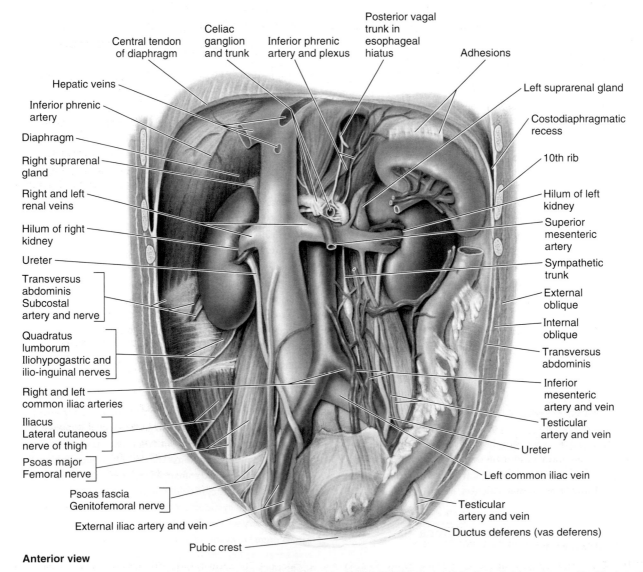

Anterior view

FIGURE 2.76. Posterior abdominal wall showing great vessels, kidneys, and suprarenal glands. Most of the fascia has been removed in this view. The ureter crosses the external iliac artery just beyond the common iliac bifurcation. The gonadal arteries (testicular arteries, as in this male, or ovarian arteries in females) cross anterior to the ureters and provide ureteric branches to them. The renal arteries are not seen here because they lie posterior to the renal veins. The superior mesenteric artery arises superior to and runs anteriorly across the left renal vein, compressing the vein against the abdominal aorta posteriorly.

on the posterior abdominal wall (Fig. 2.76)—that is, they were originally formed as and remain retroperitoneal viscera.

Perinephric fat (perirenal fat capsule) surrounds the kidneys and their vessels as it extends into their hollow centers, the **renal sinuses** (Fig. 2.77). The kidneys, suprarenal glands, and the fat surrounding them are enclosed (except inferiorly) by a condensed, membranous layer of **renal fascia,** which continues medially to ensheath the renal vessels, blending with the vascular sheaths of the latter. Inferomedially, a delicate extension of the renal fascia is prolonged along the ureter as the **peri-ureteric fascia.** External to the renal fascia is **paranephric fat** (pararenal fat body), the extraperitoneal fat of the lumbar region that is most obvious posterior to the kidney. The renal fascia sends collagen bundles through the paranephric fat.

The collagen bundles, renal fascia, and perinephric and paranephric fat, along with the tethering provided by the renal vessels and ureter, hold the kidneys in a relatively fixed position. However, movement of the kidneys occurs during respiration and when changing from the supine to the erect position, and vice versa. Normal renal mobility is

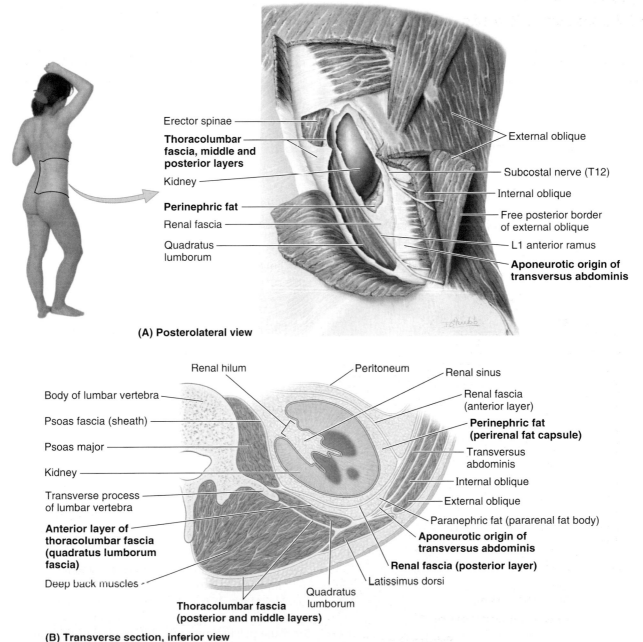

(A) Posterolateral view

Erector spinae
Thoracolumbar fascia, middle and posterior layers
Kidney
Perinephric fat
Renal fascia
Quadratus lumborum

External oblique
Subcostal nerve (T12)
Internal oblique
Free posterior border of external oblique
L1 anterior ramus
Aponeurotic origin of transversus abdominis

(B) Transverse section, inferior view

Renal hilum
Peritoneum
Renal sinus
Body of lumbar vertebra
Psoas fascia (sheath)
Psoas major
Kidney
Transverse process of lumbar vertebra
Anterior layer of thoracolumbar fascia (quadratus lumborum fascia)
Deep back muscles

Renal fascia (anterior layer)
Perinephric fat (perirenal fat capsule)
Transversus abdominis
Internal oblique
External oblique
Paranephric fat (pararenal fat body)
Aponeurotic origin of transversus abdominis
Renal fascia (posterior layer)
Latissimus dorsi
Quadratus lumborum
Thoracolumbar fascia (posterior and middle layers)

FIGURE 2.77. Lumbar approach to kidney and musculofascial relationships of kidney. A. The external aspect of the right posterior abdominal wall is shown. The posterolateral abdominal wall has been incised between the muscles of the anterolateral abdominal wall and the muscles of the back. The kidney and perinephric fat surrounding it inside the renal fascia are exposed. See Figure. 2.95A for an earlier stage of this dissection. B. This transverse section of the kidney shows the relationships of the muscles and fascia. Because the renal fascia surrounds the kidney as a separate sheath, it must be incised in any surgical operation on the kidney, whether from an anterior or a posterior approach.

approximately 3 cm, approximately the height of one vertebral body. Superiorly, the renal fascia is continuous with the fascia on the inferior surface of the diaphragm (diaphragmatic fascia); thus the primary attachment of the suprarenal glands is to the diaphragm. Inferiorly, the anterior and posterior layers of renal fascia are only loosely united, if attached at all. (See the blue boxes "Perinephric Abscess" and "Nephroptosis" on p. 298.)

KIDNEYS

The ovoid **kidneys** remove excess water, salts, and wastes of protein metabolism from the blood while returning nutrients and chemicals to the blood. They lie retroperitoneally on the posterior abdominal wall, one on each side of the vertebral column at the level of the T12–L3 vertebrae (Fig. 2.76).

At the concave medial margin of each kidney is a vertical cleft, the **renal hilum** (Figs. 2.76 and 2.77B). The renal hilum is the entrance to a space within the kidney, the **renal sinus.** Structures that serve the kidneys (vessels, nerves, and structures that drain urine from the kidney) enter and exit the renal sinus through the renal hilum. The hilum of the left kidney lies near the transpyloric plane, approximately 5 cm from the median plane (Fig. 2.78). The transpyloric plane passes through the superior pole of the right kidney, which is approximately 2.5 cm lower than the left pole, probably due to the presence of the liver. Posteriorly, the superior parts of the kidneys lie deep to the 11th and 12th ribs. The levels of the kidneys change during respiration and with changes in posture. Each kidney moves 2–3 cm in a vertical direction during the movement of the diaphragm that occurs with deep breathing. Because the usual surgical approach to the kidneys is through the posterior abdominal

wall, it is helpful to know that the inferior pole of the right kidney is approximately a finger's breadth superior to the iliac crest.

During life, the kidneys are reddish brown and measure approximately 10 cm in length, 5 cm in width, and 2.5 cm in thickness. Superiorly, the posterior aspects of the kidneys are associated with the diaphragm, which separates them from the pleural cavities and the 12th pair of ribs (Fig. 2.76). More inferiorly, the posterior surfaces of the kidney are related to the psoas major muscles medially and the quadratus lumborum muscle (Figs. 2.76 and 2.77). See the blue box "Pain in Pararenal Region," p. 298. The subcostal nerve and vessels and the iliohypogastric and ilio-inguinal nerves descend diagonally across the posterior surfaces of the kidneys. The liver, duodenum, and ascending colon are anterior to the right kidney (Figs. 2.75B and 2.79). This kidney is separated from the liver by the *hepatorenal recess.* The left kidney is related to the stomach, spleen, pancreas, jejunum, and descending colon.

At the hilum, the *renal vein* is anterior to the *renal artery,* which is anterior to the renal pelvis (Figs. 2.76 and 2.80A). Within the kidney, the *renal sinus* is occupied by the renal pelvis, calices, vessels, and nerves, and a variable amount of fat (Fig. 2.80C & D). Each kidney has anterior and posterior surfaces, medial and lateral margins, and superior and inferior poles. However, because of the protrusion of the lumbar vertebral column into the abdominal cavity, the kidneys are obliquely placed, lying at an angle to each other (Fig. 2.77B). Consequently, the transverse diameter of the kidneys is foreshortened in anterior views (Fig. 2.76A) and anteroposterior (AP) radiographs (Fig. 2.81). The lateral margin of each kidney is convex, and the medial margin is concave where the renal sinus and renal pelvis are located. The indented medial margin gives the kidney a somewhat bean-shaped appearance.

The **renal pelvis** is the flattened, funnel-shaped expansion of the superior end of the ureter (Figs. 2.80B–D, 2.81, and 2.82). The **apex of the renal pelvis** is continuous with the ureter. The renal pelvis receives two or three **major calices** (calyces), each of which divides into two or three **minor calices.** Each minor calyx is indented by a **renal papilla,** the apex of the *renal pyramid,* from which the urine is excreted. In living persons, the renal pelvis and its calices are usually collapsed (empty). The pyramids and their associated cortex form the lobes of the kidney. The lobes are visible on the external surfaces of the kidneys in fetuses, and evidence of the lobes may persist for some time after birth.

URETERS

The **ureters** are muscular ducts (25–30 cm long) with narrow lumina that carry urine from the kidneys to the urinary bladder (Figs. 2.76 and 2.82). They run inferiorly from the apices of the renal pelves at the hila of the kidneys, passing over the pelvic brim at the bifurcation of the common iliac arteries. They then run along the lateral wall of the pelvis and enter the urinary bladder.

The abdominal parts of the ureters adhere closely to the parietal peritoneum and are retroperitoneal throughout their

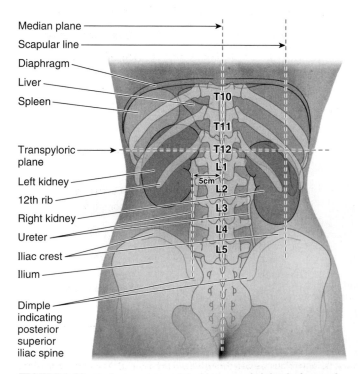

Median plane
Scapular line
Diaphragm
Liver
Spleen
T10
T11
Transpyloric plane
T12
L1
Left kidney
5cm
L2
12th rib
L3
Right kidney
L4
Ureter
L5
Iliac crest
Ilium
Dimple indicating posterior superior iliac spine

FIGURE 2.78. Surface anatomy of the kidneys and abdominal part of ureters.

Inferior vena cava (IVC)

Contacts bare area of liver

Right suprarenal gland

Hepatorenal recess

Contacts right lobe of liver

Duodenum

Contacts ascending colon

Contacts small intestine (ileum)

Root of mesentery of small intestine

Contacts caudate lobe of liver

Esophagus and left gastric artery

Left suprarenal gland

Contacts spleen

Contacts stomach

Root of transverse mesocolon

Contacts descending colon

Contacts small intestine (jejunum)

Superior mesenteric artery and vein

Ureter

Anterior view

FIGURE 2.79. Relationships of kidneys, suprarenal glands, pancreas, and duodenum. The right suprarenal gland is at the level of the omental foramen (*black arrow*).

Superior pole

Medial margin

Renal hilum

Renal artery

Renal vein

Renal pelvis

Ureter

Lateral margin

Anterior surface

Inferior pole

(A) Anterior view

Anterior surface

Renal sinus

Posterior and anterior lips of renal hilum

Renal hilum

Pelvis

Apex of renal pelvis

Medial margin

Posterior surface

Ureter

(B) Anteromedial view

Fibrous capsule

Cortex

Minor calyx ⎫
            ⎬ Calices
Major calyx ⎭

Medulla and renal column

Pyramid

Renal pelvis

Papilla

Renal sinus

Medullary ray

Ureter

(C) Anterior view exposing calices

Renal cortex

Renal papilla

Minor calyx ⎫
            ⎬ Calices
Major calyx ⎭

Renal pelvis

Ureter

Renal columns

Renal pyramids

(D) Anterior view, coronal section

FIGURE 2.80. External and internal appearance of kidneys. A. The right kidney. **B.** Renal sinus, as seen through the renal hilum. **C.** The anterior lip of the renal hilum has been cut away to expose the renal pelvis and calices within the renal sinus. **D.** This coronal section of the kidney shows the organ's internal structure. The renal pyramids contain the collecting tubules and form the medulla of the kidney. The renal cortex contains the renal corpuscles.

Anteroposterior view

FIGURE 2.81. Intravenous urogram (pyelogram). The contrast medium was injected intravenously and was concentrated and excreted by the kidneys. This AP projection shows the calices, renal pelvis, and ureter outlined by the contrast medium filling their lumina. (Courtesy of Dr. John Campbell, Department of Medical Imaging, Sunnybrook Medical Centre, University of Toronto, Toronto, ON, Canada.)

course. From the back, the surface marking of the ureter is a line joining a point 5 cm lateral to the L1 spinous process and the posterior superior iliac spine (Fig. 2.78). The ureters occupy a sagittal plane that intersects the tips of the transverse processes of the lumbar vertebrae. When examining

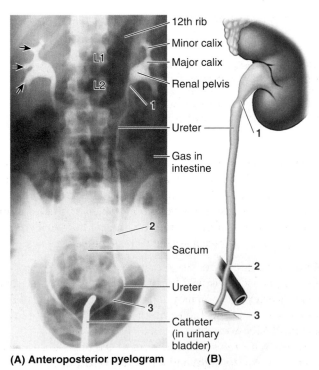

(A) Anteroposterior pyelogram   (B)

FIGURE 2.82. Normal constrictions of ureters demonstrated by retrograde pyelogram. A. Contrast medium was injected into the ureters from a flexible endoscope (urethroscope) in the bladder. The *arrows* represent papillae bulging into the minor calices. **B.** Sites at which relative constrictions in the ureters normally appear: (1) at the ureteropelvic junction, (2) crossing the external iliac artery and/or pelvic brim, and (3) as the ureter traverses the bladder wall.

the ureters radiographically using contrast medium (Figs. 2.81 and 2.82), the ureters normally demonstrate relative constrictions in three places: (1) at the junction of the ureters and renal pelves, (2) where the ureters cross the brim of the pelvic inlet, and (3) during their passage through the wall of the urinary bladder (Fig. 2.82). These constricted areas are potential sites of obstruction by ureteric stones (calculi).

Congenital anomalies of the kidneys and ureters are fairly common. (See the blue box "Congenital Anomalies of Kidneys and Ureters" on p. 299.)

SUPRARENAL GLANDS

The **suprarenal (adrenal) glands,** yellowish in living persons, are located between the superomedial aspects of the kidneys and the diaphragm (Fig. 2.83), where they are surrounded by connective tissue containing considerable perinephric fat. The suprarenal glands are enclosed by renal fascia by which they are attached to the *crura of the diaphragm.* Although the name "suprarenal" implies that the kidneys are their primary relationship, their major attachment is to the diaphragmatic crura. They are separated from the kidneys by a thin septum (part of the renal fascia—see the blue box "Renal Transplantation," p. 298).

The shape and relations of the suprarenal glands differ on the two sides. The *pyramidal right gland* is more apical (situated over the superior pole) relative to the left kidney, lies anterolateral to the right crus of the diaphragm, and makes contact with the IVC anteromedially (Fig. 2.79) and the liver anterolaterally. The *crescent-shaped left gland* is medial to the superior half of the left kidney and is related to the spleen, stomach, pancreas, and the left crus of the diaphragm.

Each gland has a *hilum,* where the veins and lymphatic vessels exit the gland, whereas, the arteries and nerves enter the glands at multiple sites. The medial borders of the suprarenal glands are 4–5 cm apart. In this area, from right to left, are the IVC, right crus of the diaphragm, celiac ganglion, celiac trunk, SMA, and the left crus of the diaphragm.

Each suprarenal gland has two parts: the *suprarenal cortex* and *suprarenal medulla* (Fig. 2.83, *inset*); these parts have different embryological origins and different functions.

The **suprarenal cortex** derives from mesoderm and secretes corticosteroids and androgens. These hormones cause the kidneys to retain sodium and water in response to stress, increasing the blood volume and blood pressure. They also affect muscles and organs such as the heart and lungs.

The **suprarenal medulla** is a mass of nervous tissue permeated with capillaries and sinusoids that derives from *neural crest cells* associated with the sympathetic nervous system (see Fig. 2.87). The *chromaffin cells* of the medulla are related to sympathetic ganglion (postsynaptic) neurons in both derivation (neural crest cells) and function. These cells secrete catecholamines (mostly epinephrine) into the bloodstream in response to signals from presynaptic neurons. Powerful medullary hormones, epinephrine (adrenaline) and norepinephrine (noradrenaline), activate the body to a flight-or-fight status in response to traumatic stress. They also increase heart

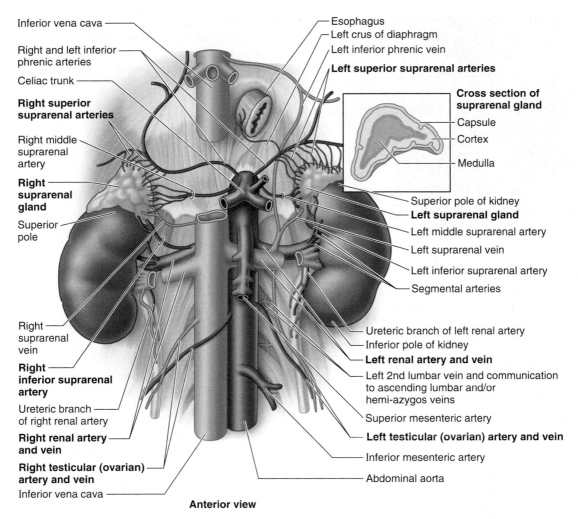

Anterior view

FIGURE 2.83. Blood vessels of suprarenal glands, kidneys, and superior parts of ureters. The celiac plexus of nerves and ganglia that surrounds the celiac trunk has been removed. The inferior vena cava has been transected, and its superior part has been elevated from its normal position to reveal the arteries that pass posterior to it. The renal veins have been cut so that the kidneys could be moved laterally. For the normal relationships of the kidneys and suprarenal glands with the great vessels, see Figure 2.76. A cross section of the suprarenal gland (*inset*) shows that it is composed of two distinct parts: the cortex and medulla, which are two separate endocrine glands that became closely related during embryonic development.

rate and blood pressure, dilate the bronchioles, and change blood flow patterns, preparing for physical exertion.

VESSELS AND NERVES OF KIDNEYS, URETERS, AND SUPRARENAL GLANDS

Renal Arteries and Veins. The *renal arteries* arise at the level of the IV disc between the L1 and L2 vertebrae (Figs. 2.83 and 2.84). The longer **right renal artery** passes posterior to the IVC. Typically, each artery divides close to the hilum into five *segmental arteries* that are end arteries (i.e., they do not anastomose significantly with other segmental arteries, so that the area supplied by each segmental artery is an independent, surgically resectable unit or **renal segment**). Segmental arteries are distributed to the renal segments as follows (Fig. 2.85):

- The superior (apical) segment is supplied by the **superior (apical) segmental artery;** the anterosuperior and anteroinferior segments are supplied by the **anterosuperior segmental** and **antero-inferior segmental arter-**

ies; and the inferior segment is supplied by the **inferior segmental artery.** These arteries originate from the anterior branch of the renal artery.

- The **posterior segmental artery,** which originates from a continuation of the posterior branch of the renal artery, supplies the posterior segment of the kidney.

Multiple renal arteries are common and usually enter the hilum of the kidney (Fig. 2.84). Extrahilar renal arteries from the renal artery or aorta may enter the external surface of the kidney, commonly at their poles ("polar arteries"—see the blue box "Accessory Renal Vessels" on p. 298).

Several *renal veins* drain each kidney and unite in a variable fashion to form the **right** and **left renal veins;** these veins lie anterior to the right and left renal arteries. The longer left renal vein receives the *left suprarenal vein*, the *left gonadal (testicular or ovarian) vein*, and a communication with the *ascending lumbar vein*; it then traverses the acute angle between the SMA anteriorly and the aorta posteriorly (see the blue box "Renal Vein Entrapment Syndrome" on p. 298). Each renal vein drains into the IVC.

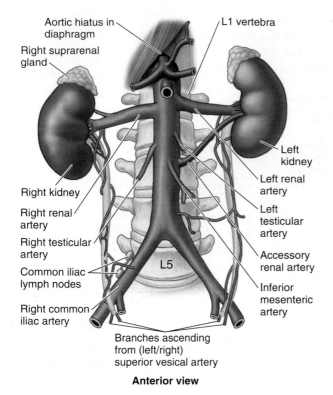

FIGURE 2.84. Arterial supply of kidneys and ureters. The abdominal aorta lies anterior to the L1-L4 vertebral bodies, usually immediately to the left of the midline. An accessory left renal artery is present.

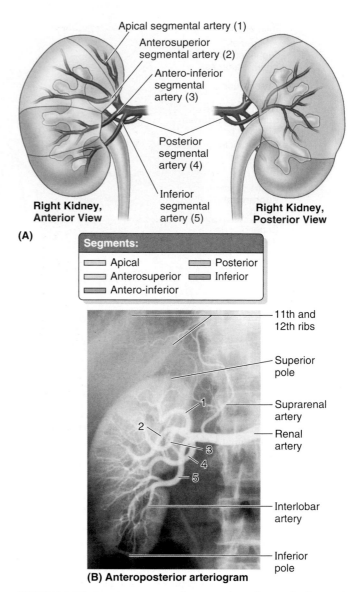

FIGURE 2.85. Renal segments and segmental arteries. A. The five renal segments and segmental renal arteries. (Numbers in parentheses identify arteries in **B.**) **B.** Renal arteriogram (*1–5,* segmental renal arteries). Although the veins of the kidney anastomose freely, segmental arteries are end arteries. (**B** courtesy of Dr. E. L. Lansdown, Professor of Medical Imaging, University of Toronto, Toronto, ON, Canada.)

Arterial Supply and Venous Drainage of Ureters. *Arterial branches to the abdominal portion of the ureter* arise consistently from the *renal arteries,* with less constant branches arising from the *testicular* or *ovarian arteries,* the *abdominal aorta,* and the *common iliac arteries* (Fig. 2.84). The branches approach the ureters medially and divide into ascending and descending branches, forming a longitudinal anastomosis on the ureteric wall. However, ureteric branches are small and relatively delicate, and disruption may lead to ischemia in spite of the continuous anastomotic channel formed. In operations in the posterior abdominal region, surgeons pay special attention to the location of ureters and are careful not to retract them laterally or unnecessarily. The arteries supplying the pelvic portion of the ureter are discussed in Chapter 3.

Veins draining the abdominal part of the ureters drain into the renal and gonadal (testicular or ovarian) veins (see Fig. 2.83).

Suprarenal Arteries and Veins. The endocrine function of the suprarenal glands makes their abundant blood supply necessary. The suprarenal arteries branch freely before entering each gland so that 50–60 branches penetrate the capsule covering the entire surface of the glands. Suprarenal arteries arise from three sources (Fig. 2.83):

- **Superior suprarenal arteries** (6–8) from the *inferior phrenic arteries.*
- **Middle suprarenal arteries** (£ 1) from the *abdominal aorta* near the level of origin of the SMA.
- **Inferior suprarenal arteries** (£ 1) from the renal arteries.

The *venous drainage of the suprarenal glands* occurs via large *suprarenal veins.* The short **right suprarenal vein** drains into the IVC, whereas the longer **left suprarenal vein,** often joined by the *inferior phrenic vein,* empties into the left renal vein.

Lymphatics of Kidneys, Ureters, and Suprarenal Glands. The *renal lymphatic vessels* follow the renal veins and drain into the *right* and *left lumbar* (*caval* and *aortic*) *lymph nodes* (Fig. 2.86). Lymphatic vessels from the superior part of the ureter may join those from the kidney or pass directly to the lumbar nodes. Lymphatic vessels from the middle part of the ureter usually drain into the *common iliac lymph nodes,* whereas vessels from its inferior part drain into the *common, external,* or *internal iliac lymph nodes.*

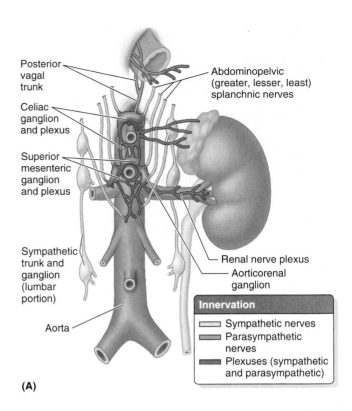

FIGURE 2.86. Lymphatics of kidneys and suprarenal glands. The lymphatic vessels of the kidneys form three plexuses: one in the substance of the kidney, one under the fibrous capsule, and one in the perirenal fat. Four or five lymphatic trunks leave the renal hilum and are joined by vessels from the capsule (*arrows*). The lymphatic vessels follow the renal vein to the lumbar (caval and aortic) lymph nodes. Lymph from the suprarenal glands also drains to the lumbar nodes. Lymphatic drainage of the ureters is also illustrated. The lumbar lymph nodes drain through the lumbar lymphatic trunks to the cisterna chyli.

The *suprarenal lymphatic vessels* arise from a plexus deep to the capsule of the gland and from one in its medulla. The lymph passes to the *lumbar lymph nodes.* Many lymphatic vessels leave the suprarenal glands.

Nerves of Kidneys, Ureters, and Suprarenal Glands. The *nerves to the kidneys* arise from the renal nerve plexus and consist of sympathetic and parasympathetic fibers (Fig. 2.87B). The **renal nerve plexus** is supplied by fibers from the abdominopelvic (especially the least) splanchnic nerves. The *nerves of the abdominal part of the ureters* derive from the renal, abdominal aortic, and superior hypogastric plexuses (Fig. 2.87A). Visceral afferent fibers conveying pain sensation (e.g., resulting from obstruction and consequent distension) follow the sympathetic fibers retrograde to spinal ganglia and cord segments T11–L2. Ureteric pain is usually referred to the ipsilateral lower quadrant of the anterior abdominal wall and especially to the groin (see the blue box "Renal and Ureteric Calculi," p. 300).

The rich *nerve supply of the suprarenal glands* is from the *celiac plexus* and abdominopelvic (greater, lesser, and least) splanchnic nerves. Myelinated presynaptic sympathetic fibers—mainly derived from the intermediolateral cell column (IML), or lateral horn, of gray matter of the spinal cord segments T10–L1—traverse both the paravertebral and the prevertebral ganglia, without synapse, to be distributed to the chromaffin cells in the suprarenal medulla (Fig. 2.87B).

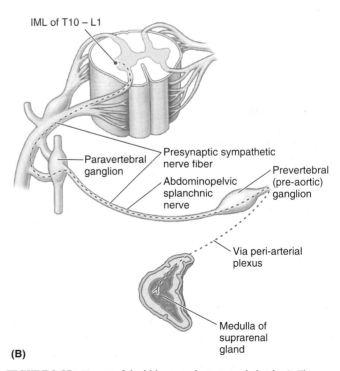

FIGURE 2.87. Nerves of the kidneys and suprarenal glands. A. The nerves of the kidneys and suprarenal glands are derived from the celiac plexus, abdominopelvic (lesser and least) splanchnic nerves, and the aorticorenal ganglion. The main efferent innervation of the kidney is vasomotor, autonomic nerves supplying the afferent and efferent arterioles. **B.** Exclusively in the case of the suprarenal medulla, the presynaptic sympathetic fibers pass through both the paravertebral and prevertebral ganglia without synapsing to end directly on the secretory cells of the suprarenal medulla. *IML,* intermediolateral cell column.

KIDNEYS, URETERS, AND SUPRARENAL GLANDS

Palpation of Kidneys

The kidneys are often impalpable. In lean adults, the inferior pole of the right kidney is palpable by bimanual examination as a firm, smooth, somewhat rounded mass that descends during inspiration. Palpation of the right kidney is possible because it is 1–2 cm inferior to the left one. To palpate the kidneys, press the *flank* (side of the trunk between the 11th and 12th ribs and the iliac crest) anteriorly with one hand while palpating deeply at the *costal margin* with the other. The left kidney is usually not palpable unless it is enlarged or a retroperitoneal mass has displaced it inferiorly.

Perinephric Abscess

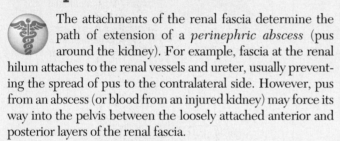 The attachments of the renal fascia determine the path of extension of a *perinephric abscess* (pus around the kidney). For example, fascia at the renal hilum attaches to the renal vessels and ureter, usually preventing the spread of pus to the contralateral side. However, pus from an abscess (or blood from an injured kidney) may force its way into the pelvis between the loosely attached anterior and posterior layers of the renal fascia.

Nephroptosis

Because the layers of renal fascia do not fuse firmly inferiorly to offer resistance, abnormally mobile kidneys may descend more than the normal 3 cm when the body is erect. When kidneys descend, the suprarenal glands remain in place because they lie in a separate fascial compartment and are firmly attached to the diaphragm. *Nephroptosis* (dropped kidney) is distinguished from an *ectopic kidney* (congenital misplaced kidney) by a ureter of normal length that has loose coiling or kinks because the distance to the bladder has been reduced. The kinks do not seem to be of significance. Symptoms of intermittent pain in the renal region, relieved by lying down, appear to result from traction on the renal vessels. The lack of inferior support for the kidneys in the lumbar region is one of the reasons transplanted kidneys are placed in the iliac fossa of the greater pelvis. Other reasons for this placement are the availability of major blood vessels and convenient access to the nearby bladder.

Renal Transplantation

Renal transplantation is the preferred treatment for selected cases of chronic renal failure. The kidney can be removed from the donor without damaging the suprarenal gland because of the weak septum of renal fascia that separates the kidney from this gland. The site for transplanting a kidney is in the iliac fossa of the greater pelvis. This site supports the transplanted kidney, so that traction is not placed on the surgically anastomosed vessels. The renal artery and vein are joined to the external iliac artery and vein, respectively, and the ureter is sutured into the urinary bladder.

Renal Cysts

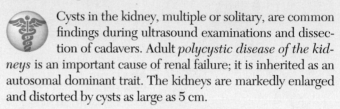 Cysts in the kidney, multiple or solitary, are common findings during ultrasound examinations and dissection of cadavers. Adult *polycystic disease of the kidneys* is an important cause of renal failure; it is inherited as an autosomal dominant trait. The kidneys are markedly enlarged and distorted by cysts as large as 5 cm.

Pain in Pararenal Region

The close relationship of the kidneys to the psoas major muscles explains why extension of the hip joints may increase pain resulting from inflammation in the pararenal areas. These muscles flex the thighs at the hip joints.

Accessory Renal Vessels

During their "ascent" to their final site, the embryonic kidneys receive their blood supply and venous drainage from successively more superior vessels. Usually the inferior vessels degenerate as superior ones take over. Failure of these vessels to degenerate results in *accessory renal arteries* (Fig. 2.84) and *veins*. Some accessory arteries ("polar arteries") enter/exit the poles of the kidneys. An inferior polar artery crosses the ureter and may obstruct it. Variations in the number and position of these vessels occur in approximately 30% of people.

Renal Vein Entrapment Syndrome

In crossing the midline to reach the IVC, the longer left renal vein traverses an acute angle between the SMA anteriorly and the abdominal aorta posteriorly (Fig. B2.31). Downward traction on the SMA may compress the left renal vein (and perhaps the third part of the duodenum) resulting in a *renal vein entrapment syndrome* (mesoaortic compression of the left renal vein), also known as "nutcracker syndrome" based on the appearance of the vein in the acute arterial angle in a sagittal view. The syndrome may include hematuria or proteinuria (blood or protein in the urine), abdominal (left flank) pain, nausea and vomiting (indicating compression of the duodenum), and left testicular pain in men (related to the left testicular vein draining into the left renal vein proximal to the compression). Uncommonly, a left-sided varicocele may occur.

Celiac trunk

Left renal { Artery / Vein }

Superior mesenteric artery

3rd part of duodenum

Small intestine

Aorta

Lateral view (from left)

FIGURE B2.31.

Congenital Anomalies of Kidneys and Ureters

Bifid renal pelvis and ureter are fairly common (Fig. B2.32A & B). These anomalies result from division of the *ureteric bud* (metanephric diverticulum), the primordium of the renal pelvis and ureter. The extent of ureteral duplication depends on the completeness of embryonic division of the ureteric bud. The bifid renal pelvis and/or ureter may be unilateral or bilateral; however, separate openings into the bladder are uncommon. Incomplete division of the ureteric bud results in a bifid ureter; complete division results in a *supernumerary kidney* (Moore, Persaud and Torchia, 2012).

An uncommon anomaly is a *retrocaval ureter* (Fig. B2.32C), which leaves the kidney and passes posterior to the IVC.

Bifid pelvis

(A) Bifid renal pelvis

Bifid ureter

Unilateral duplicated ureter

Bladder

(B) Bifid ureter and unilateral duplicated ureter

Ureter

Ureter

Junction of bifid ureter

Right kidney

Inferior vena cava

Right ureter

(C) Retrocaval ureter

Inferior mesenteric artery

(D) Horseshoe kidney

Inferior vena cava

Aorta

Anomalous renal vessels

Ectopic kidney

Left ureter

Right ureter

(E) Ectopic pelvic kidney

FIGURE B2.32.

The kidneys are close together in the embryonic pelvis. In approximately 1 in 600 fetuses, the inferior poles (rarely, the superior poles) of the kidneys fuse to form a *horseshoe kidney* (Fig. B2.32D). This U-shaped kidney usually lies at the level of L3–L5 vertebrae because the root of the *inferior mesenteric artery* prevented normal relocation of the kidneys. Horseshoe kidney usually produces no symptoms; however, associated abnormalities of the kidney and renal pelvis may be present, obstructing the ureter.

Sometimes the embryonic kidney on one or both sides fails to enter the abdomen and lies anterior to the sacrum. Although uncommon, awareness of the possibility of an *ectopic pelvic kidney* (Fig. B2.32E) should prevent it from being mistaken for a pelvic tumor and removed. A pelvic kidney in a woman also can be injured by or cause obstruction during childbirth. Pelvic kidneys usually receive their blood supply from the aortic bifurcation or a common iliac artery.

Renal and Ureteric Calculi

 Calculi (L. pebbles) are composed of salts of inorganic or organic acids or of other materials. They may form and become located in the calices of the kidneys, ureters, or urinary bladder (Fig. B2.33). A *renal calculus* (kidney stone) may pass from the kidney into the renal pelvis and then into the ureter. If the stone is sharp or larger than the normal lumen of the ureter (approximately 3 mm), it causes excessive distension of this muscular tube, the *ureteric calculus* will cause severe intermittent pain (*ureteric colic*) as it is gradually forced down the ureter by waves of contraction. The calculus may cause complete or intermittent obstruction of urinary flow. Depending on the level of obstruction, which changes, the pain may be referred to the lumbar or inguinal regions, or to the external genitalia and/or testis.

The pain is referred to the cutaneous areas innervated by spinal cord segments and sensory ganglia, which also receive visceral afferents from the ureter, mainly T11–L2. The pain passes inferoanteriorly "from the loin to the groin" as the

Stone in minor calyces

Stone in major calyx

Staghorn stone in minor and major calyces

Loose stone in renal pelvis

FIGURE B2.33.

stone progresses through the ureter. (The loin is the lumbar region, and the groin is the inguinal region.) The pain may extend into the proximal anterior aspect of the thigh by projection through the genitofemoral nerve (L1, L2), the scrotum in males and the labia majora in females. The extreme pain may be accompanied by marked digestive upset (nausea, vomiting, cramping, and diarrhea) and a generalized sympathetic response that may to various degrees mask the more specific symptoms.

Ureteric calculi can be observed and removed with a *nephroscope*, an instrument that is inserted through a small incision. Another technique, *lithotripsy*, focuses a shockwave through the body that breaks the calculus into small fragments that pass with the urine.

The Bottom Line

RETROPERITONEAL VISCERA AND THEIR NEUROVASCULATURE

Kidneys: The abdominal urinary organs and the suprarenal glands are primary retroperitoneal structures, embedded within perinephric fat that is separated from the surrounding extraperitoneal paranephric fat by a membranous condensation, the renal fascia. ♦ The kidneys are bean-shaped structures located between the T12 and the L3 vertebral levels, deep (anterior) to the 12th ribs. ♦ Closely related to the diaphragm, the kidneys move with its excursions. ♦ The suprarenal glands are located superomedially to the kidneys but are not attached to them. ♦ The kidneys are hollow. The central renal sinus

is occupied by the renal calices and renal pelvis, segmental arteries, and renal veins that are embedded in perinephric fat. ♦ The papillae of the renal pyramids, from which urine is excreted, evaginate into and are surrounded by minor calices. ♦ The minor calices merge to form major calices that in turn merge to form the renal pelvis. ♦ The vascular structures and renal pelvis exit the renal sinus at the medially directed hilum.

Ureters: The abdominal portions of the ureters descend on the anterior surface of the psoas muscles from the apex of the renal pelvis to the pelvic brim. ♦ The ureters normally have three sites of relative constriction, where kidney stones may lodge: the ureteropelvic junction, pelvic brim, and bladder wall. ♦ The abdominal portions of the ureters receive multiple, relatively delicate ureteric branches from the renal, testicular or ovarian, and common iliac arteries and from the abdominal aorta, which approach the ureters medially. ♦ A vertical line 5 cm lateral to the lumbar spinous processes, intersecting the posterior superior iliac spine, approximates the position of the ureter.

Suprarenal glands: The suprarenal glands are located superomedially to the kidneys but are attached primarily to the diaphragmatic crura by the surrounding renal fascia. ♦ Each suprarenal gland is actually two endocrine glands of different origin and function: suprarenal cortex and suprarenal medulla (the latter surrounded by the former). ♦ The suprarenal cortex derives from mesoderm and secretes corticosteroids and androgens; the suprarenal medulla derives from neural crest cells and secretes catecholamines (mostly epinephrine). ♦ The right suprarenal gland is more pyramidal in shape and apical in position relative to the right kidney, whereas the left gland is more crescentic and lies more medial to the superior half of the kidney.

Neurovasculature: The renal arteries arise from the abdominal aorta at the level of the L1–L2 IV disc. They lie anterior to the renal veins, with the right renal artery being longer than the left, and the left renal vein being longer than the right. ♦ Both renal veins receive renal and superior ureteric veins

and drain into the IVC, but the long left vein also receives the left suprarenal vein, the left gonadal vein, and a communication with the left ascending lumbar vein. ♦ Near the hilum, the renal arteries divide into anterior and posterior branches, the anterior branches giving rise to four segmental renal arteries. ♦ The segmental renal arteries are end arteries, each supplying a surgically resectable renal segment.

Suprarenal arteries arise from three sources: superior suprarenal arteries from the inferior phrenic arteries, middle suprarenal arteries from the abdominal aorta, and inferior suprarenal arteries from the renal arteries. ♦ The suprarenal glands drain via one large suprarenal vein, the right entering the IVC and the left entering the left renal vein.

Lymphatics from the suprarenal glands, kidneys, and upper ureters follow the venous drainage to the right or left lumbar (caval or aortic) lymph nodes.

Visceral afferent fibers (accompanying the sympathetic fibers) conduct pain sensation from the ureters to spinal cord segments T11–L2, with sensation referred to the corresponding dermatomes overlying the loin and groin. The suprarenal glands receive a rich nerve supply via presynaptic sympathetic fibers originating in the IMLs of the T10–L1 spinal cord segments. These fibers traverse both the paravertebral (sympathetic trunks) and prevertebral (celiac) ganglia without synapsing. They terminate directly on the chromaffin cells of the suprarenal medulla.

Summary of Innervation of Abdominal Viscera

For autonomic innervation of the abdominal viscera, several different splanchnic nerves and one cranial nerve (the vagus, CN X) deliver presynaptic sympathetic and parasympathetic fibers, respectively, to the abdominal aortic plexus and its associated sympathetic ganglia (Figs. 2.88 and 2.89; Table 2.12). The peri-arterial extensions of these plexuses deliver postsynaptic sympathetic fibers and the continuations of parasympathetic fibers to the abdominal viscera, where intrinsic parasympathetic ganglia occur.

SYMPATHETIC INNERVATION

The sympathetic part of the autonomic innervation of the abdominal viscera consists of the:

- Abdominopelvic splanchnic nerves from the thoracic and abdominal sympathetic trunks.
- Prevertebral sympathetic ganglia.
- Abdominal aortic plexus and its extensions, the peri-arterial plexuses.

The nerve plexuses are mixed, shared with the parasympathetic nervous system and visceral afferent fibers.

The **abdominopelvic splanchnic nerves** convey presynaptic sympathetic fibers to the abdominopelvic cavity. The fibers arise from cell bodies in the IMLs (or lateral horns) of

the gray matter of spinal cord segments T5–L2 or L3. The fibers pass successively through the anterior roots, anterior rami, and white communicating branches of thoracic and upper lumbar spinal nerves to reach the sympathetic trunks. They pass through the paravertebral ganglia of the trunks without synapsing to enter the abdominopelvic splanchnic nerves, which convey them to the prevertebral ganglia of the abdominal cavity. The abdominopelvic splanchnic nerves include the:

- *Lower thoracic splanchnic nerves* (greater, lesser, and least): from the thoracic part of the sympathetic trunks.
- *Lumbar splanchnic nerves:* from the lumbar part of the sympathetic trunks.

The *lower thoracic splanchnic nerves* are the main source of presynaptic sympathetic fibers serving abdominal viscera. The **greater splanchnic nerve** (from the sympathetic trunk at T5 through T9 or T10 vertebral levels), **lesser splanchnic nerve** (from T10 and T11 levels), and **least splanchnic nerve** (from the T12 level) are the specific abdominopelvic splanchnic nerves that arise from the thoracic part of the sympathetic trunks. They pierce the corresponding crus of the diaphragm to convey presynaptic sympathetic fibers to the celiac, superior mesenteric, and aorticorenal (prevertebral) sympathetic ganglia, respectively.

The **lumbar splanchnic nerves** arise from the abdominal part of the sympathetic trunks. Medially, the lumbar sympathetic trunks give off three to four lumbar splanchnic nerves, which pass to the *intermesenteric, inferior mesenteric,* and *superior*

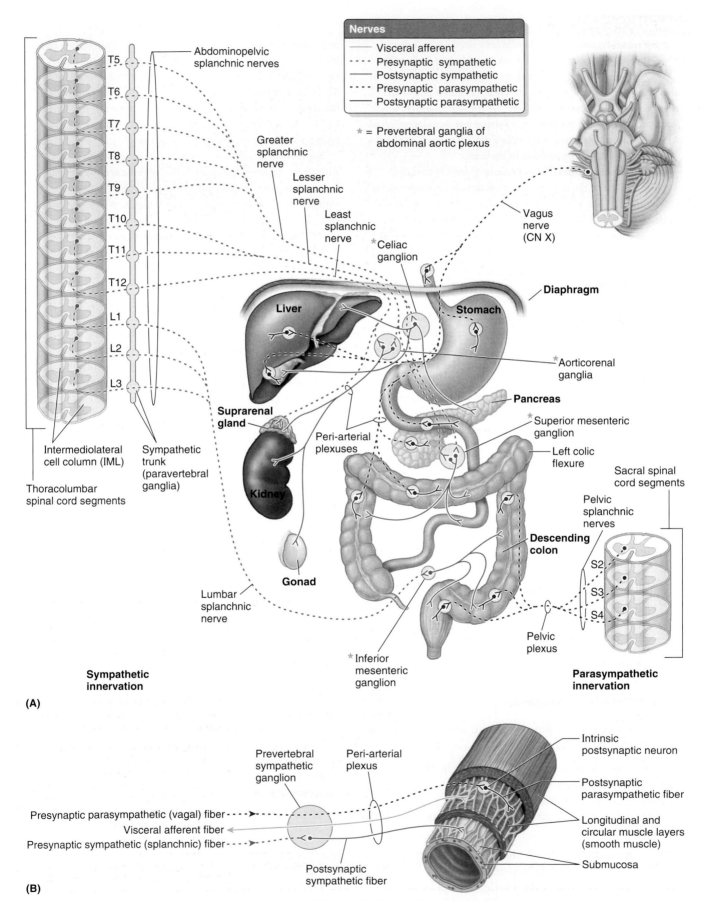

Sympathetic innervation

(A)

Parasympathetic innervation

(B)

FIGURE 2.88. Autonomic nerves of posterior abdominal wall. A. Origin and distribution of presynaptic and postsynaptic sympathetic and parasympathetic fibers, and the ganglia involved in supplying abdominal viscera are shown. **B.** The fibers supplying the intrinsic plexuses of abdominal viscera are demonstrated.

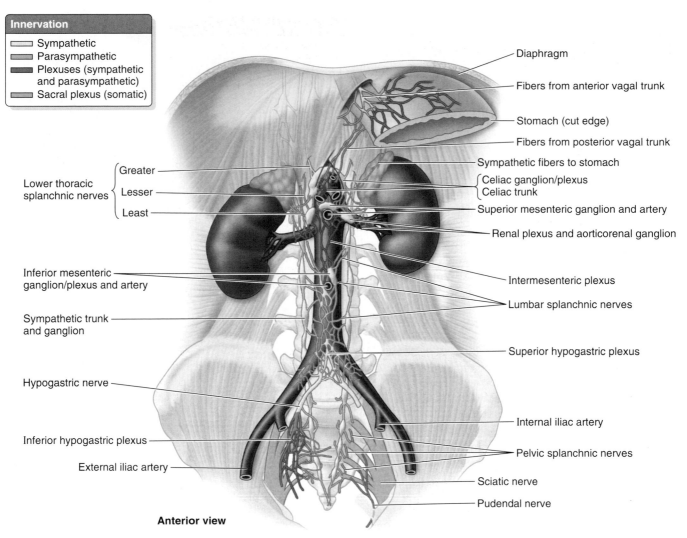

Innervation

- ⬜ Sympathetic
- ⬜ Parasympathetic
- ⬛ Plexuses (sympathetic and parasympathetic)
- ⬛ Sacral plexus (somatic)

Diaphragm

Fibers from anterior vagal trunk

Stomach (cut edge)

Fibers from posterior vagal trunk

Sympathetic fibers to stomach

Celiac ganglion/plexus
Celiac trunk

Superior mesenteric ganglion and artery

Renal plexus and aorticorenal ganglion

Intermesenteric plexus

Lumbar splanchnic nerves

Superior hypogastric plexus

Internal iliac artery

Pelvic splanchnic nerves

Sciatic nerve

Pudendal nerve

Lower thoracic splanchnic nerves
{ Greater
Lesser
Least }

Inferior mesenteric ganglion/plexus and artery

Sympathetic trunk and ganglion

Hypogastric nerve

Inferior hypogastric plexus

External iliac artery

Anterior view

FIGURE 2.89. Splanchnic nerves, nerve plexuses, and sympathetic ganglia in the abdomen.

TABLE 2.12. AUTONOMIC INNERVATION OF ABDOMINAL VISCERA (SPLANCHNIC NERVES)

Splanchnic Nerves	Autonomic Fiber Type[a]	System	Origin	Destination
A. Cardiopulmonary (cervical and upper thoracic)	Postsynaptic		Cervical and upper thoracic sympathetic trunk	Thoracic cavity (viscera superior to level of diaphragm)

B. Abdominopelvic
 	
1. Lower thoracic
  a. Greater
  b. Lesser
  c. Least
2. Lumbar
3. Sacral
	Presynaptic	Sympathetic	Lower thoracic and abdomino-pelvic sympathetic trunk:
			
			1. Thoracic sympathetic trunk:
			  a. T5–T9 or T10 level
			  b. T10–T11 level
			  c. T12 level
			
			2. Abdominal sympathetic trunk
			
			3. Pelvic (sacral) sympathetic trunk
				Abdominopelvic cavity (prevertebral ganglia serving viscera and suprarenal glands inferior to level of diaphragm)
				
				1. Abdominal prevertebral ganglia:
				  a. Celiac ganglia
				  b. Aorticorenal ganglia
				  c. and 2. Other abdominal prevertebral ganglia (superior and inferior mesenteric, and of intermesenteric/hypogastric plexuses)
				
				3. Pelvic prevertebral ganglia

C. Pelvic	Presynaptic	Parasympathetic	Anterior rami of S2–S4 spinal nerves	Intrinsic ganglia of descending and sigmoid colon, rectum, and pelvic viscera

[a]Splanchnic nerves also convey visceral afferent fibers, which are not part of the autonomic nervous system.

hypogastric plexuses, conveying presynaptic sympathetic fibers to the associated prevertebral ganglia of those plexuses.

The cell bodies of postsynaptic sympathetic neurons constitute the major prevertebral ganglia that cluster around the roots of the major branches of the abdominal aorta: the **celiac, aorticorenal, superior mesenteric,** and **inferior mesenteric ganglia.** Minor, unnamed prevertebral ganglia occur within the intermesenteric and superior hypogastric plexuses. With the exception of the innervation of the suprarenal medulla (discussed on p. 294), the synapse between presynaptic and postsynaptic sympathetic neurons occurs in the prevertebral ganglia (Fig. 2.88B). Postsynaptic sympathetic nerve fibers pass from the prevertebral ganglia to the abdominal viscera by means of the peri-arterial plexuses associated with the branches of the abdominal aorta. Sympathetic innervation in the abdomen, as elsewhere, is primarily involved in producing vasoconstriction. With regard to the gastrointestinal tract, it acts to inhibit (slow down or stop) peristalsis.

VISCERAL SENSORY INNERVATION

Visceral afferent fibers conveying pain sensations accompany the sympathetic (visceral motor) fibers. The pain impulses pass retrogradely to those of the motor fibers along the splanchnic nerves to the sympathetic trunk, through white communicating branches to the anterior rami of the spinal nerves. Then they pass into the posterior root to the spinal sensory ganglia and spinal cord. Progressively lower spinal sensory ganglia and spinal cord segments are involved in innervating the abdominal viscera as the tract proceeds caudally. The stomach (foregut) receives innervation from the T6 to T9 levels, small intestine through transverse colon (midgut) from the T8 to 12 levels, and descending colon (hindgut) from the T12 to L2 levels (Fig. 2.90). Starting from the midpoint of the sigmoid colon, visceral pain fibers run with parasympathetic fibers, the sensory impulses being conducted to S2–S4 sensory ganglia and spinal cord levels. These are the same spinal cord segments involved in the sympathetic innervation of those portions of alimentary tract.

Visceral afferent fibers conveying reflex sensations (that generally do not reach levels of consciousness) accompany the parasympathetic (visceral motor) fibers.

PARASYMPATHETIC INNERVATION

The parasympathetic part of the autonomic innervation of the abdominal viscera (Figs. 2.88 and 2.89) consists of the following:

- *Anterior* and *posterior vagal trunks.*
- *Pelvic splanchnic nerves.*
- *Abdominal* (para-aortic) *autonomic plexuses* and their extensions, the peri-arterial plexuses.
- *Intrinsic* (enteric) *parasympathetic ganglia.*

The nerve plexuses are mixed, shared with the sympathetic nervous system and visceral afferent fibers.

The *anterior* and *posterior vagal trunks* are the continuation of the left and right vagus nerves that emerge from the

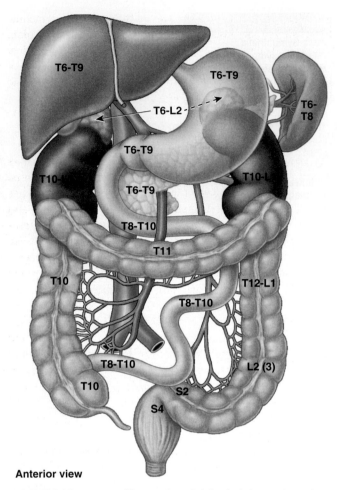

Anterior view

FIGURE 2.90. Segmental innervation of abdominal viscera. Approximate spinal cord segments and spinal sensory ganglia involved in sympathetic and visceral afferent (pain) innervation of abdominal viscera are shown.

esophageal plexus and pass through the esophageal hiatus on the anterior and posterior aspects of the esophagus and stomach (see Figs. 2.35 and 2.88A). The vagus nerves convey presynaptic parasympathetic and visceral afferent fibers (mainly for unconscious sensations associated with reflexes) to the abdominal aortic plexuses and the peri-arterial plexuses, which extend along the branches of the aorta.

The **pelvic splanchnic nerves** are distinct from other splanchnic nerves (Table 2.12) in that they:

- Have nothing to do with the sympathetic trunks.
- Derive directly from anterior rami of spinal nerves S2–S4.
- Convey presynaptic parasympathetic fibers to the inferior hypogastric (pelvic) plexus.

Presynaptic fibers terminate on the isolated and widely scattered cell bodies of postsynaptic neurons lying on or within the abdominal viscera, constituting *intrinsic (or, in the case of the GI tract, enteric) ganglia* (Fig. 2.88B).

The presynaptic parasympathetic and visceral afferent reflex fibers conveyed by the vagus nerves extend to intrinsic ganglia of the lower esophagus, stomach, small intestine, including the duodenum, ascending colon, and most of the transverse colon (see Fig. 2.88A). The fibers conveyed by the pelvic splanchnic nerves supply the descending and sigmoid parts of the colon, rectum, and pelvic organs. Thus, in terms of the gastrointestinal tract, the vagus nerves provide parasympathetic innervation of the smooth muscle and glands of the gut as far as the left colic flexure; the pelvic splanchnic nerves provide the remainder.

AUTONOMIC PLEXUSES

The **abdominal autonomic plexuses** are nerve networks consisting of both sympathetic and parasympathetic fibers, which surround the abdominal aorta and its major branches (Figs. 2.88 and 2.89). The celiac, superior mesenteric, and inferior mesenteric plexuses are interconnected. The *prevertebral sympathetic ganglia* are scattered among the celiac and mesenteric plexuses. The *intrinsic (enteric) parasympathetic ganglia,* such as the **myenteric plexus** (Auerbach plexus) in the muscular coat of the stomach and intestine, are in the walls of the viscera (see Figs. 2.48A and 2.88B).

The **celiac plexus,** surrounding the root of the celiac (arterial) trunk, contains irregular right and left **celiac ganglia** (approximately 2 cm long) that unite superior and inferior to the celiac trunk (Figs. 2.88A and 2.89). The *parasympathetic root* of the celiac plexus is a branch of the *posterior vagal trunk,* which contains fibers from the right and left vagus nerves. The *sympathetic roots* of the plexus are the greater and lesser splanchnic nerves.

The **superior mesenteric plexus** and ganglion or ganglia surround the origin of the SMA. The plexus has one median and two lateral roots. The median root is a branch of the celiac plexus, and the lateral roots arise from the lesser and least splanchnic nerves, sometimes with a contribution from the first lumbar ganglion of the sympathetic trunk.

The **inferior mesenteric plexus** surrounds the inferior mesenteric artery and gives offshoots to its branches. It receives a medial root from the intermesenteric plexus and lateral roots from the lumbar ganglia of the sympathetic trunks. An **inferior mesenteric ganglion** may also appear just inferior to the root of the inferior mesenteric artery.

The **intermesenteric plexus** is part of the aortic plexus of nerves between the superior and the inferior mesenteric arteries. It gives rise to renal, testicular or ovarian, and ureteric plexuses.

The **superior hypogastric plexus** is continuous with the intermesenteric plexus and the inferior mesenteric plexus and lies anterior to the inferior part of the abdominal aorta at its bifurcation (Table 2.12). Right and left **hypogastric nerves** join the superior hypogastric plexus to the inferior hypogastric plexus. The superior hypogastric plexus supplies *ureteric* and *testicular plexuses* and a plexus on each common iliac artery.

The **inferior hypogastric plexus** is formed on each side by a hypogastric nerve from the superior hypogastric plexus. The right and left plexuses are situated on the sides of the rectum, cervix of the uterus, and urinary bladder. The plexuses receive small branches from the superior sacral sympathetic ganglia and the sacral parasympathetic outflow from S2 through S4 sacral spinal nerves (*pelvic [parasympathetic] splanchnic nerves*). Extensions of the inferior hypogastric plexus send autonomic fibers along the blood vessels, which form visceral plexuses on the walls of the pelvic viscera (e.g., *rectal* and *vesical plexuses*).

The Bottom Line

INNERVATION OF ABDOMINAL VISCERA

Sympathetic innervation: Presynaptic sympathetic nerve fibers involved in innervating abdominal viscera arise from cell bodies in the lower two thirds of the IMLs (T5–T6 to L2–L3 spinal cord levels) and travel via spinal nerves, anterior rami, and white communicating branches to the sympathetic trunks. ♦ The fibers traverse the paravertebral ganglia of the trunks without synapsing, continuing as components of abdominopelvic splanchnic nerves. These nerves convey them to the abdominal aortic plexus, where they are joined by presynaptic parasympathetic fibers delivered by the vagus nerve. ♦ The sympathetic fibers pass to prevertebral ganglia, most of which are clustered around the major branches of the abdominal aorta. After synapsing within the ganglia, the postsynaptic sympathetic fibers join the presynaptic parasympathetic fibers, traveling via peri-arterial plexuses around the branches of the abdominal aorta to reach the viscera. ♦ A continuation of the abdominal aortic plexus inferior to the aortic bifurcation (the superior and inferior hypogastric plexuses) convey sympathetic innervation to most of the pelvic viscera. The sympathetic fibers mainly innervate the blood vessels of abdominal viscera and are inhibitory to the parasympathetic stimulation.

♦ The parasympathetic fibers synapse on or in the walls of the viscera with intrinsic postsynaptic parasympathetic neurons, which terminate on the smooth muscle or glands of the viscera.

Parasympathetic innervation: The vagus nerves supplies parasympathetic fibers to the digestive tract from the esophagus through the transverse colon. ♦ Pelvic splanchnic nerves supply the descending and sigmoid colon and rectum. ♦ Parasympathetic stimulation promotes peristalsis and secretion (although much of the latter is usually hormonally regulated).

Sensory innervation: Visceral afferent fibers follow the autonomic fibers retrograde to sensory ganglia. ♦ Afferent fibers conveying pain sensation from abdominal viscera orad (proximal) to the middle of the sigmoid colon run with the sympathetic fibers to thoracolumbar spinal sensory ganglia; all other visceral afferent fibers run with the parasympathetic fibers. Thus, visceral afferent fibers conveying reflex information from the gut orad to the middle of the sigmoid colon pass to vagal sensory ganglia; fibers conveying both pain and reflex information from the gut aborad (distal) to the middle of the sigmoid colon pass to spinal sensory ganglia S2–S4.

DIAPHRAGM

The **diaphragm** is a double-domed, musculotendinous partition separating the thoracic and abdominal cavities. Its mainly convex superior surface faces the thoracic cavity, and its concave inferior surface faces the abdominal cavity (Fig. 2.91A & B). The diaphragm is the chief muscle of inspiration (actually, of respiration altogether, because expiration is largely passive). It descends during inspiration; however, only its central part moves because its periphery, as the fixed origin of the muscle, attaches to the inferior margin of the thoracic cage and the superior lumbar vertebrae.

The *pericardium,* containing the heart, lies on the central part of the diaphragm, depressing it slightly (Fig. 2.92A). The diaphragm curves superiorly into **right** and **left domes;** normally the right dome is higher than the left dome owing to the presence of the liver. During expiration, the right dome reaches as high as the 5th rib and the left dome ascends to the 5th intercostal space. The level of the domes of the diaphragm varies according to the:

- Phase of respiration (inspiration or expiration).
- Posture (e.g., supine or standing).
- Size and degree of distension of the abdominal viscera.

The **muscular part of the diaphragm** is situated peripherally with fibers that converge radially on the trifoliate central aponeurotic part, the **central tendon** (see Fig. 2.91). The central tendon has no bony attachments and is incompletely divided into three leaves, resembling a wide cloverleaf (Fig. 2.91B). Although it lies near the center of the diaphragm, the central tendon is closer to the anterior part of the thorax.

The *caval opening* (vena caval foramen), through which the terminal part of the IVC passes to enter the heart, perforates the central tendon. The surrounding muscular part of the diaphragm forms a continuous sheet; however, for descriptive purposes it is divided into three parts, based on the peripheral attachments:

- **Sternal part:** consisting of two muscular slips that attach to the posterior aspect of the xiphoid process; this part is not always present.
- **Costal part:** consisting of wide muscular slips that attach to the internal surfaces of the inferior six costal cartilages and their adjoining ribs on each side; the costal parts form the right and left domes.
- **Lumbar part:** arising from two aponeurotic arches, the *medial* and *lateral arcuate ligaments,* and the three superior lumbar vertebrae; the lumbar part forms right and left muscular crura that ascend to the central tendon.

The **crura of the diaphragm** are musculotendinous bands that arise from the anterior surfaces of the bodies of the superior three lumbar vertebrae, the anterior longitudinal ligament, and the IV discs. The **right crus,** larger and longer than the left crus, arises from the first three or four lumbar vertebrae. The **left crus** arises from the first two or three lumbar vertebrae. Because it lies to the left of the midline, it is surprising to find that the *esophageal hiatus* is a formation

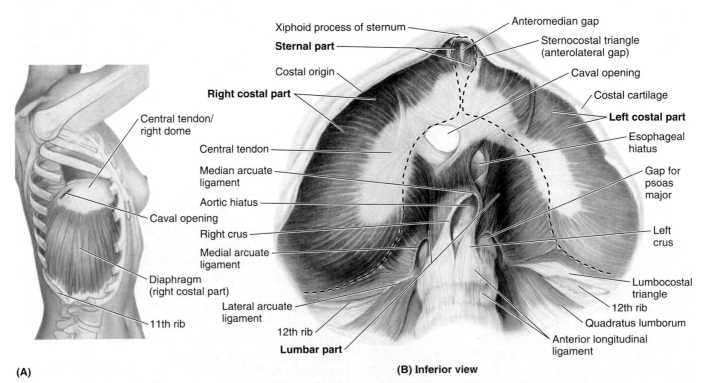

(A)

(B) Inferior view

FIGURE 2.91. Attachments, disposition, and features of the abdominal aspect of the diaphragm. A. The thoracic wall and cage have been removed to demonstrate the attachments and convexity of the right dome of the diaphragm. **B.** The fleshy sternal, costal, and lumbar parts of the diaphragm (outlined with broken lines) attach centrally to the trefoil-shaped central tendon, the aponeurotic insertion of the diaphragmatic muscle fibers.

**(A) Arteries and veins of superior
surface of diaphragm, posterior view**

Right and left
internal thoracic
arteries

Right internal
thoracic vein

Pericardiaco-
phrenic artery
and vein

Thoracic aorta

Heart inside
pericardium

Internal thoracic
artery and vein

Superior phrenic
artery

Right and left domes
of diaphragm

Right and left
superior epigastric
arteries and veins

Right and left
musculophrenic
arteries
and veins

**(B) Arteries and veins of inferior
surface of diaphragm, anterior view**

Right inferior phrenic
artery and vein

Thoracic
aorta

Superior phrenic
arteries

Left inferior phrenic
artery and vein

Inferior vena
cava

Abdominal aorta

Suprarenal vein
and artery

FIGURE 2.92.   Blood vessels of diaphragm. A. The arteries and veins of the superior surface of the diaphragm. **B.** The arteries and veins of the inferior surface of the diaphragm.

in the right crus; however, if the muscular fibers bounding each side of the hiatus are traced inferiorly, it will be seen that they pass to the right of the aortic hiatus.

The right and left crura and the fibrous **median arcuate ligament,** which unites them as it arches over the anterior aspect of the aorta, form the *aortic hiatus.* The diaphragm is also attached on each side to the *medial* and *lateral arcuate ligaments.* The **medial arcuate ligament** is a thickening of the fascia covering the psoas major, spanning between the lumbar vertebral bodies and the tip of the transverse process of L1. The **lateral arcuate ligament** covers the quadratus lumborum muscles, continuing from the L12 transverse process to the tip of the 12th rib.

The superior aspect of the central tendon of the diaphragm is fused with the inferior surface of the fibrous pericardium, the strong, external part of the fibroserous *pericardial sac* that encloses the heart.

Vessels and Nerves of Diaphragm

The arteries of the diaphragm form a branch-like pattern on both its superior (thoracic) and inferior (abdominal) surfaces. The *arteries supplying the superior surface of the diaphragm* (Fig. 2.92; Table 2.13) are the *pericardiacophrenic* and *musculophrenic arteries,* branches of the internal thoracic artery, and the **superior phrenic arteries,** arising from the thoracic aorta. The *arteries supplying the inferior surface of the diaphragm* are the **inferior phrenic arteries,** which typically are the first branches of the *abdominal aorta;* however, they may arise from the celiac trunk.

The *veins draining the superior surface of the diaphragm* are the **pericardiacophrenic** and **musculophrenic veins,** which empty into the *internal thoracic veins* and, on the right side, a **superior phrenic vein,** which drains into the IVC. Some veins from the posterior curvature of the diaphragm drain into the *azygos and hemi-azygos veins* (see Chapter 1). The *veins draining the inferior surface of the diaphragm* are the *inferior phrenic veins.* The **right inferior phrenic vein** usually opens into the IVC, whereas the **left inferior phrenic vein** is usually double, with one branch passing anterior to the esophageal hiatus to end in the IVC and the other, more posterior branch usually joining the left suprarenal vein. The right and left phrenic veins may anastomose with each other.

The *lymphatic plexuses on the superior and inferior surfaces of the diaphragm* communicate freely (Fig. 2.93A). The **anterior** and **posterior diaphragmatic lymph nodes** are on the superior surface of the diaphragm. Lymph from these nodes drains into the *parasternal, posterior mediastinal,* and *phrenic lymph nodes.* Lymphatic vessels from the inferior surface of the diaphragm drain into the anterior diaphragmatic, phrenic, and superior *lumbar (caval/aortic) lymph nodes.* Lymphatic capillaries are dense on the inferior surface of the diaphragm, constituting the primary means for absorption of peritoneal fluid and substances introduced by intraperitoneal (I.P.) injection.

The entire *motor supply to the diaphragm* is from the *right* and *left phrenic nerves,* each of which arises from the anterior rami of C3–C5 segments of the spinal cord and is distributed to the ipsilateral half of the diaphragm from its

TABLE 2.13. NEUROVASCULAR STRUCTURES OF DIAPHRAGM

Vessels and Nerves	Superior Surface of Diaphragm	Inferior Surface of Diaphragm
Arterial supply	Superior phrenic arteries from thoracic aorta Musculophrenic and pericardiophrenic arteries from internal thoracic arteries	Inferior phrenic arteries from abdominal aorta
Venous drainage	Musculophrenic and pericardiacophrenic veins drain into internal thoracic veins; superior phrenic vein (right side) drains into IVC	Inferior phrenic veins; right vein drains into IVC; left vein is doubled and drains into IVC and suprarenal vein
Lymphatic drainage	Diaphragmatic lymph nodes to phrenic nodes, then to parasternal and posterior mediastinal nodes	Superior lumbar lymph nodes; lymphatic plexuses on superior and inferior surfaces communicate freely
Innervation	Motor supply: phrenic nerves (C3–C5) Sensory supply: centrally by phrenic nerves (C3–C5), peripherally by intercostal nerves (T5–T11) and subcostal nerves (T12)	

IVC, inferior vena cava.

inferior surface (Fig. 2.93B). *Sensory innervation (pain and proprioception) to the diaphragm* is also mostly from the *phrenic nerves.* Peripheral parts of the diaphragm receive their sensory nerve supply from the *intercostal nerves* (lower six or seven) and the subcostal nerves.

Diaphragmatic Apertures

The **diaphragmatic apertures** (openings, hiatus) permit structures (vessels, nerves, and lymphatics) to pass between the thorax and abdomen (Figs. 2.91, 2.92, and 2.94). There are three large apertures for the IVC, esophagus, and aorta and a number of small ones.

CAVAL OPENING

The **caval opening** is an aperture in the central tendon primarily for the IVC. Also passing through the caval opening are terminal branches of the right phrenic nerve and a few lymphatic vessels on their way from the liver to the middle phrenic and mediastinal lymph nodes. The caval opening is located to the right of the median plane at the junction of the central tendon's right and middle leaves. The most superior of the three large diaphragmatic apertures, the caval opening lies at the level of the IV disc between the T8 and T9 vertebrae. The IVC is adherent to the margin of the opening; consequently, when the diaphragm contracts during inspiration,

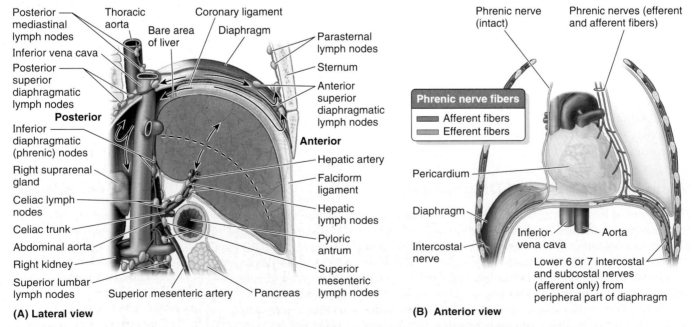

(A) Lateral view

(B) Anterior view

FIGURE 2.93. Lymphatic vessels, lymph nodes, and nerves of diaphragm. A. Lymphatic vessels are formed in two plexuses, one on the superior surface of the diaphragm and the other on its inferior surface; the plexuses communicate freely. **B.** The phrenic nerves supply all of the motor and most of the sensory innervation to the diaphragm. The lower six or seven intercostal and subcostal nerves provide sensory innervation peripherally.

Caval opening
Esophageal hiatus
Aortic hiatus
T8
T10
T12
Sternum
Diaphragm
Inferior vena cava
Esophagus
Aorta
Celiac trunk
Superior mesenteric artery

Lateral view from left

FIGURE 2.94. Apertures of diaphragm. "8-10-12" is a convenient memory device, referring to the thoracic vertebral levels at which the inferior vena cava, esophagus, and aorta penetrate the diaphragm.

it widens the opening and dilates the IVC. These changes facilitate blood flow through this large vein to the heart.

ESOPHAGEAL HIATUS

The **esophageal hiatus** is an oval opening for the esophagus in the muscle of the right crus of the diaphragm at the level of the T10 vertebra. The esophageal hiatus also transmits the anterior and posterior vagal trunks, esophageal branches of the left gastric vessels, and a few lymphatic vessels. The fibers of the right crus of the diaphragm decussate (cross one another) inferior to the hiatus, forming a muscular sphincter for the esophagus that constricts it when the diaphragm contracts. The esophageal hiatus is superior to and to the left of the aortic hiatus. In most individuals (70%), both margins of the hiatus are formed by muscular bundles of the right crus. In others (30%), a superficial muscular bundle from the left crus contributes to the formation of the right margin of the hiatus.

AORTIC HIATUS

The **aortic hiatus** is the opening posterior in the diaphragm for the descending aorta. Because the aorta does not pierce the diaphragm, movements of the diaphragm do not affect blood flow through the aorta during respiration. The aorta passes between the crura of the diaphragm posterior to the median arcuate ligament, which is at the level of the inferior border of the T12 vertebra. The aortic hiatus also transmits the thoracic duct and sometimes the azygos and hemi-azygos veins.

SMALL OPENINGS IN DIAPHRAGM

In addition to the three main apertures, there is a small opening, the **sternocostal triangle** (foramen), between the sternal and costal attachments of the diaphragm. This triangle transmits lymphatic vessels from the diaphragmatic surface of the liver and the superior epigastric vessels. The sympathetic trunks pass deep to the medial arcuate ligament, accompanied by the least splanchnic nerves. There are two small apertures in each crus of the diaphragm; one transmits the greater splanchnic nerve and the other the lesser splanchnic nerve.

Actions of Diaphragm

When the diaphragm contracts, its domes are pulled inferiorly so that the convexity of the diaphragm is somewhat flattened. Although this movement is often described as the "descent of the diaphragm," only the domes of the diaphragm descend. The diaphragm's periphery remains attached to the ribs and cartilages of the inferior six ribs. As the diaphragm descends, it pushes the abdominal viscera inferiorly. This increases the volume of the thoracic cavity and decreases the intrathoracic pressure, resulting in air being taken into the lungs. In addition, the volume of the abdominal cavity decreases slightly and intra-abdominal pressure increases somewhat.

Movements of the diaphragm are also important in circulation because the increased intra-abdominal pressure and decreased intrathoracic pressure help return venous blood to the heart. When the diaphragm contracts, compressing the abdominal viscera, blood in the IVC is forced superiorly into the heart.

The diaphragm is at its most superior level when a person is supine (with the upper body lowered, the *Trendelenburg position*). In this position, the abdominal viscera push the diaphragm superiorly in the thoracic cavity. When a person lies on one side, the hemidiaphragm rises to a more superior level because of the greater push of the viscera on that side. Conversely, the diaphragm assumes an inferior level when a person is sitting or standing. For this reason, people with dyspnea (difficult breathing) prefer to sit up, not lie down; non-tidal (reserve) lung volume is increased, and the diaphragm is working with gravity rather than opposing it.

POSTERIOR ABDOMINAL WALL

The posterior abdominal wall (Figs. 2.95–2.97) is mainly composed of the:

- Five lumbar vertebrae and associated IV discs (centrally).
- Posterior abdominal wall muscles, including the psoas, quadratus lumborum, iliacus, transversus abdominis, and oblique muscles (laterally).
- Diaphragm, which contributes to the superior part of the posterior wall.
- Fascia, including the thoracolumbar fascia.
- Lumbar plexus, composed of the anterior rami of lumbar spinal nerves.
- Fat, nerves, vessels (e.g., aorta and IVC), and lymph nodes.

If observing the anatomy of the posterior abdominal wall in only two-dimensional diagrams, such as Figure 2.97, it would be easy to suppose that it is flat. In observing a dissected cadaver or a transverse cross section such as that in Figures 2.95A & B, it is apparent that the lumbar vertebral column is a marked central prominence in the posterior wall, creating two paravertebral "gutters" on each side. The deepest (most posterior) part of these gutters is occupied by the kidneys and their surrounding fat. The abdominal aorta lies on the anterior aspect of the anteriorly protruding vertebral column. It is usually surprising

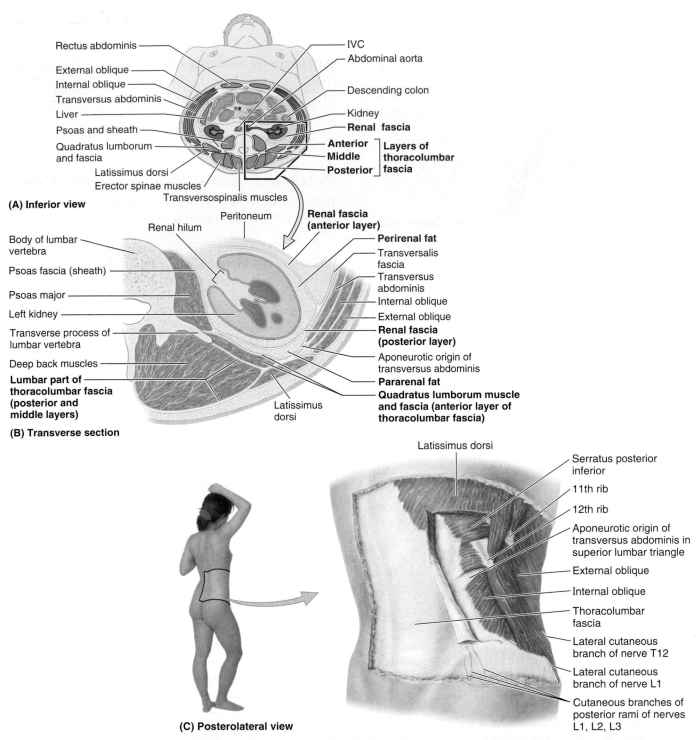

(A) Inferior view

Rectus abdominis
External oblique
Internal oblique
Transversus abdominis
Liver
Psoas and sheath
Quadratus lumborum and fascia
Latissimus dorsi
Erector spinae muscles
Transversospinalis muscles

IVC
Abdominal aorta
Descending colon
Kidney
Renal fascia
Anterior ⎫ Layers of
Middle ⎬ thoracolumbar
Posterior ⎭ fascia

(B) Transverse section

Peritoneum
Renal hilum
Body of lumbar vertebra
Psoas fascia (sheath)
Psoas major
Left kidney
Transverse process of lumbar vertebra
Deep back muscles
Lumbar part of thoracolumbar fascia (posterior and middle layers)
Latissimus dorsi

Renal fascia (anterior layer)
Perirenal fat
Transversalis fascia
Transversus abdominis
Internal oblique
External oblique
Renal fascia (posterior layer)
Aponeurotic origin of transversus abdominis
Pararenal fat
Quadratus lumborum muscle and fascia (anterior layer of thoracolumbar fascia)

(C) Posterolateral view

Latissimus dorsi
Serratus posterior inferior
11th rib
12th rib
Aponeurotic origin of transversus abdominis in superior lumbar triangle
External oblique
Internal oblique
Thoracolumbar fascia
Lateral cutaneous branch of nerve T12
Lateral cutaneous branch of nerve L1
Cutaneous branches of posterior rami of nerves L1, L2, L3

FIGURE 2.95. Fascia and aponeuroses of abdominal wall at level of renal hila. A. The relationships of the muscles, aponeurotic muscle sheaths, and fascia of the abdominal wall are demonstrated in transverse section. The three flat abdominal muscles forming the lateral walls span between complex anterior and posterior aponeurotic formations that ensheath vertically disposed muscles. The thin anterolateral walls (appearing disproportionately thick here) are distensible. Although flexible, the posterior abdominal wall is weight bearing and so is reinforced by the vertebral column and muscles that act on it; thus it is not distensible. *IVC,* inferior vena cava. **B.** Details of the disposition of the aponeurotic and fascial layers of the posterior abdominal wall. For details concerning those of the anterior abdominal wall, see Figure 2.5B. **C.** Dimensional view of the region demonstrated in section in **B.**

to find how close the lower abdominal aorta lies to the anterior abdominal wall in lean individuals (see Fig. B2.37C). Of course, many structures lie anterior to the aorta (SMA, parts of the duodenum, pancreas and left renal vein, etc.) and so these "posterior abdominal structures" may approach the anterior abdominal wall closer than might be expected in thin persons, especially when they are in the supine position.

Fascia of Posterior Abdominal Wall

The posterior abdominal wall is covered with a continuous layer of *endoabdominal fascia* that lies between the parietal peritoneum and the muscles (Fig. 2.95B). The fascia lining the posterior abdominal wall is continuous with the transversalis fascia that lines the transversus abdominis muscle. It is customary to name the fascia according to the structure it covers.

The *psoas fascia* covering the psoas major muscle (*psoas sheath*) is attached medially to the lumbar vertebrae and pelvic brim. The psoas fascia (sheath) is thickened superiorly to form the *medial arcuate ligament* (Fig. 2.91). The psoas fascia fuses laterally with the *quadratus lumborum* and *thoracolumbar fascias* (Fig. 2.95B). Inferior to the iliac crest, the psoas fascia is continuous with the part of the iliac fascia covering the iliacus.

The **thoracolumbar fascia** is an extensive fascial complex attached to the vertebral column medially that, in the lumbar region, has posterior, middle, and anterior layers with muscles enclosed between them (Fig. 2.95B & C). It is thin and transparent where it covers the thoracic parts of the deep muscles, but it is thick and strong in the lumbar region. The enclosure of the vertical deep back muscles (erector spinae) by the **posterior** and **middle layers of the thoracolumbar fascia** on the posterior aspect of the trunk is comparable to the enclosure of the rectus abdominis by the rectus sheath on the anterior aspect (Fig. 2.95A). This posterior sheath is even more formidable than the rectus sheath, however, because of the thickness of its posterior layer and the central attachment to the lumbar vertebrae, as opposed to the rectus sheaths, which lack bony support where they fuse to each other at the linea alba. The lumbar part of this posterior sheath, extending between the 12th rib and the iliac crest, attaches laterally to the internal oblique and transversus abdominis muscles, as does the rectus sheath. However, in contrast to the rectus sheath, the thoracolumbar fascia is not attached to the external oblique; it is attached to the latissimus dorsi (Fig. 2.95B & C).

The **anterior layer of the thoracolumbar fascia** (quadratus lumborum fascia), covering the anterior surface of the quadratus lumborum—a thinner, more transparent layer than the other two layers—attaches to the anterior surfaces

of the transverse processes of the lumbar vertebrae, the iliac crest, and the 12th rib (Figs. 2.95B and 2.97). The anterior layer is continuous laterally with the aponeurotic origin of the transversus abdominis muscle. It thickens superiorly to form the *lateral arcuate ligament* and is adherent inferiorly to the **iliolumbar ligaments** (Fig. 2.97).

Muscles of Posterior Abdominal Wall

The main paired muscles in the posterior abdominal wall (Fig. 2.96; Table 2.14) are the:

- *Psoas major:* passing inferolaterally.
- *Iliacus:* lying along the lateral sides of the inferior part of the psoas major.
- *Quadratus lumborum:* lying adjacent to the transverse processes of the lumbar vertebrae and lateral to superior parts of the psoas major.

The attachments, nerve supply, and main actions of these muscles are summarized in Table 2.14.

PSOAS MAJOR

The long, thick, fusiform **psoas major** lies lateral to the lumbar vertebrae (Figs. 2.96A and 2.97). *Psoas* is a Greek word meaning "muscle of the loin." (Butchers refer to the psoas of animals as the *tenderloin*.) The psoas major passes inferolaterally, deep to the inguinal ligament to reach the lesser trochanter of the femur. The lumbar plexus of nerves is embedded in the posterior part of the psoas major, anterior to the lumbar transverse processes.

ILIACUS

The **iliacus** is a large triangular muscle that lies along the lateral side of the inferior part of the psoas major. Most of

Anterior view **Posterior view**

FIGURE 2.96. Muscles of posterior abdominal wall.

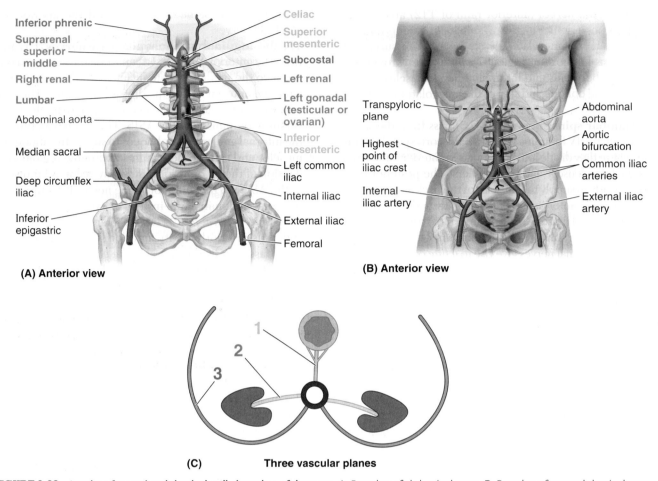

(A) Anterior view

(B) Anterior view

(C)   Three vascular planes

FIGURE 2.98. Arteries of posterior abdominal wall—branches of the aorta. A. Branches of abdominal aorta. **B.** Branches of upper abdominal aorta. **C.** Vascular planes in which branches of abdominal aorta are distributed.

TABLE 2.15. BRANCHES OF ABDOMINAL AORTA

Vascular Plane	Class	Distribution	Abdominal Branches (Arteries)	Vertebral Level
1. Anterior midline	Unpaired visceral	Digestive tract	Celiac	T12
			Superior mesenteric	L1
			Inferior mesenteric	L3
2. Lateral	Paired visceral	Urogenital and endocrine organs	Suprarenal	L1
			Renal	L1
			Gonadal (testicular or ovarian)	L2
3. Posterolateral	Paired parietal (segmental)	Diaphragm; body wall	Subcostal	L2
			Inferior phrenic	T12
			L umbar	L1–L4

abdominal aorta is sufficiently close to the anterior abdominal wall that its pulsations may be detected or apparent when the wall is relaxed (see the blue box "Pulsations of Aorta and Abdominal Aortic Aneurysm" on p. 319).

The **common iliac arteries** diverge and run inferolaterally, following the medial border of the psoas muscles to the pelvic brim. Here each common iliac artery divides into the *internal* and *external iliac arteries.* The internal iliac artery enters the pelvis. (Its course and branches are described in Chapter 3.) The external iliac artery follows the iliopsoas muscle. Just before leaving the abdomen, the external iliac artery gives rise to the *inferior epigastric* and **deep circumflex iliac arteries**, which supply the anterolateral abdominal wall.

Relations of Abdominal Aorta. From superior to inferior, the important anterior relations of the abdominal aorta are the:

- *Celiac plexus* and *ganglion* (see Figs. 2.55B and 2.71).
- Body of the *pancreas* and *splenic vein* (see Fig. 2.71).
- *Left renal vein* (see Figs. 2.83 and 2.92B).
- Horizontal part of the *duodenum*.
- Coils of *small intestine*.

The abdominal aorta descends anterior to the bodies of the T12–L4 vertebrae (Fig. 2.98A). The left lumbar veins pass posterior to the aorta to reach the IVC (Fig. 2.99). On the right, the aorta is related to the azygos vein, cisterna chyi, thoracic duct, right crus of the diaphragm, and right celiac ganglion. On the left, the aorta is related to the left crus of the diaphragm and the left celiac ganglion.

Branches of the Abdominal Aorta. The branches of the descending (thoracic and abdominal) aorta may be described as arising and coursing in three "vascular planes" and can be classified as being visceral or parietal and paired or unpaired (Fig. 2.98A & C; Table 2.15). *Paired parietal branches* of the aorta serve the diaphragm and posterior abdominal wall.

The **median sacral artery,** an *unpaired parietal branch,* may be said to occupy a fourth (posterior) plane because it arises from the posterior aspect of the aorta just proximal to its bifurcation. Although markedly smaller, it could also be considered a midline "continuation" of the aorta, in which case its lateral branches, the **small lumbar arteries** and **lateral sacral branches,** would also be included as part of the paired parietal branches.

VEINS OF POSTERIOR ABDOMINAL WALL

The veins of the posterior abdominal wall are tributaries of the IVC, except for the *left testicular* or *ovarian vein,* which enters the left renal vein instead of entering the IVC (Fig. 2.99). The IVC, the largest vein in the body, has no valves except for a variable, non-functional one at its orifice in the right atrium of the heart. The IVC returns poorly oxygenated blood from the lower limbs, most of the back, the abdominal walls, and the abdominopelvic viscera. Blood from the abdominal viscera passes through the *portal venous system* and the liver before entering the IVC via the *hepatic veins.*

The **inferior vena cava** (IVC) begins anterior to the L5 vertebra by the union of the common iliac veins. The union occurs approximately 2.5 cm to the right of the median plane, inferior to the aortic bifurcation and posterior to the proximal part of the right common iliac artery (see Fig. 2.76). The IVC ascends on the right side of the bodies of the L3–L5 vertebrae and on the right psoas major to the right of the aorta.

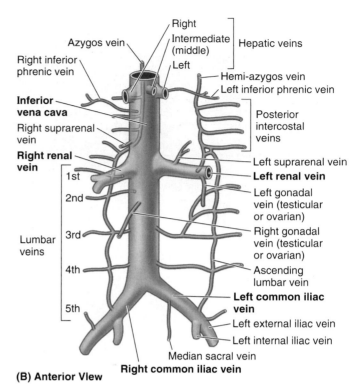

(B) Anterior View

FIGURE 2.99. Inferior vena cava and its tributaries. The asymmetry in the renal and common iliac veins reflects the placement of the IVC to the right of the midline.

The IVC leaves the abdomen by passing through the *caval opening* in the diaphragm and enters the thorax at the T8 vertebral level. Because it is formed one vertebral level inferior to the aortic bifurcation, and traverses the diaphragm four vertebral levels superior to the aortic hiatus, the overall length of the IVC is 7 cm greater than that of the abdominal aorta, although most of the additional length is intrahepatic. The IVC collects poorly oxygenated blood from the lower limbs and non-portal blood from the abdomen and pelvis. Almost all the blood from the gastrointestinal tract is collected by the hepatic portal system and passes through the hepatic veins to the IVC.

The tributaries of the IVC correspond to the paired visceral and parietal branches of the abdominal aorta. The veins that correspond to the unpaired visceral branches of the aorta are instead tributaries of the hepatic portal vein. The blood they carry does ultimately enter the IVC via the hepatic veins, after traversing the liver.

The branches corresponding to the paired visceral branches of the abdominal aorta include the right suprarenal vein, the right and left renal veins, and the right gonadal (testicular or ovarian) vein. The left suprarenal and gonadal veins drain indirectly into the IVC because they are tributaries of the left renal vein.

Paired parietal branches of the IVC include the inferior phrenic veins, the 3rd (L3) and 4th (L4) lumbar veins, and the common iliac veins. The ascending lumbar and azygos veins connect the IVC and SVC, either directly or indirectly sels, esophageal branches of the left gastric vessels) may be injured in surgical procedures on the esophageal hiatus (e.g., repair of a hiatus hernia).

Congenital Diaphragmatic Hernia

In **congenital diaphragmatic hernia** (**CDH**), part of the stomach and intestine herniate through a large posterolateral defect (foramen of Bochdalek) in the region of the lumbocostal trigone of the diaphragm (Fig. B2.34). Herniation almost always occurs on the left owing to the presence of the liver on the right. This type of hernia results from the complex development of the diaphragm. *Posterolateral defect of the diaphragm* is the only relatively common congenital anomaly of the diaphragm, occurring approximately once in 2200 newborn infants (Moore, Persaud, and Torchia, 2012). With abdominal viscera in the limited space of the prenatal pulmonary cavity, one lung (usually the left lung) does not have room to develop normally or to inflate after birth. Because of the consequent *pulmonary hypoplasia*, the mortality rate in these infants is high (approximately 76%).

POSTERIOR ABDOMINAL WALL

Psoas Abscess

Although the prevalence of *tuberculosis* (TB) has been greatly reduced, there is currently a resurgence of TB, especially in Africa and Asia, sometimes in pandemic proportions, owing to AIDS and drug resistance. TB of the vertebral column is quite common. An infection may spread through the blood to the vertebrae (*hematogenous spread*), particularly during childhood. An abscess resulting from tuberculosis in the lumbar region tends to spread from the vertebrae into the psoas fascia (sheath), where it produces a *psoas abscess* (Fig. B2.35). As a consequence, the psoas fascia thickens to form a strong stocking-like tube. Pus from the psoas abscess passes inferiorly along the psoas muscle within this fascial tube over the pelvic brim and deep to the inguinal ligament. The pus usually surfaces in the superior part of the thigh.

Pus can also reach the psoas fascia by passing from the posterior mediastinum when the thoracic vertebrae are diseased.

The inferior part of the *iliac fascia* is often tense and raises a fold that passes to the internal aspect of the iliac crest. The superior part of this fascia is loose and may form a pocket, the *iliacosubfascial fossa*, posterior to the above-mentioned fold. Part of the large intestine, such as the cecum and/or appendix on the right side and the sigmoid colon on the left side, may become trapped in this fossa, causing considerable pain.

Posterior Abdominal Pain

The iliopsoas muscle has extensive, clinically important relations to the kidneys, ureters, cecum, appendix, sigmoid colon, pancreas, lumbar lymph nodes, and nerves of the posterior abdominal wall. When any of these structures is diseased, movement of the iliopsoas usually causes pain. When intra-abdominal inflammation is suspected, the *iliopsoas test* is performed. The person is asked to lie on the unaffected side and extend the thigh on the affected side against the resistance of the examiner's hand (Bickley, 2009). The elicitation of pain with this maneuver is a *positive psoas sign*. An acutely inflamed appendix, for example, will produce a positive right psoas sign (Fig. B2.36).

Because the psoas lies along the vertebral column and the iliacus crosses the sacro-iliac joint, disease of the intervertebral and sacro-iliac joints may cause *spasm of the iliopsoas*, a protective reflex. *Adenocarcinoma of the pancreas* in advanced stages invades the muscles and nerves of the posterior abdominal wall, producing excruciating pain because of the close relationship of the pancreas to the posterior abdominal wall.

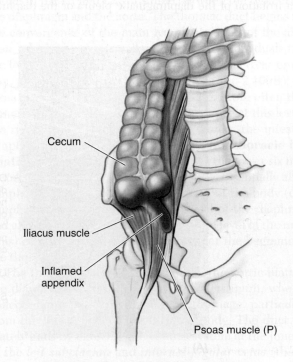

Cecum

Iliacus muscle

Inflamed appendix

Psoas muscle (P)

FIGURE B2.36. Anatomical basis of psoas sign.

FIGURE B2.35. Psoas abscess (*arrow*).

Partial Lumbar Sympathectomy

The treatment of some patients with arterial disease in the lower limbs may include a *partial lumbar sympathectomy,* the surgical removal of two or more lumbar sympathetic ganglia by division of their rami communicantes. Surgical access to the sympathetic trunks is commonly through a lateral extraperitoneal approach because the sympathetic trunks lie retroperitoneally in the extraperitoneal fatty tissue (Fig. 2.97). The surgeon splits the muscles of the anterior abdominal wall and moves the peritoneum medially and anteriorly to expose the medial edge of the psoas major, along which the sympathetic trunk lies. The left trunk is often overlapped slightly by the aorta. The right sympathetic trunk is covered by the IVC. The intimate relationship of the sympathetic trunks to the aorta and IVC also makes these large vessels vulnerable to injury during lumbar sympathectomy. Consequently, the surgeon carefully retracts them to expose the sympathetic trunks that usually lie in the groove between the psoas major laterally and the lumbar vertebral bodies medially. These trunks are often obscured by fat and lymphatic tissue. Knowing that identification of the sympathetic trunks is not easy, great care is taken not to remove inadvertently part of the genitofemoral nerve, lumbar lymphatics, or ureter.

Pulsations of Aorta and Abdominal Aortic Aneurysm

Because the aorta lies posterior to the pancreas and stomach, a tumor of these organs may transmit pulsations of the aorta that could be mistaken for an *abdominal aortic aneurysm,* a localized enlargement of the aorta (Fig. B2.37A & B). Deep palpation of the midabdomen can detect an aneurysm, which usually results from a congenital or acquired weakness of the arterial wall (Fig. B2.37C & D). Pulsations of a large aneurysm can be detected to the left of the midline; the pulsatile mass can be moved easily from side to side. Medical imaging can confirm the diagnosis in doubtful cases.

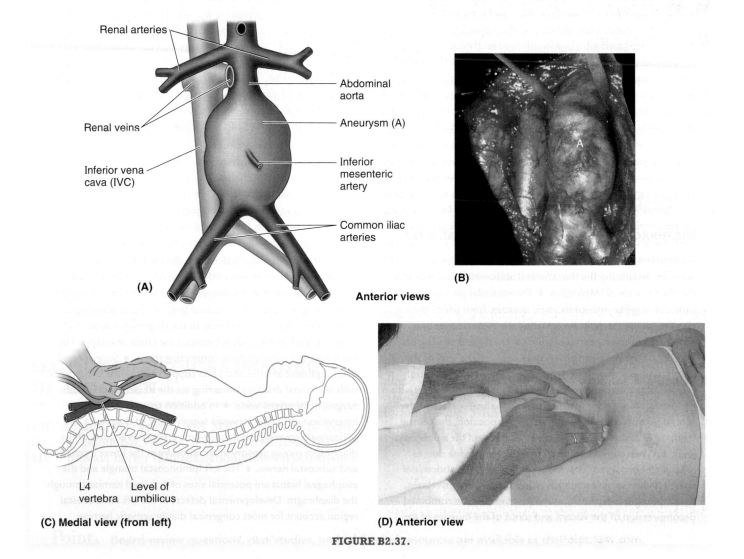

Renal arteries

Abdominal aorta

Aneurysm (A)

Renal veins

Inferior mesenteric artery

Inferior vena cava (IVC)

Common iliac arteries

(A)

(B)

Anterior views

L4 vertebra   Level of umbilicus

(C) Medial view (from left)

(D) Anterior view

FIGURE B2.37.

INTRODUCTION TO PELVIS AND PERINEUM

In common usage, the *pelvis* (L. basin) is the part of the trunk that is inferoposterior to the abdomen, and is the area of transition between the trunk and the lower limbs. The *pelvic cavity* is the inferiormost part of the abdominopelvic cavity. Anatomically, the pelvis is the part of the body surrounded by the *pelvic girdle* (bony pelvis), part of the appendicular skeleton of the lower limb (Fig. 3.1).

The pelvis is subdivided into greater and lesser pelves. The *greater pelvis* is surrounded by the superior pelvic girdle. The greater pelvis is occupied by inferior abdominal viscera, affording them protection similar to the way the superior abdominal viscera are protected by the inferior thoracic cage. The *lesser pelvis* is surrounded by the inferior pelvic girdle, which provides the skeletal framework for both the pelvic cavity and the perineum—compartments of the trunk separated by the musculofascial pelvic diaphragm. Externally, the pelvis is covered or overlapped by the inferior anterolateral abdominal wall anteriorly, the gluteal region of the lower limb posterolaterally, and the perineum inferiorly.

The term *perineum*[1] refers both to the area of the surface of the trunk between the thighs and the buttocks, extending from the coccyx to the pubis, and to the shallow compartment lying deep (superior) to this area but inferior to the pelvic diaphragm. The perineum includes the anus and external genitalia: the penis and scrotum of the male and the vulva of the female.

PELVIC GIRDLE

The **pelvic girdle** is a basin-shaped ring of bones that connects the vertebral column to the two femurs. The primary *functions of the pelvic girdle* are to:

- Bear the weight of the upper body when sitting and standing.
- Transfer that weight from the axial to the lower appendicular skeleton for standing and walking.
- Provide attachment for the powerful muscles of locomotion and posture and those of the abdominal wall, withstanding the forces generated by their actions.

Consequently, the pelvic girdle is strong and rigid, especially compared to the pectoral (shoulder) girdle. Other functions of the pelvic girdle are to:

- Contain and protect the pelvic viscera (inferior parts of the urinary tracts and the internal reproductive organs) and the inferior abdominal viscera (intestines), while permitting passage of their terminal parts (and, in females, a full-term fetus) via the perineum.
- Provide support for the abdominopelvic viscera and gravid (pregnant) uterus.
- Provide attachment for the erectile bodies of the external genitalia.
- Provide attachment for the muscles and membranes that assist the functions listed above by forming the pelvic floor and filling gaps that exist in or around it.

---

[1]The term *perineum* has been used in different ways, in different languages, and in different circumstances. In its most restricted sense, and in obstetrics, it has been used to refer to the area superficial to the perineal body, between the vulva or scrotum and the anus or to the perineal body itself. In an intermediate sense, it has included only the *perineal region*, a superficial (surface) area bounded by the thighs laterally, the mons pubis anteriorly, and the coccyx posteriorly. In its widest sense, as used in *Terminologia Anatomica* (the international anatomical terminology) and in this book, it refers to the region of the body that includes all structures of the anal and urogenital triangles, superficial and deep, extending as far superiorly as the inferior fascia of the pelvic diaphragm.

pelvic aperture) (Figs. 3.1A and 3.2A). The bony edge (rim) surrounding and defining the pelvic inlet is the **pelvic brim,** formed by the:

- *Promontory* and *ala of the sacrum* (superior surface of its lateral part, adjacent to the body of the sacrum).
- A **right** and **left linea terminalis** (terminal line) together form a continuous oblique ridge consisting of the:
  - **Arcuate line** on the inner surface of the ilium.
  - *Pecten pubis* (pectineal line) and *pubic crest,* forming the superior border of the superior ramus and body of the pubis.

The **pubic arch** is formed by the **ischiopubic rami** (conjoined inferior rami of the pubis and ischium) of the two sides (Fig. 3.2A & C). These rami meet at the *pubic symphysis,* their inferior borders defining the **subpubic angle** (Fig. 3.3). The width of the subpubic angle is determined by the distance between the right and the left ischial tuberosities, which can be measured with the gloved fingers in the vagina during a pelvic examination.

The **pelvic outlet** (inferior pelvic aperture) is bounded by the (Figs. 3.1A and 3.2A):

- *Pubic arch* anteriorly.
- *Ischial tuberosities* laterally.
- Inferior margin of the *sacrotuberous ligament* (running between the coccyx and the ischial tuberosity) *posterolaterally.*
- *Tip of the coccyx* posteriorly.

The **greater pelvis** (false pelvis) is the part of the pelvis (Fig. 3.1):

- Superior to the pelvic inlet.
- Bounded by the iliac alae posterolaterally and the antero-superior aspect of the S1 vertebra posteriorly.
- Occupied by abdominal viscera (e.g., the ileum and sigmoid colon).

The **lesser pelvis** (true pelvis) is the part of the pelvis:

- Between the *pelvic inlet* and the *pelvic outlet.*
- Bounded by the pelvic surfaces of the hip bones, sacrum, and coccyx.
- That includes the true *pelvic cavity* and the deep parts of the *perineum* (perineal compartment), specifically the ischio-anal fossae (Fig. 3.1B).
- That is of major obstetrical and gynecological significance.

The concave superior surface of the musculofascial *pelvic diaphragm* forms the floor of the true pelvic cavity, which is thus deepest centrally. The convex inferior surface of the pelvic diaphragm forms the roof of the perineum, which is therefore shallow centrally and deep peripherally. Its lateral parts (ischio-anal fossae) extending well up into the lesser pelvis. The terms *pelvis, lesser pelvis,* and *pelvic cavity* are commonly used incorrectly, as if they were synonymous terms.

Orientation of Pelvic Girdle

When a person is in the anatomical position, the right and left anterior superior iliac spines (ASISs) and the anterior aspect of the pubic symphysis lie in the same vertical plane (Fig. 3.2B & C). When a pelvic girdle in this position is viewed anteriorly (Fig. 3.2A), the tip of the coccyx appears close to the center of the pelvic inlet, and the pubic bones and pubic symphysis constitute more of a weight-bearing floor than an anterior wall. In the median view (Fig. 3.1A), the *sacral promontory* is located directly superior to the center of the pelvic outlet (site of the perineal body). Consequently, the curved axis of the pelvis intersects the axis of the abdominal cavity at an oblique angle.

The pelvic girdles of males and females differ in several respects (Fig. 3.3; Table 3.1). These sexual differences are related mainly to the heavier build and larger muscles of most men and to the adaptation of the pelvis (particularly the lesser pelvis) in women for parturition (childbearing). See the blue box "Variations in Male and Female Pelves," on p. 334.

Joints and Ligaments of Pelvic Girdle

The primary joints of the pelvic girdle are the *sacro-iliac joints* and the *pubic symphysis* (Fig. 3.4A). The sacro-iliac joints link the **axial skeleton** (skeleton of the trunk, composed of the vertebral column at this level) and the **inferior appendicular skeleton** (skeleton of the lower limb). The lumbosacral and sacrococcygeal joints, although joints of the axial skeleton, are directly related to the pelvic girdle. Strong ligaments support and strengthen these joints.

SACRO-ILIAC JOINTS

The **sacro-iliac joints** are strong, weight-bearing compound joints, consisting of an anterior synovial joint (between the ear-shaped *auricular surfaces* of the sacrum and ilium, covered with articular cartilage) and a posterior syndesmosis (between the *tuberosities* of these bones) (Fig. 3.4B). The auricular surfaces of this synovial joint have irregular but congruent elevations and depressions that interlock (Figs. 3.5A-C). The sacro-iliac joints differ from most synovial joints in that limited mobility is allowed, a consequence of their role in transmitting the weight of most of the body to the hip bones.

Weight is transferred from the axial skeleton to the ilia via the sacro-iliac ligaments (Fig. 3.4A), and then to the femurs during standing, and to the ischial tuberosities during sitting. As long as tight apposition is maintained between the articular surfaces, the sacro-iliac joints remain stable. Unlike a keystone at the top of an arch, the sacrum is actually suspended between the iliac bones and is firmly attached to them by posterior and interosseous sacro-iliac ligaments (Fig. 3.5A).

The thin **anterior sacro-iliac ligaments** are merely the anterior part of the fibrous capsule of the synovial part of the joint (Figs. 3.5A and 3.6). The abundant **interosseous sacro-iliac ligaments** (lying deep between the tuberosities of the sacrum and ilium and occupying an area of approximately 10 cm²) are the primary structures involved in transferring

Antero-inferior Views

FIGURE 3.3. Pelvic girdles of male and female. Pubic arches, or subpubic angles typical for each gender (male = *red;* female = *green*) can be approximated by spreading index and middle finger (demonstrating narrow subpubic angle of male pelvis) or thumb and index finger (demonstrating wider subpubic angle of female pelvis).

TABLE 3.1. COMPARISON OF MALE AND FEMALE BONY PELVES

Bony Pelvis	Male (♂)	Female (♀)
General structure	Thick and heavy	Thin and light
Greater pelvis (false pelvis)	Deep	Shallow
Lesser pelvis (true pelvis)	Narrow and deep, tapering	Wide and shallow, cylindrical
Pelvic inlet (superior pelvic aperture)	Heart-shaped, narrow	Oval and rounded; wide
Pelvic outlet (inferior pelvic aperture)	Comparatively small	Comparatively large
Pubic arch and subpubic angle	Narrow (<70°)	Wide (>80°)
Obturator foramen	Round	Oval
Acetabulum	Large	Small
Greater sciatic notch	Narrow (~70°); inverted V	Almost 90°

5th lumbar vertebra (L5)
Lumbosacral joint
Ilium
Sacro-iliac joint
Sacrum
Sacro-coccygeal joint
Coccyx
Acetabulum
Head of femur
Femur
Pubic symphysis

(A) Anterior view—joints of pelvic girdle

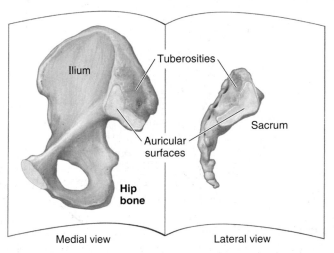

Ilium
Tuberosities
Sacrum
Auricular surfaces
Hip bone
Medial view
Lateral view

(B) Open book view of articulating surfaces of sacro-iliac joint

FIGURE 3.4. **Joints of pelvic girdle. A.** The sacro-iliac joints unite the axial and inferior appendicular skeletons. The lumbosacral and sacrococcygeal joints are joints of the axial skeleton directly related to the pelvic girdle. **B.** The auricular surfaces and tuberosities of the ilium and sacrum are demonstrated in an "opened book" view.

the weight of the upper body from the axial skeleton to the two ilia of the appendicular skeleton (Fig. 3.5A).

The **posterior sacro-iliac ligaments** are the posterior external continuation of the same mass of fibrous tissue (Figs. 3.5A and 3.6). Because the fibers of the interosseous and posterior sacro-iliac ligaments run obliquely upward and outward from the sacrum, the axial weight pushing down on the sacrum actually pulls the ilia inward (medially) so that they compress the sacrum between them, locking the irregular but congruent surfaces of the sacro-iliac joints together. The *iliolumbar ligaments* are accessory ligaments to this mechanism (Fig. 3.6).

Inferiorly, the posterior sacro-iliac ligaments are joined by fibers extending from the posterior margin of the ilium (between the posterior superior and posterior inferior iliac spines) and the base of the coccyx to form the massive *sacrotuberous ligament* (Fig. 3.6). This ligament passes from the posterior ilium and lateral sacrum and coccyx to the ischial tuberosity, transforming the sciatic notch of the hip bone into a

large sciatic foramen. The *sacrospinous ligament*, passing from lateral sacrum and coccyx to the ischial spine, further subdivides this foramen into *greater* and *lesser sciatic foramina*.

Most of the time, movement at the sacro-iliac joint is limited by interlocking of the articulating bones and the sacro-iliac ligaments to slight gliding and rotary movements (Fig. 3.5D). When landing after a high jump or when weightlifting in the standing position, exceptional force is transmitted through the bodies of the lumbar vertebrae to the superior end of the sacrum. Because this transfer of weight occurs anterior to the axis of the sacro-iliac joints, the superior end of the sacrum is pushed inferiorly and anteriorly. However, rotation of the superior sacrum is counterbalanced by the strong sacrotuberous and sacrospinous ligaments that anchor the inferior end of the sacrum to the ischium, preventing its superior and posterior rotation (Figs. 3.5D and 3.6). By allowing only slight upward movement of the inferior end of the sacrum relative to the hip bones, resilience is provided to the sacro-iliac region when the vertebral column sustains sudden increases in force or weight.

PUBIC SYMPHYSIS

The **pubic symphysis** consists of a fibrocartilaginous interpubic disc and surrounding ligaments uniting the bodies of the pubic bones in the median plane (Fig. 3.7). The **interpubic disc** is generally wider in women. The ligaments joining the bones are thickened at the superior and inferior margins of the symphysis, forming superior and inferior pubic ligaments. The **superior pubic ligament** connects the superior aspects of the pubic bodies and interpubic disc, extending as far laterally as the pubic tubercles. The **inferior** (arcuate) **pubic ligament** is a thick arch of fibers that connects the inferior aspects of the joint components, rounding off the *subpubic angle* as it forms the apex of the *pubic arch* (Fig. 3.3). The decussating, fibers of the tendinous attachments of the rectus abdominis and external oblique muscles also strengthen the pubic symphysis anteriorly (see Chapter 2).

LUMBOSACRAL JOINTS

L5 and S1 vertebrae articulate at the anterior *intervertebral (IV) joint* formed by the L5/S1 *IV disc* between their bodies (Fig. 3.4A) and at two posterior *zygapophysial joints* (facet joints) between the articular processes of these vertebrae (Fig. 3.1). The facets on the S1 vertebra face posteromedially, interlocking with the anterolaterally facing inferior articular facets of the L5 vertebra, preventing the lumbar vertebra from sliding anteriorly down the incline of the sacrum. These joints are further strengthened by fan-like **iliolumbar ligaments** radiating from the transverse processes of the L5 vertebra to the ilia (Fig. 3.6).

SACROCOCCYGEAL JOINT

The **sacrococcygeal joint** is a secondary cartilaginous joint (Fig. 3.4A) with an IV disc. Fibrocartilage and ligaments join the apex of the sacrum to the base of the coccyx. The **anterior** and **posterior sacrococcygeal ligaments** are long strands that reinforce the joint (Fig. 3.6).

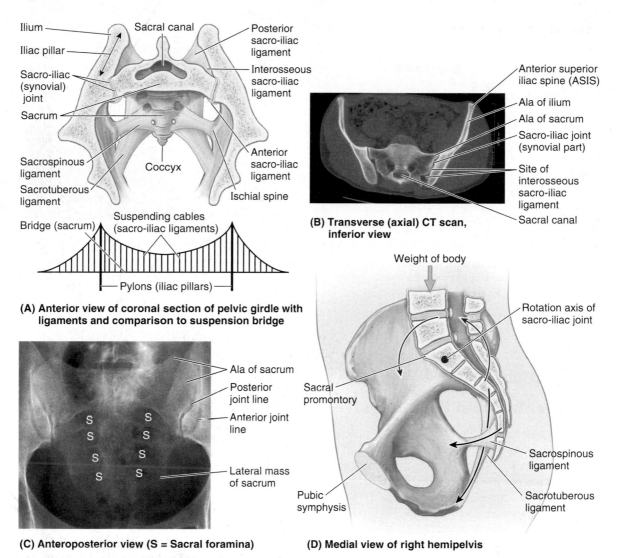

FIGURE 3.5. Sacro-iliac joints and pubic symphysis with associated ligaments. A. The posterior half of a coronally sectioned pelvic girdle and its sacro-iliac joints are shown. The strong interosseous sacro-iliac ligaments lie deep (antero-inferior) to the posterior sacro-iliac ligaments and consist of shorter fibers connecting the tuberosity of the sacrum to the tuberosity of the ilium, suspending the sacrum from the ilia (left and right ilium) like the central portion of a suspension bridge is suspended from the pylons at each end. **B.** CT scan of the synovial and syndesmotic portions of the sacro-iliac joint. **C.** Because the articulating surfaces are irregular and slightly oblique, the anterior and posterior parts of the joint appear separately in an AP radiograph. **D.** The weight of the body is transmitted to the sacrum anterior to the axis of rotation at the sacro-iliac joint. The tendency for increased weight or force to rotate the upper sacrum anteriorly and inferiorly is resisted by the strong sacrotuberous and sacrospinous ligaments anchoring the inferior sacrum and coccyx to the ischium.

FIGURE 3.6. Ligaments of pelvic girdle. The ligaments of hip joint (shown but not labeled) are identified in Chapter 5 (Lower Limb).

(A) Antero-inferior view of pubic bones and pubic symphysis   **(B) Anteroposterior radiograph of pubic bones and symphysis**

FIGURE 3.7. Pubic symphysis. A. The pubic symphysis is a secondary cartilaginous joint between the bodies of the pubic bones. **B.** Radiographic appearance of the pubic symphysis in the anatomical position. In this position, the bodies of the pubic bones are nearly horizontal, and the joint appears foreshortened.

PELVIC GIRDLE

Variations in Male and Female Pelves

Although anatomical differences between male and female pelves are usually clear cut, the pelvis of any person may have some features of the opposite sex. The pelvic types shown in Figure B3.1A and C are most common in males, B and A in white females, and B and C in black females, whereas D is uncommon in both sexes. The **gynecoid pelvis** is the normal female type (Fig. B3.1B); its pelvic inlet typically has a rounded oval shape and a wide transverse diameter. An **platypelloid** or markedly **android** (masculine or funnel-shaped) **pelvis** in a woman may present hazards to successful vaginal delivery of a fetus (Fig. B3.1A).

In *forensic medicine* (the application of medical and anatomical knowledge for the purposes of law), identification of human skeletal remains usually involves the diagnosis of sex. A prime focus of attention is the pelvic girdle because sexual differences usually are clearly visible. Even fragments of the pelvic girdle are useful in determining sex.

Pelvic Diameters (Conjugates)

The size of the lesser pelvis is particularly important in obstetrics because it is the bony canal through which the fetus passes during normal child birth. To determine the capacity of the female pelvis for childbearing, the diameters of the lesser pelvis are noted radiographically or manually during a pelvic examination. The minimum

FIGURE B3.1.

anteroposterior (AP) diameter of the lesser pelvis, the **true** (obstetrical) **conjugate** from the middle of the sacral promontory to the posterosuperior margin (closest point) of the pubic symphysis (Fig. B3.2A & B), is the narrowest *fixed distance* through which the baby's head must pass in a vaginal delivery. This distance, however, cannot be measured directly during a pelvic examination because of the presence of the

bladder. Consequently, the **diagonal conjugate** (Fig. B3.2B) is measured by palpating the sacral promontory with the tip of the *middle finger,* using the other hand to mark the level of the inferior margin of the pubic symphysis on the examining hand (Fig. B3.2C). After the examining hand is withdrawn, the distance between the tip of the *index finger* (1.5 cm shorter than the middle finger) and the marked level of the pubic symphysis is measured to estimate the true conjugate, which should be 11.0 cm or greater.

In all pelvic girdles, the ischial spines extend toward each other, and the **interspinous distance** between them is normally the narrowest part of the **pelvic canal** (the passageway through the pelvic inlet, lesser pelvis, and pelvic outlet) through which a baby's head must pass at birth (Fig. B3.2B), but it is not a fixed distance (see the blue box "Relaxation of Pelvic Ligaments and Increased Joint Mobility During Pregnancy," p. 336). During a pelvic examination, if the ischial tuberosities are far enough apart to permit three fingers to enter the vagina side by side, the subpubic angle is considered sufficiently wide to permit passage of an average fetal head at full term.

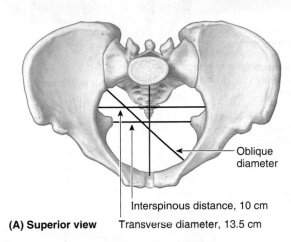

(A) Superior view
- Oblique diameter
- Interspinous distance, 10 cm
- Transverse diameter, 13.5 cm

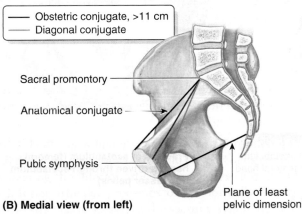

— Obstetric conjugate, >11 cm
— Diagonal conjugate

- Sacral promontory
- Anatomical conjugate
- Pubic symphysis
- Plane of least pelvic dimension

(B) Medial view (from left)

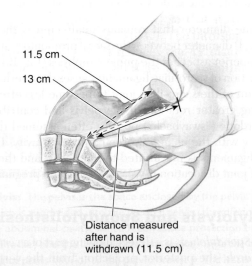

- 11.5 cm
- 13 cm
- Distance measured after hand is withdrawn (11.5 cm)

(C) Medial view (from right)

FIGURE B3.2.

Pelvic Fractures

Anteroposterior compression of the pelvis occurs during crush accidents (as when a heavy object falls on the pelvis, Fig. B3.3A). This type of trauma commonly produces *fractures of the pubic rami.* When the pelvis is compressed laterally, the acetabula and ilia are squeezed toward each other and may be broken.

Fractures of the bony pelvic ring are almost always multiple fractures or a fracture combined with a joint dislocation. To illustrate this, try breaking a pretzel ring at just one point. Some pelvic fractures result from the tearing away of bone by the strong ligaments associated with the sacro-iliac joints. (These ligaments are shown in Figs 3.3 and 3.4A.)

Pelvic fractures can result from direct trauma to the pelvic bones, such as occurs during an automobile accident (Fig. B3.3A), or be caused by forces transmitted to these bones from the lower limbs during falls on the feet (Fig. B3.3B). Weak areas of the pelvis, where fractures often occur, are the pubic rami, the acetabula (or the area immediately surrounding them), the region of the sacro-iliac joints, and the alae of the ilium.

Pelvic fractures may cause injury to pelvic soft tissues, blood vessels, nerves, and organs. Fractures in the pubo-obturator area are relatively common and are often complicated because of their relationship to the urinary bladder and urethra, which may be ruptured or torn.

Falls on the feet or buttocks from a high ladder may drive the head of the femur through the acetabulum into the pelvic cavity, injuring pelvic viscera, nerves, and vessels. In individuals younger than 17 years of age, the acetabulum may fracture through the triradiate cartilage into its three developmental parts (Fig. 3.2C) or the bony acetabular margins may be torn away.

Pelvic diaphragm
Pubic symphysis
Levator ani
 Puborectalis
 Pubococcygeus
 Iliococcygeus
Coccygeus
Sacro-iliac joint

Urogenital hiatus
Perineal body
Ischial tuberosity
External anal sphincter
Anococcygeal ligament (body)
Greater sciatic foramen
Sacrospinous ligament

(A) Inferior view of perineum, lithotomy position

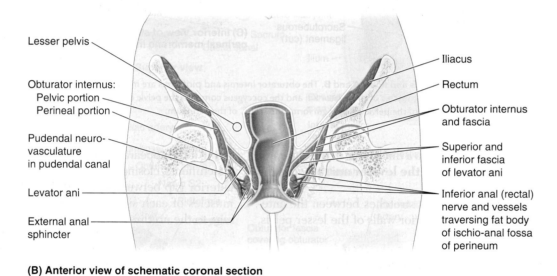

Lesser pelvis
Obturator internus:
 Pelvic portion
 Perineal portion
Pudendal neuro-vasculature in pudendal canal
Levator ani
External anal sphincter

Iliacus
Rectum
Obturator internus and fascia
Superior and inferior fascia of levator ani
Inferior anal (rectal) nerve and vessels traversing fat body of ischio-anal fossa of perineum

(B) Anterior view of schematic coronal section

FIGURE 3.11. Pelvic diaphragm and anorectum in situ. A and **B.** The components of the pelvic diaphragm (levator ani and coccygeus) form the floor of the pelvic cavity and the roof of the perineum. **B.** The basin-like nature for which the pelvis was named is evident in this coronal section. The fat-filled ischio-anal fossae of the perineum also lie within the bony ring of the lesser pelvis.

The levator ani consists of three parts, often poorly demarcated but designated according to attachments and fiber course (Figs. 3.9A & D, 3.10C, and 3.11):

- **Puborectalis:** the thicker, narrower, medial part of the levator ani, consisting of muscle fibers that are continuous between the posterior aspects of the bodies of the right and left pubic bones. It forms a U-shaped muscular sling (*puborectal sling*) that passes posterior to the anorectal junction (Fig. 3.12), bounding the urogenital hiatus. This part plays a major role in maintaining fecal continence.

- **Pubococcygeus:** the wider but thinner intermediate part of the levator ani, which arises lateral to the puborectalis

from the posterior aspect of the body of the pubis and anterior tendinous arch (Figs. 3.9A & D, 3.10C, and 3.11). It passes posteriorly in a nearly horizontal plane; its lateral fibers attach to the coccyx and its medial fibers merge with those of the contralateral muscle to form a fibrous raphe or tendinous plate, part of the **anococcygeal body** or ligament between the anus and the coccyx (often referred to clinically as the "levator plate").

Shorter muscular slips of the pubococcygeus extending medially and blending with the fascia around midline structures are named for the structure near their termination: *pubovaginalis* (females), *puboprostaticus* (males), *puboperinealis*, and *pubo-analis*.

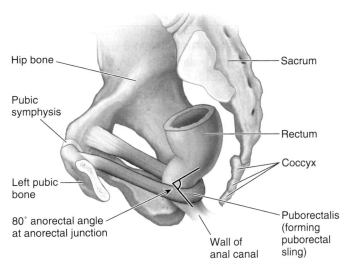

Hip bone

Pubic symphysis

Left pubic bone

80° anorectal angle at anorectal junction

Sacrum

Rectum

Coccyx

Puborectalis (forming puborectal sling)

Wall of anal canal

Medial view from left

FIGURE 3.12. Puborectalis muscle. Most of the left hip bone has been removed to demonstrate that this part of the levator ani is formed by continuous muscle fibers following a U-shaped course around the ano-rectal junction. The puborectalis thus forms a puborectal sling, the tonus of which is responsible for maintaining the anorectal angle (perineal flexure).

- **Iliococcygeus:** the posterolateral part of the levator ani, which arises from the posterior tendinous arch and ischial spine. It is thin and often poorly developed (appearing more aponeurotic than muscular), and also blends with the anococcygeal body posteriorly.

The levator ani forms a dynamic floor for supporting the abdominopelvic viscera. It is tonically contracted most of the time to support the abdominopelvic viscera, and to assist in maintaining urinary and fecal continence. It is actively contracted during activities such as forced expiration, coughing, sneezing, vomiting, and fixation of the trunk during strong movements of the upper limbs (e.g., when lifting heavy objects), primarily to increase support of the viscera during periods of increased intra-abdominal pressure, and perhaps secondarily to contribute to the increased pressure (to aid expulsion).

Penetrated centrally by the anal canal, the levator ani is funnel shaped, with the U-shaped puborectalis looping around the "funnel spout"; its tonic contraction bends the anorectum anteriorly. Active contraction of the (voluntary) puborectalis portion is important in maintaining fecal continence immediately after rectal filling or during peristalsis when the rectum is full and the involuntary sphincter muscle is inhibited (relaxed).

The levator ani must relax to allow urination and defecation. The increased intra-abdominal pressure for defecation is provided by contraction of the (thoracic) diaphragm and muscles of the anterolateral abdominal wall. Acting together, the parts of the levator ani elevate the pelvic floor after their relaxation and the consequent descent of the pelvic diaphragm that occurs during urination and defecation.

Peritoneum and Peritoneal Cavity of Pelvis

The parietal peritoneum lining the abdominal cavity continues inferiorly into the pelvic cavity, but does not reach the pelvic floor. Instead, it reflects onto the pelvic viscera, remaining separated from the pelvic floor by the pelvic viscera and the surrounding pelvic fascia (Table 3.3). Except for the ovaries and uterine tubes, the pelvic viscera are not completely ensheathed by the peritoneum, lying inferior to it for the main part. Only their superior and superolateral surfaces are covered with peritoneum. Only the uterine tubes (except for their ostia, which are open) are intraperitoneal and suspended by a mesentery. The ovaries, although suspended in the peritoneal cavity by a mesentery, are not covered with glistening peritoneum; instead a special, relatively dull epithelium of cuboidal cells (*germinal epithelium*) covers them.

A loose areolar (fatty) layer between the transversalis fascia and the parietal peritoneum of the inferior part of the anterior abdominal wall allows the bladder to expand between these layers as it becomes distended with urine. The region superior to the bladder (*1* in Table 3.3) is the only site where the parietal peritoneum is not firmly bound to the underlying structures. Consequently, the level at which the peritoneum reflects onto the superior surface of the bladder, creating the **supravesical fossa** (*2* in Table 3.3), is variable, depending on the fullness of the bladder. When the peritoneum reflects from the abdominopelvic wall onto the pelvic viscera and fascia, a series of folds and fossae is created (*2–7* in Table 3.3).

In the female, as the peritoneum at or near the midline reaches the posterior border of the roof of the bladder, it reflects onto the anterior aspect of the uterus at the isthmus of the uterus (see "Female Internal Genital Organs," p. 382); thus it is not related to the anterior vaginal fornix, which is subperitoneal in location. The peritoneum passes over the fundus of the uterus and descends the entire posterior aspect of the uterus onto the posterior vaginal wall before reflecting superiorly onto the anterior wall of the inferior rectum (rectal ampulla). The "pocket" thus formed between the uterus and the rectum is the **recto-uterine pouch** (cul-de-sac of Douglas) (*6* in Table 3.3C). The median recto-uterine pouch is often described as being the inferiormost extent of the peritoneal cavity in the female, but often its lateral extensions on each side of the rectum, the **pararectal fossae,** are deeper.

Prominent peritoneal ridges, the **recto-uterine folds,** formed by underlying fascial ligaments demarcate the lateral boundaries of the pararectal fossae (Table 3.3A). As the peritoneum passes up and over the uterus in the middle of the pelvic cavity, a double peritoneal fold, the *broad ligament of the uterus,* extends between the uterus and the lateral pelvic wall on each side, forming a partition that separates the paravesical fossae and pararectal fossae of each side. The uterine tubes, ovaries, ligaments of the ovaries, and round ligaments of the uterus are enclosed within the broad ligaments. Subdivisions of the broad ligament related to these structures will be discussed with the uterus later in this chapter. Recall that in

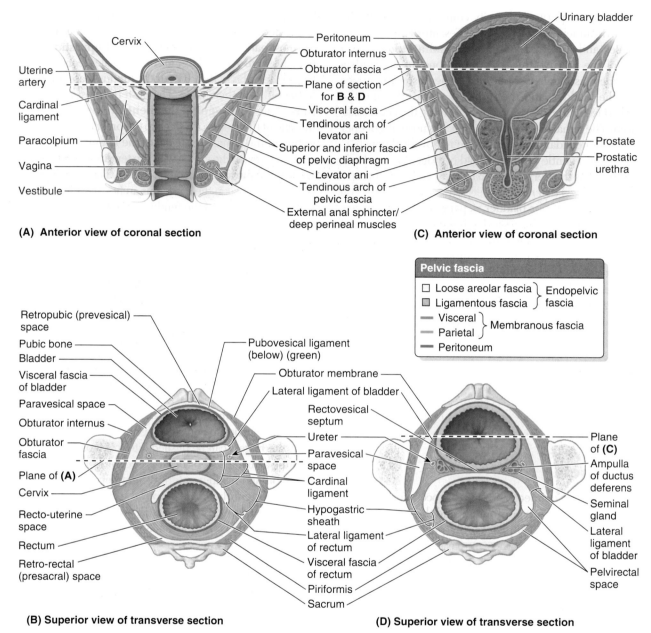

(A) Anterior view of coronal section

(C) Anterior view of coronal section

(B) Superior view of transverse section

(D) Superior view of transverse section

FIGURE 3.13. Pelvic fascia: endopelvic fascia and fascial ligaments. Coronal and transverse sections of female (**A** and **B**) and male (**C** and **D**) pelves demonstrating the parietal and visceral pelvic fascia and the endopelvic fascia between them, with its ligamentous and loose areolar components.

they are also referred to as ligaments. The anteriormost lamina, the **lateral ligament of the bladder,** passes to the bladder, conveying the superior vesical arteries and veins. The posteriormost lamina (*lateral rectal ligament*) passes to the rectum, conveying the middle rectal artery and vein.

In the male, the middle lamina forms a relatively thin fascial partition, the **rectovesical septum** (Fig. 3.13D), between the posterior surface of the bladder and the prostate anteriorly and the rectum posteriorly. In the female, the middle lamina is markedly more substantial than the other two, passing medially to the uterine cervix and vagina as the **cardinal ligament** (transverse cervical ligament) (Figs. 3.13B and 3.14A & B).

In its superiormost portion, at the base of the peritoneal broad ligament, the uterine artery runs medially toward the

cervix while the ureters pass immediately inferior to them. The ureters pass on each side of the cervix heading anteriorly toward the bladder. This relationship ("water passing under the bridge") is an especially important one for surgeons (see the blue box "Iatrogenic Injury of the Ureters" on p. 361). The cardinal ligament, and the way in which the uterus normally "rests" on top of the bladder, provide the main passive support for the uterus. The perineal muscles provide dynamic support for the uterus by contracting during moments of increased intra-abdominal pressure (sneezing, coughing, etc.). Passive and dynamic supports together resist the tendency for the uterus to fall or be pushed through the hollow tube formed by the vagina (uterine prolapse). The cardinal ligament has enough fibrous content to anchor wide loops of suture during surgical repairs.

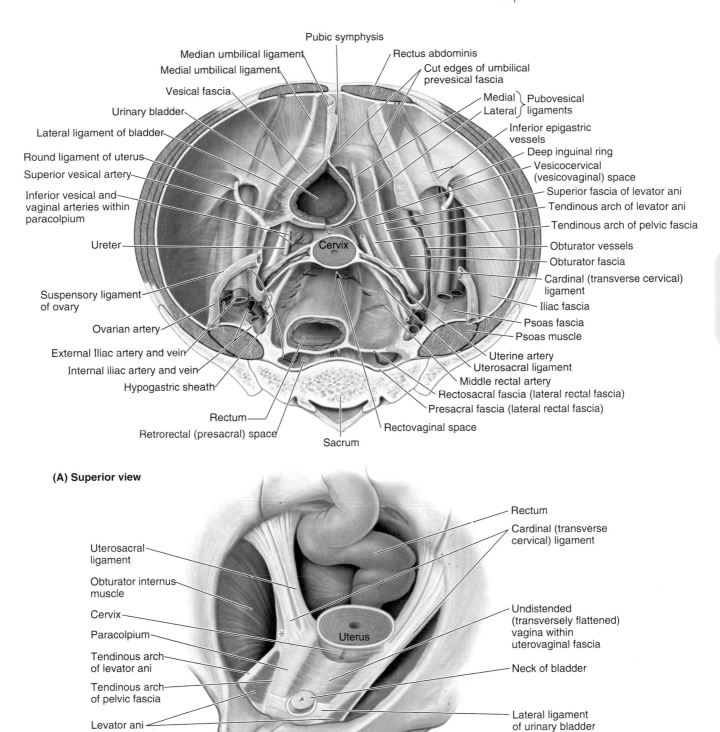

(A) Superior view

(B) Left anterolateral view

∗ Ischial spine

FIGURE 3.14. Pelvic fascial ligaments. A. Peritoneum and loose areolar endopelvic fascia have been removed to demonstrate the pelvic fascial ligaments found inferior to the peritoneum but superior to the female pelvic floor (pelvic diaphragm). The tendinous arch of the levator ani is a thickening of the obturator (parietal) fascia, providing the anterolateral attachment of the levator ani. The tendinous arch of the pelvic fascia (highlighted in *green*) is a thickening at the point of reflection of parietal membranous fascia onto the pelvic viscera, where it becomes visceral membranous fascia. **B.** Fascial ligaments supporting the vagina and cervix of the uterus. Since the posterior part of the urinary bladder rests on the anterior wall of the vagina, the paracolpium supports the vagina and contributes to the support of the bladder.

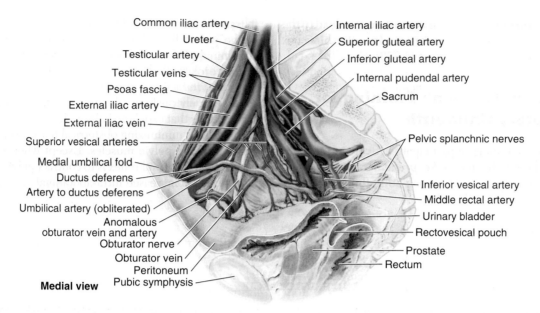

FIGURE 3.15. Neurovascular relationships of pelvis. The neurovascular structures of the male pelvis are shown. Generally, the pelvic veins lie between the pelvic arteries (which lie medially or internally), and the somatic nerves (which lie laterally or externally).

first, followed by the associated pelvic veins, and then the somatic nerves of the pelvis.

Pelvic Arteries

The pelvis is richly supplied with arteries, among which multiple anastomoses occur, providing an extensive collateral circulation. Information concerning the origin, course, distribution, and anastomoses of the arteries of the pelvis is provided in Figure 3.16 and Table 3.4. The following text provides additional information not provided in the table.

Six main arteries enter the lesser pelvis of females: the paired internal iliac and ovarian arteries, and the unpaired median sacral and superior rectal arteries. Since the testicular arteries do not enter the lesser pelvis, only four main arteries enter the lesser pelvis of males.

INTERNAL ILIAC ARTERY

The **internal iliac artery** is the principal artery of the pelvis, supplying most of the blood to the pelvic viscera and some to the musculoskeletal part of the pelvis; however, it also supplies branches to the gluteal region, medial thigh regions, and the perineum (Fig. 3.15).

Each internal iliac artery, approximately 4 cm long, begins as the *common iliac artery* and bifurcates into the internal and external iliac arteries at the level of the IV disc between the L5 and S1 vertebrae. The ureter crosses the common iliac artery or its terminal branches at or immediately distal to the bifurcation. The internal iliac artery is separated from the sacro-iliac joint by the internal iliac vein and the lumbosacral trunk. It descends posteromedially into the lesser pelvis, medial to the external iliac vein and obturator nerve, and lateral to the peritoneum.

Anterior Division of Internal Iliac Artery. Although variations are common, the internal iliac artery usually ends at the superior edge of the greater sciatic foramen by dividing into anterior and posterior divisions (trunks). The branches of the **anterior division of the internal iliac artery** are mainly visceral (i.e., they supply the bladder, rectum, and reproductive organs), but they also include parietal branches that pass to the thigh and buttocks (Fig. 3.17A & B). The arrangement of the visceral branches is variable.

Umbilical Artery. Before birth, the umbilical arteries are the main continuation of the internal iliac arteries, passing along the lateral pelvic wall and then ascending the anterior abdominal wall to and through the umbilical ring into the umbilical cord.

Prenatally, the **umbilical arteries** conduct oxygen- and nutrient-deficient blood to the placenta for replenishment. When the umbilical cord is cut, the distal parts of these vessels no longer function and become occluded distal to branches that pass to the bladder. The *occluded parts* form fibrous cords called the *medial umbilical ligaments* (Figs. 3.16 and 3.17A & B). The ligaments raise folds of peritoneum (*medial umbilical folds*) on the deep surface of the anterior abdominal wall (see Chapter 2).

Postnatally, the *patent parts of the umbilical arteries* run antero-inferiorly between the urinary bladder and the lateral wall of the pelvis.

Obturator Artery. The origin of the **obturator artery** is variable; usually it arises close to the origin of the umbilical artery, where it is crossed by the ureter. It runs antero-inferiorly on the obturator fascia on the lateral wall of the pelvis, and passes between the obturator nerve and vein (Figs. 3.16 and 3.17A & B).

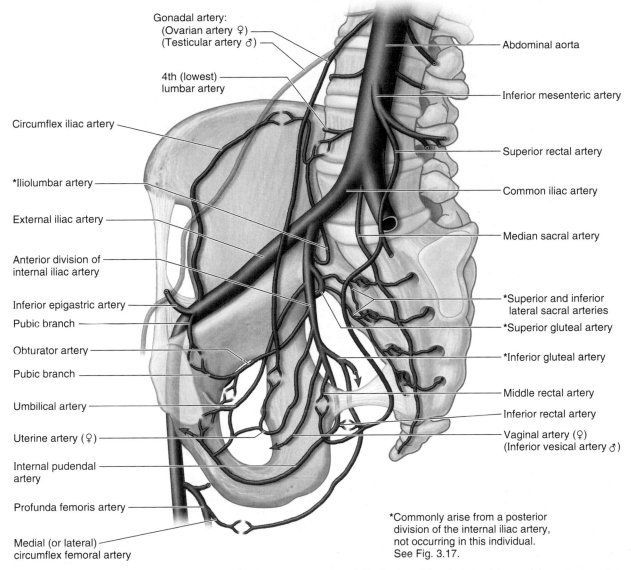

Gonadal artery:
(Ovarian artery ♀)
(Testicular artery ♂)

4th (lowest) lumbar artery

Circumflex iliac artery

*Iliolumbar artery

External iliac artery

Anterior division of internal iliac artery

Inferior epigastric artery
Pubic branch

Obturator artery
Pubic branch

Umbilical artery

Uterine artery (♀)

Internal pudendal artery

Profunda femoris artery

Medial (or lateral) circumflex femoral artery

Abdominal aorta

Inferior mesenteric artery

Superior rectal artery

Common iliac artery

Median sacral artery

*Superior and inferior lateral sacral arteries
*Superior gluteal artery

*Inferior gluteal artery

Middle rectal artery
Inferior rectal artery
Vaginal artery (♀)
(Inferior vesical artery ♂)

*Commonly arise from a posterior division of the internal iliac artery, not occurring in this individual. See Fig. 3.17.

FIGURE 3.16. Arteries and arterial anastomoses in pelvis. The origins, courses, and distribution of the arteries and the arterial anastomoses formed are described in Table 3.4.

Within the pelvis, the obturator artery gives off muscular branches, a nutrient artery to the ilium, and a pubic branch. The **pubic branch** arises just before the obturator artery leaves the pelvis. It ascends on the pelvic surface of the pubis to anastomose with its fellow of the opposite side, and the *pubic branch of the inferior epigastric artery,* a branch of the external iliac artery.

In a common variation (20%), an **aberrant** or **accessory obturator artery** arises from the inferior epigastric artery and descends into the pelvis along the usual route of the pubic branch (Figs. 3.15 and 3.16). Surgeons performing hernia repairs must keep this common variation in mind. The extrapelvic distribution of the obturator artery is described with the lower limb.

Inferior Vesical Artery. The **inferior vesical artery** occurs only in males (Figs. 3.16 and 3.17A), being replaced by the vaginal artery in females (Figs. 3.16 and 3.17B).

Uterine Artery. The **uterine artery** is an additional branch of the internal iliac artery in females, usually arising separately and directly from the internal iliac artery (Figs. 3.16 and 3.17B). It may arise from the umbilical artery. Developmentally, it is the homolog of the artery to the ductus deferens in the male. It descends on the lateral wall of the pelvis, anterior to the internal iliac artery, and passes medially to reach the junction of the uterus and vagina, where the cervix (neck) of the uterus protrudes into the superior vagina (Fig. 3.18A & B). As it passes medially, the uterine artery passes directly superior to the ureter. The relationship of ureter to artery is often remembered by the phrase *"water (urine) passes under the bridge (uterine artery)."* On reaching the side of the cervix, the uterine artery divides into a smaller descending **vaginal branch,** which supplies the cervix and vagina, and a larger **ascending branch,** which runs along the lateral margin of the uterus, supplying it. The ascending branch bifurcates into

TABLE 3.4. ARTERIES OF PELVIS

Artery	Origin	Course	Distribution	Anastomoses
Gonadal	Abdominal aorta	Descends retroperitoneally;		
Testicular (♂)		traverses inguinal canal and enters scrotum	Abdominal ureter, testis, and epididymis	Cremasteric artery, artery of ductus deferens
Ovarian (♀)		crosses pelvic brim, descends in suspensory ligament of ovary	Abdominal and/or pelvic ureter, ovary, and ampullary end of uterine tube	Uterine artery via tubal and ovarian branches
Superior rectal	Continuation of inferior mesenteric artery	Crosses left common iliac vessels and descends into pelvis between layers of sigmoid mesocolon	Superior part of rectum	Middle rectal artery; inferior rectal (internal pudendal) artery
Median sacral	Posterior aspect of abdominal aorta	Descends close to midline over L4 and L5 vertebrae, sacrum, and coccyx	Inferior lumbar vertebrae, sacrum, and coccyx	Lateral sacral artery (via medial sacral branches)
Internal iliac	Common iliac artery	Passes medially over pelvic brim and descends into pelvic cavity; often forms anterior and posterior divisions	Main blood supply to pelvic organs, gluteal muscles, and perineum	
Anterior division of internal iliac	Internal iliac artery	Passes anteriorly along lateral wall of pelvis, dividing into visceral, obturator, and internal pudendal arteries	Pelvic viscera, muscles of superior medial thigh, and perineum	
Umbilical	Anterior division of internal iliac artery	Runs a short pelvic course, gives off superior vesical arteries, then obliterates, becoming medial umbilical ligament	Superior aspect of urinary bladder and, in some males, ductus deferens (via superior vesical arteries and artery to ductus deferens)	(Occasionally the patent part of the umbilical artery)
Superior vesical	(Patent proximal umbilical artery)	Usually multiple; pass to superior aspect of urinary bladder	Superior aspect of urinary bladder; in some males, ductus deferens (via artery to ductus deferens)	Inferior vesical (♂); vaginal artery (♀)
Obturator		Runs antero-inferiorly on obturator fascia of lateral pelvic wall, exiting pelvis via obturator canal	Pelvic muscles, nutrient artery to ilium, head of femur, and muscles of medial compartment of thigh	Inferior epigastric (via pubic branch); umbilical artery
Inferior vesical (♂)		Passes subperitoneally in lateral ligament of bladder, giving rise to prostatic artery (♂) and occasionally the artery to the ductus deferens	Inferior aspect of male urinary bladder, pelvic part of ureter; prostate, and seminal glands; occasionally ductus deferens	Superior vesical artery
Artery to ductus deferens (♂)	(Superior or inferior vesical artery)	Runs subperitoneally to ductus deferens	Ductus deferens	Testicular artery; cremasteric artery
Prostatic branches (♂)	(Inferior vesical artery)	Descends on posterolateral aspects of prostate	Prostate and prostatic urethra	Deep perineal (internal pudendal)
Uterine (♀)		Runs anteromedially in base of broad ligament/superior cardinal ligament, gives rise to vaginal branch, then crosses ureter superiorly to reach lateral aspect of uterine cervix	Uterus, ligaments of uterus, medial parts of uterine tube and ovary, and superior vagina	Ovarian artery (via tubal and ovarian branches); vaginal artery

TABLE 3.4. ARTERIES OF PELVIS (Continued)

Artery	Origin	Course	Distribution	Anastomoses
Vaginal (♀)	(Uterine artery)	Divides into vaginal and inferior vesical branches, the former descending on the vagina, the latter passing to the urinary bladder	Vaginal branch: lower vagina, vestibular bulb, and adjacent rectum; inferior vesical branch: fundus of urinary bladder	Vaginal branch of uterine artery, superior vesical artery
Internal pudendal	Anterior division of internal iliac artery	Exits pelvis via infrapiriform part of greater sciatic foramen, enters perineum (ischio-anal fossa) via lesser sciatic foramen, passes via pudendal canal to UG triangle	Main artery of perineum, including muscles and skin of anal and urogenital triangles, erectile bodies	(Umbilical artery; prostatic branches of inferior vesical artery in males)
Middle rectal		Descends in pelvis to inferior part of rectum	Inferior part of rectum, seminal glands, prostate (vagina)	Superior and inferior rectal arteries
Inferior gluteal[a]		Exits pelvis via infrapiriform part of greater sciatic foramen	Pelvic diaphragm (coccygeus and levator ani), piriformis, quadratus femoris, superiormost hamstrings, gluteus maximus, and sciatic nerve	Profunda femoris artery (via medial and lateral circumflex femoral arteries)
Posterior division of internal iliac	Internal iliac artery	Passes posteriorly and gives rise to parietal branches	Pelvic wall and gluteal region	
Iliolumbar[b]	Posterior division of internal iliac artery	Ascends anterior to sacro-iliac joint and posterior to common iliac vessels and psoas major, dividing into iliac and lumbar branches	Psoas major, iliacus, and quadratus lumborum muscles; cauda equina in vertebral canal	Circumflex iliac artery and 4th (and lowest) lumbar artery
Lateral sacral (superior and inferior)		Runs on anteromedial aspect of piriformis to send branches into pelvic sacral foramina	Piriformis, structures in sacral canal, erector spinae, and overlying skin	Medial sacral arteries (from median sacral artery)
Superior gluteal		Passes between lumbosacral trunk and anterior ramus of S1 spinal nerve to exit pelvis via suprapiriform portion of greater sciatic foramen	Piriformis, all three gluteal muscles, and tensor fasciae latae	Lateral sacral, inferior gluteal, internal pudendal, deep circumflex femoral, lateral circumflex femoral

[a]May occur as terminal branch of posterior division of internal iliac artery.
[b]Often arises directly from internal iliac artery, proximal to divisions.

ovarian and **tubal branches,** which continue to supply the medial ends of the ovary and uterine tube, and anastomose with the ovarian and tubal branches of the ovarian artery.

Vaginal Artery. The **vaginal artery** is the homolog to the inferior vesical artery in males. It often arises from the initial part of the uterine artery instead of arising directly from the anterior division. The vaginal artery supplies numerous branches to the anterior and posterior surfaces of the vagina (Figs 3.16, 3.17B, and 3.18).

Middle Rectal Artery. The **middle rectal artery** may arise independently from the internal iliac artery, or it may arise in common with the inferior vesical artery or the internal pudendal artery (Figs. 3.16 and 3.17).

Internal Pudendal Artery. The **internal pudendal artery,** larger in males than in females, passes inferolaterally, anterior to the piriformis muscle and sacral plexus. It

leaves the pelvis between the piriformis and coccygeus muscles by passing through the inferior part of the *greater sciatic foramen.* The internal pudendal artery then passes around the posterior aspect of the ischial spine or the sacrospinous ligament and enters the *ischio-anal fossa* through the *lesser sciatic foramen.*

The internal pudendal artery, along with the internal pudendal veins and branches of the pudendal nerve, passes through the pudendal canal in the lateral wall of the ischio-anal fossa (Fig. 3.11B). As it exits the pudendal canal, medial to the ischial tuberosity, the internal pudendal artery divides into its terminal branches, the *perineal artery* and *dorsal arteries of the penis or clitoris.*

Inferior Gluteal Artery. The **inferior gluteal artery** is the larger terminal branch of the anterior division of the internal iliac artery (Fig. 3.18A), but may arise from the posterior

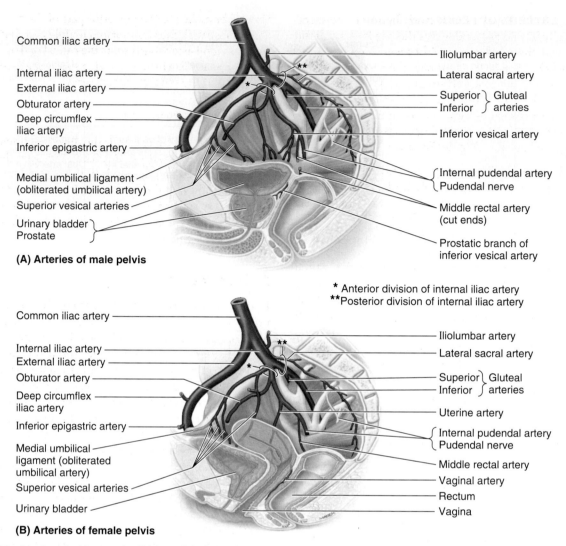

Common iliac artery

Internal iliac artery
External iliac artery
Obturator artery
Deep circumflex
iliac artery
Inferior epigastric artery

Medial umbilical ligament
(obliterated umbilical artery)
Superior vesical arteries
Urinary bladder
Prostate

Iliolumbar artery
Lateral sacral artery
Superior ⎱ Gluteal
Inferior ⎰ arteries
Inferior vesical artery
Internal pudendal artery
Pudendal nerve
Middle rectal artery
(cut ends)
Prostatic branch of
inferior vesical artery

(A) Arteries of male pelvis

* Anterior division of internal iliac artery
**Posterior division of internal iliac artery

Common iliac artery

Internal iliac artery
External iliac artery
Obturator artery
Deep circumflex
iliac artery
Inferior epigastric artery

Medial umbilical
ligament (obliterated
umbilical artery)
Superior vesical arteries
Urinary bladder

Iliolumbar artery
Lateral sacral artery
Superior ⎱ Gluteal
Inferior ⎰ arteries
Uterine artery
Internal pudendal artery
Pudendal nerve
Middle rectal artery
Vaginal artery
Rectum
Vagina

(B) Arteries of female pelvis

FIGURE 3.17.   Arteries of pelvis. Anterior divisions of the internal iliac arteries usually supply most of the blood to pelvic structures.

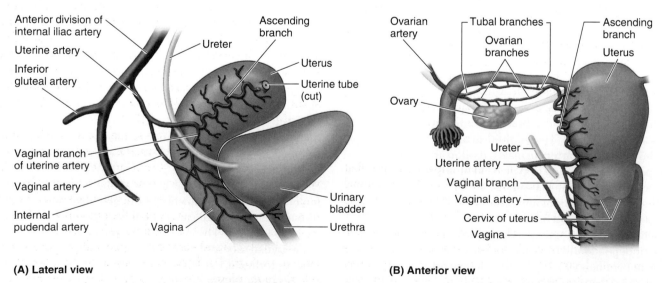

Anterior division of
internal iliac artery
Uterine artery
Inferior
gluteal artery

Ureter
Ascending
branch
Uterus
Uterine tube
(cut)

Vaginal branch
of uterine artery
Vaginal artery
Internal
pudendal artery

Vagina

Urinary
bladder
Urethra

(A) Lateral view

Ovarian
artery

Ovary

Tubal branches
Ovarian
branches

Ascending
branch
Uterus

Ureter
Uterine artery
Vaginal branch
Vaginal artery
Cervix of uterus
Vagina

(B) Anterior view

FIGURE 3.18.   Uterine and vaginal arteries. A. The origin of the arteries from the anterior division of the internal iliac artery and distribution to the uterus and vagina are shown. **B.** The anastomoses between the ovarian and tubal branches of the ovarian and uterine arteries and between the vaginal branch of the uterine artery and the vaginal artery provide potential pathways of collateral circulation. These communications occur, and the ascending branch courses, between the layers of the broad ligament.

division (Fig. 3.17). It passes posteriorly between the sacral nerves (usually S2 and S3), and leaves the pelvis through the inferior part of the *greater sciatic foramen,* inferior to the piriformis muscle (Fig. 3.16). It supplies the muscles and skin of the buttock, and the posterior surface of the thigh.

Posterior Division of Internal Iliac Artery. When the internal iliac artery divides into anterior and posterior divisions, the posterior division typically gives rise to the following three parietal arteries (Fig. 3.17A & B):

- **Iliolumbar artery:** This artery runs superolaterally in a *recurrent fashion* (turning sharply backward relative to its source) to the iliac fossa. Within the fossa, the artery divides into an *iliac branch,* which supplies the iliacus muscle and ilium, and a *lumbar branch,* which supplies the psoas major and quadratus lumborum muscles.
- **Lateral sacral arteries:** Superior and inferior lateral sacral arteries may arise as independent branches or via a common trunk. The lateral sacral arteries pass medially and descend anterior to the sacral anterior rami, giving off *spinal branches,* which pass through the anterior sacral foramina, and supply the spinal meninges enclosing the roots of the sacral nerves. Some branches of these arteries pass from the sacral canal through the posterior sacral foramina and supply the erector spinae muscles of the back and the skin overlying the sacrum.
- **Superior gluteal artery:** The largest branch of the posterior division, the superior gluteal artery supplies the gluteal muscles in the buttocks.

OVARIAN ARTERY

The **ovarian artery** arises from the abdominal aorta inferior to the renal artery but considerably superior to the inferior mesenteric artery (Fig. 3.16). As it passes inferiorly, the ovarian artery adheres to the parietal peritoneum and runs anterior to the ureter on the posterior abdominal wall, usually giving branches to it. As the ovarian artery enters the lesser pelvis, it crosses the origin of the external iliac vessels. It then runs medially, dividing into an **ovarian branch** and a **tubal branch,** which supply the ovary and uterine tube, respectively (Fig. 3.18B). These branches anastomose with the corresponding branches of the uterine artery.

MEDIAN SACRAL ARTERY

The **median sacral artery** is a small unpaired artery that usually arises from the posterior surface of the abdominal aorta, just superior to its bifurcation, but it may arise from its anterior surface (Fig. 3.16). This vessel runs anterior to the bodies of the last one or two lumbar vertebrae, the sacrum, and the coccyx, its terminal branches participating in a series of anastomotic loops. Before the median sacral artery enters the lesser pelvis, it sometimes gives rise to a pair of *L5 arteries.*

As it descends over the sacrum, the median sacral artery gives off small parietal (lateral sacral) branches that anastomose with the lateral sacral arteries. It also gives rise to small visceral branches to the posterior part of the rectum, which anastomose with the superior and middle rectal arteries. The median sacral artery represents the caudal end of the embryonic dorsal aorta, which reduced in size as the tail-like caudal eminence of the embryo disappeared.

SUPERIOR RECTAL ARTERY

The **superior rectal artery** is the direct continuation of the inferior mesenteric artery (Fig. 3.16). It crosses the left common iliac vessels and descends in the sigmoid mesocolon to the lesser pelvis. At the level of the S3 vertebra, the superior rectal artery divides into two branches, which descend on each side of the rectum and supply it as far inferiorly as the internal anal sphincter.

Pelvic Veins

Pelvic venous plexuses are formed by the interjoining veins surrounding the pelvic viscera (Fig. 3.19B & C). These intercommunicating networks of veins are clinically important. The various plexuses within the lesser pelvis (rectal, vesical, prostatic, uterine, and vaginal) unite and are drained mainly by tributaries of the *internal iliac veins,* but some of them drain through the superior rectal vein into the inferior mesenteric vein of the hepatic portal system (Fig. 3.19A), or through lateral sacral veins into the *internal vertebral venous plexus* (see Chapter 4). Additional relatively minor paths of venous drainage from the lesser pelvis include the parietal **median sacral vein** and, in females, the ovarian veins.

The **internal iliac veins** form superior to the greater sciatic foramen and lie postero-inferior to the internal iliac arteries (Fig. 3.19A & B). Tributaries of the internal iliac veins are more variable than the branches of the internal iliac artery with which they share names, but roughly accompany them, draining the same territories that the arteries supply. However, there are no veins accompanying the umbilical arteries between the pelvis and the umbilicus, and the **iliolumbar veins** from the iliac fossae of the greater pelvis usually drain into the common iliac veins instead. The internal iliac veins merge with the external iliac veins to form the **common iliac veins,** which unite at the level of vertebra L4 or L5 to form the **inferior vena cava** (Fig. 3.19A).

The **superior gluteal veins,** the accompanying veins (L. *venae comitantes*) of the superior gluteal arteries of the gluteal region, are the largest tributaries of the internal iliac veins except during pregnancy, when the uterine veins become larger. Testicular veins traverse the greater pelvis as they pass from the deep inguinal ring toward their posterior abdominal terminations but do not usually drain pelvic structures.

The **lateral sacral veins** often appear disproportionately large in angiographs. They anastomose with the internal vertebral venous plexus (Chapter 4), providing an alternate collateral pathway to reach either the inferior or superior vena cava. It may also provide a pathway for metastasis of prostatic or ovarian cancer cells to vertebral or cranial sites.

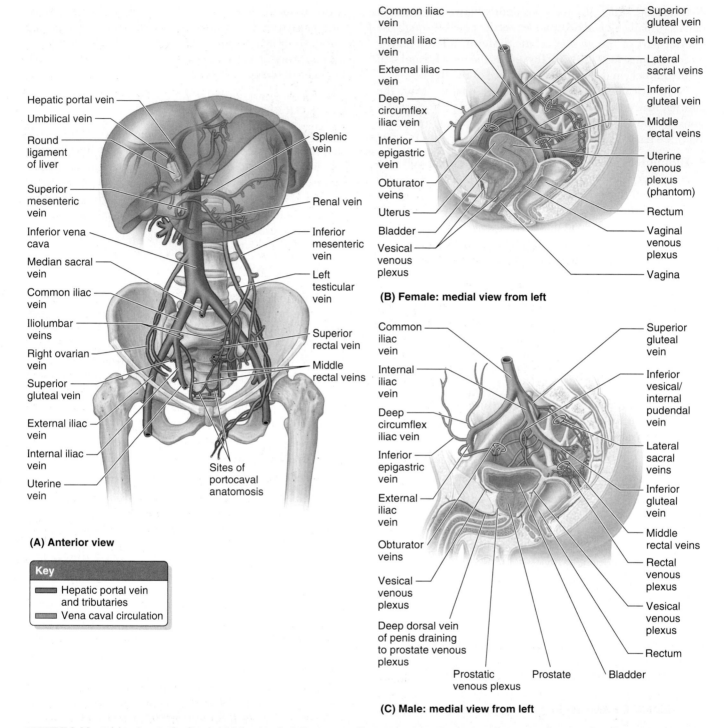

(A) Anterior view

(B) Female: medial view from left

(C) Male: medial view from left

Key
- Hepatic portal vein and tributaries
- Vena caval circulation

FIGURE 3.19. Pelvic veins. A. The female (*right*) and male (*left*) patterns of hepatic portal and systemic (vena caval) venous systems of the abdominopelvic cavity are shown. Venous drainage from pelvic organs flows mainly to the caval system via the internal iliac veins. The superior rectum normally drains into the hepatic portal system, although the superior rectal veins anastomose with the middle and inferior rectal veins, which are tributaries of the internal iliac veins. The female (**B**) and male (**C**) pelvic veins and venous plexuses are demonstrated.

Lymph Nodes of Pelvis

The lymph nodes receiving lymph drainage from pelvic organs are variable in number, size, and location. Dividing them into definite groups is often somewhat arbitrary. Four primary groups of nodes are located in or adjacent to the pelvis, named for the blood vessels with which they are associated (Fig. 3.20):

- **External iliac lymph nodes:** lie above the pelvic brim, along the external iliac vessels. They receive lymph mainly from the inguinal lymph nodes; however, they receive lymph

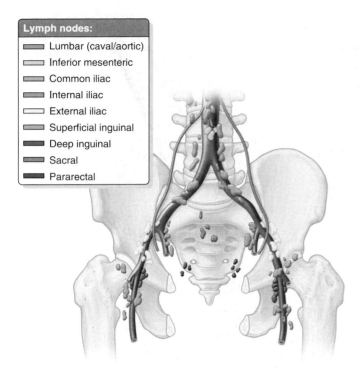

Lymph nodes:
- Lumbar (caval/aortic)
- Inferior mesenteric
- Common iliac
- Internal iliac
- External iliac
- Superficial inguinal
- Deep inguinal
- Sacral
- Pararectal

FIGURE 3.20. Lymph nodes of pelvis.

from pelvic viscera, especially the superior parts of the middle to anterior pelvic organs. Whereas most of the lymphatic drainage from the pelvis tends to parallel routes of venous drainage, the lymphatic drainage to the external iliac nodes does not. These nodes drain into the common iliac nodes.

- **Internal iliac lymph nodes:** clustered around the anterior and posterior divisions of the internal iliac artery and the origins of the gluteal arteries. They receive drainage from the inferior pelvic viscera, deep perineum, and gluteal region and drain into the common iliac nodes.
- **Sacral lymph nodes:** lie in the concavity of the sacrum, adjacent to the median sacral vessels. They receive lymph from postero-inferior pelvic viscera and drain either to internal or common iliac nodes.
- **Common iliac lymph nodes:** lie superior to the pelvic brim, along the common iliac blood vessels (Fig. 3.20), and receive drainage from the three main groups listed above. These nodes begin a common route for drainage from the pelvis that passes next to the lumbar (caval/aortic) nodes. Inconstant direct drainage to the common iliac nodes occurs from some pelvic organs (e.g., from the neck of the bladder and inferior vagina).

Additional minor groups of nodes (e.g., the **pararectal nodes**) occupy the connective tissue along the branches of the internal iliac vessels.

Both primary and minor groups of pelvic nodes are highly interconnected, so that many nodes can be removed without disturbing drainage. The interconnections also allow cancer to spread in virtually any direction, to any pelvic or abdominal viscus. While the lymphatic drainage tends to parallel the venous drainage (except for that to the external iliac nodes, where

proximity provides a rough guide), the pattern is not sufficiently predictable to allow the progress of metastatic cancer from pelvic organs to be anticipated or staged in a manner comparable to that of breast cancer progressing though the axillary nodes. Lymphatic drainage from the specific pelvic organs is described following the description of the pelvic viscera (p. 400).

Pelvic Nerves

The pelvis is innervated mainly by the **sacral** and **coccygeal spinal nerves** and the *pelvic part of the autonomic nervous system*. The piriformis and coccygeus muscles form a bed for the sacral and coccygeal nerve plexuses (Fig. 3.21). The anterior rami of the S2 and S3 nerves emerge between the digitations of these muscles.

OBTURATOR NERVE

The *obturator nerve* arises from the anterior rami of spinal nerves L2–L4 of the *lumbar plexus* in the abdomen (greater pelvis) and enters the lesser pelvis. It runs in the extraperitoneal fat along the lateral wall of the pelvis to the *obturator canal*, an opening in the obturator membrane that otherwise fills the obturator foramen. Here it divides into anterior and posterior parts, which leave the pelvis through this canal and supply the medial thigh muscles. No pelvic structures are supplied by the obturator nerve.

LUMBOSACRAL TRUNK

At or immediately superior to the pelvic brim, the descending part of the L4 nerve unites with the anterior ramus of the L5 nerve to form the thick, cord-like **lumbosacral trunk** (see Figs. 3.9D, 3.21, and 3.22). The trunk passes inferiorly, on the anterior surface of the ala of the sacrum, and joins the sacral plexus.

SACRAL PLEXUS

The plexus is demonstrated in Figure 3.22, and the segmental composition and distribution of the nerves derived from it are listed in Table 3.5. The following text provides additional information about the formation of the nerves and their courses.

The **sacral plexus** is located on the posterolateral wall of the lesser pelvis. The two main nerves arising from the sacral plexus, the *sciatic* and *pudendal nerves*, lie external to the parietal pelvic fascia. Most branches of the sacral plexus leave the pelvis through the *greater sciatic foramen*.

The *sciatic nerve* is the largest nerve in the body. It is formed as the large anterior rami of spinal nerves L4–S3 converge on the anterior surface of the piriformis (Figs. 3.21 and 3.22). As it is formed, the sciatic nerve passes through the greater sciatic foramen, usually inferior to the piriformis, to enter the gluteal region. It then descends along the posterior aspect of the thigh to supply the posterior aspect of the thigh and the entire leg and foot.

The **pudendal nerve** is the main nerve of the perineum and the chief sensory nerve of the external genitalia.

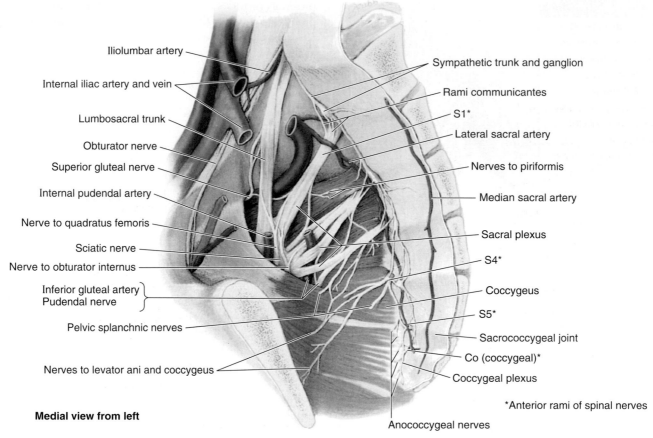

Iliolumbar artery

Internal iliac artery and vein

Lumbosacral trunk

Obturator nerve

Superior gluteal nerve

Internal pudendal artery

Nerve to quadratus femoris

Sciatic nerve

Nerve to obturator internus

Inferior gluteal artery
Pudendal nerve

Pelvic splanchnic nerves

Nerves to levator ani and coccygeus

Sympathetic trunk and ganglion

Rami communicantes

S1*

Lateral sacral artery

Nerves to piriformis

Median sacral artery

Sacral plexus

S4*

Coccygeus

S5*

Sacrococcygeal joint

Co (coccygeal)*

Coccygeal plexus

*Anterior rami of spinal nerves

Anococcygeal nerves

Medial view from left

FIGURE 3.21. Nerves and nerve plexuses of pelvis. Somatic nerves (sacral and coccygeal nerve plexuses) and the pelvic (sacral) part of the sympathetic trunk are shown. Although located in the pelvis, most of the nerves seen here are involved with the innervation of the lower limb rather than the pelvic structures.

Accompanied by the internal pudendal artery, it leaves the pelvis through the greater sciatic foramen between the piriformis and coccygeus muscles. It then hooks around the ischial spine and sacrospinous ligament and enters the perineum through the lesser sciatic foramen (Fig. 3.22).

The *superior gluteal nerve* leaves the pelvis through the greater sciatic foramen, superior to the piriformis to supply muscles in the gluteal region (Figs. 3.21 and 3.22).

The *inferior gluteal nerve* leaves the pelvis through the greater sciatic foramen (Fig. 3.22), inferior to the piriformis and superficial to the sciatic nerve, accompanying the inferior gluteal artery. Both break up into several branches that enter the deep surface of the overlying gluteus maximus muscle.

COCCYGEAL PLEXUS

The **coccygeal plexus** is a small network of nerve fibers formed by the anterior rami of S4 and S5 and the **coccygeal nerves** (Fig. 3.21). It lies on the pelvic surface of the coccygeus and supplies this muscle, part of the levator ani, and the sacrococcygeal joint. The **anococcygeal nerves** arising from this plexus pierce the coccygeus and anococcygeal ligament to supply a small area of skin between the tip of the coccyx and the anus.

PELVIC AUTONOMIC NERVES

Autonomic nerves enter the pelvic cavity via four routes (Fig. 3.23):

- *Sacral sympathetic trunks:* primarily provide sympathetic innervation to the lower limbs.
- *Peri-arterial plexuses:* postsynaptic, sympathetic, vasomotor fibers to superior rectal, ovarian, and internal iliac arteries and their derivative branches.
- *Hypogastric plexuses:* most important route by which sympathetic fibers are conveyed to the pelvic viscera.
- *Pelvic splanchnic nerves:* pathway for parasympathetic innervation of pelvic viscera and descending and sigmoid colon.

The **sacral sympathetic trunks** are the inferior continuation of the lumbar sympathetic trunks (Figs. 3.21 and 3.23). Each of the sacral trunks is diminished in size from that of the lumbar trunks and usually has four sympathetic ganglia. The sacral trunks descend on the pelvic surface of the sacrum just medial to the pelvic sacral foramina and converge to form the small median **ganglion impar** (coccygeal ganglion) anterior to the coccyx. The sacral sympathetic trunks descend posterior to the rectum in the extraperitoneal connective tissue and send communicating branches (gray rami communicantes) to each of the anterior rami of the sacral and coccygeal nerves.

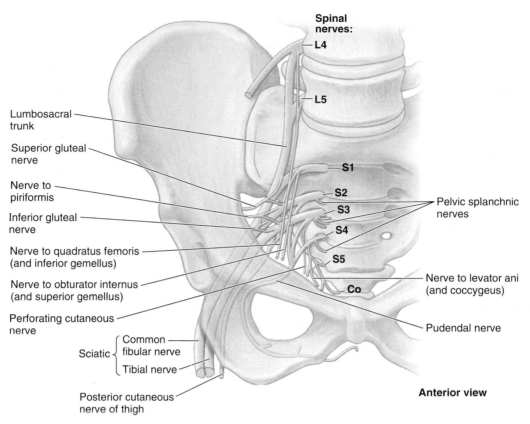

FIGURE 3.22. Somatic nerves of pelvis—the sacral plexus.

TABLE 3.5. SOMATIC NERVES OF PELVIS

Nerve	Origin	Distribution
Sciatic	L4, L5, S1, S2, S3	Articular branches to hip joint and muscular branches to flexors of knee in thigh and all muscles in leg and foot
Superior gluteal	L4, L5, S1	Gluteus medius and gluteus minimus muscles
Nerve to quadratus femoris (and inferior gemellus)	L4, L5, S1	Quadratus femoris and inferior gemellus muscles
Inferior gluteal	L5, S1, S2	Gluteus maximus
Nerve to obturator internus (and superior gemellus)	L5, S1, S2	Obturator internus and superior gemellus muscles
Nerve to piriformis	S1, S2	Piriformis muscle
Posterior cutaneous nerve of thigh	S2, S3	Cutaneous branches to buttocks and uppermost medial and posterior surfaces of thigh
Perforating cutaneous	S2, S3	Cutaneous branches to medial part of buttocks
Pudendal	S2, S3, S4	Structures in perineum: sensory to genitalia; muscular branches to perineal muscles, external urethral sphincter, and external anal sphincter
Pelvic splanchnic	S2, S3, S4	Pelvic viscera via inferior hypogastric and pelvic plexuses
Nerves to levator ani and coccygeus	S3, S4	Levator ani and coccygeus muscles

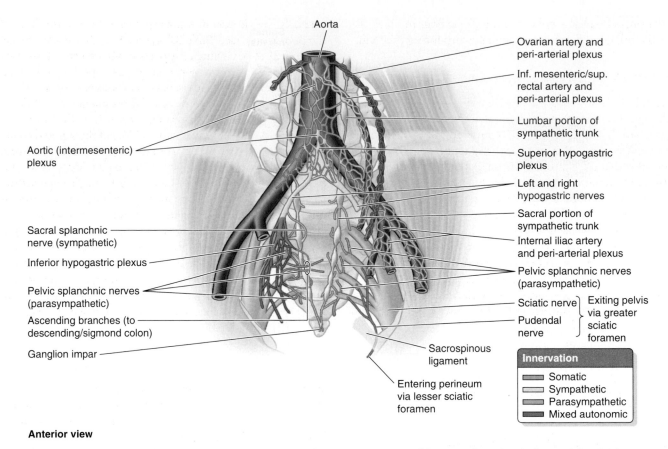

FIGURE 3.23. Autonomic nerves of pelvis. The superior hypogastric plexus is a continuation of the aortic plexus that divides into left and right hypogastric nerves as it enters the pelvis. The hypogastric and pelvic splanchnic nerves merge to form the inferior hypogastric plexuses, which thus consist of both sympathetic and parasympathetic fibers. Autonomic (sympathetic) fibers also enter the pelvis via the sympathetic trunks and peri-arterial plexuses.

They also send small branches to the median sacral artery and the inferior hypogastric plexus. The primary function of the sacral sympathetic trunks is to provide postsynaptic fibers to the sacral plexus for sympathetic (vasomotor, pilomotor, and sudomotor) innervation of the lower limb.

The *peri-arterial plexuses of the ovarian, superior rectal, and internal iliac arteries* are minor routes by which sympathetic fibers enter the pelvis. Their primary function is vasomotion of the arteries they accompany.

The **hypogastric plexuses** (superior and inferior) are networks of sympathetic and visceral afferent nerve fibers. The main part of the *superior hypogastric plexus* is a prolongation of the *intermesenteric plexus* (see Chapter 2), which lies inferior to the bifurcation of the aorta (Fig. 3.23). It carries fibers conveyed to and from the intermesenteric plexus by the L3 and L4 splanchnic nerves. The superior hypogastric plexus enters the pelvis, dividing into **right** and **left hypogastric nerves,** which descend on the anterior surface of the sacrum. These nerves descend lateral to the rectum within *hypogastric sheaths* and then spread in a fan-like fashion as they merge with the pelvic splanchnic nerves to form the right and left *inferior hypogastric plexuses.*

The **inferior hypogastric plexuses** thus contain both sympathetic and parasympathetic fibers as well as visceral afferent fibers, which continue through the lamina of the hypogastric sheath to the pelvic viscera, upon which they form sub-plexuses collectively referred to as the **pelvic plexuses.** In both sexes, sub-plexuses are associated with the lateral aspects of the rectum and inferolateral surfaces of the bladder. In addition, sub-plexuses in the male are also associated with the prostate and seminal glands. In females, sub-plexuses are also associated with the cervix of the uterus and the lateral fornices of the vagina.

Pelvic splanchnic nerves arise in the pelvis from the anterior rami of spinal nerves S2–S4 of the sacral plexus (Figs 3.21– 3.23). They convey presynaptic parasympathetic fibers derived from the S2–S4 spinal cord segments, which make up the sacral outflow of the parasympathetic (craniosacral) nervous system, and visceral afferent fibers from cell bodies in the spinal ganglia of the corresponding spinal nerves. The greatest contribution of these fibers is usually from the S3 nerve.

The hypogastric/pelvic system of plexuses, receiving sympathetic fibers via lumbar splanchnic nerves and parasympathetic fibers via pelvic splanchnic nerves, innervate the pelvic viscera. Although the sympathetic component largely produces vasomotion as elsewhere, here it also inhibits peristaltic contraction of the rectum and stimulates contraction of the internal genital organs during orgasm, producing ejaculation in the male.

Because the pelvis does not include a cutaneous area, pelvic sympathetic fibers do not produce pilomotion or vasomotion functions. The parasympathetic fibers distributed within the pelvis stimulate contraction of the rectum and bladder for defecation and urination, respectively. Parasympathetic fibers in the prostatic plexus penetrate the pelvic floor to reach the erectile bodies of the external genitalia, producing erection.

VISCERAL AFFERENT INNERVATION IN PELVIS

Visceral afferent fibers travel with autonomic nerve fibers, although the sensory impulses are conducted centrally, retrograde to the efferent impulses conveyed by the autonomic fibers. All visceral afferent fibers conducting reflexive sensation (information that does not reach consciousness) travel with parasympathetic fibers. Thus, in the case of the pelvis, they travel through the pelvic and inferior hypogastric plexuses and the pelvic splanchnic nerves to the spinal sensory ganglia of spinal nerves S2–S4.

The paths followed by visceral afferent fibers conducting pain from the pelvic viscera differ in terms of course and destination, depending on whether the viscus or part of the viscus from which the pain is emanating is located superior or inferior to the **pelvic pain line.** Except in the case of the alimentary canal, the pelvic pain line corresponds to the inferior limit of the peritoneum (see Table 3.3 figures B & C). Intraperitoneal abdominopelvic viscera, or aspects of visceral structures that are in contact with the peritoneum, are superior to the pain line; subperitoneal pelvic viscera or portions of viscera are inferior to the pain line. In the case of the alimentary tract (large intestine), the pain line does not correlate with the peritoneum; the pain line occurs in the middle of the sigmoid colon.

Visceral afferent fibers conducting pain impulses from abdominopelvic viscera superior to the pain line follow sympathetic fibers retrograde, ascending through hypogastric/aortic plexuses, abdominopelvic splanchnic nerves, lumbar sympathetic trunks, and white rami communicantes to reach cell bodies in the inferior thoracic/upper lumbar spinal ganglia. Afferent fibers conducting pain impulses from the viscera or portions of viscera inferior to the pain line follow the parasympathetic fibers retrograde through the pelvic and inferior hypogastric plexuses and pelvic splanchnic nerves to reach cell bodies in the spinal sensory ganglia of S2–S4.

NEUROVASCULAR STRUCTURES OF PELVIS

Iatrogenic Injury of Ureters

INJURY DURING LIGATION OF UTERINE ARTERY

The fact that the ureter passes immediately inferior to the uterine artery near the lateral part of the fornix of the vagina is clinically important. The ureter is in danger of being inadvertently clamped (crushed), ligated, or transected during a *hysterectomy* (excision of uterus) when the uterine artery is ligated and severed to remove the uterus. The point at which the uterine artery and ureter cross lies approximately 2 cm superior to the ischial spine.

INJURY DURING LIGATION OF OVARIAN ARTERY

The ureters are vulnerable to injury when the ovarian vessels are ligated during an *ovariectomy* (excision of ovary) because these structures are close to each other as they cross the pelvic brim.

Ligation of Internal Iliac Artery and Collateral Circulation in Pelvis

Occasionally the internal iliac artery becomes stenotic (the lumen becomes narrow) due to atherosclerotic cholesterol deposit (Fig. B3.6), or is surgically ligated to control pelvic hemorrhage. Because of the numerous anastomoses between the artery's branches and adjacent arteries (see Fig. 3.16; Table 3.4), ligation does not stop blood flow but it does reduce blood pressure, allowing *hemostasis* (arrest of bleeding) to occur. Examples of collateral pathways to the internal iliac artery include the following pairs of anastomosing arteries: lumbar and iliolumbar, median sacral and lateral sacral, superior rectal and middle rectal, and inferior gluteal and profunda femoris artery. Blood flow in the artery is maintained, although it may be reversed in the anastomotic branch. The collateral pathways may maintain the blood supply to the pelvic viscera, gluteal region, and genital organs.

Injury to Pelvic Nerves

During childbirth, the fetal head may compress the nerves of the mother's sacral plexus, producing pain in the lower limbs. The *obturator nerve* is vulnerable to injury during surgery (e.g., during removal of cancerous lymph nodes from the lateral pelvic wall). Injury to this nerve may cause painful spasms of the adductor muscles of the thigh and sensory deficits in the medial thigh region.

Abdominal aorta
Stenotic segment of right common iliac artery
Left common iliac artery
Median sacral artery
Superior gluteal artery
Internal iliac artery
External iliac artery
Femoral artery
Obturator artery

AP view

FIGURE B3.6. Iliac arteriogram. Radiopaque dye was injected into the abdominal aorta in the lumbar region. There is a site of narrowing (stenosis) of the right common iliac artery (*circled area*). (Courtesy of Dr. D. Sniderman, Associate Professor of Medical Imaging, University of Toronto, Toronto, ON, Canada.)

The Bottom Line

NEUROVASCULAR STRUCTURES OF PELVIS

Progressing from the pelvic cavity outward, as when dissecting the pelvis, the retroperitoneal hypogastric/pelvic autonomic nerve plexuses are encountered first (nearest the viscera), then pelvic arteries, pelvic veins, and finally the pelvic somatic nerves and sympathetic trunks, the latter two being adjacent to the pelvic walls.

Pelvic arteries: Multiple anastomosing arteries provide a collateral circulatory system that helps ensure an adequate blood supply to the greater and lesser pelves. Most arterial blood is delivered to the lesser pelvis by the internal iliac arteries, which commonly bifurcate into an anterior division (providing all the visceral branches) and a posterior division (usually exclusively parietal). ♦ Postnatally, the umbilical arteries become occluded distal to the origin of the superior vesical arteries and, in the male, the arteries to the ductus deferens. ♦ The inferior vesical (males) and vaginal arteries (females) supply the inferior bladder and pelvic urethra. The inferior vesical artery also supplies the prostate; the vaginal artery supplies the superior vagina. ♦ The uterine artery is exclusively female, but both sexes have middle rectal arteries.

Parietal branches of the anterior division of the internal iliac in both sexes include the obturator, inferior gluteal, and internal pudendal arteries, the main branches of which arise outside of the lesser pelvis. ♦ A clinically significant aberrant obturator artery arises from the inferior epigastric vessels in approximately 20% of the population. ♦ The iliolumbar, superior gluteal, and lateral sacral arteries are parietal branches of the posterior division of the internal iliac artery, distributed outside of the lesser pelvis. ♦ The iliolumbar artery is a major supplier to structures of the iliac fossae (greater pelvis). ♦ The gonadal arteries of both sexes descend into the greater pelvis from the abdominal aorta, but only the ovarian arteries enter the lesser pelvis.

Pelvic veins: The venous plexuses associated with and named for the various pelvic viscera intercommunicate with each other and the internal vertebral (epidural) venous plexuses of the vertebral canal. However, most venous blood exits the pelvis via the internal iliac veins.

Pelvic lymph drainage and nodes: Lymphatic drainage from the pelvis follows a pattern that mainly, but not completely, follows the pattern of venous drainage through variable minor and major groups of lymph nodes, the latter including the sacral and internal, external, and common iliac nodes. ♦ Aspects of the anterior to middle pelvic organs, approximately at the level of (and including) the roof of the undistended urinary bladder, drain to the external iliac nodes, independent of the venous drainage. ♦ The pelvic lymph nodes are highly interconnected, so that lymphatic drainage (and metastatic cancer cells) can pass in almost any direction, to any pelvic or abdominal organ.

Pelvic nerves: Somatic nerves within the pelvis form the sacral plexus, primarily concerned with innervation of the lower limbs and perineum. ♦ The pelvic portions of the sympathetic trunks are also primarily concerned with innervation of the lower limbs. ♦ Autonomic nerves are primarily brought to the pelvis via the superior hypogastric plexus (sympathetic fibers) and pelvic splanchnic nerves (parasympathetic fibers), the two merging to form the inferior hypogastric and pelvic plexuses. ♦ Sympathetic fibers to the pelvis produce vasomotion and contraction of internal genital organs during orgasm; they also inhibit rectal peristalsis. ♦ Pelvic parasympathetic fibers stimulate bladder and rectal emptying and extend to the erectile bodies of the external genitalia to produce erection. ♦ Visceral afferent fibers travel retrogradely along the autonomic nerve fibers. ♦ Visceral afferents conveying unconscious reflex sensation follow the course of the parasympathetic fibers to the spinal sensory ganglia of S2–S4, as do those transmitting pain sensations from the viscera inferior to the pelvic pain line (structures that do not contact the peritoneum plus the distal sigmoid colon and rectum). ♦ Visceral afferent fibers conducting pain from structures superior to the pelvic pain line (structures in contact with the peritoneum, except for the distal sigmoid colon and rectum) follow the sympathetic fibers retrogradely to inferior thoracic and superior lumbar spinal ganglia.

PELVIC VISCERA

The **pelvic viscera** include the distal parts of the urinary system and gastrointestinal tract, and the reproductive system. Although the sigmoid colon and parts of the small bowel extend into the pelvic cavity, they are abdominal rather than pelvic viscera. The bladder and rectum—true pelvic viscera—are inferior continuations of systems encountered in the abdomen. Except for features related to sharing of the male urethra by the urinary and reproductive tracts, and physical relationships to the respective reproductive organs,

there are relatively few distinctions between the male and female pelvic urinary and gastrointestinal organs.

Urinary Organs

The pelvic urinary organs (Fig. 3.24A) are the:

- Pelvic portions of the ureters, which carry urine from the kidneys.
- Urinary bladder, which temporarily stores urine.
- Urethra, which conducts urine from the bladder to the exterior.

Inferior vena cava
11th rib
12th rib
Common iliac artery
Bifurcation of common iliac artery
Internal iliac artery
External iliac artery
Urethra

Left supra-renal gland
Left kidney
Uretopelvic junction*
Abdominal aorta
Ureter
Crossing iliac vessels and pelvic brim*
Urinary bladder
Traversing bladder wall*

*Normal sites of relative constriction of ureter

(A) Anterior view

Crest of ilium
Ilium
Dilated segment of pelvic part of ureter
Contracted segment of pelvic part of ureter
Urinary bladder

L5

(B) Anteroposterior view

FIGURE 3.24. Genito-urinary viscera. A. The course and normal sites of relative constriction of the ureters. **B.** Normal intravenous urogram. The *arrows* indicate transient narrowing of the lumina of the ureters resulting from peristaltic contraction.

URETERS

The **ureters** are muscular tubes, 25–30 cm long, that connect the kidneys to the urinary bladder. The ureters are retroperitoneal; their superior abdominal portions are described in Chapter 2. As the ureters cross the bifurcation of the common iliac artery (or the beginning of the external iliac artery), they pass over the pelvic brim, thus leaving the abdomen and entering the lesser pelvis (Fig. 3.24A & B). The pelvic parts of the ureters run on the lateral walls of the pelvis, parallel to the anterior margin of the greater sciatic notch, between

the parietal pelvic peritoneum and the internal iliac arteries. Opposite the ischial spine, they curve anteromedially, superior to the levator ani, and enter the urinary bladder. The inferior ends of the ureters are surrounded by the *vesical venous plexus* (Fig. 3.19B & C).

The ureters pass obliquely through the muscular wall of the urinary bladder in an inferomedial direction, entering the outer surface of the bladder approximately 5 cm apart, but their internal openings into the lumen of the empty bladder are separated by only half that distance. This oblique passage through the bladder wall forms a one-way "flap valve," the internal pressure of the filling bladder causing the intramural passage to collapse. In addition, contractions of the bladder musculature act as a sphincter preventing the reflux of urine into the ureters when the bladder contracts, increasing internal pressure during micturition. Urine is transported down the ureters by means of peristaltic contractions, a few drops being transported at intervals of 12–20 sec (Fig. 3.24B).

In males, the only structure that passes between the ureter and the peritoneum is the *ductus deferens* (see Fig. 3.34); it crosses the ureter within the ureteric fold of peritoneum. The ureter lies posterolateral to the ductus deferens and enters the posterosuperior angle of the bladder, just superior to the seminal gland.

In females, the ureter passes medial to the origin of the uterine artery and continues to the level of the ischial spine, where it is crossed superiorly by the uterine artery (see the blue box "Iatrogenic Injury of the Ureters" on p. 361). It then passes close to the lateral part of the fornix of the vagina and enters the posterosuperior angle of the bladder.

Arterial Supply and Venous Drainage of Pelvic Portion of Ureters. The *arterial supply* to the pelvic parts of the ureters is variable, with ureteric branches extending from the common iliac, internal iliac, and ovarian arteries (Fig. 3.25; Table 3.4). The ureteric branches anastomose along the length of the ureter forming a continuous blood supply, although not necessarily effective collateral pathways. The most constant arteries supplying the terminal parts of the ureter in females are branches of the *uterine arteries*. The source of similar branches in males are the *inferior vesical arteries*. The blood supply of the ureters is a matter of great concern to surgeons operating in the region (see the blue box "Iatrogenic Compromise of Ureteric Blood Supply," p. 373).

The *venous drainage* from the pelvic parts of the ureters generally parallels the arterial supply, draining to veins with corresponding names. *Lymphatic vessels* pass primarily to common and internal iliac nodes (Fig. 3.20).

Innervation of Ureters. The nerves to the ureters derive from adjacent autonomic plexuses (renal, aortic, superior and inferior hypogastric—Fig. 3.26). The ureters are primarily superior to the pelvic pain line. Afferent (pain) fibers from the ureters follow sympathetic fibers in a retrograde direction to reach the spinal ganglia and spinal cord segments of T10–L2 or L3. *Ureteric pain* is usually referred to the ipsilateral lower quadrant of the abdomen, especially to the groin (inguinal region). See the blue box "Ureteric Calculi" on page 373.

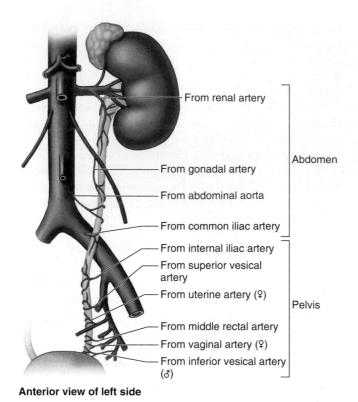

Anterior view of left side

FIGURE 3.25. Blood supply of ureter. Branches supplying the abdominal half of the ureter approach medially, while those supplying the pelvic half approach laterally. During surgery, the ureters are avoided and left undisturbed when possible. If necessary, traction of the ureters is applied gently and only toward the blood supply to avoid disruption of the small branches.

URINARY BLADDER

The **urinary bladder,** a hollow viscus with strong muscular walls, is characterized by its distensibility (Fig. 3.27A). The bladder is a temporary reservoir for urine, and varies in size, shape, position, and relationships according to its content, and the state of neighboring viscera. When empty, the adult urinary bladder is located in the lesser pelvis, lying partially superior to and partially posterior to the pubic bones (Fig. 3.27B). It is separated from these bones by the potential *retropubic space* (of Retzius) and lies mostly inferior to the peritoneum, resting on the pubic bones and pubic symphysis anteriorly and the prostate (males) or anterior wall of the vagina (females) posteriorly (Fig. 3.27A & B). The bladder is relatively free within the extraperitoneal subcutaneous fatty tissue, except for its neck, which is held firmly by the *lateral ligaments of bladder* and the *tendinous arch of the pelvic fascia*—especially its anterior component, the *puboprostatic ligament* in males and the *pubovesical ligament* in females (see also Fig. 3.14A). In females, since the posterior aspect of the bladder rests directly upon the anterior wall of the vagina, the lateral attachment of the vagina to the tendinous arch of the pelvic fascia, the *paracolpium,* is an indirect but important factor in supporting the urinary bladder (see Fig. 3.14B; DeLancey, 1992; Ashton-Miller and DeLancey, 2007).

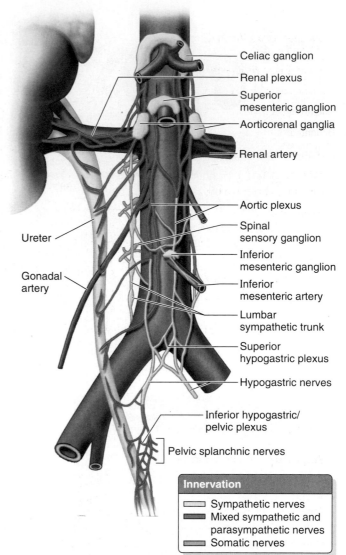

Anterior view

FIGURE 3.26. Innervation of ureters. Nerve fibers from the renal, aortic, and superior and inferior hypogastric plexuses extend to the ureter, carrying visceral afferent and sympathetic fibers to the T10–L2(3) spinal sensory ganglia and cord segments. Parasympathetic fibers, from the S2–S4 spinal cord segments, are distributed to the pelvic part of the ureter. Extrinsic ANS fibers are not essential for the initiation and propagation of ureteric peristalsis.

In infants and young children, the urinary bladder is in the abdomen even when empty (Fig. 3.28A). The bladder usually enters the greater pelvis by 6 years of age; however, it is not located entirely within the lesser pelvis until after puberty. An empty bladder in adults lies almost entirely in the lesser pelvis, its superior surface level with the superior margin of the pubic symphysis (Fig. 3.28B). As the bladder fills, it enters the greater pelvis as it ascends in the extraperitoneal fatty tissue of the anterior abdominal wall (Fig. 3.27A). In some individuals, a full bladder may ascend to the level of the umbilicus.

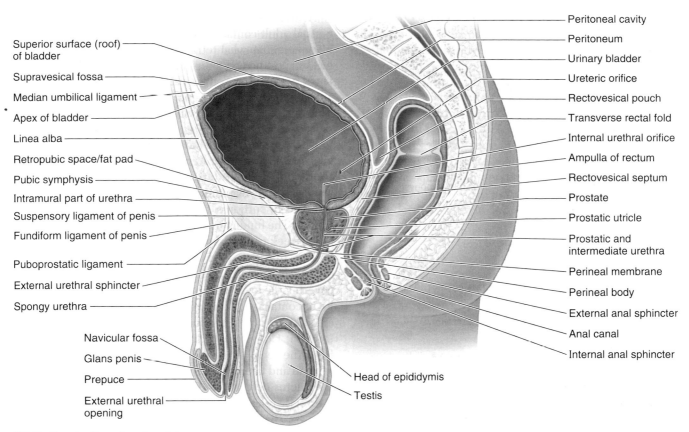

Peritoneal cavity

Peritoneum

Urinary bladder

Ureteric orifice

Rectovesical pouch

Transverse rectal fold

Internal urethral orifice

Ampulla of rectum

Rectovesical septum

Prostate

Prostatic utricle

Prostatic and intermediate urethra

Perineal membrane

Perineal body

External anal sphincter

Anal canal

Internal anal sphincter

Superior surface (roof) of bladder

Supravesical fossa

Median umbilical ligament

Apex of bladder

Linea alba

Retropubic space/fat pad

Pubic symphysis

Intramural part of urethra

Suspensory ligament of penis

Fundiform ligament of penis

Puboprostatic ligament

External urethral sphincter

Spongy urethra

Navicular fossa

Glans penis

Prepuce

External urethral opening

Head of epididymis

Testis

(A) Median section of male pelvis

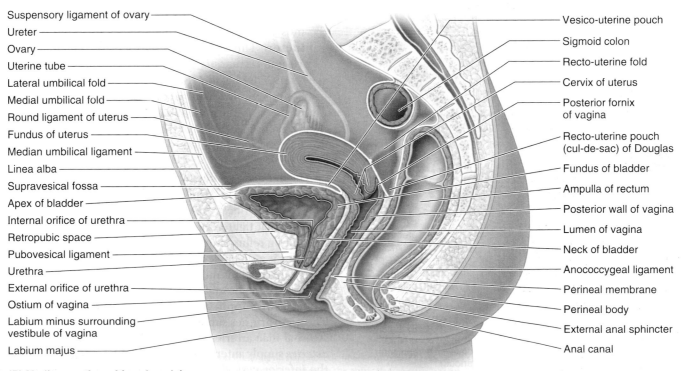

Suspensory ligament of ovary

Ureter

Ovary

Uterine tube

Lateral umbilical fold

Medial umbilical fold

Round ligament of uterus

Fundus of uterus

Median umbilical ligament

Linea alba

Supravesical fossa

Apex of bladder

Internal orifice of urethra

Retropubic space

Pubovesical ligament

Urethra

External orifice of urethra

Ostium of vagina

Labium minus surrounding vestibule of vagina

Labium majus

Vesico-uterine pouch

Sigmoid colon

Recto-uterine fold

Cervix of uterus

Posterior fornix of vagina

Recto-uterine pouch (cul-de-sac) of Douglas

Fundus of bladder

Ampulla of rectum

Posterior wall of vagina

Lumen of vagina

Neck of bladder

Anococcygeal ligament

Perineal membrane

Perineal body

External anal sphincter

Anal canal

(B) Median section of female pelvis

FIGURE 3.27. Viscera in hemisected male and female pelves. A. In this male pelvis, the urinary bladder is distended, as if full. Compare its relation to the anterior abdominal wall, pubic symphysis, and level of the supravesical fossa to that of the non-distended (empty) bladder in part **B. B.** In this female pelvis, the uterus was sectioned in its own median plane and is depicted as though it coincided with the median plane of the body, which is seldom the case. With the bladder empty, the normal disposition of the uterus shown here—bent on itself (anteflexed) at the junction of the body and cervix and tipped anteriorly (anteverted)—causes its weight to be borne mainly by the bladder. The urethra lies anterior and parallel to the lower half of the vagina.

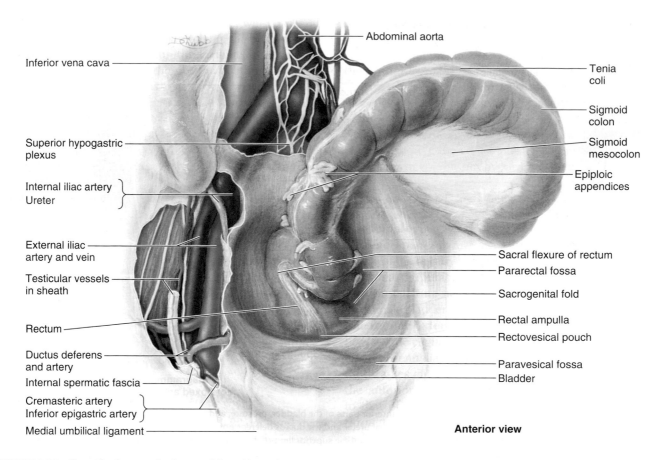

- Abdominal aorta
- Inferior vena cava
- Superior hypogastric plexus
- Internal iliac artery
- Ureter
- External iliac artery and vein
- Testicular vessels in sheath
- Rectum
- Ductus deferens and artery
- Internal spermatic fascia
- Cremasteric artery
- Inferior epigastric artery
- Medial umbilical ligament
- Tenia coli
- Sigmoid colon
- Sigmoid mesocolon
- Epiploic appendices
- Sacral flexure of rectum
- Pararectal fossa
- Sacrogenital fold
- Rectal ampulla
- Rectovesical pouch
- Paravesical fossa
- Bladder

Anterior view

FIGURE 3.31. Sigmoid colon entering lesser pelvis and becoming rectum. The sigmoid colon is intraperitoneal, suspended by the sigmoid mesocolon, but the rectum becomes retroperitoneal and then subperitoneal as it descends. The peritoneum has been removed superior to sacral promontory and right iliac fossa, revealing the superior hypogastric plexus lying in the bifurcation of the abdominal aorta and the internal iliac artery, ureter, and ductus deferens crossing the pelvic brim to enter the lesser pelvis.

layer of smooth muscle, and the fatty omental appendices are discontinued (see also Fig. 3.56).

Although its name is derived from the Latin term for "straight" (*rectus*), the term was coined during ancient studies on animals to describe the distal part of the colon; the human rectum is characterized by a number of flexures. The rectum follows the curve of the sacrum and coccyx, forming the **sacral flexure of the rectum.** The rectum ends antero-inferior to the tip of the coccyx, immediately before a sharp postero-inferior angle (the **anorectal flexure of the anal canal**) that occurs as the gut perforates the pelvic diaphragm (levator ani). The roughly 80° anorectal flexure is an important mechanism for fecal continence, being maintained during the resting state by the tonus of the puborectalis muscle, and by its active contraction during peristaltic contractions if defecation is not to occur. With the flexures of the rectosigmoid junction superiorly and the anorectal junction inferiorly, the rectum has an S shape when viewed laterally.

Three sharp **lateral flexures of the rectum** (**superior** and **inferior** on the left side, and **intermediate** on the right) are apparent when the rectum is viewed anteriorly (Fig. 3.32). The flexures are formed in relation to three internal

infoldings (**transverse rectal folds**): two on the left and one on the right side. The folds overlie thickened parts of the circular muscle layer of the rectal wall. The dilated terminal part of the rectum, lying directly superior to and supported by the pelvic diaphragm (levator ani) and anococcygeal ligament, is the **ampulla of the rectum** (Figs. 3.27, 3.31, and 3.32). The ampulla receives and holds an accumulating fecal mass until it is expelled during defecation. The ability of the ampulla to relax to accommodate the initial and subsequent arrivals of fecal material is another essential element of maintaining fecal continence.

Peritoneum covers the anterior and lateral surfaces of the superior third of the rectum, only the anterior surface of the middle third, and no surface of the inferior third because it is subperitoneal (see Table 3.3). In males, the peritoneum reflects from the rectum to the posterior wall of the bladder, where it forms the floor of the *rectovesical pouch*. In females, the peritoneum reflects from the rectum to the posterior part of the fornix of the vagina, where it forms the floor of the *recto-uterine pouch*. In both sexes, lateral reflections of peritoneum from the superior third of the rectum form *pararectal fossae* (Fig. 3.31), which permit the rectum to distend as it fills with feces.

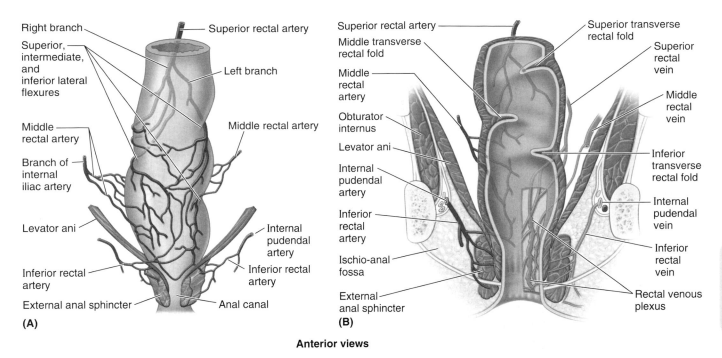

Anterior views

FIGURE 3.32. **Arteries and veins of rectum and anal canal. A.** Despite their name, the inferior rectal arteries, which are branches of the internal pudendal arteries, mainly supply the anal canal. The three sharp lateral flexures of the rectum reflect the way in which the lumen navigates the transverse rectal folds (shown in part **B**) on the internal surface. **B.** This coronal section of the rectum and anal canal demonstrates the arterial supply and venous drainage. The internal and external rectal venous plexuses are most directly related to the anal canal. The flexures and transverse rectal folds help support the weight of the feces.

The rectum lies posteriorly against the inferior three sacral vertebrae and the coccyx, anococcygeal ligament, median sacral vessels, and inferior ends of the sympathetic trunks and sacral plexuses. In males, the rectum is related anteriorly to the fundus of the urinary bladder, terminal parts of the ureters, ductus deferentes, seminal glands, and prostate (see Figs. 3.13D and 3.27A). The *rectovesical septum* lies between the fundus of the bladder and the ampulla of the rectum and is closely associated with the seminal glands and prostate. In females, the rectum is related anteriorly to the vagina and is separated from the posterior part of the fornix and the cervix by the *recto-uterine pouch* (see Figs. 3.13D and 3.27B). Inferior to this pouch, the weak rectovaginal septum separates the superior half of the posterior wall of the vagina from the rectum.

ARTERIAL SUPPLY AND VENOUS DRAINAGE OF RECTUM

The *superior rectal artery,* the continuation of the abdominal inferior mesenteric artery, supplies the proximal part of the rectum (Fig. 3.32). The right and left *middle rectal arteries,* which often arise from the anterior divisions of the internal iliac arteries in the pelvis, supply the middle and inferior parts of the rectum. The **inferior rectal arteries,** arising from the internal pudendal arteries in the perineum, supply the anorectal junction and anal canal. Anastomoses between the superior and inferior rectal arteries may provide potential collateral circulation, but anastomoses with the middle rectal arteries are sparse.

Blood from the rectum drains through the *superior, middle,* and *inferior rectal veins* (Fig. 3.32B). Anastomoses

occur between the portal and systemic veins in the wall of the anal canal. Because the superior rectal vein drains into the portal venous system and the middle and inferior rectal veins drain into the systemic system, these anastomoses are clinically important areas of portocaval anastomosis (see Fig. 2.75A). The submucosal rectal venous plexus surrounds the rectum, communicating with the vesical venous plexus in males and the uterovaginal venous plexus in females. The **rectal venous plexus** consists of two parts (Fig. 3.32B): the **internal rectal venous plexus** just deep to the mucosa of the anorectal junction and the subcutaneous **external rectal venous plexus** external to the muscular wall of the rectum. Although these plexuses bear the term *rectal,* they are primarily "anal" in terms of location, function, and clinical significance (see "Venous and Lymphatic Drainage of Anal Canal," p. 413).

INNERVATION OF RECTUM

The nerve supply to the rectum is from the sympathetic and parasympathetic systems (Fig. 3.33). The *sympathetic supply* is from the lumbar spinal cord, conveyed via lumbar splanchnic nerves and the hypogastric/pelvic plexuses, and through the peri-arterial plexus of the inferior mesenteric and superior rectal arteries. The *parasympathetic supply* is from the S2–S4 spinal cord level, passing via the pelvic splanchnic nerves and the left and right inferior hypogastric plexuses to the rectal (pelvic) plexus. Because the rectum is inferior (distal) to the pelvic pain line, all visceral afferent fibers follow the parasympathetic fibers retrogradely to the S2–S4 spinal sensory ganglia.

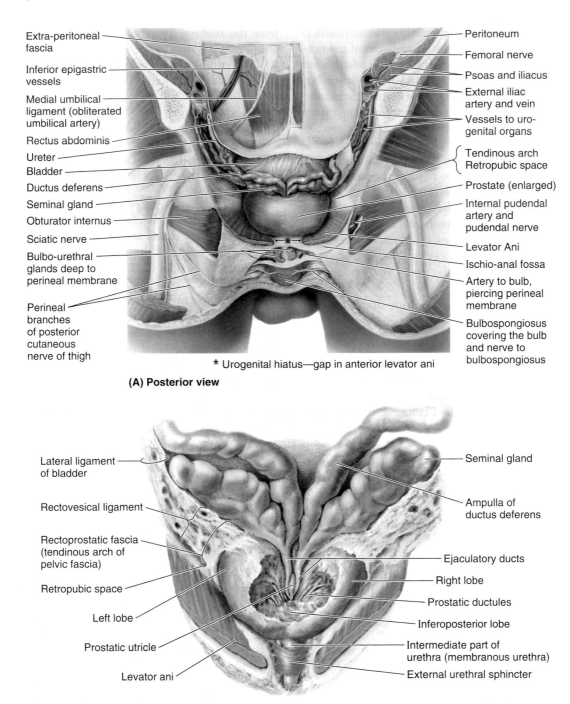

(A) Posterior view

Extra-peritoneal fascia

Inferior epigastric vessels

Medial umbilical ligament (obliterated umbilical artery)

Rectus abdominis

Ureter

Bladder

Ductus deferens

Seminal gland

Obturator internus

Sciatic nerve

Bulbo-urethral glands deep to perineal membrane

Perineal branches of posterior cutaneous nerve of thigh

Peritoneum

Femoral nerve

Psoas and iliacus

External iliac artery and vein

Vessels to uro-genital organs

Tendinous arch Retropubic space

Prostate (enlarged)

Internal pudendal artery and pudendal nerve

Levator Ani

Ischio-anal fossa

Artery to bulb, piercing perineal membrane

Bulbospongiosus covering the bulb and nerve to bulbospongiosus

* Urogenital hiatus—gap in anterior levator ani

(B) Posterior view

Lateral ligament of bladder

Rectovesical ligament

Rectoprostatic fascia (tendinous arch of pelvic fascia)

Retropubic space

Left lobe

Prostatic utricle

Levator ani

Seminal gland

Ampulla of ductus deferens

Ejaculatory ducts

Right lobe

Prostatic ductules

Inferoposterior lobe

Intermediate part of urethra (membranous urethra)

External urethral sphincter

FIGURE 3.36. Posterior aspect of male pelvic viscera and posterior dissection of prostate. A. The posterior pelvic wall, rectum, and rectovesical septum have been removed. The umbilical ligaments, like the urinary bladder, are embedded in extraperitoneal or subperitoneal fascia (mostly removed in this dissection). **B.** The ejaculatory ducts are formed by the merger of the duct of the seminal gland and the ductus deferens. The vestigial prostatic utricle, usually seen as an invagination in an anterior view, appears in this posterior dissection as an evagination lying between the ejaculatory ducts.

- A posterior surface that is related to the ampulla of the rectum.
- Inferolateral surfaces that are related to the levator ani.

Although not clearly distinct anatomically, the following lobes of the prostate are traditionally described (Fig. 3.38A):

- The **isthmus of the prostate** (commissure of prostate; historically, the anterior "lobe") lies anterior to the ure-

thra. It is fibromuscular, the muscle fibers representing a superior continuation of the external urethral sphincter muscle to the neck of the bladder, and contains little, if any, glandular tissue.

- **Right** and **left lobes of the prostate,** separated anteriorly by the isthmus and posteriorly by a central, shallow longitudinal furrow, may each be subdivided for descriptive purposes into four indistinct lobules defined by their

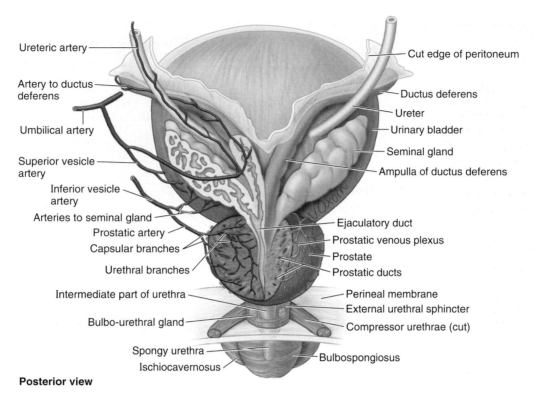

Ureteric artery

Artery to ductus deferens

Umbilical artery

Superior vesicle artery

Inferior vesicle artery

Arteries to seminal gland

Prostatic artery

Capsular branches

Urethral branches

Intermediate part of urethra

Bulbo-urethral gland

Spongy urethra

Ischiocavernosus

Cut edge of peritoneum

Ductus deferens

Ureter

Urinary bladder

Seminal gland

Ampulla of ductus deferens

Ejaculatory duct

Prostatic venous plexus

Prostate

Prostatic ducts

Perineal membrane

External urethral sphincter

Compressor urethrae (cut)

Bulbospongiosus

Posterior view

FIGURE 3.37. Pelvic part of ureters, urinary bladder, seminal glands, terminal parts of ductus deferens, and prostate. The left seminal gland and ampulla of the ductus deferens are dissected free and sliced open. Part of the prostate is also cut away to expose the ejaculatory duct. The perineal membrane lies between the external genitalia and the deep part of the perineum (anterior recess of ischio-anal fossa). It is pierced by the urethra, ducts of the bulbo-urethral glands, dorsal and deep arteries of the penis, cavernous nerves, and the dorsal nerve of the penis.

relationship to the urethra and ejaculatory ducts, and—although less apparent—by the arrangement of the ducts and connective tissue:

(1) an **inferoposterior** (lower posterior) **lobule** that lies posterior to the urethra and inferior to the ejaculatory ducts. This lobule constitutes the aspect of the prostate palpable by digital rectal examination.

(2) an **inferolateral** (lower lateral) **lobule** directly lateral to the urethra, forming the major part of the right or left lobe.

(3) a **superomedial lobule,** deep to the inferoposterior lobule, surrounding the ipsilateral ejaculatory duct.

(4) an **anteromedial lobule,** deep to the inferolateral lobule, directly lateral to the proximal prostatic urethra.

An embryonic *middle (median) lobe* gives rise to (3) and (4) above. This region tends to undergo hormone-induced hypertrophy in advanced age, forming a *middle lobule* that lies between the urethra and the ejaculatory ducts and is closely related to the neck of the bladder. Enlargement of the middle lobule is believed to be at least partially responsible for the formation of the *uvula* that may project into the internal urethral orifice (Fig. 3.30).

Some clinicians, especially urologists and sonographers, divide the prostate into peripheral and central (internal) zones (Fig. 3.38B). The central zone is comparable to the middle lobe.

The **prostatic ducts** (20–30) open chiefly into the *prostatic sinuses* that lie on either side of the seminal colliculus on the posterior wall of the prostatic urethra (Fig. 3.37). Prostatic fluid, a thin, milky fluid, provides approximately 20% of the volume of **semen** (a mixture of secretions produced by the testes, seminal glands, prostate, and bulbo-urethral glands that provides the vehicle by which sperms are transported) and plays a role in activating the sperms.

Arterial Supply and Venous Drainage of Prostate. The prostatic arteries are mainly branches of the internal iliac artery (see Table 3.4; Figs. 3.17A and 3.37), especially the *inferior vesical arteries,* but also the internal pudendal and middle rectal arteries. The veins join to form a plexus around the sides and base of the prostate (Figs. 3.19C and 3.37). This **prostatic venous plexus,** between the fibrous capsule of the prostate and the prostatic sheath, drains into the *internal iliac veins.* The prostatic venous plexus is continuous superiorly with the *vesical venous plexus* and communicates posteriorly with the *internal vertebral venous plexus.*

BULBO-URETHRAL GLANDS

The two pea-size **bulbo-urethral glands** (Cowper glands) lie posterolateral to the intermediate part of the urethra, largely embedded within the external urethral sphincter (Figs. 3.30B, 3.34, 3.36, and 3.37). The **ducts of the**

(A) Transverse anatomic section of prostate (left) at level of red line in median section (right)

- Isthmus of prostate
- Inferolateral lobule
- Prostatic urethra
- Anteromedial lobule
- Seminal colliculus
- Ejaculatory ducts
- Superomedial lobule
- Inferoposterior lobule
- Furrow in posterior surface

- Internal urethral sphincter
- Seminal gland
- Superomedial lobule
- Ejaculatory duct
- Prostatic urethra
- Inferoposterior lobule
- Isthmus of prostate
- Apex of prostate
- Intermediate urethra
- External urethral sphincter

- Prostatic venous plexus
- Prostatic capsule
- AMZ
- PZ
- CZ
- PZ

- Anterior muscular zone (AMZ)
- Prostatic urethra
- Seminal colliculus
- Prostatic sinus (receiving openings of prostatic ducts)
- Peripheral zone of prostate (PZ)
- Prostatic utricle
- Ejaculatory ducts
- Central (internal) zone of prostate (CZ)
- Anterior wall of rectum
- Rectum

- AMZ
- PZ
- CZ
- PZ
- SIZE 1 .5 CM/DIV

(B) Graphic interpretation (left) of transverse ultrasound image (rt.) at level of green line in (A-rt).

FIGURE 3.38. **Lobules and zones of prostate demonstrated by anatomical section and ultrasonographic imaging. A.** Poorly demarcated lobules demonstrated in anatomic sections. **B.** The ultrasound (US) transducer was inserted into the rectum to scan the anteriorly located prostate. The ducts of the glands in the peripheral zone open into the prostatic sinuses, whereas the ducts of the glands in the central (internal) zone open into the prostatic sinuses and the seminal colliculus.

bulbo-urethral glands pass through the perineal membrane with the intermediate urethra, and open through minute apertures into the proximal part of the spongy urethra in the bulb of the penis. Their mucus-like secretion enters the urethra during sexual arousal.

INNERVATION OF INTERNAL GENITAL ORGANS OF MALE PELVIS

The ductus deferens, seminal glands, ejaculatory ducts, and prostate are richly innervated by sympathetic nerve fibers. *Presynaptic sympathetic fibers* originate from cell bodies in the intermediolateral cell column of the T12–L2 (or L3) spinal cord segments. They traverse the paravertebral ganglia of the sympathetic trunks to become components of lumbar (abdominopelvic) splanchnic nerves and the hypogastric and pelvic plexuses (see Fig. 3.29, p. 367).

Presynaptic parasympathetic fibers from S2 and S3 spinal cord segments traverse *pelvic splanchnic nerves*, which also join the inferior hypogastric/pelvic plexuses. Synapses with postsynaptic sympathetic and parasympathetic neurons occur within the plexuses, en route to or near the pelvic viscera. As part of an orgasm, the sympathetic system stimulates contraction of the internal urethral sphincter to prevent retrograde ejaculation. Simultaneously, it stimulates rapid peristaltic-like contractions of the ductus deferens, and the combined contraction of and secretion from the seminal glands and prostate that provide the vehicle (semen), and the expulsive force to discharge the sperms during ejaculation. The function of the parasympathetic innervation of the internal genital organs is unclear. However, parasympathetic fibers traversing the prostatic nerve plexus form the *cavernous nerves* that pass to the erectile bodies of the penis, which are responsible for producing penile erection.

MALE INTERNAL GENITAL ORGANS

Male Sterilization

The common method of sterilizing males is a *deferentectomy*, popularly called a *vasectomy*. During this procedure, part of the ductus deferens is ligated and/or excised through an incision in the superior part of the scrotum (Fig. B3.11). Hence, the subsequent ejaculated fluid from the seminal glands, prostate, and bulbo-urethral glands contains no sperms. The unexpelled sperms degenerate in the epididymis and the proximal part of the ductus deferens.

Reversal of a deferentectomy is successful in favorable cases (patients < 30 years of age and < 7 years postoperation) in most instances. The ends of the sectioned ductus deferentes are reattached under an operating microscope.

Abscesses in Seminal Glands

Localized collections of pus (abscesses) in the seminal glands may rupture, allowing pus to enter the peritoneal cavity. Seminal glands can be palpated during a rectal examination, especially if enlarged or full. They are palpated most easily when the bladder is moderately full. They can also be massaged to release their secretions for microscopic examination to detect *gonococci* (organisms that cause gonorrhea), for example.

Hypertrophy of Prostate

The prostate is of considerable medical interest because enlargement or *benign hypertrophy of the prostate (BHP)* is common after middle age, affecting virtually every male who lives long enough. An enlarged prostate projects into the urinary bladder and impedes urination by distorting the prostatic urethra. The middle lobule usually enlarges the most and obstructs the internal urethral orifice. The more the person strains, the more the valve-like prostatic mass occludes the urethra.

BHP is a common cause of urethral obstruction, leading to *nocturia* (need to void during the night), *dysuria* (difficulty and/or pain during urination), and *urgency* (sudden desire to void). BHP also increases the risk of bladder infections (cystitis) as well as kidney damage.

The prostate is examined for enlargement and tumors (focal masses or asymmetry) by *digital rectal examination* (Fig. B3.12). The palpability of the prostate depends on the fullness of the bladder. A full bladder offers resistance, holding the gland in place and making it more readily palpable. The malignant prostate feels hard and often irregular. In advanced stages, cancer cells metastasize both via lymphatic routes (initially to the internal iliac and sacral lymph nodes and later to distant nodes), and via venous routes (by way of the internal vertebral venous plexus, to the vertebrae and brain).

Because of the close relationship of the prostate to the prostatic urethra, obstructions may be relieved endoscopically. The instrument is inserted transurethrally through the external urethral orifice and spongy urethra into the prostatic urethra. All or part of the prostate, or just the hypertrophied part, is removed (*transurethral resection of the prostate; TURP*). In more serious cases, the entire prostate is removed along with the seminal glands, ejaculatory ducts, and terminal parts of the deferent ducts (*radical prostatectomy*).

TURP and improved open operative techniques attempt to preserve the nerves and blood vessels associated with the capsule of the prostate that pass to and from the penis, increasing the possibility for patients to retain sexual function after surgery, as well as restoring normal urinary control.

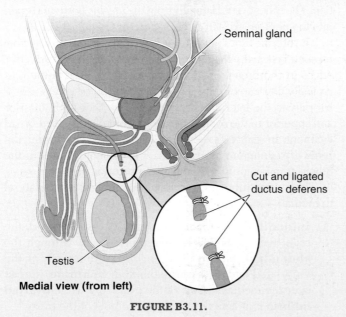

Medial view (from left)

FIGURE B3.11.

Medial view (from left)

FIGURE B3.12.

The Bottom Line

MALE INTERNAL GENITAL ORGANS

Ductus deferens: The cord-like ductus deferens is the primary component of the spermatic cord, conducting sperms from the epididymis to the ejaculatory duct. ◆ The distal portion of the ductus is superficial within the scrotum (and, therefore, easily accessible for deferentectomy or vasectomy) before it penetrates the anterior abdominal wall via the inguinal canal. ◆ The pelvic portion of the ductus lies immediately external to the peritoneum, with its terminal portion enlarging externally as its lumen becomes tortuous internally, forming the ampulla of the ductus deferens.

Seminal glands, ejaculatory ducts, and prostate: Obliquely placed seminal glands converge at the base of the bladder, where each of their ducts merges with the ipsilateral ductus deferens to form an ejaculatory duct. ◆ The two ejaculatory ducts immediately enter the posterior aspect of the prostate, running closely parallel through the gland to open on the seminal colliculus. ◆ Prostatic ducts open into prostatic sinuses, adjacent to the seminal colliculus. Thus, the major glandular secretions and sperms are delivered to the prostatic urethra. ◆ The seminal glands and prostate produce by far the greatest portion of the seminal fluid, indispensable for transport and delivery of sperms. ◆ These internal genital organs, located within the anterior male pelvis, receive blood from the inferior vesicle and middle rectal arteries, which drain into the continuous prostatic/vesicle venous plexus. ◆ Sympathetic fibers from lumbar levels stimulate the contraction and secretion resulting in ejaculation. ◆ The function of parasympathetic fibers from S2–S4 to the internal genital organs is unclear, but those traversing the prostatic nerve plexus to form the cavernous nerves produce erection.

Female Internal Genital Organs

The female internal genital organs include the ovaries, uterine tubes, uterus, and vagina.

OVARIES

The **ovaries** are almond-shaped and -sized female gonads in which the *oocytes* (female gametes or germ cells) develop. They are also endocrine glands that produce reproductive hormones. Each ovary is suspended by a short peritoneal fold or mesentery, the *mesovarium* (Fig. 3.39A). The mesovarium is a subdivision of a larger mesentery of the uterus, *the broad ligament.*

In prepubertal females, the connective tissue capsule (*tunica albuginea of the ovary*) comprising the surface of the ovary is covered by a smooth layer of **ovarian mesothelium** or **surface (germinal) epithelium,** a single layer of cuboidal cells that gives the surface a dull, grayish appearance, contrasting with the shiny surface of the adjacent peritoneal mesovarium with which it is continuous (Fig. 3.39B). After puberty, the ovarian surface epithelium becomes progressively scarred and distorted because of the repeated rupture of ovarian follicles and discharge of oocytes during ovulation. The scarring is less in women who have been taking oral contraceptives that inhibit ovulation.

The ovarian vessels, lymphatics, and nerves cross the pelvic brim, passing to and from the superolateral aspect of the ovary within a peritoneal fold, the **suspensory ligament of the ovary,** which becomes continuous with the mesovarium of the broad ligament. Medially within the mesovarium, a short *ligament of ovary* tethers the ovary to the uterus. Consequently the ovaries are typically found laterally between the uterus and the lateral pelvic wall during a manual or ultrasonic pelvic examination (Fig. 3.40). The ligament of ovary is a remnant of the superior part of the ovarian gubernaculum of the fetus (see Fig. 2.17B, p. 206). The ligament of the ovary connects the proximal (uterine) end of the ovary to the lateral angle of the uterus, just inferior to the entrance of the uterine tube (Fig. 3.39A). Because the ovary is suspended in the peritoneal cavity and its surface is not covered by peritoneum, the oocyte expelled at ovulation passes into the peritoneal cavity. However, its intraperitoneal life is short because it is normally trapped by the fimbriae of the infundibulum of the uterine tube and carried into the ampulla, where it may be fertilized.

UTERINE TUBES

The **uterine tubes** (formerly called oviducts or fallopian tubes) conduct the oocyte, discharged monthly from an ovary during child-bearing years, from the peri-ovarian peritoneal cavity to the uterine cavity. They also provide the usual site of fertilization. The tubes extend laterally from the *uterine horns* and open into the peritoneal cavity near the ovaries (Fig. 3.39A & B).

The uterine tubes (approximately 10 cm long) lie in a narrow mesentery, the **mesosalpinx,** forming the free anterosuperior edges of the broad ligaments. In the "ideal" disposition, as typically illustrated, the tubes extend symmetrically posterolaterally to the lateral pelvic walls, where they arch anterior and superior to the ovaries in the horizontally disposed broad ligament. In reality, as seen in an ultrasound examination, the tubes are commonly asymmetrically arranged with one or the other often lying superior and even posterior to the uterus.

The uterine tubes are divisible into four parts, from lateral to medial:

(1) **Infundibulum:** the funnel-shaped distal end of the tube that opens into the peritoneal cavity through the **abdominal ostium.** The finger-like processes of the fimbriated end of the infundibulum (**fimbriae**) spread over the medial surface of the ovary; one large **ovarian fimbria** is attached to the superior pole of the ovary.

(A) Posterior view

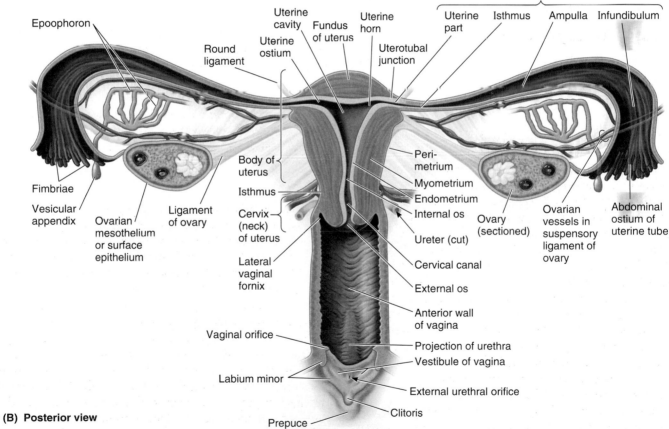

(B) Posterior view

FIGURE 3.39. Internal female genital organs. A. Isolated dissection specimen consisting of the ovaries, uterine tubes, uterus, and related structures. The broad ligament is removed on the left side. **B.** This coronal section demonstrates the internal structure of the female genital organs. The epoophoron is a collection of rudimentary tubules in the mesosalpinx (mesentery of uterine tube). The epoophoron and vesicular appendage are vestiges of the embryonic mesonephros.

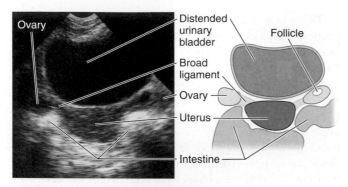

FIGURE 3.40. Ovaries and uterus as revealed by ultrasound scanning. The diagram on the right is a graphic interpretation of the image.

(2) **Ampulla:** the widest and longest part of the tube, which begins at the medial end of the infundibulum; fertilization of the oocyte usually occurs in the ampulla.

(3) **Isthmus:** the thick-walled part of the tube, which enters the uterine horn.

(4) **Uterine part:** the short intramural segment of the tube that passes through the wall of the uterus and opens via the uterine ostium into the uterine cavity at the uterine horn.

Arterial Supply and Venous Drainage of Ovaries and Uterine Tubes. The *ovarian arteries* arise from the abdominal aorta (see Fig. 3.16; Table 3.4) and descend along the posterior abdominal wall. At the pelvic brim, they cross over the external iliac vessels and enter the suspensory ligaments (Fig. 3.39A), approaching the lateral aspects of the ovaries and uterine tubes. The ascending branches of the *uterine arteries* (branches of the internal iliac arteries) course along the lateral aspects of the uterus to approach the medial aspects of the ovaries and tubes (Figs. 3.18B and 3.41). Both the ovarian and ascending uterine arteries terminate by bifurcating into *ovarian* and *tubal branches*, which supply the ovaries and tubes from opposite ends and anastomose with each other, providing a collateral circulation from abdominal and pelvic sources to both structures.

Veins draining the ovary form a vine-like **pampiniform plexus of veins** in the broad ligament near the ovary and uterine tube (Fig. 3.41). The veins of the plexus usually merge to form a singular **ovarian vein,** which leaves the lesser pelvis with the ovarian artery. The right ovarian vein ascends to enter the *inferior vena cava;* the left ovarian vein drains into the *left renal vein* (Fig. 3.19). The *tubal veins* drain into the *ovarian veins* and *uterine (uterovaginal) venous plexus* (Fig. 3.41).

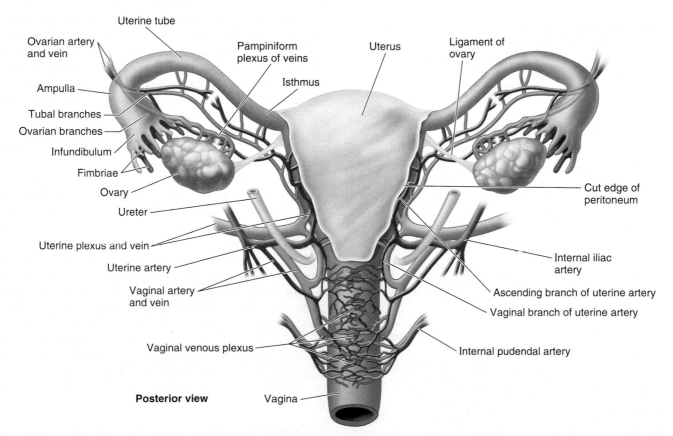

FIGURE 3.41. Blood supply and venous drainage of uterus, vagina, and ovaries. The broad ligament of the uterus is removed on each side of the uterus to show the anastomosing branches of the ovarian artery from the aorta and the uterine artery from the internal iliac artery supplying the ovary, uterine tube, and uterus. The veins follow a similar pattern, flowing retrograde to the arteries, but are more plexiform, including a pampiniform plexus related to the ovary and continuous uterine and vaginal plexuses (collectively, the uterovaginal plexus).

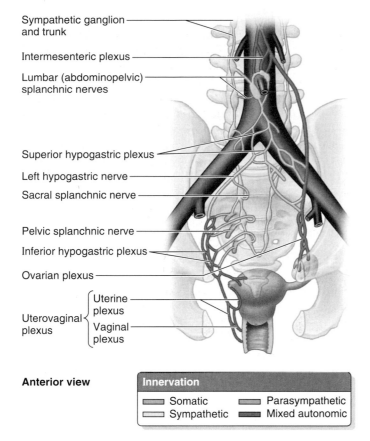

Sympathetic ganglion and trunk

Intermesenteric plexus

Lumbar (abdominopelvic) splanchnic nerves

Superior hypogastric plexus

Left hypogastric nerve

Sacral splanchnic nerve

Pelvic splanchnic nerve

Inferior hypogastric plexus

Ovarian plexus

Uterovaginal plexus { Uterine plexus / Vaginal plexus }

Anterior view

Innervation	
▭ Somatic	▭ Parasympathetic
▭ Sympathetic	▭ Mixed autonomic

FIGURE 3.42. Nerve supply of ovaries and female internal genital organs. In addition to autonomic (visceral motor) fibers, these nerves convey visceral afferent fibers from these organs. The inferior part of the vagina is not depicted because it receives somatic innervation.

Innervation of Ovaries and Uterine Tubes. The nerve supply derives partly from the *ovarian plexus*, descending with the ovarian vessels, and partly from the *uterine (pelvic) plexus* (Fig. 3.42). The ovaries and uterine tubes are intraperitoneal and, therefore, are superior to the *pelvic pain line* (see Table 3.3). Thus, visceral afferent pain fibers ascend retrogradely with the descending sympathetic fibers of the ovarian plexus and lumbar splanchnic nerves to cell bodies in the T11–L1 spinal sensory ganglia. Visceral afferent reflex fibers follow parasympathetic fibers retrogradely through the uterine (pelvic) and inferior hypogastric plexuses and the pelvic splanchnic nerves to cell bodies in the S2–S4 spinal sensory ganglia.

UTERUS

The **uterus** (womb) is a thick-walled, pear-shaped, hollow muscular organ. The embryo and fetus develop in the uterus. Its muscular walls adapt to the growth of the fetus and then provide the power for its expulsion during childbirth. The non-gravid (non-pregnant) uterus usually lies in the lesser pelvis, with its body lying on the urinary bladder and its cervix between the urinary bladder and rectum (Fig. 3.43A).

The uterus is a very dynamic structure, the size and proportions of which change during the various changes of life (see the blue box "Lifetime Change in Normal Anatomy of Uterus," on p. 393).

The adult uterus is usually *anteverted* (tipped antero-superiorly relative to the axis of the vagina) and *anteflexed* (flexed or bent anteriorly relative to the cervix, creating the *angle of flexion*) so that its mass lies over the bladder. Consequently, when the bladder is empty, the uterus typically lies in a nearly transverse plane (Figs. 3.43AB & 3.44A). The position of the uterus changes with the degree of fullness of the bladder (Fig. 3.44B) and rectum, and stage of pregnancy. Although its size varies considerably, the non-gravid uterus is approximately 7.5 cm long, 5 cm wide, and 2 cm thick and weighs approximately 90 g. The uterus is divisible into two main parts (Fig. 3.43B): the body and cervix.

The **body of the uterus,** forming the superior two thirds of the organ, includes the **fundus of the uterus,** the rounded part that lies superior to the uterine ostia (Fig. 3.39B). The body lies between the layers of the broad ligament and is freely movable (Fig. 3.39A). It has two surfaces: vesical (related to the bladder) and intestinal. The body is demarcated from the cervix by the **isthmus of the uterus,** a relatively constricted segment, approximately 1 cm long (Figs. 3.39A & B and 3.43B).

The **cervix of the uterus** is the cylindrical, relatively narrow inferior third of the uterus, approximately 2.5 cm long in an adult non-pregnant woman. For descriptive purposes, two parts are described: a **supravaginal part** between the isthmus and the vagina, and a **vaginal part,** which protrudes into the superiormost anterior vaginal wall (Fig. 3.43B). The rounded vaginal part surrounds the **external os of the uterus** and is surrounded in turn by a narrow recess, the *vaginal fornix* (Fig. 3.43C). The supravaginal part is separated from the bladder anteriorly by loose connective tissue and from the rectum posteriorly by the *recto-uterine pouch* (Fig. 3.43A).

The slit-like **uterine cavity** is approximately 6 cm in length from the external os to the wall of the fundus (Fig. 3.39B). The **uterine horns** (L. *cornua*) are the superolateral regions of the uterine cavity, where the uterine tubes enter. The uterine cavity continues inferiorly as the **cervical canal.** The fusiform canal extends from a narrowing inside the isthmus of the uterine body, the **anatomical internal os,** through the supravaginal and vaginal parts of the cervix, communicating with the lumen of the vagina through the external os. The uterine cavity (in particular, the cervical canal) and the lumen of the vagina together constitute the **birth canal,** through which the fetus passes at the end of gestation.

The wall of the body of the uterus consists of three coats, or layers:

- **Perimetrium**—the serosa or outer serous coat—consists of peritoneum supported by a thin layer of connective tissue.
- **Myometrium**—the middle coat of smooth muscle—becomes greatly distended (more extensive but much

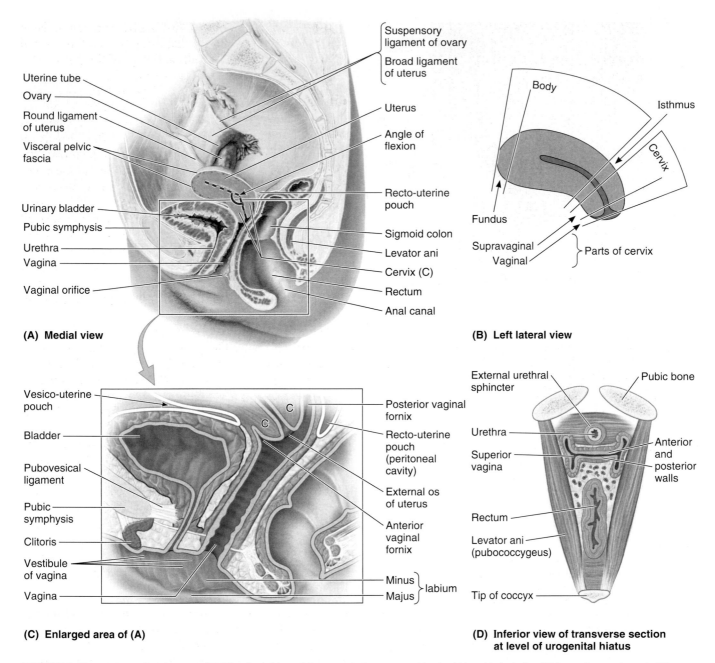

(A) Medial view

Suspensory ligament of ovary
Broad ligament of uterus
Uterine tube
Ovary
Round ligament of uterus
Visceral pelvic fascia
Uterus
Angle of flexion
Urinary bladder
Pubic symphysis
Urethra
Vagina
Vaginal orifice
Recto-uterine pouch
Sigmoid colon
Levator ani
Cervix (C)
Rectum
Anal canal

(B) Left lateral view

Body
Isthmus
Cervix
Fundus
Supravaginal
Vaginal
Parts of cervix

(C) Enlarged area of (A)

Vesico-uterine pouch
Bladder
Pubovesical ligament
Pubic symphysis
Clitoris
Vestibule of vagina
Vagina
C
C
Posterior vaginal fornix
Recto-uterine pouch (peritoneal cavity)
External os of uterus
Anterior vaginal fornix
Minus
Majus } labium

(D) Inferior view of transverse section at level of urogenital hiatus

External urethral sphincter
Pubic bone
Urethra
Superior vagina
Anterior and posterior walls
Rectum
Levator ani (pubococcygeus)
Tip of coccyx

FIGURE 3.43. Uterus and vagina. A and **B.** The disposition of the uterus is demonstrated in situ (**A**) and in isolation (**B**) in median sections. **A.** When the bladder is empty, the typical uterus is anteverted and anteflexed. **B.** The two main parts of the uterus, the body and cervix, are separated by the isthmus. Knowledge of further subdivisions of the main parts is especially important for such things as describing the location of tumors, sites of attachment of the placenta, and considering the consequences. **C** is an enlarged view of the outlined area in **A**. Note in (**A**) and (**C**) that the axes of the urethra and vagina are parallel, and the urethra is adherent to the anterior vaginal wall. Placing a gloved finger in the vagina can help direct the insertion of a catheter through the urethra into the bladder. **D.** A transverse section through the inferior female pelvic organs as they penetrate the pelvic floor through the urogenital hiatus (the gap between the right and the left sides of the levator ani) demonstrates the typical disposition of the non-distended lumina.

thinner) during pregnancy. The main branches of the blood vessels and nerves of the uterus are located in this coat. During childbirth, contraction of the myometrium is hormonally stimulated at intervals of decreasing length to dilate the cervical os and expel the fetus and placenta. During the menses, myometrial contractions may produce cramping.

• **Endometrium**—the inner mucous coat—is firmly adhered to the underlying myometrium. The endometrium is actively involved in the menstrual cycle, differing in structure with each stage of the cycle. If conception occurs, the blastocyst becomes implanted in this layer; if conception does not occur, the inner surface of this coat is shed during menstruation.

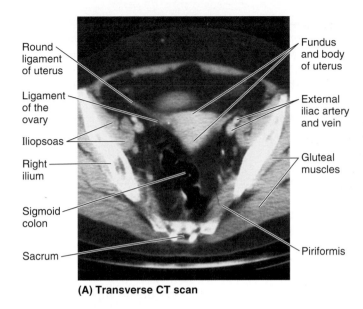

Round ligament of uterus
Ligament of the ovary
Iliopsoas
Right ilium
Sigmoid colon
Sacrum

Fundus and body of uterus
External iliac artery and vein
Gluteal muscles
Piriformis

(A) Transverse CT scan

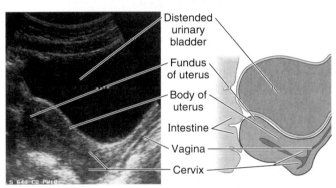

Distended urinary bladder
Fundus of uterus
Body of uterus
Intestine
Vagina
Cervix

(B) Longitudinal (median) ultrasound image

FIGURE 3.44. Imaging of female pelvic viscera. A. Because the uterus is nearly horizontally disposed when anteverted and anteflexed over the bladder, most of its body, including the fundus, appears in this transverse CT scan. (Courtesy of Dr. Donald R. Cahill, Department of Anatomy, Mayo Medical School, Rochester, MN.) **B.** Temporary retroversion and retroflexion result when a fully distended urinary bladder temporarily retroverts the uterus and decreases its angle of flexion. Compare with Figure 3.43A. (Courtesy of Dr. A. M. Arenson, Assistant Professor of Medical Imaging, University of Toronto, Toronto, ON, Canada.)

The amount of muscular tissue in the cervix is markedly less than in the body of the uterus. The cervix is mostly fibrous and is composed mainly of collagen with a small amount of smooth muscle and elastin.

Ligaments of Uterus. Externally, the **ligament of the ovary** attaches to the uterus postero-inferior to the uterotubal junction (Fig. 3.39A & B). The **round ligament of the uterus** (L. *ligamentum teres uteri*) attaches antero-inferiorly to this junction. These two ligaments are vestiges of the *ovarian gubernaculum,* related to the relocation of the gonad from its developmental position on the posterior abdominal wall (Fig. 2.17A).

The **broad ligament of the uterus** is a double layer of peritoneum (mesentery) that extends from the sides of the uterus to the lateral walls and floor of the pelvis (Fig. 3.39A). This ligament assists in keeping the uterus in position. The two layers of the broad ligament are continuous with each other at a free edge that surrounds the uterine tube. Laterally, the peritoneum of the broad ligament is prolonged superiorly over the vessels as the *suspensory ligament of the ovary.* Between the layers of the broad ligament on each side of the uterus, the *ligament of the ovary* lies posterosuperiorly and the *round ligament of the uterus* lies antero-inferiorly. The uterine tube lies in the anterosuperior free border of the broad ligament, within a small mesentery called the *mesosalpinx.* Similarly, the ovary lies within a small mesentery called the *mesovarium* on the posterior aspect of the broad ligament. The largest part of the broad ligament, inferior to the mesosalpinx and mesovarium, which serves as a mesentery for the uterus itself, is the **mesometrium.**

The uterus is a dense structure located in the center of the pelvic cavity. The principal supports of the uterus holding it in this position are both passive and active or dynamic. *Dynamic support of the uterus* is provided by the pelvic diaphragm. Its tone during sitting and standing and active contraction during periods of increased intraabdominal pressure (sneezing, coughing, etc.) is transmitted through the surrounding pelvic organs and the endopelvic fascia in which they are embedded. *Passive support of the uterus* is provided by its position—the way in which the normally *anteverted* and *anteflexed* uterus rests on top of the bladder. When intra-abdominal pressure is increased, the uterus is pressed against the bladder. The cervix is the least mobile part of the uterus because of the passive support provided by attached condensations of endopelvic fascia (ligaments), which may also contain smooth muscle (Figs. 3.13 and 3.14):

- *Cardinal (transverse cervical) ligaments* extend from the supravaginal cervix and lateral parts of the fornix of the vagina to the lateral walls of the pelvis (Fig. 3.14).
- *Uterosacral ligaments* pass superiorly and slightly posteriorly from the sides of the cervix to the middle of the sacrum; they are palpable during a rectal examination.

Together these passive and active supports keep the uterus centered in the pelvic cavity and resist the tendency for the uterus to fall or be pushed through the vagina (see the blue box "Disposition of Uterus and Uterine Prolapse," p. 392).

Relations of Uterus. Peritoneum covers the uterus anteriorly and superiorly, except for the cervix (Fig. 3.39A). The peritoneum is reflected anteriorly from the uterus onto the bladder and posteriorly over the posterior part of the fornix of the vagina to the rectum (Fig. 3.43A). Anteriorly, the uterine body is separated from the urinary bladder by the **vesico-uterine pouch,** where the peritoneum is reflected from the uterus onto the posterior margin of the superior surface of the bladder. Posteriorly, the uterine body and supravaginal part of the cervix are separated from the sigmoid colon by a layer of peritoneum, and the peritoneal cavity and from the rectum by the *recto-uterine pouch*. Laterally, the uterine artery crosses the ureter superiorly, near the cervix (Fig. 3.41).

Summary of the relations of the uterus (Fig. 3.45):

- *Anteriorly* (antero-inferiorly in its normal anteverted position): the vesico-uterine pouch and superior surface of the bladder; the supravaginal part of the cervix is related to the bladder and is separated from it by only fibrous connective tissue.
- *Posteriorly:* the recto-uterine pouch containing loops of small intestine and the anterior surface of rectum; only the visceral pelvic fascia uniting the rectum and uterus here resists increased intra-abdominal pressure.
- *Laterally:* the peritoneal broad ligament flanking the uterine body and the fascial cardinal ligaments on each side of the cervix and vagina; in the transition between the two ligaments, the ureters run anteriorly slightly superior to the lateral part of the vaginal fornix and inferior to the uterine arteries, usually approximately 2 cm lateral to the supravaginal part of the cervix (see Fig. 3.13A).

Arterial Supply and Venous Drainage of Uterus. The blood supply of the uterus derives mainly from the *uterine arteries*, with potential collateral supply from the ovarian arteries (Fig. 3.41). The *uterine veins* enter the broad ligaments with the arteries and form a **uterine venous plexus** on each side of the cervix. Veins from the uterine plexus drain into the internal iliac veins.

VAGINA

The **vagina**, a distensible musculomembranous tube (7–9 cm long), extends from the middle cervix of the uterus to the **vaginal orifice,** the opening at the inferior end of the vagina (Figs. 3.39B and 3.43A & C). The vaginal orifice, external urethral orifice, and ducts of the greater and lesser vestibular glands open into the **vestibule of the vagina,** the cleft between the labia minora. The vaginal part of the cervix lies anteriorly in the superior vagina. The vagina:

- serves as a canal for menstrual fluid,
- forms the inferior part of the birth canal,
- receives the penis and ejaculate during sexual intercourse, and
- communicates superiorly with the *cervical canal* and inferiorly with the vestibule of the vagina.

Median umbilical fold — Supravesical fossa
Medial umbilical fold — Urinary bladder
Transverse vesical fold — Paravesical fossa
Vesico-uterine pouch — Deep inguinal ring
of Uterus { Fundus — Round ligament of uterus
Body — Broad ligament of uterus
Mesosalpinx — Uterine tube
Recto-uterine pouch — Rectum
Uterosacral fold — Pararectal fossa
Sigmoid colon — Ovarian artery
— Ovarian vein
Sigmoid mesocolon — Right ureter

FIGURE 3.45. Relationship of the female pelvic viscera. The peritoneum is intact, lining the pelvic cavity and covering the superior aspect of the bladder, fundus and body of uterus, and much of the rectum. In this supine cadaver, the uterine tube and meso salpinx on each side are hanging down, obscuring the ovaries from view. The uterus is typically asymmetrically placed, as it is here. The round ligament of the uterus follows the same subperitoneal course as the ductus deferens of the male.

The vagina is usually collapsed. The orifice is usually collapsed toward the midline so that its lateral walls are in contact on each side of an anteroposterior slit. Superior to the orifice, however, the anterior and posterior walls are in contact on each side of a transverse potential cavity, H-shaped in cross section (Fig. 3.43D), except at its superior end where the cervix holds them apart. The vagina lies posterior to the urinary bladder and urethra, the latter projecting along the midline of its inferior anterior wall (Fig. 3.39B). The vagina lies anterior to the rectum, passing between the medial margins of the levator ani (puborectalis) muscles. The **vaginal fornix,** the recess around the cervix, has *anterior, posterior,* and *lateral parts* (Figs. 3.39A and 3.43C). The **posterior vaginal fornix** is the deepest part and is closely related to the recto-uterine pouch. Four muscles compress the vagina and act as sphincters: **pubovaginalis,** *external urethral sphincter*, **urethrovaginal sphincter,** and *bulbospongiosus* (Fig. 3.46).

The vagina is related (Fig. 3.27):

- anteriorly to the fundus of the urinary bladder and urethra;
- laterally to the levator ani, visceral pelvic fascia, and ureters; and
- posteriorly (from inferior to superior) to the anal canal, rectum, and recto-uterine pouch.

ARTERIAL SUPPLY AND VENOUS DRAINAGE OF VAGINA

The arteries supplying the superior part of the vagina derive from the *uterine arteries.* The arteries supplying the middle

and inferior parts of the vagina derive from the *vaginal* and *internal pudendal arteries* (Figs. 3.18 and 3.41).

The vaginal veins form **vaginal venous plexuses** along the sides of the vagina and within the vaginal mucosa (Fig. 3.41). These veins are continuous with the *uterine venous plexus* as the **uterovaginal venous plexus,** and drain into the internal iliac veins through the uterine vein. This plexus also communicates with the vesical and rectal venous plexuses.

INNERVATION OF VAGINA AND UTERUS

Only the inferior one fifth to one quarter of the vagina is somatic in terms of innervation. Innervation of this part of the vagina is from the *deep perineal nerve,* a branch of the *pudendal nerve,* which conveys sympathetic and visceral afferent fibers but no parasympathetic fibers (Fig. 3.47). Only this somatically innervated part is sensitive to touch and temperature, even though the somatic and visceral afferent fibers have their cell bodies in the same (S2–S4) spinal ganglia.

Most of the vagina (superior three quarters to four fifths) is visceral in terms of its innervation. Nerves to this part of the vagina and to the uterus are derived from the **uterovaginal nerve plexus,** which travels with the uterine artery at the junction of the base of the (peritoneal) broad ligament and the superior part of the (fascial) transverse cervical ligament. The uterovaginal nerve plexus is one of the pelvic plexuses that extends to the pelvic viscera from the inferior hypogastric plexus. Sympathetic, parasympathetic, and visceral afferent fibers pass through this plexus.

Sympathetic innervation originates in the inferior thoracic spinal cord segments and passes through *lumbar splanchnic nerves* and the intermesenteric-hypogastric-pelvic series of plexuses. *Parasympathetic innervation* originates in the S2–S4 spinal cord segments and passes through the *pelvic splanchnic nerves* to the inferior hypogastric-uterovaginal plexus. The *visceral afferent innervation* of the superior (intraperitoneal; fundus and body) and inferior (subperitoneal; cervical) parts of the uterus and vagina differ in terms of course and destination. Visceral afferent fibers conducting pain impulses from the intraperitoneal uterine fundus and body (superior to the *pelvic pain line*) follow the sympathetic innervation retrograde to reach cell bodies in the inferior thoracic-superior lumbar spinal ganglia. Afferent fibers conducting pain impulses from the subperitoneal uterine cervix and vagina (inferior to the pelvic pain line) follow the parasympathetic fibers retrograde through the uterovaginal and inferior hypogastric plexuses and pelvic splanchnic nerves to reach cell bodies in the spinal sensory ganglia of S2–S4. The two different routes followed by visceral pain fibers is clinically significant in that it offers mothers a variety of types of anesthesia for childbirth (see the blue box "Anesthesia for Childbirth," on p. 397). All visceral afferent fibers from the uterus and vagina not concerned with pain (those conveying unconscious sensations) also follow the latter route.

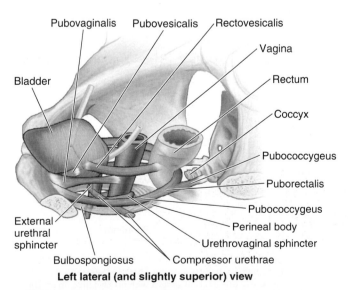

Pubovaginalis   Pubovesicalis   Rectovesicalis
Vagina
Bladder
Rectum
Coccyx
Pubococcygeus
Puborectalis
Pubococcygeus
External urethral sphincter
Perineal body
Bulbospongiosus   Compressor urethrae   Urethrovaginal sphincter

Left lateral (and slightly superior) view

FIGURE 3.46. Muscles compressing urethra and vagina. Muscles that compress the vagina and act as sphincters include the pubovaginalis, external urethral sphincter (especially its urethrovaginal sphincter part), and bulbospongiosus. The compressor urethrae and external urethral sphincter compress the urethra.

FIGURE 3.47. Innervation of female internal genital organs. Pelvic splanchnic nerves, arising from the S2–S4 anterior rami, supply parasympathetic motor fibers to the uterus and vagina (and vasodilator fibers to the erectile tissue of the clitoris and bulb of the vestibule; not shown). Presynaptic sympathetic fibers traverse the sympathetic trunk and pass through the lumbar splanchnic nerves to synapse in prevertebral ganglia with postsynaptic fibers; the latter fibers travel through the superior and inferior hypogastric plexuses to reach the pelvic viscera. Visceral afferent fibers conducting pain from intraperitoneal structures (such as the uterine body) travel with the sympathetic fibers to the T12–L2 spinal ganglia. Visceral afferent fibers conducting pain from subperitoneal structures, such as the cervix and vagina (i.e., the birth canal), travel with parasympathetic fibers to the S2–S4 spinal ganglia. Somatic sensation from the opening of the vagina also passes to the S2–S4 spinal ganglia via the pudendal nerve. In addition, muscular contractions of the uterus are hormonally induced.

FEMALE INTERNAL GENITAL ORGANS

Infections of Female Genital Tract

 Because the female genital tract communicates with the peritoneal cavity through the abdominal ostia of the uterine tubes, infections of the vagina, uterus, and tubes may result in *peritonitis*. Conversely, inflammation of a tube (*salpingitis*) may result from infections that spread from the peritoneal cavity. A major cause of infertility in women is blockage of the uterine tubes, often the result of salpingitis.

Patency of Uterine Tubes

HYSTEROSALPINGOGRAPHY

Patency of the uterine tubes may be determined by a radiographic procedure involving injection of a water-soluble radiopaque material or carbon dioxide gas into the uterus and tubes through the external os of the uterus (*hysterosalpingography*). The contrast medium travels through the uterine cavity and tubes (*arrowheads* in Fig. B3.13). Accumulation of radiopaque fluid or the appearance of gas bubbles in the pararectal fossae region of the peritoneal cavity indicates that the tubes are patent.

ENDOSCOPY

Patency of the uterine tubes can also be determined by *hysteroscopy*, examination of the interior of the tubes using a narrow endoscopic instrument (*hysteroscope*), which is introduced through the vagina and uterus.

Ligation of Uterine Tubes

Ligation of the uterine tubes is a surgical method of birth control. Oocytes discharged from the ovaries that enter the tubes of these patients degenerate and are soon absorbed. Most surgical sterilizations are done by either abdominal tubal ligation or laparoscopic tubal ligation. *Open abdominal tubal ligation* is usually performed through a short suprapubic incision made at the pubic hairline (Fig. B3.14A) and involves interruption, often with removal of a segment of the tube, and tubal closure by suture ligation. *Laparoscopic tubal ligation* is done with a fiber optic laparoscope inserted through a small incision, usually near the umbilicus (Fig. B3.14B). In this procedure, tubal continuity is interrupted by applying cautery, rings, or clips.

(A) Abdominal tubal ligation

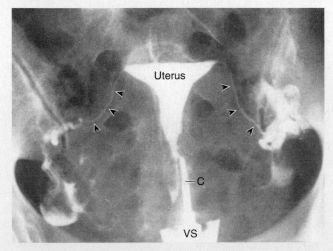

FIGURE B3.13. Hysterosalpingogram. Arrowheads, uterine tubes; c, catheter in the cervical canal, vs, vaginal speculum.

(B) Laparoscopic tubal ligation

FIGURE B3.14.

Ectopic Tubal Pregnancy

In some women, collections of pus may develop in a uterine tube (*pyosalpinx*) and the tube may be partly occluded by adhesions. In these cases, the morula (early embryo) may not be able to pass along the tube to the uterus, although sperms have obviously done so. When the blastocyst forms, it may implant in the mucosa of the uterine tube, producing an *ectopic tubal pregnancy*. Although implantation may occur in any part of the tube, the common site is in the ampulla (Fig. B3.15). Tubal pregnancy is the most common type of ectopic gestation; it occurs in approximately 1 of every 250 pregnancies in North America (Moore et al., 2012). If not diagnosed early, ectopic tubal pregnancies may result in rupture of the uterine tube, and severe hemorrhage into the abdominopelvic cavity during the first 8 weeks of gestation. Tubal rupture and hemorrhage constitute a threat to the mother's life and result in death of the embryo.

On the right side, the appendix often lies close to the ovary and uterine tube. This close relationship explains why a *ruptured tubal pregnancy* and the resulting peritonitis may be misdiagnosed as acute appendicitis. In both cases, the parietal peritoneum is inflamed in the same general area, and the pain is referred to the right lower quadrant of the abdomen.

FIGURE B3.15. Sites of ectopic pregnancy.

Remnants of Embryonic Ducts

Occasionally the mesosalpinx between the uterine tube and the ovary contains embryonic remnants (Fig. 3.39B). The *epoophoron* forms from remnants of the mesonephric tubules of the *mesonephros*, the transitory embryonic kidney. There may also be a persistent *duct of the epoophoron* (duct of Gartner), a remnant of the mesonephric duct that forms the ductus deferens and ejaculatory duct in the male. It lies between layers of the broad ligament along each side of the uterus and/or vagina. A *vesicular appendage* is sometimes attached to the infundibulum of the uterine tube. It is the remains of the cranial end of the mesonephric duct that forms the *ductus epididymis*. Although these vestigial structures are mostly of embryological and morphological interest, they occasionally accumulate fluid and form cysts (e.g., Gartner duct cysts).

Bicornate Uterus

Incomplete fusion of the embryonic paramesonephric ducts, from which the uterus is formed, results in a variety of congenital anomalies, ranging from formation of a unicornate uterus (receiving a uterine duct only from the right or left) to duplication in the form of a bicornate uterus (Fig. B3.16), doubled uterine cavites, or a completely doubled uterus (*uterus didelphys*).

FIGURE B3.16. **Bicornate uterus.** *1* and *2*, uterine cavity; *E*, cervical canal; *F*, uterine tube; *I*, isthmus of tube, *R*, right side marker. (Reprinted with permission from Stuart GCE, Reid DF. Diagnostic studies. In: Copeland LJ, ed. Textbook of Gynecology, 2nd ed. Philadelphia: Saunders, 2000.)

Disposition of Uterus and Uterine Prolapse

When intra-abdominal pressure is increased, the normally anteverted and anteflexed uterus is pressed against the bladder (Fig. B3.17A). However, the uterus may assume other dispositions, including excessive anteflexion (Fig. B3.17B), anteflexion with retroversion (Fig. B3.17C), and retroflexion with retroversion (Fig. B3.17D). Instead of pressing the uterus against the bladder, increased intra-abdominal pressure tends to push the retroverted uterus, a solid mass positioned upright over the vagina (a flexible, hollow tube), into or even through the vagina (Fig. B3.17E–G). A retroverted uterus will not necessarily prolapse, but is more likely to do so. The situation is exacerbated in the presence of a disrupted perineal body or with atrophic ("relaxed") pelvic floor ligaments and muscles (see the blue box "Disruption of Perineal Body," p. 414).

(E) First degree prolapse

(A) Normal (anteverted, anteflexed)

(B) Excessive anteflexion

(D) Retroverted and retroflexed

(F) Second degree prolapse

(C) Retroverted

Everted vaginal wall

(G) Third degree prolapse

FIGURE B3.17.

Manual Examination of Uterus

The size and disposition of the uterus may be examined by *bimanual palpation* (Fig. B3.18A). Two gloved fingers of the right hand are passed superiorly in the vagina, while the other hand is pressed inferoposteriorly on the pubic region of the anterior abdominal wall. The size and other characteristics of the uterus can be determined in this way (e.g., whether the uterus is in its normal anteverted position). When softening of the uterine isthmus occurs (*Hegar sign*), the cervix feels as though it were separated from the body. Softening of the isthmus is an early sign of pregnancy. The uterus can be further stabilized through rectovaginal examination, which is used if examination via the vagina alone does not yield clear findings (Fig. B3.18B).

Lifetime Changes in Anatomy of Uterus

The uterus is possibly the most dynamic structure in human anatomy (Fig. B3.19). At birth, the uterus is relatively large and has adult proportions (body to

Bimanual palpation; uterus anteverted and anteflexed

(A)

Medial view (from left)

(B)

Rectovaginal examination; uterus retroverted and retroflexed

FIGURE B3.18.

Newborn   4-year-old   Puberty   Nulliparous* adult

2:1   1:1
(A)   **(B)**

Multiparous** adult

Postmenopausal

2:1
(C)

2:1
(D)

(E) 3:1   **(F)** 1:1

* Has never given birth
** Has given birth two
   or more times

(A–F) Anterior views of coronally-sectioned uteri

Placenta

Umbilical
cord

Uterus

Cervix

(H) Uterus at end of pregnancy

9
10
8
7
6
5
4
3

**(G) Monthly changes in size
of uterus during pregnancy**

**(I) Postpartum uterus
(immediately following childbirth)**

(J) Multiparous uterus**

FIGURE B3.19.

cervical ratio = 2:1) due to the *prepartum* (before childbirth) influence of the maternal hormones (Fig. B3.19A). Several weeks *postpartum* (after childbirth), childhood dimensions and proportions are obtained: The body and cervix are approximately of equal length (body to cervical ratio = 1:1), with the cervix being of greater diameter (thickness) (Fig. B3.19B). Because of the small size of the pelvic cavity during infancy, the uterus is mainly an abdominal organ. The cervix remains relatively large (approximately 50% of total uterus) throughout childhood. During *puberty,* the uterus (especially its body) grows rapidly in size, once again assuming adult proportions (Fig. B3.19C). In the postpubertal, premenopausal, non-pregnant woman, the body of the uterus is pear shaped; the thick-walled superior two thirds of the uterus lies within the pelvic cavity (Fig. B3.19D). During this phase of life, the uterus

undergoes monthly changes in size, weight, and density in relation to the menstrual cycle.

Over the 9 months of pregnancy, the *gravid* uterus expands greatly to accommodate the fetus, becoming larger and increasingly thin walled (Fig. B3.19G). At the end of pregnancy (B3.19G, line 10), the fetus "drops," as the head becomes engaged in the lesser pelvis. The uterus becomes nearly membranous, with the fundus dropping below its highest level (achieved in the 9th month), at which time it extends superiorly to the costal margin, occupying most of the abdominopelvic cavity (Fig. B3.19H).

Immediately after delivery, the large uterus becomes thick walled and edematous (Fig. B3.19I), but its size reduces rapidly. The *multiparous* non-gravid uterus has a large and nodular body and usually extends into the lower abdominal cavity, often causing a slight protrusion of the inferior abdominal wall in lean women (Figs. B3.19E & J and 3.73B, p. 437).

During *menopause* (46–52 years of age), the uterus (again, especially the body) decreases in size. *Postmenopause,* the uterus is involuted and regresses to a markedly smaller size, once again assuming childhood proportions (Fig. B3.19F). All these stages represent normal anatomy for the particular age and reproductive status of the woman.

Cervical Cancer, Cervical Examination and Pap Smear

Until 1940, cervical cancer was the leading cause of death in North American women (Krebs, 2000). The decline in the incidence and number of women dying from cervical cancer is related to the accessibility of the cervix to direct visualization, and to cell and tissue study by means of Pap (Papanicolaou) smears, leading to the detection of premalignant cervical conditions (Copeland, 2000; Morris and Burke, 2000). The vagina can be distended with a *vaginal speculum* to enable inspection of the cervix (Fig. B3.20A & B). To prepare a Pap smear, a spatula is placed in the external os of the uterus (Fig. B3.20A). The spatula is rotated to scrape cellular material from the mucosa of the vaginal cervix (Fig. B3.20C), followed by insertion of a cytobrush into the cervical canal that is rotated to gather cellular material from the supravaginal cervical mucosa. The cellular material is then placed on glass slides for microscopic examination (Fig. B3.20D & E).

Because no peritoneum intervenes between the anterior cervix and the base of the bladder, cervical cancer may spread by contiguity to the bladder. It may also spread by lymphogenous (lymph borne) metastasis to external or internal iliac or sacral nodes. Hematogenous (blood borne) metastasis may occur via iliac veins or via the internal vertebral venous plexus.

Hysterectomy

Owing to the frequency of uterine and cervical cancer, hysterectomy, excision of the uterus (G. *hystera*), is a relatively common procedure. The uterus may be surgically approached and removed (A) through the anterior abdominal wall, or (B) through the vagina (Fig. B3.21).

(A) Abdominal hysterectomy

(B) Vaginal hysterectomy

FIGURE B3.21.

Speculum

Cervix

External os of uterus

Vagina

Spatula

(A)

Speculum

Vagina

Cervix

(B)

(C)

(D)

(E)

FIGURE B3.20.

Distension of Vagina

The vagina can be markedly distended, particularly in the region of the posterior part of the fornix. For example, distension of this part allows palpation of the sacral promontory during a pelvic examination (see the blue box "Pelvic Diameters (Conjugates)," p. 334). The distension also accommodates the erect penis during intercourse.

The vagina is especially distended by the fetus during parturition, particularly in an AP direction when the fetus's shoulders are delivered (Fig. B3.22). Lateral distension is limited by the ischial spines, which project posteromedially, and the sacrospinous ligaments extending from these spines to the lateral margins of the sacrum and coccyx. The birth canal is thus deep anteroposteriorly and narrow transversely at this point, causing the fetus's shoulders to rotate into the AP plane.

Delivery of right shoulder

Delivery of left shoulder

FIGURE B3.22.

Digital Pelvic Examination

Because of its relatively thin, distensible walls and central location within the pelvis, the cervix, ischial spines, and sacral promontory can be palpated with the gloved digits in the vagina and/or rectum (*manual pelvic examination*). Pulsations of the uterine arteries may also be felt through the lateral parts of the fornix, as may irregularities of the ovaries, such as cysts (Fig. B3.23).

Manual digital examination of vagina

Bimanual palpation of uterine adnexa (accessory structures e.g., ovaries)

Palm of right hand on abdominal wall, with fingers pressing into abdominal wall to resist movement of uterus and adnexa away from palpating fingertips of left hand

Medial views (from left)

FIGURE B3.23.

Vaginal Fistulae

Because of the close relationship of the vagina to adjacent pelvic organs, obstetrical trauma during long and difficult labor may result in weaknesses, necrosis, or tears in the vaginal wall and sometimes beyond. These may form or subsequently develop into abnormal passages (*fistulas*) between the vaginal lumen and the lumina of the adjacent bladder, urethra, and rectum, or the perineum (Fig. B3.24). Urine enters the vagina from both *vesicovaginal* and *urethrovaginal fistulas*, but the flow is continuous from the former and occurs only during micturition from the latter. Fecal matter may be discharged from the vagina when there is a *rectovaginal fistula*.

Vesicovaginal fistula   Rectovaginal fistula

Urethrovaginal fistula   Vaginoperineal fistula

Medial view (from left)

FIGURE B3.24.

Culdoscopy and Culdocentesis

An endoscopic instrument (*culdoscope*) can be inserted through the posterior part of the vaginal fornix to examine the ovaries or uterine tubes (e.g., for the presence of a tubal pregnancy). Although it involves less disruption of tissue, *culdoscopy* has been largely replaced by *laparoscopy,* which, however, provides greater flexibility for operative procedures and better visualization of pelvic organs (see the blue box "Laparoscopic Examination of Pelvic Viscera," p. 397). There is also less risk of bacterial contamination of the peritoneal cavity.

A pelvic abscess in the recto-uterine pouch can be drained through an incision made in the posterior part of the vaginal fornix (*culdocentesis*). Similarly, fluid in the peritoneal cavity (e.g., blood) can be aspirated by this technique (Fig. B3.25).

(A) Laparoscopy of pelvic viscera

Medial view (from left)

FIGURE B3.25.

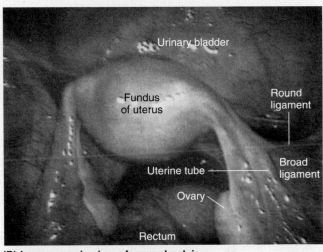

(B) Laparoscopic view of normal pelvis

FIGURE B3.26.

Laparoscopic Examination of Pelvic Viscera

Visual examination of the pelvic viscera is especially useful in diagnosing many conditions affecting the pelvic viscera, such as *ovarian cysts* and tumors, *endometriosis* (the presence of functioning endometrial tissue outside the uterus), and ectopic pregnancies. *Laparoscopy* involves inserting a *laparoscope* into the peritoneal cavity through a small (approximately 2 cm) incision below the umbilicus (Fig. B3.26). Insufflation of inert gas creates a pneumoperitoneum to provide space to visualize, and the pelvis is elevated so that gravity will pull the intestines into the abdomen. The uterus can be externally manipulated to facilitate visualization, or additional openings (ports) can be made to introduce other instruments for manipulation or to enable therapeutic procedures (e.g., ligation of the uterine tubes).

Anesthesia for Childbirth

Several options are available to women to reduce the pain and discomfort experienced during childbirth. *General anesthesia* has advantages for emergency procedures and for women who choose it over regional anesthesia. General anesthesia renders the mother unconscious; she is unaware of the labor and delivery. Clinicians monitor and regulate maternal respiration and both maternal and fetal cardiac function. Childbirth occurs passively under the control of maternal hormones with the assistance of an obstetrician. The mother is spared pain and discomfort but is unaware of the earliest moments of her baby's life.

Women who choose *regional anesthesia,* such as a spinal, pudendal nerve, or caudal epidural block, often wish to participate actively (e.g., using the Lamaze method) and be conscious of their uterine contractions to "bear down," or push, to assist the contractions and expel the fetus, yet do not wish to experience all the pain of labor.

Spinal anesthesia, in which the anesthetic agent is introduced with a needle into the spinal subarachnoid space at the L3–L4 vertebral level (A in Fig. B3.27), produces complete anesthesia inferior to approximately the waist level. The perineum, pelvic floor, and birth canal are anesthetized, and motor and sensory functions of the entire lower limbs, as well as sensation of uterine contractions, are temporarily eliminated. The mother is conscious, but she must depend on electronic monitoring of uterine contractions. If labor is extended or the level of anesthesia is inadequate, it may be difficult or impossible to re-administer the anesthesia. Because the anesthetic agent is heavier than cerebrospinal fluid, it remains in the inferior spinal subarachnoid space while the patient is inclined. The anesthetic agent circulates into the cerebral subarachnoid space in the cranial cavity when the patient lies flat following the delivery. A severe headache is a common sequel to spinal anesthesia.

A *pudendal nerve block* is a peripheral nerve block that provides local anesthesia over the S2–S4 dermatomes (the majority of the perineum) and the inferior quarter of the vagina (C in Fig. B3.27). It does not block pain from the superior birth canal (uterine cervix and superior vagina), so the mother is able to feel uterine contractions. It can be re-administered, but to do so may be disruptive and involve the use of a sharp instrument in close proximity to the infant's head. The anatomical basis of the administration of a pudendal block is provided in the blue box "Pudendal and Ilio-inguinal Nerve Blocks," p. 433.

The *caudal epidural block* is a popular choice for participatory childbirth (B in Fig. B3.27). It must be administered in advance of the actual delivery, which is not possible with a precipitous birth. The anesthetic agent is administered using an in-dwelling catheter in the sacral canal, enabling administration of more anesthetic agent for a deeper or more prolonged anesthesia, if necessary. Within the sacral canal, the

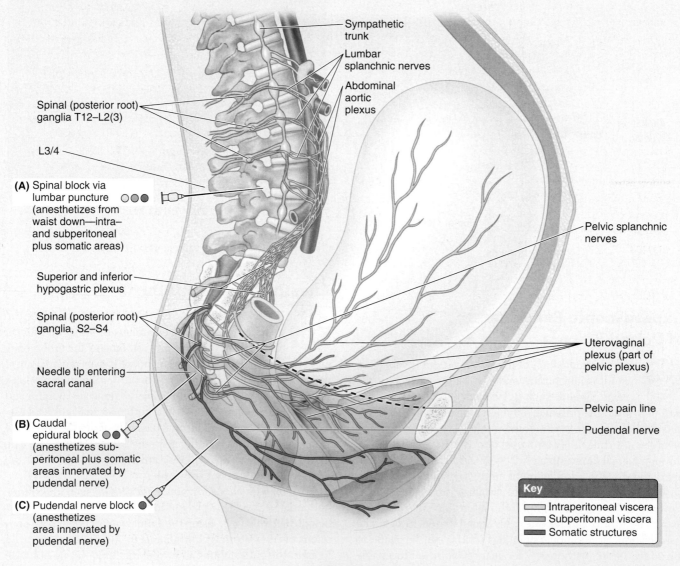

Sympathetic trunk

Lumbar splanchnic nerves

Abdominal aortic plexus

Spinal (posterior root) ganglia T12–L2(3)

L3/4

(A) Spinal block via lumbar puncture (anesthetizes from waist down—intra– and subperitoneal plus somatic areas)

Superior and inferior hypogastric plexus

Spinal (posterior root) ganglia, S2–S4

Needle tip entering sacral canal

(B) Caudal epidural block (anesthetizes subperitoneal plus somatic areas innervated by pudendal nerve)

(C) Pudendal nerve block (anesthetizes area innervated by pudendal nerve)

Pelvic splanchnic nerves

Uterovaginal plexus (part of pelvic plexus)

Pelvic pain line

Pudendal nerve

Key
- Intraperitoneal viscera
- Subperitoneal viscera
- Somatic structures

FIGURE B3.27.

anesthesia bathes the S2–S4 spinal nerve roots, including the pain fibers from the uterine cervix and superior vagina, and the afferent fibers from the pudendal nerve. Thus the entire birth canal, pelvic floor, and majority of the perineum are anesthetized, but the lower limbs are not usually affected. The pain fibers from the uterine body (superior to the *pel-vic pain line*) ascend to the inferior thoracic-superior lumbar levels; these and the fibers superior to them are not affected by the anesthetic, so the mother is aware of her uterine contractions. With epidural anesthesia, no "spinal headache" occurs because the vertebral epidural space is not continuous with the cranial extradural (epidural) space (see Chapter 4).

The Bottom Line

FEMALE INTERNAL GENITAL ORGANS

Ovaries and uterine tubes: The ovaries are suspended by two peritoneal folds: the mesovarium from the posterosuperior aspect of the broad ligament, and the vascular suspensory ligament of the ovary from the lateral wall of the pelvis. ♦ They are attached to the uterus by the ligaments of the ovaries. ♦ The peritoneum ends at the ovary itself. It is replaced on the surface of the ovary with a duller, cuboidal epithelium.

The uterine tubes are the conduits and the site of fertilization for oocytes discharged into the peritoneal cavity. ♦ Coursing in a peritoneal fold (mesosalpinx) that makes up the superior margin of the broad ligament, each uterine tube has a fimbriated, funnel-like infundibulum, a wide ampulla, a narrow isthmus, and a short uterine part that traverses the uterine wall to enter the cavity.

The ovaries and uterine tubes receive a double (collateral) blood supply from the abdominal aorta via the ovarian arteries and from the internal iliac arteries via the uterine arteries. ♦ This collateral circulation allows the ovaries to be spared to supply estrogen when a hysterectomy necessitates ligation of the uterine arteries. ♦ Sympathetic and visceral afferent pain fibers travel with the ovarian vessels. ♦ Parasympathetic and visceral afferent reflex fibers traverse pelvic plexuses and pelvic splanchnic nerves.

Uterus: Shaped like an inverted pear, the uterus is the organ in which the blastocyst (early embryo) implants and develops into a mature embryo and then a fetus. ♦ Although its size and proportions change during the various phases of life, the non-gravid uterus consists of a body and cervix, demarcated by a relatively narrow isthmus. ♦ The uterus has a trilaminar wall consisting of (1) an inner vascular and secretory endometrium, which undergoes cyclical changes to prepare for implantation to occur and sheds with menstrual flow if it does not; (2) a hormonally stimulated intermediate smooth muscle myometrium, which dilates the cervical canal (exit) and expels the fetus during childbirth; and (3) visceral peritoneum (perimetrium), which covers most of the fundus and body (except for a bare area abutting the bladder) and continues bilaterally as the broad ligament (mesometrium).

The uterus is normally anteverted and anteflexed so that its weight is borne largely by the urinary bladder, although it also receives significant passive support from the cardinal ligaments and active support from the muscles of the pelvic floor. ♦ The uterine artery supplies the uterus and, during pregnancy, the placenta. ♦ The uterine veins drain to the uterovaginal venous plexus.

Vagina: The vagina is a musculomembranous passage connecting the uterine cavity to the exterior, allowing the entrance/insertion of the penis, ejaculate, tampons, or examining digits and the exit of a fetus or menstrual fluid. ♦ The vagina lies between and is closely related to the urethra anteriorly and rectum posteriorly, but is separated from the latter by the peritoneal recto-uterine pouch superiorly and the fascial rectovaginal septum inferiorly. The vagina is indented (invaginated) anterosuperiorly by the uterine cervix so that an encircling pocket or vaginal fornix is formed around it. ♦ Most of the vagina is located within the pelvis, receiving blood via pelvic branches of the internal iliac arteries (uterine and vaginal arteries) and draining directly into the uterovaginal venous plexus and, via deep (pelvic) routes, to the internal and external iliac and sacral lymph nodes. ♦ The inferiormost part of the vagina is located within the perineum, receiving blood from the internal pudendal artery and draining via superficial (perineal) routes into superficial inguinal nodes. ♦ The vagina is capable of remarkable distension, enabling manual examination (palpation) of pelvic landmarks and viscera (especially the ovaries) as well as of pathology (e.g., ovarian cysts).

Innervation of uterus and vagina: The inferiormost (perineal) portion of the vagina receives somatic innervation via the pudendal nerve (S2–S4) and is, therefore, sensitive to touch and temperature. ♦ The remainder of the vagina and uterus is pelvic and thus visceral in its location, receiving innervation from autonomic and visceral afferent fibers. ♦ All unconscious, reflex-type sensation travels retrogradely along the parasympathetic pathways to the S2–S4 spinal sensory ganglia, as does pain sensation arising in the subperitoneal uterus (primarily cervix) and vagina (inferior to the pelvic pain line)—that is, from the birth canal. ♦ However, pain sensation from the intraperitoneal uterus (superior to the pelvic pain line) travels retrogradely along the sympathetic pathway to the inferiormost thoracic and superior lumbar spinal ganglia. ♦ Epidural anesthesia may be administered to take advantage of the discrepancy in the pain pathways to facilitate participatory childbirth methods; uterine contractions are felt, but the birth canal is anesthetized.

Lymphatic Drainage of Pelvic Viscera

For the main part, the lymphatic vessels of the pelvis follow the venous system, following the tributaries of the internal iliac vein to the internal iliac nodes, directly or via the sacral lymph nodes (Fig. 3.48). However, structures located superiorly in the anterior portion of the pelvis drain to the external iliac nodes, a lymphatic pathway that does not parallel venous drainage. From both external and internal iliac nodes, lymph flows via common iliac and lumbar (caval/aortic) lymph nodes, draining via lumbar lymphatic trunks into the cisterna chyli.

LYMPHATIC DRAINAGE FROM URINARY SYSTEM

The superior portion of the pelvic part of the ureters drains primarily to external iliac nodes, while the inferior portion drains to the internal iliac nodes (Fig. 3.48A; Table 3.7). Lymphatic vessels from the superolateral aspects of the bladder pass to the *external iliac lymph nodes*, whereas those from the fundus and neck pass to the *internal iliac lymph nodes*. Some vessels from the neck of the bladder drain into the sacral or common iliac lymph nodes. Most lymphatic vessels from the female urethra and proximal part of the male urethra pass to

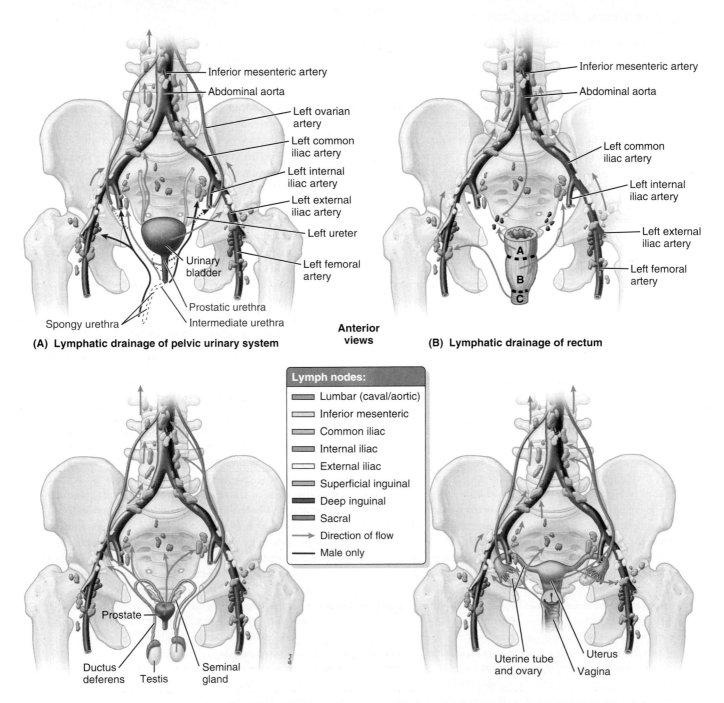

(A) Lymphatic drainage of pelvic urinary system

Anterior views

(B) Lymphatic drainage of rectum

Lymph nodes:
- Lumbar (caval/aortic)
- Inferior mesenteric
- Common iliac
- Internal iliac
- External iliac
- Superficial inguinal
- Deep inguinal
- Sacral
- → Direction of flow
- — Male only

(C) Lymphatic drainage of male internal genital organs

(D) Lymphatic drainage of female internal genital organs

FIGURE 3.48. Lymphatic drainage of pelvic viscera.

TABLE 3.7. LYMPHATIC DRAINAGE OF STRUCTURES OF PELVIS AND PERINEUM

Zones of pelvic organs initially draining to specific groups of regional nodes

Lymph Node Group		Structures Typically Draining to Lymph Node Group	
Lumbar	*Female:* along ovarian vessels	Gonads and associated structures; common iliac nodes	*Female:* ovary; uterine tube (except isthmus and intra-uterine parts); fundus of uterus
	Male: along testicular vessels		*Male urethra:* testis; epididymis
Inferior mesenteric		Superiormost rectum; sigmoid colon; descending colon; pararectal nodes	
Common iliac		External and internal iliac lymph nodes	
Internal iliac		Inferior pelvic structures; deep perineal structures; sacral nodes	*Female:* base of bladder; inferior pelvic ureter; anal canal (above pectinate line); inferior rectum; middle and upper vagina; cervix; body of uterus
			Male: prostatic urethra; prostate; base of bladder; inferior pelvic ureter; inferior seminal glands; cavernous bodies; anal canal (above pectinate line); inferior rectum
External iliac		Anterosuperior pelvic structures; deep inguinal nodes	*Female:* superior bladder; superior pelvic ureter; upper vagina; cervix; lower body of uterus
			Male: superior bladder; superior pelvic ureter; upper seminal gland; pelvic part of ductus deferens; intermediate and spongy urethra (secondary)
Superficial inguinal		Lower limb; superficial drainage of inferolateral quadrant of trunk, including anterior abdominal wall inferior to umbilicus, gluteal region, and superficial perineal structures	*Female:* superolateral uterus (near attachment of round ligament); skin of perineum including vulva; ostium of vagina (inferior to hymen); prepuce of clitoris; peri-anal skin; anal canal inferior to pectinate line
			Male: skin of perineum including skin and prepuce of penis; scrotum; peri-anal skin; anal canal inferior to pectinate line
Deep inguinal		Glans clitoris or penis; superficial inguinal nodes	*Female:* glans clitoris
			Male: glans penis; distal spongy urethra
Sacral		Postero-inferior pelvic structures: inferior rectum; inferior vagina	
Pararectal		Superior rectum	

the *internal iliac lymph node*. However, a few vessels from the female urethra may also drain into the sacral nodes and, from the distal female urethra, to the *inguinal lymph nodes*.

LYMPHATIC DRAINAGE FROM RECTUM

Lymphatic vessels from the superior rectum pass to *inferior mesenteric lymph nodes*, many passing through **pararectal lymph nodes** (located directly on the muscle layer of the rectum) and/or sacral lymph nodes en route (Fig. 3.48B; Table 3.7). The inferior mesenteric nodes drain into the *lumbar (caval/aortic) lymph nodes*. Lymphatic vessels from the inferior half of the rectum drain directly to *sacral lymph nodes* or, especially from the distal ampulla, follow the middle rectal vessels to drain into the *internal iliac lymph nodes*.

LYMPHATIC DRAINAGE FROM MALE PELVIC VISCERA

Lymphatic vessels from the ductus deferens, ejaculatory ducts, and inferior parts of the seminal glands drain to the *external iliac lymph nodes* (Fig. 3.48C; Table 3.7). The lymphatic vessels from the superior parts of the seminal glands and prostate terminate chiefly in the *internal iliac lymph nodes*, but some drainage from the latter may pass to the *sacral nodes*.

LYMPHATIC DRAINAGE FROM FEMALE PELVIC VISCERA

Lymphatic vessels from the ovaries, joined by vessels from the uterine tubes and most from the fundus of the uterus, follow the ovarian veins as they ascend to the *right* and *left lumbar (caval/aortic) lymph nodes* (Fig. 3.48D; Table 3.7).

Lymphatic vessels from the uterus drain in many directions, coursing along the blood vessels that supply it as well as the ligaments attached to it:

- Most lymphatic vessels from the fundus and superior uterine body pass along the ovarian vessels to the *lumbar (caval/aortic) lymph nodes*, but some vessels from the fundus, particularly those near the entrance of the uterine

tubes and attachments of the round ligaments, run along the round ligament of the uterus to the *superficial inguinal lymph nodes*.
- Vessels from most of the uterine body and some from the cervix pass within the broad ligament to the *external iliac lymph nodes*.
- Vessels from the uterine cervix also pass along the uterine vessels, within the transverse cervical ligaments, to the *internal iliac lymph nodes,* and along uterosacral (sacrogenital) ligaments to the *sacral lymph nodes*.

Lymphatic vessels from the vagina drain from the parts of the vagina as follows:

- Superior part: to the internal and external iliac lymph nodes.
- Middle part: to the internal iliac lymph nodes.
- Inferior part: to the sacral and common iliac nodes (Fig. 3.48; Table 3.7).
- External orifice: to the superficial inguinal lymph nodes.

PERINEUM

The **perineum** refers to a shallow compartment of the body (*perineal compartment*) bounded by the pelvic outlet and separated from the pelvic cavity by the fascia covering the inferior aspect of the pelvic diaphragm, formed by the levator ani and coccygeus muscles (Fig. 3.49). In the anatomical position, the surface of the perineum—the **perineal region**—is the narrow region between the proximal parts of the thighs; however, when the lower limbs are abducted, it is a diamond-shaped area extending from the mons pubis anteriorly in females, the medial surfaces (insides) of the thighs laterally, and the gluteal folds and superior end of the intergluteal (natal) cleft posteriorly (Fig. 3.50).

The osseofibrous structures marking the boundaries of the perineum (perineal compartment) (Fig. 3.51A & B) are the:

- *Pubic symphysis*, anteriorly.
- **Ischiopubic rami** (combined *inferior pubic rami* and *ischial rami*), anterolaterally.

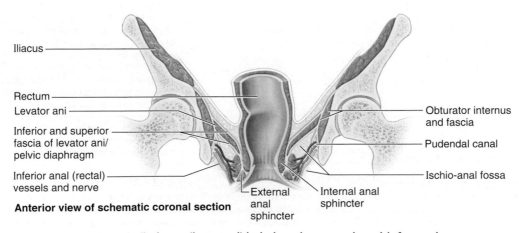

Iliacus
Rectum
Levator ani
Inferior and superior fascia of levator ani/ pelvic diaphragm
Inferior anal (rectal) vessels and nerve
Anterior view of schematic coronal section
External anal sphincter
Internal anal sphincter
Obturator internus and fascia
Pudendal canal
Ischio-anal fossa

FIGURE 3.49. The inferior fascia of the pelvic diaphragm (levator ani) is the boundary separating pelvis from perineum.

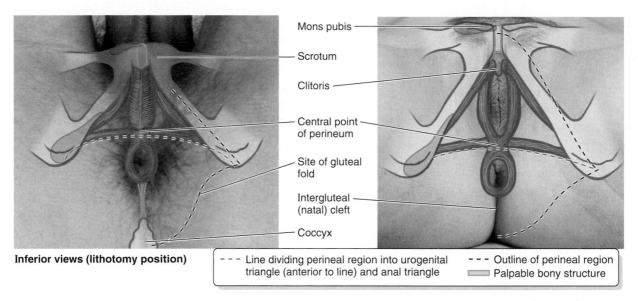

Mons pubis

Scrotum

Clitoris

Central point of perineum

Site of gluteal fold

Intergluteal (natal) cleft

Coccyx

Inferior views (lithotomy position)

- - - Line dividing perineal region into urogenital triangle (anterior to line) and anal triangle

- - - Outline of perineal region

▭ Palpable bony structure

FIGURE 3.50. Male and female perineal regions. Boundaries and surface features of the perineal region with projections of the osseous boundaries and muscles of the superficial muscles of the perineum. The penis and some of the scrotum (part of the perineal region) are retracted anteriorly and thus not shown.

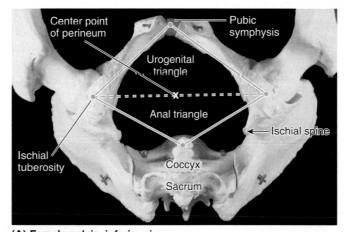

(A) Female pelvis, inferior view

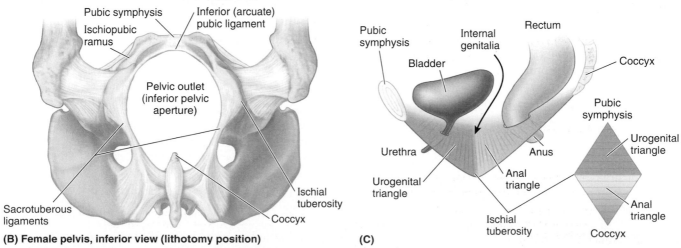

(B) Female pelvis, inferior view (lithotomy position)

(C)

FIGURE 3.51. Boundaries and disposition of perineum. A. Pelvic girdle demonstrating bony features bounding the perineum. The two triangles comprising the diamond-shaped perineum are superimposed. **B.** The osseofibrous structures bounding the pelvic outlet and perineum are identified. This view of the female pelvis is the one obstetricians visualize when the patient is on the examining table. **C.** The two triangles (urogenital and anal) that together comprise the perineum do not occupy the same plane. The plane between the bladder and rectum is occupied by internal genitalia and a septum formed during embryonic development as the urogenital sinus was partitioned into the urinary bladder and urethra anteriorly and the anorectum posteriorly.

- *Ischial tuberosities*, laterally.
- *Sacrotuberous ligaments*, posterolaterally.
- Inferiormost *sacrum* and *coccyx*, posteriorly.

A transverse line joining the anterior ends of the ischial tuberosities divides the diamond-shaped perineum into two triangles, the oblique planes of which intersect at the transverse line (Fig. 3.51B & C). The **anal triangle** lies posterior to this line. The anal canal and its orifice, the anus, constitute the major deep and superficial features of the triangle, lying centrally surrounded by ischioanal fat. The **urogenital** (UG) **triangle** is anterior to this line. In contrast to the open anal triangle, the UG triangle is "closed" by a thin sheet of tough, deep fascia, the **perineal membrane,** which stretches between the two sides of the pubic arch, covering the anterior part of the pelvic outlet (Fig. 3.52C). The perineal membrane thus fills the anterior gap in the pelvic diaphragm (the urogenital hiatus, Fig. 3.52A), but is perforated by the urethra in both sexes and by the vagina of the female. The membrane and the ischiopubic rami to which it attaches provide a foundation for the erectile bodies of the external genitalia—the penis and scrotum of males, and the pudendum or vulva of females—which are the superficial features of the triangle (Fig. 3.50).

The midpoint of the line joining the ischial tuberosities is the **central point of the perineum.** This is the location of the **perineal body**, which is an irregular mass, variable in size and consistency, and containing collagenous and elastic fibers, and both skeletal and smooth muscle (Fig. 3.52E). The perineal body lies deep to the skin, with relatively little overlying subcutaneous tissue, posterior to the vestibule of the vagina or bulb of the penis and anterior to the anus and anal canal. The perineal body is the site of convergence and interlacing of fibers of several muscles, including the:

- Bulbospongiosus.
- External anal sphincter.
- Superficial and deep transverse perineal muscles.
- Smooth and voluntary slips of muscle from the external urethral sphincter, levator ani, and muscular coats of the rectum.

Anteriorly, the perineal body blends with the posterior border of the perineal membrane and superiorly with the rectovesical or rectovaginal septum (Fig. 3.53A & B).

Fasciae and Pouches of Urogenital Triangle

PERINEAL FASCIAE[2]

The perineal fascia consists of superficial and deep layers. The **subcutaneous tissue of the perineum,** like that of the inferior anterior abdominal wall consists of a superficial *fatty layer* and a deep *membranous layer,* the (superficial) **perineal fascia** (Colles fascia).

[2]The terminology used in this section (in boldface) was recommended by the *Federative International Committee on Anatomical Terminology* (FICAT) in 1998; however, because many clinicians concerned with the perineum use eponyms, the authors have placed commonly used terms in parentheses so that the FICAT terminology will be understood by all readers.

In females, the **fatty layer of subcutaneous tissue of the perineum** makes up the substance of the labia majora and mons pubis, and is continuous anteriorly and superiorly with the fatty layer of subcutaneous tissue of the abdomen (Camper fascia) (Fig. 3.53A & C). In males, the fatty layer is greatly diminished in the urogenital triangle, being replaced altogether in the penis and scrotum with smooth (dartos) muscle. It is continuous between the penis or scrotum and thighs with the fatty layer of subcutaneous tissue of the abdomen (Fig. 3.53B & D). In both sexes, the fatty layer of subcutaneous tissue of the perineum is continuous posteriorly with the ischio-anal fat pad in the anal region (Fig. 3.53E).

The membranous **perineal fascia** does not extend into the anal triangle, being attached posteriorly to the posterior margin of the perineal membrane and perineal body (Fig. 3.53A & B). Laterally it is attached to the fascia lata (deep fascia) of the superiormost medial aspect of the thigh (Fig. 3.53C & E). Anteriorly in males, the perineal fascia is continuous with the **dartos fascia** of the penis and scrotum; however, on each side of and anterior to the scrotum, the perineal fascia becomes continuous with the membranous layer of subcutaneous tissue of the abdomen (Scarpa fascia) (Fig. 3.53B). In females, the perineal fascia passes superior to the fatty layer forming the labia majora and becomes continuous with the membranous layer of subcutaneous tissue of the abdomen (Fig. 3.53A & C).

The **deep perineal fascia** (investing or Gallaudet fascia) intimately invests the ischiocavernosus, bulbospongiosus, and superficial transverse perineal muscles (Fig. 3.53A & E). It is also attached laterally to the ischiopubic rami. Anteriorly it is fused to the suspensory ligament of the penis (see Fig. 3.63) and is continuous with the deep fascia covering the external oblique muscle of the abdomen and the rectus sheath. In females, the deep perineal fascia is fused with the suspensory ligament of the clitoris and, as in males, with the deep fascia of the abdomen.

SUPERFICIAL PERINEAL POUCH

The **superficial perineal pouch** (space or compartment) is a potential space between the perineal fascia and the perineal membrane, bounded laterally by the ischiopubic rami (Figs. 3.52D & E and 3.53).

In males, the superficial perineal pouch contains the:

- *Root* (bulb and crura) *of the penis* and associated muscles (*ischiocavernosus* and *bulbospongiosus*).
- Proximal (bulbous) part of the *spongy urethra*.
- *Superficial transverse perineal muscles.*
- *Deep perineal branches* of the internal pudendal vessels and pudendal nerves.

In females, the superficial perineal pouch contains the:

- *Clitoris* and associated muscle (ischiocavernosus).
- *Bulbs of the vestibule* and surrounding muscle (bulbospongiosus).
- *Greater vestibular glands.*
- *Superficial transverse perineal muscles.*
- Related vessels and nerves (*deep perineal branches* of the internal pudendal vessels and pudendal nerves).

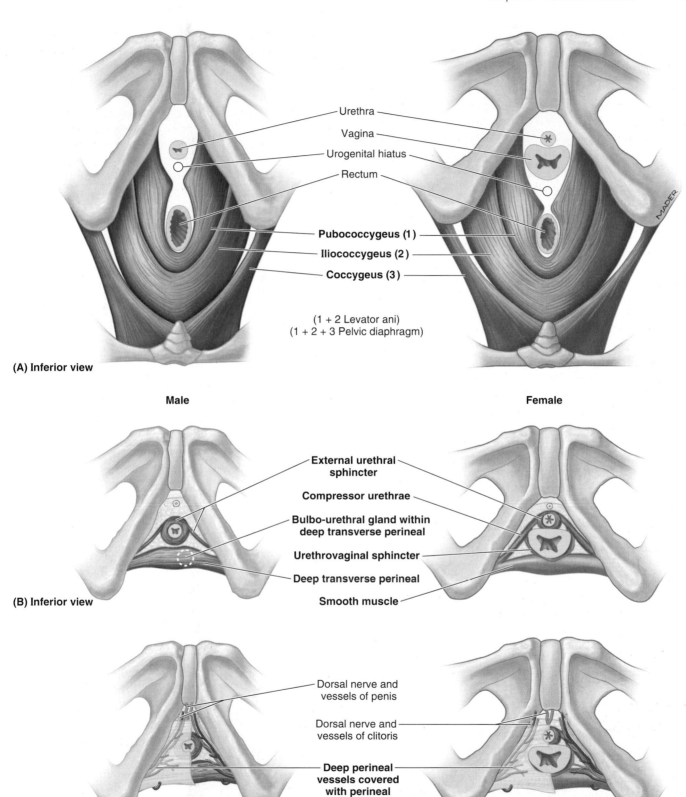

Male   **Female**

FIGURE 3.52. Layers of perineum of males and females. The layers are shown as being built up from deep (**A**) to superficial (**E**) layers. **A.** The pelvic outlet is almost closed by the pelvic diaphragm (levator ani and coccygeus muscles), forming the floor of the pelvic cavity and, as viewed here, the roof of the perineum. The urethra (and vagina in females) and rectum pass through the urogenital hiatus of the pelvic diaphragm. **B** and **C.** The external urethral sphincter and deep transverse perineal muscle span the region of the urogenital hiatus, which is closed inferiorly by the perineal membrane extending between the ischiopubic rami.

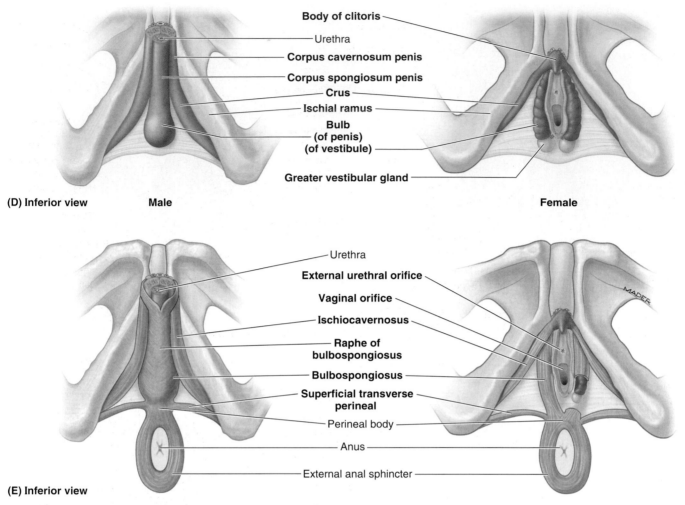

(D) Inferior view   Male

Body of clitoris
Urethra
Corpus cavernosum penis
Corpus spongiosum penis
Crus
Ischial ramus
Bulb
(of penis)
(of vestibule)
Greater vestibular gland

Female

(E) Inferior view

Urethra
External urethral orifice
Vaginal orifice
Ischiocavernosus
Raphe of
bulbospongiosus
Bulbospongiosus
Superficial transverse
perineal
Perineal body
Anus
External anal sphincter

FIGURE 3.52. (*Continued*) **D and E.** Inferior to the perineal membrane, the superficial perineal pouch (space) contains the erectile bodies and the muscles associated with them.

The structures of the superficial perineal pouch will be discussed in greater detail, specific to each sex, under "Male Perineum" and "Female Perineum," later in this chapter.

DEEP PERINEAL POUCH

The **deep perineal pouch** (space) is bounded inferiorly by the perineal membrane, superiorly by the inferior fascia of the pelvic diaphragm, and laterally by the inferior portion of the obturator fascia (covering the obturator internus muscle) (Fig. 3.53C & D). It includes the fat-filled anterior recesses of the ischio-anal fossae. The superior boundary in the region of the urogenital hiatus is indistinct.

In both sexes, the deep perineal pouch contains:

- Part of the urethra, centrally.
- The inferior part of the external urethral sphincter muscle, above the center of the perineal membrane, surrounding the urethra.
- Anterior extensions of the ischio-anal fat pads.

In males, the deep perineal pouch contains the:

- *Intermediate part of the urethra,* the narrowest part of the male urethra.
- *Deep transverse perineal muscles,* immediately superior to the perineal membrane (on its superior surface), running transversely along its posterior aspect.
- *Bulbo-urethral glands,* embedded within the deep perineal musculature.
- Dorsal neurovascular structures of the penis.

In females, the deep perineal pouch contains the:

- Proximal part of the *urethra.*
- A mass of smooth muscle in the place of deep transverse perineal muscles on the posterior edge of the perineal membrane, associated with the perineal body.
- Dorsal neurovasculature of the clitoris.

Past Concept of Deep Perineal Pouch and External Urethral Sphincter. Traditionally, a trilaminar, triangular *UG diaphragm* has been described as making up the deep

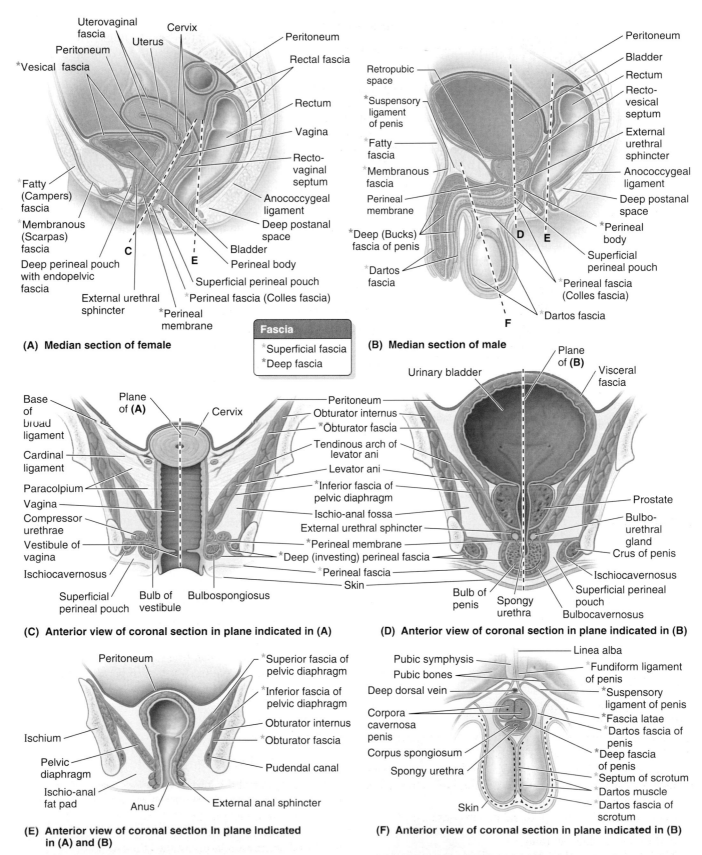

(A) Median section of female

Uterovaginal fascia
Cervix
Uterus
Peritoneum
*Vesical fascia
Peritoneum
Rectal fascia
Rectum
Vagina
Recto-vaginal septum
Anococcygeal ligament
Deep postanal space
*Fatty (Campers) fascia
*Membranous (Scarpas) fascia
Deep perineal pouch with endopelvic fascia
C
E
Bladder
Perineal body
Superficial perineal pouch
External urethral sphincter
*Perineal fascia (Colles fascia)
*Perineal membrane

Fascia
*Superficial fascia
*Deep fascia

(B) Median section of male

Peritoneum
Bladder
Rectum
Recto-vesical septum
External urethral sphincter
Anococcygeal ligament
Deep postanal space
Retropubic space
*Suspensory ligament of penis
*Fatty fascia
*Membranous fascia
Perineal membrane
*Deep (Bucks) fascia of penis
*Dartos fascia
D
E
*Perineal body
Superficial perineal pouch
*Perineal fascia (Colles fascia)
*Dartos fascia
F

(C) Anterior view of coronal section in plane indicated in (A)

Base of broad ligament
Plane of (A)
Cervix
Cardinal ligament
Paracolpium
Vagina
Compressor urethrae
Vestibule of vagina
Ischiocavernosus
Superficial perineal pouch
Bulb of vestibule
Bulbospongiosus
Peritoneum
Obturator internus
*Obturator fascia
Tendinous arch of levator ani
Levator ani
*Inferior fascia of pelvic diaphragm
Ischio-anal fossa
External urethral sphincter
*Perineal membrane
*Deep (investing) perineal fascia
*Perineal fascia
Skin

(D) Anterior view of coronal section in plane indicated in (B)

Urinary bladder
Plane of (B)
Visceral fascia
Prostate
Bulbo-urethral gland
Crus of penis
Ischiocavernosus
Superficial perineal pouch
Bulbocavernosus
Bulb of penis
Spongy urethra

(E) Anterior view of coronal section in plane indicated in (A) and (B)

Peritoneum
*Superior fascia of pelvic diaphragm
*Inferior fascia of pelvic diaphragm
Obturator internus
*Obturator fascia
Pudendal canal
Ischium
Pelvic diaphragm
Ischio-anal fat pad
Anus
External anal sphincter

(F) Anterior view of coronal section in plane indicated in (B)

Pubic symphysis
Pubic bones
Deep dorsal vein
Corpora cavernosa penis
Corpus spongiosum
Spongy urethra
Skin
Linea alba
*Fundiform ligament of penis
*Suspensory ligament of penis
*Fascia latae
*Dartos fascia of penis
*Deep fascia of penis
*Septum of scrotum
*Dartos muscle
*Dartos fascia of scrotum

FIGURE 3.53. Fasciae of perineum. A and **B.** Median sections, viewed from left, demonstrate the fasciae in the female (**A**) and male (**B**). The planes of the sections shown in parts **C–F** are indicated. **C.** This coronal section of the female urogenital triangle is in the plane of the vagina. Fibro-areolar components of the endopelvic fascia (cardinal ligament and paracolpium) are shown. **D.** This coronal section of the male urogenital triangle is in the plane of the prostatic urethra. **E.** This coronal section of the anal triangle is in the plane of the lower rectal and anal canals. **F.** This coronal section demonstrates the subcutaneous tissue of the proximal penis and scrotum. An enlarged view of the layers of the penis is provided in Figure 3.61C.

perineal pouch. Although the classical descriptions appear justified when viewing only the superficial aspect of the structures occupying the deep pouch (Fig. 3.54A), the long-held concept of a flat, essentially two-dimensional diaphragm is erroneous. According to this concept, a trilaminar "UG diaphragm" consisted of the perineal membrane (inferior fascia of the UG diaphragm) inferiorly, a superior fascia of the UG diaphragm superiorly, and deep perineal muscles in between. The deep pouch was the space between the two fascial membranes, occupied by what was perceived to be a flat muscular sheet consisting of a disc-like sphincter urethra anterior to or within an equally two-dimensional, transversely oriented deep transverse perineal muscle. In males, the bulbo-urethral glands were also considered occupants of the pouch. Only the descriptions of the perineal membrane and deep transverse perineal muscles of the male (with embedded glands)

appear to be supported by evidence, which includes medical imaging of live subjects (Myers et al., 1998a, 1998b). Many texts, atlases, and medical illustrations continue to feature the old model, and students are likely to encounter the outdated images and concepts in clinical training and practice, and need to be aware of the inaccuracies in this regard.

Current Concept of Deep Perineal Pouch and External Urethral Sphincter. In the female, the posterior edge of the perineal membrane is typically occupied by a mass of smooth muscle in the place of the deep transverse perineal muscles (Wendell-Smith, 1995). Immediately superior to the posterior half of the perineal membrane, the flat, sheet-like, deep transverse perineal muscle, when developed (typically only in males), offers dynamic support for the pelvic viscera. As described by Oelrich (1980), however, the urethral sphincter muscle is not a flat, planar structure,

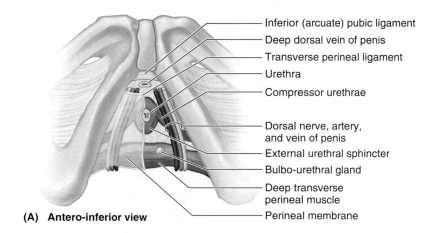

- Inferior (arcuate) pubic ligament
- Deep dorsal vein of penis
- Transverse perineal ligament
- Urethra
- Compressor urethrae
- Dorsal nerve, artery, and vein of penis
- External urethral sphincter
- Bulbo-urethral gland
- Deep transverse perineal muscle
- Perineal membrane

(A) Antero-inferior view

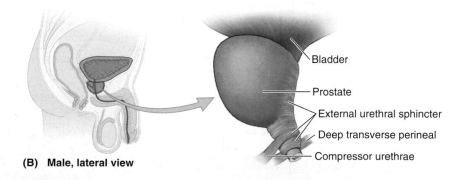

Bladder
Prostate
External urethral sphincter
Deep transverse perineal
Compressor urethrae

(B) Male, lateral view

Vaginal wall
Bladder
External urethral sphincter
Compressor urethrae
Urethrovaginal sphincter
Deep transverse perineal
Urethra
Vagina

(C) Female, lateral view

FIGURE 3.54. Deep perineal pouch and male and female external urethral sphincters. A. The deep perineal pouch is seen through (left side) and after removal of the perineal membrane (right side). **B.** The trough-like fibers of the superior male external urethral sphincter ascend to the neck of the bladder as part of the isthmus of the prostate. The inferior sphincter includes cylindrical and loop-like portions (compressor urethrae). **C.** The female urethral sphincter complex is shown.

and the only "superior fascia" is the intrinsic fascia of the external urethral sphincter muscle. Contemporary views consider the *inferior fascia of the pelvic diaphragm* to be the superior boundary of the deep pouch (Fig. 3.53C–E). In both views, the strong *perineal membrane* is the inferior boundary (floor) of the deep pouch, separating it from the superficial pouch. The perineal membrane is indeed, with the perineal body, the final passive support of the pelvic viscera.

The male **external urethral sphincter** is more like a tube or trough than a disc. In the male only the inferior part of the muscle forms an encircling investment (a true sphincter) for the intermediate part of the urethra inferior to the prostate (Fig. 3.54B). Its larger, trough-like part extends vertically to the neck of the bladder as part of the *isthmus of the prostate,* displacing glandular tissue and investing the prostatic urethra anteriorly and anterolaterally only (see also Fig. 3.38). Apparently, the muscular primordium is established around the whole length of the urethra before development of the prostate. As the prostate develops from urethral glands, the posterior and posterolateral muscle atrophies, or is displaced by the prostate. Whether this part of the muscle compresses or dilates the prostatic urethra is a matter of some controversy.

The female **external urethral sphincter** is more properly a "urogenital sphincter" (Oelrich, 1983). Here, too, a part forms a true anular sphincter around the urethra (Fig. 3.54C), with several additional parts extending from it: a superior part, extending to the neck of the bladder; a subdivision described as extending inferolaterally to the ischial ramus on each side (the compressor urethrae muscle); and yet another band-like part, which encircles both the vagina and the urethra (urethrovaginal sphincter). In both the male and female, the musculature described is oriented perpendicular to the perineal membrane, rather than lying in a plane parallel to it.

(A) Anterior view of schematic coronal section

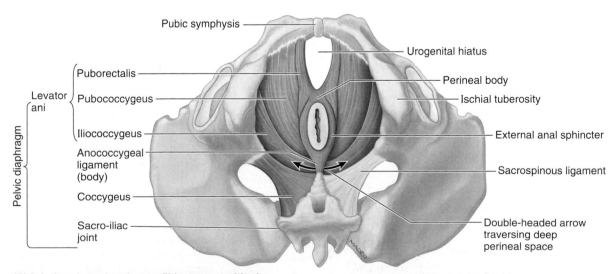

(B) Inferior view of perineum (lithotomy position)

FIGURE 3.55. Pelvic diaphragm and ischio-anal fossae. A. Coronal section of the pelvis in the plane of the rectum and anal canal, demonstrating lateral and medial walls and roof of the ischio-anal fossae. **B.** Fascia covering the inferior aspect of the pelvic diaphragm forms the roof of the ischio-anal fossae. The left sacrospinous ligament has been removed to reveal the coccygeus. Abscesses of the right or left ischio-anal fossa may extend to the contralateral fossa via the deep postanal space (*double-headed arrow*).

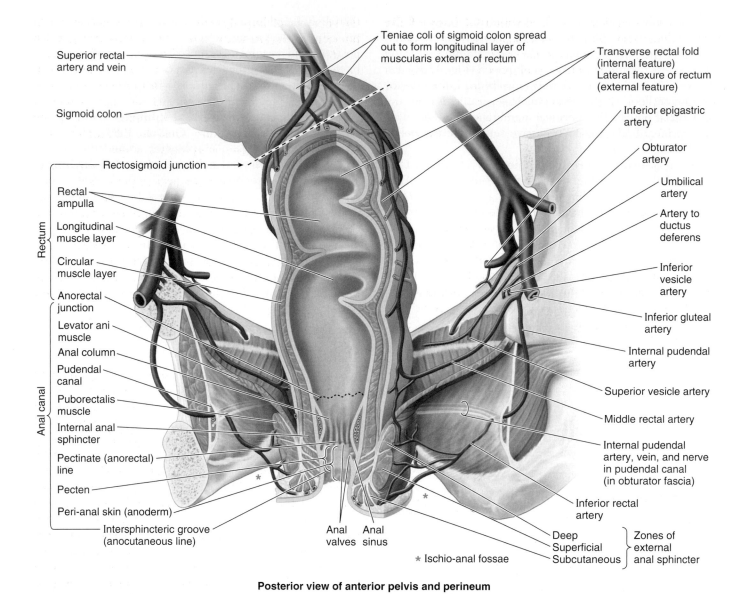

Superior rectal artery and vein

Sigmoid colon

Rectosigmoid junction

Rectal ampulla

Longitudinal muscle layer

Circular muscle layer

Anorectal junction

Levator ani muscle

Anal column

Pudendal canal

Puborectalis muscle

Internal anal sphincter

Pectinate (anorectal) line

Pecten

Peri-anal skin (anoderm)

Intersphincteric groove (anocutaneous line)

Rectum

Anal canal

Teniae coli of sigmoid colon spread out to form longitudinal layer of muscularis externa of rectum

Transverse rectal fold (internal feature)
Lateral flexure of rectum (external feature)

Inferior epigastric artery

Obturator artery

Umbilical artery

Artery to ductus deferens

Inferior vesicle artery

Inferior gluteal artery

Internal pudendal artery

Superior vesicle artery

Middle rectal artery

Internal pudendal artery, vein, and nerve in pudendal canal (in obturator fascia)

Inferior rectal artery

Anal valves   Anal sinus

* Ischio-anal fossae

Deep
Superficial
Subcutaneous

Zones of external anal sphincter

Posterior view of anterior pelvis and perineum

FIGURE 3.56. Rectum and anal canal, levator ani, and ischio-anal fossa. The left posterolateral third of the rectum and anal canal have been removed to demonstrate the luminal features. The pudendal vessels and nerves are transmitted by the pudendal canal, a space within the obturator fascia that covers the medial surface of the obturator internus, lining the lateral wall of the ischio-anal fossa.

Features of Anal Triangle

ISCHIO-ANAL FOSSAE

The **ischio-anal fossae** (formerly called ischiorectal fossae) on each side of the anal canal are large fascia-lined, wedge-shaped spaces between the skin of the anal region and the pelvic diaphragm (Figs. 3.53D, 3.55A, and 3.56). The apex of each fossa lies superiorly where the levator ani muscle arises from the obturator fascia. The ischio-anal fossae, wide inferiorly and narrow superiorly, are filled with fat and loose connective tissue. The two ischio-anal fossae communicate by means of the *deep postanal space* over the *anococcygeal ligament* (body), a fibrous mass located between the anal canal and the tip of the coccyx (Figs. 3.53A & B and 3.55B).

Each ischio-anal fossa is bounded:

- Laterally by the ischium and overlapping inferior part of the obturator internus, covered with obturator fascia.
- Medially by the external anal sphincter, with a sloping superior medial wall or roof formed by the levator ani as it descends to blend with the sphincter; both structures surround the anal canal.
- Posteriorly by the sacrotuberous ligament and gluteus maximus.
- Anteriorly by the bodies of the pubic bones, inferior to the origin of the puborectalis. These parts of the fossae, extending into the UG triangle superior to the perineal membrane (and musculature on its superior surface), are known as the **anterior recesses of the ischio-anal fossae.**

Each ischio-anal fossa is filled with a **fat body of the ischio-anal fossa.** These fat bodies support the anal canal but they are readily displaced to permit descent and expansion of the anal canal during the passage of feces. The fat bodies are traversed by tough, fibrous bands, as well as by several neurovascular structures, including the inferior anal/rectal vessels and nerves and two other cutaneous nerves, the perforating branch of S2 and S3 and the perineal branch of S4 nerve.

PUDENDAL CANAL AND ITS NEUROVASCULAR BUNDLE

The **pudendal canal** (Alcock canal) is an essentially horizontal passageway within the obturator fascia that covers the medial aspect of the obturator internus and lines the lateral wall of the ischio-anal fossa (Figs. 3.55A and 3.56). The internal pudendal artery and vein, the pudendal nerve, and the nerve to the obturator internus enter this canal at the lesser sciatic notch, inferior to the ischial spine. The internal pudendal vessels and the pudendal nerve supply and drain blood from and innervate most of the perineum. As the artery and nerve enter the canal, they give rise to the **inferior rectal artery** and **nerve,** which pass medially to supply the external anal sphincter and the peri-anal skin (Figs. 3.56–3.58; Table 3.8). Toward the distal

FIGURE 3.57. Distribution of pudendal nerve. The five regions traversed by the nerve are shown. The pudendal nerve supplies the skin, organs, and muscles of the perineum; therefore, it is concerned with micturition, defecation, erection, ejaculation, and, in the female, parturition. Although the pudendal nerve is shown here in the male, its distribution is similar in the female because the parts of the female perineum are homologs of those in the male.

(anterior) end of the pudendal canal, the artery and nerve both bifurcate, giving rise to the *perineal nerve* and *artery*, which are distributed mostly to the superficial pouch (inferior to the perineal membrane), and to the *dorsal artery* and *nerve of the penis or clitoris*, which run in the deep pouch (superior to the membrane). When the latter structures reach the dorsum of the penis or clitoris, the nerves run distally on the lateral side of the continuation of the internal pudendal artery as they both proceed to the glans penis or glans clitoris.

The perineal nerve has two branches: The **superficial perineal nerve** gives rise to posterior scrotal or labial (cutaneous) branches, and the **deep perineal nerve** supplies the muscles of the deep and superficial perineal pouches, the skin of the vestibule, and the mucosa of the inferiormost part of the vagina. The inferior rectal nerve communicates with the posterior scrotal or labial and perineal nerves. The **dorsal nerve of the penis** or **clitoris** is the primary sensory nerve serving the male or female organ, especially the sensitive glans at the distal end.

ANAL CANAL

The **anal canal** is the terminal part of the large intestine and of the entire digestive tract. It extends from the superior aspect of the pelvic diaphragm to the **anus** (Figs. 3.55B and 3.56). The canal (2.5–3.5 cm long) begins where the rectal ampulla narrows at the level of the U-shaped sling formed by the puborectalis muscle (Fig. 3.12). The anal canal ends at the anus, the external outlet of the alimentary tract. The anal canal, surrounded by internal and external anal sphincters, descends postero-inferiorly between the anococcygeal ligament and the perineal body. The canal is collapsed, except during passage of feces. Both sphincters must relax before defecation can occur.

The **internal anal sphincter** (Figs. 3.55A and 3.56) is an involuntary sphincter surrounding the superior two thirds of the anal canal. It is a thickening of the circular muscle layer. Its contraction (tonus) is stimulated and maintained by sympathetic fibers from the superior rectal (peri-arterial) and hypogastric plexuses. Its contraction is inhibited by parasympathetic fiber stimulation, both intrinsically in relation to peristalsis, and extrinsically by fibers conveyed by the pelvic splanchnic nerves. This sphincter is tonically contracted most of the time to prevent leakage of fluid or flatus; however, it relaxes (is inhibited) temporarily in response to distension of the rectal ampulla by feces or gas, requiring voluntary contraction of the puborectalis and external anal sphincter if defecation or flatulence is not to occur. The ampulla relaxes after initial distension (when peristalsis subsides) and tonus returns until the next peristalsis, or until a threshold level of distension occurs, at which point inhibition of the sphincter is continuous until distension is relieved.

The **external anal sphincter** is a large voluntary sphincter that forms a broad band on each side of the inferior two thirds of the anal canal (Figs. 3.52E, 3.55, and 3.56). This sphincter is attached anteriorly to the perineal body and posteriorly to the coccyx via the anococcygeal ligament. It blends superiorly with the puborectalis muscle.

(A) Medial view of male (from left)

(B) Left anterolateral view of female

FIGURE 3.58. Arteries of perineum.

TABLE 3.8. ARTERIES OF PERINEUM

Artery	Origin	Course	Distribution in Perineum
Internal pudendal	Anterior division of internal iliac artery	Leaves pelvis through greater sciatic foramen; hooks around ischial spine to enter perineum via lesser sciatic foramen; enters pudendal canal	Primary artery of perineum and external genital organs
Inferior rectal	Internal pudendal artery	Arises at entrance to pudendal canal; traverses ischio-anal fossa to anal canal	Anal canal inferior to pectinate line; anal sphincters; peri-anal skin
Perineal		Arises within pudendal canal; passes to superficial pouch (space) on exit	Supplies superficial perineal muscles and scrotum of male/vestibule of female
Posterior scrotal (♂) or labial (♀)	Terminal branch of perineal artery	Runs in superficial fascia of posterior scrotum or labia majora	Skin of scrotum or labia majora and minora
Artery of bulb of penis (♂) or vestibule (♀)		Pierces perineal membrane to reach bulb of penis or vestibule of vagina	Supplies bulb of penis (including bulbar urethra) and bulbo-urethral gland (male) or bulb of vestibule and greater vestibular gland (female)
Deep artery of penis (♂) or clitoris (♀)	Terminal branch of internal pudendal artery	Pierces perineal membrane to enter crura of corpora cavernosa of penis or clitoris; branches run proximally and distally	Supplies most erectile tissue of corpora cavernosa of penis or clitoris via helicine arteries
Dorsal artery of penis (♂) or clitoris (♀)		Passes to deep pouch; pierces perineal membrane and traverses suspensory ligament of penis or clitoris to run on dorsum of penis or clitoris to glans	Deep perineal pouch; skin of penis; fascia of penis or clitoris; distal corpus spongiosum of penis, including spongy urethra; glans penis or clitoris
External pudendal, superficial, and deep branches	Femoral artery	Pass medially from thigh to reach anterior aspect of the urogenital triangle of perineum	Anterior aspect of scrotum and skin at root of penis of male; mons pubis and anterior aspect of labia of female

The external anal sphincter is described as having subcutaneous, superficial, and deep parts; these are zones rather than muscle bellies and are often indistinct. The external anal sphincter is supplied mainly by S4 through the inferior rectal nerve (Fig. 3.57), although its deep part also receives fibers from the nerve to the levator ani, in common with the puborectalis, with which it contracts in unison to maintain continence when the internal sphincter is relaxed (except during defecation).

Internally, the superior half of the mucous membrane of the anal canal is characterized by a series of longitudinal ridges called **anal columns** (Fig. 3.56). These columns contain the terminal branches of the superior rectal artery and vein. The **anorectal junction,** indicated by the superior ends of the anal columns, is where the rectum joins the anal canal. At this point, the wide rectal ampulla abruptly narrows as it traverses the pelvic diaphragm. The inferior ends of the anal columns are joined by **anal valves.** Superior to the valves are small recesses called **anal sinuses.** When compressed by feces, the anal sinuses exude mucus, which aids in evacuation of feces from the anal canal.

The inferior comb-shaped limit of the anal valves forms an irregular line, the **pectinate line,** that indicates the junction of the superior part of the anal canal (visceral; derived from the embryonic hindgut), and the inferior part (somatic; derived from the embryonic proctodeum).

The anal canal superior to the pectinate line differs from the part inferior to the pectinate line in its arterial supply, innervation, and venous and lymphatic drainage (Fig. 3.59). These differences result from the different embryological origins of the superior and inferior parts of the anal canal (Moore, Persaud, and Torchiam 2012).

Arterial Supply of Anal Canal. The *superior rectal artery* supplies the anal canal *superior to the pectinate line* (Figs. 3.32A and 3.59). The two *inferior rectal arteries* supply the anal canal *inferior to the pectinate line* as well as the surrounding muscles and peri-anal skin (Figs. 3.32, 3.58, and 3.59; Table 3.8). The *middle rectal arteries* assist with the blood supply to the anal canal by forming anastomoses with the superior and inferior rectal arteries.

Venous and Lymphatic Drainage of Anal Canal. The *internal rectal venous plexus* drains in both directions from the level of the pectinate line. *Superior to the pectinate line,* the internal rectal plexus drains chiefly into the *superior rectal vein* (a tributary of the inferior mesenteric vein) and the portal system (Figs. 3.32B and 3.59). *Inferior to the pectinate line,* the internal rectal plexus drains into the *inferior rectal veins* (tributaries of the caval venous system) around the margin of the external anal sphincter. The *middle rectal veins* (tributaries of the internal iliac veins) mainly drain the muscularis externa of the ampulla and form anastomoses with the superior and inferior rectal veins. In addition to the abundant venous anastomoses, the rectal plexuses receive multiple arteriovenous anastomoses (AVAs) from the superior and middle rectal arteries.

The normal submucosa of the anorectal junction is markedly thickened, and in section has the appearance of a cavernous (erectile) tissue, owing to the presence of the sacculated veins of the internal rectal venous plexus. The vascular submucosa is especially thickened in the left lateral, right anterolateral, and right posterolateral positions, forming anal cushions, or threshold pads, at the point of closure of the anal canal. Because these cushions contain plexuses of saccular veins capable of directly receiving arterial blood via multiple

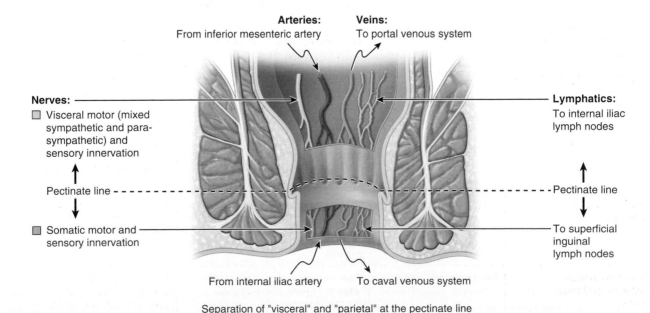

Nerves:
☐ Visceral motor (mixed sympathetic and para-sympathetic) and sensory innervation

Arteries:
From inferior mesenteric artery

Veins:
To portal venous system

Lymphatics:
To internal iliac lymph nodes

Pectinate line - Pectinate line

☐ Somatic motor and sensory innervation

To superficial inguinal lymph nodes

From internal iliac artery   To caval venous system

Separation of "visceral" and "parietal" at the pectinate line

FIGURE 3.59. **Transitions occurring at pectinate line.** Vessels and nerves superior to the pectinate line are visceral; those inferior to the pectinate line are parietal or somatic. This orientation reflects the embryological development of the anorectum.

AVAs, they are variably pliable and turgid, and form a sort of flutter valve that contributes to the normally water- and gastight closure of the anal canal.

Superior to the pectinate line, the lymphatic vessels drain deeply into the *internal iliac lymph nodes,* and through them into the common iliac and lumbar lymph nodes (Figs. 3.48B and 3.59; Table 3.7). *Inferior to the pectinate line,* the lymphatic vessels drain superficially into the **superficial inguinal lymph nodes,** as does most of the perineum.

Innervation of Anal Canal. The nerve supply to the anal canal *superior to the pectinate line* is visceral innervation from the *inferior hypogastric plexus,* involving sympathetic, parasympathetic, and visceral afferent fibers (Figs. 3.33 and 3.59). Sympathetic fibers maintain the tonus of the internal anal sphincter. Parasympathetic fibers inhibit the tonus of the internal sphincter and evoke peristaltic contraction for defecation. The superior part of the anal canal, like the rectum superior to it, is inferior to the *pelvic pain line* (see Table 3.3); all visceral afferents travel with the parasympathetic fibers to spinal sensory ganglia S2–S4. Superior to the pectinate line, the anal canal is sensitive only to stretching, which evokes sensations at both the conscious and unconscious (reflex) levels. For example, distension of the rectal ampulla inhibits (relaxes) the tonus of the internal sphincter.

The nerve supply of the anal canal *inferior to the pectinate line* is somatic innervation derived from the *inferior anal (rectal) nerves,* branches of the pudendal nerve. Therefore, this part of the anal canal is sensitive to pain, touch, and temperature. Somatic efferent fibers stimulate contraction of the voluntary external anal sphincter.

PERINEUM

Disruption of Perineal Body

The perineal body is an important structure, especially in women, because it is the final support of the pelvic viscera, linking muscles that extend across the pelvic outlet, like crossing beams supporting the overlying pelvic diaphragm. Stretching or tearing the attachments of perineal muscles from the perineal body can occur during childbirth, removing support from the pelvic floor. As a result, *prolapse of pelvic viscera,* including prolapse of the bladder (through the urethra) and prolapse of the uterus and/or vagina (through the vaginal orifice) may occur. (Various degrees of prolapse are illustrated in the blue box "Disposition of Uterus and Uterine Prolapse," p. 392).

The perineal body can also be disrupted by trauma, inflammatory disease, and infection, which can result in the formation of a *fistula* (abnormal canal) connected to the vestibule (see the blue box "Vaginal Fistulae," p. 396). Attenuation of the perineal body, associated with diastasis (separation) of the puborectalis and pubococcygeus parts of the levator ani, may also result in the formation of a *cystocele, rectocele,* and/or *enterocele,* hernial protrusions of part of the bladder, rectum, or rectovaginal pouch, respectively, into the vaginal wall (Fig. B3.28).

Episiotomy

During vaginal surgery and labor, an *episiotomy* (surgical incision of the perineum and inferoposterior vaginal wall) may be made to enlarge the vaginal orifice, with the intention of decreasing excessive traumatic tearing of the perineum and uncontrolled jagged tears of the perineal muscles. Episiotomies are still performed in a large portion of vaginal deliveries in the United States (Gabbe et al., 2007). It is generally agreed that episiotomy is indicated when

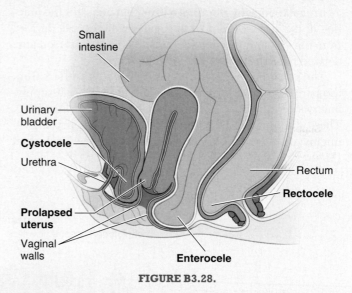

FIGURE B3.28.

descent of the fetus is arrested or protracted, when instrumentation is necessary (e.g., use of obstetrical forceps), or to expedite delivery when there are signs of fetal distress. However, routine prophylactic episiotomy is widely debated and declining in frequency.

The perineal body is the major structure incised during a *median episiotomy* (Fig. B3.29A & B). The rationale of the median incision is that the scar produced as the wound heals will not be greatly different from the fibrous tissue surrounding it. Also, because the incision extends only partially into this fibrous tissue, some surgeons believe that the incision is more likely to be self-limiting, resisting further tearing. However, when further tearing does occur, it is directed toward the anus, and sphincter damage or anovaginal fistulae are poten-

Inferior view (lithotomy position)

FIGURE B3.29.

tial sequelae. Recent studies indicate median episiotomies are associated with an increased incidence of severe lacerations, associated in turn with an increased incidence of long-term incontinence, pelvic prolapse, and anovaginal fistulae.

Mediolateral episiotomies (Fig. B3.29A) appear to result in a lower incidence of severe laceration and are less likely to be associated with damage to the anal sphincters and canal. (*Note:* The clinical use of the term *mediolateral* is technically inappropriate here; it actually refers to an incision that is initially a median incision that then turns laterally as it proceeds posteriorly, circumventing the perineal body and directing further tearing away from the anus.)

Rupture of Urethra in Males and Extravasation of Urine

Fractures of the pelvic girdle, especially those resulting from separation of the pubic symphysis and puboprostatic ligaments, often cause a *rupture of the intermediate part of the urethra*. Rupture of this part of the urethra results in the *extravasation* (escape) *of urine and blood* into the deep perineal pouch (Fig. B3.30A); the fluid may pass superiorly through the urogenital hiatus and distribute extraperitoneally around the prostate and bladder.

The common site of *rupture of the spongy urethra* and *extravasation of urine* is in the bulb of the penis (Fig. B3.30B). This injury usually results from a forceful blow to the perineum (*straddle injury*), such as falling on a metal beam or, less commonly, from the incorrect passage (*false passage*) of a transurethral catheter or device that fails to negotiate the angle of the urethra in the bulb of the penis. Rupture of the corpus spongiosum and spongy urethra results in urine passing from it (extravasating) into the superficial perineal space. The attachments of the perineal fascia determine the direction of flow of the extravasated urine. Urine may pass into the loose connec-

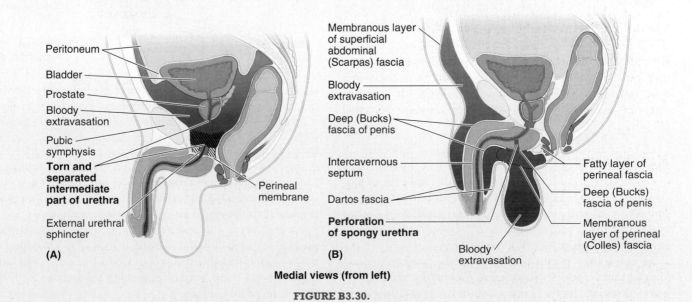

Medial views (from left)

FIGURE B3.30.

tive tissue in the scrotum, around the penis, and superiorly, deep to the membranous layer of subcutaneous connective tissue of the inferior anterior abdominal wall.

The urine cannot pass far into the thighs because the membranous layer of superficial perineal fascia blends with the fascia lata, enveloping the thigh muscles, just distal to the inguinal ligament. In addition, urine cannot pass posteriorly into the anal triangle because the superficial and deep layers of perineal fascia are continuous with each other around the superficial perineal muscles and with the posterior edge of the perineal membrane between them. Rupture of a blood vessel into the superficial perineal pouch resulting from trauma would result in a similar containment of blood in the superficial perineal pouch.

Starvation and Rectal Prolapse

The fat bodies of the ischio-anal fossae are among the last reserves of fatty tissue to disappear with starvation. In the absence of the support provided by the ischio-anal fat, rectal prolapse is relatively common.

Pectinate Line—a Clinically Important Landmark

The *pectinate line* (also called the dentate or muco-cutaneous line by some clinicians) is a particularly important landmark because it is visible and approximates the level of important anatomical changes related to the transition from visceral to parietal (Fig. 3.59), affecting such things as the types of tumors that occur, and the direction in which they metastasize.

Anal Fissures; Ischio-anal and Peri-anal Abscesses

The ischio-anal fossae are occasionally the sites of infection, which may result in the formation of *ischio-anal abscesses* (Fig. B3.31A). These collections of pus are painful. Infections may reach the ischio-anal fossae in several ways:

- After *cryptitis* (inflammation of anal sinuses).
- Extension from a pelvirectal abscess.
- After a tear in the anal mucous membrane.
- From a penetrating wound in the anal region.

Diagnostic signs of an ischio-anal abscess are fullness and tenderness between the anus and the ischial tuberosity. A peri-anal abscess may rupture spontaneously, opening into the anal canal, rectum, or peri-anal skin. Because the ischio-anal fossae communicate posteriorly through the *deep post-anal space*, an abscess in one fossa may spread to the other one, and form a semicircular "horseshoe-shaped" abscess around the posterior aspect of the anal canal.

In chronically constipated persons, the anal valves and mucosa may be torn by hard feces. An *anal fissure* (slit-like lesion) is usually located in the posterior midline, inferior to

Plane of coronal sections

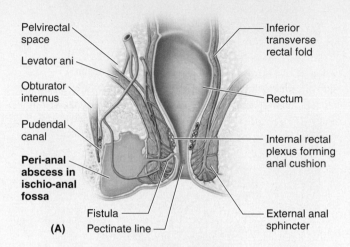

Pelvirectal space

Levator ani

Obturator internus

Pudendal canal

Peri-anal abscess in ischio-anal fossa

Fistula

(A) Pectinate line

Inferior transverse rectal fold

Rectum

Internal rectal plexus forming anal cushion

External anal sphincter

Internal iliac vein

Middle rectal vein

Internal pudendal vein

Internal rectal plexus

Inferior rectal vein

External rectal plexus

(B)

Rectum

Internal hemorrhoid

External anal sphincter

External hemorrhoid

Anterior views of coronal sections

FIGURE B3.31.

the anal valves. It is painful because this region is supplied by sensory fibers of the inferior rectal nerves. A *peri-anal abscess* may follow infection of an anal fissure, and the infection may spread to the ischio-anal fossae and form ischio-anal abscesses or spread into the pelvis and form a *pelvirectal abscess*.

An *anal fistula* may result from the spread of an anal infection and cryptitis (inflammation of an anal sinus). One end of this abnormal canal (fistula) opens into the anal canal, and the other end opens into an abscess in the ischio-anal fossa or into the peri-anal skin.

Hemorrhoids

Internal hemorrhoids (piles) are prolapses of rectal mucosa (more specifically, of the "anal cushions") containing the normally dilated veins of the *internal rectal venous plexus* (Fig. B3.31B). Internal hemorrhoids result from a breakdown of the muscularis mucosae, a smooth muscle layer deep to the mucosa. Internal hemorrhoids that prolapse into or through the anal canal are often compressed by the contracted sphincters, impeding blood flow. As a result, they tend to strangulate and ulcerate. Because of the presence of abundant arteriovenous anastomoses, bleeding from internal hemorrhoids is characteristically bright red. The current practice is to treat only prolapsed, ulcerated internal hemorrhoids. *External hemorrhoids* are thromboses (blood clots) in the veins of the *external rectal venous plexus* and are covered by skin. Predisposing factors for hemorrhoids include pregnancy, chronic constipation and prolonged toilet sitting and straining, and any disorder that impedes venous return, including increased intra-abdominal pressure.

The anastomoses between the superior, middle, and inferior rectal veins form clinically important communications between the portal and systemic venous systems (see Fig. 2.75A). The superior rectal vein drains into the inferior mesenteric vein, whereas the middle and inferior rectal veins drain through the systemic system into the inferior vena cava. Any abnormal increase in pressure in the valveless portal system or veins of the trunk may cause enlargement of the superior rectal veins, resulting in an increase in blood flow or stasis in the internal rectal venous plexus. In the *portal hypertension* that occurs in relation to *hepatic cirrhosis,* the portocaval anastomosis between the superior and the middle and inferior rectal veins, along with portocaval anastomoses elsewhere, may become varicose. It is important to note that the veins of the rectal plexuses *normally* appear varicose (dilated and tortuous), even in newborns, and that internal hemorrhoids occur most commonly in the absence of portal hypertension.

Regarding pain from and the treatment of hemorrhoids, it is important to note that the anal canal superior to the pectinate line is visceral; thus it is innervated by visceral afferent pain fibers, so that an incision or needle insertion in this region is painless. Internal hemorrhoids are not painful and can be treated without anesthesia. Inferior to the pectinate line, the anal canal is somatic, supplied by the inferior anal (rectal) nerves containing somatic sensory fibers. Therefore, it is sensitive to painful stimuli (e.g., to the prick of a hypodermic needle). External hemorrhoids can be painful but often resolve in a few days.

Anorectal Incontinence

Stretching of the pudendal nerve(s) during a traumatic childbirth can result in *pudendal nerve damage* and *anorectal incontinence.*

The Bottom Line

PERINEUM AND PERINEAL REGION

The perineum is the diamond-shaped compartment bounded peripherally by the osseofibrous pelvic outlet and deeply (superiorly) by the pelvic diaphragm. ♦ The surface area overlying this compartment is the perineal region. ♦ The urogenital (UG) triangle (anteriorly) and anal triangle (posteriorly) that together form this diamond-shaped area lie at angles to each other. ♦ The intersecting planes of the triangles define the transverse line (extending between ischial tuberosities) that is the base of each triangle. ♦ Centrally, the UG triangle is perforated by the urethra and, in females, by the vagina. ♦ The anal triangle is perforated by the anal canal. ♦ The perineal body is a musculofibrous mass between the UG and the anal perforating structures, at the center point of the perineum.

UG triangle: The subcutaneous tissue of the urogenital triangle includes a superficial fatty layer and a deeper membranous layer, the perineal fascia (Colles fascia), which are continuous with corresponding layers of the inferior anterior abdominal wall. ♦ In females, the fatty layer is thick within the mons pubis and labia majora, but in males it is replaced by smooth dartos muscle in the penis and scrotum. ♦ The perineal fascia is limited to the UG triangle, fusing with the deep fascia at the posterior border (base) of the triangle. ♦ In males, this layer extends into the penis and scrotum, where it is closely associated with the loose, mobile skin of these structures.

♦ The planar perineal membrane divides the urogenital triangle of the perineum into superficial and deep perineal pouches.

♦ The superficial perineal pouch is between the membranous layer of subcutaneous tissue of the perineum and the perineal membrane, and is bounded laterally by the ischiopubic rami.

♦ The deep perineal pouch is between the perineal membrane and the inferior fascia of the pelvic diaphragm, and is bounded laterally by the obturator fascia. ♦ The superficial perineal pouch contains the erectile bodies of the external genitalia and associated muscles, the superficial transverse perineal muscle, deep perineal nerves and vessels, and in females the greater vestibular glands. ♦ The deep pouch includes the fat-filled anterior recesses of the ischio-anal fossae (laterally), the deep perineal muscle and inferiormost part of the external urethral sphincter, the part of the urethra traversing the perineal membrane and inferiormost external urethral sphincter (the intermediate urethra of males), the dorsal nerves of the penis/clitoris, and in males the bulbo-urethral glands.

Anal triangle: The ischio-anal fossae are fascia-lined, wedge-shaped spaces occupied by ischio-anal fat bodies.

♦ The fat bodies provide supportive packing that can be compressed or pushed aside to permit the temporary descent and expansion of the anal canal or vagina for passage of feces or a fetus. ♦ The fat bodies are traversed by inferior anal/rectal neurovasculature. ♦ The pudendal canal is an important passageway in the lateral wall of the fossa, between layers of the obturator fascia, for neurovasculature passing to and from the UG triangle.

Anal canal: The anal canal is the terminal part of both the large intestine and the digestive tract, the anus being the external outlet. ♦ Closure (and thus fecal continence) is maintained by the coordinated action of the involuntary internal and voluntary external anal sphincters. ♦ The sympathetically stimulated tonus of the internal sphincter maintains closure, except during filling of the rectal ampulla and when inhibited during a parasympathetically stimulated peristaltic contraction of the rectum. ♦ During these moments, closure is maintained (unless defecation is permitted) by voluntary contraction of the puborectalis and external anal sphincter. ♦ Internally, the pectinate line demarcates the transition from visceral to somatic neurovascular supply and drainage. ♦ The anal canal is surrounded by superficial and deep venous plexuses, the veins of which normally have a varicose appearance. ♦ Thromboses in the superficial plexus and mucosal prolapse, including portions of the deep plexus, constitute painful external and insensitive internal hemorrhoids, respectively.

Male Urogenital Triangle

The **male urogenital triangle** includes the external genitalia and perineal muscles. The **male external genitalia** include the distal urethra, scrotum, and penis.

DISTAL MALE URETHRA

The male urethra is subdivided into four parts: intramural (preprostatic), prostatic, intermediate, and spongy. The intramural and prostatic parts are described with the pelvis (earlier in this chapter). Details concerning all four parts of the male urethra are provided and compared in Table 3.6.

The **intermediate (membranous) part of the urethra** begins at the apex of the prostate and traverses the deep perineal pouch, surrounded by the external urethral sphincter. It then penetrates the perineal membrane, ending as the urethra enters the bulb of the penis (Fig. 3.60). Posterolateral to this part of the urethra are the small *bulbo-urethral glands* and their slender ducts, which open into the proximal part of the spongy urethra.

The **spongy urethra** begins at the distal end of the intermediate part of the urethra and ends at the **male external urethral orifice**, which is slightly narrower than any of the other parts of the urethra. The lumen of the spongy urethra is approximately 5 mm in diameter; however, it is expanded in the bulb of the penis to form the **intrabulbar fossa,** and in the glans penis to form the **navicular fossa.** On each side, the slender *ducts of the bulbo-urethral glands* open into the proximal part of the spongy urethra; the orifices of these ducts are extremely small. There are also many minute openings of the ducts of mucus-secreting **urethral glands** into the spongy urethra.

Arterial Supply of Distal Male Urethra. The arterial supply of the intermediate and spongy parts of the urethra is from branches of the *dorsal artery of the penis* (Figs. 3.52C and 3.58; Table 3.8).

Venous and Lymphatic Drainage of Distal Male Urethra. Veins accompany the arteries and have similar names. Lymphatic vessels from the intermediate part of the urethra drain mainly into the *internal iliac lymph nodes* (Table 3.7; see Fig. 3.65), whereas most vessels from the spongy urethra pass to the *deep inguinal lymph nodes,* but some lymph passes to the external iliac nodes.

Innervation of Distal Male Urethra. The innervation of the intermediate part of the urethra is the same as that of the prostatic part: autonomic (efferent) innervation via the *prostatic nerve plexus,* arising from the *inferior hypogastric plexus.* The *sympathetic innervation* is from the lumbar spinal cord levels via the lumbar splanchnic nerves, and the *parasympathetic innervation* is from the sacral levels via the *pelvic splanchnic nerves.* The visceral afferent fibers follow the parasympathetic fibers retrogradely to sacral spinal sensory ganglia. The dorsal nerve of the penis, a branch of the *pudendal nerve,* provides somatic innervation of the spongy part of the urethra (Fig. 3.57).

SCROTUM

The **scrotum** is a cutaneous fibromuscular sac for the testes and associated structures. It is situated postero-inferior to the penis and inferior to the pubic symphysis. The bilateral embryonic formation of the scrotum is indicated by the midline **scrotal raphe** (Fig. 3.61A & E), which is continuous on the ventral surface of the penis with the **penile raphe** and posteriorly along the median line of the perineum with the **perineal raphe.** Internally, deep to the scrotal raphe, the scrotum is divided into two compartments, one for each testis, by a prolongation of the dartos fascia, the **septum of the scrotum.** The testes and epididymides and their coverings are described with the abdomen (see Chapter 2).

Arterial Supply of Scrotum. Anterior scrotal arteries, terminal branches of the **external pudendal arteries** (from the femoral artery), supply the anterior aspect of the scrotum. **Posterior scrotal arteries,** terminal branches of the superficial perineal branches of the *internal pudendal arteries,* supply the posterior aspect (Fig. 3.58A; Table 3.8).

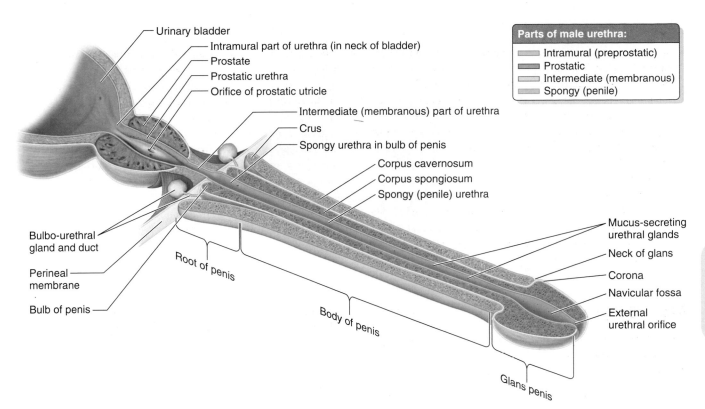

FIGURE 3.60. Male urethra and associated structures. The urethra has four parts: the vesicular part (in the bladder neck), the prostatic urethra, the intermediate part (membranous urethra), and the spongy (cavernous) urethra. The ducts of the bulbo-urethral glands open into the proximal part of the spongy urethra. The urethra is not uniform in its caliber: The external urethral orifice and intermediate part are narrowest. Attempting to approach this "straight-line" position as much as possible facilitates passage of a catheter or other transurethral device.

The scrotum also receives branches from the cremasteric arteries (branches of the inferior epigastric arteries).

Venous and Lymphatic Drainage of Scrotum. The *scrotal veins* accompany the arteries, sharing the same names but draining primarily to the *external pudendal veins*. Lymphatic vessels from the scrotum carry lymph to the *superficial inguinal lymph nodes* (Table 3.6).

Innervation of Scrotum. The *anterior aspect of the scrotum* is supplied by derivatives of the *lumbar plexus:* **anterior scrotal nerves,** derived from the *ilio-inguinal nerve,* and the *genital branch of the genitofemoral nerve* (Table 3.10). The *posterior aspect of the scrotum* is supplied by derivatives of the sacral plexus: **posterior scrotal nerves,** branches of the *superficial perineal branches* of the *pudendal nerve,* and the *perineal branch of the posterior cutaneous nerve of thigh* (Figs. 3.57, 3.62A, and 3.64). Sympathetic fibers conveyed by these nerves assist in the thermoregulation of the testes, stimulating contraction of the smooth dartos muscle in response to cold or stimulating the scrotal sweat glands while inhibiting contraction of the dartos muscle in response to excessive warmth.

PENIS

The **penis** is the male copulatory organ and, by conveying the urethra, provides the common outlet for urine and semen (Figs. 3.60–3.62). The penis consists of a *root, body,* and *glans.* It is composed of three cylindrical cavernous bodies of erectile tissue: the paired **corpora cavernosa** dorsally and the single **corpus spongiosum** ventrally. In the anatomical position, the penis is erect; when the penis is flaccid, its dorsum is directed anteriorly. Each *cavernous body* has an outer fibrous covering or capsule, the **tunica albuginea** (Fig. 3.61C). Superficial to the outer covering is the **deep fascia of the penis** (Buck fascia), the continuation of the deep perineal fascia that forms a strong membranous covering for the corpora cavernosa and corpus spongiosum, binding them together (Fig. 3.61C & D). The corpus spongiosum contains the *spongy urethra.* The corpora cavernosa are fused with each other in the median plane, except posteriorly where they separate to form the **crura of the penis** (Figs. 3.60 and 3.62B). Internally, the cavernous tissue of the corpora is separated (usually incompletely) by the **septum penis** (Fig. 3.61C).

The **root of the penis,** the attached part, consists of the crura, bulb, and ischiocavernosus and bulbospongiosus muscles (Figs. 3.60 and 3.62A & B). The root is located in the superficial perineal pouch, between the perineal membrane superiorly and the deep perineal fascia inferiorly (see Fig. 3.53B & D). The **crura** and **bulb of the penis** consist of erectile tissue. Each crus is attached to the inferior part of the internal surface of the corresponding ischial ramus (see

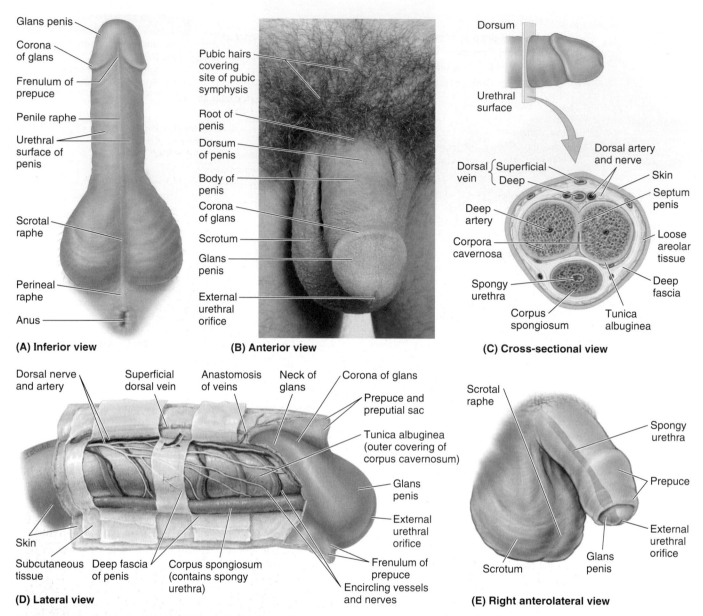

FIGURE 3.61. Penis and scrotum. A. The urethral surface of the circumcised penis is shown. The spongy urethra is deep to the cutaneous penile raphe. The scrotum is divided into right and left halves by the cutaneous scrotal raphe, which is continuous with the penile and perineal raphes. **B.** The dorsum of the circumcised penis and the anterior surface of the scrotum are shown. The penis comprises a root, body, and glans. **C.** The penis contains three erectile masses: two corpora cavernosa and a corpus spongiosum (containing the spongy urethra). **D.** The skin of the penis extends distally as the prepuce, overlapping the neck and corona of the glans. **E.** An uncircumcised penis.

Fig. 3.52D), anterior to the ischial tuberosity. The enlarged posterior part of the bulb of the penis is penetrated superiorly by the urethra, continuing from its intermediate part (Figs. 3.60 and 3.62B).

The **body of the penis** is the free pendulous part that is suspended from the pubic symphysis. Except for a few fibers of the bulbospongiosus near the root of the penis and the ischiocavernosus that embrace the crura, the body of the penis has no muscles (Fig. 3.62).

The penis consists of thin skin, connective tissue, blood and lymphatic vessels, fascia, the corpora cavernosa, and corpus spongiosum containing the spongy urethra (Fig. 3.61C). Distally, the corpus spongiosum expands to form the conical

glans penis, or head of the penis (Figs. 3.61A, B, & D and 3.62B). The margin of the glans projects beyond the ends of the corpora cavernosa to form the **corona of the glans.** The corona overhangs an obliquely grooved constriction, the **neck of the glans,** which separates the glans from the body of the penis. The slit-like opening of the spongy urethra, the *external urethral orifice* (meatus), is near the tip of the glans penis.

The skin of the penis is thin, darkly pigmented relative to adjacent skin, and connected to the tunica albuginea by loose connective tissue. At the neck of the glans, the skin and fascia of the penis are prolonged as a double layer of skin, the **prepuce** (foreskin), which in uncircumcised males

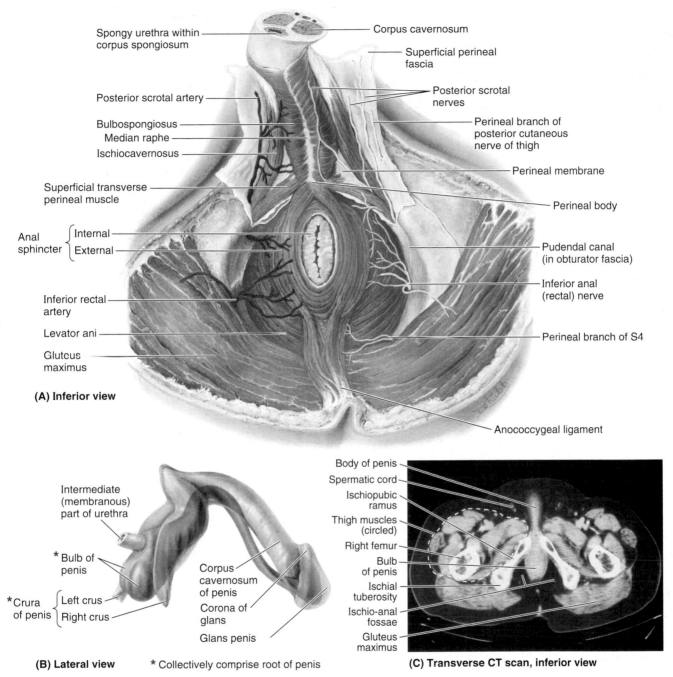

Spongy urethra within corpus spongiosum

Corpus cavernosum

Superficial perineal fascia

Posterior scrotal artery

Posterior scrotal nerves

Bulbospongiosus

Median raphe

Ischiocavernosus

Perineal branch of posterior cutaneous nerve of thigh

Superficial transverse perineal muscle

Perineal membrane

Perineal body

Anal sphincter { Internal / External }

Pudendal canal (in obturator fascia)

Inferior rectal artery

Inferior anal (rectal) nerve

Levator ani

Perineal branch of S4

Gluteus maximus

(A) Inferior view

Anococcygeal ligament

Intermediate (membranous) part of urethra

Body of penis

Spermatic cord

Ischiopubic ramus

Thigh muscles (circled)

Right femur

*Bulb of penis

Corpus cavernosum of penis

Bulb of penis

Ischial tuberosity

*Crura of penis { Left crus / Right crus }

Corona of glans

Ischio-anal fossae

Glans penis

Gluteus maximus

(B) Lateral view   * Collectively comprise root of penis

(C) Transverse CT scan, inferior view

FIGURE 3.62. Male perineum and structure of penis. A. The anal canal is surrounded by the external anal sphincter, with an ischio-anal fossa on each side. The inferior anal (rectal) nerve branches from the pudendal nerve at the entrance to the pudendal canal and, with the perineal branch of S4, supplies the external anal sphincter. **B.** The corpus spongiosum has been separated from the corpora cavernosa. The natural flexures of the penis are preserved. The glans penis fits like a cap over the blunt ends of the corpora cavernosa. **C.** CT scan at level of superficial pouch of a male. (Courtesy of Dr. Donald R. Cahill, Department of Anatomy, Mayo Medical School, Rochester, MN.)

covers the glans penis to a variable extent (Fig 3.61E). The **frenulum of the prepuce** is a median fold that passes from the deep layer of the prepuce to the urethral surface of the glans (Fig. 3.61A & D).

The **suspensory ligament of the penis** is a condensation of deep fascia that arises from the anterior surface of the pubic symphysis (Fig. 3.63). The ligament passes inferiorly and splits to form a sling that is attached to the deep fascia

of the penis at the junction of its root and body. The fibers of the suspensory ligament are short and taut, anchoring the erectile bodies of the penis to the pubic symphysis.

The **fundiform ligament of the penis** is an irregular mass or condensation of collagen and elastic fibers of the subcutaneous tissue that descends in the midline from the linea alba anterior to the pubic symphysis (see Fig. 3.53F). The ligament splits to surround the penis and then unites and

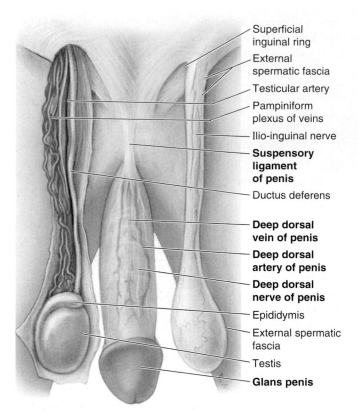

- Superficial inguinal ring
- External spermatic fascia
- Testicular artery
- Pampiniform plexus of veins
- Ilio-inguinal nerve
- **Suspensory ligament of penis**
- Ductus deferens
- **Deep dorsal vein of penis**
- **Deep dorsal artery of penis**
- **Deep dorsal nerve of penis**
- Epididymis
- External spermatic fascia
- Testis
- **Glans penis**

FIGURE 3.63. Vessels and nerves on dorsum of penis and contents of spermatic cord. The skin of the penis and scrotum has been removed. The superficial (dartos) fascia covering the penis has also been removed to expose the deep dorsal vein in the midline flanked by bilateral dorsal arteries and nerves.

blends inferiorly with the dartos fascia forming the scrotal septum. The fibers of the fundiform ligament are relatively long and loose and lie superficial (anterior) to the suspensory ligament.

Arterial Supply of Penis. The penis is supplied mainly by *branches of the internal pudendal arteries* (see Fig. 3.58A; Table 3.8).

- **Dorsal arteries of the penis** run on each side of the deep dorsal vein in the dorsal groove between the corpora cavernosa (Figs. 3.61C & D and 3.63), supplying the fibrous tissue around the corpora cavernosa, the corpus spongiosum and spongy urethra, and the penile skin.
- **Deep arteries of the penis** pierce the crura proximally and run distally near the center of the corpora cavernosa, supplying the erectile tissue in these structures (Figs. 3.58A and 3.61C).
- **Arteries of the bulb of the penis** supply the posterior (bulbous) part of the corpus spongiosum and the urethra within it as well as the bulbo-urethral gland (see Fig. 3.58A).

In addition, **superficial** and **deep branches of the external pudendal arteries** supply the penile skin, anastomosing with branches of the internal pudendal arteries.

The *deep arteries of the penis* are the main vessels supplying the cavernous spaces in the erectile tissue of the corpora cavernosa and are, therefore, involved in the erection of the penis. They give off numerous branches that open directly into the cavernous spaces. When the penis is flaccid, these arteries are coiled, restricting blood flow; they are called **helicine arteries of the penis** (G. *helix*, a coil).

Venous Drainage of Penis. Blood from the cavernous spaces is drained by a venous plexus that joins the **deep dorsal vein of the penis** in the deep fascia (Figs. 3.61C and 3.63). This vein passes between the laminae of the suspensory ligament of the penis, inferior to the inferior pubic ligament and anterior to the perineal membrane, to enter the pelvis, where it drains into the prostatic venous plexus. Blood from the skin and subcutaneous tissue of the penis drains into the **superficial dorsal vein(s),** which drain(s) into the *superficial external pudendal vein.* Some blood also passes to the internal pudendal vein.

Innervation of Penis. The nerves derive from the S2–S4 spinal cord segments and spinal ganglia, passing through the pelvic splanchnic and pudendal nerves, respectively (Fig. 3.64). Sensory and sympathetic innervation is provided

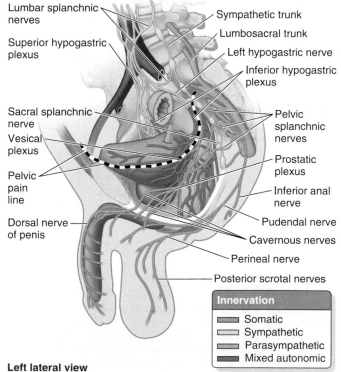

- Lumbar splanchnic nerves
- Superior hypogastric plexus
- Sacral splanchnic nerve
- Vesical plexus
- Pelvic pain line
- Dorsal nerve of penis
- Sympathetic trunk
- Lumbosacral trunk
- Left hypogastric nerve
- Inferior hypogastric plexus
- Pelvic splanchnic nerves
- Prostatic plexus
- Inferior anal nerve
- Pudendal nerve
- Cavernous nerves
- Perineal nerve
- Posterior scrotal nerves

Innervation
- Somatic
- Sympathetic
- Parasympathetic
- Mixed autonomic

Left lateral view

FIGURE 3.64. Nerves of perineum. The pudendal nerve conveys the majority of sensory, sympathetic, and somatic motor fibers to the perineum. Although originating from the same spinal cord segments from which the pudendal nerve is derived, the parasympathetic fibers of the cavernous nerves course independently of the pudendal nerve. With the exception of the cavernous nerves, parasympathetic fibers do not occur outside the head, neck, or cavities of the trunk. The cavernous nerves arise from the prostatic plexus of males and from the vesical plexus of females. They terminate on the arteriovenous anastomoses and helicine arteries of the erectile bodies, which, when stimulated, produce erection of the penis or engorgement of the clitoris and vestibular bulb in females.

primarily by the *dorsal nerve of the penis*, a terminal branch of the *pudendal nerve*, which arises in the pudendal canal and passes anteriorly into the deep perineal pouch. It then runs to the dorsum of the penis, where it runs lateral to the dorsal artery (Figs. 3.61C and 3.63). It supplies both the skin and glans penis. The penis is richly supplied with a variety of sensory nerve endings, especially the glans penis. Branches of the *ilio-inguinal nerve* supply the skin at the root of the penis. *Cavernous nerves*, conveying parasympathetic fibers independently from the prostatic nerve plexus, innervate the helicine arteries of the erectile tissue.

LYMPHATIC DRAINAGE OF MALE PERINEUM

Lymph from the skin of all parts of the perineum, including the hairless skin inferior to the pectinate line of the anorectum but excluding the glans penis, drains to the *superficial inguinal nodes* (Fig. 3.65).

Reflective of their abdominal origins, lymph from the testes follow a route, independent of the scrotal drainage, along the testicular veins to the intermesenteric portion of the *lumbar (caval/aortic)* and *pre-aortic lymph nodes*.

Lymphatic drainage from the intermediate and proximal parts of the urethra and cavernous bodies drain into the *internal iliac lymph nodes*, whereas most vessels from the distal spongy urethra and glans penis pass to the *deep inguinal nodes*, but some lymph passes to the external inguinal nodes.

PERINEAL MUSCLES OF MALE

The **superficial perineal muscles,** located in the superficial perineal pouch, include the superficial transverse peri-

neal, bulbospongiosus, and ischiocavernosus muscles (Figs. 3.62A and 3.66). Details about the attachments, innervation, and actions of these muscles are provided in Table 3.9.

The **superficial transverse perineal muscles** and the bulbospongiosus muscles join the external anal sphincter in attaching centrally to the perineal body. They cross the pelvic outlet like intersecting beams, supporting the perineal body to aid the pelvic diaphragm in supporting the pelvic viscera. Simultaneous contraction of the superficial perineal muscles (plus the deep transverse perineal muscle) during penile erection provides a firmer base for the penis.

The **bulbospongiosus muscles** form a constrictor that compresses the bulb of the penis and the corpus spongiosum, thereby aiding in emptying the spongy urethra of residual urine and/or semen. The anterior fibers of the bulbospongiosus, encircling the most proximal part of the body of the penis, also assist erection by increasing the pressure on the erectile tissue in the root of the penis (Fig. 3.62A). At the same time, they also compress the deep dorsal vein of the penis, impeding venous drainage of the cavernous spaces and helping promote enlargement and turgidity of the penis.

The **ischiocavernosus muscles** surround the crura in the root of the penis. They force blood from the cavernous spaces in the crura into the distal parts of the corpora cavernosa, which increases the turgidity (firm distension) of the penis during erection. Contraction of the ischiocavernosus muscles also compresses the tributaries of deep dorsal vein of the penis leaving the crus of the penis, thereby restricting venous outflow from the penis and helping maintain the erection.

Because of their function during erection and the activity of the bulbospongiosus subsequent to urination and ejaculation to expel the last drops of urine and semen, the perineal muscles are generally more developed in males than in females.

ERECTION, EMISSION, EJACULATION, AND REMISSION

When a male is stimulated erotically, arteriovenous anastomoses by which blood is normally able to bypass the "empty" potential spaces or sinuses of the corpora cavernosa are closed. The smooth muscle in the fibrous trabeculae and coiled helicine arteries relaxes (is inhibited) as a result of parasympathetic stimulation (S2–S4 through the cavernous nerves from the **prostatic nerve plexus**). Consequently, the *helicine arteries* straighten, enlarging their lumina and allowing blood to flow into and dilate the cavernous spaces in the corpora of the penis.

The bulbospongiosus and ischiocavernosus muscles compress veins egressing from the corpora cavernosa, impeding the return of venous blood. As a result, the corpora cavernosa and corpus spongiosum become engorged with blood near arterial pressure, causing the erectile bodies to become turgid (enlarged and rigid), and an **erection** occurs.

During **emission,** semen (sperms and other glandular secretions) is delivered to the prostatic urethra through the ejaculatory ducts after peristalsis of the ductus deferentes and seminal glands. Prostatic fluid is added to the seminal

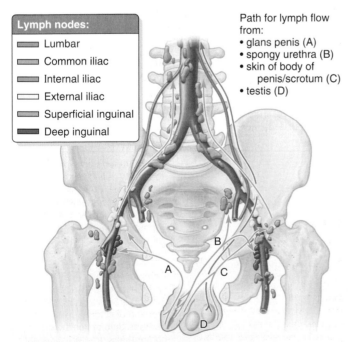

Lymph nodes:
- ▬ Lumbar
- ▬ Common iliac
- ▬ Internal iliac
- ▬ External iliac
- ▬ Superficial inguinal
- ▬ Deep inguinal

Path for lymph flow from:
- glans penis (A)
- spongy urethra (B)
- skin of body of penis/scrotum (C)
- testis (D)

FIGURE 3.65. Lymphatic drainage of male urogenital triangle—penis, spongy urethra, scrotum, and testis. The *arrows* indicate the direction of lymph flow to the lymph nodes.

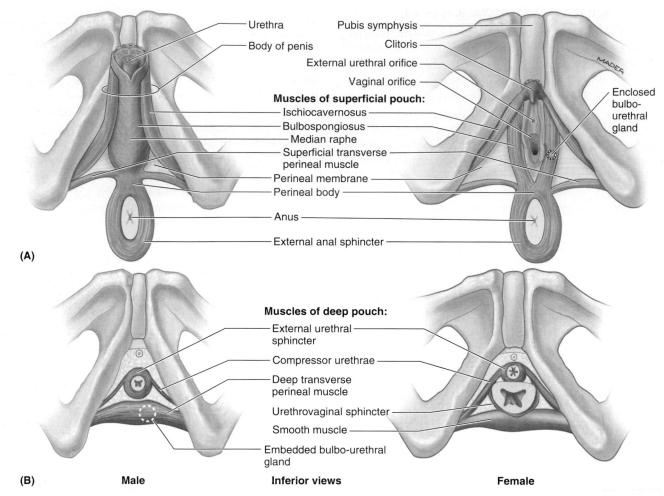

FIGURE 3.66. **Muscles of perineum. A.** Muscles of superficial perineal pouch. **B.** Muscles of deep perineal pouch.

TABLE 3.9. MUSCLES OF PERINEUM

Muscle	Origin	Course and Distribution	Innervation	Main Action
External anal sphincter	Skin and fascia surrounding anus; coccyx via anococcygeal ligament	Passes around lateral aspects of anal canal, insertion into perineal body	Inferior anal (rectal) nerve, a branch of pudendal nerve (S2–S4)	Constricts anal canal during peristalsis, resisting defecation; supports and fixes perineal body and pelvic floor
Bulbospongiosus	*Male:* median raphe on ventral surface of bulb of penis; perineal body	*Male:* surrounds lateral aspects of bulb of penis and most proximal part of body of penis, inserting into perineal membrane, dorsal aspect of corpus spongiosum and corpora cavernosa, and fascia of bulb of penis	Muscular (deep) branch of perineal nerve, a branch of pudendal nerve (S2–S4)	*Male:* supports and fixes perineal body/pelvic floor; compresses bulb of penis to expel last drops of urine/semen; assists erection by compressing outflow via deep perineal vein and by pushing blood from bulb into body of penis
	Female: perineal body	*Female:* passes on each side of lower vagina, enclosing bulb and greater vestibular gland; inserts into pubic arch and fascia of corpora cavernosa of clitoris		*Female:* supports and fixes perineal body/pelvic floor; "sphincter" of vagina; assists in erection of clitoris (and perhaps bulb of vestibule); compresses greater vestibular gland

TABLE 3.9. MUSCLES OF PERINEUM (Continued)

Muscle	Origin	Course and Distribution	Innervation	Main Action
Ischiocavernosus	Internal surface of ischiopubic ramus and ischial tuberosity	Embraces crus of penis or clitoris, inserting onto inferior and medial aspects of crus and to perineal membrane medial to crus	Muscular (deep) branch of perineal nerve, a branch of pudendal nerve (S2–S4)	Maintains erection of penis or clitoris by compressing outflow veins and pushing blood from the root of penis or clitoris into the body of penis or clitoris
Superficial transverse perineal muscle		Passes along inferior aspect of posterior border of perineal membrane to perineal body		Supports and fixes perineal body/pelvic floor to support abdominopelvic viscera and resist increased intra-abdominal pressure
Deep transverse perineal muscle		Passes along superior aspect of posterior border of perineal membrane to perineal body and external anal sphincter		
External urethral sphincter	(Compressor urethra portion only)	Surrounds urethra superior to perineal membrane; in males, it also ascends anterior aspect of prostate; in females, some fibers also enclose vagina (urethrovaginal sphincter)	Dorsal nerve of penis or clitoris, the terminal branch of the pudendal nerve (S2–S4)	Compresses urethra to maintain urinary continence; in females, urethrovaginal sphincter portion also compresses vagina

fluid as the smooth muscle in the prostate contracts. Emission is a sympathetic response (L1–L2 nerves). During **ejaculation,** semen is expelled from the urethra through the external urethral orifice.

Ejaculation results from:

- Closure of the internal urethral sphincter at the neck of the urinary bladder, *a sympathetic response* (L1–L2 nerves).
- Contraction of the urethral muscle, *a parasympathetic response* (S2–S4 nerves).

- Contraction of the bulbospongiosus muscles, from the pudendal nerves (S2–S4).

After ejaculation, the penis gradually returns to a flaccid state (**remission**), resulting from sympathetic stimulation, which causes constriction of the smooth muscle in the coiled helicine arteries. The bulbospongiosus and ischiocavernosus muscles relax, allowing more blood to be drained from the cavernous spaces in the corpora cavernosa into the deep dorsal vein.

MALE UROGENITAL TRIANGLE

Urethral Catheterization

Urethral catheterization is done to remove urine from a person who is unable to micturate. It is also performed to irrigate the bladder and to obtain an uncontaminated sample of urine. When inserting catheters and *urethral sounds* (slightly conical instruments for exploring and dilating a constricted urethra), the curves of the male urethra must be considered. Just distal to the perineal membrane, the spongy urethra is well covered inferiorly and posteriorly by erectile tissue of the bulb of the penis; however, a short segment of the intermediate part of the urethra is unprotected (Fig. B3.32). Because the urethral wall is thin and the angle that must be negotiated to enter the intermediate part of the spongy urethra, the wall is vulnerable to rupture during the insertion of urethral catheters and sounds. The intermediate part, the least distensible part, runs infero-

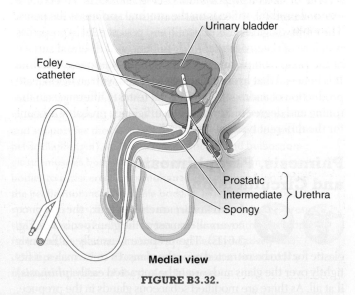

Medial view

FIGURE B3.32.

Female Urogenital Triangle

The **female urogenital triangle** includes the female external genitalia, perineal muscles, and anal canal.

FEMALE EXTERNAL GENITALIA

The **female external genitalia** (Fig. 3.67) include the mons pubis, labia majora (enclosing the pudendal cleft), labia minora (enclosing the vestibule of vagina), clitoris, bulbs of vestibule, and greater and lesser vestibular glands. The synonymous terms **vulva** and **pudendum** include all these parts; the term *pudendum* is commonly used clinically. The vulva serves:

- As sensory and erectile tissue for sexual arousal and intercourse.
- To direct the flow of urine.
- To prevent entry of foreign material into the urogenital tract.

Mons Pubis. The **mons pubis** is the rounded, fatty eminence anterior to the pubic symphysis, pubic tubercles, and superior pubic rami. The eminence is formed by a mass of fatty subcutaneous tissue. The amount of

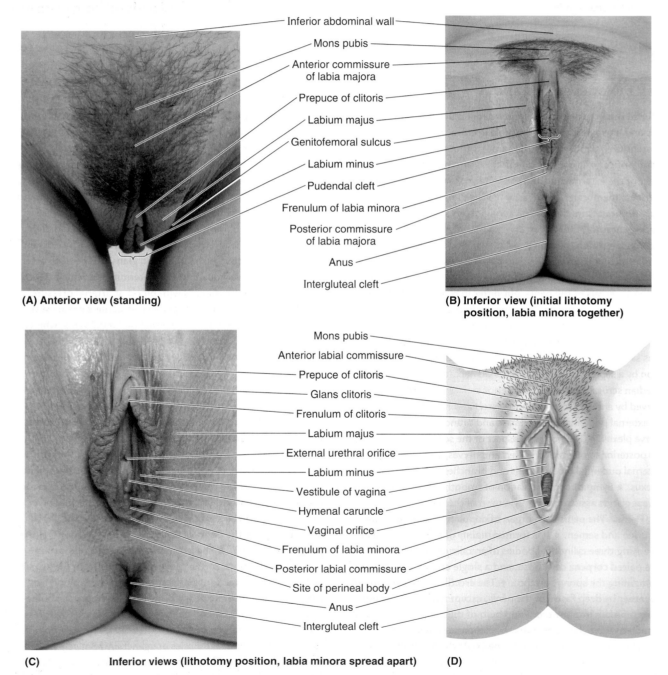

(A) Anterior view (standing)

(B) Inferior view (initial lithotomy position, labia minora together)

(C)   Inferior views (lithotomy position, labia minora spread apart)   **(D)**

Labels: Inferior abdominal wall · Mons pubis · Anterior commissure of labia majora · Prepuce of clitoris · Labium majus · Genitofemoral sulcus · Labium minus · Pudendal cleft · Frenulum of labia minora · Posterior commissure of labia majora · Anus · Intergluteal cleft · Mons pubis · Anterior labial commissure · Prepuce of clitoris · Glans clitoris · Frenulum of clitoris · Labium majus · External urethral orifice · Labium minus · Vestibule of vagina · Hymenal caruncle · Vaginal orifice · Frenulum of labia minora · Posterior labial commissure · Site of perineal body · Anus · Intergluteal cleft

FIGURE 3.67. Female external genitalia. A–C. Surface anatomy of vulva (pudendum) of vagina demonstrated in three positions. **D.** Illustration of vulva, similar to (**C**). Moisture typically keeps the labia minora passively apposed, keeping the vestibule of vagina closed (**B**) unless spread apart as in (**C**).

fat increases at puberty and decreases after menopause. The surface of the mons is continuous with the anterior abdominal wall. After puberty, the mons pubis is covered with coarse pubic hairs.

Labia Majora. The **labia majora** are prominent folds of skin that indirectly protect the clitoris and urethral and vaginal orifices (Fig. 3.67). Each labium majus is largely filled with a finger-like "digital process" of loose subcutaneous tissue containing smooth muscle, and the termination of the round ligament of the uterus (Fig. 3.68). The labium majus passes inferoposteriorly from the mons pubis toward the anus (Fig. 3.67D).

The labia majora lie on the sides of a central depression (a narrow slit when the thighs are adducted—Fig. 3.67A),

the **pudendal cleft,** within which are the labia minora and vestibule (Fig. 3.67C & D). The external aspects of the labia majora in the adult are covered with pigmented skin containing many sebaceous glands, and are covered with crisp pubic hairs. The internal aspects of the labia are smooth, pink, and hairless.

The labia majora are thicker anteriorly where they join to form the **anterior commissure.** Posteriorly, in nulliparous women (those never having borne children), they merge to form a ridge, the **posterior commissure,** which overlies the perineal body and is the posterior limit of the vulva. This commissure usually disappears after the first vaginal birth.

Labia Minora. The **labia minora** are rounded folds of fat-free, hairless skin. They are enclosed in the pudendal

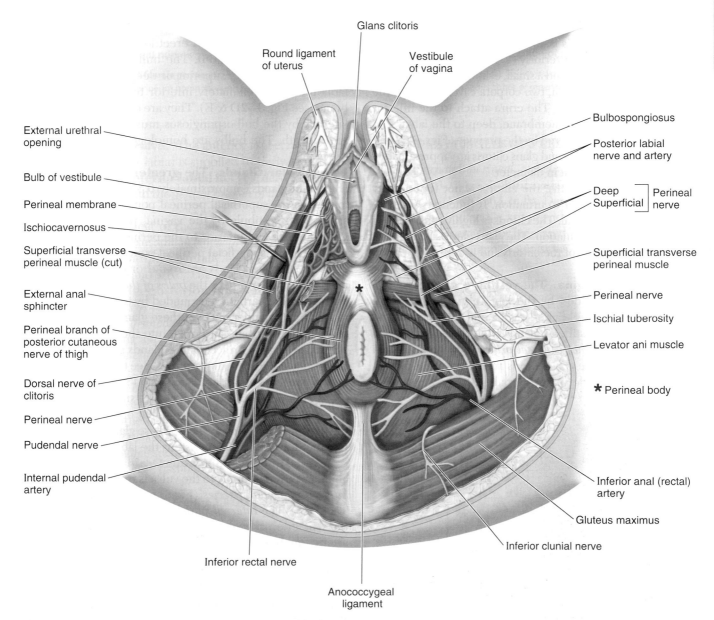

FIGURE 3.68. Female perineum. Skin, subcutaneous tissue (including perineal fascia and ischio-anal fat bodies), and the investing fascia of the muscles have been removed. On the right side, the bulbospongiosus muscle has been resected to reveal the bulb of the vestibule. Deeper dissection of the superficial pouch (right side) reveals the bulbs of the vestibule and the greater vestibular glands.

TABLE 3.10. NERVES OF PERINEUM

Nerve	Origin	Course	Distribution
Anterior labial nerves (♀); anterior scrotal nerves (♂)	Terminal part of ilio-inguinal nerve (L1)	Arise as ilio-inguinal exits superficial inguinal ring; pass anteriorly and inferiorly	*In females,* sensory to mons pubis and anterior part of labium majus; *in males,* sensory to pubic region, skin of proximal penis, and anterior aspect of scrotum, and adjacent thigh
Genital branch of genitofemoral nerve	Genitofemoral nerve (L1 and L2)	Emerges through or near superficial inguinal ring	*In females,* sensory to anterior labia majora; *in males,* motor to cremaster muscle, sensory to anterior aspect of scrotum and adjacent thigh
Perineal branch of posterior cutaneous nerve of thigh	Posterior cutaneous nerve of thigh (S1–S3)	Arises deep to inferior border of gluteus maximus; passes medially over sacrotuberous ligament to parallel ischiopubic ramus	Sensory to lateral perineum (labia majora in ♀, scrotum in ♂), genitofemoral sulcus, and superiormost medial thigh; may overlap lateral parts of perineum supplied by pudendal nerve
Inferior clunial nerves	Posterior cutaneous nerve of thigh (S1–S3)	Arise deep to and emerge from inferior border of gluteus maximus, ascending in subcutaneous tissue	Skin of inferior and inferolateral gluteal region (buttocks)—gluteal fold and area superior to it
Pudendal nerve (S2–S4)	Sacral plexus (anterior rami of S2–S4)	Exits pelvis via infrapiriform part of greater sciatic foramen; passes posterior to sacrospinous ligament; enters perineum via lesser sciatic foramen, immediately dividing into branches as it enters pudendal canal	Motor to muscles of perineum and sensory to majority of perineal region via its branches, the inferior rectal and perineal nerves, and the dorsal nerve of clitoris or penis
Inferior anal (rectal) nerve	Pudendal nerve (S3–4)	Passes medially from area of ischial spine (entrance to pudendal canal), traversing ischio-anal fat body	External anal sphincter; participates in innervation of inferior and medial-most part of levator ani (puborectalis); sensory to anal canal inferior to pectinate line and circumanal skin
Perineal nerve	Pudendal nerve	Arises near entrance to pudendal canal, paralleling parent nerve to end of canal, then passes medially	Divides into superficial and deep branches, the posterior labial or scrotal nerve and the deep perineal nerve
Posterior labial nerves (♀), posterior scrotal nerves (♂)	Superficial terminal branch of perineal nerve	Arise in anterior (terminal) end of pudendal canal, passing medially and superficially	*In females,* labia minora and all but anterior labia majora; *in males,* posterior aspect of scrotum
Deep perineal nerve	Deep terminal branch of perineal nerve	Arise in anterior (terminal) end of pudendal canal, passing medially then deeply in superficial perineal pouch	Motor to muscles of superficial perineal pouch (ischiocavernosus, bulbospongiosus, and superficial perineal muscles); *in females,* sensory to vestibule of vagina and inferior part of vagina

FEMALE UROGENITAL TRIANGLE

Female Circumcision

Although illegal and now being actively discouraged in most countries, *female circumcision* is widely practiced in some cultures. The operation performed during childhood removes the prepuce of the clitoris and commonly also removes part or all of the clitoris and labia minora. This disfiguring procedure is erroneously thought to inhibit sexual arousal and gratification.

Vulvar Trauma

The highly vascular bulbs of the vestibule are susceptible to disruption of vessels as the result of trauma (e.g., athletic injuries such as jumping hurdles, sexual assault, and obstetrical injury). These injuries often result in *vulvar hematomas* (localized collection of blood) in the labia majora, for example.

Infection of Greater Vestibular Glands

The greater vestibular glands are usually not palpable, but are so when infected. Occlusion of the vestibular gland duct can predispose the individual to *infection of the greater vestibular gland*. The gland is the site or origin of most vulvar adenocarcinomas (cancers). *Bartholinitis*, inflammation of the greater vestibular (Bartholin) glands, may result from a number of pathogenic organisms. Infected glands may enlarge to a diameter of 4–5 cm and impinge on the wall of the rectum. Occlusion of the vestibular gland duct without infection can result in the accumulation of mucin (*Bartholin gland cyst*) (Fig. B3.34).

Pudendal and Ilio-inguinal Nerve Blocks

To relieve perineal pain during childbirth, *pudendal nerve block anesthesia* may be performed by injecting a local anesthetic agent into the tissues surrounding the pudendal nerve (Fig. B3.35). The injection is made where the pudendal nerve crosses the lateral aspect of the sacrospinous ligament, near its attachment to the ischial spine. The needle may be passed through the overlying skin (as illustrated) or, more commonly perhaps, through the vagina parallel to the palpating finger. Because the fetus's head is usually stationed within the lesser pelvis at this stage, it is important that the physician's finger is always positioned between the needle tip and the baby's head during the procedure.

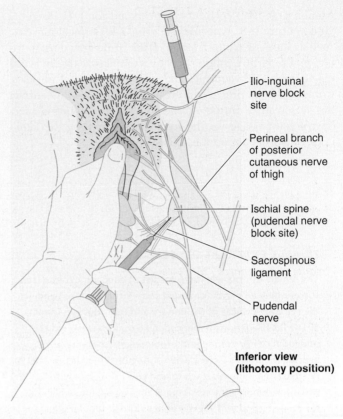

- Ilio-inguinal nerve block site
- Perineal branch of posterior cutaneous nerve of thigh
- Ischial spine (pudendal nerve block site)
- Sacrospinous ligament
- Pudendal nerve

Inferior view (lithotomy position)

FIGURE B3.35.

To abolish sensation from the anterior part of the perineum, an *ilio-inguinal nerve block* is performed. When patients continue to complain of pain sensation after proper administration of a pudendal or pudendal and ilio-inguinal nerve blocks, it is usually the result of overlapping innervation by the perineal branch at the posterior cutaneous nerve of the thigh. Other types of anesthesia for childbirth are explained and compared in the blue box "Anesthesia for Childbirth," p. 397.

Exercises for Increased Development of Female Perineal Muscles

The superficial transverse perineal muscle, bulbospongiosus, and external anal sphincter, through their common attachment to the perineal body, form crossing beams over the pelvic outlet to support the perineal body, as in males. In the absence of the functional demands related to urination, penile erection, and ejaculation in males, the muscles are commonly relatively underdeveloped in women. However, when developed, they contribute to the support of the pelvic viscera, and help prevent urinary stress incontinence and postpartum prolapse of pelvic viscera. Therefore, many gynecologists as well as prepartum classes for participatory childbirth recommend that

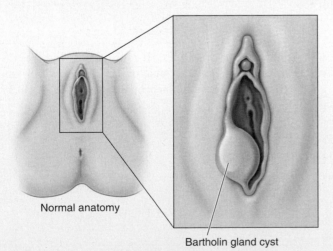

Normal anatomy

Bartholin gland cyst

FIGURE B3.34.

women practice *Kegel exercises* (named for J. H. Kegel, a 20th-century U.S. gynecologist) using the perineal muscles, such as successive interruption of the urine flow during urination. Prepartum childbirth classes emphasize that in learning to voluntarily contract and relax the perineal muscles, women become prepared to resist the tendency to contract the musculature during uterine contractions, allowing a less obstructed passage for the fetus and decreasing the likelihood of tearing the perineal muscles.

Vaginismus

The initial distension of the bulbospongiosus and transverse perineal muscles are thought to trigger the involuntary spasms of the perivaginal and levator ani muscles of *vaginismus*, an emotional (psychosomatic) gynecological disorder. Vaginismus is encountered clinically when pelvic examination is attempted. In mild forms, it causes *dyspareunia* (painful intercourse); in severe forms, it prevents vaginal entry.

The Bottom Line

FEMALE EXTERNAL GENITALIA

The female external genitalia consist of concentric folds (labia) surrounding an organ for sexual stimulation (clitoris) and the separate orifices of the urinary and reproductive systems. ♦ The fat-filled mons pubis and labia majora surround the pudendal cleft, covering and protecting its contents (e.g., bearing the body's weight when sitting on a bicycle). ♦ The fat-free labia minora attach to and cover the glans clitoris while surrounding the vestibule of the vagina, into which the external urethral and vaginal orifices and vestibular glands open. ♦ The erectile clitoris, consisting of a highly sensitive glans, short body, and crura that attach to the pubic rami and perineal membrane, functions solely as a tactile sensory organ. ♦ A hymen or its remnants, hymenal caruncles, demarcate the vagina from the vestibule and vaginal orifice. ♦ Immediately superior to the bases of the labia minora on each side of the vaginal orifice, the bulbs of the vestibule are paired masses of erectile tissue, homologous with the bulb of the penis. ♦ The internal pudendal vessels serve most of the vulva, with the external pudendal vessels serving a smaller anterior area. ♦ Except for the glans clitoris and associated structures (which

drain to deep inguinal and external iliac nodes), lymph from the perineum drains to the superficial inguinal nodes.

Innervation of the perineum is primarily from the pudendal nerve, with additional cutaneous innervation anteriorly from anterior labial nerves (ilio-inguinal and genitofemoral nerves), and laterally from the posterior cutaneous nerve of the thigh. ♦ Parasympathetic fibers, passing independently from the pelvis to the perineum as cavernous nerves, innervate the erectile tissues.

Female perineal muscles: Although homologous to the muscles of the male, the perineal muscles of the female are generally less well developed. ♦ In addition to the sphincteric functions of the external anal and urethral sphincters for maintaining fecal and urinary continence, the female perineal muscles are also capable of supporting the perineal body (which in turn supports the pelvic diaphragm). ♦ Learning to control perineal muscles through routine (Kegel) exercises may reduce the risk of obstetrical laceration of perineal muscles, and subsequent prolapse of pelvic viscera. ♦ The perineal muscles are innervated by muscular branches of the pudendal nerve.

SECTIONAL IMAGING OF PELVIS AND PERINEUM

Magnetic Resonance Imaging

MRI provides excellent evaluation of pelvic structures in any plane (Fig. 3.72) and permits outstanding delineation of the

uterus and ovaries (Fig. 3.73). It also permits the identification of tumors (e.g., a myoma, or benign neoplasm) and congenital anomalies (e.g., bicornuate uterus—Fig. B3.16, p. 392).

(A) Anatomical median section

(B) Median MRI

A	Anus	P	Prostate
B	Bulb of penis	PC	Peritoneal cavity
Co	Coccyx	PP	Prostatic venous plexus
Cav	Corpus cavernosum of penis	Ps	Psoas muscle
Cs	Corpus spongiosum of penis	R	Rectum
F	Femur	RA	Rectus abdominis
FN	Femoral nerve	RF	Retropubic fat
IL	Ilium	RVP	Rectovesical pouch
IM	Iliacus muscle	S	Sacrum
IR	Ischiopubic ramus	SG	Seminal gland
LA	Levator ani	SN	Sacral nerves
Oe	Obturator externus	Sy	Pubic symphysis
Oi	Obturator internus	UB	Urinary bladder

——— Sections on this page
——— Sections on next page

(C) Dissection, posterior view

(D) Coronal MRI

FIGURE 3.72. MRI scans of male pelvis and perineum.

(E) Anatomical transverse section

(F) Transverse MRI scan

AC	Anal canal	IT	Ischial tuberosity	Pm	Perineal membrane
Ad	Adductor muscles	LA	Levator ani	PR	Puborectalis
CC	Crus of clitoris	LM	Labium majus	Pu	Pubic bone
FA	Femoral artery	MP	Mons pubis	QF	Quadratus femoris
FV	Femoral vein	Max	Gluteus maximus	R	Rectum
GC	Gluteal cleft	OE	Obturator externus	Sy	Pubic symphysis
IAF	Ischio-anal fossa	OI	Obturator internus	Ur	Urethra
IPR	Ischiopubic ramus	Pec	Pectineus	V	Vagina
				Ve	Vestibule of vagina

(G) Anatomical transverse section

(H) Transverse MRI scan

FIGURE 3.73. *(Continued)*

Back

4 CHAPTER

OVERVIEW OF BACK AND VERTEBRAL COLUMN

The **back** comprises the posterior aspect of the trunk, inferior to the neck and superior to the buttocks. It is the region of the body to which the head, neck, and limbs are attached. The back includes the:

- Skin and subcutaneous tissue.
- Muscles: a superficial layer, primarily concerned with positioning and moving the upper limbs, and deeper layers ("true back muscles"), specifically concerned with moving or maintaining the position of the axial skeleton (posture).
- Vertebral column: the vertebrae, intervertebral (IV) discs, and associated ligaments (Fig. 4.1).
- Ribs (in the thoracic region): particularly their posterior portions, medial to the angles of the ribs.
- Spinal cord and meninges (membranes that cover the spinal cord).
- Various segmental nerves and vessels.

Because of their close association with the trunk, the back of the neck and the posterior and deep cervical muscles and vertebrae are also described in this chapter. The scapulae, although located in the back, are part of the appendicular skeleton and are considered with the upper limb (Chapter 6).

Study of the soft tissues of the back is best preceded by examination of the *vertebrae* and the fibrocartilaginous *intervertebral discs* that are interposed between the bodies of adjacent vertebrae. The vertebrae and IV discs collectively make up the **vertebral column** (spine), the skeleton of the neck and back that is the main part of the *axial skeleton* (i.e., articulated bones of the cranium, vertebral column, ribs, and sternum) (Fig. 4.1D). The vertebral column extends from the cranium (skull) to the apex of the coccyx. In adults, it is 72–75 cm long, of which approximately one quarter is formed by the IV discs that separate and bind the vertebrae together. The vertebral column:

- Protects the spinal cord and spinal nerves.
- Supports the weight of the body superior to the level of the pelvis.
- Provides a partly rigid and flexible axis for the body and an extended base on which the head is placed and pivots.
- Plays an important role in posture and *locomotion* (the movement from one place to another).

VERTEBRAE

The vertebral column in an adult typically consists of 33 vertebrae arranged in five regions: 7 cervical, 12 thoracic, 5 lumbar, 5 sacral, and 4 coccygeal (Fig. 4.1A–D). Significant motion occurs only between the 25 superior vertebrae. Of the 9 inferior vertebrae, the 5 sacral vertebrae are fused in adults to form the *sacrum,* and after approximately age 30, the 4 coccygeal vertebrae fuse to form the *coccyx.* The **lumbosacral angle** occurs at the junction of the long axes of the lumbar region of the vertebral column and the sacrum (Fig. 4.1D). The vertebrae gradually become larger as the vertebral column descends to the sacrum and then become progressively smaller toward the apex of the coccyx (Fig. 4.1A–D). The change in size is related to the fact that successive vertebrae bear increasing amounts of the body's weight as the column descends. The vertebrae reach maximum size immediately superior to the sacrum, which transfers the weight to the pelvic girdle at the sacro-iliac joints.

The vertebral column is flexible because it consists of many relatively small bones, called **vertebrae** (singular = **vertebra**), that are separated by resilient IV discs (Fig. 4.1D). The 25 cervical, thoracic, lumbar, and first sacral vertebrae also articulate at synovial *zygapophysial (facet) joints* (Fig. 4.2D), which facilitate and control the vertebral column's flexibility. Although the movement between two adjacent vertebrae is small, in aggregate the vertebrae and IV discs uniting them form a remarkably flexible yet rigid column that protects the spinal cord it surrounds.

Structure and Function of Vertebrae

Vertebrae vary in size and other characteristics from one region of the vertebral column to another, and to a lesser degree within each region; however, their basic structure is

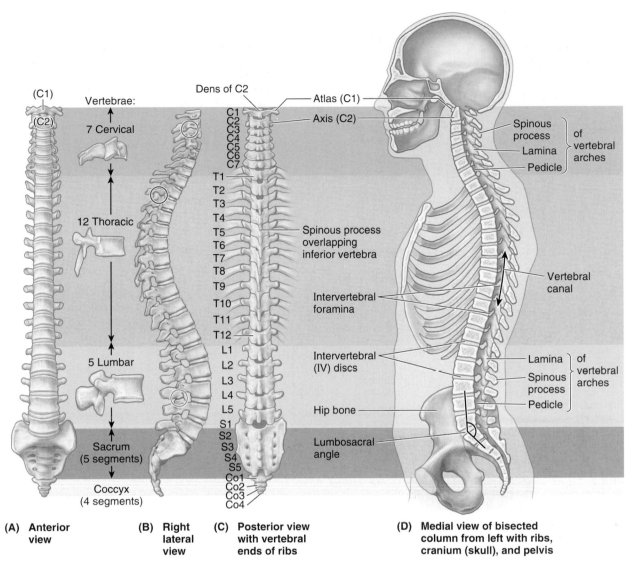

(A) Anterior view

(B) Right lateral view

(C) Posterior view with vertebral ends of ribs

(D) Medial view of bisected column from left with ribs, cranium (skull), and pelvis

FIGURE 4.1. Vertebral column and its five regions. The isolated vertebrae between (**A**) and (**B**) are typical of each of the three mobile regions of the vertebral column. The continuous, weight-bearing column of vertebral bodies and IV discs increases in size as the column descends. Zygapophysial (facet) joints representative of each region are circled. The posterior view (**C**) includes the vertebral ends of ribs, representing the skeleton of the back. The bisected vertebral column in (**D**) demonstrates the vertebral canal. The intervertebral (IV) foramina (also seen in **B**) are openings in the lateral wall of the vertebral canal through which spinal nerves exit.

the same. A **typical vertebra** (Fig. 4.2) consists of a vertebral body, a vertebral arch, and seven processes.[1]

The **vertebral body** is the more massive, roughly cylindrical, anterior part of the bone that gives strength to the vertebral column and supports body weight. The size of the vertebral bodies increases as the column descends, most markedly from T4 inferiorly, as each bears progressively greater body weight.

The vertebral body consists of vascular, trabecular (spongy, cancellous) bone enclosed by a thin external layer of compact bone (Fig. 4.3). The *trabecular bone* is a meshwork of mostly tall vertical trabeculae intersecting with short, horizontal trabeculae. The spaces between the trabeculae are occupied by red bone marrow that is among the most actively hematopoietic (blood-forming) tissues of the mature individual. One or more large foramina in the posterior surface of the vertebral body accommodate basivertebral veins that drain the marrow (see Fig. 4.26).

In life, most of the superior and inferior surfaces of the vertebral body are covered with discs of hyaline cartilage (vertebral "end plates"), which are remnants of the cartilaginous model from which the bone develops. In dried laboratory and museum skeletal specimens, this cartilage is absent, and the exposed bone appears spongy, except at the periphery where an **epiphysial rim** or ring of smooth bone, derived from an *anular epiphysis,* is fused to the body (Fig. 4.2B).

[1] In contemporary usage, the terms *vertebral body* and *centrum* and the terms *vertebral arch* and *neural arch* are often erroneously used as synonyms. Technically, however, in each case the former is a gross anatomy term applied to parts of the adult vertebrae, and the latter is an embryology term referring to parts of a developing vertebra ossifying from primary centers. The vertebral body includes the centrum and part of the neural arch; the vertebral arch is thus less extensive than the neural arch, and the centrum is less extensive than the vertebral body (O'Rahilly, 1986; Standring, 2008).

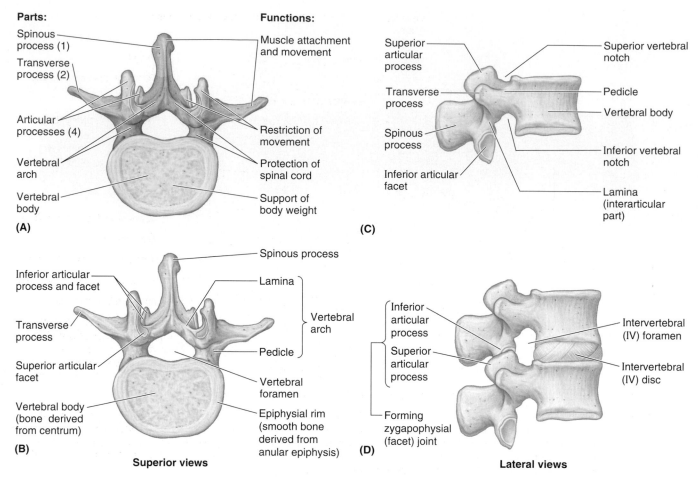

Parts:

Spinous process (1)
Transverse process (2)
Articular processes (4)
Vertebral arch
Vertebral body

Functions:

Muscle attachment and movement
Restriction of movement
Protection of spinal cord
Support of body weight

(A)

Superior articular process
Transverse process
Spinous process
Inferior articular facet

Superior vertebral notch
Pedicle
Vertebral body
Inferior vertebral notch
Lamina (interarticular part)

(C)

Inferior articular process and facet
Transverse process
Superior articular facet
Vertebral body (bone derived from centrum)

Spinous process
Lamina
Pedicle
Vertebral foramen
Epiphysial rim (smooth bone derived from anular epiphysis)

Vertebral arch

(B)

Superior views

Inferior articular process
Superior articular process
Forming zygapophysial (facet) joint

Intervertebral (IV) foramen
Intervertebral (IV) disc

(D)

Lateral views

FIGURE 4.2. Typical vertebra, represented by the 2nd lumbar vertebra. A. Functional components include the vertebral body (*bone color*), a vertebral arch (*red*), and seven processes: three for muscle attachment and leverage (*blue*) and four that participate in synovial joints with adjacent vertebrae (*yellow*). **B and C.** Bony formations of vertebrae are demonstrated. The vertebral foramen is bounded by the vertebral arch and body. A small superior vertebral notch and a larger inferior vertebral notch flank the pedicle. **D.** The superior and inferior notches of adjacent vertebrae plus the IV disc that unites them form the IV foramen for passage of a spinal nerve and its accompanying vessels. Each articular process has an articular facet where contact occurs with the articular facets of adjacent vertebrae (**B–D**).

In addition to serving as growth zones, the anular epiphyses and their cartilaginous remnants provide some protection to the vertebral bodies and permit some diffusion of fluid between the IV disc and the blood vessels (capillaries) in the vertebral body (see Fig. 4.26). The superior and inferior epiphyses usually unite with the **centrum,** the primary ossification center for the central mass of the vertebral body (Fig. 4.2B), early in adult life (at approximately age 25) (see "Ossification of Vertebrae," p. 453).

The **vertebral arch** is posterior to the vertebral body and consists of two (right and left) pedicles and laminae (Fig. 4.2A & C). The **pedicles** are short, stout cylindrical processes that project posteriorly from the vertebral body to meet two broad, flat plates of bone, called **laminae,** which unite in the midline. The vertebral arch and the posterior surface of the vertebral body form the walls of the **vertebral foramen** (Fig. 4.2A & B). The succession of vertebral foramina in the articulated vertebral column forms the **vertebral canal** (spinal canal). The canal contains the spinal cord and the roots of the spinal nerves, along with the membranes (meninges), fat, and vessels that surround and serve them (Figs. 4.1D and 4.3). (See the blue box "Laminectomy," p. 457.)

The **vertebral notches** are indentations observed in lateral views of the vertebrae superior and inferior to each pedicle between the superior and inferior articular processes posteriorly and the corresponding projections of the body anteriorly (Fig. 4.2C). The **superior** and **inferior vertebral notches** of adjacent vertebrae and the IV discs connecting them form **intervertebral foramina** (Fig. 4.2D) through which the spinal nerves emerge from the vertebral column (see Fig. 4.27). Also, the spinal (posterior root) ganglia are located in these foramina.

Seven processes arise from the vertebral arch of a typical vertebra (Fig. 4.2A–C):

- One median **spinous process** projects posteriorly (and usually inferiorly, typically overlapping the vertebra below) from the vertebral arch at the junction of the laminae.
- Two **transverse processes** project posterolaterally from the junctions of the pedicles and laminae.
- Four **articular processes** (G. *zygapophyses*)—two **superior** and two **inferior**—also arise from the junctions of the pedicles and laminae, each bearing an **articular surface (facet).**

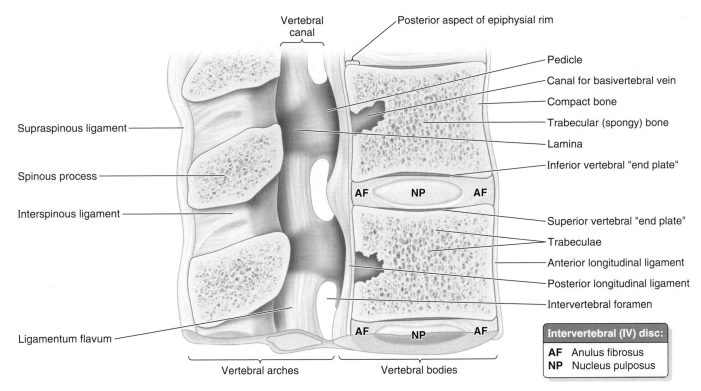

Medial view of left halves of two adjacent hemisected vertebrae and associated IV discs

FIGURE 4.3. Internal aspects of vertebral bodies and vertebral canal. The bodies consist largely of trabecular (spongy) bone—with tall, vertical supporting trabeculae linked by short horizontal trabeculae—covered by a relatively thin layer of compact bone. Hyaline cartilage "end plates" cover the superior and inferior surfaces of the bodies, surrounded by smooth bony epiphysial rims. The posterior longitudinal ligament, covering the posterior aspect of the bodies and linking the IV discs, forms the anterior wall of the vertebral canal. Lateral and posterior walls of the vertebral canal are formed by vertebral arches (pedicles and laminae) alternating with IV foramina and ligamenta flava.

The spinous and transverse processes provide attachment for deep back muscles and serve as levers, facilitating the muscles that fix or change the position of the vertebrae.

The articular processes are in apposition with corresponding processes of vertebrae adjacent (superior and inferior) to them, forming *zygapophysial (facet) joints* (Figs. 4.1B and 4.2D). Through their participation in these joints, these processes determine the types of movement permitted and restricted between the adjacent vertebrae of each region.

The articular processes also assist in keeping adjacent vertebrae aligned, particularly preventing one vertebra from slipping anteriorly on the vertebra below. Generally, the articular processes bear weight only temporarily, as when one rises from the flexed position, and unilaterally when the cervical vertebrae are laterally flexed to their limit. However, the inferior articular processes of the L5 vertebra bear weight even in the erect posture.

Regional Characteristics of Vertebrae

Each of the 33 vertebrae is unique; however, most of the vertebrae demonstrate characteristic features identifying them as belonging to one of the five regions of the vertebral column (e.g., vertebrae having foramina in their transverse processes are cervical vertebrae) (Fig. 4.4). In addition, certain individual vertebrae have distinguishing features; the C7 vertebra, for example, has the longest spinous process. It

forms a prominence under the skin at the back of the neck, especially when the neck is flexed (see Fig. 4.8A).

In each region, the **articular facets** are oriented on the articular processes of the vertebrae in a characteristic direction that determines the type of movement permitted between the adjacent vertebrae and, in aggregate, for the region. For example, the articular facets of thoracic vertebrae are nearly vertical, and together define an arc centered in the IV disc; this arrangement permits rotation and lateral flexion of the vertebral column in this region (Fig. 4.7). Regional variations in the size and shape of the vertebral canal accommodate the varying thickness of the spinal cord (Fig. 4.1D).

CERVICAL VERTEBRAE

Cervical vertebrae form the skeleton of the neck (Fig. 4.1). The smallest of the 24 movable vertebrae, the cervical vertebrae are located between the cranium and the thoracic vertebrae. Their smaller size reflects the fact that they bear less weight than do the larger inferior vertebrae. Although the cervical IV discs are thinner than those of inferior regions, they are relatively thick compared to the size of the vertebral bodies they connect. The relative thickness of the IV discs, the nearly horizontal orientation of the articular facets, and the small amount of surrounding body mass give the cervical region the greatest range and variety of movement of all the vertebral regions.

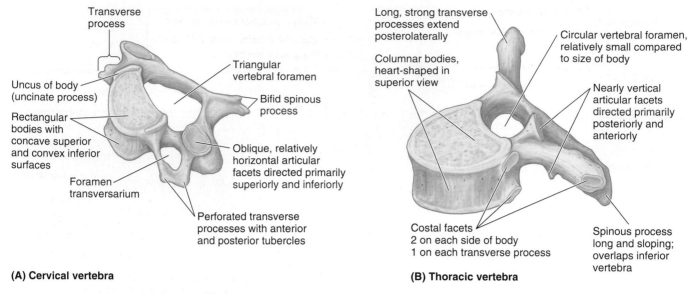

(A) Cervical vertebra

Transverse process

Uncus of body (uncinate process)

Rectangular bodies with concave superior and convex inferior surfaces

Foramen transversarium

Triangular vertebral foramen

Bifid spinous process

Oblique, relatively horizontal articular facets directed primarily superiorly and inferiorly

Perforated transverse processes with anterior and posterior tubercles

(B) Thoracic vertebra

Long, strong transverse processes extend posterolaterally

Columnar bodies, heart-shaped in superior view

Circular vertebral foramen, relatively small compared to size of body

Nearly vertical articular facets directed primarily posteriorly and anteriorly

Costal facets 2 on each side of body 1 on each transverse process

Spinous process long and sloping; overlaps inferior vertebra

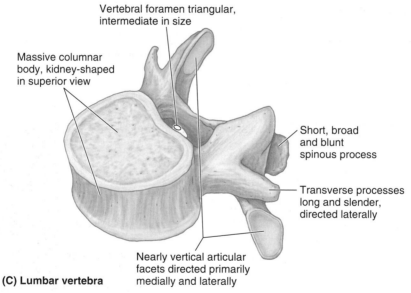

(C) Lumbar vertebra

Vertebral foramen triangular, intermediate in size

Massive columnar body, kidney-shaped in superior view

Short, broad and blunt spinous process

Transverse processes long and slender, directed laterally

Nearly vertical articular facets directed primarily medially and laterally

Left anterior superior oblique views of "typical" presacral vertebrae

FIGURE 4.4. Comparison of presacral vertebrae. As the vertebral column descends, bodies increase in size in relationship to increased weight-bearing. The size of the vertebral canal changes in relationship to the diameter of the spinal cord.

The distinctive features of cervical vertebrae are illustrated in Figures 4.4A and 4.5 and described in Table 4.1. The most distinctive feature of each cervical vertebra is the oval **foramen transversarium** (transverse foramen) in the *transverse process.* The vertebral arteries and their accompanying veins pass through the transverse foramina, except those in C7, which transmit only small accessory veins. Thus the foramina are smaller in C7 than those in other cervical vertebrae, and occasionally they are absent.

The *transverse processes of cervical vertebrae* end laterally in two projections: an **anterior tubercle** and a **posterior tubercle.** The tubercles provide attachment for a laterally

placed group of cervical muscles (levator scapulae and scalenes). The anterior rami of the cervical spinal nerves course initially on the transverse processes in **grooves for spinal nerves** between the tubercles (Fig. 4.5A & B). The anterior tubercles of vertebra C6 are called **carotid tubercles** (Fig. 4.5A) because the common carotid arteries may be compressed here, in the groove between the tubercle and body, to control bleeding from these vessels. Bleeding may continue because of the carotid's multiple anastomoses of distal branches with adjacent and contralateral branches, but at a slower rate.

Vertebrae C3–C7 are typical cervical vertebrae (Figs. 4.4A and 4.5A; Table 4.1). They have large vertebral foramina to

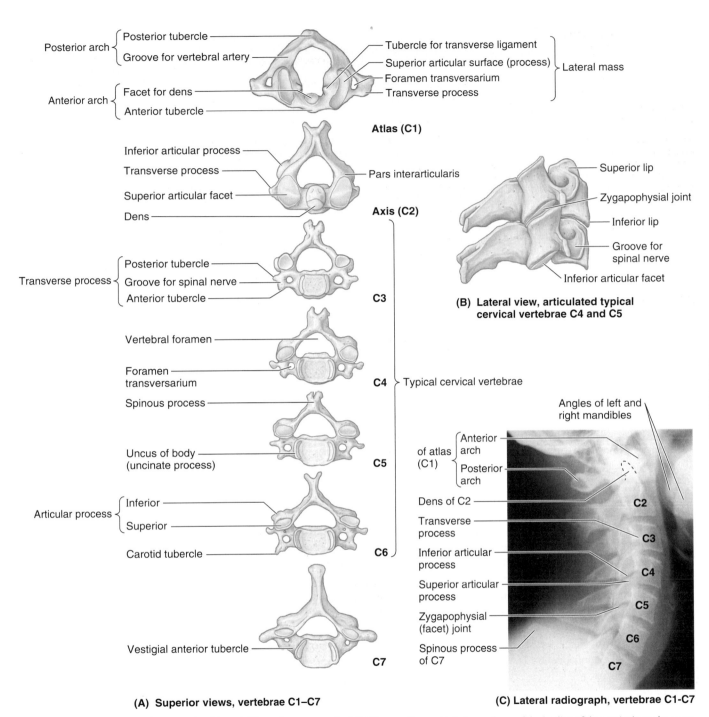

(A) Superior views, vertebrae C1–C7

(B) Lateral view, articulated typical cervical vertebrae C4 and C5

(C) Lateral radiograph, vertebrae C1-C7

FIGURE 4.5. Cervical vertebrae. A. C1, C2, and C3 vertebrae are atypical. **B.** The superior and inferior surfaces of the bodies of the cervical vertebrae are reciprocally convex and concave. Combined with the oblique orientation of the articular facets, this facilitates flexion and extension as well as lateral flexion. **C.** The anterior arch of the atlas lies anterior to the continuous curved line formed by the anterior surfaces of the C2–C7 vertebral bodies. (Courtesy of Dr. J. Heslin, Toronto, Ontario, Canada.)

accommodate the *cervical enlargement of the spinal cord* as a consequence of this region's role in the innervation of the upper limbs. The superior borders of the transversely elongated bodies of the cervical vertebrae are elevated posteriorly and especially laterally, but they are depressed anteriorly, resembling somewhat a sculpted seat.

The inferior border of the body of the superiorly placed vertebra is reciprocally shaped. The adjacent cervical

vertebrae articulate in a way that permits free flexion and extension and some lateral flexion but restricted rotation. The planar, nearly horizontal articular facets of the articular processes are also favorable for these movements. The elevated superolateral margin is the **uncus of the body** (uncinate process) (Fig. 4.4A).

The spinous processes of the C3–C6 vertebrae are short and usually bifid in white people, especially males, but usually

TABLE 4.1. CERVICAL VERTEBRAE[a]

Part	Characteristics
Vertebral body	Small and wider from side to side than anteroposteriorly; superior surface concave with uncus of body (uncinate process); inferior surface convex
Vertebral foramen	Large and triangular
Transverse processes	Foramina transversarii and anterior and posterior tubercles; vertebral arteries and accompanying venous and sympathetic plexuses pass through foramina transversarii of all cervical vertebrae except C7, which transmits only small accessory vertebral veins.
Articular processes	Superior facets directed superoposteriorly; inferior facets directed infero-anteriorly; obliquely placed facets are most nearly horizontal in this region
Spinous processes	Short (C3–C5) and bifid (C3–C6); process of C6 long, that of C7 is longer (thus C 7 is called "vertebra prominens")

[a]The C1, C2, and C7 vertebrae are atypical.

not as commonly in people of African descent or in females (Duray et al., 1999). C7 is a prominent vertebra that is characterized by a long spinous process. Because of this prominent process, C7 is called the **vertebra prominens.** Run your finger along the midline of the posterior aspect of your neck until you feel the prominent C7 spinous process. It is the most prominent spinous process in 70% of people (Fig. 4.8A).

The two superior-most cervical vertebrae are atypical. **Vertebra C1,** also called the **atlas,** is unique in that it has neither a body nor a spinous process (Figs. 4.5A and 4.6B). This ring-shaped bone has paired **lateral masses** that serve the place of a body by bearing the weight of the globe-like cranium in a manner similar to the way that Atlas of Greek mythology bore the weight of the world on his shoulders (Fig. 4.6E). The transverse processes of the atlas arise from the lateral masses, causing them to be more laterally placed than those of the inferior vertebrae. This feature makes the atlas the widest of the cervical vertebrae, thus providing increased leverage for attached muscles.

The kidney-shaped, concave **superior articular surfaces** of the lateral masses articulate with two large cranial protuberances, the **occipital condyles,** at the sides of the foramen magnum (Fig. 4.6A). **Anterior** and **posterior arches,** each of which bears a **tubercle** in the center of its external aspect, extend between the lateral masses, forming a complete ring (Fig. 4.6B). The posterior arch, which corresponds to the lamina of a typical vertebra, has a wide **groove for the vertebral artery** on its superior surface. The C1 nerve also runs in this groove.

Vertebra C2, also called the **axis,** is the strongest of the cervical vertebrae (Figs. 4.5A and 4.6C). C1, carrying the cranium, rotates on C2 (e.g., when a person turns the head to indicate "no"). The axis has two large, flat bearing surfaces, the **superior articular facets,** on which the atlas rotates. The distinguishing feature of C2 is the blunt tooth-like **dens** (odontoid process), which projects superiorly from its body. Both the dens (G. tooth) and the spinal cord inside its coverings (meninges) are encircled by the atlas. The dens lies anterior to the spinal cord and serves as the pivot about which the rotation of the head occurs.

The dens is held in position against the posterior aspect of the anterior arch of the atlas by the **transverse ligament of the atlas** (Fig. 4.6B). This ligament extends from one lateral mass of the atlas to the other, passing between the dens and spinal cord, forming the posterior wall of the "socket" that receives the dens. Thus it prevents posterior (horizontal) displacement of the dens and anterior displacement of the atlas. Either displacement would compromise the portion of the vertebral foramen of C1 that gives passage to the spinal cord. C2 has a large bifid spinous process (Fig. 4.6C & D) that can be felt deep in the *nuchal groove,* the superficial vertical groove at the back of the neck.

THORACIC VERTEBRAE

The **thoracic vertebrae** are in the upper back and provide attachment for the ribs (Fig. 4.1). Thus the primary characteristic features of thoracic vertebrae are the **costal facets** for articulation with ribs. The costal facets and other characteristic features of thoracic vertebrae are illustrated in Figures 4.4B and 4.7 and listed in Table 4.2.

The middle four thoracic vertebrae (T5–T8) demonstrate all the features typical of thoracic vertebrae. The articular processes extend vertically with paired, nearly coronally oriented articular facets that define an arc centered in the IV disc. This arc permits rotation and some lateral flexion of the vertebral column in this region. In fact, the greatest degree of rotation is permitted here (Fig. 4.7A). Attachment of the rib cage, combined with the vertical orientation of articular facets and overlapping spinous processes, limits flexion and extension as well as lateral flexion.

The T1–T4 vertebrae share some features of cervical vertebrae. T1 is atypical of thoracic vertebrae in that it has a long, almost horizontal spinous process that may be nearly as prominent as that of the vertebra prominens. T1 also has a complete costal facet on the superior edge of its body for the 1st rib and a demifacet on its inferior edge that contributes to the articular surface for the 2nd rib.

The T9–T12 vertebrae have some features of lumbar vertebrae (e.g., tubercles similar to the accessory processes).

(A) Cranial base, external surface (inferior view)

Occipital condyles
Foramen magnum

(B) Atlas (C1 vertebra), superior view

Anterior arch
Foramen for dens of axis
Lateral mass
Vertebral foramen (for spinal cord)
Posterior arch
Anterior tubercle
Facet for dens
Superior articular surface
Transverse ligament of atlas
Transverse process
Foramen transversarium
Groove for vertebral artery
Posterior tubercle

X-ray beam

(C) Axis (C2 vertebra), posterosuperior view

Dens of axis
Posterior articular facet for transverse ligament of atlas
Body
Vertebral foramen (for spinal cord)
Grooves for attachment of alar ligaments
Superior articular facet
Foramen transversarium
Transverse process
Pars interarticularis
Inferior articular process
Lamina
Spinous process (bifid)

Occipital condyles
Lateral mass of atlas (C1)
Dens of axis (C2)
Body of axis (C2)
Lower row of teeth
Cranium
Lateral atlanto-axial joint

Anteroposterior radiograph of C1 and C2 (taken through open mouth)

(D) Axis (C2 vertebra), superior view

Body
Dens of axis
Vertebral foramen (for spinal cord)
Facet for atlas
Superior articular facet
Transverse process
Inferior articular process
Lamina
Spinous process (bifid)

Lateral mass of atlas (C1)
Dens of axis (C2)
Body of axis (C2)
C3 vertebra
Anterior view

(E) Articulating atlas and axis (C1 and C2 vertebra) as viewed radiographically

FIGURE 4.6. Cranial base and C1 and C2 vertebrae. A. The occipital condyles articulate with the superior articular facets of the atlas (vertebra C1). **B.** The atlas, on which the cranium rests, has neither a spinous process nor a body. It consists of two lateral masses connected by anterior and posterior arches. **C and D.** The tooth-like dens characterizes the axis (vertebra C2) and provides a pivot around which the atlas turns and carries the cranium. It articulates anteriorly with the anterior arch of the atlas ("Facet for dens of axis," in part **B**), and posteriorly with the transverse ligament of the atlas (see part **B**). **E.** Radiograph and articulated atlas and axis showing the dens projecting superiorly from the body of the axis between the lateral masses of the atlas. Since the atlas and axis lie posterior to the mandible (Fig. 4.5C), anteroposterior radiographs must be taken through the open mouth as indicated in the orientation figure.

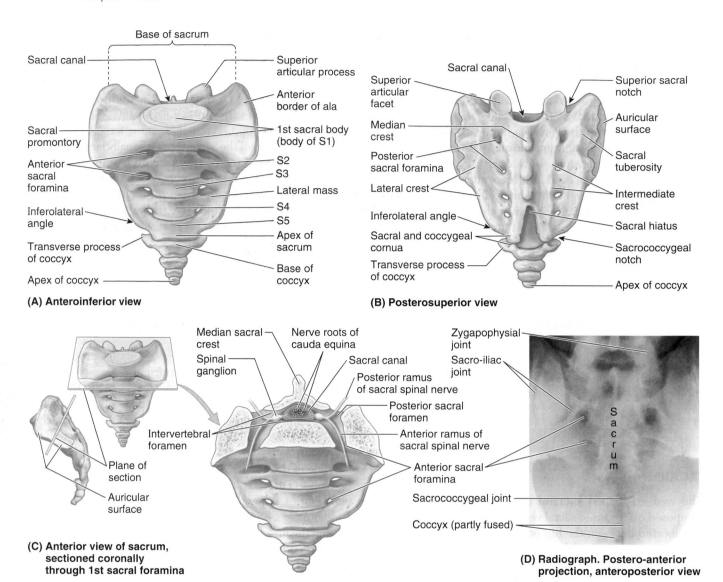

(A) Anteroinferior view

(B) Posterosuperior view

(C) Anterior view of sacrum, sectioned coronally through 1st sacral foramina

(D) Radiograph. Postero-anterior projection, anteroposterior view

FIGURE 4.10. Sacrum and coccyx. A. Base and pelvic surface of sacrum and coccyx. **B.** Dorsal surface of sacrum and coccyx. **C.** Lateral and anterior orientation drawings of the sacrum in its anatomical position demonstrate the essentially frontal plane and level at which the sacrum has been sectioned to reveal the sacral canal containing the cauda equina. Spinal ganglia lie within the IV foramina, as they do at superior vertebral levels. However, the sacral posterior and anterior rami of the spinal nerves exit via posterior and anterior (pelvic) sacral foramina, respectively. The lateral orientation drawing demonstrates the auricular surface that joins the ilium to form the synovial part of the sacro-iliac joint. In the anatomical position, the S1–S3 vertebrae lie in an essentially transverse plane, forming a roof for the posterior pelvic cavity. **D.** In anteroposterior radiographs the oblique plane of the auricular surfaces creates two lines indicating each sacro-iliac joint. The lateral line is the anterior aspect of the joint, the medial line is the posterior aspect.

articular processes form **coccygeal cornua,** which articulate with the sacral cornua. The last three coccygeal vertebrae often fuse during middle life, forming a beak-like coccyx; this accounts for its name (G. *coccyx,* cuckoo). With increasing age, Co1 often fuses with the sacrum, and the remaining coccygeal vertebrae usually fuse to form a single bone.

The coccyx does not participate with the other vertebrae in support of the body weight when standing; however, when sitting it may flex anteriorly somewhat, indicating that it is receiving some weight. The coccyx provides attachments for parts of the gluteus maximus and coccygeus muscles and the *anococcygeal ligament,* the median fibrous band of the pubococcygeus muscles (see Chapter 3).

SURFACE ANATOMY OF LUMBAR VERTEBRAE, SACRUM, AND COCCYX

The spinous processes of lumbar vertebrae are large and easy to observe when the trunk is flexed (Fig. 4.11A). They can also be palpated in the *posterior median furrow* (Fig. 4.11B & C). The *L2 spinous process* provides an estimate of the position of the inferior end of the spinal cord. A horizontal line joining the highest points of the iliac crests passes through the tip of the L4 spinous process and the L4–L5 IV disc. This is a useful landmark when performing a lumbar puncture to obtain a sample of cerebrospinal fluid (CSF) (see the blue box "Lumbar Spinal Puncture," p. 505).

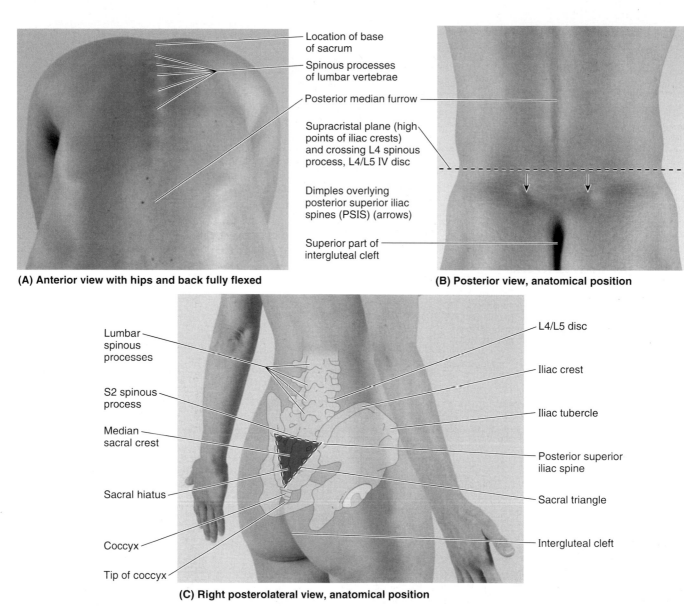

Location of base of sacrum

Spinous processes of lumbar vertebrae

Posterior median furrow

Supracristal plane (high points of iliac crests) and crossing L4 spinous process, L4/L5 IV disc

Dimples overlying posterior superior iliac spines (PSIS) (arrows)

Superior part of intergluteal cleft

(A) Anterior view with hips and back fully flexed

(B) Posterior view, anatomical position

Lumbar spinous processes

S2 spinous process

Median sacral crest

Sacral hiatus

Coccyx

Tip of coccyx

L4/L5 disc

Iliac crest

Iliac tubercle

Posterior superior iliac spine

Sacral triangle

Intergluteal cleft

(C) Right posterolateral view, anatomical position

FIGURE 4.11. Surface anatomy of lumbar vertebrae, sacrum, and coccyx.

The *S2 spinous process* lies at the middle of a line drawn between the *posterior superior iliac spines,* indicated by the *skin dimples* (Fig. 4.11B). The dimples are formed by the attachment of skin and deep fascia to these spines. This level indicates the inferior extent of the subarachnoid space (lumbar cistern). The *median sacral crest* can be felt inferior to the L5 spinous process. The **sacral triangle** is formed by the lines joining the two posterior superior iliac spines and the superior part of the **intergluteal** (natal) **cleft** between the buttocks. The sacral triangle outlining the sacrum is a common area of pain resulting from low back sprains. The *sacral hiatus* can be palpated at the inferior end of the sacrum located in the superior part of the intergluteal cleft.

The transverse processes of thoracic and lumbar vertebrae are covered with thick muscles and may or may not be palpable. The *coccyx* can be palpated in the intergluteal cleft,

inferior to the apex of the sacral triangle. The **apex of the coccyx** can be palpated approximately 2.5 cm posterosuperior to the anus. Clinically, the coccyx is examined with a gloved finger in the anal canal.

Ossification of Vertebrae

Vertebrae begin to develop during the embryonic period as mesenchymal condensations around the notochord. Later, these mesenchymal bone models chondrify and cartilaginous vertebrae form. Typically, vertebrae begin to ossify toward the end of the embryonic period (8th week), with three **primary ossification centers** developing in each cartilaginous vertebra: an endochondral **centrum,** which will eventually constitute most of the body of the vertebra, and two perichondral centers, one in each half of the **neural arch** (Fig. 4.12A–J & M).

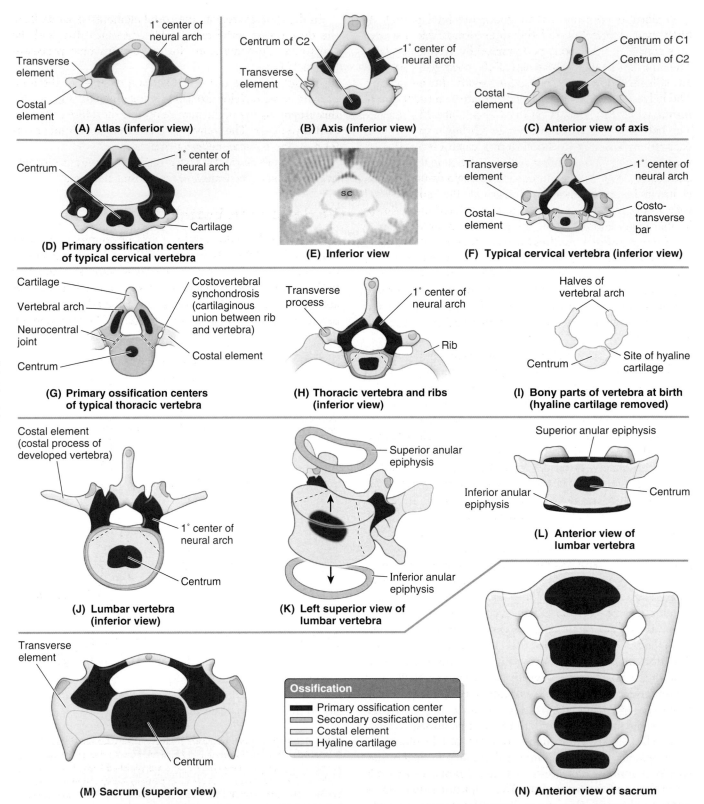

FIGURE 4.12. Ossification of vertebrae. A. Vertebra C1 (atlas) lacks a centrum. **B and C.** Vertebra C2 (axis) has two centra, one of which forms most of the dens. **D–F.** The development of "typical" cervical vertebrae is shown, including (**D**) the primary ossification centers within the hyaline cartilage, (**E**) a CT scan of the vertebra shown in part **D** (*SC*, spinal cord), and (**F**) the primary and secondary ossification centers. **G–I.** The development of thoracic vertebrae is shown, including (**G**) the three primary ossification centers in a cartilaginous vertebra of a 7-week-old embryo (observe the joints present at this stage), (**H**) the primary and secondary ossification centers (with ribs developed from costal elements), and (**I**) the bony parts of a thoracic vertebra after skeletonization (cartilage removed). **J–L.** The development of the lumbar vertebrae is shown, including (**J**) the primary and secondary ossification centers, (**K**) the anular epiphyses separated from the body, and (**L**) the anular epiphyses in place. **M and N.** The development of the sacrum is shown. Note that the ossification and fusion of sacral vertebrae may not be completed until age 35.

Ossification continues throughout the fetal period. At birth, typical vertebra and the superiormost sacral vertebrae consist of three bony parts united by hyaline cartilage. The inferior sacral vertebrae and all the coccygeal vertebrae are still entirely cartilaginous; they ossify during infancy. The halves of the neural arches articulate at **neurocentral joints,** which are primary cartilaginous joints (Fig. 4.12G). The halves of the neural/vertebral arch begin to fuse with each other posterior to the vertebral canal during the 1st year, beginning in the lumbar region and then in the thoracic and cervical regions. The neural arches begin fusing with the centra in the upper cervical region around the end of the 3rd year, but usually the process is not completed in the lower lumbar region until after the 6th year (Moore et al., 2012).

Five **secondary ossification centers** develop during puberty in each typical vertebra: one at the tip of the spinous process; one at the tip of each transverse process; and two anular epiphyses (ring epiphyses), one on the superior and one on the inferior edges of each vertebral body (i.e., around the margins of the superior and inferior surfaces of the vertebral body) (Fig. 4.12F & I–L).

The hyaline **anular epiphyses,** to which the IV discs attach, are sometimes referred to as *epiphysial growth plates* and form the zone from which the vertebral body grows in height. When growth ceases early in the adult period, the epiphyses usually unite with the vertebral body. This union results in the characteristic smooth raised margin, the **epiphysial rim,** around the edges of the superior and inferior surfaces of the body of the adult vertebra (Figs. 4.2B and 4.3). All secondary ossification centers have usually united with the vertebrae by age 25; however, the ages at which specific unions occur vary.

Exceptions to the typical pattern of ossification occur in vertebrae C1, C2, and C7 (Fig. 4.12A–C) and in the sacrum (Fig. 4.12M & N) and coccyx. In addition, at all levels, primordial "ribs" (**costal elements**) appear in association with the secondary ossification centers of the transverse processes (**transverse elements**). The costal elements normally develop into ribs only in the thoracic region; they become part of the transverse process or its equivalent at other levels.

In the cervical region, the costal element normally remains diminutive as part of the transverse process. *Foramina transversarii* develop as gaps between the two lateral ossification centers, medial to a linking **costotransverse bar,** which forms the lateral boundary of the foramina (Fig. 4.12A–F). Also, as a result of the cervical transverse processes being formed from the two developmental elements, the transverse processes of cervical vertebrae end laterally in an *anterior tubercle* (from the costal element) and a *posterior tubercle* (from the transverse element). The atypical morphology of vertebrae C1 and C2 is also established during development. The centrum of C1 becomes fused to that of C2 and loses its peripheral connection to the remainder of C1, thus forming the *dens* (Fig. 4.12C). Since these first two centra are fused and are now part of C2, no IV disc is formed between C1 and C2 to connect them. The part of the body that remains with C1 is represented by the *anterior arch* and *tubercle of C1.*

In the thoracic region, the costal elements separate from the developing vertebrae and elongate into ribs, and the transverse elements alone form the transverse processes (Fig. 4.12I).

All but the base of the transverse processes of the lumbar vertebrae develop from the costal element (Fig. 4.12J); this projecting bar of the mature bone is therefore called the **costal process.** The transverse elements of the lumbar vertebrae form the *mammillary processes.*

The ala and auricular surfaces of the sacrum are formed by the fusion of the transverse and costal elements.

Variations in Vertebrae

Most people have 33 vertebrae, but developmental errors may result in 32 or 34 vertebrae (Fig. 4.13). Estimates of the frequency of abnormal numbers of vertebrae superior to the sacrum (the normal number is 24) range between 5% and 12%. Variations in vertebrae are affected by race, gender, and developmental factors (genetic and environmental).

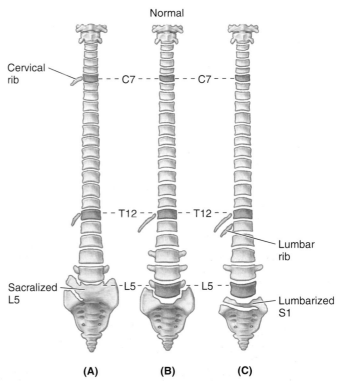

FIGURE 4.13. Variations in vertebrae and their relationship to ribs. A. A "cranial shift" is demonstrated, in which there are 13 ribs, including a cervical rib articulating with vertebra C7, and a diminished 12th rib articulating with vertebra T12. Vertebra L5 is shown partially incorporated into the sacrum, but such "sacralization" can also be complete. The lowest sacral segment (S5) is partially segmented. **B.** The common arrangement of the vertebrae and the position of the 1st and 12th ribs are shown. **C.** A "caudal shift" is shown, in which the 12th rib is increased in size, and there is a small lumbar rib. The transverse process of vertebra L4 is increased in size, whereas that of vertebra L5 is greatly reduced. The first sacral segment is shown partially separated from the rest of the sacrum, but such "lumbarization" can also be complete. The 1st coccygeal segment is incorporated into the sacrum—that is, it is "sacralized."

Zygapophysial joints

Normal

Following bilateral dislocation

C6

C7

(F) Median MRI scan

Bilateral facet dislocation (locked facets)

C6

C7

Ant

Rt ←→ Left

Post

(G) Transverse CT scan – inferior view

i = inferior articular processes of C6
s = superior articular processes of C7

Normally, the superior articular processes are anterior to the inferior processes, with their flat articular facets in contact as a zygapophysial joint.

FIGURE B4.3. Dislocations of cervical vertebrae. Four stages of injury are shown: (**A**) stage I, flexion sprain; (**B**) stage II, anterior subluxation with 25% anterior translation; (**C**) stage III, 50% translation; and (**D**) stage IV, complete dislocation. **E.** This lateral view radiograph shows a stage III dislocation with 50% translation. **F.** This MRI study of a stage IV dislocation with cord injury reveals that the body of C7 is fractured (*open white arrowhead*). The ligamentum flavum is disrupted (*curved black arrow*), and the spinous process is avulsed (*straight black arrow*). **G.** This transverse CT scan (same individual shown in **F**) reveals the reversed position of the articular processes of the C6 and C7 vertebrae owing to "facet jumping."

Fracture and Dislocation of Atlas

The atlas (vertebra C1) is a bony ring, with two wedge-shaped lateral masses, connected by relatively thin anterior and posterior arches and a transverse ligament (Fig. 4.4A). Because the taller side of the lateral mass is directed laterally, vertical forces (as would result from striking the bottom of a pool in a diving accident) compressing the lateral masses between the occipital condyles and the axis drive them apart, fracturing one or both of the anterior or posterior arches (Fig. B4.4B).

If the force is sufficient, *rupture of the transverse ligament* that links them will also occur (Fig. B4.4C). The resulting *Jefferson* or *burst fracture* (Fig. B4.4C–E) in itself does not

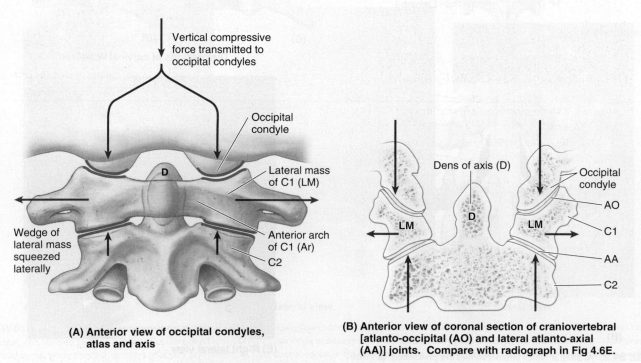

Vertical compressive force transmitted to occipital condyles

Occipital condyle

Lateral mass of C1 (LM)

D

Wedge of lateral mass squeezed laterally

Anterior arch of C1 (Ar)

C2

(A) Anterior view of occipital condyles, atlas and axis

Dens of axis (D)

Occipital condyle

AO

LM   D   LM

C1

AA

C2

(B) Anterior view of coronal section of craniovertebral [atlanto-occipital (AO) and lateral atlanto-axial (AA)] joints. Compare with radiograph in Fig 4.6E.

FIGURE B4.4 A-B. Jefferson fracture of atlas. (*Continued on next page*)

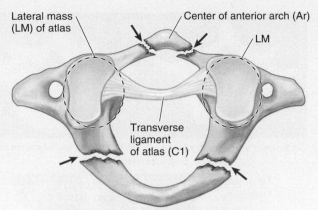

(C) Inferior view of Jefferson (burst) fracture of C1

Labels: Lateral mass (LM) of atlas; Center of anterior arch (Ar); LM; Transverse ligament of atlas (C1)

(D) Inferior view of CT scan of Jefferson fracture

(E) Anterior view of reconstructed CT image of Jefferson fracture showing fragment of anterior arch (Ar) and outward (lateral) shift of lateral masses of C1 (LM)

FIGURE B4.4 C-E. Jefferson fracture of atlas.

necessarily result in spinal cord injury, because the dimensions of the bony ring actually increase. Spinal cord injury is more likely, however, if the transverse ligament has also been ruptured (see the blue box "Rupture of Transverse Ligament of Atlas" on p. 477) indicated radiographically by widely spread lateral masses.

Fracture and Dislocation of Axis

Fractures of the vertebral arch of the axis (vertebra C2) are one of the most common injuries of the cervical vertebrae (up to 40%) (Yochum and Rowe, 2004). Usually the fracture occurs in the bony column formed by the superior and inferior articular processes of the axis, the **pars interarticularis** (Fig. 4.5A). A fracture in this location, called a *traumatic spondylolysis of C2* (Fig. B4.5A, B, & D), usually occurs as a result of *hyperextension of the head on the neck,* rather than the combined hyperextension of the head and neck, which may result in *whiplash injury.*

Such hyperextension of the head was used to execute criminals by hanging, in which the knot was placed under the chin before the body suddenly dropped its length through the gallows floor (Fig. B4.5C); thus, this fracture has been called a *hangman's fracture.*

In more severe injuries, the body of the C2 vertebra is displaced anteriorly with respect to the body of the C3 vertebra. With or without such subluxation (incomplete dislocation) of

(A) Posterosuperior view

Labels: Dens (D) of axis (C2); Body of axis (B); Superior articular facet; Foramen transversarium; Transverse process; **Pars interarticularis (fractured)**; Inferior articular process; Lamina; Spinous process (SP)

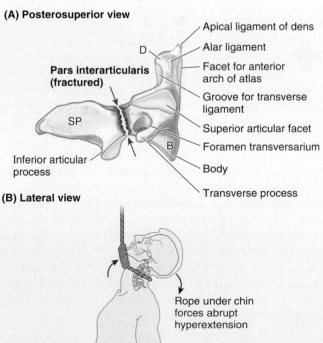

(B) Lateral view

Labels: Apical ligament of dens; Alar ligament; Facet for anterior arch of atlas; Groove for transverse ligament; Superior articular facet; Foramen transversarium; Body; Transverse process; **Pars interarticularis (fractured)**; D; SP; B; Inferior articular process

(C)

Rope under chin forces abrupt hyperextension

FIGURE B4.5 A-C. Fracture and dislocation of axis. Posterosuperior (**A**) and lateral (**B**) views of a hangman's fracture of the C2 vertebra are shown (*arrows*). **C.** The position of the knot produces hyperextension during hanging (*arrows*). (*Continued on next page*)

Cranium

Posterior
arch of
atlas
(C1)

Anterior
arch of
atlas
(C1)

D

SP

B

(D) Lateral view

FIGURE B4.5 D. Fracture and dislocation of axis. (*continued*)
D. Right lateral view radiograph demonstrating a hangman's fracture
(*arrow*) of C2.

the axis, injury of the spinal cord and/or of the brainstem is
likely, sometimes resulting in *quadriplegia* (paralysis of all
four limbs) or death.

Fractures of the dens are also common axis injuries
(40–50%), which may result from a horizontal blow to
the head or as a complication of *osteopenia* (pathological
loss of bone mass) (see the blue box "Fracture of Dens,"
p. 476).

Lumbar Spinal Stenosis

 Lumbar spinal stenosis describes a *stenotic* (narrow) vertebral foramen in one or more lumbar
vertebrae (Fig. B4.6B). This condition may be a
hereditary anomaly that can make a person more vulnerable to age-related degenerative changes such as IV disc
bulging. Lumbar spinal nerves increase in size as the vertebral column descends, but paradoxically, the IV foramina decrease in size. Narrowing is usually maximal at the
level of the IV discs. However, stenosis of a lumbar vertebral foramen alone may cause compression of one or
more spinal nerve roots occupying the inferior vertebral
canal (Fig. 4.1). Surgical treatment of lumbar stenosis
may consist of decompressive laminectomy (see the blue
box "Laminectomy," p. 457). When IV disc protrusion
occurs in a patient with spinal stenosis (Fig. B4.6B), it
further compromises a vertebral canal that is already limited, as does arthritic proliferation and ligamentous
degeneration.

Cervical Ribs

A *cervical rib* is a relatively common anomaly. In
1–2% of people, the developmental costal element of C7, which normally becomes a small part
of the transverse process that lies anterior to the

(A) Normal vertebral foramen **(B) Stenotic vertebral foramen**
Superior views

Tip of conus
medullaris

Nerve roots of
cauda equina

**Region of lumbar
spinal stenosis
(arrow)**

Sacrum

(C) Sagittal MRI, viewed from left

Aorta

**L4/L5 IV disc
(bulging)**

Psoas major
muscle

**Lateral recess
stenosis (arrow)
and nerve roots
of cauda equina**

**Hypertrophic
articular
processes**

(D) Transverse MRI, inferior view

FIGURE B4.6. Lumbar spinal stenosis. Normal (**A**) and stenotic (**B**)
vertebral foramina are compared. The sagittal (**C**) and transverse (**D**)
lumbar MRIs demonstrate a high-grade stenosis caused by hypertrophic
articular processes and ligamenta flava and moderate peripheral bulging of the L4–L5 IV disc.

foramen transversarium (Fig. 4.5A), becomes abnormally
enlarged. This structure may vary in size from a small protuberance to a complete rib that occurs bilaterally about
60% of the time.

The *supernumerary (extra) rib* or a fibrous connection
extending from its tip to the first thoracic rib may elevate and
place pressure on structures that emerge from the superior
thoracic aperture, notably the subclavian artery or inferior
trunk of the brachial plexus, and may cause *thoracic outlet
syndrome.*

Caudal Epidural Anesthesia

In living persons, the sacral hiatus is closed by the membranous **sacrococcygeal ligament,** which is pierced by the *filum terminale* (a connective tissue strand extending from the tip of the spinal cord to the coccyx). Deep (superior) to the ligament, the epidural space of the sacral canal is filled with fatty connective tissue (Fig. B4.7A). In *caudal epidural anesthesia* or *caudal analgesia,* a local anesthetic agent is injected into the fat of the sacral canal that surrounds the proximal portions of the sacral nerves. This can be accomplished by several routes, including the sacral hiatus (Fig. B4.7B & C). Because the sacral hiatus is located between the sacral cornua and inferior to the S4 spinous process or median sacral crest, these palpable bony landmarks are important for locating the hiatus (Fig. B4.7A). The anesthetic solution spreads superiorly and extradurally, where it acts on the S2–Co1 spinal nerves of the cauda equina. The height to which the anesthetic ascends is controlled by the amount injected and the position of the patient. Sensation is lost inferior to the epidural block. Anesthetic agents can also be injected through the posterior sacral foramina into the sacral canal around the spinal nerve roots (*transsacral epidural anesthesia*) (Fig. B4.7B). Epidural anesthesia during childbirth is discussed in Chapter 3.

Injury of Coccyx

An abrupt fall onto the buttocks may cause a painful subperiosteal bruising or fracture of the coccyx, or a fracture—dislocation of the sacrococcygeal joint. Displacement is common, and surgical removal of the fractured bone may be required to relieve pain. An especially difficult childbirth occasionally injures the mother's coccyx. A troublesome syndrome, *coccygodynia* (or coccydynia), often follows coccygeal trauma; pain relief is commonly difficult.

(A) Posterior view

Sacrococcygeal ligament
4th sacral spinous process
Sacral cornua
Sacral hiatus

(B) Posterior view

Lumbar cistern of subarachnoid space
Pia mater (transparent, covering nerve roots of cauda equina)
Arachnoid mater (purple)
Dura mater (gray) of dural sac
Cauda equina in CSF
Epidural space
S1 vertebral level
S2 vertebral level
S1 spinal nerve
Sacral foramina
Trans-sacral (epidural) anesthesia
S5 spinal nerve
Sacral cornua
Sacral canal
Filum terminale externum
Caudal-epidural anesthesia

(C) Median section

Filum terminale internum
Dural sac
Subarachnoid space
Dura mater
Filum terminale externum
Epidural space

(D) Transsacral (epidural) anesthesia

FIGURE B4.7.

Abnormal Fusion of Vertebrae

In approximately 5% of people, L5 is partly or completely incorporated into the sacrum—conditions known as *hemisacralization* and *sacralization of the L5 vertebra* (Fig. B4.8A), respectively. In others, S1 is more or less separated from the sacrum and is partly or completely fused with L5 vertebra, which is called *lumbarization of the S1 vertebra* (Fig. B4.8B). When L5 is sacralized, the L5–S1 level is strong and the L4–L5 level degenerates, often producing painful symptoms.

Pelvic surface   **Dorsal surface**

(A) Sacralization of L5 vertebra

Pelvic surface   **Dorsal surface**

**(B) Lumbarization of S1 vertebra
(S1 is not part of sacrum)**

FIGURE B4.8.

Effect of Aging on Vertebrae

Between birth and age 5, the body of a typical lumbar vertebra increases in height threefold (from 5–6 mm to 15–18 mm), and between ages 5 and 13, it increases another 45–50%. Longitudinal growth continues throughout adolescence, but the rate decreases and is completed between ages 18 and 25.

During middle and older age, there is an overall decrease in bone density and strength, particularly centrally within the vertebral body. Consequently, the articular surfaces gradually bow inward so that both the superior and inferior surfaces of the vertebrae become increasingly concave (Fig. B4.9A), and the IV discs become increasingly convex. The bone loss and consequent change in shape of the vertebral bodies may account in part for the slight loss in height that occurs with aging. The development of these concavities may cause an apparent narrowing of the intervertebral "space" on radiographs based on the distance between the margins of the vertebral bodies; however, this should not be interpreted as a loss of IV disc thickness.

Aging of the IV discs combined with the changing shape of the vertebrae results in an increase in compressive forces at the periphery of the vertebral bodies, where the discs attach. In response, *osteophytes* (bony spurs) commonly develop around the margins of the vertebral body (along the attach-

(A) Medial view of right half of lumbar vertebra

(B) Left anterior superior oblique view   *****osteophytes**

FIGURE B4.9. Effects of aging on vertebrae.

ments of the fibers of the outer part of the disc), especially anteriorly and posteriorly (Fig. B4.9B). Similarly, as altered mechanics place greater stresses on the zygapophysial joints, osteophytes develop along the attachments of the joint capsules and accessory ligaments, especially those of the superior articular process, whereas extensions of the articular cartilage develop around the articular facets of the inferior processes.

This bony or cartilaginous growth during advanced age has traditionally been viewed as a disease process (*spondylosis* in the case of the vertebral bodies, *osteoarthrosis* in the case of the zygapophysial joints), but it may be more realistic to view it as an expected morphological change with age, representing normal anatomy for a particular age range.

Correlation of these findings with pain is often difficult. Some people with these manifestations present with pain, others demonstrate the same age-related changes but have no pain, and still others exhibit little morphological change but complain of the same types of pain as those with evident change. In view of this and the typical occurrence of these findings, some clinicians have suggested that such age-related changes should not be considered pathological, but as the normal anatomy of aging (Bogduk, 2012).

Anomalies of Vertebrae

Sometimes the epiphysis of a transverse process fails to fuse. Therefore, caution must be exercised so that a persistent epiphysis is not mistaken for a vertebral fracture in a radiograph or computed tomographic (CT) scan.

A common birth defect of the vertebral column is *spina bifida occulta,* in which the neural arches of L5 and/or S1 fail to develop normally and fuse posterior to the vertebral canal. This bony defect, present in up to 24% of the population (Greer, 2009), usually occurs in the vertebral arch of L5 and/or S1. The defect is concealed by the overlying skin, but its location is often indicated by a tuft of hair. Most people with spina bifida occulta have no back problems. When examining a newborn, adjacent vertebrae should be palpated in sequence to be certain the vertebral arches are intact and continuous from the cervical to the sacral regions.

In severe types of spina bifida, *spina bifida cystica,* one or more vertebral arches may fail to develop completely. Spina bifida cystica is associated with herniation of the meninges (*meningocele,* a spina bifida associated with a meningeal cyst) and/or the spinal cord (*meningomyelocele*) (Fig. B4.10). Neurological symptoms are usually present in severe cases of meningomyelocele (e.g., paralysis of the limbs and disturbances in bladder and bowel control). Severe forms of spina bifida result from *neural tube defects,* such as the defective closure of the neural tube during the 4th week of embryonic development (Moore, et al., 2012).

FIGURE B4.10. Infant with spina bifida cystica.

The Bottom Line

VERTEBRAE

Typical vertebrae: Vertebrae consist of vertebral bodies, which bear weight and increase in size proportionately, and vertebral arches, which collectively house and protect the spinal cord and the roots of the spinal nerves. ♦ Processes extending from the vertebral arch provide attachment and leverage for muscles, or direct movements between vertebrae.

Regional characteristics of vertebrae: The chief regional characteristics of vertebrae are ♦ foramina transversarii for cervical vertebrae, ♦ costal facets for thoracic vertebrae, ♦ the absence of foramina transversarii and costal facets for lumbar vertebrae, ♦ the fusion of adjacent sacral vertebrae, and ♦ the rudimentary nature of coccygeal vertebrae.

Ossification of vertebrae: Vertebrae typically ossify from three primary ossification centers within a cartilaginous model: a centrum that will form most of the body and a center in each half of the neural arch. ♦ Thus, by the time of birth, most vertebrae consist of three bony parts united by hyaline cartilage. ♦ Fusion occurs during the first 6 years in a centrifugal pattern from the lumbar region. ♦ During puberty, five secondary ossification centers appear: three related to the spinous and transverse processes and two anular epiphyses around the superior and inferior margins of the vertebral body. ♦ Costal elements formed in association with the ossification center of the transverse process usually form ribs only in the thoracic region. They form components of the transverse processes or their equivalents in other regions. ♦ Knowledge of the pattern of ossification of vertebrae allows understanding of the normal structure of typical and atypical vertebrae, as well as variations and malformations.

VERTEBRAL COLUMN

The **vertebral column** (spine) is an aggregate structure, normally made up of 33 vertebrae and the components that unite them into a single structural, functional entity—the "axis" of the axial skeleton. Because it provides the semirigid, central "core" about which movements of the trunk occur, "soft" or hollow structures that run a longitudinal course are subject to damage or kinking (e.g., the spinal cord, descending aorta, venae cavae, thoracic duct, and esophagus). Thus they lie in close proximity to the vertebral axis, where they receive its semirigid support and torsional stresses on them are minimized.

Joints of Vertebral Column

The joints of the vertebral column include the:

- Joints of the vertebral bodies.
- Joints of the vertebral arches.
- Craniovertebral (atlanto-axial and atlanto-occipital) joints.
- Costovertebral joints (see Chapter 1).
- Sacro-iliac joints (see Chapter 3).

JOINTS OF VERTEBRAL BODIES

The joints of the vertebral bodies are *symphyses* (*secondary cartilaginous joints*) designed for weight-bearing and strength. The articulating surfaces of adjacent vertebrae are connected by **IV discs** and ligaments (Fig. 4.14).

The IV discs provide strong attachments between the vertebral bodies, uniting them into a continuous semirigid column and forming the inferior half of the anterior border of the IV foramen. In aggregate, the discs account for 20–25%

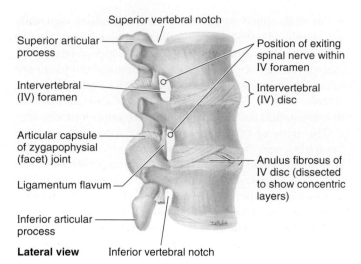

FIGURE 4.14. Lumbar vertebrae and IV discs. This view of the superior lumbar region shows the structure of the anuli fibrosi of the discs and the structures involved in formation of IV foramina. The disc forms the inferior half of the anterior boundary of an IV foramen (except in the cervical region). Thus herniation of the disc will not affect the spinal nerve exiting from the superior part of that foramen, bounded by bone.

of the length (height) of the vertebral column (Fig. 4.1). As well as permitting movement between adjacent vertebrae, their resilient deformability allows them to serve as shock absorbers. Each IV disc consists of an *anulus fibrosus,* an outer fibrous part, composed of concentric lamellae of fibrocartilage, and a gelatinous central mass, the *nucleus pulposus.*

The **anulus fibrosus** (L. *anus,* a ring) is a bulging fibrous ring consisting of concentric lamellae (layers) of fibrocartilage forming the circumference of the IV disc (Figs. 4.14 and

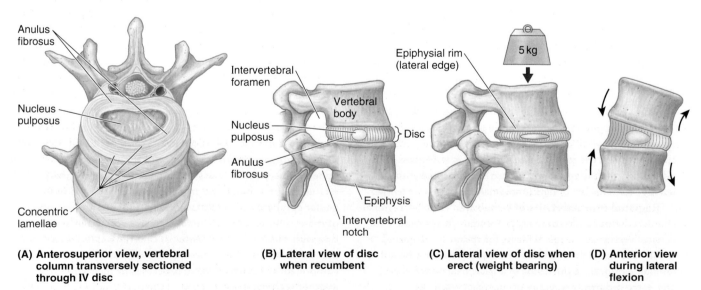

(A) Anterosuperior view, vertebral column transversely sectioned through IV disc

(B) Lateral view of disc when recumbent

(C) Lateral view of disc when erect (weight bearing)

(D) Anterior view during lateral flexion

FIGURE 4.15. Structure and function of IV discs. A. The disc consists of a nucleus pulposus and an anulus fibrosus. The superficial layers of the anulus have been cut and spread apart to show the direction of the fibers. Note that the combined thickness of the rings of the anulus is diminished posteriorly—that is, the anulus is thinner posteriorly. **B.** The fibrogelatinous nucleus pulposus occupies the center of the disc and acts as a cushion and shock-absorbing mechanism. **C.** The pulpy nucleus flattens and the anulus bulges when weight is applied, as occurs during standing and more so during lifting. **D.** During flexion and extension movements, the nucleus pulposus serves as a fulcrum. The anulus is simultaneously placed under compression on one side and tension on the other.

4.15A). The anuli insert into the smooth, rounded *epiphysial rims* on the articular surfaces of the vertebral bodies formed by the fused *anular epiphyses* (Figs. 4.2B and 4.15B & C). The fibers forming each lamella run obliquely from one vertebra to another, about 30 or more degrees from vertical. The fibers of adjacent lamellae cross each other obliquely in opposite directions at angles of more than 60 degrees (Fig. 4.14). This arrangement allows limited rotation between adjacent vertebrae, while providing a strong bond between them. The anulus is thinner posteriorly and may be incomplete posteriorly in the adult in the cervical region (Mercer and Bogduk, 1999). The anulus becomes decreasingly vascularized centrally, and only the outer third of the anulus receives sensory innervation.

The **nucleus pulposus** (L. *pulpa*, fleshy) is the core of the IV disc (Fig. 4.15A). At birth, these pulpy nuclei are about 88% water and are initially more cartilaginous than fibrous. Their semifluid nature is responsible for much of the flexibility and resilience of the IV disc and of the vertebral column as a whole.

Vertical forces deform the IV discs, which thus serve as shock absorbers. The nuclei become broader when compressed and thinner when tensed or stretched (as when hanging or suspended) (Fig. 4.15C). Compression and tension occur simultaneously in the same disc during anterior and lateral flexion and extension of the vertebral column (Fig. 4.15D). During these movements, as well as during rotation, the turgid nucleus acts as a semifluid fulcrum. Because the lamellae of the anulus fibrosus are thinner and less numerous posteriorly than they are anteriorly or laterally, the nucleus pulposus is not centered in the disc but is positioned between the center and posterior aspect of the disc (Fig. 4.15A). The nucleus pulposus is avascular; it receives its nourishment by diffusion from blood vessels at the periphery of the anulus fibrosus and vertebral body.

There is no IV disc between C1 and C2 vertebrae; the most inferior functional disc is between L5 and S1 vertebrae. The discs vary in thickness in different regions. The thickness of the discs increases as the vertebral column descends. However, their thickness relative to the size of the bodies they connect is most clearly related to the range of movement, and relative thickness is greatest in the cervical and lumbar regions. Their thickness is most uniform in the thoracic region. The discs are thicker anteriorly in the cervical and lumbar regions, their varying shapes producing the secondary curvatures of the vertebral column (see Fig. 4.1B).

Uncovertebral "joints" or **clefts** (of Luschka) commonly develop between the unci of the bodies of C3 or 4–C6 or 7 vertebrae and the beveled inferolateral surfaces of the vertebral bodies superior to them after 10 years of age (Fig. 4.16). The joints are at the lateral and posterolateral margins of the IV discs. The articulating surfaces of these joint-like structures are covered with cartilage moistened by fluid contained within an interposed potential space, or "capsule." They are considered synovial joints by some; others consider them to be degenerative spaces (clefts) in the discs occupied by extracellular fluid. The uncovertebral "joints" are frequent sites of bone spur formation in later years, which may cause neck pain.

The **anterior longitudinal ligament** is a strong, broad fibrous band that covers and connects the anterolateral

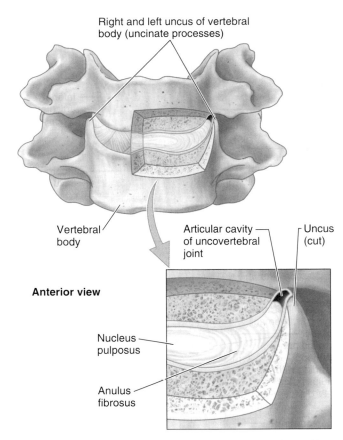

Right and left uncus of vertebral body (uncinate processes)

Vertebral body

Anterior view

Articular cavity of uncovertebral joint

Uncus (cut)

Nucleus pulposus

Anulus fibrosus

FIGURE 4.16. Uncovertebral joints. These small, synovial joint-like structures are between the unci of the bodies of the lower vertebrae and the beveled surfaces of the vertebral bodies superior to them. These joints are at the posterolateral margins of the IV discs.

aspects of the vertebral bodies and IV discs (Fig. 4.17). The ligament extends longitudinally from the pelvic surface of the sacrum to the anterior tubercle of vertebra C1 and the occipital bone anterior to the foramen magnum are the superiormost parts, the anterior atlanto-axial and atlanto-occipital ligaments. Although thickest on the anterior aspect of the vertebral bodies (illustrations often depict only this portion), the anterior longitudinal ligament also covers the lateral aspects of the bodies to the IV foramen. This ligament prevents hyperextension of the vertebral column, maintaining stability of the joints between the vertebral bodies. *The anterior longitudinal ligament is the only ligament that limits extension;* all other IV ligaments limit forms of flexion.

The **posterior longitudinal ligament** is a much narrower, somewhat weaker band than the anterior longitudinal ligament (Fig. 4.17; see also 4.18B). The posterior longitudinal ligament runs within the vertebral canal along the posterior aspect of the vertebral bodies. It is attached mainly to the IV discs and less so to the posterior aspects of the vertebral bodies from C2 to the sacrum, often bridging fat and vessels between the ligament and the bony surface. This ligament weakly resists hyperflexion of the vertebral column and helps prevent or redirect posterior herniation of the nucleus pulposus. It is well provided with nociceptive (pain) nerve endings.

Movements of Vertebral Column

The range of movement of the vertebral column varies according to the region and the individual. Contortionists, who begin their training during early childhood, become capable of extraordinary movements. The normal range of movement possible in healthy young adults is typically reduced by 50% or more as they age.

The mobility of the vertebral column results primarily from the compressibility and elasticity of the IV discs. The vertebral column is capable of flexion, extension, lateral flexion and extension, and rotation (torsion) (Fig. 4.22). Bending of the vertebral column to the right or left from the neutral (erect) position is *lateral flexion;* returning to the erect posture from a position of lateral flexion is *lateral extension.*

The range of movement of the vertebral column is limited by the:

- Thickness, elasticity, and compressibility of the IV discs.
- Shape and orientation of the zygapophysial joints.
- Tension of the joint capsules of the zygapophysial joints.
- Resistance of the back muscles and ligaments (e.g., the ligamenta flava and the posterior longitudinal ligament).
- Attachment to the thoracic (rib) cage.
- Bulk of surrounding tissue.

Movements are not produced exclusively by the back muscles. They are assisted by gravity and the action of the anterolateral abdominal muscles. Movements between adjacent vertebrae occur at the resilient nuclei pulposi of the IV discs (serving as the axis of movement) and at the zygapophysial joints (Figs. 4.14 and 4.15).

The orientation of the latter joints permits some movements and restricts others. With the exception perhaps of C1–C2, movement never occurs at a single segment of the column. Although movements between adjacent vertebrae are relatively small, especially in the thoracic region, the summation of all the small movements produces a considerable range of movement of the vertebral column as a whole (e.g., when flexing to touch the floor; Fig. 4.22A). Movements of the vertebral column are freer in the cervical and lumbar regions than elsewhere. Flexion, extension, lateral flexion, and rotation of the neck are especially free because the:

- IV discs, although thin relative to most other discs, are thick relative to the size of the vertebral bodies at this level.
- Articular surfaces of the zygapophysial joints are relatively large and the joint planes are almost horizontal.
- Joint capsules of the zygapophysial joints are loose.
- Neck is relatively slender (with less surrounding soft tissue bulk compared with the trunk).

Flexion of the vertebral column is greatest in the cervical region. The sagittally oriented joint planes of the lumbar region are conducive to flexion and extension. Extension of the vertebral column is most marked in the lumbar region and is usually more extensive than flexion; however, the interlocking articular processes here prevent rotation (Fig. 4.9). The lumbar region, like the cervical region, has IV discs that are large relative to the size of the vertebral bodies. Lateral flexion of the vertebral column is greatest in the cervical and lumbar regions (Fig. 4.22B).

The thoracic region, in contrast, has IV discs that are thin relative to the size of the vertebral bodies. Relative stability is also conferred on this part of the vertebral column through its connection to the sternum by the ribs and costal cartilages. The joint planes here lie on an arc that is centered on the vertebral body, permitting rotation in the thoracic region (Fig. 4.22C). This rotation of the upper trunk, in combination with the rotation permitted in the cervical region and that at the atlanto-axial joints, enables the torsion of the axial skeleton that occurs as one looks back over the shoulder. However, flexion is limited in the thoracic region, including lateral flexion.

Curvatures of Vertebral Column

The vertebral column in adults has four *curvatures* that occur in the cervical, thoracic, lumbar, and sacral regions (Fig. 4.23). The **thoracic** and **sacral kyphoses** (singular = **kyphosis**) are concave anteriorly, whereas the **cervical** and **lumbar lordoses** (singular = **lordosis**) are concave posteriorly. When the posterior surface of the trunk is observed, especially in a lateral view, the normal curvatures of the vertebral column are especially apparent (Fig. 4.24).

The thoracic and sacral kyphoses are **primary curvatures** that develop during the fetal period in relationship

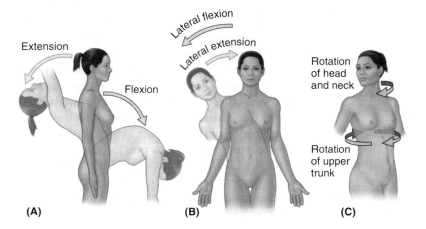

FIGURE 4.22. Movements of vertebral column. A. Flexion and extension, both in the median plane, are shown. Flexion and extension are occurring primarily in the cervical and lumbar regions. **B.** Lateral flexion (to the right or left in a frontal plane) is shown, also occurring mostly in the cervical and lumbar regions. **C.** Rotation around a longitudinal axis, which occurs primarily at the craniovertebral joints (augmented by the cervical region) and the thoracic region, is shown.

Curvatures:

Cervical (2°)

Thoracic (1°)

Lumbar (2°)

Sacral (1°)

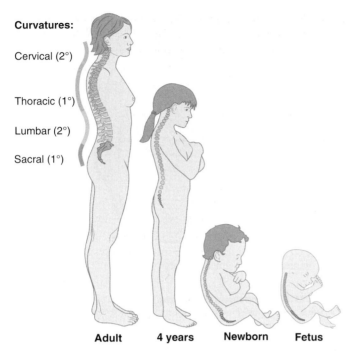

Adult   4 years   Newborn   Fetus

FIGURE 4.23. Curvatures of vertebral column. The four curvatures of the adult vertebral column—cervical, thoracic, lumbar, and sacral—are contrasted with the C-shaped curvature of the column during fetal life, when only the primary (1°) curvatures exist. The secondary (2°) curvatures develop during infancy and childhood.

to the (flexed) fetal position (Moore et al., 2012). Compare the curvatures in Figure 4.23, noting that the primary curvatures are in the same direction as the main curvatures of the fetal vertebral column. The primary curvatures are retained throughout life as a consequence of differences in height between the anterior and posterior parts of the vertebrae.

The cervical and lumbar lordoses are **secondary curvatures** that result from extension from the flexed fetal position. They begin to appear during the late fetal period but do not become obvious until infancy. Secondary curvatures are maintained primarily by differences in thickness between the anterior and the posterior parts of the IV discs.

The *cervical lordosis* becomes fully evident when an infant begins to raise (extend) the head while prone and to hold the head erect while sitting. The *lumbar lordosis* becomes apparent when toddlers begin to assume the upright posture, standing and walking. This curvature, generally more pronounced in females, ends at the *lumbosacral angle* formed at the junction of L5 vertebra with the sacrum (Fig. 4.1D). The *sacral kyphosis* also differs in males and females, that of the female reduced so that the coccyx protrudes less into the pelvic outlet (see Chapter 3).

The curvatures of the vertebral column provide additional flexibility (shock-absorbing resilience), further augmenting that provided by the IV discs. When the load borne by the vertebral column is markedly increased (as by carrying a heavy backpack), both the IV discs and the flexible curvatures are compressed (i.e., the curvatures tend to increase).

While the flexibility provided by the IV discs is passive and limited primarily by the zygapophysial joints and

Cervical lordosis (2° curvature)

Thoracic kyphosis (1° curvature)

Lumbar lordosis (2° curvature)

Sacral kyphosis (1° curvature)

Lateral view

FIGURE 4.24. Surface anatomy of curvatures of vertebral column.

longitudinal ligaments, that provided by the curvatures is actively (dynamically) resisted by the contraction of muscle groups antagonistic to the movement (e.g., the long extensors of the back resist excessive thoracic kyphosis, whereas the abdominal flexors resist excessive lumbar lordosis).

Carrying additional weight anterior to the body's normal gravitational axis (e.g., abnormally large breasts, a pendulous abdomen in men or during late pregnancy, or carrying a young child) also tends to increase these curvatures. The muscles that provide resistance to the increase in curvature often ache when the weight is borne for extended periods.

When sitting, especially in the absence of back support for long periods of time, one usually "cycles" between back flexion (slumping) and extension (sitting up straight) to minimize stiffness and fatigue. This allows alternation between the active support provided by the extensor muscles of the back and the passive resistance to flexion provided by ligaments.

Vasculature of Vertebral Column

Vertebrae are supplied by *periosteal* and *equatorial branches* of the major cervical and *segmental arteries* and their **spinal branches** (Fig. 4.25). Parent arteries of periosteal, equatorial, and spinal branches occur at all levels of the vertebral column, in close association with it, and include the following arteries (described in detail in other chapters):

- *Vertebral* and *ascending cervical arteries* in the neck (Chapter 8).
- The major *segmental arteries* of the trunk:
  - *Posterior intercostal arteries* in the thoracic region (Chapter 1).
  - *Subcostal* and *lumbar arteries* in the abdomen (Chapter 2).
  - *Iliolumbar* and *lateral and medial sacral arteries* in the pelvis (Chapter 3).

Periosteal and **equatorial branches** arise from these arteries as they cross the external (anterolateral) surfaces of the vertebrae. Spinal branches enter the IV foramina and divide. Smaller **anterior** and **posterior vertebral canal branches** pass to the vertebral body and vertebral arch, respectively, and give rise to ascending and descending branches that anastomose with the spinal canal branches of adjacent levels (Fig. 4.25). Anterior vertebral canal branches send **nutrient arteries** anteriorly into the vertebral bodies that supply most of the red marrow of the central vertebral body (Bogduk, 2012). The larger branches of the spinal branches continue as terminal *radicular* or *segmental medullary arteries* distributed to the posterior and anterior roots of the spinal nerves and their coverings and to the spinal cord, respectively (see "Vasculature of Spinal Cord and Spinal Nerve Roots," p. 501).

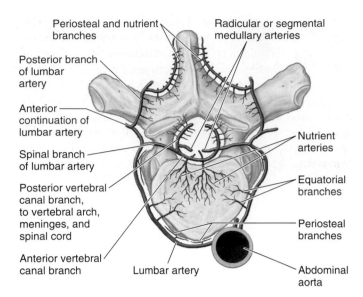

FIGURE 4.25. Blood supply of vertebrae. Typical vertebrae are supplied by segmental arteries—here lumbar arteries. In the thoracic and lumbar regions, each vertebra is encircled on three sides by paired intercostal or lumbar arteries that arise from the aorta. The segmental arteries supply equatorial branches to the vertebral body, and posterior branches supply the vertebral arch structures and the back muscles. Spinal branches enter the vertebral canal through the IV foramina to supply the bones, periosteum, ligaments, and meninges that bound the epidural space and radicular or segmental medullary arteries that supply nervous tissue (spinal nerve roots and spinal cord).

Spinal veins form venous plexuses along the vertebral column both inside and outside the vertebral canal. These plexuses are the **internal vertebral venous plexuses** (epidural venous plexuses) and **external vertebral venous plexuses,** respectively (Fig. 4.26). These plexuses communicate through the intervertebral foramina. Both plexuses are densest

(A) Superior view

(B) Median section

FIGURE 4.26. Venous drainage of vertebral column. A. The venous drainage parallels the arterial supply and enters the external and internal vertebral venous plexuses. There is also anterolateral drainage from the external aspects of the vertebrae into segmental veins. **B.** The dense plexus of thin-walled vessels within the vertebral canal, the internal vertebral venous plexuses, consists of valveless anastomoses between anterior and posterior longitudinal venous sinuses.

anteriorly and posteriorly and relatively sparse laterally. The large, tortuous **basivertebral veins** form within the vertebral bodies. They emerge from foramina on the surfaces of the vertebral bodies (mostly the posterior aspect) and drain into the anterior external and especially the anterior internal vertebral venous plexuses, which may form large longitudinal sinuses. The **intervertebral veins** receive veins from the spinal cord and vertebral venous plexuses as they accompany the spinal nerves through the IV foramina to drain into the *vertebral veins* of the neck and *segmental* (*intercostal, lumbar,* and *sacral*) *veins* of the trunk (Figs. 4.26A and 4.27).

Nerves of Vertebral Column

Other than the zygapophysial joints (innervated by *articular branches of the medial branches of the posterior rami,* as described with these joints), the vertebral column is innervated by (**recurrent**) **meningeal branches of the spinal nerves** (Fig. 4.27). These small branches are the only branches to arise from the *mixed spinal nerve,* arising immediately after it is formed and before its division into anterior and posterior rami, or from the anterior ramus immediately after its formation.

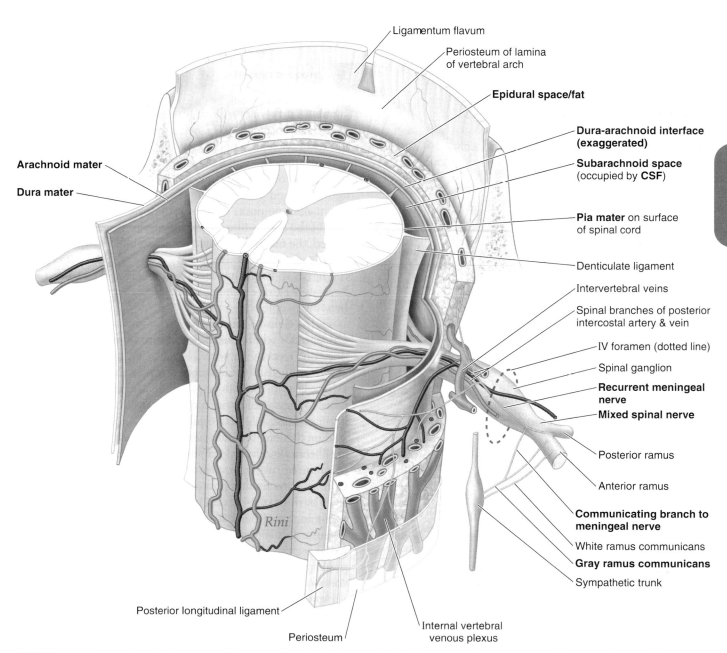

FIGURE 4.27. Innervation of periosteum and ligaments of vertebral column and of meninges. Except for the zygapophysial joints and external elements of the vertebral arch, the fibroskeletal structures of the vertebral column (and the meninges) are supplied by the (recurrent) meningeal nerves. Although usually omitted from diagrams and illustrations of spinal nerves, these fine nerves are the first branches to arise from all 31 pairs of spinal nerves and are the nerves that initially convey localized pain sensation from the back produced by acute herniation of an IV disc or from sprains, contusions, fractures, or tumors of the vertebral column itself. (Based on Frick H, Kummer B, Putz R. *Wolf-Heidegger's atlas of human anatomy,* 4th ed. Basel: Karger AG, 1990:476.)

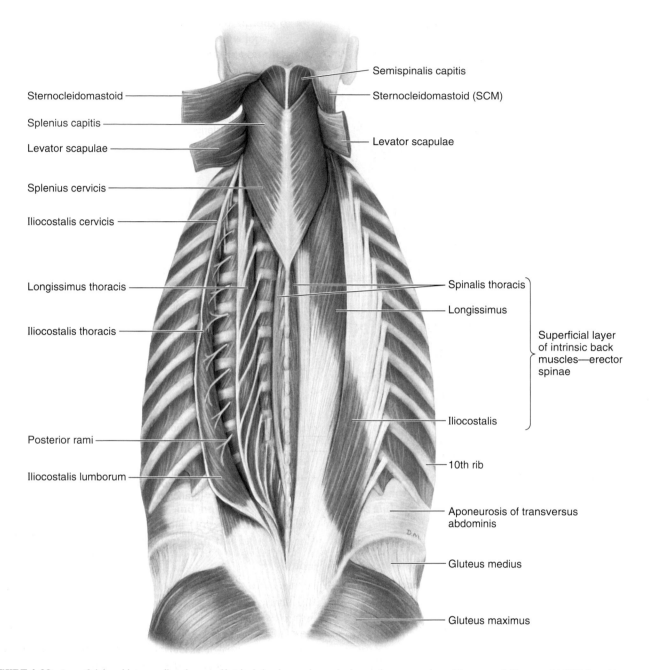

FIGURE 4.29. Superficial and intermediate layers of intrinsic back muscles: splenius and erector spinae. The sternocleidomastoid (SCM) and levator scapulae muscles are reflected to reveal the splenius capitis and splenius cervicis muscles. On the right side, the erector spinae is undisturbed (in situ) and shows the three columns of this massive muscle. On the left side, the spinalis muscle, the thinnest and most medial of the erector spinae columns, is displayed as a separate muscle by reflecting the longissimus and iliocostalis columns of the erector spinae. As they ascend, the direction of fibers is different in the three main groups of muscles: the superficial (splenius) muscles run from medial to lateral, the intermediate (erector spinae) muscles run mostly vertically, and the deep (transversospinalis) muscles run mainly from lateral to medial (see Fig. 4.32).

by *deep fascia* that attaches medially to the nuchal ligament, the tips of the spinous processes of the vertebrae, the supraspinous ligament, and the median crest of the sacrum. The fascia attaches laterally to the cervical and lumbar transverse processes and the angles of the ribs. The thoracic and lumbar parts of the deep fascia constitute the *thoracolumbar fascia*.

It extends laterally from the spinous processes and forms a thin covering over the intrinsic back muscles in the thoracic region and a strong thick covering for muscles in the lumbar region. The intrinsic back muscles are grouped into superficial, intermediate, and deep layers according to their relationship to the surface.

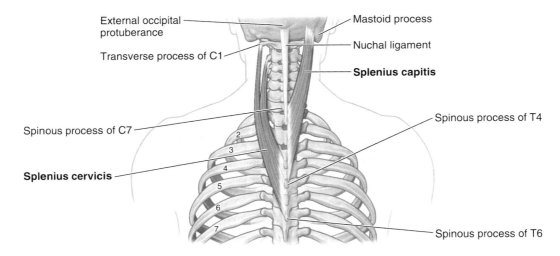

External occipital protuberance

Transverse process of C1

Spinous process of C7

Splenius cervicis

Mastoid process

Nuchal ligament

Splenius capitis

Spinous process of T4

Spinous process of T6

2
3
4
5
6
7

FIGURE 4.30. Superficial layer of intrinsic back muscles (splenius muscles).

TABLE 4.4. SUPERFICIAL LAYER OF INTRINSIC BACK MUSCLES

Muscle	Proximal Attachment	Distal Attachment	Nerve Supply	Main Action(s)
Splenius	Nuchal ligament and spinous processes of C7–T6 vertebrae	*Splenius capitis:* fibers run superolaterally to mastoid process of temporal bone and lateral third of superior nuchal line of occipital bone. *Splenius cervicis:* tubercles of transverse processes of C1–C3 or C4 vertebrae	Posterior rami of spinal nerves	*Acting alone:* laterally flex neck and rotate head to side of active muscles. *Acting together:* extend head and neck

SUPERFICIAL LAYER

The **splenius muscles** (L. *musculi splenii*) are thick and flat and lie on the lateral and posterior aspects of the neck, covering the vertical muscles somewhat like a bandage, which explains their name (L. *splenion,* bandage) (Figs. 4.29 and 4.30). The splenius muscles arise from the midline and extend superolaterally to the cervical vertebrae (**splenius cervicis**) and cranium (**splenius capitis**). The splenius muscles cover and hold the deep neck muscles in position. The superficial layer of intrinsic muscles is illustrated in Figure 4.30, and information on their attachments, nerve supply, and actions is provided in Table 4.4.

INTERMEDIATE LAYER

The massive **erector spinae muscles** lie in a "groove" on each side of the vertebral column between the spinous processes centrally and the angles of the ribs laterally (Fig. 4.29). The erector spinae are the *chief extensors of the vertebral column* and are divided into three columns: The **iliocostalis** forms the lateral column, the **longissimus** forms the intermediate column, and the **spinalis** forms the medial column. Each column is divided regionally into three parts according to the superior attachments (e.g., iliocostalis lumborum, iliocostalis thoracis, and iliocostalis cervicis). The common

origin of the three erector spinae columns is through a broad tendon that attaches inferiorly to the posterior part of the iliac crest, the posterior aspect of the sacrum, the sacro-iliac ligaments, and the sacral and inferior lumbar spinous processes.

The erector spinae are often referred to as the "long muscles" of the back. In general, they are dynamic (motion-producing) muscles, acting bilaterally to extend (straighten) the flexed trunk. The muscles of the intermediate layer of intrinsic muscles are illustrated in isolation in Figure 4.31, and information on their attachments, nerve supply, and actions is provided in Table 4.5.

DEEP LAYER

Deep to the erector spinae is an obliquely disposed group of much shorter muscles, the **transversospinalis muscle group** consisting of the semispinalis, multifidus, and rotatores. These muscles originate from transverse processes of vertebrae and pass to spinous processes of more superior vertebrae. They occupy the "gutter" between the transverse and the spinous processes and are attached to these processes, the laminae between them, and the ligaments linking them together (Fig. 4.32).

(text continues on p. 488)

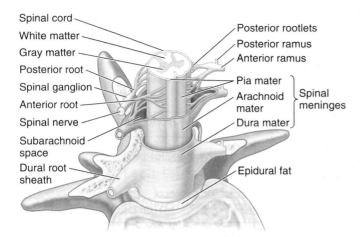

Spinal cord
White matter
Gray matter
Posterior root
Spinal ganglion
Anterior root
Spinal nerve
Subarachnoid space
Dural root sheath

Posterior rootlets
Posterior ramus
Anterior ramus
Pia mater
Arachnoid mater
Dura mater
} Spinal meninges
Epidural fat

FIGURE 4.41. Spinal cord, spinal nerves, and spinal meninges. Three membranes (the spinal meninges) cover the spinal cord: dura mater, arachnoid mater, and pia mater. As the spinal nerve roots extend toward an IV foramen, they are surrounded by a dural root sheath (sleeve) that is continuous distally with the epineurium of the spinal nerve.

posterior and anterior nerve roots as **dural root sheaths,** or sleeves (Figs. 4.41 and 4.44). Distal to the spinal ganglia, these sheaths blend with the **epineurium** (outer connective tissue covering of spinal nerves) that adheres to the periosteum lining the IV foramina.

Innervation of Dura Mater. Nerve fibers are distributed to the spinal dura by the (*recurrent*) *meningeal nerves* (see Fig. 4.27). The function of these afferent and sympathetic fibers is unclear, although it is known that the afferent fibers supply pain receptors that are involved in the referred pain characteristic of spinal disorders and become irritated when there is inflammation of the meninges (*meningitis*).

SPINAL ARACHNOID MATER

The **spinal arachnoid mater** is a delicate, avascular membrane composed of fibrous and elastic tissue that lines the spinal dural sac and its dural root sheaths. It encloses the CSF-filled subarachnoid space containing the spinal cord,

Extradural (epidural) space occupied by fat
Arachnoid mater
Posterior root
Spinal dural sac
Spinal nerve
Intervertebral foramen (above pedicle)
Intervertebral vein

Dura-arachnoid interface [subdural (potential) "space"]–**Schematically exaggerated; see note in table**

Posterior spinal arteries
Periosteum covering surface of compact bone
Internal vertebral venous plexus

CSF in subarachnoid space
Denticulate ligament (pia mater)
Anterior root
Spinal dura mater
Pia mater
Vertebral body
Anterior spinal artery
Spinal cord
Arachnoid trabeculae

FIGURE 4.42. Cross-section of spinal cord in situ demonstrating meninges and associated spaces.

TABLE 4.14. SPACES ASSOCIATED WITH SPINAL MENINGES[a]

Space	Location	Contents
Epidural	Space between periosteum lining bony wall of vertebral canal and spinal dura mater	Fat (loose connective tissue); internal vertebral venous plexuses; inferior to L2 vertebra, ensheathed roots of spinal nerves
Subarachnoid (leptomeningeal)	Naturally occurring space between arachnoid mater and pia mater	CSF; radicular, segmental, medullary, and spinal arteries; veins; arachnoid trabeculae

[a]Although it is common to refer to a "subdural space," there is no naturally occurring space at the arachnoid–dura junction (Haines, 2006).

spinal nerve roots, and spinal ganglia (Figs. 4.41, 4.42, and 4.43).

The spinal arachnoid is not attached to the spinal dura but is held against its inner surface by the pressure of the CSF. In a lumbar spinal puncture, the needle traverses the spinal dura and arachnoid simultaneously. Their apposition is the **dura–arachnoid interface** (Fig. 4.42), often erroneously referred to as the "subdural space." No actual space occurs naturally at this site; it is, rather, a weak cell layer (Haines, 2006). Bleeding into this layer creates a pathological space at the dura–arachnoid junction in which a *subdural hematoma* is formed. In the cadaver, because of the absence of CSF, the spinal arachnoid falls away from the inner surface of the dura and lies loosely on the spinal cord.

The spinal arachnoid is separated from the pia mater on the surface of the spinal cord by the *subarachnoid space* containing CSF. Delicate strands of connective tissue, the **arachnoid trabeculae,** span the subarachnoid space connecting the spinal arachnoid and pia.

SPINAL PIA MATER

The **spinal pia mater,** the innermost covering membrane of the spinal cord, is thin and transparent, and closely follows all the surface features of the spinal cord (Haines, 2006). The spinal pia also directly covers the roots of the spinal nerves and the spinal blood vessels. Inferior to the conus medullaris, the spinal pia continues as the filum terminale (Fig. 4.39).

The spinal cord is suspended in the dural sac by the *filum terminale* and the right and left **denticulate ligaments** (L. *denticulus,* small tooth), which run longitudinally along each side of the spinal cord (Figs. 4.43–4.45). The denticulate ligaments consist of a fibrous sheet of pia extending midway between the posterior and anterior nerve roots from the lateral surfaces of the spinal cord. The 20–22 sawtooth-like processes attach to the inner surface of the arachnoid-lined dural sac. The most superior process of the right and left denticulate ligaments attaches to the cranial dura immediately superior to the foramen magnum, and the inferior process extends from the conus medullaris, passing between the T12 and the L1 nerve roots.

SUBARACHNOID SPACE

The **subarachnoid space** is located between the arachnoid and pia mater and is filled with CSF (Figs. 4.41–4.43). The enlargement of the subarachnoid space in the dural sac, caudal to the conus medullaris and containing CSF and the cauda equina, is the **lumbar cistern** (Figs. 4.39 and 4.40). It extends from the L2 vertebra to the second segment of the sacrum. Dural root sheaths, enclosing spinal nerve roots in extensions of the subarachnoid space, protrude from the sides of the lumbar cistern (Fig. 4.44A & B).

Vasculature of Spinal Cord and Spinal Nerve Roots

ARTERIES OF SPINAL CORD AND NERVE ROOTS

The arteries supplying the spinal cord are branches of the vertebral, ascending cervical, deep cervical, intercostal, lumbar, and lateral sacral arteries (Figs. 4.46 and 4.47). Three longitudinal arteries supply the spinal cord: an *anterior*

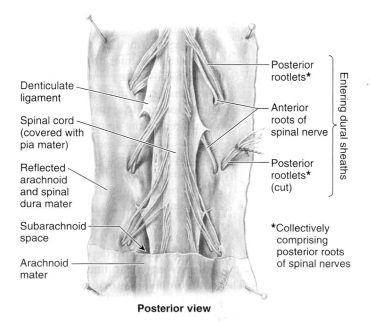

Denticulate ligament

Spinal cord (covered with pia mater)

Reflected arachnoid and spinal dura mater

Subarachnoid space

Arachnoid mater

Posterior rootlets*

Anterior roots of spinal nerve

Posterior rootlets* (cut)

Entering dural sheaths

*Collectively comprising posterior roots of spinal nerves

Posterior view

FIGURE 4.43. Spinal cord within its meninges. The spinal dura and arachnoid mater have been split and pinned flat to expose the spinal cord and denticulate ligaments between posterior and anterior spinal nerve roots.

Lumbar puncture is not performed in the presence of increased intracranial pressure (within the cranial cavity). The intracranial pressure is generally previously determined by CT scanning, but may also be determined by examination of the fundus (back) of the interior of the eyeball with an ophthalmoscope (see blue box "Papilledema," p. 911).

Spinal Anesthesia

An anesthetic agent is injected into the subarachnoid space. Anesthesia usually occurs within 1 minute. A headache may follow *spinal anesthesia,* which likely results from the leakage of CSF through the lumbar puncture. (See also the blue box "Anesthesia for Childbirth," p. 397.)

Epidural Anesthesia (Blocks)

An anesthetic agent is injected into the epidural space using the position described for lumbar spinal puncture, or through the sacral hiatus (caudal epidural anesthesia/block). (See also the blue box "Anesthesia for Childbirth," p. 397.)

Ischemia of Spinal Cord

The segmental reinforcements of the blood supply to the spinal cord from the segmental medullary arteries are important in supplying blood to the anterior and posterior spinal arteries. Fractures, dislocations, and fracture–dislocations may interfere with the blood supply to the spinal cord from the spinal and medullary arteries.

Deficient blood supply (ischemia) of the spinal cord affects its function and can lead to muscle weakness and paralysis. The spinal cord may also suffer circulatory impairment if the segmental medullary arteries, particularly the great anterior segmental medullary artery (of Adamkiewicz), are narrowed by *obstructive arterial disease.*

Sometimes the aorta is purposely occluded (cross clamped) during surgery. Patients undergoing such surgeries, and those with ruptured aneurysms of the aorta or occlusion of the great anterior segmental medullary artery, may lose all sensation and voluntary movement inferior to the level of impaired blood supply to the spinal cord (*paraplegia*) secondary to death of neurons in the part of the spinal cord supplied by the anterior spinal artery (Figs. 4.46 and 4.47).

Neurons with cell bodies distant from the site of ischemia of the spinal cord will also die, secondary to the degeneration of axons traversing the site. The likelihood of *iatrogenic paraplegia* depends on such factors as the age of the patient,

the extent of the disease, and the length of time the aorta is cross clamped.

When systemic blood pressure drops severely for 3–6 min, blood flow from the segmental medullary arteries to the anterior spinal artery supplying the midthoracic region of the spinal cord may be reduced or stopped. These people may also lose sensation and voluntary movement in the areas supplied by the affected level of the spinal cord.

Spinal Cord Injuries

The vertebral canal varies considerably in size and shape from level to level, particularly in the cervical and lumbar regions. A narrow vertebral canal in the cervical region, into which the spinal cord fits tightly, is potentially dangerous because a minor fracture and/or dislocation of a cervical vertebra may damage the spinal cord. The protrusion of a cervical IV disc into the vertebral canal after a neck injury may cause *spinal cord shock* associated with paralysis inferior to the site of the lesion.

In some people, no fracture or dislocation of cervical vertebrae can be found. If the individual dies and an autopsy is performed, a softening of the spinal cord may be detected at the site of the cervical disc protrusion. Encroachment of the vertebral canal by a protruding IV disc, by swollen ligamenta flava, or resulting from *osteoarthritis of the zygapophysial joints* may exert pressure on one or more of the spinal nerve roots of the cauda equina. Pressure may produce sensory and motor symptoms in the area of distribution of the involved spinal nerve. This group of bone and joint abnormalities, called *lumbar spondylosis* (degenerative joint disease), also causes localized pain and stiffness.

Transection of the spinal cord results in loss of all sensation and voluntary movement inferior to the lesion. Transection between the following levels will result in the indicated effects:

- C1–C3: no function below head level; a ventilator is required to maintain respiration.
- C4–C5: *quadriplegia* (no function of upper and lower limbs); respiration occurs.
- C6–C8: loss of lower limb function combined with a loss of hand and a variable amount of upper limb function; the individual may be able to self-feed or propel a wheelchair.
- T1–T9 *paraplegia* (paralysis of both lower limbs); the amount of trunk control varies with the height of the lesion.
- T10–L1: some thigh muscle function, which may allow walking with long leg braces.
- L2–L3: retention of most leg muscle function; short leg braces may be required for walking.

The Bottom Line

CONTENTS OF VERTEBRAL CANAL

The spinal cord, spinal nerve roots, CSF, and meninges that surround them are the main contents of the vertebral canal.

Spinal cord: In adults, the spinal cord occupies only the superior two thirds of the vertebral canal and has two (cervical and lumbosacral) enlargements related to innervation of the limbs. ♦ The inferior, tapering end of the spinal cord, the conus medullaris, ends at the level of the L1 or L2 vertebra. ♦ However, the filum terminale and spinal nerve roots from the lumbosacral part of the spinal cord that form the cauda equina continue inferiorly within the lumbar cistern containing CSF.

Spinal meninges and CSF: Nerve tissues and neurovascular structures of the vertebral canal are suspended in CSF contained within the dural sac and dural root sheaths. ♦ The fluid-filled subarachnoid space is lined with pia and arachnoid mater, which are continuous membranes (leptomeninges). ♦ Because the spinal cord does not extend into the lumbar cistern (the inferior part of the subarachnoid space), it is an ideal site for sampling CSF or for injection of anesthetic agents.

Vasculature of spinal cord and spinal nerve roots: Longitudinal spinal arteries supplying the spinal cord are reinforced by asymmetric segmental medullary arteries occurring at irregular levels (mostly in association with the cervical and lumbar enlargements) that also supply the spinal nerve roots at those levels ♦ At levels and on the sides where segmental medullary arteries do not occur, radicular arteries supply the nerve roots. ♦ The veins draining the spinal cord have a distribution and drainage generally reflective of the spinal arteries, although there are normally three longitudinal spinal veins both anteriorly and posteriorly.

thePoint   **Board-review questions, case studies, and additional resources are available at thePoint.lww.com.**

for the upper limbs) (Fig. 5.2A). Both limbs initially extend from the trunk with their developing thumbs and great toes directed superiorly and the palms and soles directed anteriorly. Both limbs then undergo torsion around their long axes, but in opposite directions (Fig. 5.2B–D).

The medial rotation and permanent pronation of the lower limb explain how:

- the knee, unlike the joints superior to it, extends anteriorly and flexes posteriorly, as do the joints inferior to the knee (e.g., interphalangeal joints of the toes);
- the foot becomes oriented with the great toe on the medial side (Fig. 5.2D), whereas the hand (in the anatomical position) becomes oriented with the thumb on the lateral side; and
- the "barber-pole" pattern of the segmental innervation of the skin (dermatomes) of the lower limb develops (see "Cutaneous Innervation of Lower Limb," p. 536).

The torsion and twisting of the lower limb is still in progress at birth (note that babies' feet tend to meet sole to sole when they are brought together, like clapping). Completion of the process coincides with the mastering of walking skills.

BONES OF LOWER LIMB

The skeleton of the lower limb (inferior appendicular skeleton) may be divided into two functional components: the pelvic girdle and the bones of the free lower limb (Fig. 5.1). The **pelvic girdle** (bony pelvis) is a bony ring composed of the sacrum and right and left hip bones joined anteriorly at the pubic symphysis.

The pelvic girdle attaches the free lower limb to the axial skeleton, the sacrum being common to the axial skeleton and the pelvic girdle. The pelvic girdle also makes up the skeleton of the lower part of the trunk. Its protective and supportive functions serve the abdomen, pelvis, and perineum as well as the lower limbs. The *bones of the free lower limb* are contained within and specifically serve that part of the limb.

Arrangement of Lower Limb Bones

Body weight is transferred from the vertebral column through the *sacro-iliac joints* to the pelvic girdle and from the pelvic girdle through the hip joints to the femurs (L. *femora*) (Fig. 5.3A).

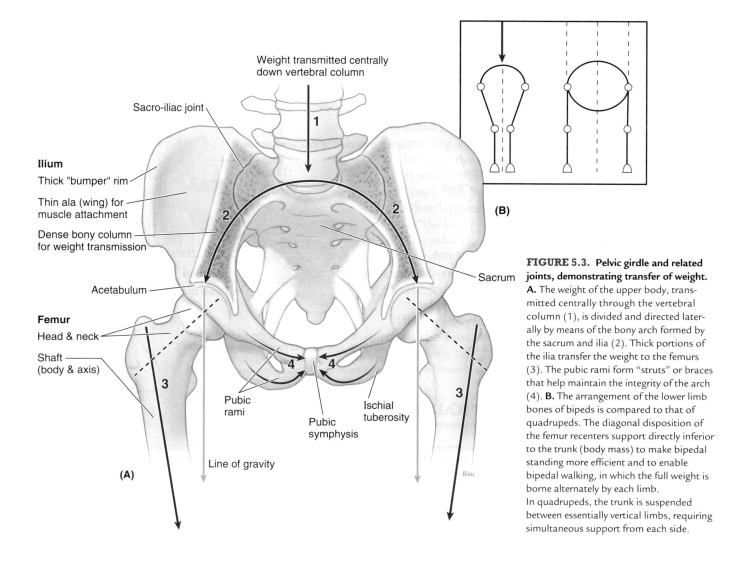

FIGURE 5.3. Pelvic girdle and related joints, demonstrating transfer of weight. **A.** The weight of the upper body, transmitted centrally through the vertebral column (1), is divided and directed laterally by means of the bony arch formed by the sacrum and ilia (2). Thick portions of the ilia transfer the weight to the femurs (3). The pubic rami form "struts" or braces that help maintain the integrity of the arch (4). **B.** The arrangement of the lower limb bones of bipeds is compared to that of quadrupeds. The diagonal disposition of the femur recenters support directly inferior to the trunk (body mass) to make bipedal standing more efficient and to enable bipedal walking, in which the full weight is borne alternately by each limb.

In quadrupeds, the trunk is suspended between essentially vertical limbs, requiring simultaneous support from each side.

To support the erect bipedal posture better, the femurs are oblique (directed inferomedially) within the thighs so that when standing the knees are adjacent and placed directly inferior to the trunk, returning the center of gravity to the vertical lines of the supporting legs and feet (Figs. 5.1, 5.3, and 5.4). Compare this oblique position of the femurs with that of quadrupeds, in whom the femurs are vertical and the knees are apart, with the trunk mass suspended between the limbs (Fig. 5.3B).

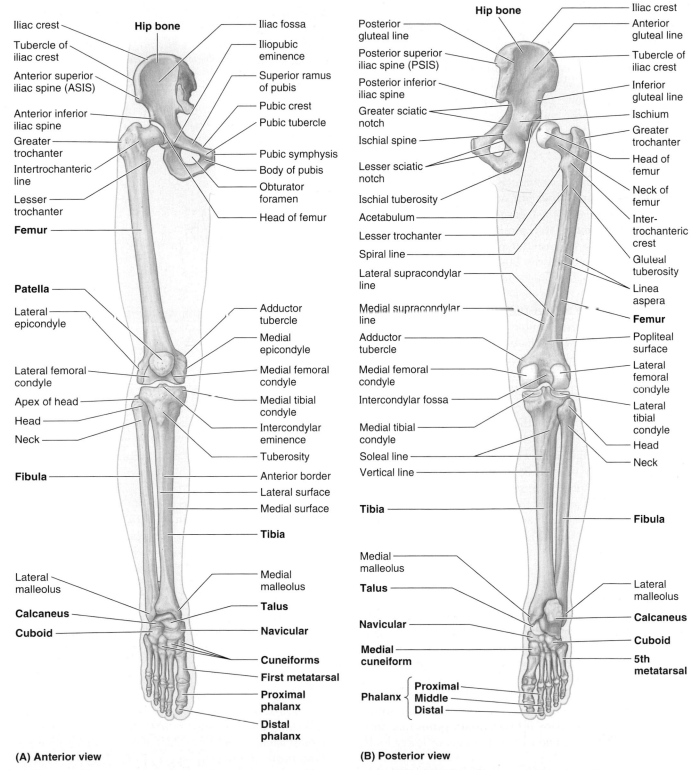

(A) Anterior view

(B) Posterior view

FIGURE 5.4. Bones of lower limb. A and B. Individual bones and bony formations are identified. The foot is in full plantarflexion. The hip joint is disarticulated (**B**) to demonstrate the acetabulum of the hip bone, which receives the head of the femur.

The femurs of human females are slightly more oblique than those of males, reflecting the greater width of their pelves. At the knees, the distal end of each femur articulates with the patella and tibia of the corresponding leg. Weight is transferred from the knee joint to the ankle joint by the tibia. The fibula does not articulate with the femur and does not bear or transfer weight, but it provides for muscle attachment and contributes to the formation of the ankle joint.

At the ankle, the weight borne by the tibia is transferred to the *talus* (Fig. 5.4). The talus is the keystone of a longitudinal arch formed by the tarsal and metatarsal bones of each foot that distributes the weight evenly between the heel and forefoot when standing, creating a flexible but stable bony platform to support the body.

Hip Bone

The mature **hip bone** (L. *os coxae*) is the large, flat pelvic bone formed by the fusion of three primary bones—*ilium, ischium,* and *pubis*—at the end of the teenage years. Each of the three bones is formed from its own primary center of ossification; five secondary centers of ossification appear later.

At birth, the three primary bones are joined by hyaline cartilage; in children, they are incompletely ossified (Fig. 5.5). At puberty, the three bones are still separated by a Y-shaped **triradiate cartilage** centered in the acetabulum, although the two parts of the ischiopubic rami fuse by the 9th year (Fig. 5.5B). The bones begin to fuse between 15 and 17 years of age; fusion is complete between 20 and 25 years of age. Little or no trace of the lines of fusion of the primary bones is visible in older adults (Fig. 5.6). Although the bony components are rigidly fused, their names are still used in adults to describe the three parts of the hip bone.

Because much of the medial aspect of the hip bones/bony pelvis is primarily concerned with pelvic and perineal structures and functions (Chapter 3) or their union with the vertebral column (Chapter 4), it is described more thoroughly in those chapters. Aspects of the hip bones concerned with lower limb structures and functions, mainly involving their lateral aspects, are described in this chapter.

ILIUM

The **ilium** forms the largest part of the hip bone and contributes the superior part of the acetabulum (Fig. 5.5B). The ilium has thick medial portions (columns) for weight bearing and thin, wing-like, posterolateral portions, the **alae** (L. wings), that provide broad surfaces for the fleshy attachment of muscles (Fig. 5.3).

The **body of the ilium** joins the pubis and ischium to form the acetabulum. Anteriorly, the ilium has stout **anterior superior** and **anterior inferior iliac spines** that provide attachment for ligaments and tendons of lower limb muscles (Fig. 5.6).

Beginning at the anterior superior iliac spine (ASIS), the long curved and thickened superior border of the ala of the

(A) Anterior view

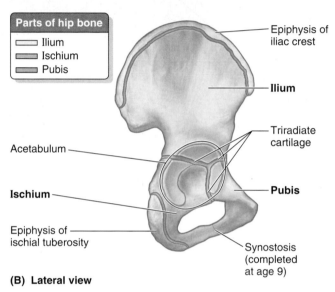

(B) Lateral view

FIGURE 5.5. Parts of hip bones. A. An anteroposterior radiograph of an infant's hips shows the three parts of the incompletely ossified hip bones (ilium, ischium, and pubis). **B.** The right hip bone of a 13-year-old demonstrating the Y-shaped triradiate cartilage.

ilium, the **iliac crest,** extends posteriorly, terminating at the **posterior superior iliac spine** (PSIS). The crest serves as a protective "bumper" and is an important site of aponeurotic attachment for thin, sheet-like muscles and deep fascia. A prominence on the external lip of the crest, the **tubercle of the iliac crest** (iliac tubercle), lies 5–6 cm posterior to the ASIS. The **posterior inferior iliac spine** marks the superior end of the *greater sciatic notch.*

The lateral surface of the ala of the ilium has three rough curved lines—the posterior, anterior, and inferior **gluteal lines**—that demarcate the proximal attachments of the three large gluteal muscles (pl., *glutei*). Medially, each ala has a large, smooth depression, the **iliac fossa** (Fig. 5.6B), that provides proximal attachment for the iliacus muscle. The bone forming the superior part of this fossa may become thin and translucent, especially in older women with osteoporosis.

Posteriorly, the medial aspect of the ilium has a rough, ear-shaped articular area called the **auricular surface** (L. *auricula,* a little ear), and an even rougher **iliac tuberosity**

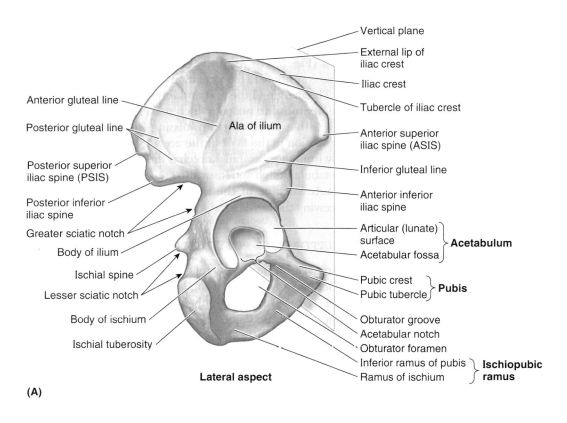

Anterior gluteal line

Posterior gluteal line

Posterior superior iliac spine (PSIS)

Posterior inferior iliac spine

Greater sciatic notch

Body of ilium

Ischial spine

Lesser sciatic notch

Body of ischium

Ischial tuberosity

Ala of ilium

Vertical plane

External lip of iliac crest

Iliac crest

Tubercle of iliac crest

Anterior superior iliac spine (ASIS)

Inferior gluteal line

Anterior inferior iliac spine

Articular (lunate) surface
Acetabular fossa } **Acetabulum**

Pubic crest
Pubic tubercle } **Pubis**

Obturator groove
Acetabular notch
Obturator foramen

Inferior ramus of pubis
Ramus of ischium } **Ischiopubic ramus**

Lateral aspect

(A)

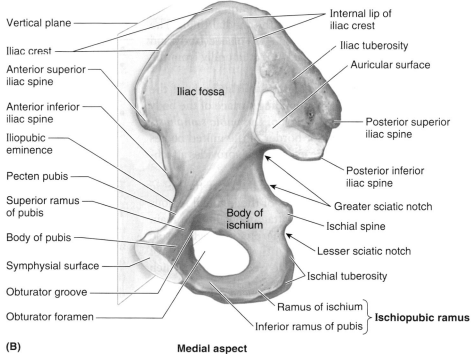

Vertical plane

Iliac crest

Anterior superior iliac spine

Anterior inferior iliac spine

Iliopubic eminence

Pecten pubis

Superior ramus of pubis

Body of pubis

Symphysial surface

Obturator groove

Obturator foramen

Iliac fossa

Body of ischium

Internal lip of iliac crest

Iliac tuberosity

Auricular surface

Posterior superior iliac spine

Posterior inferior iliac spine

Greater sciatic notch

Ischial spine

Lesser sciatic notch

Ischial tuberosity

Ramus of ischium
Inferior ramus of pubis } **Ischiopubic ramus**

(B)   **Medial aspect**

FIGURE 5.6. Right hip bone of adult in anatomical position. In this position, the anterior superior iliac spine (ASIS) and the anterior aspect of the pubis lie in the same coronal plane (blue). **A.** The large hip bone is constricted in the middle and expanded at its superior and inferior ends. **B.** The symphysial surface of the pubis articulates with the corresponding surface of the contralateral hip bone. The auricular surface of the ilium articulates with a corresponding surface of the sacrum to form the sacro-iliac joint.

"hammock" that receives the rounded and anteromedially directed **head of talus.** The hammock (spring ligament) is suspended across a gap between a shelf-like medial projection of the calcaneus (sustentaculum tali) and the navicular bone, which lies anteriorly (Fig. 5.11B & E).

The talus is the only tarsal bone that has no muscular or tendinous attachments. Most of its surface is covered with articular cartilage. The talar body bears the trochlea superiorly and narrows into a *posterior process* that features a **groove for the tendon of the flexor hallucis longus** (Fig. 5.11E), flanked by a prominent **lateral tubercle** and a less prominent **medial tubercle** (Fig. 5.11A & D).

The **calcaneus** (L., heel bone) is the largest and strongest bone in the foot (Fig. 5.11). When standing, the calcaneus transmits the majority of the body's weight from the talus to the ground. The anterior two thirds of the calcaneus's superior surface articulates with the talus and its anterior surface articulates with the cuboid.

The lateral surface of the calcaneus has an oblique ridge (Fig. 5.11D), the **fibular trochlea,** that lies between the tendons of the fibularis longus and brevis. This trochlea anchors a tendon pulley for the evertors of the foot (muscles that move the sole of the foot away from the median plane). The **sustentaculum tali** (L., talar shelf), the shelf-like support of the head of the talus, projects from the superior border of the medial surface of the calcaneus (Fig. 5.11B & E). The posterior part of the calcaneus has a massive, weight-bearing prominence, the **calcaneal tuberosity** (L. *tuber calcanei*), which has **medial, lateral,** and **anterior tubercles.** Only the medial tubercle contacts the ground during standing.

The **navicular** (L., little ship) is a flattened, boat-shaped bone located between the head of the talus posteriorly and the three cuneiforms anteriorly (Fig. 5.11). The medial surface of the navicular projects inferiorly to form the **navicular tuberosity,** an important site for tendon attachment because the medial border of the foot does not rest on the ground, as does the lateral border. Instead, it forms a *longitudinal arch of the foot*, which must be supported centrally. If this tuberosity is too prominent, it may press against the medial part of the shoe and cause foot pain.

The **cuboid,** approximately cubical in shape, is the most lateral bone in the distal row of the tarsus (Fig. 5.11A & D). Anterior to the **tuberosity of the cuboid** on the lateral and inferior surfaces of the bone is a **groove for the tendon of the fibularis** (peroneus) **longus** muscle.

The three cuneiform bones (Fig. 5.11A, D, & E) are the medial (1st), intermediate (2nd), and lateral (3rd). The **medial cuneiform** is the largest bone, and the **intermediate cuneiform** is the smallest. Each cuneiform (L. *cuneus*, wedge shaped) articulates with the navicular posteriorly and the base of its appropriate metatarsal anteriorly. The **lateral cuneiform** also articulates with the cuboid.

METATARSUS

The **metatarsus** (anterior or distal foot, forefoot—Fig. 5.11C) consists of five metatarsals that are numbered from the medial side of the foot (Fig. 5.11A). In the articulated skeleton of the foot (Figs. 5.1, 5.4, and 5.11), the tarsometatarsal joints form an oblique **tarsometatarsal line** joining the midpoints of the medial and shorter lateral borders of the foot. Thus, the metatarsals and phalanges are located in the anterior half (forefoot) and the tarsals are in the posterior half (hindfoot) (Fig. 5.11A & C).

The **1st metatarsal** is shorter and stouter than the others. The **2nd metatarsal** is the longest. Each metatarsal has a base proximally, a shaft, and a head distally (Fig. 5.11C). The base of each metatarsal is the larger, proximal end. The bases of the metatarsals articulate with the cuneiform and cuboid bones, and the heads articulate with the proximal phalanges. The bases of the 1st and 5th metatarsals have large tuberosities that provide for tendon attachment; the **tuberosity of the 5th metatarsal** projects laterally over the cuboid (Fig. 5.11A & D). On the plantar surface of the head of the 1st metatarsal are prominent **medial** and **lateral sesamoid bones** (Fig. 5.11E); they are embedded in the tendons passing along the plantar surface (see the following section on Surface Anatomy).

PHALANGES

The 14 **phalanges** of the lower limb are as follows: the 1st digit (great toe) has 2 phalanges (proximal and distal); the other four digits have 3 phalanges each: proximal, middle, and distal (Fig. 5.11A & D). Each **phalanx** has a **base** (proximally), a **shaft,** and a **head** (distally). The phalanges of the 1st digit are short, broad, and strong. The middle and distal phalanges of the 5th digit may be fused in elderly people.

Surface Anatomy of Bones of Foot

The *head of the talus* is palpable anteromedial to the proximal part of the lateral malleolus when the foot is inverted, and anterior to the medial malleolus when the foot is everted (Fig. 5.12A). Eversion of the foot makes the talar head more prominent as it moves away from the navicular. The head of the talus occupies the space between the sustentaculum tali and the navicular tuberosity. If the talar head is difficult to palpate, draw a line from the tip of the medial malleolus to the navicular tuberosity; the head of the talus lies deep to the center of this line. When the foot is plantarflexed, the superior surface of the body of the talus can be palpated on the anterior aspect of the ankle, anterior to the inferior end of the tibia.

The weight-bearing *medial tubercle of the calcaneus* on the plantar surface of the foot is broad and large (Fig. 5.12D), but often it is not palpable because of the overlying skin and subcutaneous tissue. The *sustentaculum tali* is the only part of the medial aspect of the calcaneus that may be palpated as a small prominence approximately a finger's breadth distal to the tip of the medial malleolus (Fig. 5.12B). The entire lateral surface of the calcaneus is subcutaneous. The *fibular trochlea*, a small lateral extension of the calcaneus, may be detectable as a small tubercle on the lateral aspect of the calcaneus, antero-inferior to the tip of the lateral malleolus (Fig 5.12C).

Usually, palpation of bony prominences on the plantar surface of the foot is difficult because of the thick skin, fascia, and

FIGURE 5.12. Surface projection and palpation of bony prominences of foot.

pads of fat. The medial and lateral *sesamoid bones* inferior to the head of the 1st metatarsal can be felt to slide when the great toe is moved passively. The *heads of the metatarsals* can be palpated by placing the thumb on their plantar surfaces and the index finger on their dorsal surfaces. If *callosities* (calluses), thickenings of the keratin layer of the epidermis, are present, the metatarsal heads are difficult to palpate.

The *tuberosity of the 5th metatarsal* forms a prominent landmark on the lateral aspect of the foot (Fig. 5.12C & D), that can easily be palpated at the midpoint of the lateral border of the foot. The *shafts of the metatarsals and phalanges*

can be felt on the dorsum of the foot between the extensor tendons.

The *cuboid* can be felt on the lateral aspect of the foot, posterior to the base of the 5th metatarsal. The *medial cuneiform* can be palpated between the tuberosity of the navicular and the base of the 1st metatarsal (Fig. 5.12B). The *head of the 1st metatarsal* forms a prominence on the medial aspect of the foot. The *tuberosity of the navicular* is easily seen and palpated on the medial aspect of the foot (Fig. 5.12B), inferoanterior to the tip of the medial malleolus. The cuboid and cuneiforms are difficult to identify individually by palpation.

BONES OF LOWER LIMB

Lower Limb Injuries

Knee, leg, and foot injuries are the most common lower limb injuries. Injuries to the hips make up less than 3% of lower limb injuries. In general, most injuries result from acute trauma during contact sports such as hockey and football and from overuse during endurance sports such as marathon races.

Adolescents are most vulnerable to these injuries because of the demands of sports on their maturing musculoskeletal systems. The cartilaginous models of the bones in the developing lower limbs are transformed into bone by endochondral ossification (Fig. 5.2E & F). Because the process is not completed until early adulthood, cartilaginous epiphysial plates still exist during the teenage years, when physical activity often peaks and involvement in competitive sports is most common.

Lateral view   **Anterior view**

(A) Compound (open) fracture with external bleeding

(B) March (stress) fracture of tibia (*arrows*), most apparent in the MRI study at the right

(C) Diagonal fracture with shortening

(E) Transverse "boot top" fracture with shortening due to over-riding of fracture fragments

(D) Transverse "boot top" fracture

A - E Anterior views

FIGURE B5.4.

In addition, severe torsion during skiing may produce a *diagonal fracture* (Fig. B5.4C) of the tibial shaft at the junction of the middle and inferior thirds, as well as a *fracture of the fibula*. Diagonal fractures are often associated with limb shortening caused by overriding of the fractured ends. Frequently during skiing, a fracture results from a high-speed forward fall, which angles the leg over the rigid ski boot, producing a "boot-top fracture" (Fig. B5.4D & E).

Fractures Involving Epiphysial Plates

  The primary ossification center for the superior end of the tibia appears shortly after birth and joins the shaft of the tibia during adolescence (usually 16–18 years of age). Tibial fractures in children are more serious if they involve the epiphysial plates because continued normal growth of the bone may be jeopardized. The tibial tuberosity usually forms by inferior bone growth from the superior epiphysial center at approximately 10 years of age, but a separate center for the tibial tuberosity may appear at approximately 12 years of age. Disruption of the epiphysial plate at the tibial tuberosity may cause inflammation of the tuberosity and chronic recurring pain during adolescence (*Osgood-Schlatter disease*), especially in young athletes (Fig. B5.5).

Osgood-Schlatter Disease

Prominence of tibial tuberosity (*double arrow*) elongated and fragmented (*single arrow*), with overlying soft tissue swelling

FIGURE B5.5.

Fibular Fractures

Fibular fractures commonly occur 2–6 cm proximal to the distal end of the lateral malleolus and are often associated with *fracture–dislocations of the ankle joint*, which are combined with tibial fractures (Fig. B5.6B). When a person slips and the foot is forced into an excessively inverted position, the ankle ligaments tear, forcibly tilting the talus against the lateral malleolus, and may shear it off (Fig. B5.6C).

Fractures of the lateral and medial malleoli are relatively common in soccer and basketball players. Fibular fractures can be painful owing to disrupted muscle attachments. Walking is compromised because of the bone's role in ankle stability.

Eversion

(A) Tibial and fibular fractures

Inversion

(B) Fibular fracture with excessive inversion of foot

Posterior views

FIGURE B5.6.

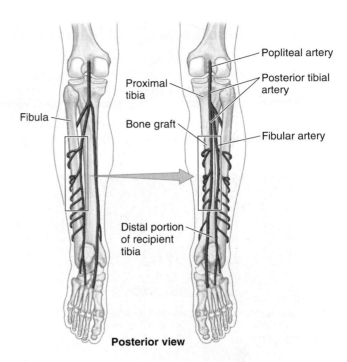

Popliteal artery

Posterior tibial artery

Proximal tibia

Fibula

Bone graft

Fibular artery

Distal portion of recipient tibia

Posterior view

Section of left fibula grafted into right tibia

FIGURE B5.7.

Bone Grafts

If a part of a major bone is destroyed by injury or disease, the limb becomes useless. Replacement of the affected segment by a bone transplant may avoid amputation. The fibula is a common source of bone for grafting. Even after a segment of the shaft has been removed, walking, running, and jumping can be normal.

Free vascularized fibulas have been used to restore skeletal integrity to upper and lower limbs in which congenital bone defects exist and to replace segments of bone after trauma or excision of a malignant tumor (Fig. B5.7). The remaining parts of the fibula usually do not regenerate because the periosteum and nutrient artery are generally removed with the piece of bone, so that the graft will remain alive and grow when transplanted to another site. Secured in its new site, the fibular segment restores the blood supply of the bone to

which it is now attached. Healing proceeds as if a fracture had occurred at each of its ends.

Awareness of the location of the nutrient foramen in the fibula is important when performing free vascularized fibular transfers. Because the nutrient foramen is located in the middle third of the fibula in most cases (Fig. 5.9, posterior view), this segment of the bone is used for transplanting when the graft must include a blood supply to the medullary cavity as well as to the compact bone of the surface (via the periosteum).

Because of its extensive subcutaneous location, the anterior tibia is accessible for obtaining pieces of bone for grafting in children; it is also used as a site for *intramedullary infusion* in dehydrated or shocked children.

Calcaneal Fractures

A hard fall onto the heel, from a ladder for example, may fracture the calcaneus into several pieces, producing a *comminuted fracture* (Fig. B5.8A). A calcaneal fracture is usually disabling because it disrupts the subtalar (talocalcaneal) joint, where the talus articulates with the calcaneus.

Fractures of Talar Neck

Fractures of the talar neck (Fig. B5.8B) may occur during severe dorsiflexion of the ankle (e.g., when a person is pressing extremely hard on the brake pedal of a vehicle during a head-on collision). In some cases, the body of the talus dislocates posteriorly.

POSTURE AND GAIT

The lower limbs function primarily in standing and walking. Typically the actions of lower limb muscles are described as if the muscle were acting in isolation, which rarely occurs.

In this book, including the comments in the tables, the role of each muscle (or of the functional group of which it is a member) is described in typical activities, especially standing and walking. It is important to be familiar with lower limb movements and concentric and eccentric contractions of muscles, as described in the Introduction (p. 29), and to have a basic understanding of the processes of standing and walking.

Standing at Ease

When a person is standing at ease with the feet slightly apart and rotated laterally so the toes point outward, only a few of the back and lower limb muscles are active (Fig. 5.19). The mechanical arrangement of the joints and muscles are such that a minimum of muscular activity is required to keep from falling. In the stand-easy position, the hip and knee joints are extended and are in their most stable positions (maximal contact of articular surfaces for weight transfer, with supporting ligaments taut).

The ankle joint is less stable than the hip and knee joints, and the line of gravity falls between the two limbs, just anterior to the axis of rotation of the ankle joints. Consequently, a tendency to fall forward (*forward sway*) must be countered periodically by bilateral contraction of the calf muscles (plantarflexion). The spread or splay of the feet increases lateral stability. However, when *lateral sway* occurs, it is countered by the hip abductors (acting through the iliotibial tract). The fibular collateral ligament of the knee joint and the evertor muscles of one side act with the thigh adductors, tibial collateral ligament, and invertor muscles of the contralateral side.

Walking: The Gait Cycle

Locomotion is a complex function. The movements of the lower limbs during walking on a level surface may be divided into alternating swing and stance phases, illustrated in Figure 5.20 and described in Table 5.2. The **gait cycle** consists of one cycle of swing and stance by one limb. The **stance phase** begins with a **heel strike** (Fig. 5.20A), when the heel strikes the ground and begins to assume the body's full weight (loading response), and ends with a *push off* by the forefoot (Fig 5.20G)—a result of plantarflexion. (See the blue box "Absence of Plantarflexion," p. 607).

The **swing phase** begins after push off when the toes leave the ground and ends when the heel strikes the ground. The swing phase occupies approximately 40% of the walking cycle and the stance phase, 60%. The stance phase of walking is longer than the swing phase because

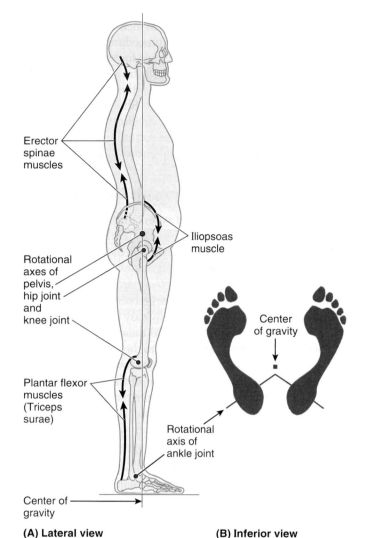

Erector spinae muscles

Iliopsoas muscle

Rotational axes of pelvis, hip joint and knee joint

Plantar flexor muscles (Triceps surae)

Rotational axis of ankle joint

Center of gravity

Center of gravity

(A) Lateral view

(B) Inferior view

FIGURE 5.19. Relaxed standing. A. The relationship of the line of gravity to the transverse rotational axes of the pelvis and lower limb in the relaxed standing (stand-easy) position is demonstrated. Only minor postural adjustments, mainly by the extensors of the back and the plantarflexors of the ankle, are necessary to maintain this position because the ligaments of the hip and knee are being tightly stretched to provide passive support. **B.** A bipedal platform is formed by the feet during relaxed standing. The weight of the body is symmetrically distributed around the center of gravity, which falls in the posterior third of a median plane between the slightly parted and laterally rotated feet, anterior to the rotational axes of the ankle joints.

it begins and ends with relatively short periods (each 10% of the cycle) of double support (both feet are contacting the ground) as the weight is transferred from one side to the other, with a more extended period of single support (only one foot on the ground bearing all body weight) in between as the contralateral limb swings forward. In **running,** there is no period of double support; consequently, the time and percentage of the gait cycle represented by the stance phase are reduced.

Walking is a remarkably efficient activity, taking advantage of gravity and momentum so that a minimum

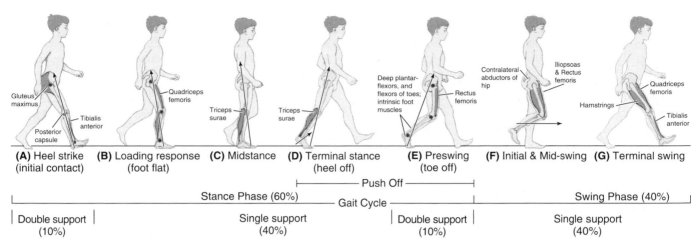

(A) Heel strike (initial contact) **(B)** Loading response (foot flat) **(C)** Midstance **(D)** Terminal stance (heel off) **(E)** Preswing (toe off) **(F)** Initial & Mid-swing **(G)** Terminal swing

Push Off

Stance Phase (60%) ── Gait Cycle ── Swing Phase (40%)

| Double support (10%) | Single support (40%) | Double support (10%) | Single support (40%) |

FIGURE 5.20. Gait cycle. The activity of one limb between two repeated events of walking. Eight phases are typically described, two of which have been combined in (**F**) for simplification.

TABLE 5.2. MUSCLE ACTION DURING GAIT CYCLE

	Phase of Gait	Mechanical Goals	Active Muscle Groups	Examples
STANCE PHASE	**Heel strike** (initial contact)	**Lower forefoot to ground**	Ankle dorsiflexors (eccentric contraction)	**Tibialis anterior**
		Continue doooloration (reverse forward swing)	Hip extensors	Gluteus maximus
		Preserve longitudinal arch of foot	Intrinsic muscles of foot	Flexor digitorum brevis
			Long tendons of foot	Tibialis anterior
	Loading response (flat foot)	**Accept weight**	Knee extensors	**Quadriceps**
		Decelerate mass (slow dorsiflexion)	Ankle plantarflexors	Triceps surae (soleus and gastrocnemius)
		Stabilize pelvis	Hip abductors	**Gluteus medius and minimus; tensor fasciae latae**
		Preserve longitudinal arch of foot	Intrinsic muscles of foot	Flexor digitorum brevis
			Long tendons of foot	Tibialis posterior; long flexors of digits
	Midstance	Stabilize knee	Knee extensors	Quadriceps
		Control dorsiflexion (preserve momentum)	Ankle plantarflexors (eccentric contraction)	Triceps surae (soleus and gastrocnemius)
		Stabilize pelvis	Hip abductors	**Gluteus medius and minimus; tensor fasciae latae**
		Preserve longitudinal arch of foot	Intrinsic muscles of foot	Flexor digitorum brevis
			Long tendons of foot	Tibialis posterior; long flexors of digits
	Terminal stance (heel off)	**Accelerate mass**	Ankle plantarflexors (concentric contraction)	**Triceps surae (soleus and gastrocnemius)**
		Stabilize pelvis	Hip abductors	**Gluteus medius and minimus; tensor fasciae latae**
		Preserve arches of foot; fix forefoot	Intrinsic muscles of foot	Adductor hallucis
			Long tendons of foot	Tibialis posterior; long flexors of digits

TABLE 5.2. MUSCLE ACTION DURING GAIT CYCLE (Continued)

	Phase of Gait	Mechanical Goals	Active Muscle Groups	Examples
STANCE PHASE (cont'd.)	**Preswing** (toe off)	Accelerate mass	Long flexors of digits	Flexor hallucis longus; flexor digitorum longus
		Preserve arches of foot; fix forefoot	Intrinsic muscles of foot	Adductor hallucis
			Long tendons of foot	Tibialis posterior; long flexors of digits
		Decelerate thigh; prepare for swing	Flexor of hip (eccentric contraction)	Iliopsoas; rectus femoris
SWING PHASE	**Initial swing**	**Accelerate thigh; vary cadence**	**Flexor of hip (concentric contraction)**	**Iliopsoas; rectus femoris**
		Clear foot	**Ankle dorsiflexors**	**Tibialis anterior**
	Midswing	**Clear foot**	**Ankle dorsiflexors**	**Tibialis anterior**
	Terminal swing	Decelerate thigh	Hip extensors (eccentric contraction)	Gluteus maximus; hamstrings
		Decelerate leg	Knee flexors (eccentric contraction)	Hamstrings
		Position foot	**Ankle dorsiflexors**	Tibialis anterior
		Extend knee to place foot (control stride); prepare for contact	**Knee extensors**	Quadriceps

of physical exertion is required. Most energy is used (1) in the eccentric contraction of the dorsiflexors during the beginning (**loading response**) phase of stance (Fig. 5.20B) as the heel is lowered to the ground following heel strike, and (2) especially at the end of stance (**terminal stance;** Fig. 5.20D) as the plantarflexors concentrically contract, pushing the forefoot (metatarsals and phalanges) down to produce push off, thus providing most of the propulsive force.

During the last part of the stance phase (**push off** or *toe off;* Fig. 5.20E), the toes flex to grip the ground and augment the push off initiated from the ball of the foot (sole underlying the heads of the medial two metatarsals). The long flexors and intrinsic muscles of the foot stabilize the forefoot and toes so that the effect of plantarflexion at the ankle and flexion of the toes is maximized.

The swing phase also involves flexion of the hip so that the free limb accelerates faster than the forward movement of the body. During **initial swing** (Fig. 5.20F), the knee flexes almost simultaneously, owing to momentum (without expenditure of energy), followed by dorsiflexion (lifting the forefoot up) at the ankle joint. The latter two movements have the effect of shortening the free limb so that it will clear the ground as it swings forward. By **midswing,** knee extension is added to the flexion and momentum of the thigh to realize anterior swing fully.

The extensors of the hip and flexors of the knee contract eccentrically at the end of swing phase (**terminal swing;** Fig. 5.20G) to decelerate the forward movement, while extensors of the knee (quadriceps) contract as necessary to extend the

leg for the desired length of stride and to position the foot (present the heel) for heel strike.

Contraction of the knee extensors is maintained through the heel strike into the loading phase to absorb shock and keep the knee from buckling until it reaches full extension. Because the unsupported side of the hip tends to drop during the swing phase (which would negate the effect of limb shortening), abductor muscles on the supported side contract strongly during the single support part of the stance phase (Fig. 5.20F & G), pulling on the fixed femur to resist the tilting and keep the pelvis level. The same muscles also rotate (advance) the contralateral side of the pelvis forward, concurrent with the swing of its free limb.

Of course, all these actions alternate from side to side with each step. The extensors of the hip normally make only minor contributions to level walking. Primarily, the hip is passively extended by momentum during stance, except when accelerating or walking fast, and becomes increasingly active with increase in slope (steepness) during walking uphill or up stairs. Concentric hip flexion and knee extension are used during the swing phase of level walking and so are not weight-bearing actions; however, they are affected by body weight when their eccentric contraction is necessary for deceleration or walking downhill or down stairs.

Stabilization and resilience are important during locomotion. The invertors and evertors of the foot are principal stabilizers of the foot during the stance phase. Their long tendons, plus those of the flexors of the digits, also help support the arches of the foot during the stance phase, assisting the intrinsic muscles of the sole.

ANTERIOR AND MEDIAL REGIONS OF THIGH

Organization of Proximal Lower Limb

During evolution, the development of a prominent gluteal region is closely associated with the assumption of bipedalism and an erect posture. The prominent gluteal region is unique to humans. Modification of the shape of the femur necessary for bipedal walking and running (specifically the "bending" of the bone, creating the angle of inclination and the trochanters, p. 518) allows the superior placement of the abductors of the thigh into the gluteal region.

The remaining thigh muscles are organized into three compartments by intermuscular septa that pass deeply between the muscle groups from the inner surface of the fascia lata to the linea aspera of the femur (see Fig. 5.13D). The compartments are *anterior* or *extensor, medial* or *adductor,* and *posterior* or *flexor,* so named on the basis of their location or action at the knee joint. Generally, the anterior group is innervated by the femoral nerve, the medial group by the obturator nerve, and the posterior group by the tibial portion of the sciatic nerve. Although the compartments vary in absolute and relative size depending on the level, the anterior compartment is the largest overall and includes the femur.

To facilitate continuity and follow an approach commonly used in dissection courses, the anterior and medial compartments of the thigh are addressed initially, followed by continuous examination of the posterior aspect of the proximal limb: gluteal region and posterior thigh. This approach is then continued by consideration of the popliteal fossa and leg.

Anterior Thigh Muscles

The large **anterior compartment of the thigh** contains the **anterior thigh muscles,** the *flexors of the hip* (Fig. 5.21A–D) and *extensors of the knee* (Fig. 5.21E–I). For attachments, nerve supply, and main actions of these muscles, see Tables 5.3.I and 5.3.II. The anterior thigh muscles include the pectineus, iliopsoas, sartorius, and quadriceps femoris.[1]

The major muscles of the anterior compartment tend to atrophy (diminish) rapidly with disease, and physical therapy is often necessary to restore strength, tone, and symmetry with the opposite limb after immobilization of the thigh or leg.

PECTINEUS

The **pectineus** is a flat quadrangular muscle located in the anterior part of the superomedial aspect of the thigh (Fig. 5.21A & B; Table 5.3.I). It often appears to be composed of two layers, superficial and deep, and these are generally

[1]Because of its anterior position, the tensor fasciae latae is often studied with the anterior thigh muscles for convenience (i.e., when the cadaver is supine); however, it is actually part of the gluteal group and will be included with that group in this book.

innervated by two different nerves. Because of the dual nerve supply and the muscle's actions (the pectineus adducts and flexes the thigh and assists in medial rotation of the thigh), it is actually a transitional muscle between the anterior and medial compartments.

ILIOPSOAS

The **iliopsoas,** the chief flexor of the thigh, is the most powerful of the hip flexors with the longest range. Although it is one of the body's most powerful muscles, it is relatively hidden, with most of its mass located in the posterior wall of the abdomen and greater pelvis. Its broad lateral part, the **iliacus,** and its long medial part, the **psoas major,** arise from the iliac fossa and lumbar vertebrae, respectively (Fig. 5.21C; Table 5.3.I). Thus, it is the only muscle attached to the vertebral column, pelvis, and femur. It is in a unique position not only to produce movement but to stabilize (fixate). However, it can also perpetuate and even contribute to deformity and disability when it is malformed (especially if it is shortened), dysfunctional, or diseased.

Concentric contraction of the iliopsoas typically moves the free limb, producing flexion at the hip to lift the limb and initiate its forward swing during walking (i.e., during the pre-swing and initial swing phases) as the opposite limb accepts weight (Fig. 5.20E & F), or to elevate the limb during climbing. However, it is also capable of moving the trunk. Bilateral contraction of the iliopsoas muscles initiates flexion of the trunk at the hip on the fixed thigh—as when (incorrectly) doing sit-ups—and decreases the lumbar lordosis (curvature) of the vertebral column. It is active during walking downhill, its eccentric contraction resisting acceleration.

The iliopsoas is also a postural muscle, active during standing in maintaining normal lumbar lordosis (and indirectly the compensatory thoracic kyphosis; see Chapter 4) and resisting hyperextension of the hip joint (see Fig. 5.19).

SARTORIUS

The **sartorius,** the "tailor's muscle" (L. *sartus,* patched or repaired), is long and ribbon-like. It passes lateral to medial across the superoanterior part of the thigh (Fig. 5.21D; Table 5.3.I). The sartorius lies superficially in the anterior compartment, within its own relatively distinct fascial sheath. It descends inferiorly as far as the medial side of the knee.

The sartorius, the longest muscle in the body, acts across two joints. It flexes the hip joint and participates in flexion of the knee joint. It also weakly abducts the thigh and laterally rotates it. The actions of both sartorius muscles bring the lower limbs into the cross-legged sitting position. None of the actions of the sartorius is strong; therefore, it is mainly a synergist, acting with other thigh muscles that produce these movements.

QUADRICEPS FEMORIS

The **quadriceps femoris** (L., four-headed femoral muscle) forms the main bulk of the anterior thigh muscles, and

Anterior views

FIGURE 5.21. Muscles of anterior thigh: flexors of hip joint.

TABLE 5.3.I. MUSCLES OF ANTERIOR THIGH: FLEXORS OF HIP JOINT

Muscle	Proximal Attachment[a]	Distal Attachment	Innervation[b]	Main Action(s)
Pectineus (Fig. 5.21A & B)	Superior ramus of pubis	Pectineal line of femur, just inferior to lesser trochanter	Femoral nerve (**L2**, L3); may receive a branch from obturator nerve	Adducts and flexes thigh; assists with medial rotation of thigh
Iliopsoas (Fig. 5.21A & C) **Psoas major**	Sides of T12–L5 vertebrae and discs between them; transverse processes of all lumbar vertebrae	Lesser trochanter of femur	Anterior rami of lumbar nerves (**L1, L2,** L3)	Act conjointly in flexing thigh at hip joint and in stabilizing this joint[c]
Psoas minor	Sides of T12–L1 vertebrae and intervertebral discs	Pectineal line, iliopectineal eminence via iliopectineal arch	Anterior rami of lumbar nerves (L1, L2)	
Iliacus	Iliac crest, iliac fossa, ala of sacrum, and anterior sacro-iliac ligaments	Tendon of psoas major, lesser trochanter, and femur distal to it	Femoral nerve (**L2**, L3)	
Sartorius (Fig. 5.21A & D)	Anterior superior iliac spine and superior part of notch inferior to it	Superior part of medial surface of tibia	Femoral nerve (L2, L3)	Flexes, abducts, and laterally rotates thigh at hip joint; flexes leg at knee joint, (medially rotating leg when knee is flexed)[d]

[a] The Latin word *insertio* means *attachment*. The terms insertion and origin (L. *origo*) have not been used here (or elsewhere) since they change with function.

[b] The spinal cord segmental innervation is indicated (e.g., "L1, L2, L3" means that the nerves supplying the psoas major are derived from the first three lumbar segments of the spinal cord). Numbers in boldface (**L1, L2**) indicate the main segmental innervation. Damage to one or more of the listed spinal cord segments, or to the motor nerve roots arising from them, results in paralysis of the muscles concerned.

[c] The psoas major is also a postural muscle that helps control the deviation of the trunk and is active during standing.

[d] The four actions of the sartorius (L. *sartor,* tailor) produce the once common cross-legged sitting position used by tailors, hence the name.

collectively constitutes the largest and one of the most powerful muscles in the body. It covers almost all the anterior aspect and sides of the femur (Fig. 5-21E–I). The quadriceps femoris (usually shortened to quadriceps) consists of four parts: (1) rectus femoris, (2) vastus lateralis, (3) vastus intermedius, and (4) vastus medialis. Collectively, the quadriceps is a two-joint muscle capable of producing action at both the hip and knee.

The quadriceps is the great extensor of the leg. Concentric contraction of the quadriceps to extend the knee against gravity is important during rising from sitting or squatting, climbing and walking up stairs, and for acceleration and projection (running and jumping) when it is lifting or moving the body's weight. Consequently, it may be three times stronger than its antagonistic muscle group, the hamstrings.

FIGURE 5.21. Muscles of anterior thigh *(continued)*: extensors of knee.

TABLE 5.3.II. MUSCLES OF ANTERIOR THIGH: EXTENSORS OF KNEE

Muscle	Proximal Attachment	Distal Attachment	Innervation[a]	Main Action
Quadriceps femoris (Fig. 5.21E–H)				
Rectus femoris	Anterior inferior iliac spine and ilium superior to acetabulum	Via common tendinous (quadriceps tendon) and independent attachments to base of patella; indirectly via patellar ligament to tibial tuberosity; medial and lateral vasti also attach to tibia and patella via aponeuroses (medial and lateral patellar retinacula)	Femoral nerve (L2, **L3, L4**)	Extend leg at knee joint; rectus femoris also steadies hip joint and helps iliopsoas flex thigh
Vastus lateralis	Greater trochanter and lateral lip of linea aspera of femur			
Vastus medialis	Intertrochanteric line and medial lip of linea aspera of femur			
Vastus intermedius	Anterior and lateral surfaces of shaft of femur			

[a] The spinal cord segmental innervation is indicated (e.g., "L1, L2, L3" means that the nerves supplying the quadriceps femoris are derived from the first three lumbar segments of the spinal cord). Numbers in boldface (**L3, L4**) indicate the main segmental innervation. Damage to one or more of the listed spinal cord segments or to the motor nerve roots arising from them results in paralysis of the muscles concerned.

In level walking, the quadriceps muscles become active during the termination of the swing phase, preparing the knee to accept weight (Fig. 5.20G; Table 5.2). The quadriceps is primarily responsible for absorbing the jarring shock of heel strike, and its activity continues as the weight is assumed during the early stance phase (loading response). It also functions as a fixator during bent-knee sports, such as skiing and tennis, and contracts eccentrically during downhill walking and descending stairs.

The tendons of the four parts of the quadriceps unite in the distal portion of the thigh to form a single, strong, broad **quadriceps tendon** (Fig.5.21F). The **patellar ligament** (L. *ligamentum patellae*), attached to the tibial tuberosity, is the continuation of the quadriceps tendon in which the patella is embedded. The *patella* is thus the largest sesamoid bone in the body.

The medial and lateral vasti muscles also attach independently to the patella and form aponeuroses, the **medial** and **lateral patellar retinacula,** which reinforce the joint capsule of the knee joint on each side of the patella en route to attachment to the anterior border of the tibial plateau. The retinacula also play a role in keeping the patella aligned over the patellar surface of the femur.

The **patella** provides a bony surface that is able to withstand the compression placed on the quadriceps tendon during kneeling and the friction occurring when the knee is flexed and extended during running. The patella also provides additional leverage for the quadriceps in placing the tendon more anteriorly, farther from the joint's axis, causing it to approach the tibia from a position of greater mechanical advantage. The inferiorly directed apex of the patella indicates the level of the joint plane of the knee when the leg is extended and the patellar ligament is taut (Fig. 5.22C).

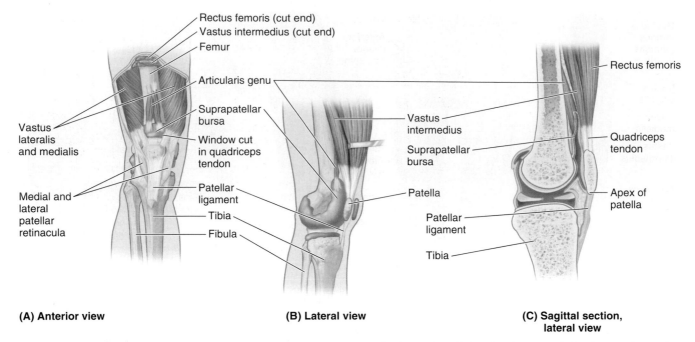

FIGURE 5.22. Suprapatellar bursa and articularis genu. In **A** and **B,** the suprapatellar bursa, normally a potential space extending between the quadriceps and the femur (exaggerated for schematic purposes in **C**), is depicted as if injected with latex.

Testing the quadriceps[2] is performed with the person in the supine position with the knee partly flexed. The person extends the knee against resistance. During the test, contraction of the rectus femoris should be observable and palpable if the muscle is acting normally, indicating that its nerve supply is intact.

Rectus Femoris. The **rectus femoris** received its name because it runs straight down the thigh (L. *rectus,* straight). Because of its attachments to the hip bone and tibia via the patellar ligament (Fig. 5.21E & F), *it crosses two joints;* hence it is capable of flexing the thigh at the hip joint and extending the leg at the knee joint. The rectus femoris is the only part of the quadriceps that crosses the hip joint, and as a hip flexor it acts with and like the iliopsoas during the preswing and initial swing phases of walking (Fig. 5.20F; Table 5.2).

The ability of the rectus femoris to extend the knee is compromised during hip flexion, but it does contribute to the extension force during the toe off phase of walking, when the thigh is extended. It is particularly efficient in movements combining knee extension and hip flexion from a position of hip hyperextension and knee flexion, as in the preparatory position for kicking a soccer ball. The rectus femoris is susceptible to injury and avulsion from the anterior inferior iliac spine during kicking, hence the name "kicking muscle." A loss of function of the rectus femoris may reduce thigh flexion strength by as much as 17%.

Vastus Muscles. The names of the three large **vastus muscles** (pl., vasti) indicate their position around the femoral shaft (Fig. 5.21E–I; Table 5.3.II):

- **Vastus lateralis,** the largest component of the quadriceps, lies on the lateral side of the thigh.
- **Vastus medialis** covers the medial side of the thigh.
- **Vastus intermedius** lies deep to the rectus femoris, between the vastus medialis and vastus lateralis.

It is difficult to isolate the function of the three vastus muscles.

The small, flat **articularis genu** (articular muscle of the knee), a derivative of the vastus intermedius, usually consists of a variable number of muscular slips that attach superiorly to the inferior part of the anterior aspect of the femur, and inferiorly to the synovial membrane of the knee joint and the wall of the *suprapatellar bursa* (Figs. 5.21E and 5.22). The articularis genu muscle pulls the synovial membrane superiorly during extension of the leg, thereby preventing folds of the membrane from being compressed between the femur and the patella within the knee joint.

Medial Thigh Muscles

The muscles of the medial compartment of the thigh comprise the **adductor group,** consisting of the adductor longus, adductor brevis, adductor magnus, gracilis, and obturator externus (Fig. 5.23). In general, they attach proximally to the antero-inferior external surface of the bony pelvis (pubic bone, ischiopubic ramus, and ischial tuberosity), and adjacent obturator membrane, and distally to the linea aspera of the femur (Fig. 5.23A; Table 5.4)

All adductor muscles, except the "hamstring part" of the adductor magnus and part of the pectineus are supplied by the *obturator nerve* (L2–L4). The hamstring part of the adductor magnus is supplied by the tibial part of the sciatic

[2]There are entire texts dedicated to the testing of muscles. We are providing only a few important examples useful to primary care health professionals.

FIGURE 5.23. Muscles of medial thigh: adductors of thigh.

TABLE 5.4. MUSCLES OF MEDIAL THIGH: ADDUCTORS OF THIGH

Muscle[a]	Proximal Attachment	Distal Attachment	Innervation[b]	Main Action
Adductor longus (Fig. 5.23E & G)	Body of pubis inferior to pubic crest	Middle third of linea aspera of femur	Obturator nerve, branch of, anterior division (L2, **L3**, L4)	Adducts thigh
Adductor brevis (Fig. 5.23F & G)	Body and inferior ramus of pubis	Pectineal line and proximal part of linea aspera of femur		Adducts thigh; to some extent flexes it
Adductor magnus (Fig. 5.23C, D, & G)	Adductor part: inferior ramus of pubis, ramus of ischium Hamstrings part: ischial tuberosity	Adductor part: gluteal tuberosity, linea aspera, medial supracondylar line Hamstring part: adductor tubercle of femur	Adductor part: obturator nerve (L2, **L3, L4**), branches of posterior division Hamstring part: tibial part of sciatic nerve (**L4**)	Adducts thigh Adductor part: flexes thigh Hamstrings part: extends thigh
Gracilis (Fig. 5.23H)	Body and inferior ramus of pubis	Superior part of medial surface of tibia.	Obturator nerve (**L2**, L3)	Adducts thigh; flexes leg; helps rotate leg medially
Obturator externus	Margins of obturator foramen and obturator membrane	Trochanteric fossa of femur	Obturator nerve (L3, **L4**)	Laterally rotates thigh; steadies head of femur in acetabulum

[a]Collectively, the five muscles listed are the adductors of the thigh, but their actions are more complex (e.g., they act as flexors of the hip joint during flexion of the knee joint and are active during walking).

[b]The spinal cord segmental innervation is indicated (e.g., "L2, L3, L4" means that the nerves supplying the adductor longus are derived from the second to fourth lumbar segments of the spinal cord). Numbers in boldface (**L3**) indicate the main segmental innervation. Damage to one or more of the listed spinal cord segments or to the motor nerve roots arising from them results in paralysis of the muscles concerned.

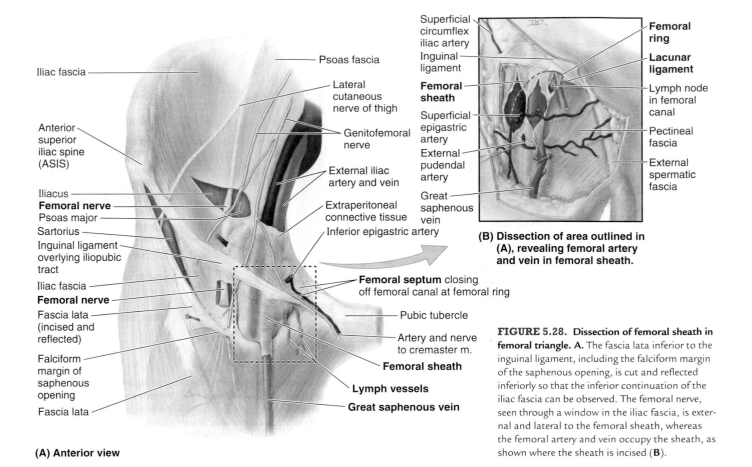

Iliac fascia

Anterior superior iliac spine (ASIS)

Iliacus
Femoral nerve
Psoas major
Sartorius
Inguinal ligament overlying iliopubic tract
Iliac fascia
Femoral nerve
Fascia lata (incised and reflected)
Falciform margin of saphenous opening
Fascia lata

Psoas fascia

Lateral cutaneous nerve of thigh

Genitofemoral nerve

External iliac artery and vein

Extraperitoneal connective tissue
Inferior epigastric artery

Femoral septum closing off femoral canal at femoral ring

Pubic tubercle

Artery and nerve to cremaster m.

Femoral sheath

Lymph vessels

Great saphenous vein

(A) Anterior view

Superficial circumflex iliac artery
Inguinal ligament
Femoral sheath
Superficial epigastric artery
External pudendal artery
Great saphenous vein

Femoral ring
Lacunar ligament
Lymph node in femoral canal
Pectineal fascia
External spermatic fascia

(B) Dissection of area outlined in (A), revealing femoral artery and vein in femoral sheath.

FIGURE 5.28. **Dissection of femoral sheath in femoral triangle. A.** The fascia lata inferior to the inguinal ligament, including the falciform margin of the saphenous opening, is cut and reflected inferiorly so that the inferior continuation of the iliac fascia can be observed. The femoral nerve, seen through a window in the iliac fascia, is external and lateral to the femoral sheath, whereas the femoral artery and vein occupy the sheath, as shown where the sheath is incised (**B**).

The *base of the femoral canal* is the oval **femoral ring** formed by the small (approximately 1 cm wide) proximal opening at its abdominal end. This opening is closed by extraperitoneal fatty tissue that forms the transversely oriented **femoral septum** (Fig. 5.28A). The abdominal surface of the septum is covered by parietal peritoneum. The femoral septum is pierced by lymphatic vessels connecting the inguinal and external iliac lymph nodes.

The *boundaries of the femoral ring* are (Fig. 5.26B):

• *Laterally,* the vertical septum between the femoral canal and femoral vein.
• *Posteriorly,* the superior ramus of the pubis covered by the pectineus muscle and its fascia.
• *Medially,* the lacunar ligament.
• *Anteriorly,* the medial part of the inguinal ligament.

FEMORAL ARTERY

Details concerning the origin, course, and distribution of the arteries of the thigh are illustrated in Figure 5.29 and described in Table 5.5.

The **femoral artery,** the continuation of the external iliac artery distal to the inguinal ligament, is the primary artery of the lower limb (Figs. 5.26–29; Table 5.5). It enters the *femoral triangle* deep to the midpoint of the inguinal ligament (midway between the ASIS and the pubic tubercle),

lateral to the femoral vein (Fig. 5.30A). The pulsations of the femoral artery are palpable within the triangle because of its relatively superficial position deep (posterior) to the fascia lata. The artery lies and descends on the adjacent borders of the iliopsoas and pectineus muscles that form the floor of the triangle. The superficial epigastric artery, superficial (and sometimes the deep) circumflex iliac arteries, and the superficial and deep external pudendal arteries arise from the anterior aspect of the proximal part of the femoral artery.

The **profunda femoris artery** (deep artery of thigh) is the largest branch of the femoral artery and the chief artery to the thigh (Fig 5.29). It arises from the lateral or posterior side of the femoral artery in the femoral triangle. In the middle third of the thigh, where it is separated from the femoral artery and vein by the adductor longus (Figs. 5.27B and 5.30B), it gives off 3–4 *perforating arteries* that wrap around the posterior aspect of the femur (Fig. 5.29; Table 5.5). The perforating arteries supply muscles of all three fascial compartments (adductor magnus, hamstrings, and vastus lateralis).

The **circumflex femoral arteries** encircle the uppermost shaft of the femur and anastomose with each other and other arteries, supplying the thigh muscles and the superior (proximal) end of the femur. The **medial circumflex femoral artery** is especially important because it supplies

FIGURE 5.29. Arteries of anterior and medial thigh.

TABLE 5.5. ARTERIES OF ANTERIOR AND MEDIAL THIGH

Artery	Origin	Course	Distribution
Femoral	Continuation of external iliac artery distal to inguinal ligament	Descends through femoral triangle bisecting it; then courses through adductor canal; terminates as it traverses adductor hiatus, where its name becomes popliteal artery	Branches supply anterior and anteromedial aspects of thigh
Profunda femoris artery (deep artery of thigh)	Femoral artery 1–5 cm inferior to inguinal ligament	Passes deeply between pectineus and adductor longus; descending posterior to latter on medial side of femur	Three to four perforating arteries pass through adductor magnus muscle, winding around femur to supply muscles in medial, posterior, and lateral part of anterior compartments
Medial circumflex femoral	Profunda femoris artery; may arise from femoral artery	Passes medially and posteriorly between pectineus and iliopsoas; enters gluteal region and gives rise to posterior retinacular arteries; then terminates by dividing into transverse and ascending branches	Supplies most of blood to head and neck of femur; transverse branch takes part in cruciate anastomosis of thigh; ascending branch joins inferior gluteal artery
Lateral circumflex femoral		Passes laterally deep to sartorius and rectus femoris, dividing into ascending, transverse, and descending arteries	Ascending branch supplies anterior part of gluteal region; transverse branch winds around femur; descending branch joins genicular peri-articular anastomosis
Obturator	Internal iliac artery or (in ~20%) as an accessory or replaced obturator artery from the inferior epigastric artery	Passes through obturator foramen; enters medial compartment of thigh and divides into anterior and posterior branches, which pass on respective sides of adductor brevis	Anterior branch supplies obturator externus, pectineus, adductors of thigh, and gracilis; posterior branch supplies muscles attached to ischial tuberosity

femoral triangle, whereas the middle third represents the artery while it is in the *adductor canal*. Approximately 3.75 cm along this line distal to the inguinal ligament, the profunda femoris artery arises from the femoral artery.

The *femoral vein* is (Figs. 5.26B & 5.27A):

• Medial to the femoral artery at the base of the femoral triangle (indicated by inguinal ligament).
• Posterior to the femoral artery at the apex of the femoral triangle.
• Posterolateral to the artery in the adductor canal.

The *femoral triangle*, in the supero-anterior aspect of the thigh, is not a prominent surface feature in most people. When some people sit cross-legged, the sartorius and adductor longus stand out, delineating the femoral triangle. The surface anatomy of the femoral triangle is clinically important because of its contents (Fig. 5.26B).

The *femoral artery* can be felt pulsating just inferior to the midinguinal point. When you palpate the femoral pulse, the *femoral vein* is just medial, the femoral nerve is a finger's breadth lateral, and the *femoral head* is just posterior. The femoral artery runs a 5-cm superficial course through the femoral triangle before it is covered by the sartorius in the adductor canal.

The *great saphenous vein* enters the thigh posterior to the medial femoral condyle and passes superiorly along a line from the adductor tubercle to the *saphenous opening*. The central point of this opening, where the great saphenous vein enters the femoral vein, is located 3.75 cm inferior and 3.75 cm lateral to the pubic tubercle (Fig. 5.27A).

ANTERIOR AND MEDIAL REGIONS OF THIGH

Hip and Thigh Contusions

Sports broadcasters and trainers refer to a "hip pointer," which is a *contusion of the iliac crest* that usually occurs at its anterior part (e.g., where the sartorius attaches to the ASIS). This is one of the most common injuries to the hip region, usually occurring in association with collision sports, such as the various forms of football, ice hockey, and volleyball.

Contusions cause bleeding from ruptured capillaries and infiltration of blood into the muscles, tendons, and other soft tissues. The term *hip pointer* may also refer to avulsion of bony muscle attachments, for example, of the sartorius or rectus femoris to the anterior superior and inferior iliac spines, respectively, of the hamstrings from the ischium. However, these injuries should be called *avulsion fractures*.

Another term commonly used is "charley horse," which may refer either to the cramping of an individual thigh muscle because of ischemia or to contusion and rupture of blood vessels sufficient enough to form a *hematoma*. The injury is usually the consequence of tearing of fibers of the rectus femoris; sometimes the quadriceps tendon is also partially torn. The most common site of a thigh hematoma is in the quadriceps. A charley horse is associated with localized pain and/or muscle stiffness and commonly follows direct trauma (e.g., a stick slash in hockey or a tackle in football).

Psoas Abscess

The psoas major muscle arises in the abdomen from the intervertebral discs, the sides of the T12–L5 vertebrae, and their transverse processes (see Fig. B2.35). The medial arcuate ligament of the diaphragm arches obliquely over the proximal part of the psoas major. The transversalis fascia on the internal abdominal wall is continuous with the psoas fascia, where it forms a fascial covering for the psoas major that accompanies the muscle into the anterior region of the thigh.

There is a resurgence of tuberculosis (TB) in Africa, Asia, and elsewhere. A retroperitoneal *pyogenic infection* (pus-forming) in the abdomen or greater pelvis, characteristically occurring in association with TB of the vertebral column, or secondary to regional enteritis of the ileum (*Crohn disease*), may result in the formation of a *psoas abscess*. When the abscess passes between the psoas and its fascia to the inguinal and proximal thigh regions, severe pain may be referred to the hip, thigh, or knee joint. A psoas abscess should always be considered when edema occurs in the proximal part of the thigh. Such an abscess may be palpated or observed in the inguinal region, just inferior or superior to the inguinal ligament, and may be mistaken for an indirect inguinal hernia or a femoral hernia, an enlargement of the inguinal lymph nodes, or a saphenous varix. The lateral border of the psoas is commonly visible in radiographs of the abdomen; an obscured psoas shadow may be an indication of abdominal pathology.

Paralysis of Quadriceps

A person with *paralyzed quadriceps muscles* cannot extend the leg against resistance and usually presses on the distal end of the thigh during walking to prevent inadvertent flexion of the knee joint.

Weakness of the vastus medialis or vastus lateralis, resulting from arthritis or trauma to the knee joint, can result in abnormal patellar movement and loss of joint stability.

Chondromalacia Patellae

Chondromalacia patellae (runner's knee) is a common knee injury for marathon runners. Such overstressing of the knee region can also occur in running sports such as basketball. The soreness and aching around or deep to the patella results from *quadriceps imbalance*. Chondromalacia patellae may also result from a blow to the patella or extreme flexion of the knee (e.g., during squatting when power lifting).

Patellar Fractures

A direct blow to the patella may fracture it into two or more fragments (Fig B5.12). *Transverse patellar fractures* may result from a blow to the knee or sudden contraction of the quadriceps (e.g., when one slips and attempts to prevent a backward fall). The proximal fragment is pulled superiorly with the quadriceps tendon, and the distal fragment remains with the patellar ligament.

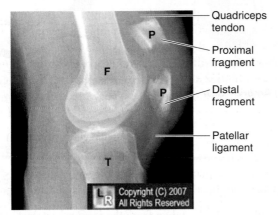

Femur (F), Patella (P), Tibia (T)

FIGURE B5.12.

Abnormal Ossification of Patella

The patella is cartilaginous at birth. It ossifies during the 3rd–6th years, frequently from more than one ossification center. Although these centers usually coalesce and form a single bone, they may remain separate on one or both sides, giving rise to a *bipartite* or *tripartite patella* (Fig. B5.13). An unwary observer might interpret this

Patella (P)

Posterior view

(A) Bipartite patella

(B) Coronal MRI image of bipartite patella (arrow = bipartate segment; arrowhead = false "fracture" line)

FIGURE B5.13.

condition on a radiograph or CT as a patellar fracture. *Ossification abnormalities* are nearly always bilateral; therefore, diagnostic images should be examined from both sides. If the defects are bilateral, the defects are likely ossification abnormalities.

Patellar Tendon Reflex

Tapping the patellar ligament with a reflex hammer (Fig. B5.14) normally elicits the *patellar tendon reflex* ("knee jerk"). This myotatic (deep tendon) reflex is routinely tested during a physical examination by having the person sit with the legs dangling. A firm strike on the ligament with a reflex hammer usually causes the leg to extend. If the reflex is normal, a hand on the person's quadriceps should feel the muscle contract. This tendon reflex tests the integrity of the femoral nerve and the L2–L4 spinal cord segments.

Tapping the ligament activates muscle spindles in the quadriceps. Afferent impulses from the spindles travel in the femoral nerve to the L2–L4 segments of the spinal cord. From here, efferent impulses are transmitted via motor fibers in the femoral nerve to the quadriceps, resulting in a jerk-like contraction of the muscle and extension of the leg at the knee joint.

Diminution or absence of the patellar tendon reflex may result from any lesion that interrupts the innervation of the quadriceps (e.g., peripheral nerve disease).

Patellar ligament

FIGURE B5.14.

Transplantation of Gracilis

Because the gracilis is a relatively weak member of the adductor group of muscles, it can be removed without noticeable loss of its actions on the leg. Surgeons often transplant the gracilis, or part of it, with its nerve and blood vessels to replace a damaged muscle in the hand, for example. Once the muscle is transplanted, it soon produces good digital flexion and extension.

Freed from its distal attachment, the muscle has also been relocated and repositioned to create a replacement for a nonfunctional external anal sphincter.

Posterior views

(C) Lateral view

(D) Superior view

(E) Superior view

FIGURE 5.39. Action of abductors/medial rotators of thigh in walking. A and B. The role of the abductors (gluteus medius and minimus, tensor fasciae latae) is demonstrated. When the weight is on both feet (**A**), the pelvis is evenly supported and does not sag. When the weight is borne by one limb (**B**), the muscles on the supported side fix the pelvis so that it does not sag to the unsupported side. Keeping the pelvis level enables the non-weight-bearing limb to clear the ground as it is brought forward during the swing phase. **C and D.** The role of the rotators of the thigh is demonstrated in lateral (**C**) and superior (**D**) views. Note that most abductors—the tensor fasciae latae, gluteus minimus, and most (the anterior fibers) of the gluteus medius—lie anterior to the lever provided by the axis of the head, neck, and greater trochanter of the femur to rotate the thigh around the vertical axis traversing the femoral head. The superior view of the right hip joint (**D**) includes the superior pubic ramus, acetabulum, and iliac crest; the inferior part of the ilium has been removed to reveal the head and neck of the femur. The lines of pull of the rotators of the hip are indicated by arrows, demonstrating the antagonistic relationship resulting from their positions relative to the lever and the center of rotation (fulcrum). The medial rotators pull the greater trochanter anteriorly and the lateral rotators pull the trochanter posteriorly, resulting in rotation of the thigh around the vertical axis. Note that all of these muscles also pull the head and neck of the femur medially into the acetabulum, strengthening the joint. In walking (**E**), the same muscles that act unilaterally during the stance phase (planted limb) to keep the pelvis level via abduction can simultaneously produce medial rotation at the hip joint, advancing the opposite unsupported side of the pelvis (augmenting advancement of the free limb). The lateral rotators of the advancing (free) limb act during the swing phase to keep the foot parallel to the direction (line) of advancement.

However, unlike the gluteus maximus, the tensor fasciae latae is served by the superior gluteal neurovascular bundle. Despite its gluteal innervation and shared attachment, this tensor is primarily a flexor of the thigh because of its anterior location; however, it generally does not act independently.

To produce flexion, the tensor fasciae latae acts in concert with the iliopsoas and rectus femoris. When the iliopsoas is paralyzed, the tensor fasciae latae undergoes hypertrophy in an attempt to compensate for the paralysis. It also works in conjunction with other abductor/medial rotator muscles (gluteus medius and minimus) (Fig. 5.39). It lies too far anteriorly to be a strong abductor and thus probably contributes primarily as a synergist or fixator.

The tensor fasciae latae tenses the fascia lata and iliotibial tract. Because the iliotibial tract is attached to the femur via the lateral intermuscular septum, the tensor produces little if any movement of the leg (Fig. 5.36B). However, when the knee is fully extended, it contributes to (increases) the extending force, adding stability, and plays a role in supporting the femur on the tibia when standing if lateral sway occurs. When the knee is flexed by other muscles, the tensor fasciae latae can synergistically augment flexion and lateral rotation of the leg.

The abductors/medial rotators of the hip joint play an essential role during locomotion, advancing and preventing the sagging of the unsupported side of the pelvis during walking, as illustrated and explained in Figure 5.39. The supportive and action-producing functions of the abductors/medial rotators depend on normal:

- Muscular activity and innervation from the superior gluteal nerve.
- Articulation of the hip joint components.
- Strength and angulation of the femoral neck.

PIRIFORMIS

The pear-shaped **piriformis** (L. *pirum,* a pear) is located partly on the posterior wall of the lesser pelvis, and partly posterior to the hip joint (Figs. 5.34F & G, 5.35, and 5.37; Table 5.6). The piriformis leaves the pelvis through the *greater sciatic foramen,* almost filling it, to reach its attachment to the superior border of the *greater trochanter.*

Because of its key position in the buttocks, the *piriformis is the landmark of the gluteal region.* The piriformis provides the key to understanding relationships in the gluteal region because it determines the names of the blood vessels and nerves (Fig. 5.38A):

- The superior gluteal vessels and nerve emerge superior to it.
- The inferior gluteal vessels and nerve emerge inferior to it.

See the blue box "Injury to Sciatic Nerve," p. 582.

OBTURATOR INTERNUS AND GEMELLI

The **obturator internus** and the **superior** and **inferior gemelli** (L. *geminus,* small twin) form a tricipital (three-headed) muscle, the **triceps coxae** (triceps of the hip), which occupies the gap between the piriformis and the quadratus femoris (Figs. 5.34H and 5.38A & B). The common tendon of these muscles lies horizontally in the buttocks as it passes to the greater trochanter of the femur.

The attachments, action, and innervation are described in Table 5.6. The *obturator internus* is located partly in the pelvis, where it covers most of the lateral wall of the lesser pelvis (Fig. 5.38B). It leaves the pelvis through the *lesser sciatic foramen,* makes a right-angle turn (Figs. 5.38B and 5.39D), becomes tendinous, and receives the distal attachments of the gemelli before attaching to the medial surface of the greater trochanter (trochanteric fossa) of the femur.

The small *gemelli* are narrow, triangular extrapelvic reinforcements of the obturator internus. Although the inferior gemellus receives separate innervation from the nerve to the quadratus femoris, it is more realistic to consider these three muscles as a unit (i.e., the *triceps coxae*) because they are incapable of independent action.

The **bursa of the obturator internus** allows free movement of the muscle over the posterior border of the ischium, where the border forms the lesser sciatic notch and the trochlea over which the tendon glides as it turns (Fig. 5.37).

QUADRATUS FEMORIS

The **quadratus femoris,** a short, flat quadrangular muscle, is located inferior to the obturator internus and gemelli (Figs. 5.34I, 5.35, 5.37, and 5.38A). True to its name, the quadratus femoris is a rectangular muscle that is a strong lateral rotator of the thigh.

OBTURATOR EXTERNUS

Based on its location (posterior to the pectineus and the superior ends of the adductor muscles), and its innervation (*obturator nerve*), the obturator externus was described earlier in this chapter (p. 550) with the medial thigh muscles (Fig. 5.23H; Table 5.4). However, it functions as a lateral rotator of the thigh, and its distal attachment is visible only during dissection of the gluteal region (Fig. 5.38B) or hip joint. That is why it is mentioned again in this context.

The belly of the obturator externus lies deep in the proximal thigh, with its tendon passing inferior to the neck of the femur and deep to the quadratus femoris, on the way to its attachment to the *trochanteric fossa of the femur* (Figs. 5.38A and 5.39D). The obturator externus, with other short muscles around the hip joint, stabilizes the head of the femur in the acetabulum. It is most effective as a lateral rotator of the thigh when the hip joint is flexed.

Posterior Thigh Region

The **posterior thigh muscles** and their attachments are illustrated in Figure 5.40, and their attachments, innervation, and actions are described in Table 5.7.

FIGURE 5.40. Muscles of posterior thigh: extensors of hip and flexors of knee.

TABLE 5.7. MUSCLES OF POSTERIOR THIGH: EXTENSORS OF HIP AND FLEXORS OF KNEE

Muscle[a]	Proximal Attachment	Distal Attachment	Innervation[b]	Main Action
Semitendinosus	Ischial tuberosity	Medial surface of superior part of tibia	Tibial division of sciatic nerve part of tibia (**L5, S1**, S2)	Extend thigh; flex leg and rotate it medially when knee is flexed; when thigh and leg are flexed, these muscles can extend trunk
Semimembranosus		Posterior part of medial condyle of tibia; reflected attachment forms oblique popliteal ligament (to lateral femoral condyle)		
Biceps femoris	Long head: ischial tuberosity Short head: linea aspera and lateral supracondylar line of femur	Lateral side of head of fibula; tendon is split at this site by fibular collateral ligament of knee	Long head: tibial division of sciatic nerve (L5, **S1**, S2) Short head: common fibular division of sciatic nerve (L5, **S1**, S2)	Flexes leg and rotates it laterally when knee is flexed; extends thigh (e.g., accelerating mass during first step of gait).

[a] Collectively these three muscles are known as hamstrings.

[b] The spinal cord segmental innervation is indicated (e.g., "L5, S1, S2" means that the nerves supplying the semitendinosus are derived from the fifth lumbar segment and first two sacral segments of the spinal cord). Numbers in boldface (**L5, S1**) indicate the main segmental innervation. Damage to one or more of the listed spinal cord segments or to the motor nerve roots arising from them results in paralysis of the muscles concerned.

Three of the four muscles in the posterior aspect of the thigh are *hamstrings*. The **hamstring muscles** (Figs. 5.40A–D and 5.41B) are: (1) *semitendinosus*, (2) *semimembranosus*, and (3) *biceps femoris* (long head). The hamstring muscles ("hamstrings" for short) share common features:

- Proximal attachment to the ischial tuberosity deep to the gluteus maximus (Fig. 5.40A , F–H).
- Distal attachment to the bones of the leg (Fig. 5.40B–E).

- Thus they span and act on two joints, producing extension at the hip joint and flexion at the knee joint.
- Innervation by the tibial division of the sciatic nerve (Fig. 5.41A).

The long head of the biceps femoris meets all these conditions, but the short head of the biceps, the fourth muscle of the posterior compartment, fails to meet any of them.

FIGURE 5.41. Muscles and fascial compartments of thigh. A. Segments of the hamstring muscles are excised to reveal the sciatic nerve. The level of the sections shown in parts **B** and **C** is indicated. **B.** An anatomical transverse section through the middle thigh, 10–15 cm inferior to the inguinal ligament. The three compartments of the thigh are demonstrated in different shades of color. Note that each has its own nerve supply and functional group(s) of muscles. **C.** Transverse MRI of the right thigh corresponding to **B.** (Courtesy of Dr. W. Kucharczyk, Chair of Medical Imaging, Faculty of Medicine, University of Toronto and Clinical Director of the Tri-Hospital Resonance Centre, Toronto, Ontario, Canada.)

The hamstrings received their name because it is common to tie hams (pork thighs) up for curing and/or smoking using the long tendons of these muscles (Fig. 5.40F). This also explains the expression "hamstringing the enemy" by slashing these tendons lateral and medial to the knees.

The two actions of the hamstrings cannot be performed maximally at the same time: full flexion of the knee requires so much shortening of the hamstrings that they cannot provide the additional contraction that would be necessary for simultaneous full extension of the thigh; similarly, full extension of the hip shortens the hamstrings so they cannot further contract to act fully on the knee. When the thighs and legs are fixed, the hamstrings can help extend the trunk at the hip joint.

The hamstrings are active in thigh extension under all situations except full flexion of the knee, including maintenance of the relaxed standing posture (standing at ease). A person with paralyzed hamstrings tends to fall forward because the gluteus maximus muscles cannot maintain the necessary muscle tone to stand straight.

The hamstrings are the hip extensors involved in walking on flat ground, when the gluteus maximus demonstrates minimal activity. However, rather than producing either hip extension or knee flexion per se during normal walking, the hamstrings demonstrate most activity when they are eccentrically contracting, resisting (decelerating) hip flexion and knee extension during terminal swing (between midswing and heel strike) (see Fig. 5.20G; Table 5.2).

The length of the hamstrings varies, but this is usually a matter of conditioning. In some people, they are not long enough to allow them to touch their toes when the knees are extended. Routine stretch exercise can lengthen these muscles and tendons.

To test the hamstrings, the person flexes their leg against resistance. Normally, these muscles—especially their tendons on each side of the popliteal fossa—should be prominent as they bend the knee (see Fig. 5.48C).

SEMITENDINOSUS

The **semitendinosus,** as its name indicates, is half tendinous (Fig. 5.40F). It has a fusiform belly that is usually interrupted by a tendinous intersection and a long, cord-like tendon that begins approximately two thirds of the way down the thigh. Distally, the tendon attaches to the medial surface of the superior part of the tibia as part of the *pes anserinus* formation in conjunction with the tendinous insertions of the sartorius and gracilis (Fig. 5.40D).

SEMIMEMBRANOSUS

The **semimembranosus** is a broad muscle that is also aptly named because of the flattened membranous form of its proximal attachment to the ischial tuberosity (Fig. 5.40G; Table 5.7). The tendon of the semimembranosus forms around the middle of the thigh and descends to the posterior part of the medial condyle of the tibia.

The semimembranous tendon divides distally into three parts: (1) a direct attachment to the posterior aspect of the medial tibial condyle, (2) a part that blends with the popliteal fascia, and (3) a reflected part that reinforces the intercondylar part of the joint capsule of the knee as the **oblique popliteal ligament** (Fig. 5.40G; see also Fig. 5.58B).

When the knee is flexed to 90°, the tendons of the medial hamstrings or "semi-" muscles (semitendinosus and semimembranosus) pass to the medial side of the tibia. In this position, contraction of the medial hamstrings (and of synergists including the gracilis, sartorius, and popliteus) produces a limited amount (about 10°) of medial rotation of the tibia at the knee. The two medial hamstrings are not as active as the lateral hamstring, the biceps femoris, which is the "workhorse" of extension at the hip (Hamill and Knutzen, 2008).

BICEPS FEMORIS

The fusiform **biceps femoris,** as its name indicates, has two heads: a *long head* and a *short head* (Fig. 5.40F–H). In the inferior part of the thigh, the long head becomes tendinous and is joined by the short head. The rounded common tendon of these heads attaches to the head of the fibula and can easily be seen and felt as it passes the knee, especially when the knee is flexed against resistance.

The **long head of the biceps femoris** crosses and provides protection for the sciatic nerve after it descends from the gluteal region into the posterior aspect of the thigh (Figs. 5.38A and 5.41A–C). When the sciatic nerve divides into its terminal branches, the lateral branch (common fibular nerve) continues this relationship, running with the biceps tendon.

The **short head of the biceps femoris** arises from the lateral lip of the inferior third of the linea aspera and supracondylar ridge of the femur (Fig. 5.40B & H). Whereas the hamstrings have a common nerve supply from the tibial division of the sciatic nerve, *the short head of the biceps is innervated by the fibular division* (Table 5.7). Because each of the two heads of the biceps femoris has a different nerve supply, a wound in the posterior thigh with nerve injury may paralyze one head and not the other.

When the knee is flexed to 90°, the tendons of the lateral hamstring (biceps), as well as the iliotibial tract, pass to the lateral side of the tibia. In this position, contraction of the biceps and tensor fasciae latae produces about 40° lateral rotation of the tibia at the knee. Rotation of the flexed knee is especially important in snow skiing.

Neurovascular Structures of Gluteal and Posterior Thigh Regions

Several important nerves arise from the *sacral plexus* and either supply the gluteal region (e.g., superior and inferior gluteal nerves) or pass through it to supply the perineum and thigh (e.g., the pudendal and sciatic nerves, respectively). Figure 5.42 depicts the nerves of the gluteal region and posterior thigh, and Table 5.8 describes their origin, course, and distribution.

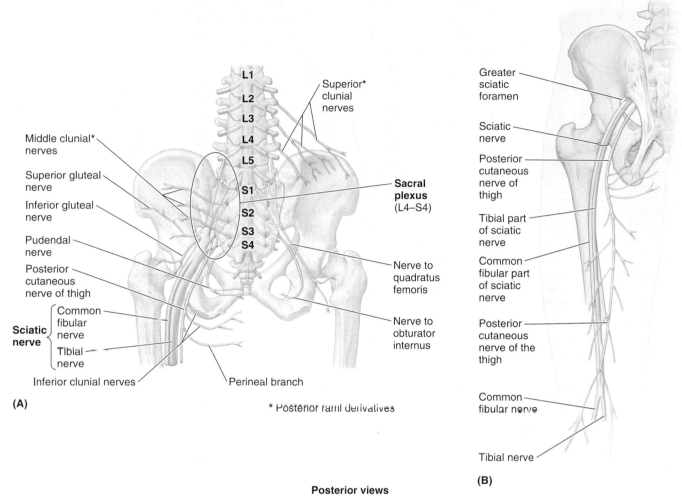

FIGURE 5.42. Nerves of the gluteal and posterior thigh regions.

TABLE 5.8. NERVES OF GLUTEAL AND POSTERIOR THIGH REGIONS

Nerve	Origin	Course	Distribution
Clunial			
Superior	As lateral cutaneous branches of posterior rami of L1–L3 spinal nerves	Pass inferolaterally across iliac crest	Supply skin of superior buttocks as far as tubercle of iliac crest
Middle	As lateral cutaneous branches of posterior rami of S1–S3 spinal nerves	Exit through posterior sacral foramina and pass laterally to gluteal region	Supply skin over sacrum and adjacent area of buttocks
Inferior	Posterior cutaneous nerve of thigh (anterior rami of S2–S3 spinal nerves)	Emerges from inferior border of gluteus maximus and ascends superficial to it	Supplies skin of inferior half of buttocks as far as greater trochanter

TABLE 5.8. NERVES OF GLUTEAL AND POSTERIOR THIGH REGIONS (Continued)

Nerve	Origin	Course	Distribution
Sciatic	Sacral plexus (anterior and posterior divisions of anterior rami of L4–S3 spinal nerves)	Enters gluteal region via greater sciatic foramen inferior to piriformis and deep to gluteus maximus; descends in posterior thigh deep to biceps femoris; bifurcates into tibial and common fibular nerves at apex of popliteal fossa	Supplies no muscles in gluteal region; supplies all muscles of posterior compartment of thigh (tibial division supplies all but short head of biceps, which is supplied by common fibular division)
Posterior cutaneous nerve of thigh	Sacral plexus (anterior and posterior divisions of anterior rami of S1–S3 spinal nerves)	Enters gluteal region via greater sciatic foramen inferior to piriformis and deep to gluteus maximus, emerging from inferior border of latter; descends in posterior thigh deep to fascia lata	Supplies skin of inferior half of buttocks (through inferior clunial nerves), skin over posterior thigh and popliteal fossa, and skin of lateral perineum and upper medial thigh (via its perineal branch)
Superior gluteal	Sacral plexus (posterior divisions of anterior rami of L4–S1 spinal nerves)	Enters gluteal region via greater sciatic foramen superior to piriformis; courses laterally between gluteus medius and minimus as far as tensor fasciae latae	Innervates gluteus medius, gluteus minimus, and tensor fasciae latae muscles
Inferior gluteal	Sacral plexus (posterior divisions of anterior rami of L5–S2 spinal nerves)	Enters gluteal region via greater sciatic foramen inferior to piriformis and deep to inferior part of gluteus maximus, dividing into several branches	Supplies gluteus maximus
Nerve to quadratus femoris	Sacral plexus (anterior divisions of anterior rami of L4–S1 spinal nerves)	Enters gluteal region via greater sciatic foramen inferior to piriformis, deep (anterior) to sciatic nerve	Innervates hip joint, inferior gemellus, and quadratus femoris
Pudendal	Sacral plexus (anterior divisions of anterior rami of S2–S4 spinal nerves)	Exits pelvis via greater sciatic foramen inferior to piriformis; descends posterior to sacrospinous ligament; enters perineum through lesser sciatic foramen	Supplies no structures in gluteal region or posterior thigh (principal nerve to perineum)
Nerve to obturator internus	Sacral plexus (posterior divisions of anterior rami of L5–S2 spinal nerves)	Exits pelvis via greater sciatic foramen inferior to piriformis; descends posterior to sacrospinous ligament; enters perineum through lesser sciatic foramen	Supplies superior gemellus and obturator internus

CLUNIAL NERVES

The skin of the gluteal region is richly innervated by **superior, middle,** and **inferior clunial nerves** (L. *clunes,* buttocks). These superficial nerves supply the skin over the iliac crest, between the posterior superior iliac spines, and over the iliac tubercles. Consequently, these nerves are vulnerable to injury when bone is taken from the ilium for grafting.

DEEP GLUTEAL NERVES

The *deep gluteal nerves* are the superior and inferior gluteal nerves, sciatic nerve, nerve to quadratus femoris, posterior cutaneous nerve of the thigh, nerve to obturator internus, and pudendal nerve (Figs. 5.38A and 5.42; Table 5.8). All of these nerves are branches of the sacral plexus and leave the pelvis through the greater sciatic foramen. Except for the superior gluteal nerve, they all emerge inferior to the piriformis.

Superior Gluteal Nerve. The **superior gluteal nerve** runs laterally between the gluteus medius and minimus with the deep branch of the superior gluteal artery. It divides into a superior branch that supplies the gluteus medius and an inferior branch that continues to pass between the gluteus medius and the gluteus minimus to supply both muscles and the tensor fasciae latae.

See the blue box "Injury to Superior Gluteal Nerve" on p. 581.

Inferior Gluteal Nerve. The **inferior gluteal nerve** leaves the pelvis through the greater sciatic foramen, inferior to the piriformis and superficial to the sciatic nerve, accompanied by multiple branches of the inferior gluteal artery and vein. The inferior gluteal nerve also divides into several branches, which provide motor innervation to the overlying gluteus maximus.

Sciatic Nerve. The **sciatic nerve** is the largest nerve in the body and is the continuation of the main part of the *sacral plexus.* The branches (rami) converge at the inferior border of the piriformis to form the sciatic nerve, a thick, flattened band approximately 2 cm wide. The sciatic nerve is the most lateral structure emerging through the greater sciatic foramen inferior to the piriformis.

Medial to the sciatic nerve are the inferior gluteal nerve and vessels, the internal pudendal vessels, and the pudendal nerve. The sciatic nerve runs inferolaterally under cover of the gluteus maximus, midway between the greater trochanter and ischial tuberosity. The nerve rests on the ischium and then passes posterior to the obturator internus, quadratus femoris, and adductor magnus muscles. The sciatic nerve is so large that it receives a named branch of the inferior gluteal artery, the **artery to the sciatic nerve.**

The sciatic nerve supplies no structures in the gluteal region. It supplies the posterior thigh muscles, all leg and foot muscles, and the skin of most of the leg and foot. It also supplies the articular branches to all joints of the lower limb. The sciatic nerve is really two nerves, the *tibial nerve,* derived from anterior (preaxial) divisions of the anterior rami, and the *common fibular nerve,* derived from posterior (postaxial) divisions of the anterior rami, which are loosely bound together in the same connective tissue sheath (Figs. 5.42 and 5.43A).

The tibial and common fibular nerves usually separate in the distal thigh (Fig. 5.42B); however, in approximately 12% of people, the nerves separate as they leave the pelvis (Fig. 5.43A). In these cases, the tibial nerve passes inferior to the piriformis, and the common fibular nerve pierces this muscle or passes superior to it (Fig. 5.43B & C).

Nerve to Quadratus Femoris. The **nerve to the quadratus femoris** leaves the pelvis anterior to the sciatic nerve and obturator internus, and passes over the posterior surface

of the hip joint (Fig. 5.42). It supplies an articular branch to this joint and innervates the inferior gemellus and quadratus femoris muscles.

Posterior Cutaneous Nerve of Thigh. The **posterior cutaneous nerve of the thigh** supplies more skin than any other cutaneous nerve (Fig. 5.42). Its fibers from the anterior divisions of S2 and S3 supply the skin of the perineum via its *perineal branch.* Some of the fibers from the posterior divisions of the anterior rami of S1 and S2 supply the skin of the inferior part of the buttocks (via the *inferior clunial nerves).* Other fibers continue inferiorly in branches that supply the skin of the posterior thigh and proximal part of the leg. Unlike most nerves bearing the name *cutaneous,* the main part of this nerve lies deep to the deep fascia (fascia lata), with only its terminal branches penetrating the subcutaneous tissue for distribution to the skin.

Pudendal Nerve. The *pudendal nerve* is the most medial structure to exit the pelvis through the greater sciatic foramen. It descends inferior to the piriformis, posterolateral to the sacrospinous ligament, and enters the perineum through the lesser sciatic foramen to supply structures in this region. The pudendal nerve supplies no structures in the gluteal region or posterior thigh, and is discussed in detail in Chapter 3.

Nerve to Obturator Internus. The **nerve to the obturator internus** arises from the anterior divisions of the anterior rami of the L5–S2 nerves and parallels the course of the pudendal nerve (Fig. 5.42A). As it passes around the base of the ischial spine, the nerve supplies the superior gemellus. After entering the perineum via the lesser sciatic foramen, the nerve supplies the obturator internus muscle.

ARTERIES OF GLUTEAL AND POSTERIOR THIGH REGIONS

The **arteries of the gluteal region** arise, directly or indirectly, from the *internal iliac arteries,* but the patterns of origin of the arteries are variable (Figs. 5.38A and 5.44; Table 5.9). The major branches of the internal iliac artery that supply or traverse the gluteal region are the (1) superior gluteal artery, (2) inferior gluteal artery, and (3) internal pudendal artery. The posterior compartment of the thigh has no major artery exclusive to the compartment; it receives blood from multiple sources: inferior gluteal, medial circumflex femoral, perforating, and popliteal arteries.

Superior Gluteal Artery. The **superior gluteal artery** is the largest branch of the internal iliac artery and passes posteriorly between the lumbosacral trunk and the S1 nerve. This artery leaves the pelvis through the greater sciatic foramen, superior to the piriformis, and divides immediately into superficial and deep branches. The *superficial branch* supplies the gluteus maximus and skin over the proximal attachment of this muscle. The *deep branch* supplies the gluteus medius, gluteus minimus, and tensor fasciae latae. The superior gluteal artery anastomoses with the inferior gluteal and medial circumflex femoral arteries.

Inferior Gluteal Artery. The **inferior gluteal artery** arises from the internal iliac artery and passes posteriorly through the parietal pelvic fascia, between the S1 and the

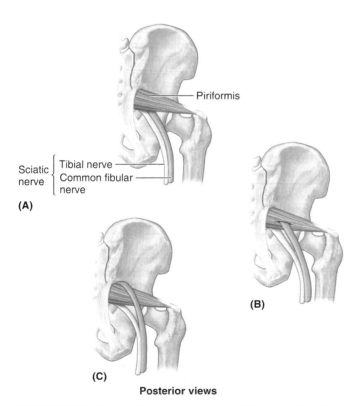

Piriformis

Sciatic nerve { Tibial nerve
Common fibular nerve

(A)

(B)

(C)

Posterior views

FIGURE 5.43. Relationship of sciatic nerve to piriformis. A. The sciatic nerve usually emerges from the greater sciatic foramen inferior to the piriformis. **B.** In 12.2% of 640 limbs studied by Dr. J. C. B. Grant, the sciatic nerve divided before exiting the greater sciatic foramen; the common fibular division (*yellow*) passed through the piriformis. **C.** In 0.5% of cases, the common fibular division passed superior to the muscle, where it is especially vulnerable to injury during intragluteal injections.

In terms of the vascular supply to the lower limb as a whole, the majority of the arterial blood coming to the limb and most of the venous blood and lymph exiting from it pass along the more protected anteromedial aspect of the limb.

Flexor muscles are generally better protected than are extensor muscles, the latter being exposed and therefore vulnerable in the flexed, defensive (fetal) position (vertebral column and limbs flexed).

Surface Anatomy of Gluteal and Posterior Thigh Regions

The skin of the gluteal region is usually thick and coarse, especially in men, whereas the skin of the thigh is relatively thin and loosely attached to the underlying subcutaneous tissue. A line joining the *highest points of the iliac crests* (Fig. 5.46A) crosses the L4–L5 intervertebral (IV) disc and is a useful landmark when a *lumbar spinal puncture* is performed (see Chapter 4), indicating the middle of the *lumbar cistern*.

The *intergluteal cleft,* beginning inferior to the apex of the sacrum, is the deep groove between the buttocks. It extends as far superiorly as the S3 or S4 segment. The *coccyx* is palpable in the superior part of the intergluteal cleft.

The *posterior superior iliac spines (PSIS)* are located at the posterior extremities of the iliac crests, and may be difficult to palpate; however, their position can always be located at the bottom of the permanent skin dimples approximately 3.75

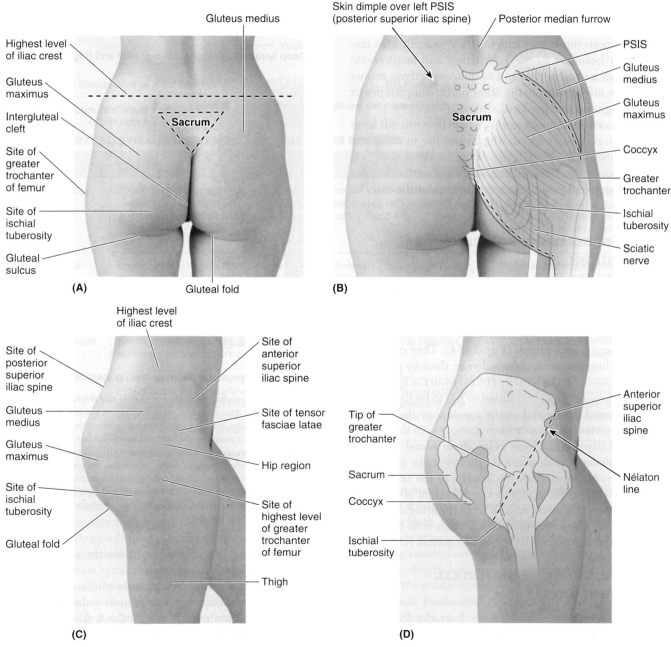

FIGURE 5.46. Surface anatomy of the gluteal region.

cm from midline (Fig. 5.46B). A line joining these dimples, often more visible in women than in men, passes through the S2 spinous process, indicating the level of the lowest limit of the *dural sac,* the middle of the sacro-iliac joints, and the bifurcation of the common iliac arteries (see Fig. 4.39).

The location of only two of the gluteal muscles can be observed. The *gluteus maximus* covering most structures in the gluteal region can be felt to contract when straightening up from bending over. The inferior edge of this large muscle is located just superior to the *gluteal fold,* which contains a variable amount of subcutaneous fat (Fig. 5.46A & C). The gluteal fold disappears when the hip joint is flexed. The degree of prominence of the gluteal fold changes in certain abnormal conditions, such as *atrophy of the gluteus maximus.* An imaginary line drawn from the coccyx to the ischial tuberosity indicates the inferior edge of the gluteus maximus (Fig. 5.46B). Another line drawn from the PSIS to a point slightly superior to the greater trochanter indicates the superior edge of this muscle.

The **gluteal sulcus,** the skin crease inferior to the gluteal fold, delineates the buttocks from the posterior aspect of the thigh (Fig. 5.46A & B). When the thigh is extended as in the figures, the *ischial tuberosity* is covered by the inferior part of the gluteus maximus; however, the tuberosity is easy to palpate when the thigh is flexed because

the gluteus maximus slips superiorly off the tuberosity, which is then subcutaneous. Feel the ischial tuberosity as you bend to sit.

The superior part of the *gluteus medius* can be palpated between the superior part of the gluteus maximus and the iliac crest (Figs. 5.46B and 5.47A & B). The gluteus medius of one buttocks can be felt when all the body weight shifts onto the ipsilateral limb (the one on the same side).

The *greater trochanter,* the most lateral bony point in the gluteal region, may be felt on the lateral aspect of the hip, especially its inferior part (Fig. 5.46A–C). It is easier to palpate when you passively abduct your lower limb to relax the gluteus medius and minimus. The top of the greater trochanter lies approximately a hand's breadth inferior to the *tubercle of the iliac crest* (Fig. 5.47).

The prominence of the trochanter increases when a dislocated hip causes atrophy of the gluteal muscles and displacement of the trochanter. A line drawn from the ASIS to the ischial tuberosity (*Nélaton line*), passing over the lateral aspect of the hip region, normally passes over or near the top of the greater trochanter (Fig. 5.46D). The trochanter can be felt superior to this line in a person with a dislocated hip or a fractured femoral neck. The *lesser trochanter* is palpable with difficulty from the posterior aspect when the thigh is extended and rotated medially.

FIGURE 5.47. Surface anatomy of the hip region and lateral thigh.

The surface marking of the superior border of the *piriformis* is indicated by a line joining the skin dimple formed by the posterior superior iliac spine to the superior border of the greater trochanter of the femur (Fig. 5.48A).

The *sciatic nerve*, the most important structure inferior to the piriformis, is represented by a line that extends from a point midway between the greater trochanter and ischial tuberosity (Fig. 5.48A) down the middle of the posterior aspect of the thigh (Fig. 5.48B). The level of the bifurcation of the sciatic nerve into the tibial and common fibular nerves varies. The separation usually occurs between the middle and inferior third of the thigh. Less commonly, the division of the sciatic nerve occurs as it

(A) **Surface anatomy of the posterior aspect of the gluteal region**

Gluteus medius
Sacrum
Gluteus maximus
Piriformis
Palpable aspect of greater trochanter
Palpable aspect of ischial tuberosity
Sciatic nerve

Adductor magnus
Semitendinosus
Gracilis
Semimembranosus
Semitendinosus tendon
Gastrocnemius, medial head

Gluteus maximus
Sciatic nerve
Iliotibial tract (over vastus lateralis)
Biceps femoris
Common fibular nerve
Biceps tendon
Gastrocnemius, lateral head
Tibial nerve

(B)

Semimembranosus
Semitendinosus tendon
Popliteal fossa
Gastrocnemius, medial head
Fibularis brevis
Calcaneal tendon

Vastus lateralis
Biceps femoris tendon
Head of fibula
Gastrocnemius, lateral head
Fibularis longus
Soleus
Fibularis longus tendon
Lateral malleolus

(C)

FIGURE 5.48. Surface anatomy of the gluteal region and posterior thigh. A. Surface projection of piriformis and sciatic nerve. **B.** The hip and knee joints are extended with muscles actively tensed following exercise, to provide muscle definition. **C.** Weight is being borne by the right limb while the hip, knee, and metatarsophalangeal joints are in a flexed position.

passes through the greater sciatic foramen. The sciatic nerve stretches when the thigh is flexed and the knee is extended, and it relaxes when the thigh is extended and the knee is flexed.

The *tibial nerve* bisects the popliteal fossa. The *common fibular nerve* follows the tendon of the biceps femoris.

The *hamstrings* can be felt as a group as they arise from the ischial tuberosity and extend along the lateral and posterior aspects of the thigh (Fig. 5.48B & C). The *iliotibial tract,* the fibrous band that reinforces the fascia lata laterally, can be observed on the lateral aspect of the thigh as it passes to the *lateral tibial condyle* (Fig. 5.47A & B).

While sitting down with your lower limb extended, raise your heel off the floor and feel the anterior border of the iliotibial tract passing a finger's breadth posterior to the lateral border of the patella. Note that the iliotibial tract is prominent and taut when the heel is raised and indistinct when the heel is lowered.

The *tendons of the hamstrings* can be observed and palpated at the borders of the *popliteal fossa,* the depression between the tendons at the back of the flexed knee (Fig. 5.48B & C). The *biceps femoris tendon* is on the lateral side of the fossa. The most lateral tendon on the medial side when the knee is flexed against resistance is the *semimembranosus tendon.*

While sitting on a chair with your knee flexed, press your heel against the leg of the chair and feel your biceps femoris tendon laterally and trace it to the head of the fibula. Also feel the narrow and more prominent *semitendinosus tendon* medially, which pulls away from the semimembranosus tendon that attaches to the superomedial part of the tibia.

See the blue box "Hamstring Injuries" below.

GLUTEAL AND POSTERIOR THIGH REGIONS

Trochanteric Bursitis

 Trochanteric bursitis, inflammation of the trochanteric bursa (see Fig. 5.37), may result from repetitive actions such as climbing stairs while carrying heavy objects, or running on a steeply elevated treadmill. These movements involve the gluteus maximus and move the superior tendinous fibers repeatedly back and forth over the bursae of the greater trochanter. Trochanteric bursitis causes deep diffuse pain in the lateral thigh region.

This type of *friction bursitis* is characterized by point tenderness over the great trochanter; however, the pain radiates along the iliotibial tract that extends from the iliac tubercle to the tibia (see Figs. 5.36 and 5.39C). This thickening of the fascia lata receives tendinous reinforcements from the tensor fasciae latae and gluteus maximus muscles. The pain from an inflamed trochanteric bursa, usually localized just posterior to the greater trochanter, is generally elicited by manually resisting abduction and lateral rotation of the thigh while the person is lying on the unaffected side.

Ischial Bursitis

 Recurrent microtrauma resulting from repeated stress (e.g., as from cycling, rowing, or other activities involving repetitive hip extension while seated) may overwhelm the ability of the ischial bursa (see Fig. 5.37) to dissipate applied stress. The recurrent trauma results in inflammation of the bursa (*ischial bursitis*).

Ischial bursitis is a *friction bursitis* resulting from excessive friction between the ischial bursae and the ischial tuberosities. Localized pain occurs over the bursa, and the pain increases with movement of the gluteus maximus. Calcification may occur in the bursa with chronic bursitis. Because the ischial tuberosities bear the body's weight during sitting, these pressure points may lead to *pressure sores* in debilitated people, particularly paraplegic persons with poor nursing care.

Hamstring Injuries

 Hamstring strains (pulled and/or torn hamstrings) are common in individuals who run and/or kick hard (e.g., in running, jumping, and quick-start sports such as baseball, basketball, football, and soccer). The violent muscular exertion required to excel in these sports may avulse (tear) part of the proximal tendinous attachments of the hamstrings to the ischial tuberosity. Hamstring strains are twice as common as quadriceps strains.

Usually thigh strains are accompanied by contusion (bruising) and tearing of muscle fibers, resulting in rupture of the blood vessels supplying the muscles. The resultant *hematoma* is contained by the dense stocking-like fascia lata.

Tearing of hamstring fibers is often so painful when the athlete moves or stretches the leg that the person falls and writhes in pain. These injuries often result from inadequate warming up before practice or competition.

Avulsion (tearing away) of the ischial tuberosity at the proximal attachment of the biceps femoris and semitendinosus may result from forcible flexion of the hip with the knee extended (e.g., kicking a football). (See Fig. B5.1 and the blue box "Injuries of Hip Bone" on p. 526.)

Injury to Superior Gluteal Nerve

Injury to this nerve results in a characteristic motor loss, resulting in a disabling *gluteus medius limp,* to compensate for weakened abduction of the thigh by

Gracilis

Semitendinosus

Semimembranosus

Popliteal artery

Popliteal vein

Tibial nerve

Medial superior
genicular artery

Semitendinosus

Semimembranosus

Bursa

Gastrocnemius

Fibrous (articular)
capsule of knee joint

Medial inferior
genicular artery

**Investing fascia of
popliteus**

Plantaris

Gastrocnemius,
medial head

Biceps femoris,
long head

Biceps femoris,
short head

Lateral intermuscular
septum

Common fibular
nerve

Biceps femoris

Lateral superior
genicular artery

**Popliteal surface
of femur**

Gastrocnemius

Plantaris

Lateral inferior
genicular artery

Popliteus

Tibial nerve

Nerve to popliteus

Soleus

Gastrocnemius,
lateral head

Posterior view

FIGURE 5.51. Deep dissection of popliteal fossa. The popliteal artery runs on the floor of the fossa, formed by the popliteal surface of the femur, the joint capsule of the knee, and the investing fascia of the popliteus.

The contents, most important the popliteal artery and lymph nodes, are most easily palpated with the knee semi-flexed. Because of the deep fascial roof and osseofibrous floor, the fossa is a relatively confined space. Many disorders produce swelling of the fossa, making knee extension painful. (See the blue boxes "Popliteal Abscess and Tumor" and "Popliteal Aneurysm and Hemorrhage" on p. 604, and "Popliteal Cysts" on p. 665.)

NEUROVASCULAR STRUCTURES AND RELATIONSHIPS IN POPLITEAL FOSSA

All important neurovascular structures that pass from the thigh to the leg do so by traversing the popliteal fossa. Progressing from superficial to deep (posterior to anterior) within the fossa, as in dissection, the nerves are encountered first, then the veins. The arteries lie deepest, directly on the popliteal surface of the femur, joint capsule, and *investing fascia of the popliteus* forming the floor of the fossa (Fig. 5.51).

Nerves in Popliteal Fossa. The *sciatic nerve* usually ends at the superior angle of the popliteal fossa by dividing into the tibial and common fibular nerves (Figs. 5.49B, 5.50, and 5.51).

The **tibial nerve** is the medial, larger terminal branch of the sciatic nerve derived from anterior (preaxial) divisions of the anterior rami of the L4–S3 spinal nerves. *The tibial nerve is the most superficial of the three main central components of the popliteal fossa* (i.e., nerve, vein, and artery); however, it is still in a deep and protected position. The tibial nerve bisects the fossa as it passes from its superior to its inferior angle.

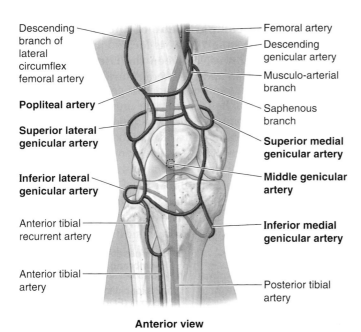

Anterior view

FIGURE 5.52. Genicular anastomosis. The many arteries making up the peri-articular anastomosis around the knee provide an important collateral circulation for bypassing the popliteal artery when the knee joint has been maintained too long in a fully flexed position or when the vessels are narrowed or occluded.

While in the fossa, the tibial nerve gives branches to the soleus, gastrocnemius, plantaris, and popliteus muscles. The **medial sural cutaneous nerve** is also derived from the tibial nerve in the popliteal fossa. It is joined by the **sural communicating branch of the common fibular nerve** at a highly variable level to form the *sural nerve*. This nerve supplies the lateral side of the leg and ankle.

The **common fibular** (peroneal) **nerve** is the lateral, smaller terminal branch of the sciatic nerve derived from posterior (postaxial) divisions of the anterior rami of the L4–S2 spinal nerves. The common fibular nerve begins at the superior angle of the popliteal fossa and follows closely the medial border of the biceps femoris and its tendon along the superolateral boundary of the fossa. The nerve leaves the fossa by passing superficial to the lateral head of the gastrocnemius and then passes over the posterior aspect of the head of the fibula. The *common fibular nerve winds around the neck of the fibula* and divides into its terminal branches.

The most inferior branches of the *posterior cutaneous nerve of the thigh* supply the skin that overlies the popliteal fossa (see Fig 5.42B). The nerve traverses most of the length of the posterior compartment of the thigh deep to the fascia lata; only its terminal branches enter the subcutaneous tissue as cutaneous nerves.

Blood Vessels in Popliteal Fossa. The **popliteal artery,** the continuation of the femoral artery (Figs. 5.51 and 5.52), begins when the latter passes through the adductor hiatus (see Fig. 5.30A). The popliteal artery passes inferolaterally through the fossa and ends at the inferior border of the popliteus by dividing into the *anterior* and *posterior*

tibial arteries. The deepest (most anterior) structure in the fossa, the popliteal artery, runs in close proximity to the joint capsule of the knee as it spans the intercondylar fossa.

Five *genicular branches of the popliteal artery* supply the capsule and ligaments of the knee joint. The genicular arteries are the **superior lateral, superior medial, middle, inferior lateral,** and **inferior medial genicular arteries** (Fig. 5.52). They participate in the formation of the periarticular **genicular anastomosis,** a network of vessels surrounding the knee that provides collateral circulation capable of maintaining blood supply to the leg during full knee flexion, which may kink the popliteal artery. Other contributors to this important genicular anastomosis are the:

- **Descending genicular artery,** a branch of the femoral artery, superomedially.
- **Descending branch of the lateral femoral circumflex artery,** superolaterally.
- **Anterior tibial recurrent artery,** a branch of the anterior tibial artery, inferolaterally.

Muscular branches of the popliteal artery supply the hamstring, gastrocnemius, soleus, and plantaris muscles. The superior muscular branches of the popliteal artery have clinically important anastomoses with the terminal part of the profunda femoris and gluteal arteries.

The **popliteal vein** begins at the distal border of the popliteus as a continuation of the *posterior tibial vein* (Fig. 5.51). Throughout its course, the vein lies close to the popliteal artery, lying superficial to it and in the same fibrous sheath. The popliteal vein is initially posteromedial to the artery and lateral to the tibial nerve. More superiorly, the popliteal vein lies posterior to the artery, between this vessel and the overlying tibial nerve. Superiorly, the popliteal vein, which has several valves, becomes the *femoral vein* as it traverses the adductor hiatus. The *small saphenous vein* passes from the posterior aspect of the lateral malleolus to the popliteal fossa, where it pierces the deep popliteal fascia and enters the popliteal vein.

Lymph Nodes in Popliteal Fossa. The **superficial popliteal lymph nodes** are usually small and lie in the subcutaneous tissue. A lymph node lies at the termination of the small saphenous vein and receives lymph from the lymphatic vessels that accompany this vein (see Fig. 5.15). The **deep popliteal lymph nodes** surround the vessels and receive lymph from the joint capsule of the knee and the lymphatic vessels that accompany the deep veins of the leg. The lymphatic vessels from the popliteal lymph nodes follow the femoral vessels to the *deep inguinal lymph nodes.*

Anterior Compartment of Leg

ORGANIZATION OF LEG

The bones of the leg (*tibia* and *fibula*) that connect the knee and ankle, and the three fascial compartments (*anterior, lateral,* and *posterior compartments of the leg*), formed by the

Superior extensor retinaculum

Anterior tibial artery

Extensor digitorum longus (EDL)

Extensor hallucis longus (EHL)

Lateral malleolus

Medial malleolus

Fibularis tertius (FT)

Tibialis anterior (TA)

Inferior fibular retinaculum

Inferior extensor retinaculum

Extensor hallucis brevis (EHB)

Deep fibular nerve

Dorsalis pedis artery
(dorsal artery of foot)

Fibularis tertius (FT)

Extensor digitorum longus (EDL)

Extensor hallucis longus (EHL)

Extensor digitorum brevis (EDB)

1st dorsal interosseous

Extensor expansion

Extensor expansion

Central band

Lateral bands

(A) Anterosuperior view of dorsum of foot

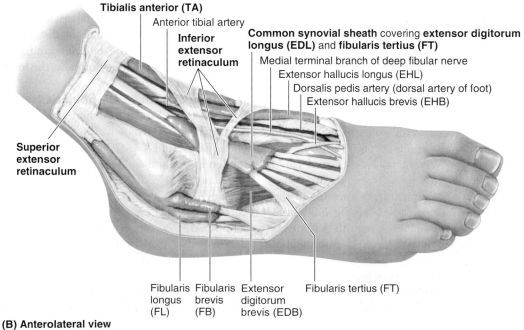

Tibialis anterior (TA)

Anterior tibial artery

Inferior
extensor
retinaculum

Common synovial sheath covering **extensor digitorum
longus (EDL)** and **fibularis tertius (FT)**

Medial terminal branch of deep fibular nerve

Extensor hallucis longus (EHL)

Dorsalis pedis artery (dorsal artery of foot)

Extensor hallucis brevis (EHB)

Superior
extensor
retinaculum

Fibularis Fibularis Extensor   Fibularis tertius (FT)
longus   brevis   digitorum
(FL)   (FB)   brevis (EDB)

(B) Anterolateral view

FIGURE 5.54. Dissections of foot. These dissections demonstrate the continuation of the anterior and lateral leg muscles into the foot. The thinner portions of the deep fascia of the leg have been removed, leaving the thicker portions that make up the extensor and fibular retinacula, which retain the tendons as they cross the ankle. **A.** The vessels and nerves are cut short. At the ankle, the vessels and the deep fibular nerve lie midway between the malleoli and between the tendons of the long dorsiflexors of the toes. **B.** Synovial sheaths surround the tendons as they pass beneath the retinacula of the ankle.

FIGURE 5.55. Muscles of anterior and lateral compartments of leg.

TABLE 5.10. MUSCLES OF ANTERIOR AND LATERAL COMPARTMENTS OF LEG

Muscle[a]	Proximal Attachment	Distal Attachment	Innervation[b]	Main Action
Anterior compartment **Tibialis anterior** (1)	Lateral condyle and superior half of lateral surface of tibia and interosseous membrane	Medial and inferior surfaces of medial cuneiform and base of 1st metatarsal	Deep fibular nerve (**L4**, L5)	Dorsiflexes ankle and inverts foot
Extensor digitorum longus (2)	Lateral condyle of tibia and superior three quarters of medial surface of fibula and interosseous membrane	Middle and distal phalanges of lateral four digits		Extends lateral four digits and dorsiflexes ankle
Extensor hallucis longus (3)	Middle part of anterior surface of fibula and interosseous membrane	Dorsal aspect of base of distal phalanx of great toe (hallux)		Extends great toe and dorsiflexes ankle
Fibularis tertius (4)	Inferior third of anterior surface of fibula and interosseous membrane	Dorsum of base of 5th metatarsal		Dorsiflexes ankle and aids in eversion of foot
Lateral compartment **Fibularis longus** (5)	Head and superior two thirds of lateral surface of fibula	Base of 1st metatarsal and medial cuneiform	Superficial fibular nerve (**L5, S1,** S2)	Everts foot and weakly plantarflexes ankle
Fibularis brevis (6)	Inferior two thirds of lateral surface of fibula	Dorsal surface of tuberosity on lateral side of base of 5th metatarsal		

[a] Numbers refer to Figure 5.55A & B.

[b] The spinal cord segmental innervation is indicated (e.g., "L4, L5" means that the nerves supplying the tibialis anterior are derived from the fourth and fifth lumbar segments of the spinal cord). Numbers in boldface (**L4**) indicate the main segmental innervation. Damage to one or more of the listed spinal cord segments or to the motor nerve roots arising from them results in paralysis of the muscles concerned.

the inferior compartment—inferior to the *fibular trochlea* on the calcaneus—and enters a groove on the antero-inferior aspect of the cuboid bone (see Fig. 5.11D). It then crosses the sole of the foot, running obliquely and distally to reach its attachment to the *1st metatarsal and medial cuneiform bones* (see Fig. 5.11B). When a person stands on one foot, the FL helps steady the leg on the foot.

Fibularis Brevis. The **fibularis brevis** (**FB**) is a fusiform muscle that lies deep to the FL, and, true to its name, the FB is shorter than its partner in the lateral compartment (Figs. 5.53, 5.55F, and 5.56A; Table 5.10). Its broad tendon grooves the posterior aspect of the lateral malleolus and can be palpated inferior to it. The narrower tendon of the FL lies posterior to the tendon of the FB and does not contact the lateral malleolus. The tendon of the FB traverses the superior compartment of the inferior fibular retinaculum, passing superior to the fibular trochlea of the calcaneus; it can be easily traced to its distal attachment to the *base of the 5th metatarsal* (Fig. 5.11D). The tendon of the *fibularis tertius*, a slip of muscle from the extensor digitorum longus, often merges with the tendon of the FB (Fig. 5.56A). Occasionally, however, the fibularis tertius passes anteriorly to attach directly to the proximal phalanx of the 5th digit.

NERVES IN LATERAL COMPARTMENT OF LEG

The **superficial fibular** (peroneal) **nerve,** a terminal branch of the common fibular nerve, is the nerve of the lateral compartment (Figs. 5.43A, 5.56A, and 5.57A; Table 5.11). After supplying the FL and FB, the superficial fibular nerve continues as a cutaneous nerve, supplying the skin on the distal part of the anterior surface of the leg and nearly all the dorsum of the foot.

BLOOD VESSELS IN LATERAL COMPARTMENT OF LEG

The lateral compartment does not have an artery coursing through it. Instead, *perforating branches* and accompanying veins supply blood to and drain blood from the compartment. Proximally, **perforating branches of the anterior tibial artery** penetrate the anterior intermuscular septum. Inferiorly, **perforating branches of the fibular artery** penetrate the posterior intermuscular septum, along with their accompanying veins (L. *venae comitantes*) (Figs. 5.58 and 5.59; Table 5.12).

Posterior Compartment of Leg

The **posterior compartment of the leg** (plantarflexor compartment) is the largest of the three leg compartments (Fig. 5.53A). The posterior compartment and the muscles within it are divided into superficial and deep subcompartments/muscle groups by the *transverse intermuscular septum.* The tibial nerve and posterior tibial and fibular vessels supply both parts of the posterior compartment but run in the deep subcompartment deep (anterior) to the transverse intermuscular septum.

The larger **superficial subcompartment** is the least confined compartmental area. The smaller **deep subcompartment,** like the anterior compartment, is bounded by the two leg bones and the *interosseous membrane* that binds them together, plus the transverse intermuscular septum. Therefore, the deep subcompartment is quite tightly confined. Because the nerve and blood vessels supplying the entire posterior compartment and the sole of the foot pass through the deep subcompartment, when swelling occurs it leads to a compartment syndrome that has serious consequences, such as muscular necrosis (tissue death) and paralysis.

Inferiorly, the deep subcompartment tapers as the muscles it contains become tendinous. The transverse intermuscular septum ends as reinforcing transverse fibers that extend between the tip of the medial malleolus and the calcaneus to form the **flexor retinaculum** (see Fig. 5.61). The retinaculum is subdivided deeply, forming separate compartments for each tendon of the deep muscle group, as well as for the tibial nerve and posterior tibial artery as they bend around the medial malleolus.

Muscles of the posterior compartment produce *plantarflexion* at the ankle, *inversion* at the subtalar and transverse tarsal joints, and *flexion* of the toes. **Plantarflexion** is a powerful movement (four times stronger than dorsiflexion) produced over a relatively long range (approximately 50° from neutral) by muscles that pass posterior to the transverse axis of the ankle joint. Plantarflexion develops thrust, applied primarily at the ball of the foot, that is used to propel the body forward and upward, and is the major component of the forces generated during the push-off (heel off and toe off) parts of the stance phase of walking and running (see Fig. 5.20D & E; Table 5.2).

SUPERFICIAL MUSCLE GROUP IN POSTERIOR COMPARTMENT

The *superficial group of calf muscles* (muscles forming prominence of "calf" of posterior leg) includes the *gastrocnemius, soleus,* and *plantaris.* Details concerning their attachments, innervation, and actions are provided in Figure 5.60A–E and Table 5.13.I). The gastrocnemius and soleus share a common tendon, the *calcaneal tendon,* which attaches to the calcaneus. Collectively these two muscles make up the three-headed **triceps surae** (L. *sura,* calf) (Figs. 5.60 and 5.61A). This powerful muscular mass tugs on the lever provided by the calcaneal tuberosity, elevating the heel and thus depressing the forefoot, generating as much as 93% of the plantarflexion force.

The large size of the gastrocnemius and soleus muscles is a human characteristic that is directly related to our upright stance. These muscles are strong and heavy because they lift, propel, and accelerate the weight of the body when walking, running, jumping, or standing on the toes.

The **calcaneal tendon** (L. *tendo calcaneus,* Achilles tendon) is the most powerful (thickest and strongest) tendon in the body. Approximately 15 cm in length, it is a continuation

FIGURE 5.60A–E. Superficial (calf) muscles of posterior compartment of leg.

TABLE 5.13.I. SUPERFICIAL MUSCLES OF POSTERIOR COMPARTMENT OF LEG

Muscle[a]	Proximal Attachment	Distal Attachment	Innervation[b]	Main Action
Gastrocnemius (1)	Lateral head: lateral aspect of lateral condyle of femur	Posterior surface of calcaneus via calcaneal tendon	Tibial nerve (S1, S2)	Plantarflexes ankle when knee is extended; raises heel during walking; flexes leg at knee joint
	Medial head: popliteal surface of femur; superior to medial condyle			
Soleus (2)	Posterior aspect of head and superior quarter of posterior surface of fibula; soleal line and middle third of medial border of tibia; and tendinous arch extending between the bony attachments			Plantarflexes ankle independent of position of knee; steadies leg on foot
Plantaris (3)	Inferior end of lateral supracondylar line of femur; oblique popliteal ligament			Weakly assists gastrocnemius in plantarflexing ankle

[a] Numbers refer to Figure 5.60A.

[b] The spinal cord segmental innervation is indicated (e.g., "S1, S2" means that the nerves supplying these muscles are derived from the first and second sacral segments of the spinal cord). Damage to one or more of the listed spinal cord segments or to the motor nerve roots arising from them results in paralysis of the muscles concerned.

of the flat aponeurosis formed halfway down the calf where the bellies of the gastrocnemius terminate (Figs. 5.60D & E and 5.61). Proximally, the aponeurosis receives fleshy fibers of the soleus directly on its deep surface but distally the soleus fibers become tendinous. The tendon thus becomes thicker (deeper) but narrower as it descends until it becomes essentially round in cross-section superior to the calcaneus. It then widens as it inserts on the posterior surface of the *calcaneal tuberosity*. The calcaneal tendon typically spirals a quarter turn (90°) during its descent, so that the gastrocnemius fibers attach laterally and the soleal fibers attach medially. This arrangement is thought to be significant to the tendon's elastic ability to absorb energy (shock) and recoil, releasing the energy as part of the propulsive force it exerts. Although they share a common tendon, the two muscles of the triceps surae are capable of acting alone, and often do so: "You stroll with the soleus but win the long jump with the gastrocnemius."

To test the triceps surae, the foot is plantarflexed against resistance (e.g., by "standing on the toes," in which case body weight [gravity] provides resistance). If normal, the calcaneal tendon and triceps surae can be observed and palpated.

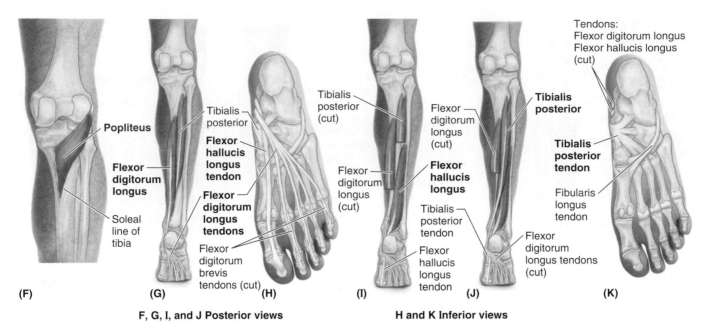

FIGURE 5.60F-K. Deep muscles of posterior compartment of leg.

TABLE 5.13.II. DEEP MUSCLES OF POSTERIOR COMPARTMENT OF LEG

Muscle[a]	Proximal Attachment	Distal Attachment	Innervation[b]	Main Action
Popliteus	Lateral surface of lateral condyle of femur and lateral meniscus	Posterior surface of tibia, superior to soleal line	Tibial nerve (L4, L5, S1)	Weakly flexes knee and unlocks it by rotating femur 5° on fixed tibia; medially rotates tibia of unplanted limb
Flexor hallucis longus (4)	Inferior two thirds of posterior surface of fibula; inferior part of interosseous membrane	Base of distal phalanx of great toe (hallux)	Tibial nerve (S2, S3)	Flexes great toe at all joints; weakly plantarflexes ankle; supports medial longitudinal arch of foot
Flexor digitorum longus (5)	Medial part of posterior surface of tibia inferior to soleal line; by a broad tendon to fibula	Bases of distal phalanges of lateral four digits		Flexes lateral four digits; plantarflexes ankle; supports longitudinal arches of foot
Tibialis posterior (6)	Interosseous membrane; posterior surface of tibia inferior to soleal line; posterior surface of fibula	Tuberosity of navicular, cuneiform, cuboid, and sustentaculum tali of calcaneus; bases of 2nd, 3rd, and 4th metatarsals	Tibial nerve (L4, L5)	Plantarflexes ankle; inverts foot

[a] Numbers refer to Figure 5.60A.

[b] The spinal cord segmental innervation is indicated (e.g., "S2, S3" means that the nerves supplying the flexor hallucis longus are derived from the second and third sacral segments of the spinal cord). Damage to one or more of the listed spinal cord segments or to the motor nerve roots arising from them results in paralysis of the muscles concerned.

A *subcutaneous calcaneal bursa,* located between the skin and the calcaneal tendon, allows the skin to move over the taut tendon. A deep *bursa of the calcaneal tendon* (retrocalcaneal bursa), located between the tendon and the calcaneus, allows the tendon to glide over the bone.

Gastrocnemius. The **gastrocnemius** is the most superficial muscle in the posterior compartment and forms the proximal, most prominent part of the *calf* (Figs. 5.60D and 5.61A; Table 5.13.I). It is a fusiform, two-headed, two-joint muscle with the medial head slightly larger and extending more distally than its lateral partner. The heads come together

at the inferior margin of the popliteal fossa, where they form the inferolateral and inferomedial boundaries of this fossa. Because its fibers are largely of the white, fast-twitch (type 2) variety, contractions of the gastrocnemius produce rapid movements during running and jumping. It is recruited into action only intermittently during symmetrical standing.

The gastrocnemius crosses and is capable of acting on both the knee and the ankle joints; however, it cannot exert its full power on both joints at the same time. It functions most effectively when the knee is extended (and is maximally activated when knee extension is combined with dorsiflexion,

(A) Posterior view

(B) Posteromedial view

FIGURE 5.61. **Dissections of posterior aspect of leg. A.** Superficial dissection. Except for the retinacula in the ankle region, the deep fascia has been removed to reveal the nerves and muscles. The three heads of the triceps surae muscle attach distally to the calcaneus via the spiraling fibers of the calcaneal tendon. **B.** Deep dissection. The gastrocnemius and most of the soleus are removed, leaving only a horseshoe-shaped section of the soleus close to its proximal attachments and the distal part of the calcaneal tendon. The transverse intermuscular septum has been split to reveal the deep muscles, vessels, and nerves.

The part/region of the foot contacting the floor or ground is the **sole** (*plantar region*, L. *regio plantaris*). The part directed superiorly is the *dorsum of the foot* (L. *dorsum pedis*), or **dorsal region of the foot** (L. *regio dorsalis pedis*). The sole of the foot underlying the calcaneus is the *heel* or **heel region** (L. *regio calcanea*), and the sole underlying the heads of the medial two metatarsals is the **ball of the foot.** The **great toe** (L. *hallux*) is also the **1st toe** (digit of foot, L. *digitus primus*), and the **little toe** (L. *digitus minimus*) is also the **5th toe.**

Skin and Fascia of Foot

Marked variations occur in the thickness (strength) and texture of skin, subcutaneous tissue (superficial fascia), and deep fascia in relationship to weight-bearing and distribution, ground contact (grip, abrasion), and the need for containment or compartmentalization.

SKIN AND SUBCUTANEOUS TISSUE

The *skin of the dorsum of the foot* is much thinner and less sensitive than skin on most of the sole. The *subcutaneous tissue* is loose deep to the dorsal skin; therefore, *edema* (swelling) is most marked over this surface, especially anterior to and around the medial malleolus. The skin over the major weight-bearing areas of the sole—the heel, lateral margin, and ball of the foot—is thick. The subcutaneous tissue in the sole is more fibrous than in other areas of the foot.

Fibrous septa—highly developed *skin ligaments* (L., retinacula cutis)—divide this tissue into fat-filled areas, making it a shock-absorbing pad, especially over the heel. The skin ligaments also anchor the skin to the underlying deep fascia (plantar aponeurosis), improving the "grip" of the sole. The skin of the sole is hairless and sweat glands are numerous; the entire sole is sensitive ("ticklish"), especially the thinner-skinned area underlying the arch of the foot.

DEEP FASCIA OF FOOT

The *deep fascia of the dorsum of the foot* is thin where it is continuous proximally with the *inferior extensor retinaculum* (Fig. 5.67A). Over the lateral and posterior aspects of the foot, the deep fascia is continuous with the **plantar fascia,** the deep fascia of the sole (Fig. 5.67B & C). The plantar fascia has a thick central part and weaker medial and lateral parts.

The thick, central part of the plantar fascia forms the strong *plantar aponeurosis*, longitudinally arranged bundles of dense fibrous connective tissue investing the central plantar muscles. It resembles the palmar aponeurosis of the palm of the hand but is tougher, denser, and elongated.

The plantar fascia holds the parts of the foot together, helps protect the sole from injury, and helps to support the longitudinal arches of the foot.

The **plantar aponeurosis** arises posteriorly from the calcaneus and functions like a superficial ligament. Distally, the longitudinal bundles of collagen fibers of the aponeurosis divide into five bands that become continuous with the **fibrous digital sheaths** that enclose the flexor tendons that pass to the toes. At the anterior end of the sole, inferior to the heads of the metatarsals, the aponeurosis is reinforced by transverse fibers forming the **superficial transverse metatarsal ligament.**

In the midfoot and forefoot, vertical *intermuscular septa* extend deeply (superiorly) from the margins of the plantar aponeurosis toward the 1st and 5th metatarsals, forming the three *compartments of the sole* (Fig. 5.67C):

1. The **medial compartment of the sole** is covered superficially by thinner *medial plantar fascia.* It contains the abductor hallucis, flexor hallucis brevis, the tendon of the flexor hallucis longus, and the medial plantar nerve and vessels.
2. The **central compartment of the sole** is covered superficially by the dense *plantar aponeurosis.* It contains the flexor digitorum brevis, the tendons of the flexor hallucis longus and flexor digitorum longus, plus the muscles associated with the latter, the quadratus plantae and lumbricals, and the adductor hallucis. The lateral plantar nerve and vessels are also located here.
3. The **lateral compartment of the sole** is covered superficially by the thinner *lateral plantar fascia* and contains the abductor and flexor digiti minimi brevis.

In the forefoot only, a fourth compartment, the **interosseous compartment of the foot,** is surrounded by the plantar and dorsal interosseous fasciae. It contains the metatarsals, the dorsal and plantar interosseous muscles, and the deep plantar and metatarsal vessels. Whereas the plantar interossei and plantar metatarsal vessels are distinctly plantar in position, the remaining structures of the compartment are located intermediate between the plantar and dorsal aspects of the foot.

A fifth compartment, the **dorsal compartment of the foot,** lies between the dorsal fascia of the foot and the tarsal bones and the dorsal interosseous fascia of the midfoot and forefoot. It contains the muscles (extensors hallucis brevis and extensor digitorum brevis) and neurovascular structures of the dorsum of the foot.

Muscles of Foot

Of the 20 individual muscles of the foot, 14 are located on the plantar aspect, 2 are on the dorsal aspect, and 4 are intermediate in position. From the plantar aspect, muscles of the sole are arranged in four layers within four compartments. The muscles of the foot are illustrated in Figures 5.68A–J and 5.69; their attachments, innervation, and actions are described in Table 5.14.

Despite their compartmental and layered arrangement, the plantar muscles function primarily as a group during the support phase of stance, maintaining the arches of the foot (see Fig 5.20B–E; Table 5.2). They basically resist forces that tend to reduce the longitudinal arch as weight is received at

**(A) Fascia of dorsum of foot
(anterolateral view)**

Inferior
extensor
retinaculum

**Dorsal fascia
of foot**

Key
- Medial compartment of sole
- Central compartment of sole
- Lateral compartment of sole
- Interosseous compartment of foot
- Dorsal compartment of foot

Dorsal fascia

Plantar fascia

**(C) Transverse section of foot
compartments (anterior view)**

Flexor digitorum
longus

**Fibrous digital
sheaths**

**Superficial
transverse
metatarsal
ligament**

**Plantar
aponeurosis**

Lateral plantar
fascia

Cutaneous
branches of
lateral plantar
vessels and
nerves

Fat pad

Flexor hallucis
longus

Site of sesamoid
bones of great
toe

Plantar digital
nerves and
arteries

**Medial plantar
fascia**

Cutaneous
branches of
medial plantar
nerve and artery

Medial
calcaneal
nerve and
artery

**(B) Sole of foot (plantar aspect)
(inferior view)**

FIGURE 5.67. Fascia and compartments of foot. A. The skin and subcutaneous tissue have been removed to demonstrate the deep fascia of the leg and dorsum of the foot. **B.** The deep plantar fascia consists of the thick plantar aponeurosis and the thinner medial and lateral plantar fascia. Thinner parts of the plantar fascia have been removed, revealing the plantar digital vessels and nerves. **C.** The bones and muscles of the foot are surrounded by the deep dorsal and plantar fascia. A large central and smaller medial and lateral compartments of the sole are created by intermuscular septa that extend deeply from the plantar aponeurosis.

the heel (posterior end of the arch) and then transferred to the ball of the foot and great toe (anterior end of the arch).

The muscles become most active in the later portion of the movement to stabilize the foot for propulsion (push off), a time when forces also tend to flatten the foot's transverse arch. Concurrently, they are also able to refine further the efforts of the long muscles, producing supination and pronation in enabling the platform of the foot to adjust to uneven ground.

The muscles of the foot are of little importance individually because fine control of the individual toes is not important to most people. Rather than producing actual movement, they are most active in fixing the foot or in increasing the pressure applied against the ground by various aspects of the sole or toes to maintain balance.

Although the adductor hallucis resembles a similar muscle of the palm that adducts the thumb, despite its name the adductor hallucis is probably most active during the push-off phase of stance in pulling the lateral four metatarsals toward the great toe, fixing the transverse arch of the foot, and resisting forces that would spread the metatarsal heads as weight and force are applied to the forefoot (Table 5.2).

In Table 5.14, note that the:

- **P**lantar interossei **AD**duct (**PAD**) and arise from a single metatarsal as unipennate muscles.
- **D**orsal interossei **AB**duct (**DAB**) and arise from two metatarsals as bipennate muscles.

FIGURE 5.72. Nerves of foot.

TABLE 5.15. NERVES OF FOOT

Nerve[a]	Origin	Course	Distribution in Foot
Saphenous (1)	Femoral nerve	Arises in femoral triangle and descends through thigh and leg; accompanies great saphenous vein anterior to medial malleolus; ends on medial side of foot	Supplies skin on medial side of foot as far anteriorly as head of 1st metatarsal
Superficial fibular (2)	Common fibular nerve	Pierces deep fascia in distal third of leg to become cutaneous; then sends branches to foot and digits	Supplies skin on dorsum of foot and all digits, except lateral side of 5th and adjoining sides of the 1st and 2nd digits
Deep fibular (3)		Passes deep to extensor retinaculum to enter dorsum of foot	Supplies extensor digitorum brevis and skin on contiguous sides of 1st and 2nd digits
Medial plantar (4)	Larger terminal branch of tibial nerve	Passes distally in foot between abductor hallucis and flexor digitorum brevis; divides into muscular and cutaneous branches	Supplies skin of medial side of sole of foot and sides of first three digits; also supplies abductor hallucis, flexor digitorum brevis, flexor hallucis brevis, and first lumbrical
Lateral plantar (5)	Smaller terminal branch of tibial nerve	Passes laterally in foot between quadratus plantae and flexor digitorum brevis muscles; divides into superficial and deep branches	Supplies quadratus plantae, abductor digiti minimi, digiti minimi brevis; deep branch supplies plantar and dorsal interossei, lateral three lumbricals, and adductor hallucis; supplies skin on sole lateral to a line splitting 4th digit
Sural (6)	Usually arises from branches of both tibial and common fibular nerves	Passes inferior to the lateral malleolus to lateral side of foot	Lateral aspect of hindfoot and midfoot
Calcaneal branches (7)	Tibial and sural nerves	Pass from distal part of the posterior aspect of leg to skin on heel	Skin of heel

[a] Numbers refer to Figure 5.72.

Sural Nerve. The **sural nerve** is formed by union of the *medial sural cutaneous nerve* (from the tibial nerve) and *sural communicating branch of the common fibular nerve*, respectively (see Fig. 5.57B; Table 5.11). The level of junction of these branches is variable; it may be high (in the popliteal fossa), or low (proximal to heel). Sometimes the branches do not join and, therefore, no sural nerve is formed. In these people, the skin normally innervated by the sural nerve is supplied by the medial and lateral sural cutaneous branches. The sural nerve accompanies the small saphenous vein and enters the foot posterior to the lateral malleolus to supply the ankle joint and skin along the lateral margin of the foot (Fig. 5.72A; Table 5.15).

ARTERIES OF FOOT

The arteries of the foot are terminal branches of the anterior and posterior tibial arteries (Figs. 5.71A and 5.73), respectively: the dorsalis pedis and plantar arteries.

Dorsalis Pedis Artery. Often a major source of blood supply to the forefoot (e.g., during extended periods of standing), the **dorsalis pedis artery** (dorsal artery of foot) is *the direct continuation of the anterior tibial artery.* The dorsalis pedis artery begins midway between the malleoli and runs anteromedially, deep to the inferior extensor retinaculum between the extensor hallucis longus and the extensor digitorum longus tendons on the dorsum of the foot.

The dorsalis pedis artery passes to the first interosseous space, where it divides into the *1st dorsal metatarsal artery* and a **deep plantar artery.** The latter passes deeply between the heads of the first dorsal interosseous muscle to enter the sole of the foot, where it joins the lateral plantar artery to form the *deep plantar arch.* The course and destination of the dorsal artery and its major continuation, the deep plantar artery, are comparable to the radial artery of the hand, which completes a deep arterial arch in the palm.

The **lateral tarsal artery,** a branch of the dorsalis pedis artery, runs laterally in an arched course beneath the EDB to supply this muscle and the underlying tarsals and joints. It anastomoses with other branches, such as the arcuate artery.

The **1st dorsal metatarsal artery** divides into branches that supply both sides of the great toe and the medial side of the 2nd toe.

The **arcuate artery** runs laterally across the bases of the lateral four metatarsals, deep to the extensor tendons, to reach the lateral aspect of the forefoot, where it may anastomose with the lateral tarsal artery to form an arterial loop. The arcuate artery gives rise to the **2nd, 3rd,** and

(A) Dorsum of foot

(B) Plantar aspect of foot

FIGURE 5.73. Arteries of foot: overview. A. The anterior tibial artery becomes the dorsalis pedis artery when it crosses the talocrural joint. **B.** The medial and lateral plantar arteries are terminal branches of the posterior tibial artery. The deep plantar artery and perforating branches of the deep plantar arch provide anastomoses between the dorsal and the plantar arteries.

The tendons on the anterior aspect of the ankle (from medial to lateral side) are easily palpated when the foot is dorsiflexed (Fig. 5.76A–C):

• The large *tendon of the tibialis anterior* leaves the cover of the superior extensor tendon, from which level the tendon is invested by a continuous synovial sheath; the tendon may be traced to its attachment to the 1st cuneiform and the base of the 1st metatarsal.

• The *tendon of the extensor hallucis longus*, obvious when the great toe is extended against resistance, may be followed to its attachment to the base of the distal phalanx of the great toe.
• The *tendons of the extensor digitorum longus* may be followed easily to their attachments to the lateral four toes.
• The *tendon of the fibularis tertius* may also be traced to its attachment to the base of the 5th metatarsal. This muscle is of minor importance and may be absent.

FOOT

Plantar Fasciitis

Inflammation of the plantar fascia—*plantar fasciitis*—is often caused by an overuse mechanism. It may result from running and high-impact aerobics, especially when inappropriate footwear is worn. Plantar fasciitis is the most common hindfoot problem in runners. It causes pain on the plantar surface of the foot and heel. The pain is often most severe after sitting, and when beginning to walk in the morning. It usually dissipates after 5–10 minutes of activity and often recurs again following rest.

Point tenderness is located at the proximal attachment of the aponeurosis to the medial tubercle of the calcaneus and on the medial surface of this bone. The pain increases with passive extension of the great toe and may be further exacerbated by dorsiflexion of the ankle and/or weight-bearing.

If a *calcaneal spur* (abnormal bony process) protrudes from the medial tubercle, plantar fasciitis is likely to cause pain on the medial side of the foot when walking (Fig. B5.26). Usually a bursa develops at the end of the spur that may also become inflamed and tender.

Infections of Foot

Foot infections are common, especially in seasons, climates, and cultures where shoes are less commonly worn. A neglected puncture wound may lead to an extensive deep infection, resulting in swelling, pain, and fever.

Deep infections of the foot often localize within the compartments between the muscular layers (Fig. 5.70B). A well-established infection in one of the enclosed fascial or muscular spaces usually requires surgical incision and drainage. When possible, the incision is made on the medial side of the foot, passing superior to the abductor hallucis to allow visualization of critical neurovascular structures, while avoiding production of a painful scar in a weight-bearing area.

Contusion of Extensor Digitorum Brevis

Functionally, the EDB and EHB muscles are relatively unimportant. Clinically, knowing the location of the belly of the EDB is important for distinguishing it from abnormal edema. Contusion and tearing of muscle fibers and associated blood vessels result in a *hematoma* (clotted extravasated blood), producing edema anteromedial to the lateral malleolus. Most people who have not seen this inflamed muscle assume they have a severely sprained ankle.

Sural Nerve Grafts

Pieces of the sural nerve are often used for nerve grafts in procedures such as repairing nerve defects resulting from wounds. The surgeon is usually able to locate this nerve in relation to the small saphenous vein (Fig. 5.74B). Because of the variations in the level of formation of the sural nerve, the surgeon may have to make incisions in both legs, and then select the better specimen.

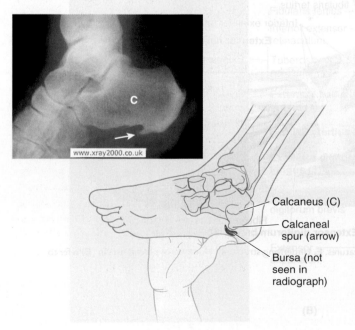

Calcaneus (C)

Calcaneal spur (arrow)

Bursa (not seen in radiograph)

FIGURE B5.26.

Anesthetic Block of Superficial Fibular Nerve

After the superficial fibular nerve pierces the deep fascia to become a cutaneous nerve, it divides into medial and intermediate cutaneous nerves (Fig. 5.72A). In thin people, these branches can often be seen or felt as ridges under the skin when the foot is plantarflexed. Injections of an anesthetic agent around these branches in the ankle region, anterior to the palpable portion of the fibula, anesthetizes the skin on the dorsum of the foot (except the web between and adjacent surfaces of the 1st and 2nd toes) more broadly and effectively than more local injections on the dorsum of the foot for superficial surgery.

Plantar Reflex

The **plantar reflex** (L4, L5, S1, and S2 nerve roots) is a myotatic (deep tendon) reflex that is routinely tested during neurologic examinations. The lateral aspect of the sole of the foot is stroked with a blunt object, such as a tongue depressor, beginning at the heel and crossing to the base of the great toe. The motion is firm and continuous but neither painful nor ticklish. Flexion of the toes is a normal response. Slight fanning of the lateral four toes and dorsiflexion of the great toe is an abnormal response (*Babinski sign*), indicating brain injury or cerebral disease, except in infants. Because the corticospinal tracts are not fully developed in newborns, a Babinski sign is usually elicited and may be present until children are 4 years of age (except in infants with a brain injury or cerebral disease).

Medial Plantar Nerve Entrapment

Compressive irritation of the medial plantar nerve as it passes deep to the flexor retinaculum, or curves deep to the abductor hallucis, may cause aching, burning, numbness, and tingling (paresthesia) on the medial side of the sole of the foot and in the region of the navicular tuberosity. *Medial plantar nerve compression* may occur during repetitive eversion of the foot (e.g., during gymnastics and running). Because of its frequency in runners, these symptoms have been called "jogger's foot."

Palpation of Dorsalis Pedis Pulse

The **dorsalis pedis artery pulse** is evaluated during a physical examination of the peripheral vascular system. Dorsalis pedis pulses may be palpated with the feet slightly dorsiflexed. The pulses are usually easy to palpate because these dorsal arteries are subcutaneous and pass along a line from the extensor retinaculum to a point just lateral to the EHL tendons (Swartz, 2009) (Fig. B5.27). A diminished or absent dorsalis pedis pulse usually suggests vascular insufficiency resulting from arterial disease. The five *P signs of acute arterial occlusion* are *pain, pallor, paresthesia, paralysis,* and *pulselessness.* Some healthy adults (and even children) have *congenitally non-palpable dorsalis pedis pulses;* the variation is usually bilateral. In these cases, the dorsalis pedis artery is replaced by an enlarged perforating fibular artery.

Extensor hallucis longus

Dorsalis pedis artery

Tibialis anterior tendon

FIGURE B5.27.

Hemorrhaging Wounds of Sole of Foot

Puncture wounds of the sole of the foot involving the deep plantar arch and its branches usually result in severe bleeding, typically from both ends of the cut artery because of the abundant anastomoses. Ligation of the deep arch is difficult because of its depth and the structures that surround it.

Lymphadenopathy

Infections of the foot may spread proximally, causing enlargement of the popliteal and inguinal lymph nodes (*lymphadenopathy*). Infections on the lateral side of the foot initially produce enlargement of popliteal lymph nodes (*popliteal lymphadenopathy*); later, the inguinal lymph nodes may enlarge.

Inguinal lymphadenopathy without popliteal lymphadenopathy can result from infection of the medial side of the foot, leg, or thigh; however, enlargement of these nodes can also result from an infection or tumor in the vulva, penis, scrotum, perineum, and gluteal region, and from terminal parts of the urethra, anal canal, and vagina.

The Bottom Line

FOOT

Muscles of foot: The intrinsic muscles of the plantar surface of the foot are arranged in four layers and divided into four fascial compartments. ♦ A tough plantar aponeurosis overlies the central compartment, passively contributing to arch maintenance and, along with firmly bound fat, protecting the vessels and nerves from compression. ♦ There is similarity to the arrangement of muscles in the palm of the hand, but the muscles of the foot generally respond as a group rather than individually, acting to maintain the longitudinal arch of the foot or push a portion of it harder against the ground to maintain balance. ♦ The movements of abduction and adduction produced by the interossei are toward or away from the 2nd digit. ♦ The foot has two intrinsic muscles on its dorsum that augment the long extensor muscles. ♦ The plantar intrinsic muscles function throughout the stance phase of gait, from heel strike to toe off, resisting forces that tend to spread the arches of the foot. ♦ These muscles are especially active in fixing the medial forefoot for the propulsive push off.

Nerves of foot: The plantar intrinsic muscles are innervated by the medial and lateral plantar nerves, whereas the dorsal muscles are innervated by the deep fibular nerve. ♦ Most of the dorsum of the foot receives cutaneous innervation from the superficial fibular nerve, the exception being the skin of the web between and the adjacent sides of the 1st and 2nd toes. The latter receives innervation from the deep fibular nerve after it supplies the muscles on the dorsum of the foot. ♦ The skin of the medial and lateral sides of the foot is innervated by the saphenous and sural nerves, respectively. ♦ The plantar aspect of the foot receives innervation from the larger medial and smaller lateral plantar nerves. ♦ The medial plantar nerve supplies more skin (the plantar aspect of the medial three and half toes and adjacent sole) but fewer muscles (the medial hallux and 1st lumbrical muscles only) than the lateral plantar nerve. ♦ The lateral planar nerve supplies the remaining muscles and skin of the plantar aspect. ♦ The distribution of the medial and lateral plantar nerves is comparable to that of the median and ulnar nerves in the palm.

Arteries of foot: The dorsal and plantar arteries of the foot are terminal branches of the anterior and posterior tibial arteries, respectively. ♦ The dorsalis pedis artery supplies all of the dorsum of the foot and, via the arcuate artery, the proximal dorsal aspect of the toes. It also contributes to formation of the deep plantar arch via its terminal deep plantar artery. ♦ The smaller medial and larger lateral plantar arteries supply the plantar aspect of the foot, the latter running in vascular planes between the 1st and 2nd layers and then, as the plantar arch, the 3rd and 4th layers of the intrinsic muscles. ♦ Anastomoses between the dorsalis pedis and plantar arteries are abundant and important for the health of the foot. ♦ Except for the scarcity of a superficial plantar arch, the arterial pattern of the foot is similar to that of the hand.

Efferent vessels of foot: Venous drainage of the foot primarily follows a superficial route, draining to the dorsum of the foot and then medially via the great saphenous vein or laterally via the small saphenous veins. ♦ From these veins, blood is shunted by perforating veins to the deep veins of the leg and thigh that participate in the musculovenous pump. ♦ The lymphatics carrying lymph from the foot drain toward and then along the superficial veins draining the foot. ♦ Lymph from the medial foot follows the great saphenous vein and drains directly to superficial inguinal lymph nodes. ♦ Lymph from the lateral foot follows the small saphenous vein and drains initially to the popliteal lymph nodes and then by deep lymphatic vessels to the deep inguinal nodes.

JOINTS OF LOWER LIMB

The joints of the lower limb include the articulations of the pelvic girdle—lumbosacral joints, sacro-iliac joints, and pubic symphysis, which are discussed in Chapter 3. The remaining joints of the lower limb are the hip joints, knee joints, tibiofibular joints, ankle joints, and foot joints (Fig. 5.77).

Hip Joint

The **hip joint** forms the connection between the lower limb and the pelvic girdle (Fig. 5.77A). It is a strong and stable *multiaxial ball and socket type of synovial joint*. The head of the femur is the ball and the acetabulum is the socket (Fig. 5.78). The hip joint is designed for stability over a wide range of movement. Next to the glenohumeral (shoulder) joint, it is the most movable of all joints. During standing, the entire weight of the upper body is transmitted through the hip bones to the heads and necks of the femora.

ARTICULAR SURFACES OF HIP JOINT

The round head of the femur articulates with the cup-like acetabulum of the hip bone (Figs. 5.77–5.80). The *head of the femur* forms approximately two thirds of a sphere. Except for the depression or *fovea for the ligament of the femoral head,* all of the head is covered with articular cartilage, which is thickest over weight-bearing areas.

The *acetabulum,* a hemispherical hollow on the lateral aspect of the hip bone, is formed by the fusion of three bony parts (see Fig. 5.5). The heavy, prominent **acetabular rim** of the acetabulum consists of a semilunar articular part covered with articular cartilage, the *lunate surface of the acetabulum*

(text continues on p. 629)

Joints:

Lumbosacral joint

Sacro-iliac joint

Hip joint

Pubic symphysis

Bones:

Lumbar vertebra

Ilium

Sacrum

Pubis

Femur

(A)

Femoropatellar joint

Knee joint

(Superior) tibiofibular joint

Interosseous membrane

Femur

Patella

Tibia

Fibula

(B)

Fibula

Tibia

Tibiofibular syndesmosis

Ankle joint

Transverse tarsal

Intertarsal

Tarsometatarsal

Metatarsophalangeal

Interphalangeal

Joints

(C)

Anterior views

FIGURE 5.77. Joints of lower limb. The lower limb joints are (**A**) those of the pelvic girdle connecting the free lower limb to the vertebral column, (**B**) the knee and tibiofibular joint, and (**C**) tibiofibular syndesmosis, ankle joint, and the many joints of the foot.

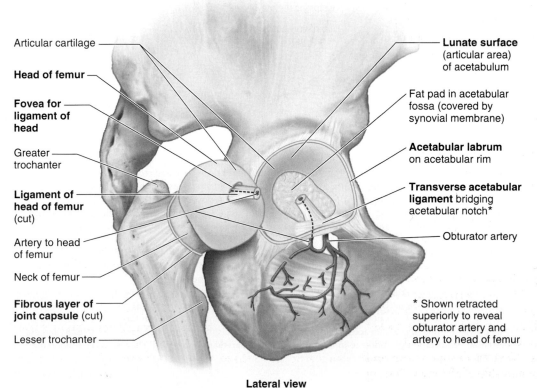

Articular cartilage

Head of femur

Fovea for ligament of head

Greater trochanter

Ligament of head of femur (cut)

Artery to head of femur

Neck of femur

Fibrous layer of joint capsule (cut)

Lesser trochanter

Lunate surface (articular area) of acetabulum

Fat pad in acetabular fossa (covered by synovial membrane)

Acetabular labrum on acetabular rim

Transverse acetabular ligament bridging acetabular notch*

Obturator artery

* Shown retracted superiorly to reveal obturator artery and artery to head of femur

Lateral view

FIGURE 5.78. Hip joint. The joint was disarticulated by cutting the ligament of the head of the femur and retracting the head from the acetabulum. The transverse acetabular ligament is retracted superiorly to show the obturator canal, which transmits the obturator nerve and vessels passing from the pelvic cavity to the medial thigh.

(A) Superior view

(B) Winding draws connected structures together

(D) AP projection

(C) Anterior view of coronal section

FIGURE 5.79. Factors increasing stability of hip joint. A. This superior view of the hip joint demonstrates the medial and reciprocal pull of the peri-articular muscles (medial and lateral rotators; *reddish brown arrows*) and intrinsic ligaments of the hip joint (*gray arrows*) on the femur. Relative strengths are indicated by arrow width: Anteriorly, the muscles are less abundant but the ligaments are robust; posteriorly, the muscles predominate. **B.** Parallel fibers linking two discs resemble those making up the tube-like fibrous layer of the hip joint capsule. When one disc (the femur) rotates relative to the other (the acetabulum), the fibers become increasingly oblique and draw the two discs together. Similarly, extension of the hip joint winds (increases the obliquity of) the fibers of the fibrous layer, pulling the head and neck of the femur tightly into the acetabulum, increasing the stability of the joint. Flexion unwinds the fibers of the capsule. **C.** In this coronal section of hip joint, the acetabular labrum and transverse acetabular ligament, spanning the acetabular notch (and included in the plane of section here), extend the acetabular rim so that a complete socket is formed. Thus the acetabular complex engulfs the head of the femur. The epiphysis of the femoral head is entirely within the joint capsule. The thick weight-bearing bone of the ilium normally lies directly superior to the head of the femur for efficient transfer of weight to the femur (Fig. 5.3). The angle of Wiberg (see text) is used radiographically to determine the degree to which the acetabulum overhangs the head of the femur. **D.** Several different lines and curvatures are used in the detection of hip abnormalities (dislocations, fractures, or slipped epiphyses). The Kohler line (*red A*) is normally tangential to the pelvic inlet and the obturator foramen. The acetabular fossa should lie lateral to this line. A fossa that crosses the line suggests an acetabular fracture with inward displacement. The Shenton line (*red B*) and the iliofemoral line (*red C*) should appear in a normal AP radiograph as smooth, continuous lines that are bilaterally symmetrical. The Shenton line is a radiographic indication of the angle of inclination (*ASIS* = anterior superior iliac spine).

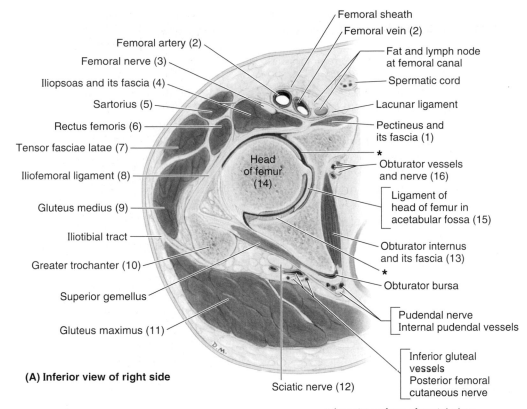

Femoral sheath
Femoral vein (2)
Femoral artery (2)
Femoral nerve (3)
Iliopsoas and its fascia (4)
Sartorius (5)
Rectus femoris (6)
Tensor fasciae latae (7)
Iliofemoral ligament (8)
Gluteus medius (9)
Iliotibial tract
Greater trochanter (10)
Superior gemellus
Gluteus maximus (11)

Fat and lymph node at femoral canal
Spermatic cord
Lacunar ligament
Pectineus and its fascia (1)
* Obturator vessels and nerve (16)
Ligament of head of femur in acetabular fossa (15)
Obturator internus and its fascia (13)
* Obturator bursa
Pudendal nerve / Internal pudendal vessels
Inferior gluteal vessels / Posterior femoral cutaneous nerve

Head of femur (14)

Sciatic nerve (12)

(A) Inferior view of right side

* Lunate surface of acetabulum

(B) Inferior view of right side

(C)

FIGURE 5.80. Sectional and radiographic anatomy of gluteal region and proximal anterior thigh at level of hip joint. A and B. A descriptive drawing and transverse (axial MRI) study of an anatomical section of the thigh are shown. Numbers in parentheses in (**A**) refer to structures identified in (**B**). **C.** The orientation drawing shows the level of the section.

(Figs. 5.78–5.80). The acetabular rim and lunate surface form approximately three quarters of a circle; the missing inferior segment of the circle is the *acetabular notch*.

The lip-shaped **acetabular labrum** (L. *labrum,* lip) is a fibrocartilaginous rim attached to the margin of the acetabulum, increasing the acetabular articular area by nearly 10%. The **transverse acetabular ligament,** a continuation of the

acetabular labrum, bridges the acetabular notch (Figs. 5.78 and 5.79C). As a result of the height of the rim and labrum, more than half of the femoral head fits within the acetabulum (Figs. 5.79C and 5.80). Thus during dissection, the femoral head must be cut from the acetabular rim to enable disarticulation of the joint. Centrally a deep non-articular part, called the *acetabular fossa,* is formed mainly by the ischium

(Figs. 5.78, 5.79C, and 5.80). This fossa is thin walled (often translucent) and continuous inferiorly with the acetabular notch.

The articular surfaces of the acetabulum and femoral head are most congruent when the hip is flexed 90°, abducted 5°, and rotated laterally 10° (the position in which the axis of the acetabulum and the axis of the femoral head and neck are aligned), which is the quadruped position!

In other words, in assuming the upright position, a relatively small degree of joint stability was sacrificed to maximize weight-bearing when erect. Even so, the hip joint is our most stable joint, owing also to its complete ball and socket construction (depth of socket), the strength of its joint capsule, and the attachments of muscles crossing the joint, many of which are located at some distance from the center of movement (Palastanga et al., 2011).

JOINT CAPSULE OF HIP JOINT

The hip joints are enclosed within strong *joint capsules,* formed of a loose external *fibrous layer* (fibrous capsule) and an internal *synovial membrane* (Fig. 5.79C). Proximally, the fibrous layer attaches to the acetabulum, just peripheral to the acetabular rim to which the labrum is attached, and to the transverse acetabular ligament (Figs. 5.79C and 5.81A, C, & D). Distally, the fibrous layer attaches to the femoral neck only anteriorly at the *intertrochanteric line* and root of the greater trochanter (Fig. 5.81B). Posteriorly, the fibrous layer crosses the neck proximal to the *intertrochanteric crest* but is not attached to it.

Most fibers of the fibrous layer of the capsule take a spiral course from the hip bone to the intertrochanteric line of the femur, but some deep fibers pass circularly around the neck, forming the **orbicular zone** (Fig. 5.79C and 5.81D). Thick parts of the fibrous layer form the **ligaments of the hip joint,** which pass in a spiral fashion from the pelvis to the femur (Fig. 5.81A, C, & D). Extension winds the spiraling ligaments and fibers more tightly, constricting the capsule and drawing the femoral head tightly into the acetabulum (Fig. 5.79B). The tightened fibrous layer increases the stability of the joint, but restricts extension of the joint to 10–20° beyond the vertical position. Flexion increasingly unwinds the spiraling ligaments and fibers. This permits considerable flexion of the hip joint with increasing mobility.

Of the three intrinsic ligaments of the joint capsule below, it is the first one that reinforces and strengthens the joint:

- *Anteriorly and superiorly* is the strong, Y-shaped **iliofemoral ligament,** which attaches to the anterior inferior iliac spine and the acetabular rim proximally and the intertrochanteric line distally (Fig. 5.81A & C). Said to be the body's strongest ligament, the iliofemoral ligament specifically prevents hyperextension of the hip joint during standing by screwing the femoral head into the acetabulum via the mechanism described above.

- *Anteriorly and inferiorly* is the **pubofemoral ligament,** which arises from the obturator crest of the pubic bone and passes laterally and inferiorly to merge with the fibrous layer of the joint capsule (Fig. 5.81A). This ligament blends with the medial part of the iliofemoral ligament, and tightens during both extension and abduction of the hip joint. The pubofemoral ligament prevents overabduction of the hip joint.

- *Posteriorly* is the **ischiofemoral ligament,** which arises from the ischial part of the acetabular rim (Fig. 5.81D). The weakest of the three ligaments, it spirals superolaterally to the femoral neck, medial to the base of the greater trochanter.

The relative size, strengths, and positions of the three ligaments of the hip joint are shown in Figure 5.79A. The ligaments and peri-articular muscles (the medial and lateral rotators of the thigh) play a vital role in maintaining the structural integrity of the joint.

Both muscles and ligaments pull the femoral head medially into the acetabulum, and they are reciprocally balanced when doing so. The medial flexors, located anteriorly, are fewer, weaker, and less mechanically advantaged, whereas the anterior ligaments are strongest. Conversely, the ligaments are weaker posteriorly where the medial rotators are abundant, stronger, and more mechanically advantaged.

In all synovial joints, a synovial membrane lines the internal surfaces of the fibrous layer, as well as any intracapsular bony surfaces not lined with articular cartilage. Thus in the hip joint, where the fibrous layer attaches to the femur distant from the articular cartilage covering the femoral head, the **synovial membrane of the hip joint** reflects proximally along the femoral neck to the edge of the femoral head. Longitudinal synovial folds (*retinacula*) occur in the synovial membrane covering the femoral neck (Fig. 5.79C). Subsynovial **retinacular arteries** (branches of the medial, and a few of the lateral, circumflex femoral artery) that supply the femoral head and neck course within the synovial folds (Fig. 5.82).

The **ligament of the head of the femur** (Figs. 5.78, 5.79C, 5.80, and 5.82), primarily a synovial fold conducting a blood vessel, is weak and of little importance in strengthening the hip joint. Its wide end attaches to the margins of the acetabular notch and the transverse acetabular ligament; its narrow end attaches to the *fovea for the ligament of the head.*

Usually, the ligament contains a small artery to the head of the femur. A *fat pad* in the acetabular fossa fills the part of the acetabular fossa that is not occupied by the ligament of the femoral head (Fig. 5.78). Both the ligament and the fat pad are covered with synovial membrane. The malleable nature of the fat pad permits it to change shape to accommodate the variations in the congruity of the femoral head and acetabulum, as well as changes in the position of the ligament of the head during joint movements. A *synovial protrusion* beyond the free margin of the joint capsule onto the posterior aspect of the femoral neck forms a bursa for the obturator externus tendon (Fig. 5.81D).

FIGURE 5.81. Ligaments of pelvis and hip joint. A. Weight transfer from the vertebral column to the pelvic girdle is a function of the sacro-iliac ligaments. Weight transfer at the hip joint is accomplished primarily by the disposition of the bones, with the ligaments limiting the range of movement and adding stability. **B.** Articulating surfaces of hip joint and sites of attachment and tendinous relationships of iliofemoral ligaments and joint capsule. **C.** Iliofemoral ligament. **D.** The ischiofemoral ligament. Because the joint capsule does not attach to the posterior aspect of the femur, the synovial membrane protrudes from the joint capsule, forming the obturator externus bursa to facilitate movement of the tendon of the obturator externus (shown in part **C**) over the bone.

FIGURE 5.82. Blood supply of head and neck of femur. Branches of the medial and lateral circumflex femoral arteries, branches of the profunda femoris artery, and the artery to the femoral head (a branch of the obturator artery) supply the head and neck of the femur. In the adult, the medial circumflex femoral artery is the most important source of blood to the femoral head and adjacent (proximal) neck.

MOVEMENTS OF HIP JOINT

Hip movements are flexion–extension, abduction–adduction, medial–lateral rotation, and circumduction (Fig. 5.83). Movements of the trunk at the hip joints are also important, such as those occurring when a person lifts their trunk from the supine position during sit-ups, or keeps the pelvis level when one foot is off the ground.

The degree of flexion and extension possible at the hip joint depends on the position of the knee. If the knee is flexed, relaxing the hamstrings, the hip joint can be actively flexed until the thigh almost reaches the anterior abdominal wall and can reach it via further passive flexion. Not all of this movement occurs at the hip joint; some results from flexion of the vertebral column. During extension of the hip joint, the fibrous layer of the joint capsule, especially the iliofemoral ligament, is taut; therefore, the hip can usually be extended only slightly beyond the vertical except by movement of the bony pelvis (flexion of lumbar vertebrae).

From the anatomical position, the range of abduction of the hip joint is usually somewhat greater than for adduction. About 60° of abduction is possible when the thigh is extended at the hip joint, and more when it is flexed. Lateral rotation is much more powerful than medial rotation.

The main muscles producing movements of the hip joint are listed in Figure 5.83B. Note that:

1. The *iliopsoas* is the strongest flexor of the hip.
2. In addition to its function as an adductor, the *adductor magnus* also serves as a flexor (anterior or aponeurotic part) and an extensor (posterior or hamstrings part).
3. Several muscles participate in both flexion and adduction (*pectineus* and *gracilis* as well all three "adductor" muscles).

4. In addition to serving as abductors, the anterior portions of the *gluteus medius* and *minimus* are also medial rotators.
5. The *gluteus maximus* serves as the primary extensor from the flexed to the straight (standing) position, and from this point posteriorly, extension is achieved primarily by the hamstrings. The gluteus maximus is also a lateral rotator.

BLOOD SUPPLY OF HIP JOINT

Arteries supplying the hip joint (Fig. 5.82) include the following:

- The *medial* and *lateral circumflex femoral arteries*, which are usually branches of the *profunda femoris artery* but occasionally they arise as branches of the *femoral artery*.
- The **artery to the head of the femur,** which is a branch of the obturator artery of variable size; it traverses the ligament of the head.

The main blood supply of the hip joint is from the *retinacular arteries* arising as branches of the circumflex femoral arteries. Retinacular arteries arising from the medial circumflex femoral artery are most abundant, bringing more blood to the head and neck of the femur because they are able to pass beneath the unattached posterior border of the joint capsule. Retinacular arteries arising from the lateral circumflex femoral must penetrate the thick iliofemoral ligament and are smaller and fewer.

NERVE SUPPLY OF HIP JOINT

Hilton's law states that the nerves supplying the muscles extending directly across and acting at a given joint also innervate the joint. Articular rami arise from the intramuscular rami

Iliac crest

Gluteus medius **(14)**

Gluteus minimus **(15)**
Gluteus maximus **(12)**
Piriformis **(9)**
Obturator internus and gemelli **(10)**
Sciatic nerve
Obturator externus **(8)**
Quadratus femoris **(11)**
Hamstrings **(13)**
Adductor brevis **(6)**
Adductor magnus **(7)**
Adductor longus **(5)**

Iliopsoas **(1)**

Acetabulum
Rectus femoris (tendon)**(3t)**
Head of femur **(H)**
Femoral nerve
Femoral artery
Pectineus **(4)**
Sartorius **(2)**
Femoral vein
Rectus femoris (3)

(A) Lateral view of sagittal section through femoral head

(B) MRI of hip joint, lateral view (Is, Ischium)

Functional groups of muscles acting at hip joint

Flexors
Iliopsoas **(1)**
Sartorius **(2)**
Tensor fasciae latae
Rectus femoris **(3)** tendon **(3t)**
Pectineus **(4)**
Adductor longus **(5)**
Adductor brevis **(6)**
Adductor magnus—anterior part **(7)**
Gracilis

Adductors
Pectineus **(4)**
Adductor longus **(5)**
Adductor brevis **(6)**
Adductor magnus **(7)**
Obturator externus **(8)**
Gracilis

Lateral rotators
Obturator externus **(8)**
Piriformis **(9)**
Obturator internus **(10)**
Gemelli **(10)**
Quadratus femoris **(11)**
Gluteus maximus **(12)**

Extensors
Gluteus maximus **(12)**
Hamstrings: **(13)**
Semitendinosus
Semimembranosus
Long head, biceps femoris
Adductor magnus—posterior part

Abductors
Gluteus medius **(14)**
Gluteus minimus **(15)**
Tensor fasciae latae

Medial rotators
Gluteus medius **(14)** } Anterior parts
Gluteus minimus **(15)** }
Tensor fasciae latae

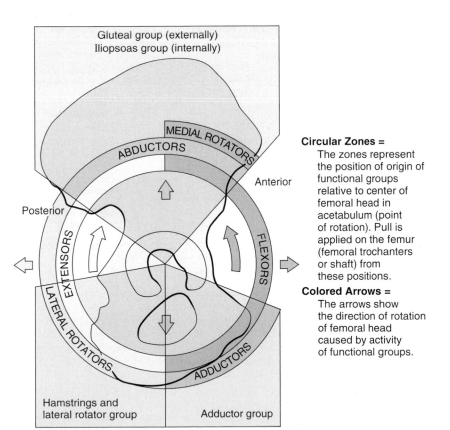

Gluteal group (externally)
Iliopsoas group (internally)

MEDIAL ROTATORS
ABDUCTORS
Anterior
Posterior
EXTENSORS
FLEXORS
LATERAL ROTATORS
ADDUCTORS

Hamstrings and lateral rotator group

Adductor group

Circular Zones =
The zones represent the position of origin of functional groups relative to center of femoral head in acetabulum (point of rotation). Pull is applied on the femur (femoral trochanters or shaft) from these positions.

Colored Arrows =
The arrows show the direction of rotation of femoral head caused by activity of functional groups.

(C) Diagrammatic lateral view

FIGURE 5.83. Relations of hip joint and muscles producing movements of joint. A. Sagittal section of the hip joint showing the muscles, vessels, and nerves related to it. The muscles are color coded to indicate their function(s). Applying Hilton's law, it is possible to deduce the innervation of the hip joint by knowing which muscles directly cross and act on the joint and their nerve supply. **B.** The relative positions of the muscles producing movements of the hip joint and the direction of the movement are demonstrated.

of the muscular branches and directly from named nerves. A knowledge of the nerve supply of the muscles and their relationship to the joints can allow one to deduce the nerve supply of many joints. Possible deductions regarding the hip joint and its muscular relationships include (Fig. 5.83):

- Flexors innervated by the femoral nerve pass anterior to the hip joint; the anterior aspect of the hip joint is innervated by the femoral nerve (directly and via articular rami of the muscular branches to the pectineus and rectus femoris).
- Lateral rotators pass inferior and posterior to the hip joint; the inferior aspect of the joint is innervated by the obturator nerve (directly and via articular rami of the muscular branch to the obturator externus), and the posterior aspect is innervated by the nerve to the quadratus femoris.
- Abductors innervated by the superior gluteal nerve pass superior to the hip joint; the superior aspect of the joint is innervated by the superior gluteal nerve.

Pain perceived as coming from the hip joint may be misleading because pain can be referred from the vertebral column.

Knee Joint

The **knee joint** is the largest and most superficial joint. It is primarily a hinge type of synovial joint, allowing flexion and extension; however, the hinge movements are combined with gliding and rolling, and with rotation about a vertical axis. Although the knee joint is well constructed, its function is commonly impaired when it is hyperextended (e.g., in body contact sports, such as ice hockey and football).

ARTICULATIONS, ARTICULAR SURFACES, AND STABILITY OF KNEE JOINT

Relevant anatomical details of the involved bones, including their articulating surfaces, were discussed in "Bones of Lower Limb," p. 512. The articular surfaces of the knee joint are characterized by their large size and their complicated and incongruent shapes. The knee joint consists of three articulations (Figs. 5.84 and 5.85):

- Two **femorotibial articulations** (**lateral** and **medial**) between the lateral and the medial femoral and tibial condyles.
- One intermediate **femoropatellar articulation** between the patella and the femur.

The fibula is not involved in the knee joint.

The knee joint is relatively weak mechanically because of the incongruence of its articular surfaces, which has been compared to two balls sitting on a warped tabletop. The stability of the knee joint depends on (1) the strength and actions of the surrounding muscles and their tendons, and (2) the ligaments that connect the femur and tibia. Of these supports, the muscles are most important; therefore, many sport injuries are preventable through appropriate conditioning and training.

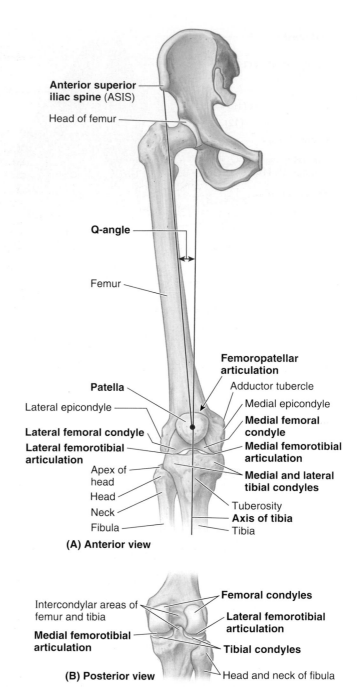

FIGURE 5.84. Bones of knee joint. A The bones articulating at the knee joint are shown. The hip bone and proximal femur are included to demonstrate the Q-angle, determined during physical examination to indicate alignment of the femur and tibia and to evaluate valgus or varus stress at the knee. **B.** The bones and bony features of the posterior aspect of the knee joint and knee are shown.

The most important muscle in stabilizing the knee joint is the large *quadriceps femoris*, particularly the inferior fibers of the vastus medialis and lateralis (Fig. 5.86A). The knee joint functions surprisingly well after a ligament strain if the quadriceps is well conditioned.

The erect, extended position is the most stable position of the knee joint. In this position, the articular surfaces are most

(A) Anterior view

Femur
Medial thigh
Patella (2)
Adductor tubercle
Medial epicondyle
Lateral condyle of femur (1)
Medial condyle of femur (3)
Lateral femorotibial articulation
Medial femorotibial articulation
Lateral condyle of tibia
Head of fibula
Medial and lateral intercondylar tubercles of intercondylar eminence
Shaft of fibula
Shaft of tibia

(B) AP projection

--- Posterior aspect of condyles

FIGURE 5.85. Radiography of knee joint. A and B. The orientation drawing depicts the structures visible in the AP radiograph of the right knee joint.

Rectus femoris (cut away)
Vastus intermedius (cut away)
Femur
Vastus lateralis
Articularis genu
Vastus medialis
Suprapatellar bursa
Quadriceps femoris tendon
Patellar retinacula
Iliotibial tract
Tibial collateral ligament
Fibular collateral ligament
Patellar ligament
Pes anserinus
Tibia

Adductor magnus
Adductor hiatus
Vastus medialis
Tendon of "hamstring" portion of adductor magnus
Medial head of gastrocnemius
Adductor tubercle
Tibial collateral ligament
Semimembranosus tendon
Fibrous layer extending across intercondylar fossa
Oblique popliteal ligament
Pes anserinus
Semimembranosus contribution to fascia of popliteus
Tendinous arch of soleus
Soleus
Linea aspera
Lateral intermuscular septum covering vastus lateralis
Popliteal surface of femur
Plantaris
Lateral head of gastrocnemius
Fibular collateral ligament
Biceps femoris tendon
Arcuate popliteal ligament and opening for popliteus tendon
Common fibular nerve
Popliteus

(A) Anterior view   **(B) Posterior view**

FIGURE 5.86. External aspect of joint capsule of knee. The fibrous layer of the joint capsule is relatively thin in some places and thickened in others to form reinforcing intrinsic (capsular) ligaments. **A.** Modifications of the anterior aspect and sides of the fibrous layer include the patellar retinacula, which attach to the sides of the quadriceps tendon, patella, and patellar ligament, and incorporation of the iliotibial tract (laterally) and the medial collateral ligament (medially). **B.** The hamstring and gastrocnemius muscles and the posterior intermuscular septum have been cut and removed to expose the adductor magnus, lateral intermuscular septum, and the floor of the popliteal fossa. Posterior modifications of the fibrous layer include the oblique and arcuate popliteal ligaments, and a perforation inferior to the arcuate popliteal ligament to allow passage of the popliteus tendon.

congruent (contact is minimized in all other positions); the primary ligaments of the joint (collateral and cruciate ligaments) are taut, and the many tendons surrounding the joint provide a splinting effect.

JOINT CAPSULE OF KNEE JOINT

The **joint capsule of the knee joint** is typical in consisting of an external *fibrous layer of the capsule* (fibrous capsule) and an internal *synovial membrane* that lines all internal surfaces of the articular cavity not covered with articular cartilage (5.87B). The fibrous layer has a few thickened parts that make up intrinsic ligaments, but for the main part, it is thin and is actually incomplete in some areas (5.86B). The fibrous layer attaches to the femur superiorly, just proximal to the articular margins of the condyles. Posteriorly, the fibrous layer encloses the condyles and the *intercondylar fossa*. The fibrous layer has an opening or gap posterior to the lateral tibial condyle to allow the tendon of the popliteus to pass out of the joint capsule to attach to the tibia (Fig. 5.87B). Inferiorly, the fibrous layer attaches to the margin of the superior articular surface (tibial plateau) of the tibia, except where the tendon of the popliteus crosses the bone (Figs. 5.86A & B and 5.87B). The quadriceps tendon, patella, and patellar ligament replace the fibrous layer anteriorly—that is, the fibrous layer is continuous with the lateral and medial margins of these structures, and there is no separate fibrous layer in the region of these structures (Figs. 5.86A and 5.87B).

The extensive *synovial membrane of the capsule* lines all surfaces bounding the articular cavity (the space containing synovial fluid) not covered by articular cartilage (Fig. 5.87A & B). Thus, it attaches to the periphery of the articular cartilage covering the femoral and tibial condyles; the posterior surface of the patella; and the edges of the *menisci*, the fibrocartilaginous discs between the tibial and femoral articular surfaces. The synovial membrane lines the internal surface of the fibrous layer laterally and medially, but centrally it becomes separated from the fibrous layer.

From the posterior aspect of the joint, the synovial membrane reflects anteriorly into the intercondylar region, covering the cruciate ligaments and the **infrapatellar fat pad,** so that they are excluded from the articular cavity. This creates a median **infrapatellar synovial fold,** a vertical fold of synovial membrane that approaches the posterior aspect of the patella, occupying all but the most anterior part of the intercondylar region. Thus, it almost subdivides the articular cavity into right and left femorotibial articular cavities; indeed, this is how arthroscopic surgeons consider the articular cavity. Fat-filled **lateral** and **medial alar folds** cover the inner surface of fat pads that occupy the space on each side of the patellar ligament internal to the fibrous layer.

Superior to the patella, the knee joint cavity extends deep to the vastus intermedius as the *suprapatellar bursa* (Figs. 5.86A and 5.88A & B). The synovial membrane of the joint capsule is continuous with the synovial lining of this bursa. This large bursa usually extends approximately 5 cm superior to the patella; however, it may extend halfway up the anterior aspect of the femur. Muscle slips deep to the vastus intermedius form the *articular muscle of the knee,* which attaches to the synovial membrane and retracts the bursa during extension of the knee (see Figs. 5.22 and 5.86A).

EXTRACAPSULAR LIGAMENTS OF KNEE JOINT

The joint capsule is strengthened by five extracapsular or capsular (intrinsic) ligaments: patellar ligament, fibular collateral ligament, tibial collateral ligament, oblique popliteal ligament, and arcuate popliteal ligament (Fig. 5.86A & B). They are sometimes called *external ligaments* to differentiate them from internal ligaments, such as the cruciate ligaments.

The *patellar ligament,* the distal part of the quadriceps femoris tendon, is a strong, thick fibrous band passing from the apex and adjoining margins of the patella to the tibial tuberosity (Fig. 5.86A). The patellar ligament is the anterior ligament of the knee joint. Laterally, it receives the *medial* and *lateral patellar retinacula,* aponeurotic expansions of the vastus medialis and lateralis and overlying deep fascia. The retinacula make up the joint capsule of the knee on each side of the patella (Figs. 5.86A and 5.87B) and play an important role in maintaining alignment of the patella relative to the patellar articular surface of the femur. The oblique placement of the femur and/or line of pull of the quadriceps femoris muscle relative to the axis of the patellar tendon and tibia, assessed clinically as the *Q-angle,* favors lateral displacement of the patella (Fig. 5.84).

The *collateral ligaments of the knee* are taut when the knee is fully extended, contributing to stability while standing (Fig. 5.88A & D). As flexion proceeds, they become increasingly slack, permitting and limiting (serving as check ligaments for) rotation at the knee.

The **fibular collateral ligament** (**FCL;** lateral collateral ligament), a cord-like extracapsular ligament, is strong. It extends inferiorly from the lateral epicondyle of the femur to the lateral surface of the fibular head (Fig. 5.88A & C). The tendon of the popliteus passes deep to the FCL, separating it from the lateral meniscus. The tendon of the biceps femoris is split into two parts by the FCL (Fig. 5.88A).

The **tibial collateral ligament** (**TCL;** medial collateral ligament) is a strong, flat, intrinsic (capsular) band that extends from the medial epicondyle of the femur to the medial condyle and the superior part of the medial surface of the tibia (Fig. 5.88D & E). At its midpoint, the deep fibers of the TCL are firmly attached to the medial meniscus. The TCL, weaker than the FCL, is more often damaged. As a result, the TCL and medial meniscus are commonly torn during contact sports such as football and ice hockey.

The **oblique popliteal ligament** is a recurrent expansion of the tendon of the semimembranosus that reinforces the joint capsule posteriorly as it spans the intracondylar fossa (Fig. 5.86B). The ligament arises posterior to the medial tibial condyle and passes superolaterally toward the lateral femoral condyle, blending with the central part of the posterior aspect of the joint capsule.

The **arcuate popliteal ligament** also strengthens the joint capsule posterolaterally. It arises from the posterior

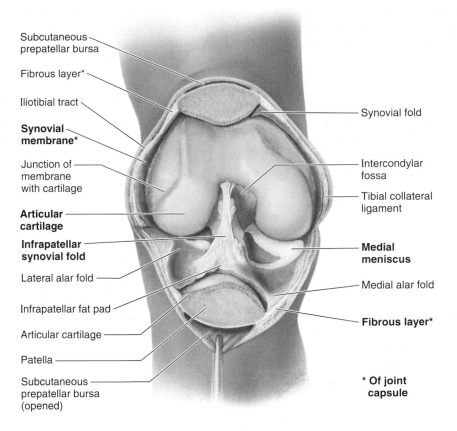

Subcutaneous prepatellar bursa

Fibrous layer*

Iliotibial tract

Synovial membrane*

Junction of membrane with cartilage

Articular cartilage

Infrapatellar synovial fold

Lateral alar fold

Infrapatellar fat pad

Articular cartilage

Patella

Subcutaneous prepatellar bursa (opened)

Synovial fold

Intercondylar fossa

Tibial collateral ligament

Medial meniscus

Medial alar fold

Fibrous layer*

* Of joint capsule

(A) Anterior view of flexed knee

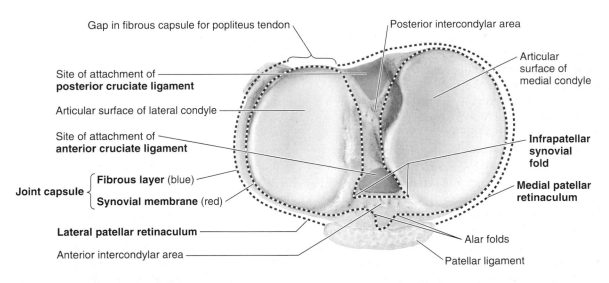

Gap in fibrous capsule for popliteus tendon

Site of attachment of **posterior cruciate ligament**

Articular surface of lateral condyle

Site of attachment of **anterior cruciate ligament**

Joint capsule {
  Fibrous layer (blue)
  Synovial membrane (red)
}

Lateral patellar retinaculum

Anterior intercondylar area

Posterior intercondylar area

Articular surface of medial condyle

Infrapatellar synovial fold

Medial patellar retinaculum

Alar folds

Patellar ligament

(B) Superior view of superior articular surface of tibia (tibial plateau)

FIGURE 5.87. Internal aspect of joint capsule of knee: layers, articular cavity, and articular surfaces. A. The joint capsule was incised transversely, the patella was sawn through, and then the knee was flexed, opening the articular cavity. The infrapatellar fold of synovial membrane encloses the cruciate ligaments, excluding them from the joint cavity. All internal surfaces not covered with or made of articular cartilage (*blue,* or *gray* in the case of the menisci) are lined with synovial membrane (mostly *purple,* but transparent and colorless where it is covering non-articular surfaces of the femur). **B.** The attachments of the fibrous layer and synovial membrane to the tibia are shown. Note that although they are adjacent on each side, they part company centrally to accommodate intercondylar and infrapatellar structures that are intracapsular (inside the fibrous layer) but extra-articular (excluded from the articular cavity by synovial membrane).

Gastrocnemius lateral head, turned superiorly

Fibular collateral ligament (FCL)

Popliteus muscle and tendon

Biceps femoris (turned inferiorly)

Iliotibial tract (turned inferiorly)

(A)

A - C Lateral views

Quadriceps femoris muscle and tendon

Suprapatellar bursa

Subcutaneous prepatellar bursa

Patella

Lateral meniscus

Patellar ligament

Fibrous layer of capsule of proximal tibiofibular joint

Gastrocnemius

Fibular collateral ligament

Popliteus

Lateral part of tibial plateau

Biceps femoris

Fibular collateral ligament

Iliotibial tract

Patellar ligament

(C)

Suprapatellar bursa

Joint cavity

Fibrous layer of joint capsule

Patella

Articular cartilage

(B)

Vastus medialis

Adductor magnus tendon

Medial superior genicular artery

Gastrocnemius tendon (of proximal attachment)

Meniscus

Semimembranosus tendon

Tibial collateral ligament (TCL)

Coronary ligament (in which a window has been cut)

Medial inferior genicular artery

Gracilis
Semitendinosus
Sartorius

Pes anserinus

Popliteus fascia overlying popliteus muscle

(D)

Adductor magnus

Gastrocnemius

Tibial collateral ligament

Tibial collateral ligament

Semi-membranosus

Patellar ligament

Sartorius
Gracilis
Semi-tendinosus

Pes anserinus

Tibial collateral ligament

(E)

D - E Medial views

FIGURE 5.88. Collateral ligaments and bursae of knee joint. A. Fibular collateral ligament. Purple latex was injected to demonstrate the extensive and complex articular cavity. The cavity/synovial membrane extends superiorly deep to the quadriceps, forming the suprapatellar bursa. **B.** Arthrogram, knee joint slightly flexed. The suprapatellar bursa is inflated with CO_2. **C.** The attachment sites of the FCL (*green*) and related muscles (*red,* proximal; *blue,* distal). **D.** Tibial collateral ligament (isolated from the fibrous layer of the joint capsule, of which it is a part). **E.** The attachment sites of the TCL and related muscles.

aspect of the fibular head, passes superomedially over the tendon of the popliteus, and spreads over the posterior surface of the knee joint. Its development appears to be inversely related to the presence and size of a *fabella* in the proximal attachment of the lateral head of gastrocnemius (see blue box "Fabella in Gastrocnemius;" Fig. B5.21 on p. 606). Both structures are thought to contribute to posterolateral stability of the knee.

INTRA-ARTICULAR LIGAMENTS OF KNEE JOINT

The intra-articular ligaments within the knee joint consist of the cruciate ligaments and menisci. The tendon of the popliteus is also intra-articular during part of its course.

The **cruciate ligaments** (L. *crux*, a cross) crisscross within the joint capsule of the joint but outside the synovial cavity (Figs. 5.89 and 5.90). The cruciate ligaments are located in

FIGURE 5.89. Cruciate ligaments of knee joint. A. Superior aspect of the superior articular surface of the tibia (tibial plateau), showing the medial and lateral condyles (articular surfaces) and the intercondylar eminence between them. The sites of attachment of the cruciate ligaments are colored *green;* those of the medial meniscus, *purple;* and those of the lateral meniscus, *orange.* **B.** The quadriceps tendon has been severed and the patella (within the tendon and its continuation, the patellar ligament) has been reflected inferiorly. The knee is flexed to demonstrate the cruciate ligaments.

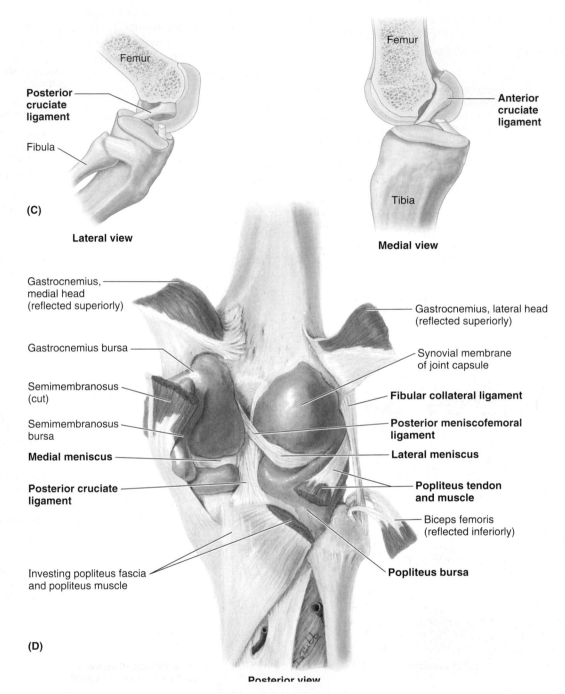

Femur

Posterior cruciate ligament

Fibula

(C)

Lateral view

Femur

Anterior cruciate ligament

Tibia

Medial view

Gastrocnemius, medial head (reflected superiorly)

Gastrocnemius bursa

Semimembranosus (cut)

Semimembranosus bursa

Medial meniscus

Posterior cruciate ligament

Investing popliteus fascia and popliteus muscle

Gastrocnemius, lateral head (reflected superiorly)

Synovial membrane of joint capsule

Fibular collateral ligament

Posterior meniscofemoral ligament

Lateral meniscus

Popliteus tendon and muscle

Biceps femoris (reflected inferiorly)

Popliteus bursa

(D)

Posterior view

FIGURE 5.89. Cruciate ligaments of knee joint (*continued*). **C.** In these lateral and medial views, the femur has been sectioned longitudinally and the near half has been removed with the proximal part of the corresponding cruciate ligament. The lateral view demonstrates how the posterior cruciate ligament resists anterior displacement of the femur on the tibial plateau. The medial view demonstrates how the anterior cruciate ligament resists posterior displacement of the femur on the tibial plateau. **D.** Both heads of the gastrocnemius are reflected superiorly, and the biceps femoris is reflected inferiorly. The articular cavity has been inflated with purple latex to demonstrate its continuity with the various bursae and the reflections and attachments of the complex synovial membrane.

FIGURE 5.90. Menisci of knee joint. A. The quadriceps tendon is cut, and the patella and patellar ligament are reflected inferiorly and anteriorly. The menisci, their attachments to the intercondylar area of the tibia, and the tibial attachments of the cruciate ligaments are shown. **B.** The band-like tibial collateral ligament is attached to the medial meniscus. The cord-like fibular collateral ligament is separated from the lateral meniscus. The posterior meniscofemoral ligament attaches the lateral meniscus to the medial femoral condyle. **C and D.** The numbers on the MRI study refer to the structures labeled in the corresponding anatomical coronal section. (Part **C** courtesy of Dr. W. Kucharczyk, Professor and Neuroradiologist Senior Scientist, Department of Medical Resonance Imaging, University Health Network, Toronto, Ontario, Canada.)

the center of the joint and cross each other obliquely, like the letter X. During medial rotation of the tibia on the femur, the cruciate ligaments wind around each other; thus the amount of medial rotation possible is limited to about 10°. Because they become unwound during lateral rotation, nearly 60° of lateral rotation is possible when the knee is flexed approximately 90°, the movement being ultimately limited by the TCL. The chiasm (crossing) of the cruciate ligaments serves as the pivot for rotatory movements at the knee. Because of their oblique orientation, in every position one cruciate ligament, or parts of one or both ligaments, is tense. It is the cruciate ligaments that maintain contact with the femoral and tibial articular surfaces during flexion of the knee (Fig. 5.89C).

The **anterior cruciate ligament** (**ACL**), the weaker of the two cruciate ligaments, arises from the anterior intercondylar area of the tibia, just posterior to the attachment of the medial meniscus (Fig. 5.89A & B). The ACL has a relatively poor blood supply. It extends superiorly, posteriorly, and laterally to attach to the posterior part of the medial side of the lateral condyle of the femur (Fig. 5.89C). It limits posterior rolling (turning and traveling) of the femoral condyles on the tibial plateau during flexion, converting it to spin (turning in place). It also prevents posterior displacement of the femur on the tibia and hyperextension of the knee joint. When the joint is flexed at a right angle, the tibia cannot be pulled anteriorly (like pulling out a drawer) because it is held by the ACL.

The **posterior cruciate ligament** (**PCL**), the stronger of the two cruciate ligaments, arises from the posterior intercondylar area of the tibia (Fig. 5.89A & D). The PCL passes superiorly and anteriorly on the medial side of the ACL to attach to the anterior part of the lateral surface of the medial condyle of the femur (Fig. 5.89B & C). The PCL limits anterior rolling of the femur on the tibial plateau during extension, converting it to spin. It also prevents anterior displacement of the femur on the tibia or posterior displacement of the tibia on the femur and helps prevent hyperflexion of the knee joint. In the weight-bearing flexed knee, the PCL is the main stabilizing factor for the femur (e.g., when walking downhill).

The **menisci of the knee joint** are crescentic plates ("wafers") of fibrocartilage on the articular surface of the tibia that deepen the surface and play a role in shock absorption (Figs. 5.89 and 5.90). The menisci (G. *meniskos*, crescent) are thicker at their external margins and taper to thin, unattached edges in the interior of the joint. Wedge shaped in transverse section, the menisci are firmly attached at their ends to the *intercondylar area of the tibia* (Fig. 5.89A). Their external margins attach to the joint capsule of the knee. The **coronary ligaments** are portions of the joint capsule extending between the margins of the menisci and most of the periphery of the tibial condyles (Figs. 5.89B and 5.90A). A slender fibrous band, the **transverse ligament of the knee,** joins the anterior edges of the menisci, crossing the anterior intercondylar area (Fig. 5.9A) and tethering the menisci to each other during knee movements.

The **medial meniscus** is C shaped, broader posteriorly than anteriorly (Fig. 5.90A). Its anterior end (horn) is attached to the anterior intercondylar area of the tibia,

anterior to the attachment of the ACL (Figs. 5.89A & B and 5.90A). Its posterior end is attached to the posterior intercondylar area, anterior to the attachment of the PCL. The medial meniscus firmly adheres to the deep surface of the TCL (Figs. 5.88D and 5.90A–D). Because of its widespread attachments laterally to the tibial intercondylar area and medially to the TCL, the medial meniscus is less mobile on the tibial plateau than is the lateral meniscus.

The lateral meniscus is nearly circular, smaller, and more freely movable than the medial meniscus (Fig. 5.90A). The tendon of the popliteus has two parts proximally. One part attaches to the lateral epicondyle of the femur and passes between the lateral meniscus and inferior part of the lateral epicondylar surface of the femur (on the tendon's medial aspect) and the FCL that overlies its lateral aspect (Figs. 5.88A and 5.89B & D). The other, more medial part of the popliteal tendon attaches to the posterior limb of the lateral meniscus. A strong tendinous slip, the posterior meniscofemoral ligament, joins the lateral meniscus to the PCL and the medial femoral condyle (Figs. 5.89D and 5.90A & B).

MOVEMENTS OF KNEE JOINT

Flexion and extension are the main knee movements; some rotation occurs when the knee is flexed. The main movements of the knee joint are illustrated in Figure 5.91, and the muscles producing them and relevant details are provided in Table 5.16.

When the knee is fully extended with the foot on the ground, the knee passively "locks" because of medial rotation of the femoral condyles on the tibial plateau (the "screw-home mechanism"). This position makes the lower limb a solid column and more adapted for weight-bearing. When the knee is "locked," the thigh and leg muscles can relax briefly without making the knee joint too unstable. To unlock the knee, the popliteus contracts, rotating the femur laterally about 5° on the tibial plateau so that flexion of the knee can occur.

Movements of Menisci. Although the rolling movement of the femoral condyles during flexion and extension is limited (converted to spin) by the cruciate ligaments, some rolling does occur, and the point of contact between the femur and the tibia moves posteriorly with flexion and returns anteriorly with extension. Furthermore, during rotation of the knee, one femoral condyle moves anteriorly on the corresponding tibial condyle while the other femoral condyle moves posteriorly, rotating about the cruciate ligaments. The menisci must be able to migrate on the tibial plateau as the points of contact between femur and tibia change.

BLOOD SUPPLY OF KNEE JOINT

The arteries supplying the knee joint are the 10 vessels that form the peri-articular **genicular anastomoses** around the knee: the genicular branches of the femoral, popliteal, and anterior and posterior recurrent branches of the anterior tibial recurrent and circumflex fibular arteries (Figs. 5.92 and 5.93B). The middle genicular branches of the popliteal artery

(A) Extension **(B) Flexion** **(C) Medial rotation of leg, knee joint flexed 90°** **(D) Lateral rotation of leg, knee joint flexed 90°**

Lateral view of knee joint

FIGURE 5.91. Movements of knee joint.

TABLE 5.16. MOVEMENTS OF KNEE JOINT AND MUSCLES PRODUCING THEM

| Movement | Degrees Possible | Muscles Producing Movement | | Factors Limiting (Checking) Movement | Comments |
		Primary	Secondary		
Extension	Normal knees extend to 0° (straight alignment of axes of tibia and femur)[a]	Quadriceps femoris	Weakly: tensor fasciae latae	Anterior edge of lateral meniscus contacts shallow groove between tibial and patellar surfaces of femoral condyles; anterior cruciate ligament contacts groove in intercondylar fossa	Ability of quadriceps to produce extension is most effective when hip joint is extended; flexion diminishes its efficiency
Flexion	120° (hip extended); 140° (hip flexed); 160° passively	Hamstrings (semitendinosus, semimembranosus, long head of biceps); short head of biceps	Gracilis, sartorius, gastrocnemius, popliteus	Calf of leg contacts thigh; length of hamstrings is also a factor—more knee flexion is possible when hip joint is flexed; cannot fully flex knee when hip is extended	Normally, role of gastrocnemius is minimal, but in presence of a supracondylar fracture, it rotates (flexes) distal fragment of femur
Medial rotation	10° with knee flexed; 5° with knee extended	Semitendinosus and semimembranosus when knee is flexed; popliteus when non-bearing knee is extended	Gracilis, sartorius	Collateral ligaments, loose during flexion without rotation, become taut at limits of rotation	When extended knee is bearing weight, action of popliteus laterally rotates femur; when not bearing weight, popliteus medially rotates patella
Lateral rotation	30°	Biceps femoris when knee is flexed		Collateral ligaments become taut; anterior cruciate ligament becomes wound around posterior cruciate ligament	At end of rotation, with no opposition, tensor fasciae latae can assist in maintaining position

[a]Straight alignment of axis of tibia with axis of femur is 0°; normal range extends to −3° (3° of hyperextension).

penetrate the fibrous layer of the joint capsule and supply the cruciate ligaments, synovial membrane, and peripheral margins of the menisci.

INNERVATION OF KNEE JOINT

Reflecting Hilton's law, the nerves supplying the muscles crossing (acting on) the knee joint also supply the joint (Fig. 5.93D); thus articular branches from the femoral (the

branches to the vasti), tibial, and common fibular nerves supply its anterior, posterior, and lateral aspects, respectively. In addition, however, the obturator and saphenous (cutaneous) nerves supply articular branches to its medial aspect.

BURSAE AROUND KNEE JOINT

There are at least 12 bursae around the knee joint because most tendons run parallel to the bones and pull lengthwise

(A) Lateral view   **(B) Medial view**

FIGURE 5.92. Arterial anastomoses around knee. In addition to providing collateral circulation, the genicular arteries of the genicular anastomosis supply blood to the structures surrounding the joint as well as to the joint itself (e.g., its joint or articular capsule). Compare these views with the anterior view in Figure 5.93B.

(A) Anterior view   **(B) Anterior view**   **Posterior view**

FIGURE 5.93. Joints and neurovascular structures of leg and foot. A. The tibiofibular articulations include the synovial tibiofibular joint and the tibiofibular syndesmosis; the latter is made up of the interosseous membrane of the leg and the anterior and posterior tibiofibular ligaments. The oblique direction of the fibers of the interosseous membrane, primarily extending inferolaterally from the tibia, allows slight upward movement of the fibula but resists downward pull on it. **B.** The arterial supply of the joints of the leg and foot is demonstrated. Peri-articular anastomoses surround the knee and ankle.

FIGURE 5.93. Joints and neurovascular structures of leg and foot (*continued*). **C.** Of the nine muscles attached to the fibula, all except one exert a downward pull on the fibula. **D.** The nerve supply of the leg and foot is demonstrated. Starting with the knee and progressing distally in the limb, cutaneous nerves become increasingly involved in providing innervation to joints, taking over completely in the distal foot and toes.

across the joint during knee movements. The main bursae of the knee are illustrated in Figure 5.94 and described in Table 5.17.

The **subcutaneous prepatellar** and **infrapatellar bursae** are located at the convex surface of the joint, allowing the skin to be able to move freely during movements of the knee (see Figs. 5.87A and 5.88A).

Four bursae communicate with the synovial cavity of the knee joint: suprapatellar bursa, popliteus bursa (deep to the distal quadriceps), anserine bursa (deep to the tendinous distal attachments of the sartorius, gracilis, and semitendinosus), and gastrocnemius bursa (Figs. 5.88A and 5.89D). The large **suprapatellar bursa** (Figs. 5.86A and 5.88A) is especially important because an infection in it may spread to the knee joint cavity. Although it develops separately from the knee joint, the bursa becomes continuous with it.

Tibiofibular Joints

The tibia and fibula are connected by two joints: the *tibiofibular joint* and the *tibiofibular syndesmosis* (inferior tibiofibular) *joint*. In addition, an *interosseous membrane* joins

the shafts of the two bones (Fig. 5.93A). The fibers of the interosseous membrane and all ligaments of both tibiofibular articulations run inferiorly from the tibia to the fibula. Thus the membrane and ligaments strongly resist the downward pull placed on the fibula by eight of the nine muscles attached to it (Fig. 5.93C). However, they allow slight upward movement of the fibula that occurs when the wide (posterior) end of the trochlea of the talus is wedged between the malleoli during dorsiflexion at the ankle. Movement at the superior tibiofibular joint is impossible without movement at the inferior tibiofibular syndesmosis.

The anterior tibial vessels pass through a hiatus at the superior end of the interosseous membrane (Fig. 5.93A & B). At the inferior end of the membrane is a smaller hiatus through which the perforating branch of the fibular artery passes.

TIBIOFIBULAR JOINT

The **tibiofibular joint** (superior tibiofibular joint) is a plane type of synovial joint between the flat facet on the fibular head and a similar articular facet located posterolaterally

(A)

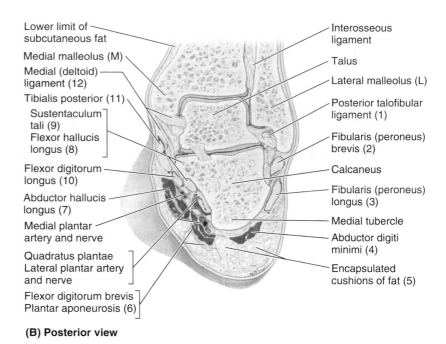

(B) Posterior view

FIGURE 5.96. Sectional anatomy of ankle region. A and B. The orientation drawing depicts the structures visible in the MRI of the ankle. (Courtesy of Dr. W. Kucharczyk, Professor and Neuroradiologist Senior Scientist, Department of Medical Resonance Imaging, University Health Network, Toronto, Ontario, Canada.)

The malleoli grip the talus tightly as it rocks in the mortise during movements of the joint. The grip of the malleoli on the trochlea is strongest during dorsiflexion of the foot (as when "digging in one's heels" when descending a steep slope or during tug-of-war) because this movement forces the wider, anterior part of the trochlea posteriorly between the malleoli, spreading the tibia and fibula slightly apart. This spreading is limited especially by the strong interosseous tibiofibular ligament as well as the anterior and posterior tibiofibular ligaments that unite the tibia and fibula (Figs. 5.96 and 5.97).

The *interosseous ligament* is deeply placed between the nearly congruent surfaces of the tibia and fibula; although demonstrated in the inset for Figure 5.93A, the ligament can actually be observed only by rupturing it or in a cross-section.

The ankle joint is relatively unstable during plantarflexion because the trochlea is narrower posteriorly and, therefore, lies relatively loosely within the mortise. It is during plantarflexion that most injuries of the ankle occur (usually as a result of sudden, unexpected—and therefore inadequately resisted—inversion of the foot).

JOINT CAPSULE OF ANKLE JOINT

The **joint capsule of the ankle joint** is thin anteriorly and posteriorly but is supported on each side by strong *lateral and medial* (collateral) *ligaments* (Figs. 5.97 and 5.98; thin

areas of the capsule have been removed in Fig. 5.97, leaving only the reinforced parts—the ligaments—and a synovial fold). Its fibrous layer is attached superiorly to the borders of the articular surfaces of the tibia and the malleoli and inferiorly to the talus. The synovial membrane is loose and lines the fibrous layer of the capsule. The synovial cavity often extends superiorly between the tibia and the fibula as far as the interosseous tibiofibular ligament.

LIGAMENTS OF ANKLE JOINT

The ankle joint is reinforced laterally by the **lateral ligament of the ankle,** a compound structure consisting of three completely separate ligaments (Fig. 5.97A & B):

1. **Anterior talofibular ligament,** a flat, weak band that extends anteromedially from the lateral malleolus to the neck of the talus.
2. **Posterior talofibular ligament,** a thick, fairly strong band that runs horizontally medially and slightly posteriorly from the malleolar fossa to the lateral tubercle of the talus.
3. **Calcaneofibular ligament,** a round cord that passes postero-inferiorly from the tip of the lateral malleolus to the lateral surface of the calcaneus.

The joint capsule is reinforced medially by the large, strong **medial ligament of the ankle** (deltoid ligament) that attaches proximally to the medial malleolus (Fig. 5.98). The

FIGURE 5.97. Dissection of ankle joint and joints of inversion and eversion. In (**A**), the foot has been inverted (by placing a wedge under the foot) to demonstrate the articular surfaces and make the lateral ligaments taut.

medial ligament fans out from the malleolus, attaching distally to the talus, calcaneus, and navicular via four adjacent and continuous parts: the **tibionavicular part**, the **tibiocalcaneal part**, and the **anterior** and **posterior tibiotalar parts**. The medial ligament stabilizes the ankle joint during eversion and prevents subluxation (partial dislocation) of the joint.

MOVEMENTS OF ANKLE JOINT

The main movements of the ankle joint are dorsiflexion and plantarflexion of the foot, which occur around a transverse axis passing through the talus (Fig. 5.99B). Because the narrow end of the trochlea of the talus lies loosely between the malleoli when the foot is plantarflexed, some "wobble" (small amounts of abduction, adduction, inversion, and eversion) is possible in this unstable position.

- *Dorsiflexion of the ankle* is produced by the muscles in the anterior compartment of the leg (see Table 5.10). Dorsiflexion is usually limited by the passive resistance of the triceps surae to stretching and by tension in the medial and lateral ligaments.
- *Plantarflexion of the ankle* is produced by the muscles in the posterior compartment of the leg (see Table 5.13). In toe dancing by ballet dancers, for example, the dorsum of the foot is in line with the anterior surface of the leg.

Calcaneal tendon
Flexor digitorum longus (FDL)
Flexor hallucis longus (FHL)
Tibialis posterior (TP)
Medial (deltoid) ligament
Bursa of calcaneal tendon
Quadratus plantae
Osseofibrous tunnel
Sustentaculum tali
Medial tubercle of talus
Attachment of abductor hallucis

(A) Medial view

Medial malleolus
Neck of talus
Ant. tibiotalar part
Medial ligament (deltoid ligament)
Post. tibiotalar part
Tibiocalcaneal part
Tibionavicular part
1st cuneiform bone
Tibialis posterior
Tibia
Groove for tibialis posterior (TP)
Calcaneal tendon
Groove for flexor hallucis longus (FHL)
Bursa of calcaneal tendon
Calcaneus
Navicular bone
Plantar calcaneonavicular ("spring") ligament and associated fibers
Sustentaculum tali
Medial tubercle of talus
*Talonavicular ligament

(B) Medial view

FIGURE 5.98. Tendons and ligaments on medial aspect of ankle and foot. A. The relationships of the flexor tendons to the medial malleolus and sustentaculum tali are shown as they descend the posterolateral aspect of the ankle region and enter the foot. Except for the part tethering the flexor hallucis longus tendon, the flexor retinaculum has been removed. **B.** The four parts of the medial (deltoid) ligament of the ankle are demonstrated in this dissection.

BLOOD SUPPLY OF ANKLE JOINT

The arteries are derived from malleolar branches of the fibular and anterior and posterior tibial arteries (Fig. 5.93B).

NERVE SUPPLY OF ANKLE JOINT

The nerves are derived from the tibial nerve and the deep fibular nerve, a division of the common fibular nerve (Fig. 5.93D).

Foot Joints

The many joints of the foot involve the tarsals, metatarsals, and phalanges (Fig. 5.99; Table 5.18). The important intertarsal joints are the *subtalar (talocalcaneal) joint* and the *transverse tarsal joint (calcaneocuboid* and *talonavicular joints)*. Inversion and eversion of the foot are the main movements involving these joints. The other intertarsal joints (e.g., *intercuneiform joints*) and the *tarsometatarsal* and *intermetatarsal joints* are relatively small and are so tightly joined by ligaments that only slight movement occurs between them. In the foot, flexion and extension occur in the forefoot at the metatarsophalangeal and interphalangeal joints (Fig. 5.100A & B; Table 5.19). Inversion is augmented by flexion of the toes (especially the great and 2nd toes), and eversion by their extension (especially of the lateral toes). All bones of the foot proximal to the metatarsophalangeal joints are united by dorsal and plantar ligaments. The bones of the metatarsophalangeal and interphalangeal joints are united by lateral and medial collateral ligaments.

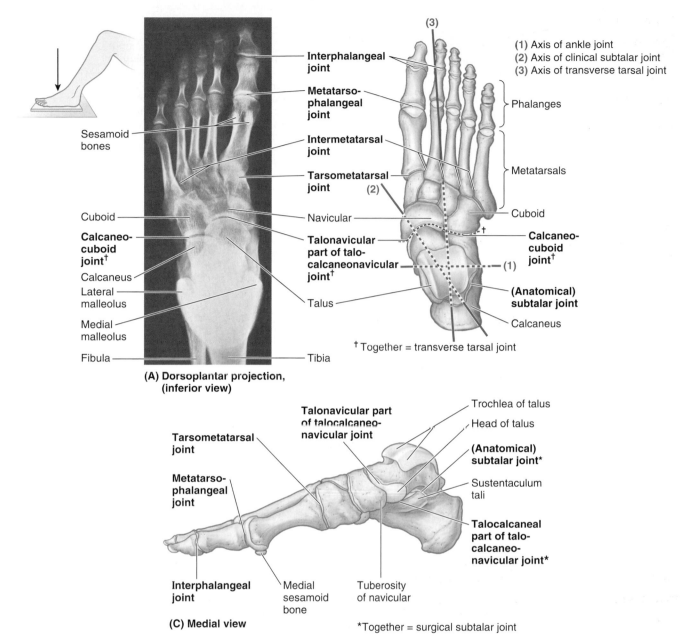

(1) Axis of ankle joint
(2) Axis of clinical subtalar joint
(3) Axis of transverse tarsal joint

Interphalangeal joint

Metatarso-phalangeal joint

Intermetatarsal joint

Tarsometatarsal joint

(2)

Sesamoid bones

Phalanges

Metatarsals

Cuboid

Navicular

Cuboid

Calcaneo-cuboid joint†

Talonavicular part of talo-calcaneonavicular joint†

Calcaneo-cuboid joint†

(1)

Calcaneus

Lateral malleolus

Talus

(Anatomical) subtalar joint

Medial malleolus

Calcaneus

Fibula

Tibia

† Together = transverse tarsal joint

(A) Dorsoplantar projection, (inferior view)

Talonavicular part of talocalcaneo-navicular joint

Trochlea of talus

Head of talus

Tarsometatarsal joint

(Anatomical) subtalar joint*

Metatarso-phalangeal joint

Sustentaculum tali

Talocalcaneal part of talo-calcaneo-navicular joint*

Interphalangeal joint

Medial sesamoid bone

Tuberosity of navicular

(C) Medial view

*Together = surgical subtalar joint

FIGURE 5.99. Joints of foot.

The **subtalar joint** occurs where the talus rests on and articulates with the calcaneus. The *anatomical subtalar joint* is a single synovial joint between the slightly concave posterior calcaneal articular surface of the talus and the convex posterior articular facet of the calcaneus (Figs. 5.96B and 5.97B). The joint capsule is weak but is supported by medial, lateral, posterior, and interosseous *talocalcaneal ligaments* (Figs. 5.96B and 5.97A). The **interosseous talocalcaneal ligament** lies within the *tarsal sinus,* which separates the subtalar and talocalcaneonavicular joints, and is especially strong. Orthopaedic surgeons use the term *subtalar joint* for the compound functional joint consisting of the anatomical subtalar joint plus the **talocalcaneal part of the talocalcaneonavicular joint.** The two separate

elements of the *clinical subtalar joint* straddle the talocalcaneal interosseous ligament. Structurally, the anatomical definition is logical because the anatomical subtalar joint is a discrete joint, having its own joint capsule and articular cavity. Functionally, however, the clinical definition is logical because the two parts of the compound joint function as a unit; it is impossible for them to function independently. The subtalar joint (by either definition) is where the majority of inversion and eversion occurs, around an axis that is oblique.

The **transverse tarsal joint** is a compound joint formed by two separate joints aligned transversely: the **talonavicular part of the talocalcaneonavicular joint**

(text continues on p. 654)

TABLE 5.18. JOINTS OF FOOT

Joint	Type	Articulating Surfaces	Joint Capsule	Ligaments	Movements	Blood Supply	Nerve Supply
Subtalar (talocalcaneal, anatomical subtalar joint)	Plane synovial joint	Inferior surface of body of talus (posterior calcaneal articular facet) articulates with superior surface (posterior talar articular surface) of calcaneus	Fibrous layer of joint capsule is attached to margins of articular surfaces	Medial, lateral, and posterior talocalcaneal ligaments support capsule; interosseous talocalcaneal ligament binds bones together	Inversion and eversion of foot	Posterior tibial and fibular arteries	Plantar aspect: medial or lateral plantar nerve Dorsal aspect: deep fibular nerve
Talocalcaneonavicular	Synovial joint; talonavicular part is ball and socket type	Head of talus articulates with calcaneus and navicular bones	Joint capsule incompletely encloses joint	Plantar calcaneonavicular (spring) ligament supports head of talus	Gliding and rotatory movements possible	Anterior tibial artery via lateral tarsal artery, a branch of dorsalis pedis artery (dorsal artery of foot)	
Calcaneocuboid	Plane synovial joint	Anterior end of calcaneus articulates with posterior surface of cuboid	Fibrous capsule encloses joint	Dorsal calcaneocuboid ligament, plantar calcaneocuboid, and long plantar ligaments support joint capsule	Inversion and eversion of foot; circumduction		
Cuneonavicular joint		Anterior navicular articulates with posterior surfaces of cuneiforms	Common capsule encloses joints	Dorsal and plantar cuneonavicular ligaments	Little movement occurs		
Tarsometatarsal		Anterior tarsal bones articulate with bases of metatarsal bones	Separate joint capsules enclose each joint	Dorsal, plantar, and interosseous tarsometatarsal ligaments bind bones together	Gliding or sliding		Deep fibular; medial and lateral plantar nerves; sural nerve
Intermetatarsal	Plane synovial joint	Bases of metatarsal bones articulate with each other		Dorsal, plantar, and interosseous intermetatarsal ligaments bind lateral four metatarsal bones together	Little individual movement occurs	Lateral metatarsal artery (a branch of dorsalis pedis artery)	Digital nerves
Metatarsophalangeal	Condyloid synovial joint	Heads of metatarsal bones articulate with bases of proximal phalanges	Separate joint capsules enclose each joint	Collateral ligaments support capsule on each side; plantar ligament supports plantar part of capsule	Flexion, extension, and some abduction, adduction, and circumduction		
Interphalangeal	Hinge synovial joint	Head of one phalanx articulates with base of one distal to it		Collateral and plantar ligaments support joints	Flexion and extension	Digital branches of plantar arch	

(A) Flexion

(B) Extension

(C) Abduction

(D) Adducted (relaxed position)

FIGURE 5.100. Movements of joints of forefoot.

TABLE 5.19. MOVEMENTS OF JOINTS OF FOREFOOT AND MUSCLES PRODUCING THEM

Movement (letters refer to Fig. 5.100)	Muscles[a]
Metatarsophalangeal joints	
Flexion (*A*)	**Flexor digitorum brevis** **Lumbricals** **Interossei** **Flexor hallucis brevis** **Flexor hallucis longus** Flexor digit minimi brevis Flexor digitorum longus
Extension (*B*)	**Extensor hallucis longus** **Extensor digitorum longus** **Extensor digitorum brevis**
Abduction (*C*)	**Abductor hallucis** **Abductor digiti minimi** **Dorsal interossei**
Adduction (*D*)	**Adductor hallucis** **Plantar interossei**
Interphalangeal joints	
Flexion (fig. *A*)	**Flexor hallucis longus** **Flexor digitorum longus** **Flexor digitorum brevis** Quadratus plantae
Extension (fig. *B*)	**Extensor hallucis longus** **Extensor digitorum longus** **Extensor digitorum brevis**

[a] Muscles in boldface are chiefly responsible for the movement; the other muscles assist them.

and the **calcaneocuboid joint** (Fig. 5.99B & C). At this joint, the midfoot and forefoot rotate as a unit on the hindfoot around a longitudinal (AP) axis, augmenting the inversion and eversion movements occurring at the clinical subtalar joint. Transection across the transverse tarsal joint is a standard method for *surgical amputation of the foot.*

MAJOR LIGAMENTS OF FOOT

The major ligaments of the plantar aspect of the foot (Fig. 5.101) are the:

- **Plantar calcaneonavicular ligament** (spring ligament), which extends across and fills a wedge-shaped gap between the sustentaculum tali and the inferior margin of the posterior articular surface of the navicular (Fig. 5.101A & B). The spring ligament supports the head of the talus and plays important roles in the transfer of weight from the talus and in maintaining the longitudinal arch of the foot, of which it is the keystone (superiormost element).
- **Long plantar ligament,** which passes from the plantar surface of the calcaneus to the groove on the cuboid. Some of its fibers extend to the bases of the metatarsals, thereby forming a tunnel for the tendon of the fibularis longus (Fig. 5.101A). The long plantar ligament is important in maintaining the longitudinal arch of the foot.
- **Plantar calcaneocuboid ligament** (short plantar ligament), which is located on a plane between the plantar calcaneonavicular and the long plantar ligaments (Fig. 5.101B). It extends from the anterior aspect of the inferior surface of the calcaneus to the inferior surface of the cuboid. It is also involved in maintaining the longitudinal arch of the foot.

ARCHES OF FOOT

If the feet were more rigid structures, each impact with the ground would generate extremely large forces of short duration (shocks) that would be propagated through the skeletal system. Because the foot is composed of numerous bones connected by ligaments, it has considerable flexibility that allows it to deform with each ground contact, thereby absorbing much of the shock. Furthermore, the tarsal and metatarsal bones are arranged in longitudinal and transverse arches passively supported and actively restrained by flexible tendons that add to the weight-bearing capabilities and resiliency of the foot. Thus, much smaller forces of longer duration are transmitted through the skeletal system.

The arches distribute weight over the pedal platform (foot), acting not only as shock absorbers but also as springboards for propelling it during walking, running, and jumping. The resilient arches add to the foot's ability to adapt to changes in surface contour. The weight of the body is transmitted to the talus from the tibia. Then it is transmitted posteriorly to the calcaneus and anteriorly to the "ball of the foot" (the sesamoids of the 1st metatarsal and the head of the 2nd metatarsal), and that weight/pressure is shared laterally with the heads of the 3rd–5th metatarsals as necessary for balance and comfort (Fig. 5.102). Between these weight-bearing points are the relatively elastic arches of the foot, which become slightly flattened by body weight during standing. They normally resume their curvature (recoil) when body weight is removed.

The **longitudinal arch of the foot** is composed of medial and lateral parts (Fig. 5.103). Functionally, both parts act as a unit with the transverse arch of the foot, spreading the weight in all directions. The **medial longitudinal arch** is higher and more important than the lateral longitudinal arch (Fig. 5.103A & B). The medial longitudinal arch is composed of the calcaneus, talus, navicular, three cuneiforms, and three metatarsals. *The talar head is the keystone of the medial longitudinal arch.* The tibialis anterior and posterior, via their tendinous attachments, help support the medial longitudinal arch. The fibularis longus tendon, passing from lateral to medial, also helps support this arch (Fig. 5.103C & E). The **lateral longitudinal arch** is much flatter than the medial part of the arch and rests on the ground during standing (Fig. 5.103B & D). It is made up of the calcaneus, cuboid, and lateral two metatarsals.

The **transverse arch of the foot** runs from side to side (Fig. 5.103C). It is formed by the cuboid, cuneiforms, and bases of the metatarsals. The medial and lateral parts of the longitudinal arch serve as pillars for the transverse arch. The tendons of the fibularis longus and tibialis posterior, crossing under the sole of the foot like a stirrup (Fig. 5.103C), help maintain the curvature of the transverse arch. The integrity of the bony arches of the foot is maintained by both passive factors and dynamic supports (Fig. 5.103E).

Passive factors involved in forming and maintaining the arches of the foot include:

- The shape of the united bones (both arches, but especially the transverse arch).
- Four successive layers of fibrous tissue that bowstring the longitudinal arch (superficial to deep):
  1. Plantar aponeurosis.
  2. Long plantar ligament.
  3. Plantar calcaneocuboid (short plantar) ligament.
  4. Plantar calcaneonavicular (spring) ligament.

Dynamic supports involved in maintaining the arches of the foot include:

- Active (reflexive) bracing action of intrinsic muscles of foot (longitudinal arch).
- Active and tonic contraction of muscles with long tendons extending into foot:
  - Flexors hallucis and digitorum longus for the longitudinal arch.
  - Fibularis longus and tibialis posterior for the transverse arch.

Plantar views

FIGURE 5.101. Plantar ligaments. A and B. Sequential stages of a deep dissection of the sole of the right foot showing the attachments of the ligaments and the tendons of the long evertor and invertor muscles.

Sesamoid bones of 1st metatarsal and head of 2nd metatarsal bones

Heads of 3rd to 5th metatarsal bones

Tuberosity of calcaneus

Plantar view

FIGURE 5.102. Weight-bearing areas of foot. Body weight is divided approximately equally between the hindfoot (calcaneus) and the forefoot (heads of the metatarsals). The forefoot has five points of contact with the ground: a large medial one that includes the two sesamoid bones associated with the head of the 1st metatarsal and the heads of the lateral four metatarsals. The 1st metatarsal supports the major share of the load, with the lateral forefoot providing balance.

Of these factors, the plantar ligaments and the plantar aponeurosis bear the greatest stress and are most important in maintaining the arches of the foot.

Surface Anatomy of Joints of Knee, Ankle, and Foot

The **knee region** is between the thigh and the leg (Fig. 5.104A). Superior to it are the large bulges formed by the *vasta lateralis* and *medialis.* Superolateral to the knee is the *iliotibial tract,* which can be followed inferiorly to the *anterolateral (Gerdy) tubercle of the tibia.* The *patella,* easily palpated and moveable from-side-to side during extension, lies anterior to the *femoral condyles* (palpable to each side of the middle of the patella). Extending from the *apex of the patella,* the *patellar ligament* is easily visible, especially in thin people, as a thick band attached to the prominent *tibial tuberosity.* The *plane of the knee joint,* between femoral condyles and tibial plateau, may be palpated on each side of the junction of patellar apex and ligament when the knee is extended. Laterally, the *head of the fibula* is readily located by following the *tendon of the biceps femoris* inferiorly. This tendon is particularly prominent when the knee is partially flexed (Fig. 5.104B). The *fibular collateral ligament* may be palpated as a cord-like structure superior to the fibular head and anterior to biceps tendon, when the knee is fully flexed.

The prominences of the *lateral and medial malleoli* provide an approximation of the *axis of the ankle joint* (Fig. 5.104C–E). When the ankle is plantarflexed, the *anterior* border of the distal end of the tibia is palpable proximal to the malleoli, providing an indication of the joint plane of the ankle joint. The *sustentaculum tali,* approximately 2 cm distal to the tip of the medial malleolus, is best felt by palpating it from below where it is somewhat obscured by the *tendon of the flexor digitorum longus,* which crosses it. On the lateral side, when the foot is inverted, the

(A) Medial longitudinal arch (medial view)

Intermediate cuneiform — Navicular — Talus — Calcaneus

Medial cuneiform

First metatarsal

(B) Lateral longitudinal arch (lateral view)

Cuboid — Lateral cuneiform — 5th metatarsal

Calcaneus

(C) Transverse arch (anterior view)

Tendon of tibialis posterior

Medial
Intermediate } Cuneiform bones
Lateral

Cuboid

Tendon of fibularis longus

(D) Superior view

Medial longitudinal arch (dark)

Lateral longitudinal arch (light)

* The calcaneus is common to both longitudinal arches

FIGURE 5.103. Arches of foot. A and B. The medial longitudinal arch is higher than the lateral longitudinal arch, which may contact the ground when standing erect. **C.** The transverse arch is demonstrated at the level of the cuneiforms, receiving stirrup-like support from a major invertor (tibialis posterior) and evertor (fibularis longus). **D.** The components of the medial (*dark gray*) and lateral (*light gray*) longitudinal arches are indicated. The calcaneus (*medium gray*) is common to both. The medial arch is primarily weight-bearing, whereas the lateral arch provides balance.

(E) Medial longitudinal arch (medial view)

FIGURE 5.103. Arches of foot (*continued*). **E.** The active (*red lines*) and passive (*gray*) supports of the longitudinal arches are represented. There are four layers of passive support (*1–4*).

lateral margin of the ***anterior surface of the calcaneus*** is uncovered and palpable. This indicates the site of the *calcaneocuboid joint*. When the foot is plantarflexed, the *head of the talus* is exposed. Palpate it dorsal to where the anterior surface of the calcaneus is felt. The *calcaneal tendon* at the posterior aspect of the ankle is easily palpated and traced to its attachment to the *calcaneal tuberosity.* In the depression on each side of the tendon, the ankle joint is superficial. When the joint is overfilled with fluid, these depressions may be obliterated. The *transverse tarsal joint* is indicated by a line from the posterior aspect of the

tuberosity of the navicular to a point halfway between the lateral malleolus and the tuberosity of the 5th metatarsal.

The ***metatarsophalangeal joint of the great toe*** lies distal to the knuckle formed by the head of the 1st metatarsal. *Gout*, a metabolic disorder, commonly causes edema and tenderness of this joint, as does *osteoarthritis* (degenerative joint disease). Severe pain in the 1st metatarsophalangeal joint is called *podagra* (from G. *pous* + G. *agra*, a seizure). Often the 1st metatarsophalangeal joint is the first one affected by arthritis.

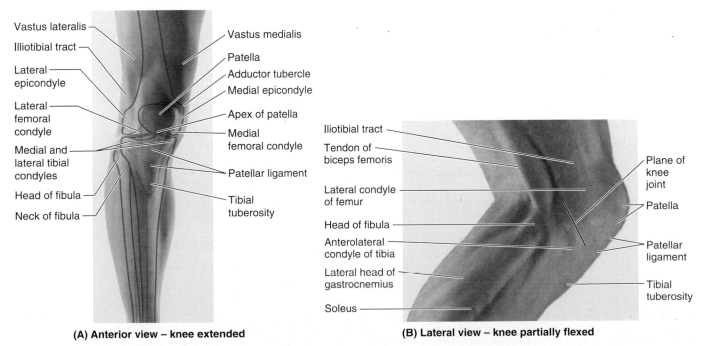

(A) Anterior view – knee extended

(B) Lateral view – knee partially flexed

FIGURE 5.104. Surface anatomy of the joints of the knee, leg, ankle, and foot.

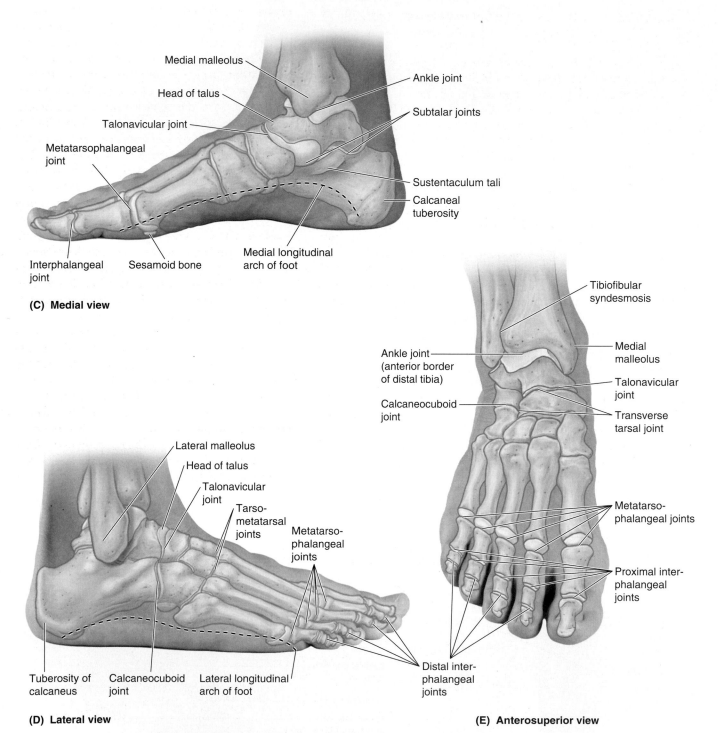

(C) Medial view

(D) Lateral view

(E) Anterosuperior view

FIGURE 5.104. Surface anatomy of the joints of the knee, leg, ankle, and foot *(continued)*.

JOINTS OF LOWER LIMB

Bipedalism and Congruity of Articular Surfaces of Hip Joint

 The acetabulum is directed inferiorly, laterally, and anteriorly in humans. The weight-bearing iliac portion of the acetabular rim overlies the femoral head, which is important for transfer of weight to the femur in the erect (standing/walking) position (Figs. 5.77A and 5.79C).

Consequently, of the positions commonly assumed by humans, the hip joint is mechanically most stable when a person is bearing weight, as when lifting a heavy object, for example. Decreases in the degree to which the ilium overlies the femoral head (detectable radiographically as the *angle of Wiberg*—Fig. 5.79C & D) may indicate joint instability.

Because of the anterior direction the axis of the acetabulum and the posterior direction of the axis of the femoral head and neck as it extends laterally (owing to the torsion angle—discussed earlier on page 518), there is an angle of 30–40° between their axes (Fig. B5.28). Consequently, the articular surfaces of the head and acetabulum are not fully congruent in the erect (bipedal) posture. The anterior part of the femoral head is "exposed" and articulates mostly with the joint capsule (Figs. 5.79C, 5.80, 5.81A & C, and 5.84). Nonetheless, rarely is >40% of the available articular surface of the femoral head in contact with the surface of the acetabulum in any position.

Relative to other joints and in view of the large size of the hip joint, this is extensive contact, contributing considerably to the joint's great stability.

Fractures of Femoral Neck

Fractures of the neck of the femur (unfortunately referred to as "fractured hips," implying that the hip bone is broken) are uncommon in most contact sports because the participants are usually young and the femoral neck is strong in people <40 years of age. When they do occur in this age group, these fractures usually result from high-energy impacts (e.g., during race-car accidents, skiing, trampoline, and equestrian events) when the lower limb is extended and the force of the impact is transmitted to the hip joint, even if applied at some distance from the joint. For example, if the foot is firmly braced against the car floor with the knee locked, or if the knee is braced against the dashboard during a head-on collision, the force of the impact may be transmitted superiorly and produce a femoral neck fracture. Femoral neck fractures are especially common in individuals >60 years, especially in women, because their femoral necks are more often weak and brittle, as a result of *osteoporosis* (Fig. B5.29). Fractures of the femoral neck are often intracapsular, and realignment of the neck fragments requires internal skeletal fixation.

Fractures of the femoral neck cause lateral rotation of the lower limb. Fractures of the femoral neck often disrupt the blood supply to the head of the femur. Most of the blood to the head and neck of the femur is supplied by the medial circumflex femoral artery (Fig. 5.82). The retinacular arteries arising from this artery are often torn when the femoral neck is fractured or the hip joint is dislocated. Following some femoral neck fractures, the artery to the ligament of the femoral head may be the only remaining source of blood to the proximal fragment. This artery is frequently inadequate for

FIGURE B5.28.

FIGURE B5.29.

maintaining the femoral head; consequently, the fragment may undergo *aseptic vascular necrosis* (tissue death).

Surgical Hip Replacement

Although the hip joint is strong and stable, it is subject to severe traumatic injury and degenerative disease. *Osteoarthritis of the hip joint,* characterized by pain, edema, limitation of motion, and erosion of articular cartilage, is a common cause of disability (Fig. B5.30A). During hip replacement, a metal prosthesis anchored to the person's femur by bone cement replaces the femoral head and neck (Fig. B5.30B). A plastic socket cemented to the hip bone replaces the acetabulum.

Hip bone

Cartilage

Femur

Normal hip

Osteophytes and eroded articular cartilage

(A) Hip with moderate arthritis   **(B)** Hip prosthesis

FIGURE B5.30.

Necrosis of Femoral Head in Children

In children, traumatic dislocations of the hip joint disrupt the artery to the head of the femur. Fractures that result in separation of the superior femoral epiphysis (the growth plate between the femoral head and neck) are also likely to result in an inadequate

blood supply to the femoral head and in *post-traumatic avascular necrosis of the head of the femur.* As a result, incongruity of the joint surfaces develops, and growth at the epiphysis is retarded. Such conditions, most common in children 3–9 years of age, produce hip pain that may radiate to the knee.

Dislocation of Hip Joint

Congenital dislocation of the hip joint is common, occurring in approximately 1.5 per 1000 neonates; it is bilateral in approximately half the cases. Girls are affected at least eight times more often than boys (Salter, 1999). Dislocation occurs when the femoral head is not properly located in the acetabulum. Inability to abduct the thigh is characteristic of congenital dislocation. In addition, the affected limb appears (and functions as if it is) shorter because the dislocated femoral head is more superior than on the normal side, resulting in a positive *Trendelenburg sign* (hip appears to drop on one side during walking). Approximately 25% of all cases of arthritis of the hip in adults are the direct result of residual defects from congenital dislocation of the hip.

Acquired dislocation of the hip joint is uncommon because this articulation is so strong and stable. Nevertheless, dislocation may occur during an automobile accident when the hip is flexed, adducted, and medially rotated, the usual position of the lower limb when a person is riding in a car.

Posterior dislocations of the hip joint are most common. A head-on collision that causes the knee to strike the dashboard

(A)

Head of femur is driven posteriorly, out of acetabulum

(B)

Posterior dislocation of the right hip joint

FIGURE B5.31.

may dislocate the hip when the femoral head is forced out of the acetabulum (Fig. B5.31A). The joint capsule ruptures inferiorly and posteriorly, allowing the femoral head to pass through the tear in the capsule, and over the posterior margin of the acetabulum onto the lateral surface of the ilium, shortening and medial rotating the limb (Fig. B5.31B).

Because of the close relationship of the *sciatic nerve* to the hip joint (Fig. 5.80A), it may be injured (stretched and/or compressed) during posterior dislocations or fracture–dislocations of the hip joint. This kind of injury may result in paralysis of the hamstrings and muscles distal to the knee supplied by the sciatic nerve. Sensory changes may also occur in the skin over the posterolateral aspects of the leg and over much of the foot because of injury to sensory branches of the sciatic nerve.

Anterior dislocation of the hip joint results from a violent injury that forces the hip into extension, abduction, and lateral rotation (e.g., catching a ski tip when snow skiing). In these cases, the femoral head is inferior to the acetabulum. Often, the acetabular margin fractures, producing a *fracture–dislocation of the hip joint.* When the femoral head dislocates, it usually carries the acetabular bone fragment and acetabular labrum with it. These injuries also occur with posterior dislocations.

Genu Valgum and Genu Varum

 The femur is placed diagonally within the thigh, whereas the tibia is almost vertical within the leg, creating an angle at the knee between the long axes of the bones (Fig. B5.32A). The angle between the two bones, referred to clinically as the **Q-angle,** is assessed by drawing a line from the ASIS to the middle of the patella and extrapolating a second (vertical) line passing through the middle of the patella and tibial tuberosity (Fig. 5.84). The Q-angle is typically greater in adult females, owing to their wider pelves. When normal, the angle of the femur within the thigh places the middle of the knee joint directly inferior to the head of the femur when standing, centering the weight-bearing line in the intercondylar region of the knee (Fig. B5.32A).

A medial angulation of the leg in relation to the thigh, in which the femur is abnormally vertical and the Q-angle is small, is a deformity called *genu varum* (bowleg) that causes unequal weight-bearing: The line of weight-bearing falls medial to the center of the knee (Fig. B5.32B). Excess pressure is placed on the medial aspect of the knee joint, which results in *arthrosis* (destruction of knee cartilages), and the fibular collateral ligament is overstressed (Fig. B.32D). A lateral angulation of the leg (large Q-angle, >17°) in relation to the thigh (exaggeration of the knee angle) is called *genu valgum* (knock-knee) (Fig. B5.32C). Because of the exaggerated knee angle in genu valgum, the weight-bearing line falls lateral to the center of the knee. Consequently, the tibial collateral ligament is overstretched, and there is excess stress on the lateral meniscus and cartilages of the lateral femoral and tibial condyles. The patella, normally pulled laterally by the tendon of the vastus lateralis, is pulled even farther laterally when the leg is extended in the presence of genu valgum so that its articulation with the femur is abnormal.

Children commonly appear bowlegged for 1–2 years after starting to walk, and knock-knees are frequently observed in children 2–4 years of age. Persistence of these abnormal knee angles in late childhood usually means congenital deformities exist that may require correction. Any irregularity of a joint eventually leads to wear and tear (arthrosis) of the articular cartilages and degenerative joint changes (*osteoarthritis [arthrosis]*).

Patellar Dislocation

When the patella is dislocated, it nearly always dislocates laterally. *Patellar dislocation* is more common in women, presumably because of their greater

(A) Normal alignment   **(B) Genu varum**   **(C) Genu valgum**   **(D) Osteoarthritis (arthrosis)**

FIGURE B5.32.

Q-angle, which, in addition to representing the oblique placement of the femur relative to the tibia, represents the angle of pull of the quadriceps relative to the axis of the patella and tibia (the term *Q-angle* was actually coined in reference to the angle of pull of the quadriceps). The tendency toward lateral dislocation is normally counterbalanced by the medial, more horizontal pull of the powerful vastus medialis. In addition, the more anterior projection of the lateral femoral condyle and deeper slope for the larger lateral patellar facet provide a mechanical deterrent to lateral dislocation. An imbalance of the lateral pull and the mechanisms resisting it result in abnormal tracking of the patella within the patellar groove and chronic patellar pain, even if actual dislocation does not occur.

Patellofemoral Syndrome

Pain deep to the patella often results from excessive running, especially downhill; hence, this type of pain is often called "runner's knee." The pain results from repetitive microtrauma caused by abnormal tracking of the patella relative to the patellar surface of the femur, a condition known as the *patellofemoral syndrome*. This syndrome may also result from a direct blow to the patella and from *osteoarthritis of the patellofemoral compartment* (degenerative wear and tear of articular cartilages). In some cases, strengthening of the vastus medialis corrects *patellofemoral dysfunction*. This muscle tends to prevent lateral dislocation of the patella resulting from the Q-angle because the vastus medialis attaches to and pulls on the medial border of the patella. Hence, weakness of the vastus medialis predisposes

the individual to the patellofemoral dysfunction and patellar dislocation.

Knee Joint Injuries

Knee joint injuries are common because the knee is a low-placed, mobile, weight-bearing joint, serving as a fulcrum between two long levers (thigh and leg). Its stability depends almost entirely on its associated ligaments and surrounding muscles.

The knee joint is essential for everyday activities such as standing, walking, and climbing stairs. It is also a main joint for sports that involve running, jumping, kicking, and changing directions. To perform these activities, the knee joint must be mobile; however, this mobility makes it susceptible to injuries.

The most common knee injury in contact sports is *ligament sprain*, which occurs when the foot is fixed in the ground (Fig. B5.33A). If a force is applied against the knee when the foot cannot move, ligament injuries are likely to occur. The tibial and fibular collateral ligaments (TCL and FCL) are tightly stretched when the leg is extended, normally preventing disruption of the sides of the knee joint.

The firm attachment of the TCL to the medial meniscus is of considerable clinical significance because tearing of this ligament frequently results in concomitant tearing of the medial meniscus. The injury is frequently caused by a blow to the lateral side of the extended knee, or excessive lateral twisting of the flexed knee that disrupts the TCL and concomitantly tears and/or detaches the medial meniscus from the joint capsule (Fig. B5.33A). This injury is common in

Twisting motion

Foot fixed

Anterior cruciate ligament (torn)

Tibial collateral ligament (torn)

Medial meniscus (torn)

Compounded knee injuries

(A)

FIGURE B5.33.

(B) Anterior drawer sign (ACL)

Half of bone is removed to show ligaments

Anterior cruciate ligament (torn)

The anterior cruciate ligament prevents the femur from sliding posteriorly on the tibia and hyperextension of the knee and limits medial rotation of the femur when the foot is on the ground, and the leg is flexed.

(C) Posterior drawer sign (PCL)

Posterior cruciate ligament (torn)

The posterior cruciate ligament prevents the femur from sliding anteriorly on the tibia, particularly when the knee is flexed.

FIGURE B5.33. (continued).

athletes who twist their flexed knees while running (e.g., in basketball, the various forms of football, and volleyball). The ACL, which serves as a pivot for rotatory movements of the knee, and is taut during flexion, may also tear subsequent to the rupture of the TCL, creating an "unhappy triad" of knee injuries.

Hyperextension and severe force directed anteriorly against the femur with the knee semiflexed (e.g., a cross-body block in football) may tear the ACL. *ACL rupture* is also a common knee injury in skiing accidents. This injury causes the free tibia to slide anteriorly under the fixed femur, known as the *anterior drawer sign* (Fig. B5.33B); it is tested clinically via the *Lachman test*. The ACL may tear away from the femur or tibia; however, tears commonly occur in the midportion of the ligament.

Although strong, *PCL ruptures* may occur when a player lands on the tibial tuberosity with the knee flexed (e.g., when knocked to the floor in basketball). PCL ruptures usually occur in conjunction with tibial or fibular ligament tears.

These injuries can also occur in head-on collisions when seat belts are not worn and the proximal end of the tibia strikes the dashboard. PCL ruptures allow the free tibia to slide posteriorly under the fixed femur, known as *the posterior drawer sign* (Fig. B5.33C).

Meniscal tears usually involve the medial meniscus. The lateral meniscus does not usually tear because of its mobility. *Pain on lateral rotation of the tibia* on the femur indicates injury of the lateral meniscus (Fig. B5.34A), whereas *pain on medial rotation of the tibia* on the femur indicates injury of the medial meniscus (Fig. B5.34B). Most meniscal tears occur in conjunction with TCL or ACL tears. Peripheral meniscal tears can often be repaired, or they may heal on their own because of the generous blood supply to this area. If tears do not heal or cannot repaired, the meniscus is removed (e.g., by arthroscopic surgery). Knee joints from which a meniscus has been removed suffer no loss of mobility; however, the knee may be less stable and the tibial plateaus often undergoes inflammatory reactions.

Pain — — Pain

(A) **(B)**

FIGURE B5.34.

(A)

(B) Normal lateral meniscus of the knee

Lateral meniscal tear

Medial meniscal tear

Transverse ligament tear

Medial meniscal tear

(C)

FIGURE B5.35.

Arthroscopy of Knee Joint

Arthroscopy is an endoscopic examination that allows visualization of the interior of the knee joint cavity with minimal disruption of tissue (Fig. B5.35). The arthroscope and one (or more) additional cannula(e) are inserted through tiny incisions, known as *portals.* The second cannula is for passage of specialized tools (e.g., manipulative probes or forceps) or equipment for trimming, shaping, or removing damaged tissue. This technique allows removal of torn menisci, loose bodies in the joint (such as bone chips), and *débridement* (the excision of devitalized articular cartilaginous material) in advanced cases of arthritis. Ligament repair or replacement may also be performed using an arthroscope. Although general anesthesia is usually preferable, knee arthroscopy can be performed using local or regional anesthesia. During arthroscopy, the articular cavity of the knee must be treated essentially as two separate (medial and lateral) femorotibial articulations, owing to the imposition of the synovial fold around the cruciate ligaments.

Aspiration of Knee Joint

Fractures of the distal end of the femur, or lacerations of the anterior thigh, may involve the suprapatellar bursa and result in infection of the knee joint. When the knee joint is infected and inflamed, the amount of synovial fluid may increase. *Joint effusions,* the escape of fluid from blood or lymphatic vessels, results in increased amounts of fluid in the joint cavity. Because the suprapatellar bursa communicates freely with the synovial cavity of the knee joint, fullness of the thigh in the region of the suprapatellar bursa may indicate increased synovial fluid. This bursa can be aspirated to remove the fluid for examination. Direct *aspiration of the knee joint* is usually performed with the patient sitting on a table with the knee flexed. The joint is approached laterally, using three bony points as landmarks for needle insertion: the anterolateral tibial (Gerdy) tubercle, the lateral epicondyle of the femur, and the apex of the patella. In addition to being the route for aspiration of serous and sanguineous (bloody) fluid, this triangular area also lends itself to drug injection for treating pathology of the knee joint.

Bursitis in Knee Region

Prepatellar bursitis is caused by friction between the skin and the patella; however, the bursa may also be injured by compressive forces resulting from a direct blow or from falling on the flexed knee. If the inflammation is chronic, the bursa becomes distended with fluid and forms a swelling anterior to the knee. This condition has been called "housemaid's knee" (Fig. B5.36); however, other people who work on their knees without knee pads, such as hardwood floor and rug installers, may also develop prepatellar bursitis.

Prepatellar bursitis (arrow)

FIGURE B5.36.

Medial view of dissection of left knee

FIGURE B5.37.

Subcutaneous infrapatellar bursitis is caused by excessive friction between the skin and the tibial tuberosity; the edema occurs over the proximal end of the tibia. This condition was formerly called "clergyman's knee" because of frequent genuflecting (L. *genu,* knee); however, it occurs more commonly in roofers and floor tilers if they do not wear knee pads. *Deep infrapatellar bursitis* results in edema between the patellar ligament and the tibia, superior to the tibial tuberosity. The inflammation is usually caused by overuse and subsequent friction between the patellar tendon and the structures posterior to it, the infrapatellar fat pad and tibia (Anderson et al., 2000). Enlargement of the deep infrapatellar bursa obliterates the dimples normally occurring on each side of the patellar ligament when the leg is extended (see Fig. 5.104A).

Abrasions or penetrating wounds may result in *suprapatellar bursitis,* an infection caused by bacteria entering the suprapatellar bursa from the torn skin (see Fig. 5.94A). The infection may spread to the cavity of the knee joint, causing localized redness and enlarged popliteal and inguinal lymph nodes.

Popliteal Cysts

Popliteal cysts (Baker cysts) are abnormal fluid-filled sacs of synovial membrane in the region of the popliteal fossa. A popliteal cyst is almost always a complication of chronic knee joint effusion. The cyst may be a herniation of the gastrocnemius or semimembranosus bursa through the fibrous layer of the joint capsule into the popliteal fossa, communicating with the synovial cavity of the knee joint by a narrow stalk (Fig. B5.37). Synovial fluid may also escape from the knee joint (*synovial effusion*) or a bursa around the knee and collect in the popliteal fossa. Here it forms a new synovial-lined sac, or popliteal cyst. Popliteal cysts are common in children but seldom cause symptoms. In adults, popliteal cysts can be large, extending as far as the midcalf, and may interfere with knee movements.

Knee Replacement

If a person's knee is diseased, resulting from osteoarthritis, for example, an artificial knee joint may be inserted (*total knee replacement arthroplasty*) (Fig. B5.38). The artificial knee joint consists of plastic and metal components that are cemented to the femoral and tibial bone ends after removal of the defective areas. The combination of metal and plastic mimics the smoothness of cartilage on cartilage and produces good results in "low-demand" people who have a relatively sedentary life. In "high-demand" people who are active in sports, the bone–cement junctions may break down, and the artificial knee components may loosen; however, improvements in bioengineering and surgical technique have provided better results.

FIGURE B5.38.

Ankle Injuries

The ankle is the most frequently injured major joint in the body. *Ankle sprains* (torn fibers of ligaments) are most common. A sprained ankle is nearly always an *inversion injury,* involving twisting of the weight-bearing plantarflexed foot. The person steps on an uneven surface and the foot is forcibly inverted. *Lateral ligament sprains* occur in running and jumping sports, particularly basketball (70–80% of players have had at least one sprained ankle). The lateral ligament is injured because it is much weaker than the medial ligament, and is the ligament that resists inversion at the talocrural joint. The *anterior talofibular ligament*—part of the lateral ligament—is most vulnerable and most commonly torn during ankle sprains, either partially or completely, resulting in instability of the ankle joint (Fig. B5.39). The *calcaneofibular ligament* may also be torn. In severe sprains, the lateral malleolus of the fibula may also be fractured. *Shearing injuries fracture the lateral malleolus* at or superior to the ankle joint. *Avulsion fractures* break the malleolus inferior to the ankle joint; a fragment of bone is pulled off by the attached ligament(s).

A *Pott fracture–dislocation of the ankle* occurs when the foot is forcibly everted (Fig. B5.40). This action pulls on the extremely strong medial ligament, often tearing off the medial malleolus. The talus then moves laterally, shearing off the lateral malleolus or, more commonly, breaking the fibula superior to the tibiofibular syndesmosis. If the tibia is carried anteriorly, the posterior margin of the distal end of the tibia is also sheared off by the talus, producing a "trimalleolar fracture." In applying this term to this injury, the entire distal end of the tibia is erroneously considered to be a "malleolus."

Tibial Nerve Entrapment

The tibial nerve leaves the posterior compartment of the leg by passing deep to the flexor retinaculum in the interval between the medial malleolus and the calcaneus (Fig. 5.71A). Entrapment and compression of the tibial nerve (*tarsal tunnel syndrome*) occurs when there

Torn fibers of anterior talofibular ligament

FIGURE B5.39.

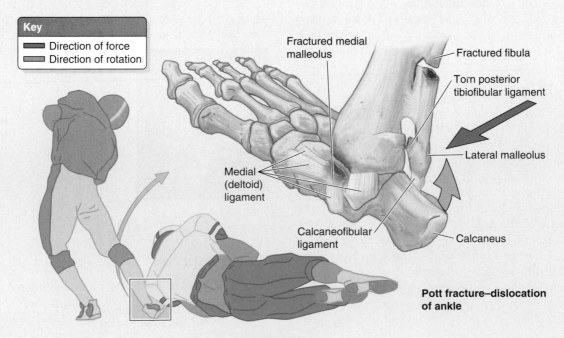

Key
- Direction of force
- Direction of rotation

Fractured medial malleolus

Fractured fibula

Torn posterior tibiofibular ligament

Lateral malleolus

Medial (deltoid) ligament

Calcaneofibular ligament

Calcaneus

Pott fracture–dislocation of ankle

FIGURE B5.40.

is edema and tightness in the ankle involving the synovial sheaths of the tendons of muscles in the posterior compartment of the leg. The area involved is from the medial malleolus to the calcaneus, and the heel pain results from compression of the tibial nerve by the flexor retinaculum.

Hallux Valgus

Hallux valgus is a foot deformity caused by pressure from footwear and degenerative joint disease; it is characterized by lateral deviation of the great toe (Fig. B5.41). The *L* in va*l*gus indicates *lateral deviation.* In some people, the painful deviation is so large that the great toe overlaps the 2nd toe (Fig. B5.41A), and there is a decrease in the medial longitudinal arch. Such deviation occurs especially in females, and its frequency increases with age. These individuals cannot move their 1st digit away from their 2nd digit because the sesamoids under the head of the 1st metatarsal are usually displaced, and lie in the space between the heads of the 1st and 2nd metatarsals (Fig. B5.41B). The 1st metatarsal shifts medially and the sesamoids shift laterally. Often the surrounding tissues swell and the resultant pressure and friction against the shoe cause a subcutaneous bursa to form; when tender and inflamed, the bursa is called a *bunion* (Fig. B5.41A). Often hard *corns* (inflamed areas of thick skin) also form over the proximal interphalangeal joints, especially of the little toe.

Hammer Toe

Hammer toe is a foot deformity in which the proximal phalanx is permanently and markedly dorsiflexed (hyperextended) at the metatarsophalangeal joint, and the middle phalanx strongly plantarflexed at the proximal interphalangeal joint. The distal phalanx of the digit is often also hyperextended. This gives the digit (usually the 2nd) a hammer-like appearance (Fig. B5.42A). This deformity of one or more toes may result from weakness of the lumbrical and interosseous muscles, which flex the metatarsophalangeal joints and extend the interphalangeal joints. A *callosity* or *callus*, hard thickening of the keratin layer of the skin, often develops where the dorsal surface of the toe repeatedly rubs on the shoe.

Claw Toes

Claw toes are characterized by hyperextension of the metatarsophalangeal joints and flexion of the distal interphalangeal joints (Fig. B5.42B). Usually, the lateral four toes are involved. Callosities develop on the dorsal surfaces of the toes because of pressure of the shoe. They may also form on the plantar surfaces of the metatarsal heads and the toe tips because they bear extra weight when claw toes are present.

Pes Planus (Flatfeet)

The flat appearance of the sole of the foot before age 3 is normal; it results from the thick subcutaneous fat pad in the sole. As children get older, the fat is lost, and a normal medial longitudinal arch becomes visible (Fig. B5.42C). Flatfeet can either be *flexible* (flat, lacking a medial arch, when weight-bearing but normal in appearance when not bearing weight [Fig. B5.42D]), or *rigid* (flat even when not bearing weight). The more common *flexible flatfeet* result from loose or degenerated intrinsic ligaments (inadequate passive arch support). Flexible flatfeet is common in childhood but usually resolves with age as the ligaments grow and mature. The condition occasionally persists into adulthood and may or may not be symptomatic.

Rigid flatfeet with a history that goes back to childhood are likely to result from a bone deformity (such as a fusion of adjacent tarsal bones). *Acquired flatfeet* ("fallen arches") are likely to be secondary to dysfunction of the tibialis posterior (dynamic arch support) owing to trauma, degeneration with age, or denervation. In the absence of normal passive or dynamic support, the plantar calcaneonavicular ligament fails to support the head of the talus. Consequently, the head of the talus displaces inferomedially and becomes prominent

(A) Hallux valgus bunion and corns

Bunion
Corns
Hallux valgus

1st metatarsal
Bunion
Hallux valgus
Normal axis of hallux

(B) Displacement of sesamoid bones

FIGURE B5.41.

(A) Hammer toe

(B) Claw toes

Normal footprint

Flatfoot footprint

(C) View of normal arch

(D) View of fallen arch

FIGURE B5.42.

(Fig. B5.42D, red arrows). As a result, some flattening of the medial part of the longitudinal arch occurs, along with lateral deviation of the forefoot. Flatfeet are common in older people, particularly if they undertake much unaccustomed standing or gain weight rapidly, adding stress on the muscles and increasing the strain on the ligaments supporting the arches.

Clubfoot (Talipes equinovarus)

 Clubfoot refers to a foot that is twisted out of position. Of the several types, all are *congenital* (present at birth). *Talipes equinovarus*, the common type

(2 per 1000 neonates), involves the subtalar joint; boys are affected twice as often as girls. The foot is inverted, the ankle is plantarflexed, and the forefoot is adducted (turned toward the midline in an abnormal manner) (Fig. B5.43A). The foot assumes the position of a horse's hoof, hence the prefix "equino" (L. *equinus*, horse). In half of those affected, both feet are malformed. A person with an uncorrected clubfoot cannot put the heel and sole flat and must bear the weight on the lateral surface of the forefoot. Consequently, walking is painful. The main abnormality is shortness and tightness of the muscles, tendons, ligaments, and joint capsules on the medial side and posterior aspect of the foot and ankle (Fig. B5.43B).

Ankle joint (plantarflexed)

Talus (deformed)

Tibionavicular ligament and tendons of extensor digitorum longus, tibialis anterior, and extensor hallucis longus (note tightness)

Calcaneus (inverted)

Bones of forefoot (in extreme varus position)

(A)

(B)

FIGURE B5.43.

The Bottom Line

JOINTS OF LOWER LIMB

Hip joint: The hip joint is the strongest and most stable joint. ♦ Its stability results from (1) the mechanical strength of its ball and (deep) socket construction, allowing extensive articular sur-face contact; (2) its strong joint capsule; and (3) its many surrounding muscles. ♦ However, it remains vulnerable, especially in older age, because of the angle of the femoral neck (inclination) and close association of the blood supply of the femoral head to the neck. Thus fractures result in avascular necrosis of the femoral head. ♦ Major movements of the hip joint include flexion and extension, possible over a wide range; medial and lateral rotation with abduction are part of every step of normal, bipedal walking.

Knee joint: The knee is a hinge joint with a wide range of motion (primarily flexion and extension, with rotation increasingly possible with flexion). ♦ It is our most vulnerable joint, owing to its incongruous articular surfaces and the mechanical disadvantage resulting from bearing the body's weight plus momentum while serving as a fulcrum between two long levers. ♦ Compensation is attempted by several features, including (1) strong intrinsic, extracapsular, and intracapsular ligaments; (2) splinting by many surrounding tendons (including the iliotibial tract); and (3) menisci that fill the spatial void, providing mobile articular surfaces. ♦ Of particular clinical importance are (1) collateral ligaments that are taut during (and limit) extension and are relaxed during flexion, allowing rotation for which they serve as check ligaments; (2) cruciate ligaments that maintain the joint during flexion, providing the pivot for rotation; and (3) the medial meniscus that is attached to the tibial collateral ligament, and is frequently injured because of this attachment.

Tibiofibular joints: The tibiofibular joints include a proximal synovial joint, an interosseous membrane, and a distal tibiofibular syndesmosis, consisting of anterior, interosseous, and posterior tibiofibular ligaments. ♦ Together these joints make up a compensatory system that allows a slight upward movement of the fibula owing to forced transverse expansion of the malleolar mortise (deep square socket) during maximal dorsiflexion of the ankle. ♦ All fibrous tibiofibular connections run downward from tibia to fibula, allowing this slight upward movement while strongly resisting the downward pull applied to the fibula by the contraction of eight of the nine muscles attached to it.

Ankle joint: The ankle (talocrural) joint is composed of a superior mortise, formed by the weight-bearing inferior surface of the tibia and the two malleoli, which receive the trochlea of the talus. ♦ The ankle joint is maintained medially by a strong, medial (deltoid) ligament, and a much weaker lateral ligament. ♦ The lateral ligament (specifically its anterior talofibular ligament component) is the most frequently injured ligament of the body. ♦ Injury occurs primarily by inadvertent inversion of the plantarflexed, weight-bearing foot. ♦ About 70° of dorsiflexion and plantarflexion is possible at the ankle joint, in addition to which small amounts of wobble occur in the less stable plantarflexed position.

Joints of foot: Functionally, there are three compound joints in the foot: (1) the clinical subtalar joint between the talus and the calcaneus, where inversion and eversion occur about an oblique axis; (2) the transverse tarsal joint, where the midfoot and forefoot rotate as a unit on the hindfoot around a longitudinal axis, augmenting inversion and eversion; and (3) the remaining joints of the foot, which allow the pedal platform (foot) to form dynamic longitudinal and transverse arches. ♦ The arches provide the resilience necessary for walking, running, and jumping, and are maintained by four layers of passive, fibrous support, plus the dynamic support provided by the intrinsic muscles of the foot, and the long fibular, tibial, and flexor tendons.

the**Point**   **Board-review questions, case studies, and additional resources are available at thePoint.lww.com.**

6 Upper Limb

OVERVIEW OF UPPER LIMB

The upper limb is characterized by its mobility and ability to grasp, strike, and conduct fine motor skills (*manipulation*). These characteristics are especially marked in the hand when performing manual activities, such as buttoning a shirt.

Synchronized interplay occurs between the joints of the upper limb to coordinate the intervening segments to perform smooth, efficient motion at the most workable distance or position required for a specific task. Efficiency of hand function results in large part from the ability to place it in the proper position by movements at the scapulothoracic, glenohumeral, elbow, radio-ulnar, and wrist joints.

The upper limb consists of four major segments, which are further subdivided into regions for precise description (Figs. 6.1 and 6.2):

1. **Shoulder:** proximal segment of the limb that overlaps parts of the trunk (thorax and back) and lower lateral neck.

It includes the **pectoral, scapular,** and **deltoid regions** of the upper limb, and the lateral part (greater supraclavicular fossa) of the lateral cervical region. It overlies half of the pectoral girdle. The **pectoral girdle (shoulder girdle)** is a bony ring, incomplete posteriorly, formed by the *scapulae* and *clavicles,* and completed anteriorly by the *manubrium of the sternum* (part of the axial skeleton).

2. **Arm** (L. *brachium*): first segment of the free upper limb (more mobile part of the upper limb independent of the trunk) and the longest segment of the limb. It extends between and connects the shoulder and the elbow, and consists of **anterior** and **posterior regions of the arm,** centered around the humerus.

3. **Forearm** (L. *antebrachium*): second longest segment of the limb. It extends between and connects the elbow and wrist and includes **anterior** and **posterior regions of the forearm** overlying the radius and ulna.

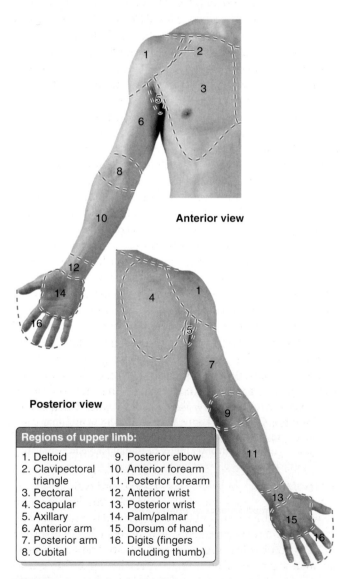

FIGURE 6.1. Segments and bones of upper limb. The joints divide the superior appendicular skeleton, and thus the limb itself, into four main segments: shoulder, arm, forearm, and hand.

Labels for Figure 6.1:
- ½ Pectoral girdle
- Clavicle
- Acromioclavicular joint
- Glenohumeral (shoulder) joint
- Scapula
- Humerus
- Arm
- Elbow joint
- Radius
- Ulna
- Forearm
- Proximal radio-ulnar joint
- Distal radio-ulnar joint
- Wrist (radio-carpal) joint
- Midcarpal joint
- Hand
- Carpus
- Metacarpus
- Phalanges
- Carpo-metacarpal joint
- Metacarpo-phalangeal joints
- Interphalangeal joints
- Anterior view

FIGURE 6.2. Regions of upper limb. For exact description, the upper limb is divided into regions based on the external features (surface anatomy) of the underlying muscular formations, bones, and joints.

Anterior view
Posterior view

Regions of upper limb:
1. Deltoid
2. Clavipectoral triangle
3. Pectoral
4. Scapular
5. Axillary
6. Anterior arm
7. Posterior arm
8. Cubital
9. Posterior elbow
10. Anterior forearm
11. Posterior forearm
12. Anterior wrist
13. Posterior wrist
14. Palm/palmar
15. Dorsum of hand
16. Digits (fingers including thumb)

4. **Hand** (L. *manus*): part of the upper limb distal to the forearm that is formed around the carpus, metacarpus, and phalanges. It is composed of the **wrist, palm, dorsum of hand,** and **digits** (fingers, including an opposable thumb), and is richly supplied with sensory endings for touch, pain, and temperature.

COMPARISON OF UPPER AND LOWER LIMBS

Developing in a similar fashion, the upper and lower limbs share many common features (see Chapter 5). However, they are sufficiently distinct in structure to enable markedly different functions and abilities. Because the upper limb is not usually involved in weight bearing or motility, its stability has been sacrificed to gain mobility. The upper limb still possesses remarkable strength; and because of the hand's ability to conform to a paddle or assume a gripping or platform configuration, it may assume a role in motility in certain circumstances.

Both the upper and the lower limbs are connected to the **axial skeleton** (cranium, vertebral column, and associated thoracic cage) via the bony pectoral and pelvic girdles, respectively. The *pelvic girdle* consists of the two hip bones connected to the sacrum (see Chapter 5). The *pectoral girdle* consists of the scapulae and clavicles, connected to the manubrium of the sternum. Both girdles possess a large flat bone located posteriorly, which provides for attachment of proximal muscles, and connects with its contralateral partner anteriorly via small bony braces, the pubic rami and clavicles. However, the flat iliac bones of the pelvic girdle are also connected posteriorly through their primary attachment to the sacrum via the essentially rigid, weight-transferring sacro-iliac joints. This posterior connection to the axial skeleton places the lower limbs inferior to the trunk, enabling them to be supportive as they function primarily in relation to the line of gravity. Furthermore, because the two sides are connected both anteriorly and posteriorly, the pelvic girdle forms a complete rigid ring that limits mobility, making the movements of one limb markedly affect the movements of the other. The pectoral girdle, however, is connected to the trunk only anteriorly, via the sternum, by flexible joints with 3 degrees of freedom. It is an incomplete ring because the scapulae are not connected with each other posteriorly. Thus, the motion of one upper limb is independent of the other, and the limbs are able to operate effectively anterior to the body, at a distance and level that enable precise eye–hand coordination.

In both the upper and the lower limbs, the long bone of the most proximal segment is the largest and is unpaired. The long bones increase progressively in number but decrease in size in the more distal segments of the limb. The second most proximal segment of both limbs (i.e., the leg and forearm) has two parallel bones, although only in the forearm do both articulate with the bone of the proximal segment, and only in the leg do both articulate directly with the distal segment.

Although the paired bones of both the leg and forearm flex and extend as a unit, only those of the upper limb are able to move (supinate and pronate) relative to each other; the bones of the leg are fixed in the pronated position.

The wrist and ankle have a similar number of short bones (eight and seven, respectively). Both groups of short bones interrupt a series of long bones that resumes distally with several sets of long bones of similar lengths, with a similar number of joints of essentially the same type. The digits of the upper limb (fingers including the thumb) are the most mobile parts of either limb. However, all other parts of the upper limb are more mobile than the comparable parts of the lower limb.

BONES OF UPPER LIMB

The pectoral girdle and bones of the free part of the upper limb form the **superior appendicular skeleton** (Fig. 6.3); the pelvic girdle and bones of the free part of the lower limb form the **inferior appendicular skeleton.** The superior appendicular skeleton articulates with the axial skeleton only at the *sternoclavicular joint*, allowing great mobility. The clavicles and scapulae of the pectoral girdle are supported, stabilized, and moved by **axio-appendicular muscles** that attach to the relatively fixed ribs, sternum, and vertebrae of the *axial skeleton*.

Clavicle

The **clavicle** (collar bone) connects the upper limb to the trunk (Figs. 6.3 and 6.4). The **shaft of the clavicle** has a double curve in a horizontal plane. Its medial half is convex anteriorly, and its **sternal end** is enlarged and triangular where it articulates with the *manubrium of the sternum* at the *sternoclavicular* (SC) *joint*. Its lateral half is concave anteriorly, and its **acromial end** is flat where it articulates with the **acromion** of the scapula at the *acromioclavicular* (AC) *joint* (Figs. 6.3B and 6.4). The medial two thirds of the shaft of the clavicle are convex anteriorly, whereas the lateral third is flattened and concave anteriorly. These curvatures increase the resilience of the clavicle, and give it the appearance of an elongated capital *S*.

The clavicle:

• Serves as a moveable, crane-like strut (rigid support) from which the scapula and free limb are suspended, keeping them away from the trunk so that the limb has maximum freedom of motion. The strut is movable and allows the scapula to move on the thoracic wall at the "*scapulothoracic joint*,"[1] increasing the range of motion of the limb.

---

[1]The **scapulothoracic joint** is a physiological "joint," in which movement occurs between musculoskeletal structures (between the scapula and associated muscles and the thoracic wall), rather than an anatomical joint, in which movement occurs between directly articulating skeletal elements. The scapulothoracic joint is where the scapular movements of elevation–depression, protraction–retraction, and rotation occur.

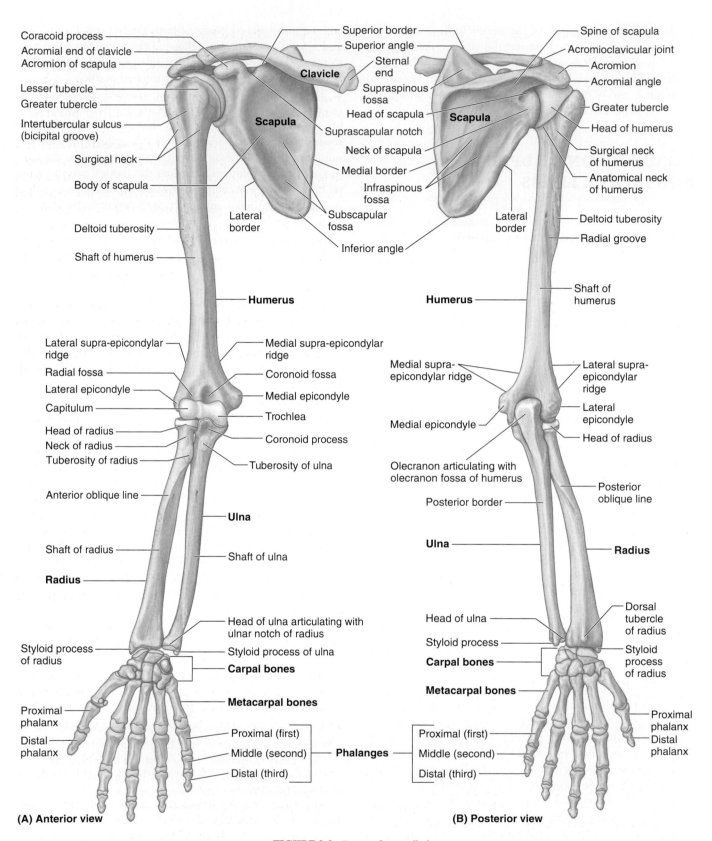

Coracoid process
Acromial end of clavicle
Acromion of scapula
Lesser tubercle
Greater tubercle
Intertubercular sulcus (bicipital groove)
Surgical neck
Body of scapula
Deltoid tuberosity
Shaft of humerus
Humerus
Lateral supra-epicondylar ridge
Radial fossa
Lateral epicondyle
Capitulum
Head of radius
Neck of radius
Tuberosity of radius
Anterior oblique line
Shaft of radius
Radius
Styloid process of radius
Proximal phalanx
Distal phalanx

Superior border
Superior angle
Sternal end
Clavicle
Supraspinous fossa
Head of scapula
Scapula
Suprascapular notch
Neck of scapula
Medial border
Infraspinous fossa
Subscapular fossa
Inferior angle
Lateral border
Medial supra-epicondylar ridge
Coronoid fossa
Medial epicondyle
Trochlea
Coronoid process
Tuberosity of ulna
Ulna
Shaft of ulna
Head of ulna articulating with ulnar notch of radius
Styloid process of ulna
Carpal bones
Metacarpal bones
Proximal (first)
Middle (second)
Distal (third)
Phalanges

(A) Anterior view

Spine of scapula
Acromioclavicular joint
Acromion
Acromial angle
Greater tubercle
Head of humerus
Surgical neck of humerus
Anatomical neck of humerus
Deltoid tuberosity
Radial groove
Shaft of humerus
Humerus
Medial supra-epicondylar ridge
Medial epicondyle
Olecranon articulating with olecranon fossa of humerus
Posterior border
Ulna
Head of ulna
Styloid process
Carpal bones
Metacarpal bones
Proximal (first)
Middle (second)
Distal (third)

Scapula
Lateral border
Lateral supra-epicondylar ridge
Lateral epicondyle
Head of radius
Posterior oblique line
Radius
Dorsal tubercle of radius
Styloid process of radius
Proximal phalanx
Distal phalanx

(B) Posterior view

FIGURE 6.3. Bones of upper limb.

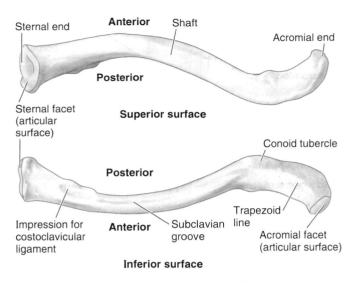

FIGURE 6.4. Right clavicle. Prominent features of the superior and inferior surfaces of the clavicle. The bone acts as a mobile strut (supporting brace) connecting the upper limb to the trunk; its length allows the limb to pivot around the trunk.

Fixing the strut in position, especially after its elevation, enables elevation of the ribs for deep inspiration.

- Forms one of the bony boundaries of the *cervico-axillary canal* (passageway between the neck and arm), affording protection to the neurovascular bundle supplying the upper limb.
- Transmits shocks (traumatic impacts) from the upper limb to the axial skeleton.

Although designated as a long bone, the clavicle has no medullary (marrow) cavity. It consists of spongy (trabecular) bone with a shell of compact bone.

The **superior surface of the clavicle,** lying just deep to the skin and platysma (G. flat plate) muscle in the subcutaneous tissue, is smooth.

The **inferior surface of the clavicle** is rough because strong ligaments bind it to the 1st rib near its sternal end and suspend the scapula from its acromial end. The **conoid tubercle,** near the acromial end of the clavicle (Fig. 6.4), gives attachment to the *conoid ligament,* the medial part of the *coracoclavicular ligament* by which the remainder of the upper limb is passively suspended from the clavicle. Also, near the acromial end of the clavicle is the **trapezoid line,** to which the *trapezoid ligament* attaches; it is the lateral part of the coracoclavicular ligament.

The **subclavian groove** (groove for the subclavius) in the medial third of the shaft of the clavicle is the site of attachment of the subclavius muscle. More medially is the **impression for the costoclavicular ligament,** a rough, often depressed, oval area that gives attachment to the ligament binding the 1st rib (L. *costa*) to the clavicle, limiting elevation of the shoulder.

Scapula

The **scapula** (shoulder blade) is a triangular flat bone that lies on the posterolateral aspect of the thorax, overlying the 2nd–7th ribs (see Fig. I.11, p. 20). The convex **posterior surface** of the scapula is unevenly divided by a thick projecting ridge of bone, the **spine of the scapula,** into a small **supraspinous fossa** and a much larger **infraspinous fossa** (Fig. 6.5A). The concave **costal surface** of most of the scapula forms a large **subscapular fossa.** The broad bony surfaces of the three fossae provide attachments for fleshy muscles. The triangular **body of the scapula** is thin and translucent superior and inferior to the spine of the scapula; although its borders, especially the lateral one, are somewhat thicker. The spine continues laterally as the flat, expanded **acromion** (G. *akros,* point), which forms the subcutaneous point of the shoulder and articulates with the acromial end of the clavicle. The **deltoid tubercle** of the scapular spine is the prominence indicating the medial point of attachment of the deltoid. The spine and acromion serve as levers for the attached muscles, particularly the trapezius.

Because the acromion is a lateral extension of the scapula, the AC joint is placed lateral to the mass of the scapula and its attached muscles (Fig. 6.5C). The *glenohumeral* (shoulder) *joint* on which these muscles operate is almost directly inferior to the AC joint; thus the scapular mass is balanced with that of the free limb, and the suspending structure (coracoclavicular ligament) lies between the two masses.

Superolaterally, the lateral surface of the scapula has a **glenoid cavity** (G. socket), which receives and articulates with the head of the humerus at the glenohumeral joint (Fig. 6.5A & C). The glenoid cavity is a shallow, concave, oval fossa (L. *fossa ovalis*), directed anterolaterally and slightly superiorly—that is considerably smaller than the ball (head of the humerus) for which it serves as a socket. The beak-like **coracoid process** (G. *korak-odés,* like a crow's beak) is superior to the glenoid cavity, and projects anterolaterally. This process also resembles in size, shape, and direction a bent finger pointing to the shoulder, the knuckle of which provides the inferior attachment for the passively supporting coracoclavicular ligament.

The scapula has medial, lateral, and superior borders and superior, lateral, and inferior angles (Fig. 6.5B). When the scapular body is in the anatomical position, the thin **medial border of the scapula** runs parallel to and approximately 5 cm lateral to the spinous processes of the thoracic vertebrae; hence it is often called the *vertebral border* (Fig. 6.5B). From the inferior angle, the **lateral border of the scapula** runs superolaterally toward the apex of the axilla; hence it is often called the *axillary border.* The lateral border is made up of a thick bar of bone that prevents buckling of this stress-bearing region of the scapula.

The lateral border terminates in the truncated **lateral angle of the scapula,** the thickest part of the bone that bears the broadened **head of the scapula** (Fig. 6.5A & B). The glenoid cavity is the primary feature of the head. The shallow constriction between the head and body defines the **neck** of the scapula. The **superior border of the scapula** is marked near the junction of its medial two thirds and lateral third by the **suprascapular notch,** which is located where the superior border joins the base of the coracoid process.

These small bones give flexibility to the wrist. The carpus is markedly convex from side to side posteriorly, and concave anteriorly. Augmenting movement at the wrist joint, the two rows of carpal bones glide on each other; in addition, each bone glides on those adjacent to it.

From lateral to medial, the four carpal bones in the proximal row (purple in Fig. 6.9A & B) are the:

- **Scaphoid** (G. *skaphé*, skiff, boat): a boat-shaped bone that articulates proximally with the radius, and has a prominent **scaphoid tubercle;** it is the largest bone in the proximal row of carpals.
- **Lunate** (L. *luna*, moon): a moon-shaped bone between the scaphoid and the triquetral bones; it articulates proximally with the radius and is broader anteriorly than posteriorly.
- **Triquetrum** (L. *triquetrus*, three-cornered): a pyramidal bone on the medial side of the carpus; it articulates proximally with the articular disc of the distal radio-ulnar joint.
- **Pisiform** (L. *pisum*, pea), a small, pea-shaped bone that lies on the palmar surface of the triquetrum.

From lateral to medial, the four carpal bones in the distal row (green in Fig. 6.9A & B) are the:

- **Trapezium** (G. *trapeze*, table): a four-sided bone on the lateral side of the carpus; it articulates with the 1st and 2nd metacarpals, scaphoid, and trapezoid bones.
- **Trapezoid:** a wedge-shaped bone that resembles the trapezium; it articulates with the 2nd metacarpal, trapezium, capitate, and scaphoid bones.
- **Capitate** (L. *caput*, head): a head-shaped bone with a rounded extremity is the largest bone in the carpus; it articulates primarily with the 3rd metacarpal distally, and with the trapezoid, scaphoid, lunate, and hamate.
- **Hamate** (L. *hamulus*, a little hook): a wedge-shaped bone on the medial side of the hand; it articulates with the 4th and 5th metacarpal, capitate, and triquetral bones; it has a distinctive hooked process, the **hook of the hamate,** that extends anteriorly.

The proximal surfaces of the distal row of carpal bones articulate with the proximal row of carpal bones, and their distal surfaces articulate with the metacarpals.

The **metacarpus** forms the skeleton of the palm of the hand between the carpus and the phalanges. It is composed of five **metacarpal bones** (metacarpals). Each metacarpal consists of a base, shaft, and head. The proximal **bases of the metacarpals** articulate with the carpal bones, and the distal **heads of the metacarpals** articulate with the proximal phalanges, and form the knuckles of the hand. The 1st metacarpal (of the thumb) is the thickest and shortest of these bones. The 3rd metacarpal is distinguished by a **styloid process** on the lateral side of its base (Fig. 6.10).

Each digit (finger) has three **phalanges** except for the first (the thumb), which has only two; however, the phalanges of the first digit are stouter than those in the other fingers. Each phalanx has a **base** proximally, a **shaft** (body), and a **head** distally (Fig. 6.9). The proximal phalanges are the largest, the middle ones are intermediate in size, and the distal ones are the smallest. The shafts of the phalanges taper distally. The terminal phalanges are flattened and expanded at their distal ends, which underlie the nail beds.

OSSIFICATION OF BONES OF HAND

Radiographs of the wrist and hand are commonly used to assess skeletal age. For clinical studies, the radiographs are compared with a series of standards in a radiographic atlas of skeletal development to determine the skeletal age. Ossification centers are usually obvious during the 1st year; however, they may appear before birth. Each carpal bone usually ossifies from one center postnatally (Fig. 6.9D). The centers for the capitate and hamate appear first.

The shaft of each metacarpal begins to ossify during fetal life, and ossification centers appear postnatally in the heads of the four medial metacarpals and in the base of the 1st metacarpal. By age 11, ossification centers of all carpal bones are visible (Fig. 6.9E).

Surface Anatomy of Upper Limb Bones

Most bones of the upper limb offer a palpable segment or surface (notable exceptions being the lunate and trapezoid), enabling the skilled examiner to discern abnormalities owing to trauma (fracture or dislocation) or malformation (Fig. 6.10).

The *clavicle* is subcutaneous and can be easily palpated throughout its length. Its sternal end projects superior to the manubrium (Fig. 6.10). Between the elevated sternal ends of the clavicles is the **jugular notch** (suprasternal notch). The acromial end of the clavicle often rises higher than the acromion, forming a palpable elevation at the *acromioclavicular (AC) joint*. The acromial end can be palpated 2–3 cm medial to the lateral border of the acromion, particularly when the arm is alternately flexed and extended. Either or both ends of the clavicle may be prominent; when present, this condition is usually bilateral.

Note the elasticity of the skin over the clavicle and how easily it can be pinched into a mobile fold. This property of the skin is useful when ligating (tying a knot around) the third part of the subclavian artery: The skin lying superior to the clavicle is pulled down onto the clavicle and then incised; after the incision is made, the skin is allowed to return to its position superior to the clavicle, where it overlies the artery (thus not endangering it during the incision).

As the clavicle passes laterally, its medial part can be felt to be convex anteriorly. The large vessels and nerves to the upper limb pass posterior to this convexity. The flattened acromial end of the clavicle does not reach the point of the shoulder, formed by the lateral tip of the acromion of the scapula.

The *acromion* of the scapula is easily felt and often visible, especially when the deltoid contracts against resistance. The superior surface of the acromion is subcutaneous and may be traced medially to the AC joint. The lateral and posterior borders of the acromion meet to form the **acromial**

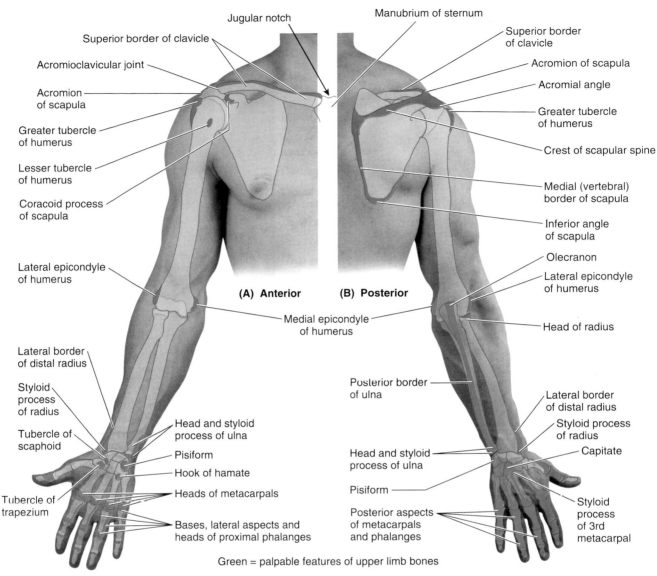

Jugular notch

Superior border of clavicle

Acromioclavicular joint

Acromion of scapula

Greater tubercle of humerus

Lesser tubercle of humerus

Coracoid process of scapula

Lateral epicondyle of humerus

Lateral border of distal radius

Styloid process of radius

Tubercle of scaphoid

Tubercle of trapezium

Manubrium of sternum

Superior border of clavicle

Acromion of scapula

Acromial angle

Greater tubercle of humerus

Crest of scapular spine

Medial (vertebral) border of scapula

Inferior angle of scapula

Olecranon

Lateral epicondyle of humerus

Head of radius

Posterior border of ulna

Lateral border of distal radius

Styloid process of radius

Capitate

Head and styloid process of ulna

Pisiform

Styloid process of 3rd metacarpal

Posterior aspects of metacarpals and phalanges

(A) Anterior   **(B) Posterior**

Medial epicondyle of humerus

Head and styloid process of ulna

Pisiform

Hook of hamate

Heads of metacarpals

Bases, lateral aspects and heads of proximal phalanges

Green = palpable features of upper limb bones

FIGURE 6.10. Surface anatomy of bones of upper limb.

angle (Fig. 6.10B). The humerus in the glenoid cavity and the *deltoid muscle* form the rounded curve of the shoulder. The **crest of the scapular spine** is subcutaneous throughout and easily palpated.

When the upper limb is in the anatomical position, the:

- *Superior angle of the scapula* lies at the level of the T2 vertebra.
- Medial end of the root of the scapular spine is opposite the spinous process of the T3 vertebra.
- *Inferior angle of the scapula* lies at the level of T7 vertebra, near the inferior border of the 7th rib and 7th intercostal space.

The *medial border of the scapula* is palpable inferior to the root of the spine of the scapula as it crosses the 3rd–7th ribs. The lateral border of the scapula is not easily palpated because it is covered by the teres major and minor muscles. When the upper limb is abducted and the hand is placed on

the back of the head, the scapula is rotated, elevating the glenoid cavity such that the medial border of the scapula parallels the 6th rib and thus can be used to estimate its position and, deep to the rib, the oblique fissure of the lung. The inferior angle of the scapula is easily felt and is often visible. It is grasped when testing movements of the glenohumeral joint to immobilize the scapula. The *coracoid process of the scapula* can be felt by palpating deeply at the lateral side of the *clavipectoral (deltopectoral) triangle* (Fig. 6.11).

The *head of the humerus* is surrounded by muscles, except inferiorly; consequently, it can be palpated only by pushing the fingers well up into the *axillary fossa* (armpit). The arm should not be fully abducted, otherwise the fascia in the axilla will be tense and impede palpation of the humeral head. When the arm is moved and the scapula is fixed (held in place), the head of the humerus can be palpated.

The *greater tubercle of the humerus* may be felt with the person's arm by the side on deep palpation through the deltoid,

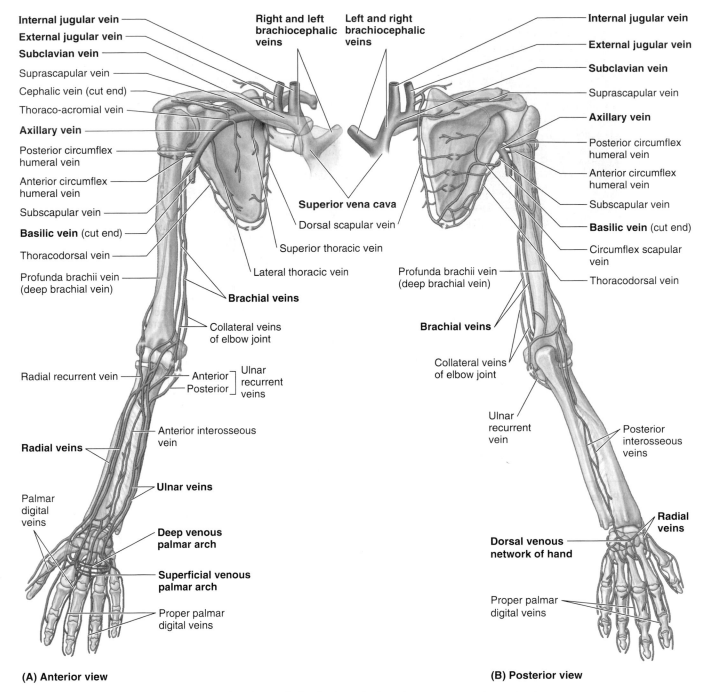

FIGURE 6.16. **Deep veins of upper limb.** The deep veins bear the same name as the arteries they accompany.

proximal to the medial epicondyle and medial to the basilic vein. Efferent vessels from these lymph nodes ascend in the arm and terminate in the **humeral** (**lateral**) **axillary lymph nodes** (see Chapter 1).

Most superficial lymphatic vessels accompanying the cephalic vein cross the proximal part of the arm and the anterior aspect of the shoulder to enter the **apical axillary lymph nodes;** however, some vessels previously enter the more superficial **deltopectoral lymph nodes.**

Deep lymphatic vessels, less numerous than superficial vessels, accompany the major deep veins in the upper limb (radial, ulnar, and brachial--Fig. 6.16) and terminate in the humeral axillary lymph nodes. They drain lymph from the joint capsules, periosteum, tendons, nerves, and muscles and ascend with the deep veins; a few deep lymph nodes may occur along their course. The axillary lymph nodes are drained by the *subclavian lymphatic trunk;* both are discussed in greater detail with the axilla, later in this chapter.

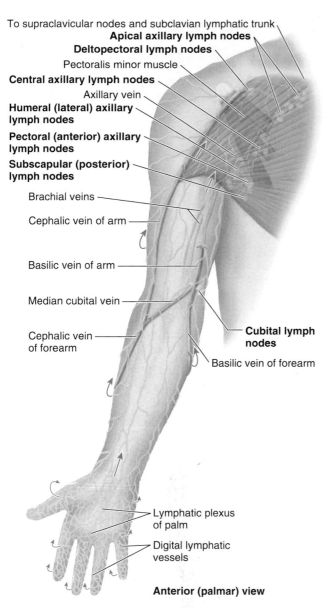

To supraclavicular nodes and subclavian lymphatic trunk
Apical axillary lymph nodes
Deltopectoral lymph nodes
Pectoralis minor muscle
Central axillary lymph nodes
Axillary vein
Humeral (lateral) axillary lymph nodes
Pectoral (anterior) axillary lymph nodes
Subscapular (posterior) lymph nodes
Brachial veins
Cephalic vein of arm
Basilic vein of arm
Median cubital vein
Cephalic vein of forearm
Cubital lymph nodes
Basilic vein of forearm
Lymphatic plexus of palm
Digital lymphatic vessels
Anterior (palmar) view

FIGURE 6.17. Lymphatic drainage of upper limb. Superficial lymphatic vessels originate from the digital lymphatic vessels of the digits and lymphatic plexus of the palm. Most drainage from the palm passes to the dorsum of the hand (*small arrows*).

Cutaneous Innervation of Upper Limb

The cutaneous nerves of the upper limb follow a general pattern that is easy to understand if it is noted that developmentally the limbs grow as lateral protrusions of the trunk, with the 1st digit (thumb or great toe) located on the cranial side (thumb is directed superiorly). Thus the lateral aspect of the upper limb is innervated by more cranial spinal cord segments or nerves than the medial aspect.

There are two *dermatome maps* in common use. One has gained popular acceptance because of its more intuitive aesthetic qualities, corresponding to concepts of limb development (Keegan and Garrett, 1948); the other is based on clinical findings and is generally preferred by neurologists (Foerster, 1933). Both maps are approximations, delineating dermatomes as distinct zones when actually there is much overlap between adjacent dermatomes and much variation (even from side to side in the same individual). In both schemes, observe the progression of the segmental innervation of the various cutaneous areas around the limb when it is placed in its "initial embryonic position" (abducted with thumb directed superiorly) (Fig. 6.18; Table 6.1).

Most cutaneous nerves of the upper limb are derived from the *brachial plexus*, a major nerve network formed by the anterior rami of the C5–T1 spinal nerves (see "Brachial Plexus" on p. 721). The nerves to the shoulder, however, are derived from the *cervical plexus*, a nerve network consisting of a series of nerve loops formed between adjacent anterior rami of the first four cervical nerves. The cervical plexus lies deep to the sternocleidomastoid muscle on the anterolateral aspect of the neck.

The cutaneous nerves of the arm and forearm[3] are illustrated in Figure 6.19, and their contributing spinal nerves, source, and course and distribution are provided in Table 6.2

Note that there are lateral, medial, and posterior (but no anterior) cutaneous nerves of the arm and forearm; as discussed later in this chapter, this pattern corresponds to that of the cords of the brachial plexus.

Motor Innervation (Myotomes) of Upper Limb

Somatic motor (general somatic efferent) fibers traveling in the same mixed peripheral nerves that convey sensory fibers to the cutaneous nerves transmit impulses to the voluntary muscles of the upper limb. The unilateral embryological muscle mass (and derived muscle) receiving innervation from a single spinal cord segment or spinal nerve constitutes a *myotome*. Upper limb muscles usually receive motor fibers from several spinal cord segments or nerves. Thus most muscles are made up of more than one myotome, and multiple spinal cord segments are usually involved in producing the movement of the upper limb (Fig. 6.20). The intrinsic muscles of the hand constitute a single myotome (T1).

(text continues on p. 697)

[3]The preferred English-equivalent terms listed by *Terminologia Anatomica* (*TA*) are used here. Official alternate *TA* terms replace *of the arm* with *brachial*, and *of the forearm* with *antebrachial*.

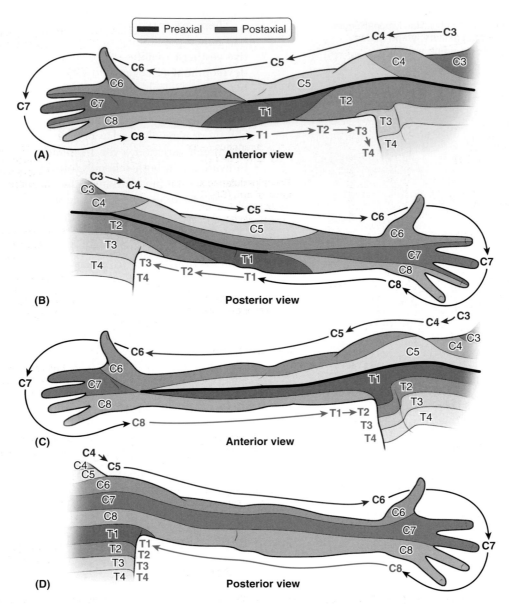

FIGURE 6.18. Segmental (dermatomal) and peripheral (cutaneous nerve) innervation of upper limb. A and B. The pattern of segmental (dermatomal) innervation of the upper limb proposed by Foerster (1933) depicts innervation of the medial aspect of the limb by upper thoracic (T1–T3) spinal cord segments, consistent with the experience of heart pain (angina pectoris) referred to that area. **C and D.** The pattern of segmental innervation proposed by Keegan and Garrett (1948) has gained popular acceptance, perhaps because of the regular progression of its stripes and correlation with developmental concepts. In both patterns, the dermatomes progress sequentially around the periphery of the outstretched limb (with the thumb directed superiorly), providing a way to approximate the segmental innervation.

TABLE 6.1. DERMATOMES OF UPPER LIMB

Spinal Segment/Nerve(s)	Description of Dermatome(s)
C3, C4	Region at base of neck, extending laterally over shoulder
C5	Lateral aspect of arm (i.e., superior aspect of abducted arm)
C6	Lateral forearm and thumb
C7	Middle and ring fingers (or middle three fingers) and center of posterior aspect of forearm
C8	Little finger, medial side of hand and forearm (i.e., inferior aspect of abducted arm)
T1	Medial aspect of forearm and inferior arm
T2	Medial aspect of superior arm and skin of axilla[a]

[a]Not indicated on the Keegan and Garrett (1948) dermatome map. However, pain experienced during a heart attack, considered to be mediated by T1 and T2, is commonly described as "radiating down the medial side of the left arm."

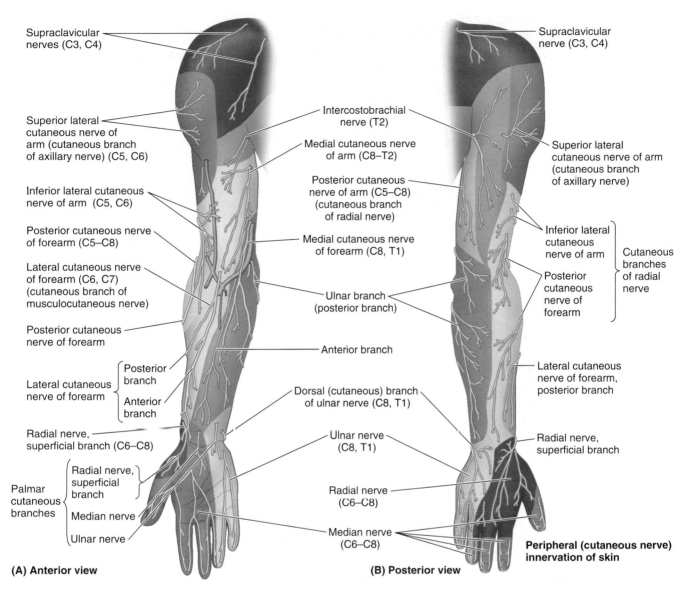

FIGURE 6.19. Distribution of peripheral (named) cutaneous nerves in upper limb. Most of the nerves are branches of nerve plexuses and, therefore, contain fibers from more than one spinal nerve or spinal cord segment.

TABLE 6.2. CUTANEOUS NERVES OF UPPER LIMB

Cutaneous Nerve	Contributing Spinal Nerves	Source	Course and Distribution
Supraclavicular nerves	C3, C4	Cervical plexus	Pass anterior to clavicle, immediately deep to platysma, and supply skin over clavicle and supero-lateral aspect of pectoralis major
Superior lateral cutaneous nerve of arm	C5, C6	Terminal branch of axillary nerve	Emerges from beneath posterior margin of deltoid and supplies skin over lower part of this muscle and on lateral side of midarm
Inferior lateral cutaneous nerve of arm	C5, C6	Radial nerve (or posterior cutaneous nerve of arm)	Perforates lateral head of triceps, passing close to cephalic vein to supply skin over inferolateral aspect of arm
Posterior cutaneous nerve of arm	C5–C8	Radial nerve (in axilla)	Crosses posterior to and communicates with intercostobrachial nerve and supplies skin on posterior arm as far as olecranon

TABLE 6.2. CUTANEOUS NERVES OF UPPER LIMB (Continued)

Cutaneous Nerve	Contributing Spinal Nerves	Source	Course and Distribution
Posterior cutaneous nerve of forearm	C5–C8	Radial nerve (with inferior lateral cutaneous nerve of arm)	Perforates lateral head of triceps, descends laterally in arm, then runs along and supplies posterior forearm to wrist.
Lateral cutaneous nerve of forearm	C6–C7	Musculocutaneous nerve (terminal branch)	Emerges lateral to biceps tendon deep to cephalic vein, supplying skin of anterolateral forearm to wrist
Medial cutaneous nerve of forearm	C8, T1	Medial cord of brachial plexus (in axilla)	Descends medial to brachial artery, pierces deep fascia with basilic vein in midarm, dividing into anterior and posterior branches that enter forearm and supply skin of anteromedial aspect to wrist
Medial cutaneous nerve of arm	C8–T2	Medial cord of brachial plexus (in axilla)	Communicates with intercostobrachial nerve, continuing to supply skin of medial aspect of distal arm
Intercostobrachial nerve	T2	Second intercostal nerve (as its lateral cutaneous branch)	Extends laterally, communicating with posterior and medial cutaneous nerves of arm, supplying skin of axilla and medial aspect of proximal arm

FIGURE 6.20. Segmental innervation of movements of the upper limb. A–F. Most movements involve portions of multiple myotomes; however, the intrinsic muscles of the hand involve a single myotome (T1).

The Bottom Line

FASCIA, EFFERENT VESSELS, CUTANEOUS INNERVATION, AND MYOTOMES OF UPPER LIMB

Fascia: The firm deep fascia of the upper limb surrounds and contains the structures of the upper limb as an expansion-limiting membrane deep to the skin and subcutaneous tissue. ♦ The deep surface of the fascia, which occasionally serves to extend the surface area available for muscular origin, is attached directly or via intermuscular septa to the enclosed bones. ♦ The deep fascia thus forms fascial compartments containing individual muscles or muscle groups of similar function and innervation. ♦ The compartments also contain or direct the spread of infection or hemorrhage.

Superficial veins: The cephalic vein courses along the cranial (cephalic) margin of the limb, while the basilic vein courses along the caudal (basic) margin of the limb. ♦ Both veins come from the dorsal venous network on the dorsum of the hand, and terminate by draining into the beginning (basilic vein) and end (cephalic vein) of the axillary vein.

Deep veins: Deep veins in the limbs usually take the form of paired accompanying veins, bearing the same name as the artery they accompany.

Lymphatic vessels: The superficial lymphatic vessels generally converge on and follow the superficial veins, and the deep lymphatics follow the deep veins. ♦ The lymph collected from the upper limb by both superficial and deep lymphatics drains into the axillary lymph nodes.

Dermatomes: As a consequence of plexus formation, two patterns of cutaneous innervation occur in the upper limb: (1) segmental innervation (dermatomes) by spinal nerves and (2) innervation by multisegmental peripheral (named) nerves. The former pattern is easiest to visualize if the limb is placed in its initial embryonic position (abducted with the thumb directed superiorly). ♦ The segments then progress in descending order around the limb (starting with C4 dermatome at the root of the neck, proceeding laterally or distally along the superior surface and then medially or proximally along the inferior surface, as the T2 dermatome continues onto the thoracic wall).

Cutaneous innervation: Like the brachial plexus, which forms posterior, lateral, and medial (but no anterior) cords, the arm and forearm have posterior, lateral, and medial (but no anterior) cutaneous nerves. ♦ The medial cutaneous nerves are branches of the medial cord of the brachial plexus. ♦ The posterior cutaneous nerves are branches of the radial nerve. ♦ Each of the lateral cutaneous nerves arise from a separate source (axillary, radial, and musculocutaneous nerves).

Myotomes: Most upper limb muscles include components of more than one myotome and thus receive motor fibers from several spinal cord segments or spinal nerves. ♦ Thus multiple spinal cord segments are involved in producing the movements of the upper limb. ♦ The intrinsic muscles of the hand constitute a single myotome (T1).

PECTORAL AND SCAPULAR REGIONS

Anterior Axio-appendicular Muscles

Four anterior axio-appendicular muscles (thoraco-appendicular or pectoral muscles) move the pectoral girdle: pectoralis major, pectoralis minor, subclavius, and serratus anterior. These muscles and their attachments are illustrated in Figure 6.21, and their attachments, nerve supply, and main actions are summarized in Table 6.3.

The **pectoralis major** is a large, fan-shaped muscle that covers the superior part of the thorax (Fig. 6.21A). It has *clavicular and sternocostal heads.* The sternocostal head is much larger, and its lateral border forms the muscular mass that makes up most of the anterior wall of the axilla. Its inferior border forms the *anterior axillary fold* (see "Axilla" on p. 713). The pectoralis major and adjacent deltoid muscles form the narrow **deltopectoral groove,** in which the cephalic vein runs (Fig. 6.15B); however, the muscles diverge slightly from each other superiorly and, along with the clavicle, form the *clavipectoral (deltopectoral) triangle* (Figs. 6.2 and 6.15B).

Producing powerful adduction and medial rotation of the arm when acting together, the two parts of the pectoralis major can also act independently: the clavicular head flexing the humerus, and the sternocostal head extending it back from the flexed position.

To test the clavicular head of pectoralis major, the arm is abducted 90°; the individual then moves the arm anteriorly against resistance. If acting normally, the clavicular head can be seen and palpated.

To test the sternocostal head of pectoralis major, the arm is abducted 60° and then adducted against resistance. If acting normally, the sternocostal head can be seen and palpated.

The **pectoralis minor** lies in the anterior wall of the axilla where it is almost completely covered by the much larger pectoralis major (Figs. 6.21B and 6.22). The pectoralis minor is triangular in shape: Its base (proximal attachment) is formed by fleshy slips attached to the anterior ends of the 3rd–5th ribs near their costal cartilages; its apex (distal attachment) is on the coracoid process of the scapula. Variations in the costal attachments of the muscle are common.

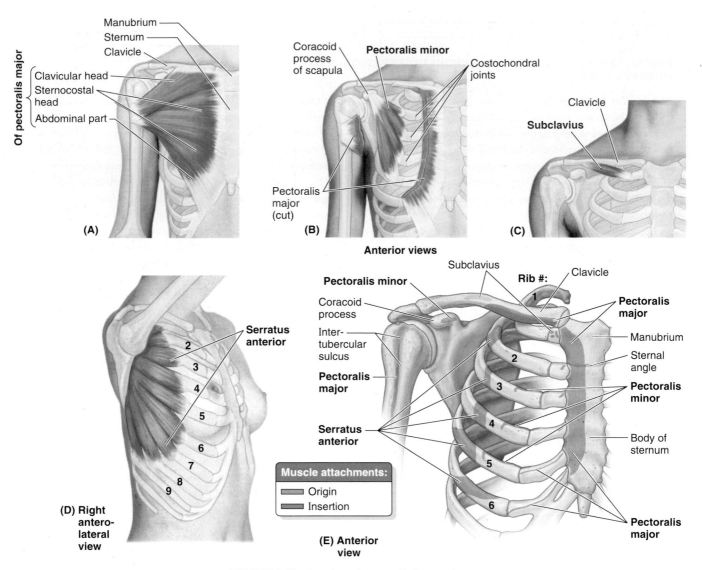

FIGURE 6.21. Anterior axio-appendicular muscles.

TABLE 6.3. ANTERIOR AXIO-APPENDICULAR MUSCLES

Muscle	Proximal Attachment	Distal Attachment	Innervation[a]	Main Action
Pectoralis major	Clavicular head: anterior surface of medial half of clavicle Sternocostal head: anterior surface of sternum, superior six costal cartilages, aponeurosis of external oblique muscle	Lateral lip of intertubercular sulcus of humerus	Lateral and medial pectoral nerves; clavicular head (C5, **C6**), sternocostal head (**C7, C8**, T1)	Adducts and medially rotates humerus; draws scapula anteriorly and inferiorly Acting alone, clavicular head flexes humerus and sternocostal head extends it from the flexed position
Pectoralis minor	3rd–5th ribs near their costal cartilages	Medial border and superior surface of coracoid process of scapula	Medial pectoral nerve (C8, T1)	Stabilizes scapula by drawing it inferiorly and anteriorly against thoracic wall
Sub-clavius	Junction of 1st rib and its costal cartilage	Inferior surface of middle third of clavicle	Nerve to subclavius (**C5**, C6)	Anchors and depresses clavicle
Serratus anterior	External surfaces of lateral parts of 1st–8th ribs	Anterior surface of medial border of scapula	Long thoracic nerve (C5, **C6, C7**)	Protracts scapula and holds it against thoracic wall; rotates scapula

[a]The spinal cord segmental innervation is indicated (e.g., "**C5**, C6" means that the nerves supplying the subclavius are derived from the fifth and sixth cervical segments of the spinal cord). Numbers in boldface (**C5**) indicate the main segmental innervation. Damage to one or more of the listed spinal cord segments or to the motor nerve roots arising from them results in paralysis of the muscles concerned.

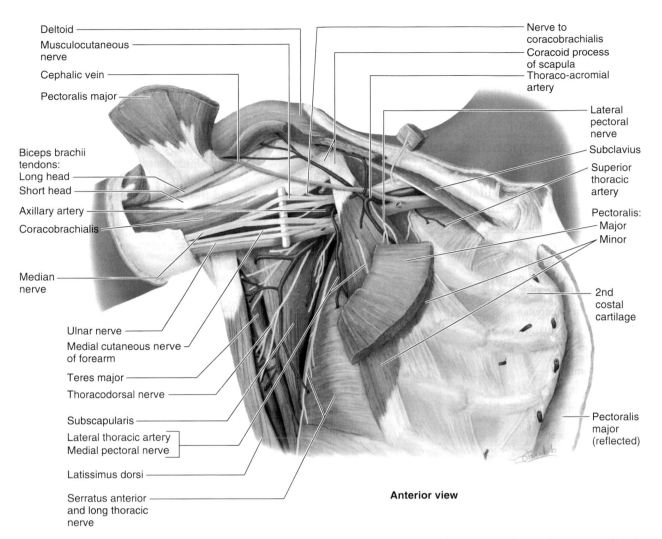

Deltoid

Musculocutaneous nerve

Cephalic vein

Pectoralis major

Biceps brachii tendons:
Long head
Short head

Axillary artery

Coracobrachialis

Median nerve

Ulnar nerve

Medial cutaneous nerve of forearm

Teres major

Thoracodorsal nerve

Subscapularis

Lateral thoracic artery
Medial pectoral nerve

Latissimus dorsi

Serratus anterior and long thoracic nerve

Nerve to coracobrachialis

Coracoid process of scapula

Thoraco-acromial artery

Lateral pectoral nerve

Subclavius

Superior thoracic artery

Pectoralis:
Major
Minor

2nd costal cartilage

Pectoralis major (reflected)

Anterior view

FIGURE 6.22. Axio-appendicular muscles contributing to walls of axilla. Of the anterior axio-appendicular muscles forming the anterior wall, only portions of the pectoralis major (attaching ends, a central part overlying the pectoralis minor, and a cube of muscle reflected superior to the clavicle), the pectoralis minor, and the subclavius remain. All the clavipectoral fascia and axillary fat have been removed, as has the axillary sheath surrounding the neurovascular bundle. This enables observation of the medial wall of the axilla, formed by the serratus anterior overlying the lateral thoracic wall, and of the latissimus dorsi contributing to the posterior wall.

The pectoralis minor stabilizes the scapula and is used when stretching the upper limb forward to touch an object that is just out of reach. It also assists in elevating the ribs for deep inspiration when the pectoral girdle is fixed or elevated. The pectoralis minor is a useful anatomical and surgical landmark for structures in the axilla (e.g., the axillary artery). With the coracoid process, the pectoralis minor forms a "bridge" under which vessels and nerves must pass to the arm.

The **subclavius** lies almost horizontally when the arm is in the anatomical position (Figs. 6.21C and 6.22). This small, round muscle is located inferior to the clavicle and affords some protection to the subclavian vessels and the superior trunk of the brachial plexus if the clavicle fractures. The subclavius anchors and depresses the clavicle, stabilizing it during movements of the upper limb. It also helps resist the tendency for the clavicle to dislocate at the sternoclavicular (SC) joint—for example, when pulling hard during a tug-of-war game.

The **serratus anterior** overlies the lateral part of the thorax and forms the medial wall of the axilla (Fig. 6.21D). This broad sheet of thick muscle was named because of the sawtoothed appearance of its fleshy slips or digitations (L. *serratus*, a saw). The muscular slips pass posteriorly and then medially to attach to the whole length of the anterior surface of the medial border of the scapula, including its inferior angle. The serratus anterior is one of the most powerful muscles of the pectoral girdle. It is a strong protractor of the scapula and is used when punching or reaching anteriorly (sometimes called the "boxer's muscle").

The strong inferior part of the serratus anterior rotates the scapula, elevating its glenoid cavity so the arm can be raised above the shoulder. It also anchors the scapula, keeping it closely applied to the thoracic wall, enabling other muscles to use it as a fixed bone for movements of the humerus. The serratus anterior holds the scapula against the thoracic wall

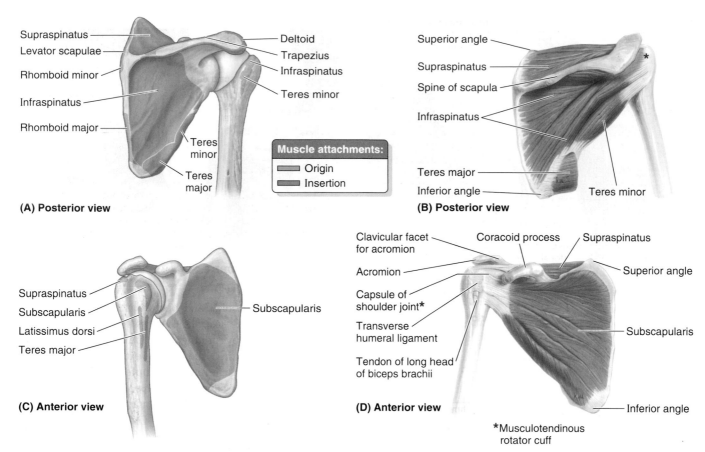

FIGURE 6.29. Scapulohumeral muscles. A–D. These muscles pass from the scapula to the humerus and act on the glenohumeral joint. Not included here is the deltoid, featured in Figure 6.30.

wall, and fixing the scapula during movements of the upper limb. The rhomboids are used when forcibly lowering the raised upper limbs (e.g., when driving a stake with a sledge hammer).

To test the rhomboids (or the function of the dorsal scapular nerve that supplies them), the individual places his or her hands posteriorly on the hips, and pushes the elbows posteriorly against resistance provided by the examiner. If the rhomboids are acting normally, they can be palpated along the medial borders of the scapulae; because they lie deep to the trapezius, they are unlikely to be visible during testing.

Scapulohumeral (Intrinsic Shoulder) Muscles

The **six scapulohumeral muscles** (deltoid, teres major, supraspinatus, infraspinatus, subscapularis, and teres minor) are relatively short muscles that pass from the scapula to the humerus and act on the glenohumeral joint. These muscles are illustrated in Figures 6.23 and 6.29, and their attachments, nerve supply, and main actions are summarized in Table 6.6.

Deltoid. The **deltoid** is a thick, powerful, coarse-textured muscle covering the shoulder and forming its rounded contour (Figs. 6.23 and 6.30; Table 6.6). As its name indicates,

TABLE 6.6. SCAPULOHUMERAL (INTRINSIC SHOULDER) MUSCLES

Muscle	Proximal Attachment	Distal Attachment	Innervation[a]	Muscle Action
Deltoid	Lateral third of clavicle; acromion and spine of scapula	Deltoid tuberosity of humerus	Axillary nerve (**C5**, C6)	Clavicular (anterior) part: flexes and medially rotates arm Acromial (middle) part: abducts arm Spinal (posterior) part: extends and laterally rotates arm
Supraspinatus[b]	Supraspinous fossa of scapula	Superior facet of greater tubercle of humerus	Suprascapular nerve (C4, **C5**, C6)	Initiates and assists deltoid in abduction of arm and acts with rotator cuff muscles[b]

TABLE 6.6. SCAPULOHUMERAL (INTRINSIC SHOULDER) MUSCLES (Continued)

Muscle	Proximal Attachment	Distal Attachment	Innervation[a]	Muscle Action
Infraspinatus[b]	Infraspinous fossa of scapula	Middle facet of greater tubercle of humerus	Suprascapular nerve (**C5**, C6)	Laterally rotates arm; and acts with rotator cuff muscles[b]
Teres minor[b]	Middle part of lateral border of scapula	Inferior facet of greater tubercle of humerus	Axillary nerve (**C5**, C6)	Laterally rotates arm; and acts with rotator cuff muscles[b]
Teres major	Posterior surface of inferior angle of scapula	Medial lip of intertubercular sulcus of humerus	Lower subscapular nerve (C5, **C6**)	Adducts and medially rotates arm
Subscapularis[b]	Subscapular fossa (most of anterior surface of scapula)	Lesser tubercle of humerus	Upper and lower subscapular nerves (C5, **C6**, C7)	Medially rotates arm; as part of rotator cuff, helps hold head of humerus in glenoid cavity

[a]The spinal cord segmental innervation is indicated (e.g., "**C5**, C6" means that the nerves supplying the deltoid are derived from the fifth and sixth cervical segments of the spinal cord). Numbers in boldface (**C5**) indicate the main segmental innervation. Damage to one or more of the listed spinal cord segments or to the motor nerve roots arising from them results in paralysis of the muscles concerned.

[b]Collectively, the supraspinatus, infraspinatus, teres minor, and subscapularis muscles are referred to as the rotator cuff, or SITS, muscles. Their primary function during all movements of the glenohumeral (shoulder) joint is to hold the humeral head in the glenoid cavity of the scapula.

the deltoid is shaped like the inverted Greek letter delta (Δ). The muscle is divided into unipennate anterior and posterior parts and a multipennate middle part (see Introduction, p. 31). The parts of the deltoid can act separately or as a whole. When all three parts of the deltoid contract simultaneously, the arm is abducted. The anterior and posterior parts act like guy ropes to steady the arm as it is abducted.

To initiate movement during the first 15° of abduction, the deltoid is assisted by the supraspinatus (Fig. 6.29B). When the arm is fully adducted, the line of pull of the deltoid coincides with the axis of the humerus; thus, it pulls directly upward on the bone and cannot initiate or produce abduction. It is, however, able to act as a shunt muscle, resisting inferior displacement of the head of the humerus from the

glenoid cavity, as when lifting and carrying suitcases. From the fully adducted position, abduction must be initiated by the supraspinatus, or by leaning to the side, allowing gravity to initiate the movement. The deltoid becomes fully effective as an abductor after the initial 15° of abduction.

The anterior and posterior parts of the deltoids are used to swing the limbs during walking. The anterior part assists the pectoralis major in flexing the arm, and the posterior part assists the latissimus dorsi in extending the arm. The deltoid also helps stabilize the glenohumeral joint and hold the head of the humerus in the glenoid cavity during movements of the upper limb.

To test the deltoid (or the function of the axillary nerve that supplies it), the arm is abducted, starting from approximately 15°, against resistance (Fig. 6.31). If acting normally, the deltoid can easily be seen and palpated. The influence of gravity is avoided when the person is supine.

Middle part of deltoid

Clavicular part of deltoid

Spinal (posterior) part of deltoid

Acromion

Clavicle

Clavicular (anterior) part of deltoid

Acromion

Acromion

Pectoralis major

Spine of scapula

Posterior view

Anterior view

Middle part of deltoid

Deltoid tuberosity (of humerus)

Right lateral view

FIGURE 6.30. Deltoid.

FIGURE 6.31. Testing deltoid muscle. The examiner resists the patient's abduction of the limb by the deltoid. If the deltoid is acting normally, contraction of the middle part of the muscle can be palpated.

FIGURE 6.32. Teres major.

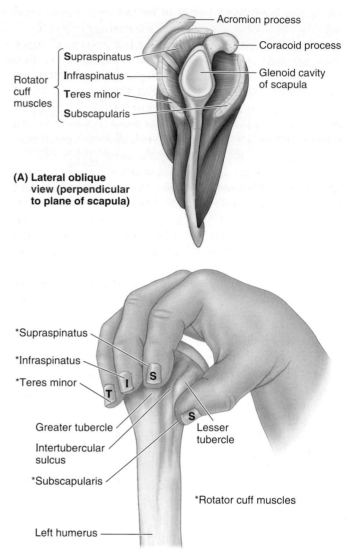

(A) Lateral oblique view (perpendicular to plane of scapula)

(B) Right anterolateral view

FIGURE 6.33. Disposition of rotator cuff muscles. A. Coming from opposite sides and three separate fossae on the scapulae, the four rotator cuff (SITS) muscles pass laterally to engulf the head of the humerus. **B.** The primary combined function of the four SITS muscles is to "grasp" and pull the relatively large head of the humerus medially, holding it against the smaller, shallow glenoid cavity of the scapula. The tendons of the muscles (represented by three fingers and the thumb) blend with the fibrous layer of the capsule of the shoulder joint to form a musculotendinous rotator cuff, which reinforces the capsule on three sides (anteriorly, superiorly, and posteriorly) as it provides active support for the joint.

Teres Major. The **teres major** (L. *teres*, round) is a thick, rounded muscle passing laterally from the inferolateral third of the scapula (Figs. 6.23, 6.29A & B, and 6.32; Table 6.6). The inferior border of the teres major forms the inferior border of the lateral part of the posterior wall of the axilla. The teres major adducts and medially rotates the arm. It can also help extend it from the flexed position, and is an important stabilizer of the humeral head in the glenoid cavity—that is, it steadies the head in its socket.

To test the teres major (or the lower subscapular nerve that supplies it), the abducted arm is adducted against resistance. If acting normally, the muscle can be easily seen and palpated in the posterior axillary fold (Fig. 6.34).

ROTATOR CUFF MUSCLES

Four of the scapulohumeral muscles (intrinsic shoulder muscles)—**s**upraspinatus, **i**nfraspinatus, **t**eres minor, and **s**ubscapularis the *SITS muscles*)—are called **rotator cuff muscles** because they form a *musculotendinous rotator cuff* around the glenohumeral joint (Figs. 6.29B & D and 6.33). All except the supraspinatus are rotators of the humerus; the supraspinatus, besides being part of the rotator cuff, initiates and assists the deltoid in the first 15° of abduction of the arm.

The tendons of the SITS muscles blend with and reinforce the fibrous layer of the joint capsule of the glenohumeral joint, thus forming the rotator cuff that protects the joint and gives it stability. The tonic contraction of the contributing muscles holds the relatively large head of the humerus in the small, shallow glenoid cavity of the scapula during arm movements. The rotator cuff (SITS) muscles and their attachments are illustrated in Figure 6.29, and their attachments, nerve supply, and main actions are listed in Table 6.6.

Supraspinatus. The **supraspinatus** occupies the supraspinous fossa of the scapula (Figs. 6.5A, 6.29A & B and 6.33A). A bursa separates it from the lateral quarter of the fossa. (See "Deltoid" on p. 704 for a discussion of this muscle's cooperative action in abducting the upper limb.)

To test the supraspinatus, abduction of the arm is attempted from the fully adducted position against resistance, while the muscle is palpated superior to the spine of the scapula.

Infraspinatus. The **infraspinatus** occupies the medial three quarters of the infraspinous fossa (Fig. 6.5A) and is partly covered by the deltoid and trapezius. In addition to helping stabilize the glenohumeral joint, the infraspinatus is a powerful lateral rotator of the humerus.

To test the infraspinatus, the person flexes the elbow and adducts the arm. The arm is then laterally rotated against resistance. If acting normally, the muscle can be palpated inferior to the scapular spine. *To test the function of the suprascapular nerve,* which supplies the supraspinatus and infraspinatus, both muscles must be tested as described.

Teres Minor. The **teres minor** is a narrow, elongate muscle that is completely hidden by the deltoid, and is often not clearly delineated from the infraspinatus. The teres minor works with the infraspinatus to rotate the arm laterally and assist in its adduction. The teres minor is most clearly distinguished from the infraspinatus by its nerve supply. The teres minor is supplied by the axillary nerve, whereas the infraspinatus is supplied by the suprascapular nerve (Table 6.6).

Subscapularis. The **subscapularis** is a thick, triangular muscle that lies on the costal surface of the scapula, and forms part of the posterior wall of the axilla (Figs. 6.29C & D and 6.33A). It crosses the anterior aspect of the scapulohumeral joint on its way to the humerus. The subscapularis is the primary medial rotator of the arm and also adducts it. It joins the other rotator cuff muscles in holding the head of the humerus in the glenoid cavity during all movements of the glenohumeral joint (i.e., it helps stabilize this joint during movements of the elbow, wrist, and hand).

Surface Anatomy of Pectoral, Scapular, and Deltoid Regions

The *clavicle* is the boundary demarcating the root of the neck from the thorax. It also indicates the "divide" between the deep cervical and axillary "lymph sheds" (like a mountain range dividing watershed areas): Lymph from structures superior to the clavicles drain via the deep cervical nodes, and lymph from structures inferior to the clavicles, as far inferiorly as the umbilicus, drain via the axillary lymph nodes.

The **infraclavicular fossa** is the depressed area just inferior to the lateral part of the clavicle (Fig. 6.34). This depression overlies the **clavipectoral (deltopectoral) triangle**—bounded by the clavicle superiorly, the pectoralis major medially, and the deltoid laterally—which may be evident in the fossa in lean individuals. The *cephalic vein,* ascending from the upper limb, enters the clavipectoral triangle and pierces the clavipectoral fascia to enter the *axillary vein.* The *coracoid process* of the scapula is not subcutaneous; it is covered by the anterior border of the deltoid; however, the tip of the process can be felt on deep palpation on the lateral aspect of the clavipectoral triangle. The coracoid process is used as a bony landmark when performing a brachial plexus block, and its position is of importance in diagnosing shoulder dislocations.

While lifting a weight, palpate the anterior sloping border of the *trapezius,* and where its superior fibers attach to the lateral third of the clavicle. When the arm is abducted and then adducted against resistance, the *sternocostal part of the pectoralis major* can be seen and palpated. If the *anterior axillary fold* bounding the axilla is grasped between the fingers and thumb, the inferior border of the *sternocostal head of the pectoralis major* can be felt. Several digitations of the *serratus anterior* are visible inferior to the anterior axillary fold. The *posterior axillary fold* is composed of skin and muscular tissue (latissimus dorsi and teres major) bounding the axilla posteriorly.

The lateral border of the acromion may be followed posteriorly with the fingers until it ends at the *acromial angle* (Fig. 6.35A). Clinically, the *length of the arm* is measured from the acromial angle to the lateral condyle of the humerus. The *spine of the scapula* is subcutaneous

Clavicular head of pectoralis major
Sternocleidomastoid
Clavicle
Jugular notch
Descending (superior) part of trapezius
Infraclavicular fossa (overlying clavipectoral triangle)
Clavicular part of deltoid
Deltopectoral groove (for cephalic vein)
Anterior axillary fold
Posterior axillary fold
Axillary fossa
Sternocostal head of pectoralis major
Digitations of serratus anterior

Anterior view

FIGURE 6.34. Surface anatomy of pectoral and deltoid regions.

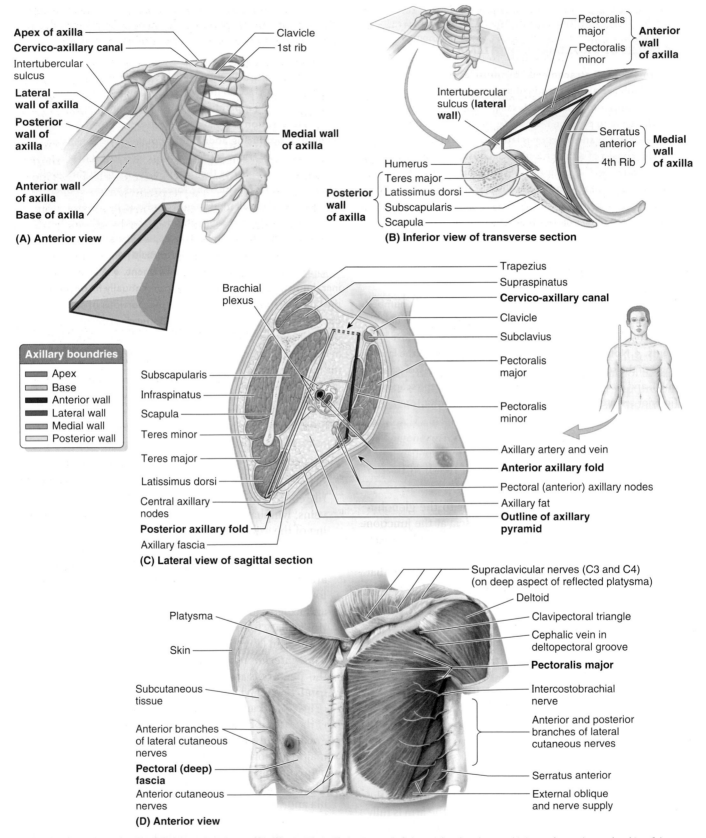

(A) Anterior view

Apex of axilla
Cervico-axillary canal
Intertubercular sulcus
Lateral wall of axilla
Posterior wall of axilla
Anterior wall of axilla
Base of axilla

Clavicle
1st rib
Medial wall of axilla

Axillary boundries
- Apex
- Base
- Anterior wall
- Lateral wall
- Medial wall
- Posterior wall

(B) Inferior view of transverse section

Intertubercular sulcus (**lateral wall**)
Humerus
Teres major
Latissimus dorsi
Subscapularis
Scapula
Posterior wall of axilla

Pectoralis major
Pectoralis minor
Anterior wall of axilla
Serratus anterior
4th Rib
Medial wall of axilla

(C) Lateral view of sagittal section

Brachial plexus
Subscapularis
Infraspinatus
Scapula
Teres minor
Teres major
Latissimus dorsi
Central axillary nodes
Posterior axillary fold
Axillary fascia

Trapezius
Supraspinatus
Cervico-axillary canal
Clavicle
Subclavius
Pectoralis major
Pectoralis minor
Axillary artery and vein
Anterior axillary fold
Pectoral (anterior) axillary nodes
Axillary fat
Outline of axillary pyramid

(D) Anterior view

Platysma
Skin
Subcutaneous tissue
Anterior branches of lateral cutaneous nerves
Pectoral (deep) fascia
Anterior cutaneous nerves

Supraclavicular nerves (C3 and C4) (on deep aspect of reflected platysma)
Deltoid
Clavipectoral triangle
Cephalic vein in deltopectoral groove
Pectoralis major
Intercostobrachial nerve
Anterior and posterior branches of lateral cutaneous nerves
Serratus anterior
External oblique and nerve supply

FIGURE 6.37. Location, boundaries, and contents of axilla. A. The axilla is a space inferior to the glenohumeral joint and superior to the skin of the axillary fossa at the junction of the arm and thorax. **B.** Note the axilla's three muscular walls. The small, lateral bony wall of the axilla is the intertubercular sulcus of the humerus. **C.** The contents of the axilla and the scapular and pectoral muscles forming its posterior and anterior walls, respectively. The inferior border of the pectoralis major forms the anterior axillary fold, and the latissimus dorsi and teres major form the posterior axillary fold. **D.** Superficial dissection of the pectoral region. Note that the subcutaneous platysma muscle is cut short on the right side. The severed muscle is reflected superiorly on the left side, together with the supraclavicular nerves, so that the clavicular attachments of the pectoralis major and deltoid can be observed.

- The *medial wall of axilla* is formed by the thoracic wall (1st–4th ribs and intercostal muscles) and the overlying serratus anterior (Fig. 6.37A & B).
- The *lateral wall of axilla* is a narrow bony wall formed by the *intertubercular sulcus* in the humerus.

The axilla contains axillary blood vessels (axillary artery and its branches, axillary vein and its tributaries), lymphatic vessels, and groups of *axillary lymph nodes,* all embedded in a matrix of *axillary fat* (Fig. 6.37C). The axilla also contains large nerves that make up the cords and branches of the *brachial plexus,* a network of interjoining nerves that pass from the neck to the upper limb (Fig. 6.38B). Proximally, these neurovascular structures are ensheathed in a sleeve-like extension of the cervical fascia, the **axillary sheath** (Fig. 6.38A).

Axillary Artery

The **axillary artery** begins at the lateral border of the 1st rib as the continuation of the *subclavian artery,* and ends at the inferior border of the teres major (Fig. 6.39). It passes posterior to the pectoralis minor into the arm, and becomes the *brachial artery* when it passes the inferior border of the teres major, at which point it usually has reached the humerus

(Fig. 6.39). For descriptive purposes, the axillary artery is divided into three parts by the pectoralis minor (the part number also indicates the number of its branches):

1. The **first part of the axillary artery** is located between the lateral border of the 1st rib and the medial border of the pectoralis minor; it is enclosed in the *axillary sheath* and has one branch—the *superior thoracic artery* (Figs. 6.38B & 6.39A; Table 6.7).
2. The **second part of the axillary artery** lies posterior to pectoralis minor and has two branches—the *thoracoacromial* and *lateral thoracic arteries*—which pass medial and lateral to the muscle, respectively.
3. The **third part of the axillary artery** extends from the lateral border of pectoralis minor to the inferior border of teres major; it has three branches. The *subscapular artery* is the largest branch of the axillary artery. Opposite the origin of this artery, the *anterior circumflex humeral and posterior circumflex humeral arteries* arise, sometimes by means of a common trunk.

The branches of the axillary artery are illustrated in Fig. 6.39, and their origin and course are described in Table 6.7.

The **superior thoracic artery** is a small, highly variable vessel that arises just inferior to the subclavius (Fig. 6.39A).

FIGURE 6.38. Contents of axilla. A. Note the axillary sheath enclosing the axillary artery and vein and the three cords of the brachial plexus. The innervation of the muscular walls of the axilla is also shown. The tendon of biceps brachii slides within the intertubercular sulcus **B.** Dissection in which most of the pectoralis major has been removed and the clavipectoral fascia, axillary fat, and axillary sheath have been completely removed. The brachial plexus of nerves surrounds the axillary artery on its lateral and medial aspects (appearing here to be its superior and inferior aspects because the limb is abducted) and on its posterior aspect (not visible from this view). Figure 6.22 on p. 699 is an enlarged view of part B.

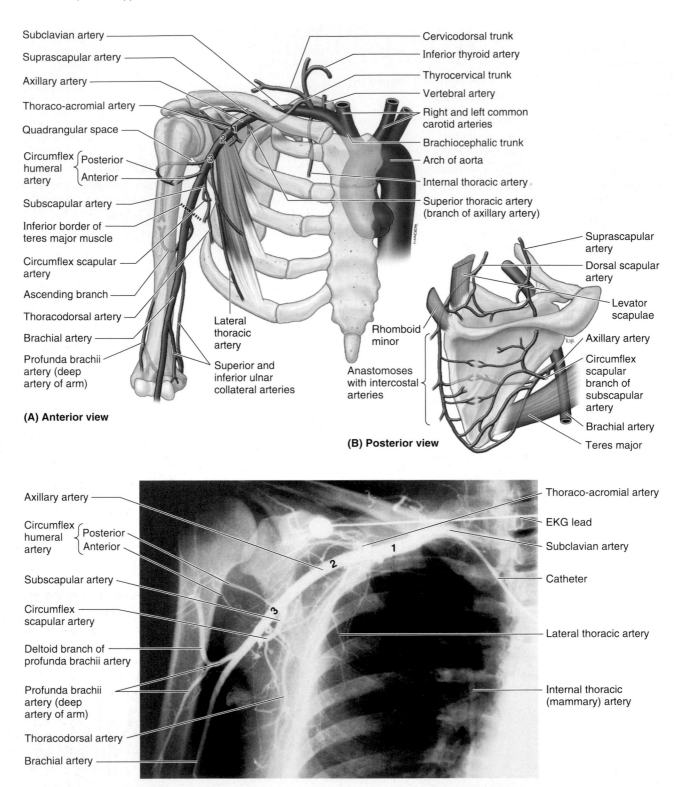

Subclavian artery
Suprascapular artery
Axillary artery
Thoraco-acromial artery
Quadrangular space
Circumflex { Posterior
humeral
artery { Anterior
Subscapular artery
Inferior border of teres major muscle
Circumflex scapular artery
Ascending branch
Thoracodorsal artery
Brachial artery
Profunda brachii artery (deep artery of arm)

Cervicodorsal trunk
Inferior thyroid artery
Thyrocervical trunk
Vertebral artery
Right and left common carotid arteries
Brachiocephalic trunk
Arch of aorta
Internal thoracic artery
Superior thoracic artery (branch of axillary artery)

Lateral thoracic artery
Superior and inferior ulnar collateral arteries

(A) Anterior view

Suprascapular artery
Dorsal scapular artery
Levator scapulae
Axillary artery
Circumflex scapular branch of subscapular artery
Brachial artery
Teres major

Rhomboid minor
Anastomoses with intercostal arteries

(B) Posterior view

Axillary artery
Circumflex { Posterior
humeral
artery { Anterior
Subscapular artery
Circumflex scapular artery
Deltoid branch of profunda brachii artery
Profunda brachii artery (deep artery of arm)
Thoracodorsal artery
Brachial artery

Thoraco-acromial artery
EKG lead
Subclavian artery
Catheter
Lateral thoracic artery
Internal thoracic (mammary) artery

(C) Anteroposterior view

1: First part of the axillary artery is located between the lateral border of the 1st rib and the medial border of pectoralis minor.
2: Second part of the axillary artery lies posterior to pectoralis minor.
3: Third part of the axillary artery extends from the lateral border of pectoralis minor to the inferior border of teres major, where it becomes the brachial artery.

FIGURE 6.39. Arteries of proximal upper limb.

TABLE 6.7. ARTERIES OF PROXIMAL UPPER LIMB (SHOULDER REGION AND ARM)

Artery	Origin		Course
Internal thoracic	Inferior surface of the first part		Descends, inclining anteromedially, posterior to sternal end of clavicle and first costal cartilage; enters thorax to descend in parasternal plane; gives rise to perforating branches, anterior intercostal, musculophrenic, and superior epigastric arteries
Thyrocervical trunk	Anterior surface of first part	Subclavian artery	Ascends as a short, stout trunk, giving rise to four branches: suprascapular, ascending cervical, inferior thyroid arteries, and the cervicodorsal trunk
Suprascapular	Thyrocervical (or as direct branch of sub-clavian artery)		Passes inferolaterally crossing anterior scalene muscle, phrenic nerve, subclavian artery, and brachial plexus running laterally posterior and parallel to clavicle; next it passes over transverse scapular ligament to supraspinous fossa; then lateral to scapular spine (deep to acromion) to infraspinous fossa on posterior surface of scapula
Superior thoracic	First part (as only branch)		Runs anteromedially along superior border of pectoralis minor; then passes between it and pectoralis major to thoracic wall; helps supply 1st and 2nd intercostal spaces and superior part of serratus anterior
Thoraco-acromial	Second part (first branch)		Curls around superomedial border of pectoralis minor; pierces costocoracoid membrane (clavipectoral fascia); divides into four branches: pectoral, deltoid, acromial, and clavicular
Lateral thoracic	Second part (second branch)	Axillary artery	Descends along axillary border of pectoralis minor; follows it onto thoracic wall, supplying lateral aspect of breast
Circumflex humeral (anterior and posterior)	Third part (sometimes via a common trunk)		Encircle surgical neck of humerus, anastomosing with each other laterally; larger posterior branch traverses quadrangular space
Subscapular	Third part (largest branch of any part)		Descends from level of inferior border of subscapularis along lateral border of scapula, dividing within 2–3 cm into terminal branches, the circumflex scapular and thoracodorsal arteries
Circumflex scapular			Curves around lateral border of scapula to enter infraspinous fossa, anastomosing with suprascapular artery
Thoracodorsal	Subscapular artery		Continues course of subscapular artery, descending with thoraco-dorsal nerve to enter apex of latissimus dorsi
Profunda brachii (deep artery of arm)	Near its origin		Accompanies radial nerve along radial groove of humerus, supplying posterior compartment of arm and participating in peri-articular arterial anastomosis around elbow joint
Superior ulnar collateral	Near middle of arm	Brachial artery	Accompanies ulnar nerve to posterior aspect of elbow; anasto-moses with posterior ulnar recurrent artery
Inferior ulnar collateral	Superior to medial epicondyle of humerus		Passes anterior to medial epicondyle of humerus to anastomose with anterior ulnar collateral artery

It commonly runs inferomedially posterior to the axillary vein and supplies the subclavius, muscles in the 1st and 2nd intercostal spaces, superior slips of the serratus anterior, and overlying pectoral muscles. It anastomoses with the intercostal and/or internal thoracic arteries.

The **thoraco-acromial artery,** a short wide trunk, pierces the costocoracoid membrane and divides into four branches (acromial, deltoid, pectoral, and clavicular), deep to the clavicular head of the pectoralis major (Fig. 6.40).

The **lateral thoracic artery** has a variable origin. It usually arises as the second branch of the second part of the axillary artery and descends along the lateral border of the pectoralis minor, following it onto the thoracic wall (Fig. 6.38B and 6.39A); however, it may arise instead from the thoraco-acromial, suprascapular, or subscapular arteries. The lateral thoracic artery supplies the pectoral, serratus anterior, and intercostal muscles, the axillary lymph nodes, and the lateral aspect of the breast.

The **subscapular artery,** the branch of the axillary artery with the greatest diameter but shortest length descends along the lateral border of the subscapularis on the posterior axillary wall. It soon terminates by dividing into the circumflex scapular and thoracodorsal arteries.

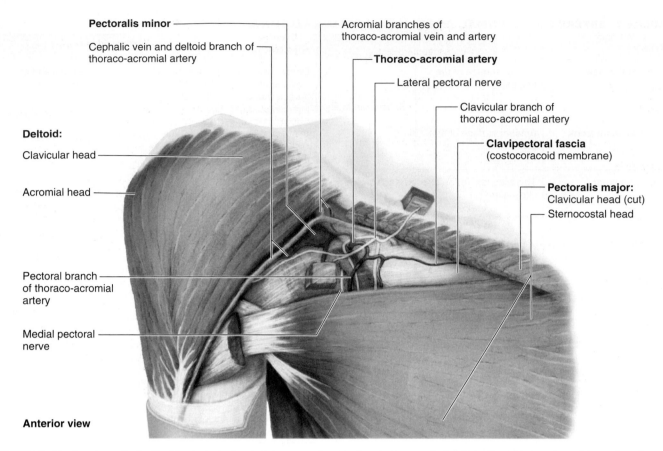

FIGURE 6.40. Anterior wall of axilla. The clavicular head of the pectoralis major is excised except for its clavicular and humeral attaching ends and two cubes, which remain to identify its nerves.

The **circumflex scapular artery,** often the larger terminal branch of the subscapular artery, curves posteriorly around the lateral border of the scapula, passing posteriorly between the subscapularis and the teres major to supply muscles on the dorsum of the scapula (Fig. 6.39B). It participates in the anastomoses around the scapula.

The **thoracodorsal artery** continues the general course of the subscapular artery to the inferior angle of the scapula and supplies adjacent muscles, principally the latissimus dorsi (Fig. 6.39A & C). It also participates in the arterial anastomoses around the scapula.

The *circumflex humeral arteries* encircle the surgical neck of the humerus, anastomosing with each other. The smaller **anterior circumflex humeral artery** passes laterally, deep to the coracobrachialis and biceps brachii. It gives off an ascending branch that supplies the shoulder. The larger **posterior circumflex humeral artery** passes medially through the posterior wall of the axilla via the **quadrangular space** with the axillary nerve to supply the glenohumeral joint and surrounding muscles (e.g., the deltoid, teres major and minor, and long head of the triceps) (Fig. 6.39A & C; Table 6.7).

Axillary Vein

The **axillary vein** lies initially (distally) on the anteromedial side of the axillary artery, with its terminal part antero-inferior to the artery (Fig. 6.41). This large vein is formed by the union of the *brachial vein* (the accompanying veins of the brachial artery) and the *basilic vein* at the inferior border of the teres major.

The axillary vein has three parts, which correspond to the three parts of the axillary artery. Thus the initial, distal end is the third part, whereas the terminal, proximal end is the first part. The axillary vein (first part) ends at the lateral border of the 1st rib, where it becomes the **subclavian vein.** The veins of the axilla are more abundant than the arteries, are highly variable, and frequently anastomose. The axillary vein receives tributaries that generally correspond to branches of the axillary artery with a few major exceptions:

- The veins corresponding to the branches of the thoraco-acromial artery do not merge to enter by a common tributary; some enter independently into the axillary vein, but others empty into the cephalic vein, which then enters the axillary vein superior to the pectoralis minor, close to its transition into the subclavian vein.
- The axillary vein receives, directly or indirectly, the *thoraco-epigastric vein*(s), which is(are) formed by the anastomoses of superficial veins from the inguinal region with tributaries of the axillary vein (usually the lateral thoracic vein). These veins constitute a collateral route that

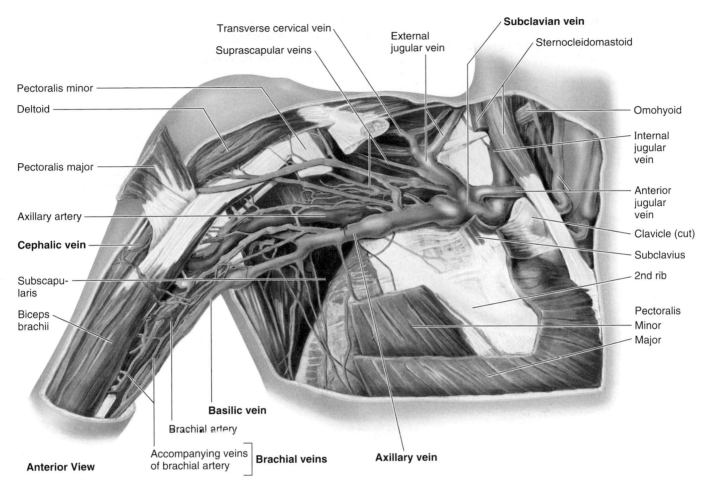

Transverse cervical vein

Suprascapular veins

External jugular vein

Subclavian vein

Sternocleidomastoid

Pectoralis minor

Deltoid

Omohyoid

Internal jugular vein

Pectoralis major

Anterior jugular vein

Axillary artery

Clavicle (cut)

Cephalic vein

Subclavius

Subscapu-laris

2nd rib

Biceps brachii

Pectoralis Minor

Major

Basilic vein

Brachial artery

Accompanying veins of brachial artery } **Brachial veins**

Axillary vein

Anterior View

FIGURE 6.41. Veins of axilla. The basilic vein parallels the brachial artery to the axilla, where it merges with the accompanying veins (L. *venae comitantes*) of the axillary artery to form the axillary vein. The large number of smaller, highly variable veins in the axilla are also tributaries of the axillary vein.

enables venous return in the presence of obstruction of the inferior vena cava (see the blue box "Collateral Routes for Abdominopelvic Venous Blood" on p. 315).

Axillary Lymph Nodes

The fibrofatty connective tissue of the axilla (axillary fat) contains many lymph nodes. The axillary lymph nodes are arranged in five principal groups: pectoral, subscapular, humeral, central, and apical. The groups are arranged in a manner that reflects the pyramidal shape of the axilla (Fig. 6.37A). Three groups of axillary nodes are related to the triangular base, one group at each corner of the pyramid (Fig. 6.42A & C).

The **pectoral (anterior) nodes** consist of three to five nodes that lie along the medial wall of the axilla, around the lateral thoracic vein and the inferior border of the pectoralis minor. The pectoral nodes receive lymph mainly from the anterior thoracic wall, including most of the breast (especially the superolateral [upper outer] quadrant and subareolar plexus; see Chapter 1).

The **subscapular (posterior) nodes** consist of six or seven nodes that lie along the posterior axillary fold and subscapular blood vessels. These nodes receive lymph

from the posterior aspect of the thoracic wall and scapular region.

The **humeral (lateral) nodes** consist of four to six nodes that lie along the lateral wall of the axilla, medial and posterior to the axillary vein. These nodes receive nearly all the lymph from the upper limb, except that carried by the lymphatic vessels accompanying the cephalic vein, which primarily drain directly to the apical axillary and infraclavicular nodes.

Efferent lymphatic vessels from these three groups pass to the **central nodes.** There are three or four of these large nodes situated deep to the pectoralis minor near the base of the axilla, in association with the second part of the axillary artery. Efferent vessels from the central nodes pass to the **apical nodes,** which are located at the apex of the axilla along the medial side of the axillary vein and the first part of the axillary artery.

The apical nodes receive lymph from all other groups of axillary nodes as well as from lymphatics accompanying the proximal cephalic vein. Efferent vessels from the apical group traverse the *cervico-axillary canal.*

These efferent vessels ultimately unite to form the **subclavian lymphatic trunk,** although some vessels may drain

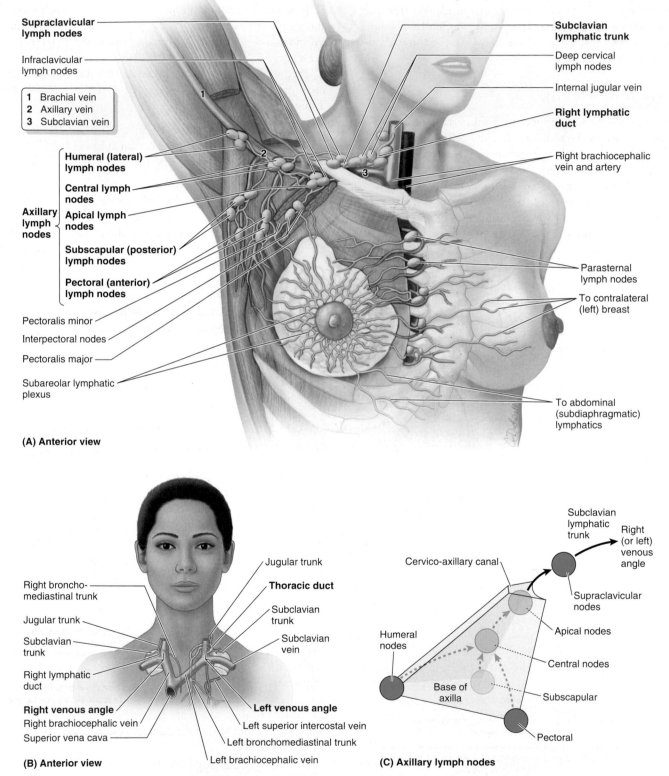

(A) Anterior view

(B) Anterior view

(C) Axillary lymph nodes

FIGURE 6.42. Axillary lymph nodes and lymphatic drainage of right upper limb and breast. A. Of the five groups of axillary lymph nodes, most lymphatic vessels from the upper limb terminate in the humeral (lateral) and central lymph nodes, but those accompanying the upper part of the cephalic vein terminate in the apical lymph nodes. The lymphatics of the breast are discussed in Chapter 1 (pp. 99–101). **B.** Lymph passing through the axillary nodes enters efferent lymphatic vessels that form the subclavian lymphatic trunk, which usually empties into the junctions of the internal jugular and subclavian veins (the venous angles). Occasionally, on the right side, this trunk merges with the jugular lymphatic and/or bronchomediastinal trunks to form a short right lymphatic duct; usually on the left side, it enters the termination of the thoracic duct. **C.** The positions of the five groups of axillary nodes, relative to each other and the pyramidal axilla. The typical pattern of drainage is indicated.

en route through the **clavicular (infraclavicular and supraclavicular) nodes.** Once formed, the subclavian trunk may be joined by the jugular and bronchomediastinal trunks on the right side to form the **right lymphatic duct,** or it may enter the right venous angle independently. On the left side, the subclavian trunk commonly joins the **thoracic duct** (Fig. 6.42A & B).

Brachial Plexus

Most nerves in the upper limb arise from the **brachial plexus,** a *major nerve network* (Figs. 6.38B and 6.43) supplying the upper limb; it begins in the neck and extends into the axilla. Almost all branches of the plexus arise in the axilla (after the plexus has crossed the 1st rib). The brachial plexus is formed by the union of the anterior rami of the last four cervical (C5–C8) and the first thoracic (T1) nerves, which constitute the **roots of the brachial plexus** (Figs. 6.43 and 6.44; Table 6.8).

The roots of the plexus usually pass through the gap between the anterior and the middle scalene (L. *scalenus anterior* and *medius*) muscles with the subclavian artery (Fig. 6.45). The sympathetic fibers carried by each root of the plexus are received from the gray rami of the middle and inferior cervical ganglia as the roots pass between the scalene muscles.

In the inferior part of the neck, the roots of the brachial plexus unite to form three trunks (Figs. 6.43–6.46A; Table 6.8):

1. A **superior trunk,** from the union of the C5 and C6 roots.
2. A **middle trunk,** which is a continuation of the C7 root.
3. An **inferior trunk,** from the union of the C8 and T1 roots.

Each trunk of the brachial plexus divides into anterior and posterior divisions as the plexus passes through the **cervico-axillary canal** posterior to the clavicle (Fig. 6.43).

(text continues on p. 724)

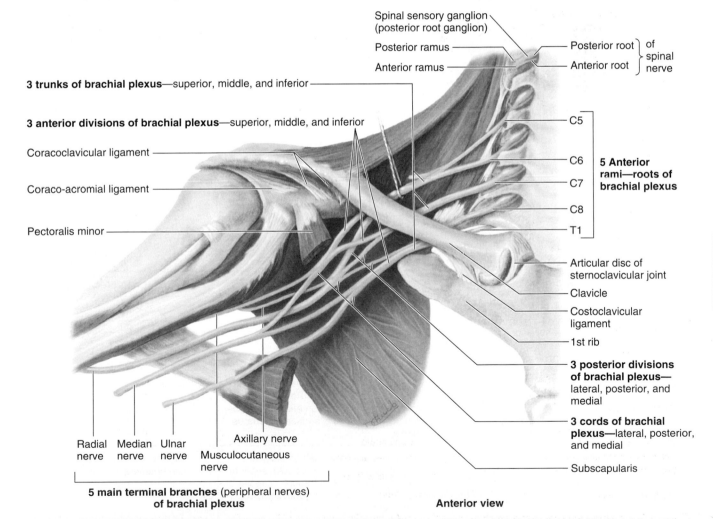

Spinal sensory ganglion (posterior root ganglion)

Posterior ramus

Anterior ramus

Posterior root ⎱ of
Anterior root ⎰ spinal nerve

3 trunks of brachial plexus—superior, middle, and inferior

3 anterior divisions of brachial plexus—superior, middle, and inferior

Coracoclavicular ligament

Coraco-acromial ligament

Pectoralis minor

C5

C6

C7

C8

T1

5 Anterior rami—roots of brachial plexus

Articular disc of sternoclavicular joint

Clavicle

Costoclavicular ligament

1st rib

3 posterior divisions of brachial plexus—lateral, posterior, and medial

3 cords of brachial plexus—lateral, posterior, and medial

Subscapularis

Radial nerve

Median nerve

Ulnar nerve

Axillary nerve

Musculocutaneous nerve

5 main terminal branches (peripheral nerves) **of brachial plexus**

Anterior view

FIGURE 6.43. Formation of brachial plexus. This large nerve network extends from the neck to the upper limb via the cervico-axillary canal (bound by the clavicle, 1st rib, and superior scapula) to provide innervation to the upper limb and shoulder region. The brachial plexus is typically formed by the anterior rami of the C5–C8 nerves and the greater part of the anterior ramus of the T1 nerve (the *roots* of the brachial plexus). Observe the merging and continuation of certain roots of the plexus to three *trunks,* the separation of each trunk into anterior and posterior *divisions,* the union of the divisions to form three *cords,* and the derivation of the main terminal branches (*peripheral nerves*) from the cords as the products of plexus formation.

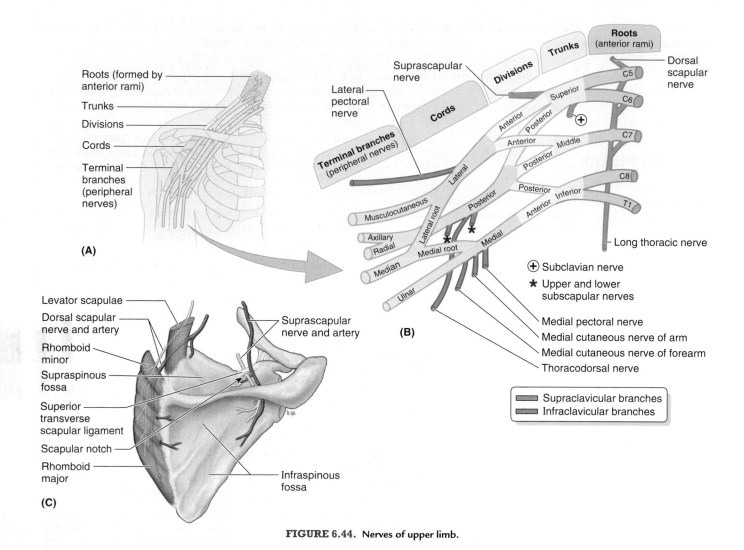

FIGURE 6.44. Nerves of upper limb.

TABLE 6.8. BRACHIAL PLEXUS AND NERVES OF UPPER LIMB

Nerve	Origin[a]	Course	Structures Innervated
Supraclavicular branches			
Dorsal scapular	Posterior aspect of anterior ramus of **C5** with a frequent contribution from C4	Pierces middle scalene; descends deep to levator scapulae and rhomboids	Rhomboids; occasionally supplies levator scapulae
Long thoracic	Posterior aspect of anterior rami of **C5, C6,** C7	Passes through cervico-axillary canal (Fig. 6.14), descending posterior to C8 and T1 roots of plexus (anterior rami); runs inferiorly on superficial surface of serratus anterior	Serratus anterior
Suprascapular	Superior trunk, receiving fibers from **C5,** C6 and often C4	Passes laterally across lateral cervical region (posterior triangle of neck), superior to brachial plexus; then through scapular notch inferior to superior transverse scapular ligament	Supraspinatus and infraspinatus muscles; glenohumeral (shoulder) joint
Subclavian nerve (nerve to subclavius)	Superior trunk, receiving fibers from C5, **C6** and often C4 (Fig. 6.44B)	Descends posterior to clavicle and anterior to brachial plexus and subclavian artery (Fig. 6.29); often giving an *accessory root to phrenic nerve*	Subclavius and sternoclavicular joint (accessory phrenic root innervates diaphragm)

TABLE 6.8. BRACHIAL PLEXUS AND NERVES OF UPPER LIMB (Continued)

Nerve	Origin[a]	Course	Structures Innervated
Infraclavicular branches			
Lateral pectoral	Side branch of lateral cord, receiving fibers from C5, **C6**, C7	Pierces costocoracoid membrane to reach deep surface of pectoral muscles; a *communicating branch to the medial pectoral nerve* passes anterior to axillary artery and vein	Primarily pectoralis major; but some lateral pectoral nerve fibers pass to pectoralis minor via branch to medial pectoral nerve (Fig. 6.46A)
Musculocutaneous	Terminal branch of lateral cord, receiving fibers from C5–C7	Exits axilla by piercing coracobrachialis (Fig. 6.43); descends between biceps brachii and brachialis (Figs. 6.47B and 6.48), supplying both; continues as *lateral cutaneous nerve of forearm*	Muscles of anterior compartment of arm (coracobrachialis, biceps brachii and brachialis) (Fig. 6.46B); skin of lateral aspect of forearm
Median	**Lateral root of median nerve** is a terminal branch of lateral cord (C6, C7) **Medial root of median nerve** is a terminal branch of medial cord (C8, T1)	Lateral and medial roots merge to form median nerve lateral to axillary artery; descends through arm adjacent to brachial artery, with nerve gradually crossing anterior to artery to lie medial to artery in cubital fossa (see Fig. 6.53, p. 738)	Muscles of anterior forearm compartment (except for flexor carpi ulnaris and ulnar half of flexor digitorum profundus), five intrinsic muscles in thenar half of palm and palmar skin (Fig. 6.46B)
Medial pectoral		Passes between axillary artery and vein; then pierces pectoralis minor and enters deep surface of pectoralis major; although it is called *medial* for its origin from medial cord, it lies lateral to lateral pectoral nerve	Pectoralis minor and sternocostal part of pectoralis major
Medial cutaneous nerve of arm	Side branches of medial cord, receiving fibers from C8, T1	Smallest nerve of plexus; runs along medial side of axillary and brachial veins; communicates with *intercostobrachial nerve*	Skin of medial side of arm, as far distal as medial epicondyle of humerus and olecranon of ulna
Median cutaneous nerve of forearm		Initially runs with ulnar nerve (with which it may be confused) but pierces deep fascia with basilic vein and enters subcutaneous tissue, dividing into anterior and posterior branches	Skin of medial side of forearm, as far distal as wrist
Ulnar	Larger terminal branch of medial cord, receiving fibers from C8, T1 and often C7	Descends medial arm; passes posterior to medial epicondyle of humerus; then descends ulnar aspect of forearm to hand (Figs. 6.46C and 6.47A)	Flexor carpi ulnaris and ulnar half of flexor digitorum profundus (forearm); most intrinsic muscles of hand; skin of hand medial to axial line of digit 4
Upper subscapular	Side branch of posterior cord, receiving fibers from **C5**	Passes posteriorly, entering subscapularis directly	Superior portion of subscapularis
Lower subscapular	Side branch of posterior cord, receiving fibers from **C6**	Passes inferolaterally, deep to subscapular artery and vein	Inferior portion of subscapularis and teres major
Thoracodorsal	Side branch of posterior cord, receiving fibers from C6, **C7**, C8	Arises between upper and lower subscapular nerves and runs inferolaterally along posterior axillary wall to apical part of latissimus dorsi	Latissimus dorsi
Axillary	Terminal branch of posterior cord, receiving fibers from **C5**, C6	Exits axillary fossa posteriorly, passing through quadrangular space[b] with posterior circumflex humeral artery (Fig. 6.48); gives rise to *superior lateral brachial cutaneous nerve;* then winds around surgical neck of humerus deep to deltoid (Fig. 6.46D)	Glenohumeral (shoulder) joint; teres minor and deltoid muscles (Fig. 6.46D); skin of superolateral arm (over inferior part of deltoid)
Radial	Larger terminal branch of posterior cord (largest branch of plexus), receiving fibers from C5–T1	Exits axillary fossa posterior to axillary artery; passes posterior to humerus in radial groove with deep brachial artery, between lateral and medial heads of triceps; perforates lateral intermuscular septum; enters cubital fossa, dividing into *superficial* (cutaneous) and *deep* (motor) *radial nerves* (Fig. 6.46D)	All muscles of posterior compartments of arm and forearm (Fig. 6.46D); skin of posterior and inferolateral arm, posterior forearm, and dorsum of hand lateral to axial line of digit 4

[a]Boldface (**C5**) indicates primary component of the nerve.

[b]Bounded superiorly by the subscapularis, head of humerus, and teres minor; inferiorly by the teres major; medially by the long head of the triceps; and laterally by the coracobrachialis and surgical neck of the humerus (Fig. 6.48).

Middle scalene

Trapezius

Levator scapulae

Branches of C5 spinal nerve

Posterior scalene

Dorsal scapular artery

Branch of C6 spinal nerve

Serratus anterior

Suprascapular nerve, artery, and vein

Brachial plexus

Deltoid

Axillary artery and vein

Pectoralis minor

Sternocleidomastoid

C5 & C6 roots of plexus

C5 and C3/C4 roots of phrenic nerve

Anterior scalene

Superior trunk

Cervicodorsal trunk (transverse cervical artery)

Internal jugular vein

Middle trunk

Brachiocephalic vein

Subclavian artery

Subclavian vein

Subclavian nerve

Subclavius

Pectoralis major (sternocostal head)

Lateral view

FIGURE 6.45. Dissection of right lateral cervical region (posterior triangle). The brachial plexus and subclavian vessels have been dissected. The anterior rami of spinal nerves C5–C8 (plus T1, concealed here by the third part of the subclavian artery) constitute the roots of the brachial plexus. Merging and subsequent splitting of the nerve fibers conveyed by the roots form the trunks and divisions at the level shown. The subclavian artery emerges between the middle and the anterior scalene muscles with the roots of the plexus.

Anterior divisions of the trunks supply *anterior (flexor) compartments* of the upper limb, and **posterior divisions of the trunks** supply *posterior (extensor) compartments.*

The divisions of the trunks form three cords of the brachial plexus (Figs. 6.43, 6.44, and 6.46, Table 6.8):

1. Anterior divisions of the superior and middle trunks unite to form the **lateral cord.**
2. Anterior division of the inferior trunk continues as the **medial cord.**
3. Posterior divisions of all three trunks unite to form the **posterior cord.**

The cords bear the relationship to the second part of the axillary artery that is indicated by their names. For example, the lateral cord is lateral to the axillary artery, although it may appear to lie superior to the artery because it is most easily seen when the limb is abducted.

The products of plexus formation are multisegmental, peripheral (named) nerves. The brachial plexus is divided into **supraclavicular** and **infraclavicular parts** by the clavicle (Fig. 6.44B; Table 6.8). Four *branches of the* *supraclavicular part of the plexus* arise from the roots (anterior rami) and trunks of the brachial plexus (dorsal scapular nerve, long thoracic nerve, nerve to subclavius, and suprascapular nerve), and are approachable through the neck. In addition, officially unnamed *muscular branches* arise from all five roots of the plexus (anterior rami C5–T1), which supply the scaleni and longus colli muscles. The C5 root of the *phrenic nerve* (considered a branch of the *cervical plexus*) arises from the C5 plexus root, joining the C3–C4 components of the nerve on the anterior surface of the anterior scalene muscle (Fig. 6.45). *Branches of the infraclavicular part of the plexus* arise from the cords of the brachial plexus and are approachable through the axilla (Figs. 6.44B and 6.46). Counting side and terminal branches, three branches arise from the lateral cord, whereas the medial and posterior cords each give rise to five branches (counting the roots of the median nerve as individual branches). The branches of the supraclavicular and infraclavicular parts of the brachial plexus are illustrated in Figs. 6.44B and 6.46 and listed in Table 6.8, along with the origin, course, and distribution of each branch.

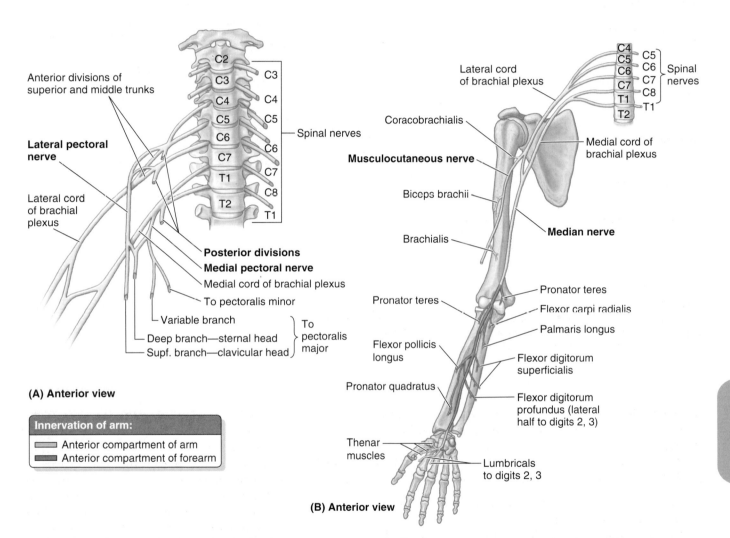

(A) Anterior view

Anterior divisions of superior and middle trunks

Lateral pectoral nerve

Lateral cord of brachial plexus

C2
C3
C4
C5
C6
C7
T1
T2

C3
C4
C5
C6
C7
C8
T1

Spinal nerves

Posterior divisions
Medial pectoral nerve
Medial cord of brachial plexus
To pectoralis minor
Variable branch
Deep branch—sternal head
Supf. branch—clavicular head

To pectoralis major

Innervation of arm:
Anterior compartment of arm
Anterior compartment of forearm

(B) Anterior view

Lateral cord of brachial plexus

Coracobrachialis

Musculocutaneous nerve

Biceps brachii

Brachialis

Pronator teres

Flexor pollicis longus

Pronator quadratus

Thenar muscles

C4
C5
C6
C7
T1
T2

C5
C6
C7
C8
T1

Spinal nerves

Medial cord of brachial plexus

Median nerve

Pronator teres
Flexor carpi radialis
Palmaris longus
Flexor digitorum superficialis
Flexor digitorum profundus (lateral half to digits 2, 3)
Lumbricals to digits 2, 3

FIGURE 6.46. Motor branches derived from cords of brachial plexus. A. The medial and lateral pectoral nerves arise from the medial and lateral cords of the brachial plexus, respectively (or from the anterior divisions of the trunks that form them, as shown here for the lateral pectoral nerve). **B.** The courses of the median and musculocutaneous nerves, and the typical pattern of branching of their motor branches are shown.

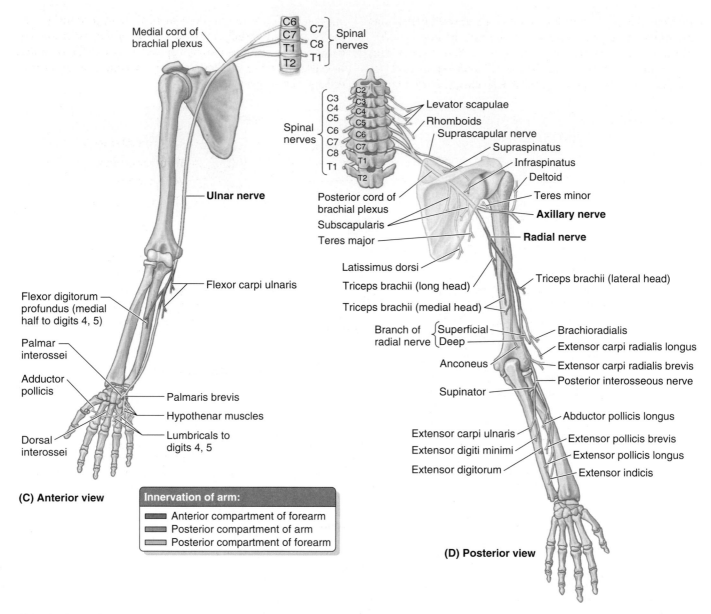

FIGURE 6.46. (*Continued*) **Motor branches derived from cords of brachial plexus. C.** The course of the ulnar nerve and the typical pattern of branching of its motor branches. **D.** The courses of the axillary and radial nerves and the typical pattern of branching of their motor branches. The posterior interosseous nerve is the continuation of the deep branch of the radial nerve, shown here bifurcating into two branches to supply all the muscles with fleshy bellies located entirely in the posterior compartment of the forearm. The dorsum of the hand has no fleshy muscle fibers; therefore, no motor nerves are distributed there.

AXILLA

Arterial Anastomoses Around Scapula

Many arterial anastomoses occur around the scapula. Several vessels join to form networks on the anterior and posterior surfaces of the scapula: the dorsal scapular, suprascapular, and (via the circumflex scapular) subscapular arteries (Fig. B6.11).

The importance of the *collateral circulation* made possible by these anastomoses becomes apparent when ligation of a lacerated subclavian or axillary artery is necessary. For example, the axillary artery may have to be ligated between the 1st rib and subscapular artery; in other cases, *vascular stenosis* of the axillary artery may result from an atherosclerotic lesion that causes reduced blood flow. In either case, the direction of blood flow in the subscapular artery is reversed, enabling blood to reach the third part of the axillary artery.

Note that the subscapular artery receives blood through several anastomoses with the suprascapular artery, dorsal scapular artery, and intercostal arteries. *Slow occlusion* of the axillary artery (e.g., resulting from disease or trauma) often enables sufficient collateral circulation to develop, preventing ischemia (loss of blood supply). *Sudden occlusion* usually does not allow sufficient time for adequate collateral circulation to develop; as a result, there is an inadequate supply of blood to the arm, forearm, and hand. While potential collateral pathways (peri-articular

anastomoses) exist around the shoulder joint proximally, and the elbow joint distally, *surgical ligation of the axillary artery* between the origins of the subscapular artery and the profunda brachii artery will cut off the blood supply to the arm because the collateral circulation is inadequate.

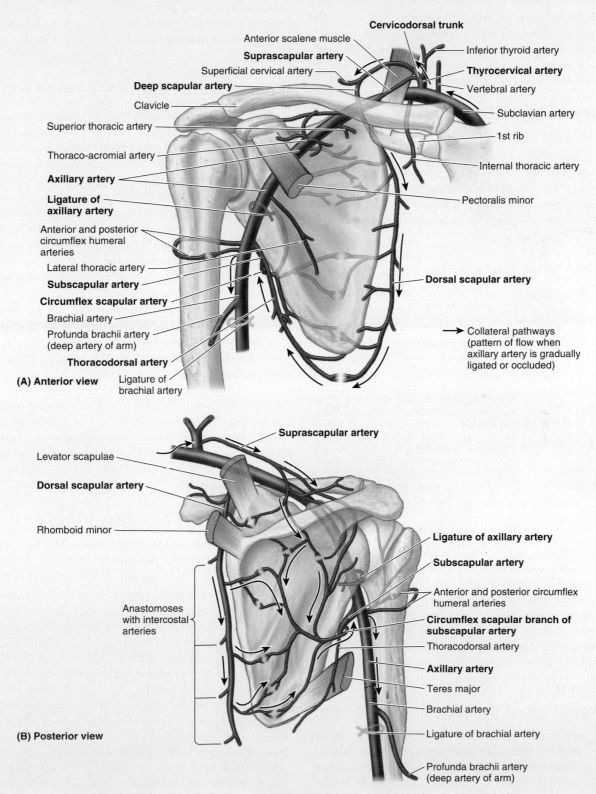

FIGURE B6.11.

Compression of Axillary Artery

The axillary artery can be palpated in the inferior part of the lateral wall of the axilla. Compression of the third part of this artery against the humerus may be necessary when profuse bleeding occurs (e.g., resulting from a stab or bullet wound in the axilla). If compression is required at a more proximal site, the axillary artery can be compressed at its origin (as the subclavian artery crosses the 1st rib) by exerting downward pressure in the angle between the clavicle and the inferior attachment of the sternocleidomastoid muscle.

Aneurysm of Axillary Artery

The first part of the axillary artery may enlarge (*aneurysm of axillary artery*) and compress the trunks of the brachial plexus, causing pain and anesthesia (loss of sensation) in the areas of the skin supplied by the affected nerves. Aneurysm of the axillary artery may occur in baseball pitchers and football quarterbacks because of their rapid and forceful arm movements.

Injuries to Axillary Vein

Wounds in the axilla often involve the axillary vein because of its large size and exposed position. When the arm is fully abducted, the axillary vein overlaps the axillary artery anteriorly. A wound in the proximal part of the axillary vein is particularly dangerous, not only because of profuse bleeding but also because of the risk of air entering it and producing *air emboli* (air bubbles) in the blood.

Role of Axillary Vein in Subclavian Vein Puncture

Subclavian vein puncture, in which a catheter is placed into the subclavian vein, has become a common clinical procedure (see blue box "Subclavian Vein Puncture" in Chapter 8, p. 1008).

The axillary vein becomes the subclavian vein as the first rib is crossed (Fig. 6.45). Because the needle is advanced medially to enter the vein as it crosses the rib, the vein actually punctured (the point of entry) in a "subclavian vein puncture" is the terminal part of the axillary vein. However, the needle tip proceeds into the lumen of the subclavian vein almost immediately. Thus it is clinically significant that the axillary vein lies anterior and inferior (i.e., superficial) to the axillary artery, and the parts of the brachial plexus that begin to surround the artery at this point.

Enlargement of Axillary Lymph Nodes

An infection in the upper limb can cause the axillary nodes to enlarge and become tender and inflamed, a condition called *lymphangitis* (inflammation of lymphatic vessels). The humeral group of nodes is usually the first to be involved.

Lymphangitis is characterized by the development of warm, red, tender streaks in the skin of the limb. Infections in the pectoral region and breast, including the superior part of the abdomen, can also produce enlargement of axillary nodes. In metastatic cancer of the apical group, the nodes often adhere to the axillary vein, which may necessitate excision of part of this vessel. Enlargement of the apical nodes may obstruct the cephalic vein superior to the pectoralis minor.

Dissection of Axillary Lymph Nodes

Excision and pathologic analysis of axillary lymph nodes are often necessary for *staging* and determining the appropriate treatment of a cancer, such as breast cancer (see p. 104). Because the axillary lymph nodes are arranged and receive lymph (and therefore metastatic breast cancer cells) in a specific order, removing and examining the lymph nodes in that order is important in determining the degree to which the cancer has developed, and is likely to have metastasized. Lymphatic drainage of the upper limb may be impeded after the removal of the axillary nodes, resulting in *lymphedema,* swelling as a result of accumulated lymph, especially in the subcutaneous tissue.

During *axillary node dissection,* two nerves are at risk of injury. During surgery, the long thoracic nerve to the serratus anterior is identified and maintained against the thoracic wall (Fig. B6.7, p. 711). As discussed earlier in this chapter, cutting the long thoracic nerve results in a winged scapula (Fig. B6.5 p. 709). If the thoracodorsal nerve to the latissimus dorsi is cut (Fig. B6.6, p. 710), medial rotation and adduction of the arm are weakened, but deformity does not result. If the nodes around this nerve are obviously malignant, sometimes the nerve has to be sacrificed as the nodes are resected to increase the likelihood of complete removal of all malignant cells.

Variations of Brachial Plexus

Variations in the formation of the brachial plexus are common (Bergman et al., 1988). In addition to the five anterior rami (C5–C8 and T1) that form the roots of the brachial plexus, small contributions may be made by the anterior rami of C4 or T2. When the superiormost root (anterior ramus) of the plexus is C4 and the inferiormost root is C8, it is a *prefixed brachial plexus.* Alternately, when the superior root is C6 and the inferior root is T2, it is a *postfixed brachial plexus.* In the latter type, the inferior trunk of the plexus may be compressed by the 1st rib, producing neurovascular symptoms in the upper limb. Variations may also occur in the formation of trunks, divisions, and cords; in the origin and/or combination of branches; and in the relationship to the axillary artery and scalene muscles. For example, the lateral or medial cords may receive fibers from anterior rami inferior or superior to the usual levels, respectively.

In some individuals, trunk divisions or cord formations may be absent in one or other parts of the plexus; however, the makeup of the terminal branches is unchanged. Because each peripheral nerve is a collection of nerve fibers bound together by connective tissue, it is understandable that the median nerve, for instance, may have two medial roots instead of one (i.e., the nerve fibers are simply grouped differently). This results from the fibers of the medial cord of the brachial plexus dividing into three branches, two forming the median nerve and the third forming the ulnar nerve. Sometimes it may be more confusing when the two medial roots are completely separate; however, understand that although the median nerve may have two medial roots the components of the nerve are the same (i.e., the impulses arise from the same place and reach the same destination whether they go through one or two roots).

Brachial Plexus Injuries

Injuries to the brachial plexus affect movements and cutaneous sensations in the upper limb. Disease, stretching, and wounds in the lateral cervical region (posterior triangle) of the neck (see Chapter 8), or in the axilla may produce brachial plexus injuries. Signs and symptoms depend on the part of the plexus involved. Injuries to the bra-

chial plexus result in *paralysis* and *anesthesia*. Testing the person's ability to perform movements assesses the degree of paralysis. In *complete paralysis,* no movement is detectable. In *incomplete paralysis,* not all muscles are paralyzed; therefore, the person can move, but the movements are weak compared with those on the normal side. Determining the ability of the person to feel pain (e.g., from a pinprick of the skin) tests the degree of anesthesia.

Injuries to superior parts of the brachial plexus (C5 and C6) usually result from an excessive increase in the angle between the neck and shoulder. These injuries can occur in a person who is thrown from a motorcycle or a horse, and lands on the shoulder in a way that widely separates the neck and shoulder (Fig. B6.12A). When thrown, the person's shoulder often hits something (e.g., a tree or the ground) and stops, but the head and trunk continue to move. This stretches or ruptures superior parts of the brachial plexus or *avulses* (tears) the roots of the plexus from the spinal cord.

Injury to the superior trunk of the plexus is apparent by the characteristic position of the limb ("waiter's tip position"), in which the limb hangs by the side in medial rotation (Fig. B6.12B; arrow). *Upper brachial plexus injuries* can also occur in a neonate when excessive stretching of the neck occurs during delivery (Fig. B6.12C).

FIGURE B6.12. Injuries to brachial plexus. A. Note the excessive increase in the angle between the head and left shoulder. **B.** The waiter's tip position (left upper limb). **C.** Observe the excessive increase in the angle between the head and the left shoulder during this delivery. **D and E.** Excessive increases in the angle between the trunk and the right upper limb. **F.** A claw hand (person is attempting to assume lightly shaded "fist" position).

FIGURE 6.49. Muscles of arm.

TABLE 6.9. MUSCLES OF ARM

Muscle	Proximal Attachment	Distal Attachment	Innervation[a]	Muscle Action
Biceps brachii	*Short head*: tip of coracoid process of scapula *Long head*: supraglenoid tubercle of scapula	Tuberosity of radius and fascia of forearm via bicipital aponeurosis	Musculocutaneous nerve (C5, **C6**, C7)	Supinates forearm and, when it is supine. flexes forearm; short head resists dislocation of shoulder
Coracobrachialis	Tip of coracoid process of scapula	Middle third of medial surface of humerus		Helps flex and adduct arm; resists dislocation of shoulder
Brachialis	Distal half of anterior surface of humerus	Coronoid process and tuberosity ulna	Musculocutaneous nerve[b] (C5, C6) and radial nerve (C5, C7)	Flexes forearm in all positions

(continued)

TABLE 6.9. MUSCLES OF ARM (Continued)

Muscle	Proximal Attachment	Distal Attachment	Innervation[a]	Muscle Action
Triceps brachii	*Long head*: infraglenoid tubercle of scapula *Lateral head*: posterior surface of humerus, superior to radial groove *Medial head*: posterior surface of humerus, inferior to radial groove	Proximal end of olecranon of ulna and fascia of forearm	Radial nerve (C6, **C7, C8**)	Chief extensor of forearm; long head resists dislocation of humerus; especially important during adduction
Anconeus	Lateral epicondyle of humerus	Lateral surface of olecranon and superior part of posterior surface of ulna	Radial nerve (C7, C8, T1)	Assists triceps in extending forearm; stabilizes elbow joint; may abduct ulna during pronation

[a]The spinal cord segmental innervation is indicated (e.g., "C5, **C6**, C7" means that the nerves supplying the biceps brachii are derived from the fifth and sixth cervical segments of the spinal cord). Numbers in boldface (**C6**) indicate the main segmental innervation. Damage to one or more of the listed spinal cord segments or to the motor nerve roots arising from them results in paralysis of the muscles concerned.

[b]Some of the lateral part of the brachialis is innervated by a branch of the radial nerve.

Table 6.9). For example, the musculocutaneous nerve pierces it, and the distal part of its attachment indicates the location of the nutrient foramen of the humerus. The coracobrachialis helps flex and adduct the arm and stabilize the glenohumeral joint. With the deltoid and long head of the triceps, it serves as a *shunt muscle*, resisting downward dislocation of the head of the humerus, as when carrying a heavy suitcase. The median nerve and/or the brachial artery may run deep to the coracobrachialis and be compressed by it.

TRICEPS BRACHII

The **triceps brachii** is a large fusiform muscle in the posterior compartment of the arm (Figs. 6.47, 6.48, 6.49F, and 6.50; Table 6.9). As indicated by its name, *the triceps has three heads:* long, lateral, and medial. The triceps is the main extensor of the forearm.

Because its **long head** crosses the glenohumeral joint, the triceps helps stabilize the adducted glenohumeral joint by serving as a shunt muscle, resisting inferior displacement of the head of the humerus. The long head also aids in extension and adduction of the arm, but it is the least active head.

The **medial head** is the workhorse of forearm extension, active at all speeds and in the presence or absence of resistance.

The **lateral head** is the strongest but is it recruited into activity primarily against resistance (Hamill and Knutzen, 2008). Pronation and supination of the forearm do not affect triceps operation. Just proximal to the distal attachment of the triceps is a friction-reducing *subtendinous olecranon bursa*, between the triceps tendon and the olecranon.

To *test the triceps* (or to determine the level of a radial nerve lesion), the arm is abducted 90° and then the flexed forearm is extended against resistance provided by the examiner. If acting normally, the triceps can be seen and palpated. Its strength should be comparable with the contralateral

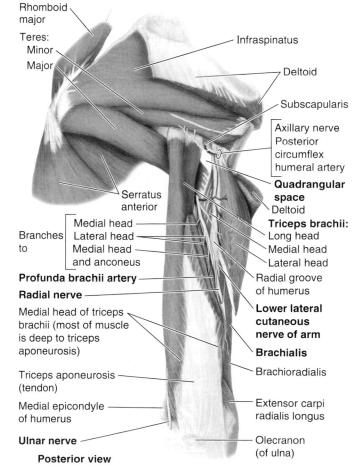

Rhomboid major

Teres:
Minor
Major

Infraspinatus

Deltoid

Subscapularis

Axillary nerve
Posterior circumflex humeral artery

Quadrangular space
Deltoid

Serratus anterior

Triceps brachii:
Long head
Medial head
Lateral head

Branches to
Medial head
Lateral head
Medial head and anconeus

Profunda brachii artery

Radial nerve

Medial head of triceps brachii (most of muscle is deep to triceps aponeurosis)

Triceps aponeurosis (tendon)

Medial epicondyle of humerus

Ulnar nerve

Posterior view

Radial groove of humerus

Lower lateral cutaneous nerve of arm

Brachialis

Brachioradialis

Extensor carpi radialis longus

Olecranon (of ulna)

FIGURE 6.50. Muscles of scapular region and posterior region of arm. The lateral head of the triceps brachii is divided and displaced to show the structures traversing the *quadrangular space* and the radial nerve and the profunda brachii artery. The exposed bone of the radial groove, which is devoid of muscular attachment, separates the humeral attachments of the lateral and medial heads of the triceps. (Bony attachments are illustrated in Figure 6.49E.)

(A) Posterior view

Deltoid

Distal attachment of deltoid

Long head

Lateral head

Medial head

Triceps brachii

Tendon

Olecranon

(B) Medial view

Deltoid

Biceps brachii

Medial bicipital groove

Biceps brachii tendon

Bicipital aponeurosis in cubital fossa

Brachialis

Location of medial intermuscular septum

Medial epicondyle of the humerus

Triceps brachii

(C) Anterolateral view

Olecranon

Medial epicondyle of humerus

Biceps brachii

Medial bicipital groove

Triceps brachii { Lateral head / Long head

Deltoid { Anterior part / Posterior part

Anterior axillary fold

Posterior axillary fold { Teres major / Latissimus dorsi

FIGURE 6.54. Surface anatomy of arm.

easily palpated at the medial and lateral aspects of the elbow. The medial epicondyle is more prominent.

In the cubital fossa, the *cephalic and basilic veins* in the subcutaneous tissue are clearly visible when a tourniquet is applied to the arm, as is the *median cubital vein*. This vein crosses the bicipital aponeurosis as it runs superomedially connecting the cephalic to the basilic vein (Fig. 6.55).

If the thumb is pressed into the cubital fossa, the muscular masses of the *long flexors of the forearm* will be felt forming the medial border, the pronator teres most directly.

The *lateral group of forearm extensors* (a soft mass that can be grasped separately), the brachioradialis (most medial) and the long and short extensors of the wrist, can be grasped between the fossa and the lateral epicondyle.

Cephalic vein of arm

Cubital fossa

Cephalic vein of forearm

Median antebrachial vein (median vein of forearm)

Skin and subcutaneous tissue

Basilic vein of arm

Median cubital vein

Medial epicondyle

Basilic vein of forearm

Brachial fascia covering biceps brachii

Cephalic vein of arm

Lateral cutaneous nerve of forearm

Median antebrachial vein

Cephalic vein of forearm

Medial cutaneous nerve of forearm

Basilic vein of arm

Cubital lymph node

Median cubital vein

Basilic vein of forearm

Perforating vein

Bicipital aponeurosis

Antebrachial fascia

(A)   **(B)**

Anterior views

FIGURE 6.55. Surface anatomy of cubital fossa.

ARM AND CUBITAL FOSSA

Bicipital Myotatic Reflex

 The *biceps reflex* is one of several deep-tendon reflexes that are routinely tested during physical examinations. The relaxed limb is passively pronated and partially extended at the elbow. The examiner's thumb is firmly placed on the biceps tendon, and the reflex hammer is briskly tapped at the base of the nail bed of the examiner's thumb (Fig. B6.13). A normal (positive) response is an involuntary contraction of the biceps, felt as a momentarily tensed tendon, usually with a brief jerk-like flexion of the elbow. A positive response confirms the integrity of the musculocutaneous nerve and the C5 and C6 spinal cord segments. Excessive, diminished, or prolonged (hung) responses may indicate central or peripheral nervous system disease, or metabolic disorders (e.g., thyroid disease).

FIGURE B6.13. Method of eliciting biceps reflex.

Biceps Tendinitis

 The tendon of the long head of the biceps is enclosed by a synovial sheath, and moves back and forth in the intertubercular sulcus (bicipital groove) of the humerus (Fig. 6.49B). Wear and tear of this mechanism can cause shoulder pain. Inflammation of the tendon (*biceps tendinitis*), usually the result of repetitive microtrauma, is common in sports involving throwing (e.g., baseball and cricket), and use of a racquet (e.g., tennis). A tight, narrow, and/or rough intertubercular sulcus may irritate and inflame the tendon, producing tenderness and *crepitus* (crackling sound).

Dislocation of Tendon of Long Head of Biceps Brachii

The tendon of the long head of the biceps can be partially or completely dislocated from the intertubercular sulcus in the humerus. This painful condition may occur in young persons during traumatic separation of the proximal epiphysis of the humerus. The injury also occurs in older persons with a history of biceps tendinitis. Usually a sensation of popping or catching is felt during arm rotation.

Rupture of Tendon of Long Head of Biceps Brachii

Rupture of the tendon usually results from wear and tear of an inflamed tendon as it moves back and forth in the intertubercular sulcus of the humerus. This injury usually occurs in individuals > 35 years of age. Typically,

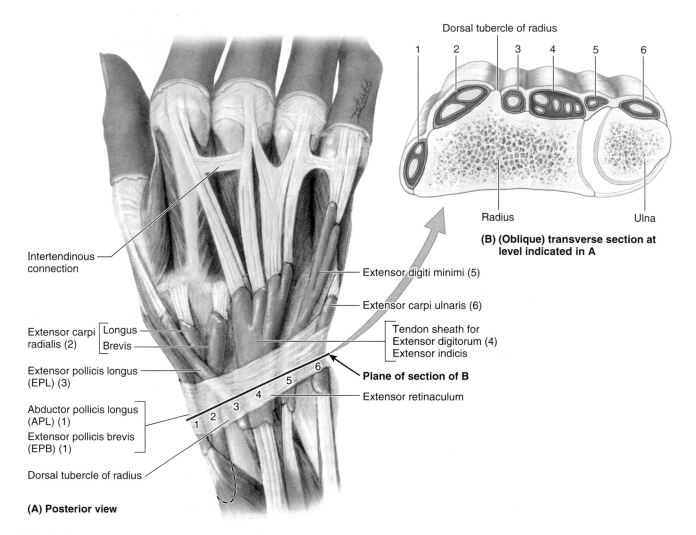

Intertendinous connection

Extensor carpi radialis (2) — Longus / Brevis

Extensor pollicis longus (EPL) (3)

Abductor pollicis longus (APL) (1)

Extensor pollicis brevis (EPB) (1)

Dorsal tubercle of radius

Extensor digiti minimi (5)

Extensor carpi ulnaris (6)

Tendon sheath for Extensor digitorum (4) Extensor indicis

Plane of section of B

Extensor retinaculum

(A) Posterior view

Dorsal tubercle of radius

Radius   Ulna

(B) (Oblique) transverse section at level indicated in A

FIGURE 6.62. Synovial sheaths and tendons on distal forearm and dorsum of hand. A. Observe that the six synovial tendon sheaths (*purple*) occupy six osseofibrous tunnels formed by attachments of the extensor retinaculum to the ulna and especially the radius, which give passage to 12 tendons of nine extensor muscles. The tendon of the extensor digitorum to the little finger is shared between the ring finger and continues to the little finger via an intertendinous connection, then receives additional fibers from the tendon of the extensor digiti minimi. Such variations are common. Numbers refer to the labeled osseofibrous tunnels shown in part **B. B.** This slightly oblique transverse section of the distal end of the forearm shows the extensor tendons traversing the six osseofibrous tunnels deep to the extensor retinaculum.

indicis to pass deep to the extensor retinaculum through the **tendinous sheath of the extensor digitorum and extensor indicis** (common extensor synovial sheath) (Fig. 6.62A & B). On the dorsum of the hand, the tendons spread out as they run toward the digits. Adjacent tendons are linked proximal to the knuckles (metacarpophalangeal joints) by three oblique *intertendinous connections* that restrict independent extension of the four medial digits (especially the ring finger). Consequently, normally none of these digits can remain fully flexed as the other ones are fully extended. Commonly, the fourth tendon is fused initially with the tendon to the ring finger and reaches the little finger by an intertendinous connection.

On the distal ends of the metacarpals and along the phalanges of the four medial digits, the four tendons flatten to form **extensor expansions** (Fig. 6.63). Each extensor digital expansion (dorsal expansion or hood) is a triangular, tendinous aponeurosis that wraps around the dorsum and sides of

a head of the metacarpal and proximal phalanx. The visor-like "hood" formed by the extensor expansion over the head of the metacarpal, holding the extensor tendon in the middle of the digit, is anchored on each side to the **palmar ligament** (a reinforced portion of the fibrous layer of the joint capsule of the metacarpophalangeal joints) (Figs. 6.63A & C).

In forming the extensor expansion, each flexor digitorum tendon divides into a **median band,** which passes to the base of the middle phalanx, and two **lateral bands,** which pass to the base of the distal phalanx (Fig. 6.63D & E). The tendons of the interosseous and lumbrical muscles of the hand join the lateral bands of the extensor expansion (Fig. 6.63).

The **retinacular ligament** is a delicate fibrous band that runs from the proximal phalanx and fibrous digital sheath obliquely across the middle phalanx and two interphalangeal joints (Fig. 6.63C). It joins the extensor expansion to the distal phalanx. During flexion of the distal interphalangeal joint,

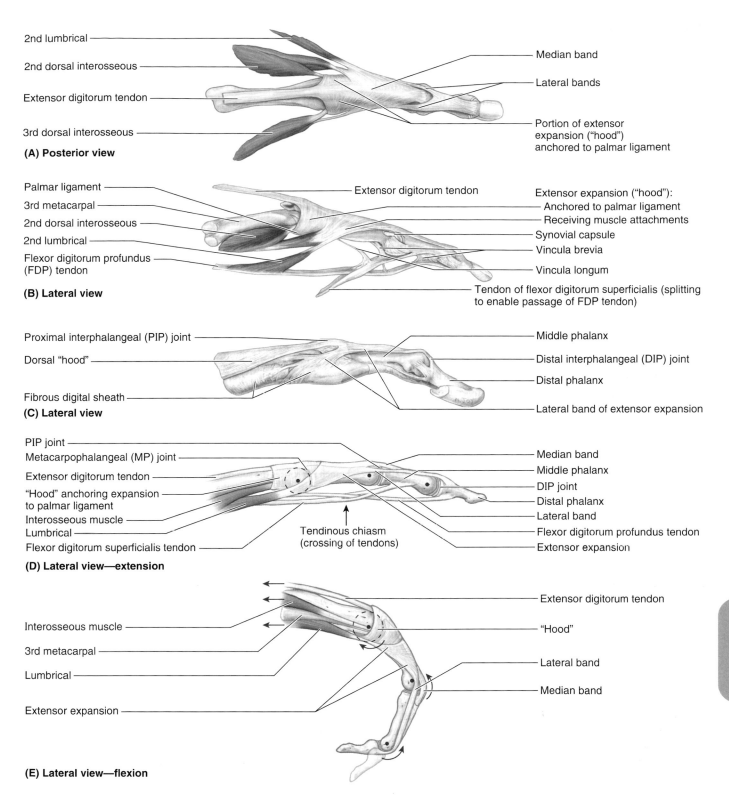

(A) Posterior view

- 2nd lumbrical
- 2nd dorsal interosseous
- Extensor digitorum tendon
- 3rd dorsal interosseous
- Median band
- Lateral bands
- Portion of extensor expansion ("hood") anchored to palmar ligament

(B) Lateral view

- Palmar ligament
- 3rd metacarpal
- 2nd dorsal interosseous
- 2nd lumbrical
- Flexor digitorum profundus (FDP) tendon
- Extensor digitorum tendon
- Extensor expansion ("hood"):
  - Anchored to palmar ligament
  - Receiving muscle attachments
- Synovial capsule
- Vincula brevia
- Vincula longum
- Tendon of flexor digitorum superficialis (splitting to enable passage of FDP tendon)

(C) Lateral view

- Proximal interphalangeal (PIP) joint
- Dorsal "hood"
- Fibrous digital sheath
- Middle phalanx
- Distal interphalangeal (DIP) joint
- Distal phalanx
- Lateral band of extensor expansion

(D) Lateral view—extension

- PIP joint
- Metacarpophalangeal (MP) joint
- Extensor digitorum tendon
- "Hood" anchoring expansion to palmar ligament
- Interosseous muscle
- Lumbrical
- Flexor digitorum superficialis tendon
- Tendinous chiasm (crossing of tendons)
- Median band
- Middle phalanx
- DIP joint
- Distal phalanx
- Lateral band
- Flexor digitorum profundus tendon
- Extensor expansion

(E) Lateral view—flexion

- Interosseous muscle
- 3rd metacarpal
- Lumbrical
- Extensor expansion
- Extensor digitorum tendon
- "Hood"
- Lateral band
- Median band

FIGURE 6.63. Dorsal digital (extensor) apparatus of 3rd digit. The metacarpal bone and all three phalanges are shown in parts **A, B, D,** and **E;** only the phalanges are shown in part **C. A.** Note the extensor digitorum tendon trifurcating (expanding) into three bands: two lateral bands that unite over the middle phalanx to insert into the base of the distal phalanx, and one median band that inserts into the base of the middle phalanx. **B.** Part of the tendon of the interosseous muscles attaches to the base of the proximal phalanx; the other part contributes to the extensor expansion, attaching primarily to the lateral bands, but also fans out into an aponeurosis. Some of the aponeurotic fibers fuse with the median band, and other fibers arch over it to blend with the aponeurosis arising from the other side. On the radial side of each digit, a lumbrical muscle attaches to the radial lateral band. The dorsal hood consists of a broad band of transversely oriented fibers attached anteriorly to the palmar ligaments of the metacarpophalangeal (MP) joints that encircle the metacarpal head and MP joint, blending with the extensor expansion to keep the apparatus centered over the dorsal aspect of the digit. **C.** Distally, retinacular ligaments extending from the fibrous digital sheath to the lateral bands also help keep the apparatus centered and coordinate movements at the proximal interphalangeal (PIP) and distal interphalangeal (DIP) joints. **D.** Contraction of the extensor digitorum alone results in extension at all joints (including the MP joint in the absence of action by the interossei and lumbricals). **E.** Because of the relationship of the tendons and the lateral bands to the rotational centers of the joints (*red dots* in parts **D** and **E**), simultaneous contraction of the interossei and lumbricals produces flexion at the MP joint but extension at the PIP and DIP joints (the so-called Z-movement).

in the forearm include unnamed muscular and articular branches, and cutaneous branches that pass to the hand:

- *Articular branches* pass to the elbow joint while the nerve is between the olecranon and the medial epicondyle.
- *Muscular branches* supply the FCU and the medial half of the FDP.
- The *palmar* and *dorsal cutaneous branches* arise from the ulnar nerve in the forearm, but their sensory fibers are distributed to the skin of the hand.

RADIAL NERVE IN FOREARM

Unlike the medial and ulnar nerves, the *radial nerve* serves motor and sensory functions in both the arm and the forearm (but only sensory functions in the hand). However, its sensory and motor fibers are distributed in the forearm by two separate branches, the superficial (sensory or cutaneous) and deep radial/posterior interosseous nerve (motor) (Fig. 6.69C & D, Table 6.13). It divides into these terminal branches as it appears in the cubital fossa, anterior to the lateral epicondyle of the humerus, between the brachialis and the brachioradialis (Fig. 6.64). The two branches immediately part company, the deep branch winding laterally around the radius, piercing the supinator en route to the posterior compartment.

The *posterior cutaneous nerve of the forearm* arises from the radial nerve in the posterior compartment of the arm, as it runs along the radial groove of the humerus. Thus it reaches the forearm independent of the radial nerve, descending in the subcutaneous tissue of the posterior aspect of the forearm to the wrist, supplying the skin (Fig. 6.69D).

The *superficial branch of the radial nerve* is also a cutaneous nerve, but it gives rise to articular branches as well. It is distributed to skin on the dorsum of the hand and to a number of joints in the hand, branching soon after it emerges from the overlying brachioradialis and crosses the roof of the anatomical snuff box (Fig. 6.65).

The *deep branch of the radial nerve*, after it pierces the supinator, runs in the fascial plane between superficial and deep extensor muscles in close proximity to the posterior interosseous artery; it is usually referred to as the *posterior interosseous nerve* (Figs. 6.64 and 6.69C). It supplies motor innervation to all the muscles with fleshy bellies located entirely in the posterior compartment of the forearm (distal to the lateral epicondyle of the humerus).

LATERAL AND MEDIAL CUTANEOUS NERVES OF FOREARM

The **lateral cutaneous nerve *of the forearm*** (lateral antebrachial cutaneous nerve) is the continuation of the musculocutaneous nerve after its motor branches have all been given off to the muscles of the anterior compartment of the arm.

The **medial cutaneous nerve of the forearm** (medial antebrachial cutaneous nerve) is an independent branch of the medial cord of the brachial plexus. With the **posterior cutaneous nerve of the forearm** from the radial nerve, each supplying the area of skin indicated by its name, these three nerves provide all the cutaneous innervation of the forearm (Fig. 6.69D). There is no "anterior cutaneous nerve of the forearm." (*Memory device:* This is similar to the brachial plexus, which has lateral, medial, and posterior cords but no anterior cord.)

Although the arteries, veins, and nerves of the forearm have been considered separately, it is important to place them into their anatomical context. Except for the superficial veins, which often course independently in the subcutaneous tissue, these neurovascular structures usually exist as components of neurovascular bundles. These bundles are composed of arteries, veins (in the limbs, usually in the form of accompanying veins), and nerves as well as lymphatic vessels, which are usually surrounded by a neurovascular sheath of varying density.

Surface Anatomy of Forearm

Three bony landmarks are easily palpated at the elbow: the *medial* and *lateral epicondyles* of the humerus and the *olecranon* of the ulna (Fig. 6.71). In the hollow located posterolaterally when the forearm is extended, the *head of the radius* can be palpated distal to the lateral epicondyle. Supinate and pronate your forearm and feel the movement of the radial head. The **posterior border of the ulna** is subcutaneous and can be palpated distally from the olecranon along the entire length of the bone. This landmark demarcates the posteromedial boundary separating the flexor–pronator (anterior) and extensor–supinator (posterior) compartments of the forearm.

The *cubital fossa*, the triangular hollow area on the anterior surface of the elbow, is bounded medially by the prominence formed by the *flexor–pronator group of muscles* that are attached to the medial epicondyle. To estimate the position of these muscles, put your thumb posterior to your medial epicondyle and then place your fingers on your forearm as shown in Figure 6.72A. The *black dot* on the dorsum of the hand indicates the position of the medial epicondyle.

The cubital fossa is bounded laterally by the prominence of the *extensor–supinator group of muscles* attached to the lateral epicondyle (Fig. 6.72B). The *pulsations of the radial artery* can be palpated throughout the forearm as it runs its superficial course from the cubital fossa to the wrist (anterior to the radial styloid process), demarcating the anterolateral boundary separating the flexor–pronator and extensor–supinator compartments of the forearm.

The *head of the ulna* is at its distal end and is easily seen and palpated. It appears as a rounded prominence at the wrist when the hand is pronated. The *ulnar styloid process* can be palpated just distal to the ulnar head. The larger *radial styloid process* can be easily palpated on the lateral side of the wrist when the hand is supinated, particularly when the tendons covering it are relaxed. The radial styloid process is located approximately 1 cm more distal than the ulnar styloid process. This relationship of the styloid processes is important in the diagnosis of certain injuries in the wrist region (e.g., fracture of the distal end of the radius). Proximal to the radial styloid process, the **surfaces of the radius** are palpable for a few centimeters. The lateral surface of the distal half of the radius is easy to palpate.

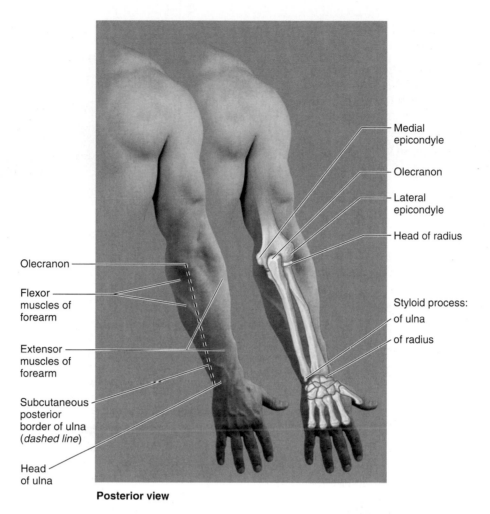

Posterior view

FIGURE 6.71. Surface anatomy of posterior forearm.

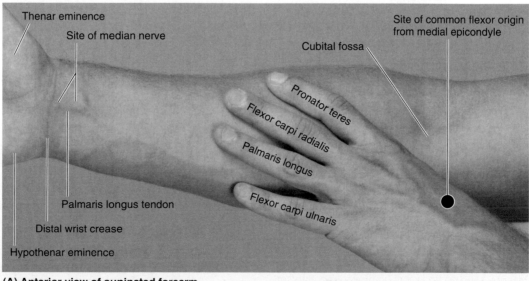

(A) Anterior view of supinated forearm

FIGURE 6.72. Surface anatomy of anterior forearm.

(B) Anterior view of pronated forearm

Dorsal venous network — Styloid process of ulna — Head of ulna — Cephalic vein — Extensor–supinator muscles of forearm

1 cm.

Styloid process of radius — Course of radial artery — Cubital fossa — Flexor–pronator muscles of forearm

FIGURE 6.72. (*Continued*) Surface anatomy of anterior forearm.

FOREARM

Elbow Tendinitis or Lateral Epicondylitis

Elbow tendinitis ("tennis elbow") is a painful musculoskeletal condition that may follow repetitive use of the superficial extensor muscles of the forearm. Pain is felt over the lateral epicondyle and radiates down the posterior surface of the forearm. People with elbow tendinitis often feel pain when they open a door or lift a glass. Repeated forceful flexion and extension of the wrist strain the attachment of the common extensor tendon, producing inflammation of the periosteum of the lateral epicondyle (*lateral epicondylitis*).

Mallet or Baseball Finger

Sudden severe tension on a long extensor tendon may avulse part of its attachment to the phalanx. The most common result of the injury is a *mallet* or *baseball finger* (Fig. B6.19A). This deformity results from the distal interphalangeal joint suddenly being forced into extreme flexion (hyperflexion) when, for example, a baseball is miscaught or a finger is jammed into the base pad (Fig. B6.19B). These actions avulse (tear away) the attachment of the tendon to the base of the distal phalanx. As a result, the person cannot extend the distal interphalangeal joint. The resultant deformity bears some resemblance to a mallet.

Fracture of Olecranon

Fracture of the olecranon, called a "fractured elbow" by laypersons, is common because the olecranon is subcutaneous and protrusive. The typical mechanism of injury is a fall on the elbow combined with sudden powerful contraction of the triceps brachii. The fractured olecranon is pulled away by the active and tonic contraction of the triceps

Mallet finger

(A)

Ruptured tendon

(B)

FIGURE B6.19. **Mallet finger. A.** The clinical appearance. **B.** Mechanism of injury.

(Fig. B6.20), and the injury is often considered to be an avulsion fracture (Salter, 1999). Because of the traction produced by the tonus of the triceps on the olecranon fragment, pinning

Triceps tendon — Humerus — Radius — Ulna

Olecranon

FIGURE B6.20.

is usually required. Healing occurs slowly, and often a cast must be worn for an extended period of time.

Synovial Cyst of Wrist

Sometimes a non-tender *cystic swelling* appears on the hand, most commonly on the dorsum of the wrist (Fig. B6.21). Usually the cyst is the size of a small grape, but it varies and may be as large as a plum. The thin-walled cyst contains clear mucinous fluid. The cause of the cyst is unknown, but it may result from mucoid degeneration (Salter, 1999). Flexion of the wrist makes the cyst enlarge, and it may be painful. Clinically, this type of swelling is called a "ganglion" (G., swelling or knot). Anatomically, a ganglion refers to a collection of nerve cell bodies (e.g., a spinal ganglion). Synovial cysts are close to and often communicate with the synovial sheaths on the dorsum of the wrist (*purple* in figure). The distal attachment of the ECRB tendon to the base of the 3rd metacarpal is another common site for such a cyst. A cystic swelling of the common flexor synovial sheath on the anterior aspect of the wrist can enlarge enough to produce compression of the median nerve by narrowing the carpal tunnel (*carpal tunnel syndrome*). This syndrome produces pain and paresthesia in the sensory distribution of the median nerve and clumsiness of finger movements (see the blue box "Carpal Tunnel Syndrome" on p. 790).

Cystic swelling

Synovial sheaths (*purple*)

Synovial cyst

Extensor tendons

FIGURE B6.21.

High Division of Brachial Artery

Sometimes the brachial artery divides at a more proximal level than usual. In this case, the ulnar and radial arteries begin in the superior or middle part of the arm, and the median nerve passes between them. The musculocutaneous and median nerves commonly communicate as shown in Figure B6.22.

Superficial Ulnar Artery

In approximately 3% of people, the ulnar artery descends superficial to the flexor muscles (Fig. B6.23). Pulsations of a superficial ulnar artery can be felt and

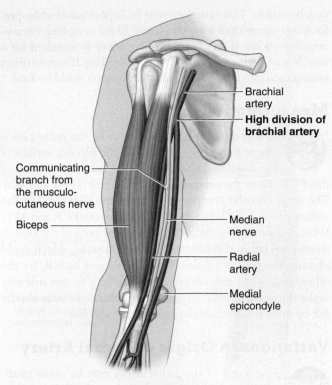

Brachial artery

High division of brachial artery

Communicating branch from the musculo-cutaneous nerve

Biceps

Median nerve

Radial artery

Medial epicondyle

FIGURE B6.22.

Deep fascia of arm

Brachial artery

Radial artery

Medial epicondyle

Bicipital aponeurosis

Superficial ulnar artery

Deep fascia of forearm

FIGURE B6.23.

Cubital Tunnel Syndrome

The ulnar nerve may be compressed (*ulnar nerve entrapment*) in the cubital tunnel formed by the tendinous arch joining the humeral and ulnar heads of attachment of the FCU (Fig. 6.59; Table 6.10). The signs and symptoms of *cubital tunnel syndrome* are the same as an ulnar nerve lesion in the ulnar groove on the posterior aspect of the medial epicondyle of the humerus.

Injury of Radial Nerve in Forearm (Superficial or Deep Branches)

The radial nerve is usually injured in the arm by a fracture of the humeral shaft. This injury is proximal to the motor branches to the long and short extensors of the wrist from the (common) radial nerve, and so *wrist-drop* is the primary clinical manifestation of an injury at this level (see the blue box "Injury to the Radial Nerve in Arm" on p. 743).

Injury to the deep branch of the radial nerve may occur when wounds of the posterior forearm are deep (penetrating). Severance of the deep branch results in an inability to extend the thumb and the metacarpophalangeal (MP) joints of the other digits. Thus the integrity of the deep branch may be tested by asking the person to extend the MP joints while the examiner provides resistance (Fig. B6.28). If the nerve is intact, the long extensor tendons should appear prominently on the dorsum of the hand, confirming that the extension is occurring at the MP joints rather than at the interphalangeal joints (movements under the control of other nerves).

Loss of sensation does not occur because the deep branch of the radial nerve is entirely muscular and articular in distribution. See Table 6.13 to determine the muscles that are paralyzed (e.g., extensor digitorum) when this nerve is severed.

When the superficial branch of the radial nerve, a cutaneous nerve, is severed, sensory loss is usually minimal. Commonly, a coin-shaped area of anesthesia occurs distal to the bases of the 1st and 2nd metacarpals. The reason the area of sensory loss is less than expected, given the areas highlighted in Figure 6.69D, is the result of the considerable overlap from cutaneous branches of the median and ulnar nerves.

FIGURE B6.28. Testing radial nerve.

The Bottom Line

FOREARM

Muscles of anterior compartment of forearm: The superficial and intermediate muscles of the anterior (flexor–pronator) compartment of the forearm are located anteromedially because they arise mainly from the common flexor attachment (medial epicondyle and supra-epicondylar ridge) of the humerus. ◆ Muscles in the superficial layer "bend" the wrist to position the hand (i.e., flex the wrist when acting exclusively and abduct or adduct the wrist when working with their extensor counterparts) and assist pronation. ◆ The only muscle of the intermediate layer (FDS) primarily flexes the proximal joints of 2nd–5th digits. ◆ Muscles of the deep layer attach to the anterior aspects of the radius and ulna, flex all (but especially the distal) joints of all five digits, and pronate the forearm. ◆ The muscles of the anterior compartment are innervated mostly by the median nerve, but one and a half muscles (the FCU and ulnar half of the FDP) are innervated by the ulnar nerve. ◆ Flexion of the wrist and hand is used for grasping, gripping, and drawing things toward one self. ◆ Pronation is

used for positioning the hand to manipulate or pick things up. Both movements are basic protective (defensive) movements.

Muscles of posterior compartment of forearm: The extensor-supinator muscles of the posterior compartment of the forearm are located posterolaterally in the proximal forearm, and are innervated by the radial nerve. ◆ The supinator acts at the radio-ulnar joint, while the remaining muscles extend and abduct the hand at the wrist joint and the thumb. The ECU may also contribute to adduction of the hand. ◆ The extensor muscles become tendinous in the distal forearm, and pass deep to the extensor retinaculum in osseofibrous tunnels. ◆ Tendons passing to the medial 4 digits are involved in complex extensor expansions on the dorsal aspects of the fingers. ◆ Extension ("cocking") of the wrist is important in enabling the flexors of the fingers to grip tightly or make a fist.

Superficial veins and cutaneous nerves of forearm: Well-developed subcutaneous veins course in the subcutaneous tissue of the forearm. These veins are subject to great variation. ♦ Once they have penetrated the deep fascia, cutaneous nerves run independently of the veins in the subcutaneous tissue, where they remain constant in location and size, with lateral, medial, and posterior cutaneous nerves of the forearm supplying the aspects of the forearm described by their names.

Neurovascular bundles of forearm: Three major (radial, median or middle, and ulnar) and two minor (anterior and posterior interosseous) neurovascular bundles occur deep to the antebrachial fascia. ♦ The radial neurovascular bundle—containing the radial artery, accompanying veins, and superficial radial nerve—courses along and defines the border between the anterior and the posterior forearm compartments (the vascular structures serving both) deep to the brachioradialis. ♦ The middle (median nerve and variable median artery and veins) and ulnar (ulnar nerve, artery, and accompanying veins) bundles course in a fascial plane between the intermediate and the deep flexor muscles. The median nerve supplies most muscles in the anterior compartment, many via its anterior interosseous branch, which courses on the interosseous membrane. ♦ The ulnar nerve supplies the one and a half exceptions (FCU and ulnar half of the FDP). ♦ The deep radial nerve penetrates the supinator to join the posterior interosseous artery in the plane between the superficial and the deep extensors. This nerve supplies all the muscles arising in the posterior compartment. ♦ The flexor muscles of the anterior compartment have approximately twice the bulk and strength of the extensor muscles of the posterior compartment. This, and the fact that the flexor aspect of the limb is the more protected aspect, accounts for the major neurovascular structures being located in the anterior compartment, with only the relatively small posterior interosseous vessels and nerve in the posterior compartment.

HAND

The **hand** is the manual part of the upper limb distal to the forearm. The **wrist** is located at the junction of the forearm and hand. Once positioned at the desired height and location relative to the body by movements at the shoulder and elbow, and the direction of action is established by pronation and supination of the forearm, the working position or attitude (tilt) of the hand is adjusted by movement at the wrist joint.

The skeleton of the hand (Fig. 6.9) consists of *carpals* in the wrist, *metacarpals* in the hand proper, and *phalanges* in the digits (fingers). The digits are numbered from one to five, beginning with the thumb: digit 1 is the thumb; digit 2, the index finger; digit 3, the middle finger; digit 4, the ring finger; and digit 5, the little finger. The palmar aspect of the hand features a central concavity that, with the crease proximal to it (over the wrist bones) separates two eminences: a lateral, larger and more prominent **thenar eminence** at the base of the thumb, and a medial, smaller **hypothenar eminence** proximal to the base of the 5th finger (Fig 6.72A).

Because of the importance of manual dexterity in occupational and recreational activities, a good understanding of the structure and function of the hand is essential for all persons involved in maintaining or restoring its activities: free motion, power grasping, precision handling, and pinching.

The **power grip** (palm grasp) refers to forcible motions of the digits acting against the palm; the fingers are wrapped around an object with counterpressure from the thumb—for example, when grasping a cylindrical structure (Fig. 6.73A). The power grip involves the long flexor muscles to the digits (acting at the interphalangeal joints), the intrinsic muscles in the palm (acting at the metacarpophalangeal joints), and the extensors of the wrist (acting at the radiocarpal and midcarpal joints). The "cocking" of the wrist by the extensors increases the distance over which the flexors of the fingers act, producing the same result as a more complete muscular contraction. Conversely, as flexion increases at the wrist, the grip becomes weaker and more insecure.

The **hook grip** is the posture of the hand that is used when carrying a briefcase (Fig. 6.73B). This grip consumes less energy, involving mainly the long flexors of the digits, which are flexed to a varying degree, depending on the size of the object that is grasped.

The **precision handling grip** involves a change in the position of a handled object that requires fine control of the movements of the digits (fingers)—for example, holding a pencil, manipulating a coin, threading a needle, or buttoning a shirt (Fig. 6.73C & D). In a precision grip, the wrist and digits are held firmly by the long flexor and extensor muscles, and the intrinsic hand muscles perform fine movements of the digits.

Pinching refers to compression of something between the thumb and the index finger—for example, handling a teacup or holding a coin on edge (Fig. 6.73E)—or between the thumb and the adjacent two fingers—for example, snapping the fingers.

The **position of rest** is assumed by an inactive hand—for example, when the forearm and hand are laid on a table (Fig. 6.73F). This position is often used when it is necessary to immobilize the wrist and hand in a cast to stabilize a fracture.

Fascia and Compartments of Palm

The *fascia of the palm* is continuous with the antebrachial fascia and the fascia of the dorsum of the hand (Fig. 6.58). The **palmar fascia** is thin over the thenar and hypothenar eminences, as **thenar** and **hypothenar fascia**, respectively (Figs. 6.74A and 6.75A). However, the palmar fascia is thick

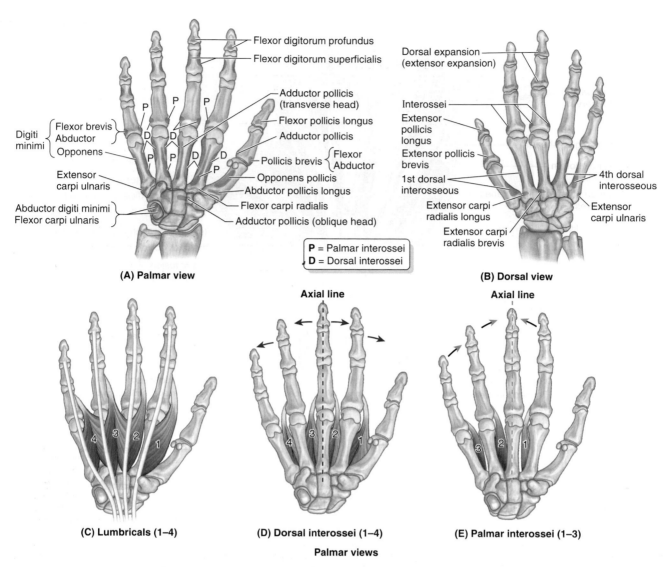

(A) Palmar view

- Flexor digitorum profundus
- Flexor digitorum superficialis
- Adductor pollicis (transverse head)
- Flexor pollicis longus
- Adductor pollicis
- Pollicis brevis { Flexor / Abductor }
- Opponens pollicis
- Abductor pollicis longus
- Flexor carpi radialis
- Adductor pollicis (oblique head)

- Digiti minimi { Flexor brevis / Abductor / Opponens }
- Extensor carpi ulnaris
- Abductor digiti minimi / Flexor carpi ulnaris

P = Palmar interossei
D = Dorsal interossei

(B) Dorsal view

- Dorsal expansion (extensor expansion)
- Interossei
- Extensor pollicis longus
- Extensor pollicis brevis
- 1st dorsal interosseous
- Extensor carpi radialis longus
- Extensor carpi radialis brevis
- 4th dorsal interosseous
- Extensor carpi ulnaris

(C) Lumbricals (1–4)

(D) Dorsal interossei (1–4) — Axial line

(E) Palmar interossei (1–3) — Axial line

Palmar views

FIGURE 6.78. Attachments of intrinsic muscles of hand and actions of interossei.

TABLE 6.14. INTRINSIC MUSCLES OF HAND

Muscle	Proximal Attachment	Distal Attachment	Innervation[a]	Main Action
Thenar muscles				
Opponens pollicis		Lateral side of 1st metacarpal	Recurrent branch of median nerve (**C8**, T1)	To oppose thumb, it draws 1st metacarpal medially to center of palm and rotates it medially
Abductor pollicis brevis	Flexor retinaculum and tubercles of scaphoid and trapezium	Lateral side of base of proximal phalanx of thumb		Abducts thumb; helps oppose it
Flexor pollicis brevis				Flexes thumb
Superficial head				
Deep head				
Adductor pollicis			Deep branch of ulnar nerve (C8, **T1**)	Adducts thumb toward lateral border of palm
Oblique head	Bases of 2nd and 3rd metacarpals, capitate, and adjacent carpals	Medial side of base of proximal phalanx of thumb		
Transverse head	Anterior surface of shaft of 3rd metacarpal			

(continued)

TABLE 6.14. INTRINSIC MUSCLES OF HAND (Continued)

Muscle	Proximal Attachment	Distal Attachment	Innervation[a]	Main Action
Hypothenar muscles				
Abductor digiti minimi	Pisiform	Medial side of base of proximal phalanx of 5th digit	Deep branch of ulnar nerve (C8, **T1**)	Abducts 5th digit; assists in flexion of its proximal phalanx
Flexor digiti minimi brevis	Hook of hamate and flexor retinaculum			Flexes proximal phalanx of 5th digit
Opponens digiti		Medial border of 5th metacarpal		Draws 5th metacarpal anterior and rotates it, bringing 5th digit into opposition with thumb
Short muscles				
Lumbricals				
1st and 2nd	Lateral two tendons of flexor digitorum profundus (as unipennate muscles)	Lateral sides of extensor expansions of 2nd–5th digits	Median nerve (C8, **T1**)	Flex metacarpophalangeal joints; extend interphalangeal joints of 2nd–5th digits
3rd and 4th	Medial three tendons of flexor digitorum profundus (as bipennate muscles)		Deep branch of ulnar nerve (C8, **T1**)	
Dorsal interossei, 1st–4th	Adjacent sides of two metacarpals (as bipennate muscles)	Bases of proximal phalanges; extensor expansions of 2nd–4th digits		Abduct 2nd–4th digits from axial line; act with lumbricals in flexing metacarpophalangeal joints and extending interphalangeal joints
Palmar interossei, 1st–3rd	Palmar surfaces of 2nd, 4th, and 5th metacarpals (as unipennate muscles)	Bases of proximal phalanges; extensor expansions of 2nd, 4th, and 5th digits		Adduct 2nd, 4th, and 5th digits toward axial line; assist lumbricals in flexing metacarpophalangeal joints and extending interphalangeal joints; extensor expansions of 2nd–4th digits

[a]The spinal cord segmental innervation is indicated (e.g., "**C8**, T1" means that the nerves supplying the opponens pollicis are derived from the eighth cervical segment and first thoracic segment of the spinal cord). Numbers in boldface (**C8**) indicate the main segmental innervation. Damage to one or more of the listed spinal cord segments or to the motor nerve roots arising from them results in paralysis of the muscles concerned.

Abductor Pollicis Brevis. The **abductor pollicis brevis (APB),** the short abductor of the thumb, forms the anterolateral part of the thenar eminence. In addition to abducting the thumb, the APB assists the opponens pollicis during the early stages of opposition by rotating its proximal phalanx slightly medially.

To test the abductor pollicis brevis, abduct the thumb against resistance. If acting normally, the muscle can be seen and palpated.

Flexor Pollicis Brevis. The **flexor pollicis brevis (FPB),** the short flexor of the thumb, is located medial to the APB (Fig. 6.77A). Its two bellies, located on opposite sides of the tendon of the FPL, share (with each other and often with the APB) a common, sesamoid-containing tendon at their distal attachment. The bellies usually differ in their innervation: The larger superficial head of the FPB is innervated by the recurrent branch of the median nerve, whereas the smaller deep head is usually innervated by the deep palmar branch of the ulnar nerve. The FPB flexes the thumb at the carpometacarpal and metacarpophalangeal joints and aids in opposition of the thumb.

To test the flexor pollicis brevis, flex the thumb against resistance. If acting normally, the muscle can be seen and palpated; however, keep in mind that the FPL also flexes the thumb.

Opponens Pollicis. The **opponens pollicis** is a quadrangular muscle that lies deep to the APB and lateral to the FPB (Fig. 6.77B). The opponens pollicis opposes the thumb, the most important thumb movement. It flexes and rotates the 1st metacarpal medially at the carpometacarpal joint during opposition; this movement occurs when picking up an object. During *opposition,* the tip of the thumb is brought into contact with the pulp (pad) of the little finger, as shown in Figure 6.76.

ADDUCTOR POLLICIS

The **adductor pollicis** is located in the adductor compartment of the hand (Fig. 6.75A). The fan-shaped muscle has two heads of origin, which are separated by the radial artery as it enters the palm to form the deep palmar arch (Figs. 6.77A and 6.79). Its tendon usually contains a sesamoid bone. The adductor pollicis adducts the thumb, moving the thumb to

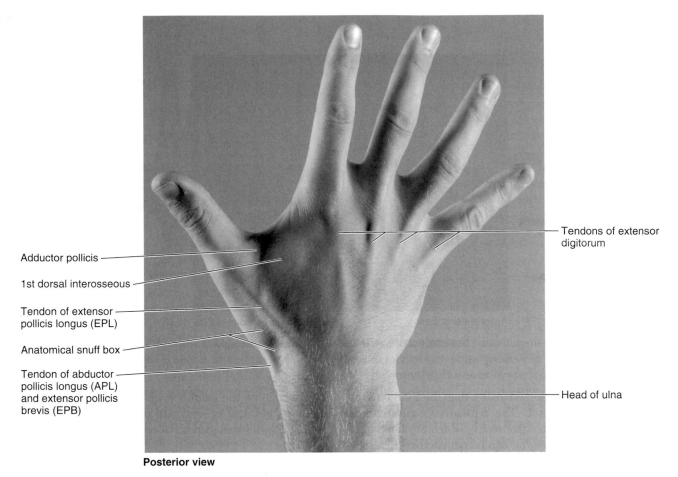

Adductor pollicis

1st dorsal interosseous

Tendon of extensor pollicis longus (EPL)

Anatomical snuff box

Tendon of abductor pollicis longus (APL) and extensor pollicis brevis (EPB)

Tendons of extensor digitorum

Head of ulna

Posterior view

FIGURE 6.88. Surface anatomy of dorsum of hand.

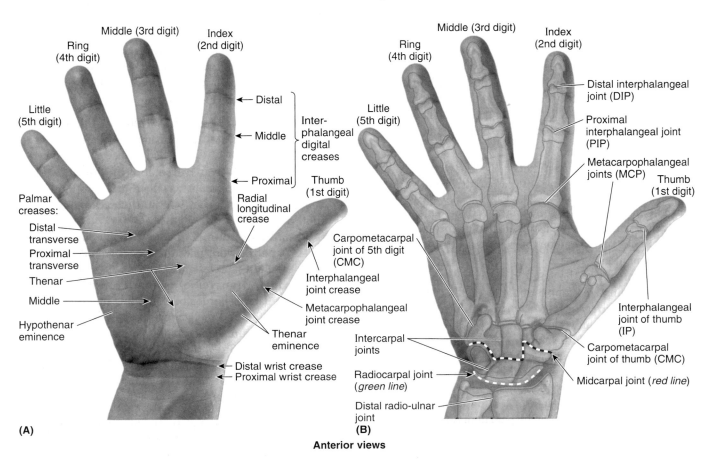

Ring (4th digit)

Middle (3rd digit)

Index (2nd digit)

Little (5th digit)

Distal

Middle

Proximal

Inter-phalangeal digital creases

Thumb (1st digit)

Radial longitudinal crease

Palmar creases:

Distal transverse

Proximal transverse

Thenar

Middle

Hypothenar eminence

Interphalangeal joint crease

Metacarpophalangeal joint crease

Thenar eminence

Distal wrist crease
Proximal wrist crease

(A)

Middle (3rd digit)

Index (2nd digit)

Ring (4th digit)

Little (5th digit)

Distal interphalangeal joint (DIP)

Proximal interphalangeal joint (PIP)

Metacarpophalangeal joints (MCP)

Thumb (1st digit)

Interphalangeal joint of thumb (IP)

Carpometacarpal joint of thumb (CMC)

Midcarpal joint (*red line*)

Carpometacarpal joint of 5th digit (CMC)

Intercarpal joints

Radiocarpal joint (*green line*)

Distal radio-ulnar joint

(B)

Anterior views

FIGURE 6.89. Surface anatomy of palmar aspect of hand.

Each of the medial four fingers usually has three *transverse digital flexion creases:*

- **Proximal digital crease:** located at the root of the finger, approximately 2 cm distal to the metacarpophalangeal joint.
- **Middle digital crease:** lies over the proximal interphalangeal joint.
- **Distal digital crease:** lies over or just proximal to the distal interphalangeal joint.

The thumb, having two phalanges, has only two flexion creases. The proximal digital crease of the thumb crosses obliquely, at or proximal to the 1st metacarpophalangeal joint. The **skin ridges** on the pulp (pads) of the digits, forming the *fingerprints,* are used for identification because of their unique patterns. The physiological function of the skin ridges is to reduce slippage when grasping objects.

HAND

Dupuytren Contracture of Palmar Fascia

 Dupuytren contracture is a disease of the palmar fascia resulting in progressive shortening, thickening, and fibrosis of the palmar fascia and aponeurosis. The fibrous degeneration of the longitudinal bands of the palmar aponeurosis on the medial side of the hand pulls the 4th and 5th fingers into partial flexion at the metacarpophalangeal and proximal interphalangeal joints (Fig. B6.29A).

(A) Longitudinal bands of palmar aponeurosis to fibrous digital sheaths of digits four and five nodular and contracted

(B)

FIGURE B6.29. Dupuytren contracture.

The contracture is frequently bilateral and is seen in some men > 50 years of age. Its cause is unknown, but evidence points to a hereditary predisposition. The disease first manifests as painless nodular thickenings of the palmar aponeurosis that adhere to the skin. Gradually, progressive contracture of the longitudinal bands produces raised ridges in the palmar skin that extend from the proximal part of the hand to the base of the 4th and 5th fingers (Fig. B6.29B). Treatment of Dupuytren contracture usually involves surgical excision of all fibrotic parts of the palmar fascia to free the fingers (Salter, 1999).

Hand Infections

 Because the palmar fascia is thick and strong, swellings resulting from hand infections usually appear on the dorsum of the hand, where the fascia is thinner. The potential fascial spaces of the palm are important because they may become infected. The fascial spaces determine the extent and direction of the spread of pus formed by these infections.

Depending on the site of infection, pus will accumulate in the thenar, hypothenar, midpalmar, or adductor compartments (Fig. 6.75A). Antibiotic therapy has made infections that spread beyond one of these fascial compartments rare; however, an untreated infection can spread proximally from the midpalmar space through the carpal tunnel into the forearm, anterior to the pronator quadratus and its fascia.

Tenosynovitis

Injuries such as a puncture of a finger by a rusty nail can cause *infection of the digital synovial sheaths* (Fig. 6.81A). When inflammation of the tendon and synovial sheath occurs (*tenosynovitis*), the digit swells and movement becomes painful. Because the tendons of the 2nd, 3rd, and 4th fingers nearly always have separate synovial sheaths, the infection is usually confined to the infected finger. If the infection is untreated, however, the proximal ends of these sheaths may rupture, allowing the infection to spread to the midpalmar space (Fig. 6.75B).

Because the synovial sheath of the little finger is usually continuous with the common flexor sheath (Fig. 6.81B), tenosynovitis in this finger may spread to the common flexor sheath and thus through the palm and carpal tunnel to the anterior forearm, draining into the space between the pronator quadratus and the overlying flexor tendons (*Parona space*). Likewise, tenosynovitis in the thumb may spread via the continuous synovial sheath of the FPL (radial bursa). How far an infection spreads from the fingers depends on variations in their connections with the common flexor sheath.

The tendons of the APL and EPB are in the same tendinous sheath on the dorsum of the wrist. Excessive friction of these tendons on their common sheath results in fibrous thickening of the sheath and stenosis of the osseofibrous tunnel. The excessive friction is caused by repetitive forceful use of the hands during gripping and wringing (e.g., squeezing water out of clothes). This condition, called *Quervain tenovaginitis stenosans*, causes pain in the wrist that radiates proximally to the forearm and distally toward the thumb. Local tenderness is felt over the common flexor sheath on the lateral side of the wrist.

Thickening of a fibrous digital sheath on the palmar aspect of the digit produces stenosis of the osseofibrous tunnel, the result of repetitive forceful use of the fingers. If the tendons of the FDS and FDP enlarge proximal to the tunnel, the person is unable to extend the finger. When the finger is extended passively, a snap is audible. Flexion produces another snap as the thickened tendon moves. This condition is called digital tenovaginitis stenosans (*trigger finger* or snapping finger).

Laceration of Palmar Arches

Bleeding is usually profuse when the palmar (arterial) arches are lacerated. It may not be sufficient to ligate only one forearm artery when the arches are lacerated, because these vessels usually have numerous communications in the forearm and hand and thus bleed from both ends. To obtain a bloodless surgical operating field for treating complicated hand injuries, it may be necessary to compress the brachial artery and its branches proximal to the elbow (e.g., using a pneumatic tourniquet). This procedure prevents blood from reaching the ulnar and radial arteries through the anastomoses around the elbow (Fig. 6.67A).

Ischemia of Digits (Fingers)

Intermittent bilateral attacks of *ischemia of the digits*, marked by cyanosis and often accompanied by paresthesia and pain, is characteristically brought on by cold and emotional stimuli. The condition may result from an anatomical abnormality or an underlying disease. When the cause of the condition is idiopathic (unknown) or primary, it is called *Raynaud syndrome* (disease).

The arteries of the upper limb are innervated by sympathetic nerves. Postsynaptic fibers from the sympathetic ganglia enter nerves that form the brachial plexus and are distributed to the digital arteries through branches arising from the plexus. When treating ischemia resulting from Raynaud syndrome, it may be necessary to perform a cervico-

dorsal *presynaptic sympathectomy* (excision of a segment of a sympathetic nerve) to dilate the digital arteries.

Lesions of Median Nerve

Lesions of the median nerve usually occur in two places: the forearm and the wrist. The most common site is where the nerve passes through the carpal tunnel.

CARPAL TUNNEL SYNDROME

Carpal tunnel syndrome results from any lesion that significantly reduces the size of the carpal tunnel (Fig. B6.30A–D) or, more commonly, increases the size of some of the nine structures or their coverings that pass through it (e.g., inflammation of synovial sheaths). Fluid retention, infection, and excessive exercise of the fingers may cause swelling of the tendons or their synovial sheaths. The median nerve is the most sensitive structure in the tunnel. The median nerve has two terminal sensory branches that supply the skin of the hand; hence *paresthesia* (tingling), *hypoesthesia* (diminished sensation), or *anesthesia* (absence of sensation) may occur in the lateral three and a half digits. The palmar cutaneous branch of the median nerve arises proximal to, and does not pass through, the carpal tunnel; thus sensation in the central palm remains unaffected. The nerve also has one terminal motor branch, the recurrent branch, which serves the three thenar muscles (Fig. 6.85A).

Progressive loss of coordination and strength of the thumb (owing to weakness of the APB and opponens pollicis) may occur if the cause of compression is not alleviated. Individuals with carpal tunnel syndrome are unable to oppose their thumbs (Fig. B6.30E) and have difficulty buttoning a shirt or blouse as well as gripping things such as a comb. As the condition progresses, sensory changes radiate into the forearm and axilla. Symptoms of compression can be reproduced by compression of the median nerve with your finger at the wrist for approximately 30 seconds. To relieve both the compression and the resulting symptoms, partial or complete surgical division of the flexor retinaculum, a procedure called *carpal tunnel release*, may be necessary. The incision for carpal tunnel release is made toward the medial side of the wrist and flexor retinaculum to avoid possible injury to the recurrent branch of the median nerve.

TRAUMA TO MEDIAN NERVE

Laceration of the wrist often causes *median nerve injury* because this nerve is relatively close to the surface. In attempted suicides by wrist slashing, the median nerve is commonly injured just proximal to the flexor retinaculum. This results in paralysis of the thenar muscles and the first two lumbricals. Hence opposition of the thumb is not possible and fine control movements of the 2nd and 3rd digits are impaired. Sensation is also lost over the thumb and adjacent two and a half fingers.

Most nerve injuries in the upper limb affect opposition of the thumb (Fig. 6.76). Undoubtedly, injuries to the nerves supplying the intrinsic muscles of the hand, especially the

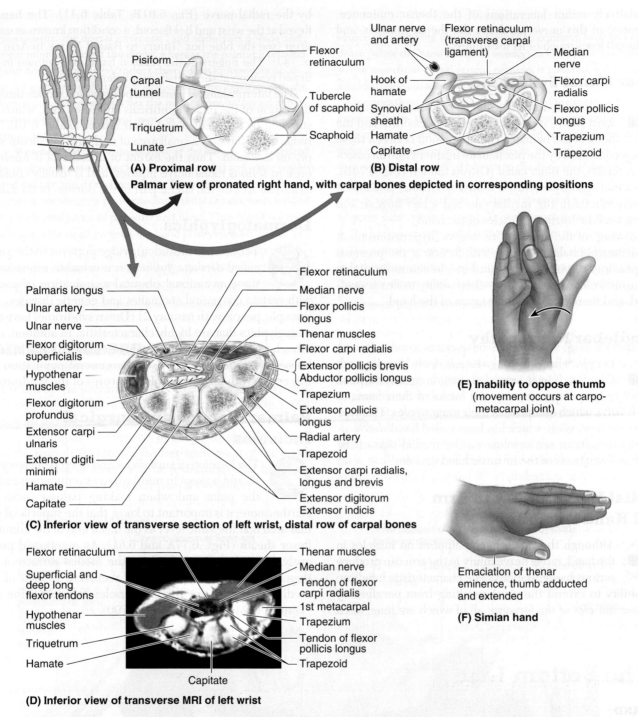

Pisiform
Carpal tunnel
Triquetrum
Lunate

Flexor retinaculum
Tubercle of scaphoid
Scaphoid

(A) Proximal row

Ulnar nerve and artery
Flexor retinaculum (transverse carpal ligament)
Median nerve
Hook of hamate
Synovial sheath
Hamate
Capitate
Flexor carpi radialis
Flexor pollicis longus
Trapezium
Trapezoid

(B) Distal row

Palmar view of pronated right hand, with carpal bones depicted in corresponding positions

Palmaris longus
Ulnar artery
Ulnar nerve
Flexor digitorum superficialis
Hypothenar muscles
Flexor digitorum profundus
Extensor carpi ulnaris
Extensor digiti minimi
Hamate
Capitate

Flexor retinaculum
Median nerve
Flexor pollicis longus
Thenar muscles
Flexor carpi radialis
Extensor pollicis brevis
Abductor pollicis longus
Trapezium
Extensor pollicis longus
Radial artery
Trapezoid
Extensor carpi radialis, longus and brevis
Extensor digitorum
Extensor indicis

(C) Inferior view of transverse section of left wrist, distal row of carpal bones

(E) Inability to oppose thumb
(movement occurs at carpo-metacarpal joint)

Flexor retinaculum
Superficial and deep long flexor tendons
Hypothenar muscles
Triquetrum
Hamate

Thenar muscles
Median nerve
Tendon of flexor carpi radialis
1st metacarpal
Trapezium
Tendon of flexor pollicis longus
Trapezoid

Capitate

(D) Inferior view of transverse MRI of left wrist

Emaciation of thenar eminence, thumb adducted and extended

(F) Simian hand

FIGURE B6.30.

median nerve, have the most severe effects on this complex movement. If the median nerve is severed in the forearm or at the wrist, the thumb cannot be opposed; however, the APL and adductor pollicis (supplied by the posterior interosseous and ulnar nerves, respectively) may imitate opposition, although ineffective.

Median nerve injury resulting from a perforating wound in the elbow region results in loss of flexion of the proximal and distal interphalangeal joints of the 2nd and 3rd digits.

The ability to flex the metacarpophalangeal joints of these fingers is also affected because digital branches of the median nerve supply the 1st and 2nd lumbricals. *Simian hand* (Fig. B6.30F) refers to a deformity in which thumb movements are limited to flexion and extension of the thumb in the plane of the palm. This condition is caused by the inability to oppose and by limited abduction of the thumb. The recurrent branch of the median nerve to the thenar muscles (Fig. 6.84A) lies subcutaneously and may be severed contacts the *coraco-acromial arch,* preventing further abduction. If the arm is then laterally rotated 180°, the tubercles are rotated posteriorly and more articular surface becomes available to continue elevation.

Circumduction at the glenohumeral joint is an orderly sequence of flexion, abduction, extension, and adduction—or the reverse (Fig. 6.91). Unless performed over a small range, these movements do not occur at the glenohumeral joint in isolation; they are accompanied by movements at the two other joints of the pectoral girdle (SC and AC). Stiffening or fixation of the joints of the pectoral girdle (*ankylosis*) results in a much more restricted range of movement, even if the glenohumeral joint is normal.

MUSCLES MOVING GLENOHUMERAL JOINT

The movements of the glenohumeral joint and the muscles that produce them—the *axio-appendicular muscles,* which may act indirectly on the joint (i.e., act on the pectoral girdle), and the *scapulohumeral muscles,* which act directly on the glenohumeral joint (Tables 6.4 and 6.5)—are illustrated in Figure 6.96 and listed in Table 6.17. Other muscles that serve the glenohumeral joint as shunt muscles, acting to resist dislocation without producing movement at the joint (e.g., when carrying a heavy suitcase), or that maintain the large head of the humerus in the relatively shallow glenoid cavity are also listed in the table.

BLOOD SUPPLY OF GLENOHUMERAL JOINT

The glenohumeral joint is supplied by the *anterior* and *posterior circumflex humeral arteries* and branches of the *suprascapular artery* (Fig. 6.39; Table 6.7).

INNERVATION OF GLENOHUMERAL JOINT

The suprascapular, axillary, and lateral pectoral nerves supply the glenohumeral joint (Table 6.8).

BURSAE AROUND GLENOHUMERAL JOINT

Several **bursae** (sac-like cavities), containing capillary films of *synovial fluid* secreted by the synovial membrane, are situated near the glenohumeral joint. Bursae are located where tendons rub against bone, ligaments, or other tendons, and where skin moves over a bony prominence. The bursae around the glenohumeral joint are of special clinical importance because some of them communicate with the joint cavity (e.g., the subscapular bursa). Consequently, opening a bursa may mean entering the cavity of the glenohumeral joint.

Subtendinous Bursa of Subscapularis. The **subtendinous bursa of subscapularis** is located between the tendon of the subscapularis and the neck of the scapula (Fig. 6.93A). The bursa protects the tendon where it passes inferior to the root of the coracoid process and over the neck

of the scapula. It usually communicates with the cavity of the glenohumeral joint through an opening in the fibrous layer of the joint capsule (Fig. 6.94A); thus it is really an extension of the glenohumeral joint cavity.

Subacromial Bursa. Sometimes referred to as the *subdeltoid bursa,* the **subacromial bursa** is located between the acromion, coraco-acromial ligament, and deltoid superiorly and the supraspinatus tendon and joint capsule of the glenohumeral joint inferiorly (Fig. 6.95A). Thus it facilitates movement of the supraspinatus tendon under the coraco-acromial arch and of the deltoid over the joint capsule of the glenohumeral joint and the greater tubercle of the humerus. Its size varies, but it does not normally communicate with the cavity of the glenohumeral joint.

Elbow Joint

The **elbow joint,** a hinge type of synovial joint, is located 2–3 cm inferior to the epicondyles of the humerus (Fig. 6.97).

ARTICULATION OF ELBOW JOINT

The spool-shaped *trochlea* and spheroidal *capitulum* of the humerus articulate with the *trochlear notch* of the ulna and the slightly concave superior aspect of the *head of the radius,* respectively; therefore, there are humero-ulnar and humero-radial articulations. The articular surfaces, covered with hyaline cartilage, are most fully congruent (in contact) when the forearm is in a position midway between pronation and supination and is flexed to a right angle.

JOINT CAPSULE OF ELBOW JOINT

The *fibrous layer of the joint capsule* surrounds the elbow joint (Fig. 6.97A & C). It is attached to the humerus at the margins of the lateral and medial ends of the articular surfaces of the capitulum and trochlea. Anteriorly and posteriorly, it is carried superiorly, proximal to the coronoid and olecranon fossae.

The *synovial membrane* lines the internal surface of the fibrous layer of the capsule and the intracapsular nonarticular parts of the humerus. It is also continuous inferiorly with the synovial membrane of the proximal radio-ulnar joint. The joint capsule is weak anteriorly and posteriorly but is strengthened on each side by collateral ligaments.

LIGAMENTS OF ELBOW JOINT

The collateral ligaments of the elbow joint are strong triangular bands that are medial and lateral thickenings of the fibrous layer of the joint capsule (Figs. 6.97A and 6.98). The lateral, fan-like **radial collateral ligament** extends from the lateral epicondyle of the humerus and blends distally with the **anular ligament of the radius,** which encircles and holds the head of the radius in the radial notch of the ulna, forming the proximal radio-ulnar joint and permitting pronation and supination of the forearm.

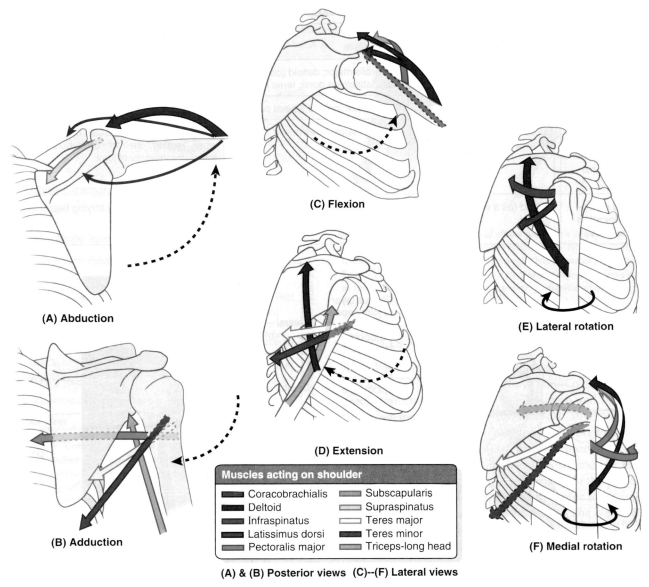

(A) Abduction

(B) Adduction

(C) Flexion

(D) Extension

(E) Lateral rotation

(F) Medial rotation

Muscles acting on shoulder

▬ Coracobrachialis	▬ Subscapularis
▬ Deltoid	▬ Supraspinatus
▬ Infraspinatus	▬ Teres major
▬ Latissimus dorsi	▬ Teres minor
▬ Pectoralis major	▬ Triceps-long head

(A) & (B) Posterior views (C)--(F) Lateral views

FIGURE 6.96. Movements of glenohumeral joint.

TABLE 6.17. MOVEMENTS OF GLENOHUMERAL JOINT

Movement (Function)	Prime Mover(s) (From Pendent Position)	Synergists	Notes
Flexion	Pectoralis major (clavicular head); deltoid (clavicular and anterior acromial parts)	Coracobrachialis (assisted by biceps brachii)	From fully extended position to its own (coronal) plane, sternocostal head of pectoralis major is major force
Extension	Deltoid (spinal part)	Teres major; latissimus dorsi; long head of triceps brachii	Latissimus dorsi, (sternocostal head of pectoralis major, and long head of triceps brachii) act from fully flexed position to their own (coronal) planes
Abduction	Deltoid (as a whole, but especially acromial part)	Supraspinatus	Supraspinatus is particularly important in initiating movement; also, upward rotation of scapula occurs throughout movement, making a significant contribution
Adduction	Pectoralis major; latissimus dorsi	Teres major; long head of triceps brachii	In upright position and in absence of resistance, gravity is prime mover

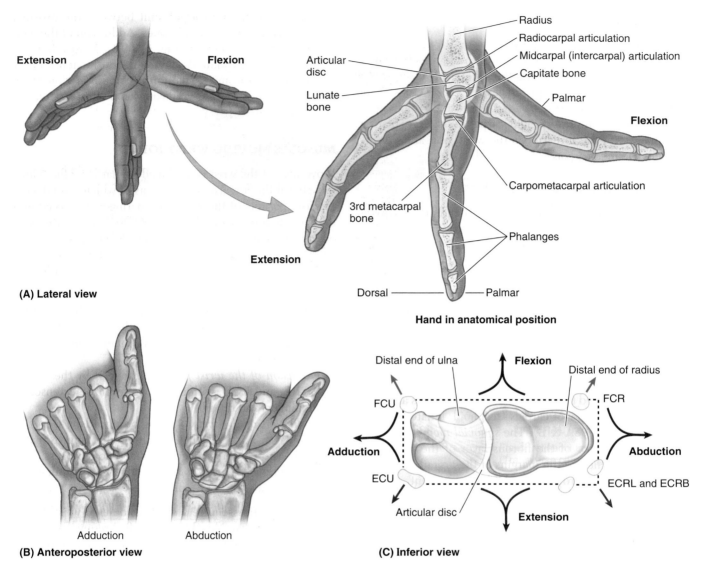

FIGURE 6.109. Movements of wrist. A. In this sagittal section of the wrist and hand during extension and flexion, observe the radiocarpal, midcarpal, and carpometacarpal articulations. Most movement occurs at the radiocarpal joint, with additional movement taking place at the midcarpal joint during full flexion and extension. **B.** Movement at the radiocarpal (RC) and midcarpal (MC) joints during adduction and abduction is demonstrated as seen in posteroanterior radiography. **C.** The *arrows* indicate the direction the hand would move when tendons of the primary ("carpi") muscles acting at the "four corners" of the joint act individually or in unison. *ECRB,* extensor carpi radialis brevis; *ECRL,* extensor carpi radialis longus; *ECU,* extensor carpi ulnaris; *FCR,* flexor carpi radialis; *FCU,* flexor carpi ulnaris.

- The **midcarpal joint,** a complex joint between the proximal and distal rows of carpal bones.
- The **pisotriquetral joint,** formed from the articulation of the pisiform with the palmar surface of the triquetrum.

JOINT CAPSULE OF INTERCARPAL JOINTS

A continuous, common articular cavity is formed by the IC and carpometacarpal joints, with the exception of the **carpometacarpal joint of the thumb,** which is independent. The wrist joint is also independent. The continuity of the articular cavities, or the lack of it, is significant in relation to the spread of infection and to *arthroscopy,* in which a flexible fiberoptic scope is inserted into the articular cavity to

view its internal surfaces and features. The *fibrous layer of the joint capsule* surrounds the IC joints, which helps unite the carpals. The *synovial membrane* lines the fibrous layer and is attached to the margins of the articular surfaces of the carpals.

LIGAMENTS OF INTERCARPAL JOINTS

The carpals are united by anterior, posterior, and interosseous ligaments (Figs. 6.108 and 6.110A).

MOVEMENTS OF INTERCARPAL JOINTS

The gliding movements possible between the carpals occur concomitantly with movements at the wrist joint, augment-

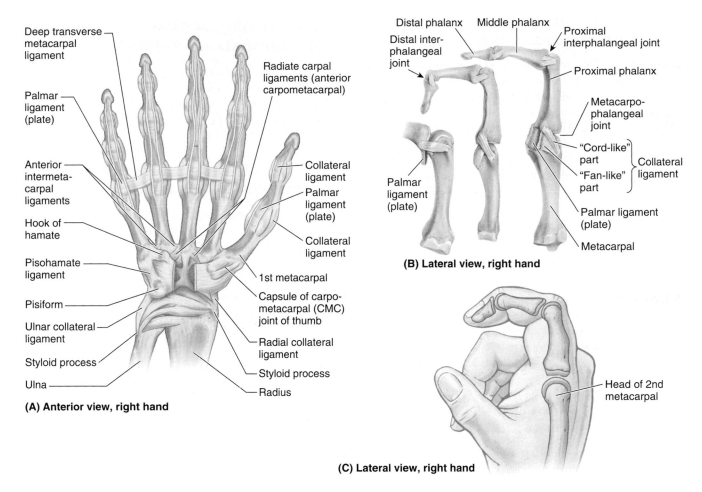

FIGURE 6.110. Joints of hand. A. Palmar ligaments of the radio-ulnar, radiocarpal, intercarpal, carpometacarpal, and interphalangeal joints. B. Meta-carpophalangeal and interphalangeal joints. The palmar ligaments (plates) are modifications of the anterior aspect of the MP and IP joint capsules. C. The flexed index finger demonstrates its phalanges and the position of the MP and IP joints. The knuckles are formed by the heads of the bones, with the joint plane lying distally.

ing them and increasing the overall range of movement. Flexion and extension of the hand are actually initiated at the *midcarpal joint,* between the proximal and the distal rows of carpals (Figs. 6.107B and 6.109A). Most flexion and adduction occur mainly at the wrist joint, whereas extension and abduction occur primarily at the midcarpal joint. Movements at the other IC joints are small, with the proximal row being more mobile than the distal row.

BLOOD SUPPLY OF INTERCARPAL JOINTS

The arteries supplying the IC joints are derived from the dorsal and palmar carpal arches (Fig. 6.82; Table 6.15).

INNERVATION OF INTERCARPAL JOINTS

The IC joints are supplied by the anterior interosseous branch of the *median nerve* and the dorsal and deep branches of the *ulnar nerve* (Fig. 6.85; Table 6.16).

Carpometacarpal and Intermetacarpal Joints

The **carpometacarpal (CMC)** and **intermetacarpal (IM) joints** are the plane type of synovial joint, except for the **CMC joint of the thumb,** which is a saddle joint (Fig. 6.107).

ARTICULATIONS OF CARPOMETACARPAL AND INTERMETACARPAL JOINTS

The distal surfaces of the carpals of the distal row articulate with the carpal surfaces of the bases of the metacarpals at the CMC joints. The important CMC joint of the thumb is between the trapezium and the base of the 1st metacarpal; it has a separate articular cavity. Like the carpals, adjacent metacarpals articulate with each other; IM joints occur between the radial and ulnar aspects of the bases of the metacarpals.

JOINT CAPSULE OF CARPOMETACARPAL AND INTERMETACARPAL JOINTS

The medial four CMC joints and three IM joints are enclosed by a *common joint capsule* on the palmar and dorsal surfaces. A *common synovial membrane* lines the internal surface of the fibrous layer of the joint capsule, surrounding a common articular cavity. The *fibrous layer of the CMC joint of the thumb* surrounds the joint and is attached to the margins of the articular surfaces. The *synovial membrane* lines the internal surface of the fibrous layer. The looseness of the capsule facilitates free movement of the joint of the thumb.

LIGAMENTS OF CARPOMETACARPAL AND INTERMETACARPAL JOINTS

The bones are united in the region of the joints by **palmar** and **dorsal CMC** and **IM ligaments** (Fig. 6.110A) and by **interosseous IM ligaments** (Fig. 6.107B). In addition, the superficial and deep **transverse metacarpal ligaments** (the former part of the palmar aponeurosis), associated with the distal ends of the metacarpals, play a role in limiting movement at the CMC and IM joints as they limit separation of the metacarpal heads.

MOVEMENTS OF CARPOMETACARPAL AND INTERMETACARPAL JOINTS

The CMC joint of the thumb permits angular movements in any plane (flexion–extension, abduction–adduction, or circumduction) and a restricted amount of axial rotation. Most important, *the movement essential to opposition of the thumb occurs here.* Although the opponens pollicis is the prime mover, all of the hypothenar muscles contribute to opposition.

Almost no movement occurs at the CMC joints of the 2nd and 3rd digits, that of the 4th digit is slightly mobile, and that of the 5th digit is moderately mobile, flexing and rotating slightly during a tight grasp (Fig. 6.73G & H). When the palm of the hand is "cupped" (as during pad-to-pad opposition of thumb and little finger), two thirds of the movement occur at the CMC joint of the thumb, and one third occurs at the CMC and IC joints of the 4th and 5th fingers.

BLOOD SUPPLY OF CARPOMETACARPAL AND INTERMETACARPAL JOINTS

The CMC and IM joints are supplied by *peri-articular arterial anastomoses of the wrist and hand* (dorsal and palmar carpal arches, deep palmar arch, and metacarpal arteries) (Figs. 6.82 and 6.83).

INNERVATION OF CARPOMETACARPAL AND INTERMETACARPAL JOINTS

The CMC and IM joints are supplied by the anterior interosseous branch of the *median nerve,* posterior interosseous branch of the *radial nerve,* and dorsal and deep branches of the *ulnar nerve* (Fig. 6.85).

Metacarpophalangeal and Interphalangeal Joints

The **metacarpophalangeal joints** are the condyloid type of synovial joint that permit movement in two planes: flexion–extension and adduction–abduction. The **interphalangeal joints** are the hinge type of synovial joint that permit flexion–extension only (Fig. 6.110B).

ARTICULATIONS OF METACARPOPHALANGEAL AND INTERPHALANGEAL JOINTS

The heads of the metacarpals articulate with the bases of the proximal phalanges in the MP joints, and the heads of the phalanges articulate with the bases of more distally located phalanges in the IP joints.

JOINT CAPSULES OF METACARPOPHALANGEAL AND INTERPHALANGEAL JOINTS

A *joint capsule* encloses each MC and IP joint with a *synovial membrane* lining a *fibrous layer* that is attached to the margins of each joint.

LIGAMENTS OF METACARPOPHALANGEAL AND INTERPHALANGEAL JOINTS

The fibrous layer of each MC and IP joint capsule is strengthened by two (medial and lateral) **collateral ligaments.** These ligaments have two parts:

- Denser *"cord-like" parts* that pass distally from the heads of the metacarpals and phalanges to the bases of the phalanges (Fig. 6.110A & B).
- Thinner *"fan-like" parts* that pass anteriorly to attach to thick, densely fibrous or fibrocartilaginous plates, the **palmar ligaments** (plates), which form the palmar aspect of the joint capsule.

The fan-like parts of the collateral ligaments cause the palmar ligaments to move like a visor over the underlying metacarpal or phalangeal heads.

The strong cord-like parts of the collateral ligaments of the MP joint, being eccentrically attached to the metacarpal heads, are slack during extension and taut during flexion. As a result, the fingers cannot usually be spread (abducted) when the MP joints are fully flexed. The interphalangeal joints have corresponding ligaments, but the distal ends of the proximal and middle phalanges, being flattened anteroposteriorly and having two small condyles, permit neither adduction or abduction.

The palmar ligaments blend with the fibrous digital sheaths and provide a smooth, longitudinal groove that allows the long flexor ligaments to glide and remain centrally placed as they cross the convexities of the joints. The palmar ligaments of the 2nd–5th MP joints are united by **deep transverse metacarpal ligaments** that hold the heads of the metacarpals together. In addition, the dorsal hood of each extensor apparatus attaches anteriorly to the sides of the palmar plates of the MP joints.

MOVEMENTS OF METACARPOPHALANGEAL AND INTERPHALANGEAL JOINTS

Flexion–extension, abduction–adduction, and circumduction of the 2nd–5th digits occur at the 2nd–5th MP joints. Movement at the MP joint of the thumb is limited to flexion–extension. Only flexion and extension occur at the IP joints.

BLOOD SUPPLY OF METACARPAL AND INTERPHALANGEAL JOINTS

Deep digital arteries that arise from the superficial palmar arches supply the MC and IP joints (Figs. 6.82 and 6.83).

INNERVATION OF METACARPAL AND INTERPHALANGEAL JOINTS

Digital nerves arising from the ulnar and median nerves supply the MC and IP joints (Figs. 6.85A & B).

JOINTS OF UPPER LIMB

Dislocation of Sternoclavicular Joint

The rarity of *dislocation of the SC joint* attests to its strength, which depends on its ligaments, its disc, and the way forces are generally transmitted along the clavicle. When a blow is received to the acromion of the scapula, or when a force is transmitted to the pectoral girdle during a fall on the outstretched hand, the force of the blow is usually transmitted along the length of the clavicle, i.e., along its long axis. The clavicle may fracture near the junction of its middle and lateral thirds, but it is rare for the SC joint to dislocate. Most dislocations of the SC joint in persons < 25 years of age result from fractures through the epiphysial plate because the epiphysis at the sternal end of the clavicle does not close until 23–25 years of age.

Ankylosis of Sternoclavicular Joint

Movement at the SC joint is critical to movement of the shoulder. When *ankylosis* (stiffening or fixation) of the joint occurs, or is necessary surgically, a section of the center of the clavicle is removed, creating a pseudojoint or "flail" joint to permit scapular movement.

Dislocation of Acromioclavicular Joint

Although its extrinsic coracoclavicular ligament is strong, the AC joint itself is weak and easily injured by a direct blow (Fig. B6.31A-D). In contact sports such as football, soccer, hockey, or the martial arts, it is not uncommon for *dislocation of the AC joint* to result from a hard fall on the shoulder or on the outstretched upper limb. Dislocation of the AC joint can also occur when an ice hockey player is driven into the boards or when a person receives a severe blow to the superolateral part of the back.

An AC joint dislocation, often called a "shoulder separation," is severe when both the AC and coracoclavicular ligaments are torn. When the coracoclavicular ligament tears, the shoulder separates from the clavicle and falls because of the weight of the upper limb. *Rupture of the coracoclavicular ligament* allows the fibrous layer of the joint capsule to be torn so that the acromion can pass inferior to the acromial end of the clavicle. Dislocation of the AC joint makes the acromion more prominent, and the clavicle may move superior to this process.

Calcific Supraspinatus Tendinitis

Inflammation and calcification of the subacromial bursa result in pain, tenderness, and limitation of movement of the glenohumeral joint. This condition is also known as *calcific scapulohumeral bursitis*. Deposition of calcium in the supraspinatus tendon is common. This causes increased local pressure that often causes excruciating pain during abduction of the arm; the pain may radiate as far as the hand. The calcium deposit may irritate the overlying subacromial bursa, producing an inflammatory reaction known as *subacromial bursitis* (Fig. B6.32).

As long as the glenohumeral joint is adducted, no pain usually results because in this position the painful lesion is away from the inferior surface of the acromion. In most people, the pain occurs during 50–130° of abduction (*painful arc syndrome*) because during this arc the supraspinatus tendon is in intimate contact with the inferior surface of the acromion. The pain usually develops in males 50 years of age and older after unusual or excessive use of the glenohumeral joint.

Rotator Cuff Injuries

The musculotendinous rotator cuff is commonly injured during repetitive use of the upper limb above the horizontal (e.g., during throwing and racquet sports, swimming, and weightlifting). Recurrent inflammation of the rotator cuff, especially the relatively avascular area of the supraspinatus tendon, is a common cause of shoulder pain and results in tears of the musculotendinous rotator cuff.

Repetitive use of the rotator cuff muscles (e.g., by baseball pitchers) may allow the humeral head and rotator cuff to impinge on the coraco-acromial arch (Fig. 6.95B), producing irritation of the arch and inflammation of the rotator cuff. As a result, *degenerative tendonitis of the rotator cuff* develops. Attrition of the supraspinatus tendon also occurs (Fig. B6.32).

To test for degenerative tendonitis of the rotator cuff, the person is asked to lower the fully abducted limb slowly and

(A) Dislocation of acromioclavicular joint without ligament rupture

(B) Dislocation of acromioclavicular joint and rupture of coracoclavicular ligament

Prominence of dislocated clavicle
Clavicle
Torn coracoclavicular ligament
Torn acromioclavicular ligament
Acromion
Coraco-acromial ligament
Coracoid process
Scapula
Humerus
(C)

(D) AP view

FIGURE B6.31.

smoothly. From approximately 90° abduction, the limb will suddenly drop to the side in an uncontrolled manner if the rotator cuff (especially its supraspinatus part) is diseased and/or torn.

Rotator cuff injuries may also occur during a sudden strain of the muscles, for example, when an older person strains to lift something, such as a window that is stuck. This strain may rupture a previously degenerated musculotendinous rotator cuff. A fall on the shoulder may also tear a previously degenerated rotator cuff. Often the intracapsular part of the tendon of the long head of the biceps brachii becomes frayed (even worn away), leaving it adherent to the intertubercular sulcus. As a result, shoulder stiffness occurs. Because they fuse, the integrity of the fibrous layer of the joint capsule of the glenohumeral joint is usually compromised when the rotator cuff is injured. As a result, the articular cavity communicates with the subacromial bursa. Because the supraspinatus muscle is no longer functional with a complete tear of the rotator cuff, the person cannot initiate abduction of the upper limb. If the arm is passively abducted 15° or more, the person can usually maintain or continue the abduction using the deltoid.

Dislocation of Glenohumeral Joint

Because of its freedom of movement and instability, the glenohumeral joint is commonly dislocated by direct or indirect injury. Because the presence of the coraco-acromial arch and support of the rotator cuff are effective in preventing upward dislocation, most dislocations of the humeral head occur in the downward (inferior)

direction. However, they are described clinically as anterior or (more rarely) posterior dislocations, indicating whether the humeral head has descended anterior or posterior to the infraglenoid tubercle and long head of the triceps. The head ends up lying anterior or posterior to the glenoid cavity.

Superiorly reflected flap including deltoid and superficial portion of synovial membrane of subacromial bursa
Deltoid
Perforation
Supraspinatus tendon blended with fibrous capsule of glenohumeral joint
Coracoid process
Tendon of long head of biceps brachii seen through perforation
Perforation
Teres minor
Cut edge of subacromial bursa
Tendon of long head of biceps brachii
Lateral view

FIGURE B6.32. Attrition of the supraspinatus tendon.

Anterior dislocation of the glenohumeral joint occurs most often in young adults, particularly athletes. It is usually caused by excessive extension and lateral rotation of the humerus (Fig. B6.33). The head of the humerus is driven infero-anteriorly, and the fibrous layer of the joint capsule and glenoid labrum may be stripped from the anterior aspect of the glenoid cavity in the process. A hard blow to the humerus when the glenohumeral joint is fully abducted tilts the head of the humerus inferiorly onto the inferior weak part of the joint capsule. This may tear the capsule and dislocate the shoulder so that the humeral head comes to lie inferior to the glenoid cavity and anterior to the infraglenoid tubercle. The strong flexor and adductor muscles of the glenohumeral joint usually subsequently pull the humeral head anterosuperiorly into a subcoracoid position. Unable to use the arm, the person commonly supports it with the other hand.

Inferior dislocation of the glenohumeral joint often occurs after an avulsion fracture of the greater tubercle of the humerus, owing to the absence of the upward and medial pull produced by muscles attaching to the tubercle (see Fig. B6.2A, p. 685).

Axillary Nerve Injury

 The axillary nerve may be injured when the glenohumeral joint dislocates because of its close relation to the inferior part of the joint capsule (Fig. B6.34). The subglenoid displacement of the head of the humerus into the quadrangular space damages the axillary nerve. *Axillary nerve injury* is indicated by paralysis of the deltoid (manifest as an inability to abduct the arm to or above the horizontal level) and loss of sensation in a small area of skin covering the central part of the deltoid (see the blue box "Injury to Axillary Nerve" on p. 710 and Fig. B6.8).

Glenoid Labrum Tears

 Tearing of the fibrocartilaginous glenoid labrum commonly occurs in athletes who throw a baseball or football and in those who have shoulder instability

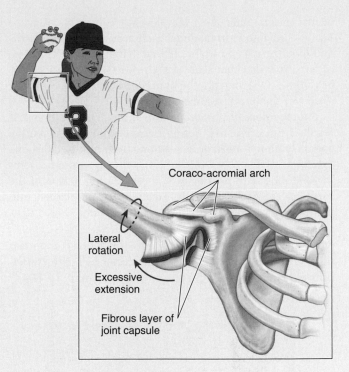

FIGURE B6.34.

and subluxation (partial dislocation) of the glenohumeral joint. The tear often results from sudden contraction of the biceps or forceful subluxation of the humeral head over the glenoid labrum (Fig. 6.95A). Usually a tear occurs in the anterosuperior part of the labrum. The typical symptom is pain while throwing, especially during the acceleration phase. A sense of popping or snapping may be felt in the glenohumeral joint during abduction and lateral rotation of the arm.

Adhesive Capsulitis of Glenohumeral Joint

 Adhesive fibrosis and scarring between the inflamed joint capsule of the glenohumeral joint, rotator cuff, subacromial bursa, and deltoid usually cause *adhesive capsulitis* ("frozen shoulder"), a condition seen in individuals 40–60 years of age. A person with this condition has difficulty abducting the arm and can obtain an apparent abduction of up to 45° by elevating and rotating the scapula. Because of the lack of movement of the glenohumeral joint, strain is placed on the AC joint, which may be painful during other movements (e.g., elevation, or shrugging, of the shoulder). Injuries that may initiate acute capsulitis are glenohumeral dislocations, calcific supraspinatus tendinitis, partial tearing of the rotator cuff, and bicipital tendinitis (Salter, 1999).

Bursitis of Elbow

The subcutaneous olecranon bursa (Figs. 6.97C and 6.101) is exposed to injury during falls on the elbow and infection from abrasions of the skin covering the olecranon. Repeated excessive pressure and friction, as

FIGURE B6.33. Dislocation of glenohumeral joint.

occurs in wrestling, for example, may cause this bursa to become inflamed, producing a friction *subcutaneous olecranon bursitis* (e.g., "student's elbow") (Fig. B6.35). This type of bursitis is also known as "dart thrower's elbow" and "miner's elbow." Occasionally, the bursa becomes infected and the area over the bursa becomes inflamed.

Subtendinous olecranon bursitis is much less common. It results from excessive friction between the triceps tendon and olecranon, for example, resulting from repeated flexion–extension of the forearm, as occurs during certain assembly-line jobs. The pain is most severe during flexion of the forearm because of pressure exerted on the inflamed subtendinous olecranon bursa by the triceps tendon (Fig. 6.101).

Bicipitoradial bursitis (*biceps bursitis*) results in pain when the forearm is pronated because this action compresses the bicipitoradial bursa against the anterior half of the tuberosity of the radius (see "Bursa around elbow joint," p. 804).

FIGURE B6.36.

FIGURE B6.35.

Avulsion of Medial Epicondyle

 Avulsion (forced separation) of the medial epicondyle in children can result from a fall that causes severe abduction of the extended elbow, an abnormal movement of this articulation. The resulting traction on the ulnar collateral ligament pulls the medial epicondyle distally (Fig. B6.36). The anatomical basis of the avulsion is that the epiphysis for the medial epicondyle may not fuse with the distal end of the humerus until up to age 20. Usually fusion is complete radiographically at age 14 in females and age 16 in males.

Traction injury of the ulnar nerve is a frequent complication of the abduction type of avulsion of the medial epicondyle of the humerus. The anatomical basis for stretching of the ulnar nerve is that it passes posterior to the medial epicondyle before entering the forearm (see Fig. 6.47A).

Ulnar Collateral Ligament Reconstruction

Rupture, tearing, or stretching of the ulnar collateral ligament (UCL; Fig. 6.107B) are increasingly common injuries related to athletic throwing—pri-

marily baseball pitching (Fig. B6-37A), but also football passing, javelin throwing, and playing water polo. *Reconstruction of the UCL*, known as a "Tommy John procedure" (after the first pitcher to undergo the surgery), involves an autologous transplant of a long tendon from the contralateral forearm or leg (e.g., the palmaris longus or plantaris tendon; Fig. B6-37B). A 10- to 15-cm length of tendon is passed through holes drilled through the medial epicondyle of the humerus and the lateral aspect of the coronoid process of the ulna (Fig. B6-37C–E).

Dislocation of Elbow Joint

 Posterior dislocation of the elbow joint may occur when children fall on their hands with their elbows flexed. Dislocations of the elbow may also result from hyperextension or a blow that drives the ulna posterior or posterolateral. The distal end of the humerus is driven through the weak anterior part of the fibrous layer of the joint capsule as the radius and ulna dislocate posteriorly (Fig. B6.38). The ulnar collateral ligament is often torn, and an associated fracture of the head of the radius, coronoid process, or olecranon process of the ulna may occur. Injury to the ulnar nerve may occur, resulting in numbness of the little finger and weakness of flexion and adduction of the wrist.

Subluxation and Dislocation of Radial Head

Preschool children, particularly girls, are vulnerable to transient *subluxation* (incomplete dislocation) of the head of the radius (also called "nursemaid's elbow" and "pulled elbow"). The history of these dislocations is typical. The child is suddenly lifted (jerked) by the upper limb while the forearm is pronated (e.g., lifting a child) (Fig. B6.39A). The child may cry out, refuse to use the limb, and protect their limb by holding it with the elbow flexed and the forearm pronated.

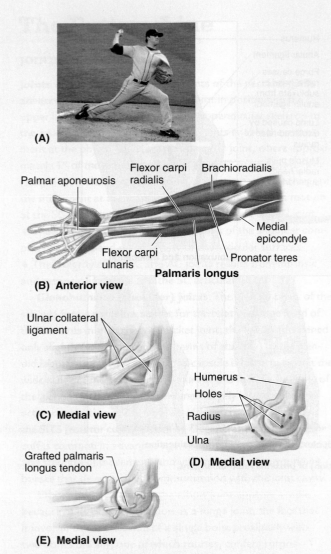

(A)

Palmar aponeurosis · Flexor carpi radialis · Brachioradialis · Medial epicondyle · Flexor carpi ulnaris · Pronator teres · **Palmaris longus**

(B) Anterior view

Ulnar collateral ligament

(C) Medial view

Humerus · Holes · Radius · Ulna

(D) Medial view

Grafted palmaris longus tendon

(E) Medial view

FIGURE B6.37.

Humerus · Fractured olecranon (of ulna) · Radius · Ulna

FIGURE B6.38. Dislocation of elbow.

The sudden pulling of the upper limb tears the distal attachment of the anular ligament, where it is loosely attached to the neck of the radius. The radial head then moves distally, partially out of the "socket" formed by the anular ligament (Fig. B6.39B). The proximal part of the torn ligament may become trapped between the head of the radius and the capitulum of the humerus.

The source of pain is the pinched anular ligament. Treatment of the subluxation consists of supination of the child's forearm while the elbow is flexed (Salter, 1999). The tear in the anular ligament heals when the limb is placed in a sling for 2 weeks.

Wrist Fractures and Dislocations

Fracture of the distal end of the radius (*Colles fracture*), the most common fracture in people >50 years of age, is discussed in the blue box "Fractures of Radius and Ulna" on p. 685. *Fracture of the scaphoid,* relatively common in young adults, is discussed in the blue box "Fracture of Scaphoid" on p. 686.

Anterior dislocation of the lunate is an uncommon but serious injury that usually results from a fall on the dorsiflexed wrist (Fig. B6.40A). The lunate is pushed out of its place in the floor of the carpal tunnel toward the palmar surface of the wrist. The displaced lunate may compress the median nerve and lead to *carpal tunnel syndrome* (discussed on p. 790). Because of its poor blood supply, *avascular necrosis of the lunate* may occur. In some cases, excision of the lunate may be required. In *degenerative joint disease of the wrist,* surgical fusion of carpals (*arthrodesis*) may be necessary to relieve the severe pain.

Fracture–separation of the distal radial epiphysis is common in children because of frequent falls in which forces are transmitted from the hand to the radius (Fig. B6.40B & C). In a lateral radiograph of a child's wrist, dorsal displacement of the distal radial epiphysis is obvious (Fig. B6.40C). When the epiphysis is placed in its normal position during reduction, the prognosis for normal bone growth is good.

Bull Rider's Thumb

Bull rider's thumb refers to a sprain of the radial collateral ligament, and an avulsion fracture of the lateral part of the proximal phalanx of the thumb. This injury is common in individuals who ride mechanical bulls.

Skier's Thumb

Skier's thumb (historically, game-keeper's thumb) refers to the rupture or chronic laxity of the collateral ligament of the 1st MP joint (Fig. B6.41). The injury results from hyperabduction of the MP joint of the thumb, which occurs when the thumb is held by the ski pole while the rest of the hand hits the ground or enters the snow. In severe injuries, the head of the metacarpal has an avulsion fracture.

OVERVIEW OF HEAD

The **head** is the superior part of the body that is attached to the trunk by the neck. It is the control and communications center as well as the "loading dock" for the body. It houses the brain; therefore, it is the site of our consciousness: ideas, creativity, imagination, responses, decision making, and memory. It includes special sensory receivers (eyes, ears, mouth, and nose), broadcast devices for voice and expression, and portals for the intake of fuel (food), water, and oxygen and the exhaust of carbon dioxide.

The head consists of the *brain* and its protective coverings (cranial vault and meninges), the *ears*, and the *face*. The face includes openings and passageways, with lubricating glands and valves (seals) to close some of them, the masticatory (chewing) devices, and the orbits that house the visual apparatus. The face also provides our identity as individuals. Disease, malformation, or trauma of structures in the head form the bases of many specialties, including dentistry, maxillofacial surgery, neurology, neuroradiology, neurosurgery, ophthalmology, oral surgery, otology, rhinology, and psychiatry.

CRANIUM

The **cranium** (skull[1]) is the skeleton of the head (Fig. 7.1A). A series of bones form its two parts, the neurocranium and viscerocranium (Fig. 7.1B). The **neurocranium** is the bony case of the brain and its membranous coverings, the cranial meninges. It also contains proximal parts of the cranial nerves and the vasculature of the brain. The neurocranium in adults is formed by a series of eight bones: four singular bones centered on the midline (*frontal, ethmoidal, sphenoidal,* and *occipital*), and two sets of bones occurring as bilateral pairs (*temporal* and *parietal*) (Figs. 7.1A, 7.2A, and 7.3).

The *neurocranium* has a dome-like roof, the **calvaria** (skullcap), and a floor or **cranial base** (basicranium). The bones forming the *calvaria* are primarily flat bones (frontal, parietal, and occipital; see Fig. 7.8A) formed by intramembranous ossification of head mesenchyme from the neural crest. The bones contributing to the *cranial base* are primarily irregular bones with substantial flat portions (sphenoidal and temporal) formed by endochondral ossification of cartilage (*chondrocranium*) or from more than one type of ossification. The *ethmoid bone* is an irregular bone that makes a relatively minor midline contribution

to the neurocranium but is primarily part of the viscerocranium (see Fig. 7.7A). The so-called flat bones and flat portions of the bones forming the neurocranium are actually curved, with convex external and concave internal surfaces.

Most calvarial bones are united by fibrous interlocking **sutures** (Fig. 7.1A & B); however, during childhood, some bones (sphenoid and occipital) are united by hyaline cartilage (**synchondroses**). The spinal cord is continuous with the brain through the *foramen magnum,* a large opening in the cranial base (Fig. 7.1C).

The **viscerocranium** (*facial skeleton*) comprises the facial bones that mainly develop in the mesenchyme of the embryonic pharyngeal arches (Moore et al., 2012). The viscerocranium forms the anterior part of the cranium and consists of the bones surrounding the mouth (upper and lower jaws), nose/nasal cavity, and most of the *orbits* (eye sockets or orbital cavities) (Figs. 7.2 and 7.3).

The *viscerocranium* consists of 15 irregular bones: 3 singular bones centered on or lying in the midline (*mandible, ethmoid,* and *vomer*), and 6 bones occurring as bilateral pairs (*maxillae; inferior nasal conchae;* and *zygomatic, palatine, nasal,* and *lacrimal bones*) (Figs. 7.1A and 7.4A). The maxillae and mandible house the teeth—that is, they provide the sockets and supporting bone for the maxillary and mandibular teeth. The *maxillae* contribute the greatest part of the upper facial skeleton, forming the skeleton of the upper jaw, which is fixed to the cranial base. The *mandible* forms the skeleton of the lower jaw, which is movable because it articulates with the cranial base at the *temporomandibular joints* (Figs. 7.1A and 7.2).

Several bones of the cranium (frontal, temporal, sphenoid, and ethmoid bones) are **pneumatized bones,** which contain **air spaces** (*air cells* or large *sinuses*), presumably to decrease their weight (Fig. 7.5). The total volume of the air spaces in these bones increases with age.

In the *anatomical position,* the cranium is oriented so that the inferior margin of the orbit and the superior margin of the external acoustic opening of the external acoustic meatus of both sides lie in the same horizontal plane (Fig. 7.1A). This standard craniometric reference is the **orbitomeatal plane** (Frankfort horizontal plane).

Facial Aspect of Cranium

Features of the anterior or **facial** (**frontal**) **aspect of the cranium** are the frontal and zygomatic bones, orbits, nasal region, maxillae, and mandible (Figs. 7.2 and 7.3).

The **frontal bone,** specifically its **squamous** (flat) **part,** forms the skeleton of the forehead, articulating inferiorly with the nasal and zygomatic bones. In some adults a *frontal suture* persists; this remnant is called a **metopic suture**. It is in the middle of the **glabella,** the smooth, slightly depressed area between the superciliary arches. The **frontal suture** divides the frontal bones of the fetal cranium (see the blue box "Development of Cranium," p. 839).

---

[1]There is confusion about exactly what the term *skull* means. It may mean the cranium (which includes the mandible), or the part of the cranium excluding the mandible. There has also been confusion because some people have used the term *cranium* for only the neurocranium. The Federative International Committee on Anatomical Terminology (FICAT) has decided to follow the Latin term *cranium* for the skeleton of the head.

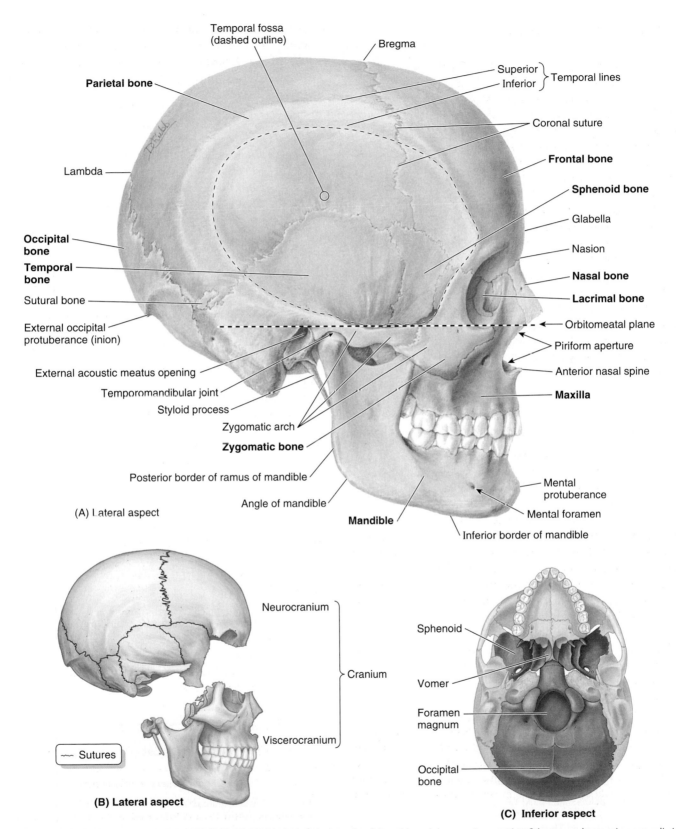

Temporal fossa (dashed outline)

Bregma

Parietal bone

Superior / Inferior } Temporal lines

Coronal suture

Frontal bone

Sphenoid bone

Glabella

Lambda

Nasion

Occipital bone

Nasal bone

Temporal bone

Lacrimal bone

Sutural bone

Orbitomeatal plane

External occipital protuberance (inion)

Piriform aperture

Anterior nasal spine

External acoustic meatus opening

Maxilla

Temporomandibular joint

Styloid process

Zygomatic arch

Zygomatic bone

Posterior border of ramus of mandible

Mental protuberance

Angle of mandible

Mental foramen

Mandible

Inferior border of mandible

(A) Lateral aspect

Neurocranium

Cranium

Sphenoid

Vomer

Foramen magnum

Occipital bone

Viscerocranium

Sutures

(B) Lateral aspect

(C) Inferior aspect

FIGURE 7.1. Adult cranium I. A. In the anatomical position, the inferior margin of the orbit and the superior margin of the external acoustic meatus lie in the same horizontal orbitomeatal (Frankfort horizontal) plane. **B.** The neurocranium and viscerocranium are the two primary functional parts of the cranium. From the lateral aspect, it is apparent that the volume of the neurocranium, housing the brain, is approximately double that of the viscerocranium. **C.** The unpaired sphenoid and occipital bones make substantial contributions to the cranial base. The spinal cord is continuous with the brain through the foramen magnum, the large opening in the basal part of the occipital bone.

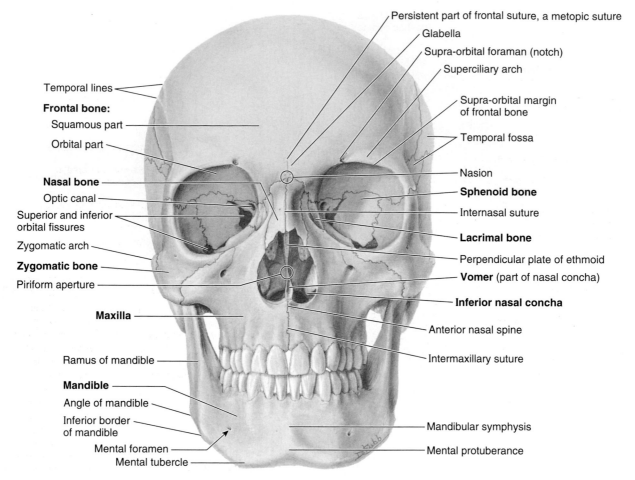

Persistent part of frontal suture, a metopic suture
Glabella
Supra-orbital foraman (notch)
Superciliary arch
Supra-orbital margin of frontal bone
Temporal fossa
Nasion
Sphenoid bone
Internasal suture
Lacrimal bone
Perpendicular plate of ethmoid
Vomer (part of nasal concha)
Inferior nasal concha
Anterior nasal spine
Intermaxillary suture
Mandibular symphysis
Mental protuberance

Temporal lines
Frontal bone:
　Squamous part
　Orbital part
Nasal bone
Optic canal
Superior and inferior orbital fissures
Zygomatic arch
Zygomatic bone
Piriform aperture
Maxilla
Ramus of mandible
Mandible
Angle of mandible
Inferior border of mandible
Mental foramen
Mental tubercle

(A) Facial (anterior) view of cranium

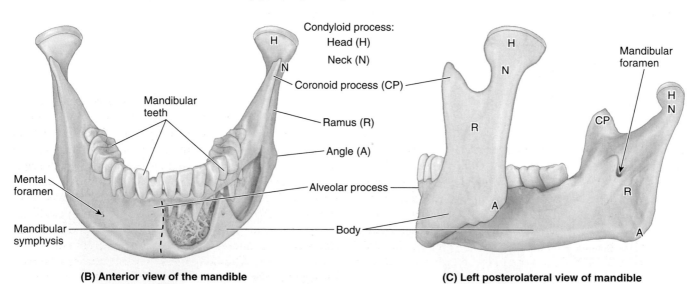

Condyloid process:
　Head (H)
　Neck (N)
Coronoid process (CP)
Ramus (R)
Angle (A)
Alveolar process
Body

Mandibular teeth
Mental foramen
Mandibular symphysis

Mandibular foramen

(B) Anterior view of the mandible

(C) Left posterolateral view of mandible

FIGURE 7.2. Adult cranium II. A. The viscerocranium, housing the optical apparatus, nasal cavity, paranasal sinuses, and oral cavity, dominates the facial aspect of the cranium. **B and C.** The mandible is a major component of the viscerocranium, articulating with the remainder of the cranium via the temporomandibular joint. The broad ramus and coronoid process of the mandible provide attachment for powerful muscles capable of generating great force in relationship to biting and chewing (mastication).

Frontal eminence
Frontal process of maxilla
Superciliary arch
Supra-orbital margin
Zygomatic process
Frontal process of zygomatic bone
Superior and inferior orbital fissures
Zygomaticofacial foramen
Zygomatic arch
Nasal septum (bony part)
Alveolar process of maxilla
Maxillary teeth
Mandibular teeth
Alveolar process of mandible

Frontal (metopic) suture
Supra-orbital foramen (notch)
Orbital cavity
Orbital surface of greater wing of sphenoid
Middle nasal concha
Nasal cavity
Infra-orbital margin
Infra-orbital foramen
Inferior nasal concha
Intermaxillary suture
Premolar teeth
Mental foramen
Mental protuberance

Bones:
- Ethmoid
- Frontal
- Inferior concha
- Lacrimal
- Mandible
- Maxilla
- Nasal
- Parietal
- Sphenoid
- Temporal
- Vomer
- Zygomatic

Facial aspect

FIGURE 7.3. Adult cranium III. The individual bones of the cranium are color coded. The supra-orbital notch, the infra-orbital foramen, and the mental foramen, giving passage to major sensory nerves of the face, are approximately in a vertical line.

The intersection of the frontal and nasal bones is the **nasion** (L. *nasus*, nose), which in most people is related to a distinctly depressed area (bridge of nose) (Figs. 7.1A and 7.2A). The nasion is one of many *craniometric points* that are used radiographically in medicine (or on dry crania in physical anthropology) to make cranial measurements, compare and describe the topography of the cranium, and document abnormal variations (Fig. 7.6; Table 7.1). The frontal bone also articulates with the lacrimal, ethmoid, and sphenoids; a horizontal portion of bone (*orbital part*) forms both the roof of the orbit and part of the floor of the anterior part of the cranial cavity (Fig. 7.3).

The **supra-orbital margin** of the frontal bone, the angular boundary between the squamous and orbital parts, has a **supra-orbital foramen (notch)** in some crania for passage of the supra-orbital nerve and vessels. Just superior to the supra-orbital margin is a ridge, the **superciliary arch,** that extends laterally on each side from the glabella. The prominence of this ridge, deep to the eyebrows, is generally greater in males (Figs. 7.2A and 7.3).

The **zygomatic bones** (cheek bones, malar bones), forming the prominences of the cheeks, lie on the inferolateral sides of the orbits and rest on the maxillae. The anterolateral rims, walls, floor, and much of the infra-orbital margins of the orbits are formed by these quadrilateral bones. A small **zygomaticofacial foramen** pierces the lateral aspect of each bone (Fig. 7.3 and 7.4A). The zygomatic bones articulate with the frontal, sphenoid, and temporal bones and the maxillae.

Inferior to the nasal bones is the pear-shaped **piriform aperture,** the anterior nasal opening in the cranium (Figs. 7.1A and 7.2A). The bony **nasal septum** can be observed through this aperture, dividing the nasal cavity into right and left parts. On the lateral wall of each nasal cavity are curved bony plates, the **nasal conchae** (Figs. 7.2A and 7.3).

The **maxillae** form the upper jaw; their **alveolar processes** include the tooth sockets (alveoli) and constitute the supporting bone for the **maxillary teeth.** The two maxillae are united at the **intermaxillary suture** in the median plane (Fig. 7.2A). The maxillae surround most of the piriform aperture and form the infra-orbital margins medially. They have a

7.11). The diploë is cancellous bone containing red bone marrow during life, through which run canals formed by diploic veins. The diploë in a dried calvaria is not red because the protein was removed during preparation of the cranium. The internal table of bone is thinner than the external table, and in some areas there is only a thin plate of compact bone with no diploë.

The bony substance of the cranium is unequally distributed. Relatively thin (but mostly curved) flat bones provide the necessary strength to maintain cavities and protect their contents. However, in addition to housing the brain, the bones of the neurocranium (and processes from them) provide proximal attachment for the strong muscles of mastication that attach distally to the mandible; consequently, high traction forces occur across the nasal cavity and orbits that are sandwiched between. Thus thickened portions of the cranial bones form stronger pillars or *buttresses* that transmit forces, bypassing the orbits and nasal cavity (Fig. 7.13). The main buttresses are the **frontonasal buttress,** extending from the region of the canine teeth between the nasal and the orbital cavities to the central frontal bone, and the **zygomatic arch–lateral orbital margin buttress** from the region of the molars to the lateral frontal and temporal bones. Similarly, **occipital buttresses** transmit forces received lateral to the foramen magnum from the vertebral column. Perhaps to compensate for the denser bone required for these buttresses, some areas of the cranium not as mechanically stressed become pneumatized (air-filled).

Regions of Head

To allow clear communications regarding the location of structures, injuries, or pathologies, the head is divided into regions (Fig. 7.14). The large number of regions into which the relatively small area of the face is divided (eight) is a reflection of both its functional complexity and personal importance, as are annual expenditures for elective aesthetic

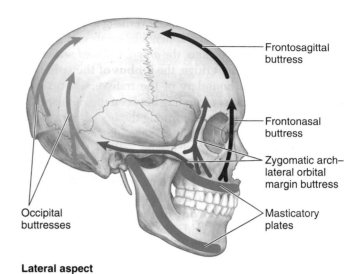

Frontosagittal buttress

Frontonasal buttress

Zygomatic arch–lateral orbital margin buttress

Masticatory plates

Occipital buttresses

Lateral aspect

FIGURE 7.13. Buttresses of cranium. The buttresses are thicker portions of cranial bone that transmit forces around weaker regions of the cranium.

surgery. With the exception of the **auricular region,** which includes the external ear, the names of the regions of the *neurocranial portion of the head* correspond to the underlying bones or bony features: **frontal, parietal, occipital, temporal,** and **mastoid regions.**

The *viscerocranial portion of the head* includes the **facial region,** which is divided into five bilateral and three median regions related to superficial features (**oral** and **buccal regions**), to deeper soft tissue formations (**parotid region**), and to skeletal features (**orbital, infra-orbital, nasal, zygomatic,** and **mental regions**). The remainder of this chapter discusses several of these regions in detail, as well as some deep regions not represented on the surface (for example, the infratemporal region and pterygopalatine fossa). The surface anatomy of these regions will be discussed with the description of each region.

Regions of the head:

1 Frontal region
2 Parietal region
3 Occipital region
4 Temporal region
5 Auricular region
6 Mastoid region

Facial region:
7 Orbital region
8 Infra-orbital region
9 Buccal region
10 Parotid region
11 Zygomatic region
12 Nasal region
13 Oral region
14 Mental region

FIGURE 7.14. Regions of head.

CRANIUM

Head Injuries

 Head injuries are a major cause of death and disability. The complications of head injuries include hemorrhage, infection, and injury to the brain (e.g., concussion) and cranial nerves. Disturbance in the level of consciousness is the most common symptom of head injury. Almost 10% of all deaths in the United States are caused by head injuries, and approximately half of traumatic deaths involve the brain (Rowland, 2010). Head injuries occur mostly in young persons between the ages of 15 and 24 years. The major cause of brain injury varies, but motor vehicle and motorcycle accidents are prominent.

Headaches and Facial Pain

Few complaints are more common than *headaches* and *facial pain*. Although usually benign and frequently associated with tension, fatigue, or mild fever, headaches may indicate a serious intracranial problem such as a brain tumor, subarachnoid hemorrhage, or meningitis. *Neuralgias* (G. *algos,* pain) are characterized by severe throbbing or stabbing pain in the course of a nerve caused by a demyelinating lesion. They are a common cause of facial pain. Terms such as *facial neuralgia* describe diffuse painful sensations. Localized aches have specific names, such as *earache* (otalgia) and *toothache* (odontalgia). A sound knowledge of the clinical anatomy of the head helps in understanding the causes of headaches and facial pain.

Injury to Superciliary Arches

The superciliary arches are relatively sharp bony ridges (see Fig. 7.3); consequently, a blow to them (e.g., during boxing) may lacerate the skin and cause bleeding. Bruising of the skin surrounding the orbit causes tissue fluid and blood to accumulate in the surrounding connective tissue, which gravitates into the superior (upper) eyelid and around the eye ("black eye"; see Fig. B7.12).

Malar Flush

The zygomatic bone was once called the malar bone; consequently, you will hear the clinical term *malar flush*. This redness of the skin covering the zygomatic process (malar eminence) is associated with a rise in temperature in various fevers occurring with certain diseases, such as *tuberculosis* and *systemic lupus erythematosus disease*.

Fractures of Maxillae and Associated Bones

Dr. Léon-Clement Le Fort (Paris surgeon and gynecologist, 1829–1893) classified three common variants of fractures of the maxillae (Fig. B7.1):

Le Fort I

Le Fort II

Le Fort III

FIGURE B7.1.

- **Le Fort I fracture:** wide variety of horizontal fractures of the maxillae, passing superior to the maxillary alveolar process (i.e., to the roots of the teeth), crossing the bony nasal septum and possibly the pterygoid plates of the sphenoid.
- **Le Fort II fracture:** passes from the posterolateral parts of the maxillary sinuses (cavities in the maxillae) superomedially through the infra-orbital foramina, lacrimals, or ethmoids to the bridge of the nose. As a result, the entire central part of the face, including the hard palate and alveolar processes, is separated from the rest of the cranium.
- **Le Fort III fracture:** horizontal fracture that passes through the superior orbital fissures and the ethmoid and nasal bones and extends laterally through the greater wings of the sphenoid and the frontozygomatic sutures. Concurrent fracturing of the zygomatic arches causes the maxillae and zygomatic bones to separate from the rest of the cranium.

Fractures of Mandible

A broken mandible usually involves two fractures, which frequently occur on opposite sides of the mandible; thus, if one fracture is observed, a search should be made for another. For example, a hard blow to the jaw often fractures the neck and body of the mandible in the region of the opposite canine tooth.

Fractures of the coronoid process of the mandible are uncommon and usually single (Fig. B7.2). *Fractures of the neck of the mandible* are often transverse and may be

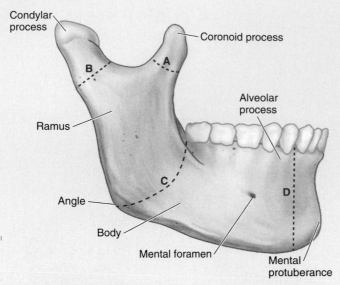

FIGURE B7.2. Fractures of mandible. *Line A,* Fracture of the coronoid process; *line B,* fracture of the neck of the mandible; *line C,* fracture of the angle of the mandible; *line D,* fracture of the body of the mandible.

associated with dislocation of the temporomandibular joint (TMJ) on the same side. *Fractures of the angle of the mandible* are usually oblique and may involve the bony socket or alveolus of the 3rd molar tooth (Fig. B7.2, *line C*). *Fractures of the body of the mandible* frequently pass through the socket of a canine tooth (Fig. B7.2, *line D*).

Resorption of Alveolar Bone

Extraction of teeth causes the alveolar bone to resorb in the affected region(s) (Fig. B7.3). Following complete loss or extraction of maxillary teeth, the tooth sockets begin to fill in with bone, and the alveolar process begins to resorb. Similarly, extraction of mandibular teeth causes the bone to resorb. Gradually, the mental foramen lies near the superior border of the body of the mandible (Fig. B7.3A-C). In some cases, the mental foramina disappear, exposing the mental nerves to injury. *Pressure from a dental prosthesis* (e.g., a denture resting on an exposed mental nerve) may produce pain during eating. Loss of all the teeth results in a decrease in the vertical facial dimension and *mandibular prognathism* (overclosure). Deep creases in the facial skin also appear that pass posteriorly from the corners of the mouth.

(A)   (B)   (C)
Mental foramen

FIGURE B7.3. Stages of resorption of edentulous (toothless) alveolar bone.

Fractures of Calvaria

The convexity of the calvaria distributes and thereby usually minimizes the effects of a blow to the head. However, hard blows in thin areas of the calvaria are likely to produce *depressed fractures,* in which a bone fragment is depressed inward, compressing and/or injuring the brain (Fig. B7.4). *Linear calvarial fractures,* the most frequent type, usually occur at the point of impact, but fracture lines often radiate away from it in two or more directions. In *comminuted fractures,* the bone is broken into several pieces. If the area of the calvaria is thick at the site of impact, the bone may bend inward without fracturing; however, a fracture may occur some distance from the site of direct trauma where the calvaria is thinner. In a *contrecoup (counterblow) fracture,* no fracture occurs at the point of impact, but one occurs on the opposite side of the cranium.

Median view

Posterosuperior view

FIGURE B7.4. Fractures of calvaria.

Surgical Access to Cranial Cavity: Bone Flaps

Surgeons access the cranial cavity and brain by performing a *craniotomy,* in which a section of the neurocranium, called a bone flap, is elevated or removed (Fig. B7.5). Because the adult pericranium (periosteum of cranium) has poor osteogenic (bone-forming) properties, little regeneration occurs after bone loss (e.g., when pieces of bone are removed during repair of a comminuted cranial fracture). Surgically produced bone flaps are put back into place and wired to other parts of the calvaria, or held in place temporarily with metal plates. Reintegration is most successful when the bone is reflected with its overlying muscle and skin, so that it retains its own blood supply during the procedure and after repositioning. If the bone flap is not replaced (i.e., a permanent plastic or metal plate replaces the flap), the procedure is called a *craniectomy*.

(A) Anterior view

Craniotomy

FIGURE B7.5.

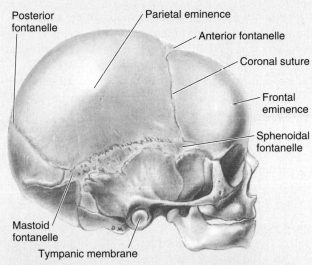

(B) Lateral view

Development of Cranium

The bones of the calvaria and some parts of the cranial base develop by *intramembranous ossification*. Most parts of the cranial base develop by *endochondral ossification*. At birth, the bones of the calvaria are smooth and unilaminar; no diploë is present. The frontal and parietal eminences are especially prominent (Fig. B7.6). The cranium of a neonate is disproportionately large compared to other parts of the skeleton; however, the facial aspect is small compared to the *calvaria*, which forms approximately one eighth of the cranium. In the adult, the facial skeleton forms one third of the cranium. The large size of the calvaria in infants results from precocious growth and development of the brain and eyes.

The rudimentary development of the face makes the orbits appear relatively large (Fig. B7.6A). The smallness of the face results from the rudimentary development of the

(C) Anterosuperior view

FIGURE B7.6. Cranial development.

maxillae, mandible, and paranasal sinuses (air-filled bone cavities), the absence of erupted teeth, and the small size of the nasal cavities.

The halves of the frontal bone in the neonate are separated by the *frontal suture,* the frontal and parietal bones are separated by the *coronal suture,* and the maxillae and mandibles are separated by the *intermaxillary suture* and *mandibular symphysis* (secondary cartilaginous joint), respectively. There are no mastoid and styloid processes (Figs. B7.6A & B). Because there are no mastoid processes at birth, the facial nerves are close to the surface when they emerge from the stylomastoid foramina. As a result, the facial nerves may be injured by forceps during a difficult delivery or later by an incision posterior to the auricle of the external ear (as for the surgical treatment of mastoiditis or middle ear problems). The mastoid processes form gradually during the 1st year as the sternocleidomastoid muscles complete their development and pull on the petromastoid parts of the temporal bones.

The bones of the calvaria of a neonate are separated by fibrous membranes; the largest occur between the angles (corners) of the flat bones (Fig. B7.6A & B). They include the *anterior* and *posterior fontanelles* and the paired *sphenoidal* and *mastoid fontanelles.* Palpation of the fontanelles during infancy, especially the anterior and posterior ones, enables physicians to determine the:

- Progress of growth of the frontal and parietal bones.
- Degree of hydration of an infant (a depressed fontanelle indicates dehydration).
- Level of intracranial pressure (a bulging fontanelle indicates increased pressure on the brain).

The **anterior fontanelle,** the largest one, is diamond or star shaped; it is bounded by the halves of the frontal bone anteriorly and the parietal bones posteriorly (Fig. B7.6). Thus it is located at the junction of the sagittal, coronal, and frontal sutures, the future site of *bregma* (Fig. 7.6; Table 7.1). By 18 months of age, the surrounding bones have fused, and the anterior fontanelle is no longer clinically palpable.

At birth, the frontal bone consists of two halves. Union of the halves begins in the 2nd year. In most cases, the *frontal suture* is obliterated by the 8th year. However, in approximately 8% of people, a remnant of the frontal suture, the **metopic suture,** persists (Figs. 7.2A and 7.3). Much less frequently, the entire suture remains (Fig. B7.6C). A persistent suture must not be interpreted as a fracture in a radiograph, or other medical image (e.g., a CT scan).

The **posterior fontanelle** is triangular and bounded by the parietal bones anteriorly, and the occipital bone posteriorly. It is located at the junction of the lambdoid and sagittal sutures, the future site of *lambda* (Fig. 7.7A and 7.8C). The posterior fontanelle begins to close during the first few months after birth, and by the end of the 1st year, it is small and no longer clinically palpable. The **sphenoidal** and **mastoid fontanelles,** overlain by the temporalis muscle (Fig. 7.16A), fuse during infancy and are less important clini-

cally than the midline fontanelles. The halves of the mandible fuse early in the 2nd year. The two maxillae and nasal bones usually do not fuse.

The softness of the cranial bones in fetuses and their loose connections at the sutures and fontanelles enable the shape of the cranium to be molded during birth (Fig. B7.7). During passage of the fetus through the birth canal, the halves of the frontal bone become flat, the occipital bone is drawn out, and one parietal bone slightly overrides the other. Within a few days after birth, the shape of the neonatal cranium returns to normal. The resilience of the cranial bones of infants allows them to resist forces that would produce fractures in adults. The fibrous sutures of the calvaria also permit the cranium to enlarge during infancy and childhood. The increase in the size of the calvaria is greatest during the first 2 years, the period of most rapid brain development. The calvaria normally increases in capacity for 15–16 years. After this, the calvaria usually increases slightly in size for 3–4 years as a result of bone thickening.

FIGURE B7.7. Molding of calvaria.

Age Changes in Face

 The mandible is the most dynamic of our bones; its size and shape and the number of teeth it normally bears, undergo considerable change with age. In the neonate, the mandible consists of two halves united in the median plane by a cartilaginous joint, the *mandibular symphysis.* Union between the halves of the mandible is effected by means of fibrocartilage; this union begins during the 1st year and the halves are fused by the end of the 2nd year. The body of the mandible in neonates is a mere shell lacking alveolar processes; each half enclosing five deciduous teeth. These teeth usually begin to erupt in infants at approximately 6 months of age. The body of the mandible elongates, particularly posterior

FIGURE B7.8. Left lateral view of dentition. *Arrows,* unerupted permanent teeth.

to the mental foramen (Fig. B7.2), to accommodate this development. Later, eight permanent teeth begin to erupt during the 6th year of life (Fig. B7.8). Eruption of the permanent teeth is not complete until early adulthood.

Rapid growth of the face during infancy and early childhood coincides with the eruption of deciduous teeth. Vertical growth of the upper face results mainly from dentoalveolar development of alveolar bone. These changes are more marked after the permanent teeth erupt. Concurrent enlargement of the frontal and facial regions is associated with the increase in the size of the *paranasal sinuses,* the air-filled extensions of the nasal cavities in certain cranial

bones (Fig. B7.9). Most paranasal sinuses are rudimentary or absent at birth. Growth of the paranasal sinuses is important in altering the shape of the face and in adding resonance to the voice.

Obliteration of Cranial Sutures

The obliteration of sutures between the bones of the calvaria usually begins between the ages of 30 and 40 years on the internal surface. Approximately 10 years later, the sutures on the external surface obliterate (Fig. B7.10; cf. Fig. 7.8B). Obliteration of sutures usually begins at the bregma and continues sequentially in the sagittal, coronal, and lambdoid sutures. Closure times vary considerably.

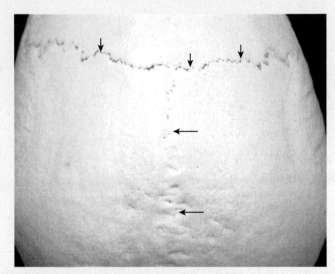

FIGURE B7.10. Obliteration (synostosis) of cranial sutures. *Arrows,* sagittal; *arrowheads,* coronal.

Age Changes in Cranium

As people age, the cranial bones normally become progressively thinner and lighter, and the diploë gradually become filled with a gray gelatinous material. In these individuals, the bone marrow has lost its blood cells and fat, giving it a gelatinous appearance.

Craniosynostosis and Cranial Malformations

Premature closure of the cranial sutures (*primary craniosynostosis*) results in several cranial malformations (Fig. B7.11). The incidence of primary craniosynostosis is approximately 1 per 2000 births (Kliegman et al., 2011). The cause of craniosynostosis is unknown, but genetic factors appear to be important. The prevailing hypothesis is that abnormal development of the cranial base creates exaggerated forces on the *dura mater* (outer covering membrane of the brain) that disrupt normal cranial sutural development. These malformations are more common in males than in

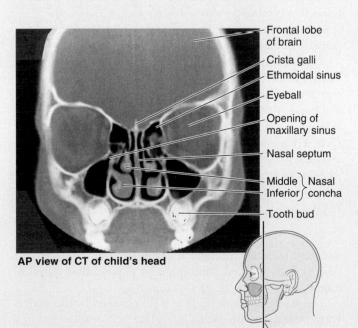

Frontal lobe of brain

Crista galli

Ethmoidal sinus

Eyeball

Opening of maxillary sinus

Nasal septum

Middle ⎫ Nasal
Inferior ⎭ concha

Tooth bud

AP view of CT of child's head

FIGURE B7.9.

(A) Scaphoncephaly   (B) Plagiocephaly   (C) Oxycephaly

FIGURE B7.11.

females, and are often associated with other skeletal anomalies. The type of malformed cranium that forms depends on which sutures close prematurely.

Premature closure of the sagittal suture, in which the anterior fontanelle is small or absent, results in a long, narrow, wedge-shaped cranium, a condition called *scaphocephaly* (Fig. B7.11A). When *premature closure of the coronal or the lambdoid suture* occurs on one side only, the cranium is twisted and asymmetrical, a condition known as *plagiocephaly* (Fig. B7.11B). *Premature closure of the coronal suture* results in a high, tower-like cranium, called *oxycephaly* or *turricephaly* (Fig. B7.11C). The latter type of cranial malformation is more common in females. Premature closure of sutures usually does not affect brain development.

The Bottom Line

CRANIUM

The cranium is the skeleton of the head, an amalgamation of functional components united to form a single skeletal formation. ♦ The basic functional components include the *neurocranium*, the container of the brain and internal ears, and *viscerocranium*, providing paired orbits, nasal cavities and teeth-bearing plates (alveolar processes) of the oral cavity. ♦ Although some mobility between cranial bones is advantageous during birth, they become fixed together by essentially immovable joints (sutures), allowing independent movement of only the mandible. ♦ Abundant fissures and foramina facilitate communication and passage of neurovascular structures between functional components. ♦ The bony substance of the cranium is unequally distributed. Relatively thin (but mostly curved) flat bones provide the necessary strength to maintain cavities and protect contents. ♦ However, the bones and processes of the neurocranium also provide proximal attachment for the strong muscles of mastication (chewing) that attach distally to the mandible. ♦ The high traction forces generated across the nasal cavity and orbits, sandwiched between the muscle attachments, are resisted by thickened portions of the bones forming stronger pillars or buttresses. ♦ The mostly superficial surface of the cranium provides both visible and palpable landmarks.

Internal features of the cranial base reflect the major formations of the brain that rest on it. ♦ Bony ridges radiating from the centrally located sella turcica divide it into three cranial fossae. ♦ The frontal lobes of the brain lie in the anterior cranial fossa. ♦ The temporal lobes lie in the middle cranial fossa. ♦ The hindbrain, consisting of the pons, cerebellum, and medulla, occupies the posterior cranial fossa, with the medulla continuing through the foramen magnum where it is continuous with the spinal cord.

FACE AND SCALP

Face

The **face** is the anterior aspect of the head from the forehead to the chin and from one ear to the other. The face provides our identity as an individual human. Thus, birth defects scarring, or other alterations resulting from pathology or trauma have marked consequences beyond their physical effects.

The basic shape of the face is determined by the underlying bones. The individuality of the face results primarily from anatomical variations in the shape and relative prominence of the features of the underlying cranium; in the deposition of fatty tissue; in the color and effects of aging on the overlying skin; and in the abundance, nature, and placement of hair on the face and scalp. The relatively large size of the **buccal fat-pads** in infants prevents collapse of the cheeks during sucking and produces their chubby-cheeked appearance. Growth of the facial bones takes longer than those of the calvaria. The ethmoid bone, orbital cavities, and superior parts of the nasal cavities have nearly completed their growth by the 7th year. Expansion of the orbits and growth of the nasal septum carry the maxillae infero-anteriorly. Considerable facial growth occurs during childhood as the paranasal sinuses develop and permanent teeth erupt.

The face plays an important role in communication. Our interactions with others take place largely via the face (including the ears); hence, the term *interface* for a site of interactions. Whereas the shape and features of the face provide our identity, much of our affect on others and their perceptions about us result from the way we use facial muscles to make the slight alterations in the features that constitute facial expression.

Scalp

The **scalp** consists of skin (normally hair bearing) and subcutaneous tissue that cover the neurocranium from the superior nuchal lines on the occipital bone to the supra-orbital margins of the frontal bone (Figs. 7.3 and 7.4A). Laterally, the scalp extends over the temporal fascia to the zygomatic arches.

The scalp is composed of five layers, the first three of which are connected intimately and move as a unit (e.g., when wrinkling the forehead and moving the scalp). Each letter in the word *scalp* serves as a memory key for one of its five layers (Fig. 7.15A):

1. **S**kin: thin, except in the occipital region, contains many sweat and sebaceous glands and hair follicles. It has an abundant arterial supply and good venous and lymphatic drainage.

FIGURE 7.15. Layers of scalp, cranium, and meninges. A. The skin is bound tightly to the epicranial aponeurosis, which moves freely over the pericranium and cranium because of the intervening loose connective tissue. *Aponeurosis* refers to the epicranial aponeurosis, the flat intermediate tendon of the occipitofrontalis muscle. The cranial meninges and the subarachnoid (leptomeningeal) space are shown. *CSF,* cerebrospinal fluid. **B.** The occipitofrontalis muscle. Innervation of the two bellies by the posterior auricular and temporal branches of the facial nerve is demonstrated.

2. **Connective tissue:** forms the thick, dense, richly vascularized subcutaneous layer that is well supplied with cutaneous nerves.

3. **Aponeurosis (epicranial aponeurosis):** the broad, strong, tendinous sheet that covers the calvaria and serves as the attachment for muscle bellies converging from the forehead and occiput (**occipitofrontalis muscle**) (Fig. 7.15B) and from the temporal bones on each side (**temporoparietalis** and **superior auricular muscles**). Collectively, these structures constitute the musculo-aponeurotic **epicranius.** The *frontal belly of the occipitofrontalis* pulls the scalp anteriorly, wrinkles the forehead, and elevates the eyebrows; the *occipital belly of the occipitofrontalis* pulls the scalp posteriorly, smoothing the skin of the forehead. The superior auricular muscle (actually a specialized posterior part of the temporoparietalis) elevates the auricle of the external ear. All parts of the epicranius (muscle and aponeurosis) are innervated by the facial nerve.

4. **Loose areolar tissue:** a sponge-like layer including potential spaces that may distend with fluid as a result of injury or infection. This layer allows free movement of the **scalp proper** (the first three layers—skin, connective tissue, and epicranial aponeurosis) over the underlying calvaria.

5. **Pericranium:** a dense layer of connective tissue that forms the external periosteum of the neurocranium. It is firmly attached but can be stripped fairly easily from the crania of living persons, except where the pericranium is continuous with the fibrous tissue in the cranial sutures.

Muscles of Face and Scalp

The facial muscles (muscles of facial expression) are in the subcutaneous tissue of the anterior and posterior scalp, face, and neck. They move the skin and change facial expressions to convey mood. Most muscles attach to bone or fascia and produce their effects by pulling the skin. The muscles of the scalp and face are illustrated in Figure 7.16, and their attachments and actions are provided in Table 7.3. Certain muscles and/or muscle groups will be discussed in further detail.

All muscles of facial expression develop from mesoderm in the second pharyngeal arches. A subcutaneous muscular sheet forms during embryonic development that spreads over the neck and face, carrying branches of the nerve of the arch (the facial nerve, CN VII) with it to supply all the muscles formed from the arch (Moore et al., 2012). The muscular sheet differentiates into muscles that surround the facial orifices (mouth, eyes, and nose), serving as sphincter and dilator mechanisms that also produce many facial expressions (Fig. 7.17). Because of their common embryological origin, the platysma and facial muscles are often fused, and their fibers are frequently intermingled.

MUSCLES OF SCALP, FOREHEAD, AND EYEBROWS

The **occipitofrontalis** is a flat digastric muscle, with **occipital** and **frontal bellies** that share a common tendon, the **epicranial aponeurosis** (Figs. 7.15 and 7.16A & B; Table 7.3). Because the aponeurosis is a layer of the scalp, independent contraction of the occipital belly retracts the scalp and contraction of the frontal belly protracts it. Acting simultaneously, the occipital belly, with bony attachments, works as a synergist with the frontal belly, which has no bony attachments, to elevate the eyebrows and produce transverse wrinkles across the forehead. This gives the face a surprised look.

MUSCLES OF MOUTH, LIPS, AND CHEEKS

The lips, shape, and degree of opening of the mouth are important for clear speech. In addition, we add emphasis to our vocal communication with our facial expressions. Several muscles alter the shape of the mouth and lips during speaking as well as during such activities as singing, whistling, and mimicry. The shape of the mouth and lips is controlled by a complex three-dimensional group of muscular slips, which include the following (Fig. 7.16B & C; Table 7.3):

- Elevators, retractors, and evertors of the upper lip.
- Depressors, retractors, and evertors of the lower lip.
- The orbicularis oris, the sphincter around the mouth.
- The buccinator in the cheek.

At rest, the lips are in gentle contact and the teeth are close together.

The **orbicularis oris,** the first of the series of sphincters associated with the alimentary system (digestive tract), encircles the mouth within the lips, controlling entry, and exit through the **oral fissure** (L. *rima oris,* the opening between the lips). The orbicularis oris is important during articulation (speech).

The **buccinator** (L. trumpeter) is a thin, flat, rectangular muscle that attaches laterally to the alveolar processes of the maxillae and mandible, opposite the molar teeth. It also attaches to the **pterygomandibular raphe,** a tendinous thickening of the buccopharyngeal fascia separating and giving origin to the superior pharyngeal constrictor posteriorly. The buccinator occupies a deeper, more medially placed plane than the other facial muscles, passing deep to the mandible so that it is more closely related to the buccal mucosa than to the skin of the face. The buccinator, active in smiling, also keeps the cheek taut, thereby preventing it from folding and being injured during chewing.

Anteriorly, the fibers of the buccinator mingle medially with those of the orbicularis oris, and the tonus of the two muscles compresses the cheeks and lips against the teeth and gums. The tonic contraction of the buccinator, and especially of the orbicularis oris, provides a gentle but continual resistance to the tendency of the teeth to tilt in an outward direction. In the presence of a short upper lip, or retractors that remove this force, crooked or protrusive ("buck") teeth develop.

The orbicularis oris (from the labial aspect) and buccinator (from the buccal aspect) work with the tongue (from the lingual aspect) to keep food between the occlusal surfaces of the teeth during mastication (chewing) and to prevent food from accumulating in the oral vestibule.

Epicranial aponeurosis
(Galea aponeurotica)

Occipitofrontalis muscle,
frontal belly

Procerus

Orbicularis oculi:
Orbital part
Palpebral part

Nasalis

Levator labii superioris
alaeque nasi

Levator labii
superioris

Zygomaticus minor

Zygomaticus major

Risorius

Depressor septi nasi

Orbicularis oris

Depressor anguli oris

Depressor labii inferioris

Platysma

Corrugator supercilii
(cut)

Temporal fascia

Palpebral fissure

Levator labii superioris
(cut)

Levator anguli oris

Parotid duct and gland

Oral fissure

Buccinator

Masseter*

Mentalis (cut)

* Not muscles of facial
expression

(A) Anterior view

FIGURE 7.16. Muscles of scalp and face.

TABLE 7.3. MUSCLES OF SCALP AND FACE

Muscle[a]	Origin	Insertion	Main Action(s)
Occipitofrontalis			
Front belly[2]	Epicranial aponeurosis	Skin and subcutaneous tissue of eyebrows and forehead	Elevates eyebrows and wrinkles skin of forehead; protracts scalp (indicating surprise or curiosity)
Occipital belly[1]	Lateral two thirds of superior nuchal line	Epicranial aponeurosis	Retracts scalp; increasing effectiveness of frontal belly
Orbicularis oculi (orbital sphincter)[2,3]	Medial orbital margin; medial palpebral ligament; lacrimal bone	Skin around margin of orbit; superior and inferior tarsal plates	Closes eyelids: palpebral part does so gently; orbital part tightly (winking)

[a] All facial muscles are innervated by the facial nerve (CN VII) via its posterior auricular branch (*1*) or via the temporal (*2*), zygomatic (*3*), buccal (*4*), marginal mandibular (*5*), or cervical (*6*) branches of the parotid plexus.

Occipitofrontalis | Corrugator supercilii | Procerus + transverse part of nasalis | Orbicularis oculi | Lev. labii sup. alaeque nasi + alar part of nasalis

Buccinator + orbicularis oris | Zygomaticus major + minor | Risorius | Risorius + depressor labii inferioris | Levator labii superioris + depressor labii

Dilators of mouth: Risorius plus levator labii superioris + depressor labii inferioris | Orbicularis oris | Depressor anguli oris | Mentalis | Platysma

FIGURE 7.17. Muscles of facial expression in action. These muscles are superficial sphincters and dilators of the orifices of the head. The facial muscles, supplied by the facial nerve (CN VII), are attached to and move the skin of the face, producing many facial expressions.

The **orbicularis oculi** closes the eyelids and wrinkles the forehead vertically (Figs. 7.16A & B and 7.18; Table 7.3). Its fibers sweep in concentric circles around the orbital margin and eyelids. Contraction of these fibers narrows the **palpebral fissure** (aperture between the eyelids) and assists the flow of lacrimal fluid (tears) by bringing the lids together laterally first, closing the palpebral fissure in a lateral to medial direction. The orbicularis oculi muscle consists of three parts:

1. *Palpebral part:* arising from the **medial palpebral ligament** and mostly located within the eyelids, gently closes the eyelids (as in blinking or sleep) to keep the cornea from drying.
2. *Lacrimal part:* passing posterior to the *lacrimal sac,* draws the eyelids medially, aiding drainage of tears.

3. *Orbital part:* overlying the orbital rim and attached to the frontal bone and maxilla medially, tightly closes the eyelids (as in winking or squinting) to protect the eyeballs against glare and dust.

When all three parts of the orbicularis oculi contract, the eyes are firmly closed (Figs. 7.17 and 7.18C).

MUSCLES OF NOSE AND EARS

As demonstrated in the blue box "Flaring of Nostrils" (p. 861), the muscles of the nose may provide evidence of breathing behaviors. Otherwise, although these muscles are functionally important in certain mammals (elephants, tapirs, rabbits,

Orbital part (O)

Palpebral part (P)

Palpebral fissure

(A)

(B)   (C)

FIGURE 7.18. Disposition and actions of orbicularis oculi muscle. A. The orbital and palpebral parts of the orbicularis oculi are demonstrated. **B.** The palpebral part gently closes the eyelids. **C.** The orbital part tightly closes the eyelids.

and some diving mammals), they are relatively unimportant in humans, except in terms of facial expression and in the specialized field of aesthetic plastic surgery. The muscles of the ears, important in animals capable of cocking or directing the ears toward the sources of sounds, are even less critical in humans.

Nerves of Face and Scalp

Cutaneous (sensory) innervation of the face and anterosuperior part of the scalp is provided primarily by the *trigeminal nerve* (CN V), whereas motor innervation to the facial muscles is provided by the *facial nerve* (CN VII).

CUTANEOUS NERVES OF FACE AND SCALP

The **trigeminal nerve** (CN V) originates from the lateral surface of the pons of the midbrain by two roots: motor and sensory. These roots are comparable to the motor (anterior) and sensory (posterior) roots of spinal nerves. The sensory root of CN V consists of the central processes of pseudounipolar neurons located in a sensory ganglion (**trigeminal ganglion**) at the distal end of the root, which is bypassed by the multipolar neuronal axons making up the motor root. CN V is the sensory nerve for the face and the motor nerve for the muscles of mastication and several small muscles (Fig. 7.19).

The peripheral processes of the neurons of the trigeminal ganglion constitute three divisions of the nerve: the *ophthalmic nerve* (CN V₁), the *maxillary nerve* (CN V₂), and the sensory component of the *mandibular nerve* (CN V₃). These nerves are named according to their main areas of termination: the eye, maxilla, and mandible, respectively. The first two divisions (ophthalmic and maxillary nerves) are wholly sensory. The mandibular nerve is largely sensory, but it also receives the motor fibers (axons) from the motor root of CN V that mainly supply the muscles of mastication. The cutaneous nerves derived from each division of CN V are illustrated in Figure 7.20, and the origin, course, and distribution of each nerve are listed and described in Table 7.4.

The cutaneous nerves of the neck overlap those of the face. Cutaneous branches of cervical nerves from the *cervical plexus* extend over the posterior aspect of the neck and scalp. The **great auricular nerve** in particular innervates the inferior aspect of the auricle (external ear) and much of

the parotid region of the face (the area overlying the angle of the jaw).

OPHTHALMIC NERVE

The **ophthalmic nerve** (CN V₁), the superior division of the trigeminal nerve, is the smallest of the three divisions of CN V. It arises from the trigeminal ganglion as a wholly sensory nerve and supplies the area of skin derived from the embryonic *frontonasal prominence* (Moore et al., 2012). As CN V₁ enters the orbit through the *superior orbital fissure*, it trifurcates into the frontal, nasociliary, and lacrimal nerves (Fig. 7.19). Except for the external nasal nerve, the cutaneous branches of CN V₁ reach the skin of the face via the orbital opening (Fig. 7.21).

The **frontal nerve,** the largest branch produced by the trifurcation of CN V₁, runs along the roof of the orbit toward the orbital opening, bifurcating approximately midway into the cutaneous **supra-orbital** and **supratrochlear nerves,** distributed to the forehead and scalp (Figs. 7.21 and 7.22).

The **nasociliary nerve,** the intermediate branch of the CN V₁ trifurcation, supplies branches to the eyeball and divides within the orbit into the posterior ethmoidal, anterior ethmoidal, and infratrochlear nerves (Fig. 7.19). The *posterior* and *anterior ethmoidal nerves* leave the orbit, the latter running a circuitous course passing through the cranial and nasal cavities. Its terminal branch, the **external nasal nerve,** is a cutaneous nerve supplying the external nose. The **infratrochlear nerve** is a terminal branch of the nasociliary nerve and its main cutaneous branch.

The **lacrimal nerve,** the smallest branch from the trifurcation of CN V₁, is primarily a cutaneous branch, but it also conveys some secretomotor fibers, sent via a communicating branch, from a ganglion associated with the maxillary nerve for innervation of the lacrimal gland (Figs. 7.20 and 7.21).

MAXILLARY NERVE

The *maxillary nerve* (CN V₂), the intermediate division of the trigeminal nerve, also arises as a wholly sensory nerve (Fig. 7.19A). CN V₂ passes anteriorly from the *trigeminal ganglion* and leaves the cranium through the *foramen rotundum* in the base of the greater wing of the sphenoid.

The lips surround the opening of the mouth, the *oral fissure.* The **vermillion border of the lip** marks the beginning of the *transitional zone* (commonly referred to as the lip) between the skin and mucous membrane of the lip. The skin of the **transitional zone** is hairless and thin, increasing its sensitivity and causing its color to be different (because of underlying capillary beds) from that of the adjacent skin of the face. The lateral junction of the lips is the **labial commissure;** the angle between the lips, medial to the commissure, that increases as the mouth opens and decreases as it closes is the **angle of the mouth.**

The median part of the upper lip features a **tubercle,** superior to which is a shallow groove, the **philtrum** (G. love charm), extending to the nasal septum. The musculofibrous folds of the lips continue laterally as the **cheek,** which also contains the buccinator muscle and buccal fat-pad. The cheek is separated from the lips by the **nasolabial sulcus,** which runs obliquely between the ala of the nose and the angle of the mouth. These grooves are easiest to observe during smiling. The lower lip is separated from the **mental protuberance** (chin) by the **mentolabial sulcus.** The lips, cheeks, and chin of the mature male grow hair as part of the secondary sex characteristics, the **beard.**

FACE AND SCALP

Facial Lacerations and Incisions

Because the face has no distinct deep fascia and the subcutaneous tissue between the cutaneous attachments of the facial muscles is loose, *facial lacerations* tend to gape (part widely). Consequently, the skin must be carefully sutured to prevent scarring. The looseness of the subcutaneous tissue also enables fluid and blood to accumulate in the loose connective tissue following bruising of the face.

Similarly, facial inflammation causes considerable swelling (e.g., a bee sting on the root of the nose may close both eyes). As a person ages, the skin loses its resiliency (elasticity). As a result, ridges and wrinkles occur in the skin perpendicular to the direction of the facial muscle fibers. Skin incisions along these cleavage or wrinkle lines (Langer lines) heal with minimal scarring (see the blue box "Skin Incisions and Scarring," p. 15).

Scalp Injuries

Because the scalp arteries arising at the sides of the head are well protected by dense connective tissue and anastomose freely, a *partially detached scalp* may be replaced with a reasonable chance of healing as long as one of the vessels supplying the scalp remains intact. During an *attached craniotomy* (surgical removal of a segment of the calvaria with a soft tissue scalp flap to expose the cranial cavity), the incisions are usually made convex and upward, and the superficial temporal artery is included in the tissue flap.

The *scalp proper,* the first three layers of the scalp (see Fig. 7.15A), is often regarded clinically as a single layer because they remain together when a scalp flap is made during a craniotomy and when part of the scalp is torn off (e.g., during an industrial accident). Nerves and vessels of the scalp enter inferiorly and ascend through layer two to the skin. Consequently, surgical pedicle scalp flaps are made so that they remain attached inferiorly to preserve the nerves and vessels, thereby promoting good healing.

The arteries of the scalp supply little blood to the calvaria, which is supplied by the middle meningeal arteries. There-

fore, loss of the scalp does not produce necrosis (death) of the calvarial bones.

Scalp Wounds

The epicranial aponeurosis is clinically important. Because of the strength of this aponeurosis, *superficial scalp wounds* do not gape, and the margins of the wound are held together. Furthermore, deep sutures are not necessary when suturing superficial wounds because the epicranial aponeurosis does not allow wide separation of the skin. *Deep scalp wounds* gape widely when the epicranial aponeurosis is lacerated in the coronal plane because of the pull of the frontal and occipital bellies of the occipitofrontalis muscle in opposite directions (anteriorly and posteriorly).

Scalp Infections

The loose connective tissue layer (layer four) of the scalp is the *danger area of the scalp* because pus or blood spreads easily in it. Infection in this layer can also pass into the cranial cavity through small *emissary veins,* which pass through parietal foramina in the calvaria, and reach intracranial structures such as the meninges (Fig. 7.8A & C). An infection cannot pass into the neck because the occipital bellies of the occipitofrontalis muscle attach to the occipital bone and mastoid parts of the temporal bones (Fig. 7.16A). Neither can a scalp infection spread laterally beyond the zygomatic arches because the epicranial aponeurosis is continuous with the temporal fascia that attaches to these arches.

An infection or fluid (e.g., pus or blood) can enter the eyelids and the root of the nose because the occipitofrontalis inserts into the skin and subcutaneous tissue and does not attach to the bone (Fig. 7.16B). The skin of the eyelid is the thinnest of the body and is delicate and sensitive. Because of the loose nature of the subcutaneous tissue within the eyelids, even a relatively slight injury or inflammation may result in an accumulation of fluid, causing the eyelids to swell. Blows to the peri-orbital region usually produce soft tissue damage because the tissues are crushed against the strong and relatively sharp margin. Consequently, "black eyes" (*peri-orbital*

FIGURE B7.12.   Ecchymosis (extravasation of blood under the skin).

ecchymosis) can result from an injury to the scalp and/or the forehead (Fig. B7.12). **Ecchymosis** (purple patches), develop as a result of extravasation of blood into the subcutaneous tissue and skin of the eyelids and surrounding regions.

Sebaceous Cysts

The ducts of sebaceous glands associated with hair follicles in the scalp may become obstructed, resulting in the retention of secretions and the formation of *sebaceous cysts* (pilar cysts). Because they are in the skin, sebaceous cysts move with the scalp.

Cephalhematoma

Sometimes after a difficult birth, bleeding occurs between the baby's pericranium (layer 5 of scalp; see Fig. 7.15A) and calvaria, usually over one parietal bone. Blood becomes trapped in this area, causing a *cephalhematoma*. This benign condition frequently results from birth trauma that ruptures multiple, minute periosteal arteries that nourish the bones of the calvaria.

Flaring of Nostrils

The actions of the nasalis muscles (Fig. 7.17, center top row) have generally been held as insignificant; however, observant clinicians study their action because of their diagnostic value. For example, true *nasal breathers* can flare their nostrils distinctly. Habitual mouth breathing, caused by chronic nasal obstruction, for example, diminishes and sometimes eliminates the ability

to flare the nostrils. Children who are *chronic mouth breathers* often develop dental malocclusion (improper bite) because the alignment of the teeth is maintained to a large degree by normal periods of occlusion and labial closure. *Anti-snoring devices* have been developed that attach to the nose to flare the nostrils and maintain a more patent air passageway.

Paralysis of Facial Muscles

Injury to the facial nerve (CN VII) or its branches produces paralysis of some or all facial muscles on the affected side (*Bell palsy*). The affected area sags, and facial expression is distorted, making it appear passive or sad (Fig. B7.13). The loss of tonus of the orbicularis oculi causes the inferior eyelid to evert (fall away from the surface of the eyeball). As a result, lacrimal fluid is not spread over the cornea, preventing adequate lubrication, hydration, and flushing of the surface of the cornea.

This makes the cornea vulnerable to ulceration. A resulting corneal scar can impair vision. If the injury weakens or paralyzes the buccinator and orbicularis oris, food will accumulate in the oral vestibule during chewing, usually requiring continual removal with a finger. When the sphincters or dilators of the mouth are affected, displacement of the mouth (drooping of its corner) is produced by contraction of unopposed contralateral facial muscles and gravity, resulting in food and saliva dribbling out of the side of the mouth. Weakened lip muscles affect speech as a result of an impaired ability to produce labial (*B, M, P,* or *W*) sounds. Affected persons cannot whistle or blow a wind instrument. They frequently dab their eyes and mouth with a handkerchief to wipe the fluid (tears and saliva), which runs from the drooping lid and mouth; the fluid and constant wiping may result in localized skin irritation.

FIGURE B7.13.

and turns supero-anteriorly on the greater wing of the sphenoid, where it divides into anterior and posterior branches (Fig. 7.28D). The **frontal branch of the middle meningeal artery** runs superiorly to the pterion and then curves posteriorly to ascend toward the vertex of the cranium. The **parietal branch of the middle meningeal artery** runs posterosuperiorly and ramifies (breaks up into distributing branches) over the posterior aspect of the cranium. Small areas of dura are supplied by other arteries: meningeal branches of the ophthalmic arteries, branches of the occipital arteries, and small branches of the vertebral arteries.

The **veins of the dura** accompany the meningeal arteries, often in pairs. The **middle meningeal veins** accompany the middle meningeal artery, leave the cranial cavity through the foramen spinosum or foramen ovale, and drain into the *pterygoid venous plexus* (Fig. 7.29B).

NERVE SUPPLY OF DURA MATER

The dura on the floors of the anterior and middle cranial fossa and the roof of the posterior cranial fossa is innervated by meningeal branches arising directly or indirectly from the trigeminal nerve (CN V) (Fig. 7.34). There are three divisions of CN V (CN V_1, CN V_2, and CN V_3), each of which contributes a meningeal branch or branches. The **anterior meningeal branches of the ethmoidal nerves** (CN V_1) and the **meningeal branches of the maxillary** (CN V_2) and **mandibular** (CN V_3) **nerves** supply the dura of the anterior cranial fossa. The latter two nerves also supply the dura of the middle cranial fossa (Fig. 7.34B). The meningeal branches of CN V_2 and CN V_3 are distributed as peri-arterial plexuses, accompanying the branches of the middle meningeal artery (Fig. 7.34A, *inset*).

The dura forming the roof of the posterior cranial fossa (tentorium cerebelli) and posterior part of the falx cerebri is supplied by the **tentorial nerve** (a branch of the ophthalmic nerve), whereas the anterior falx cerebri is innervated by ascending branches of the anterior meningeal branches (Fig. 7.34A). The dura of the floor of the posterior cranial fossa receives sensory fibers from the spinal ganglia of C2 and C3 carried by those spinal nerves or by fibers transferred to and traveling centrally with the vagus (CN X) and hypoglossal (CN XII) nerves. Sensory endings are more numerous in the dura along each side of the superior sagittal sinus and in the tentorium cerebelli than they are in the floor of the cranium.

Pain fibers are most numerous where arteries and veins course in the dura. Pain arising from the dura is generally referred, perceived as a headache arising in cutaneous or mucosal regions supplied by the involved cervical nerve or division of the trigeminal nerve.

Arachnoid Mater and Pia Mater

The *arachnoid mater* and *pia mater* (or simply *arachnoid* and *pia*; together the leptomeninges) develop from a single layer of mesenchyme surrounding the embryonic brain, becoming the parietal part (arachnoid) and visceral part (pia) of the *leptomeninx*. (Fig. 7.35). The derivation of the arachnoid–pia from a single embryonic layer is indicated in the adult by the numerous web-like *arachnoid trabeculae* passing between the arachnoid and pia, which give the arachnoid its name (G. *arachne–*, spider, cobweb + G. *eidos*, resemblance). The trabeculae are composed of flattened, irregularly shaped fibroblasts that bridge the subarachnoid space (Haines, 2006). The arachnoid and pia are in continuity immediately proximal to the exit of each cranial nerve from the dura mater. The **cranial arachnoid mater** contains fibroblasts, collagen fibers, and some elastic fibers. Although thin, the arachnoid is thick enough to be manipulated with forceps. The avascular arachnoid, although closely applied to the meningeal layer of the dura, is not attached to the dura; it is held against the inner surface of the dura by the pressure of the CSF in the subarachnoid space.

The **cranial pia mater** is an even thinner membrane than the arachnoid; it is highly vascularized by a network of fine blood vessels. The pia is difficult to see, but it gives the surface of the brain a shiny appearance. The pia adheres to the surface of the brain and follows all its contours. When the cerebral arteries penetrate the cerebral cortex, the pia follows them for a short distance, forming a **pial coat** and a **peri-arterial space** (Fig. 7.35).

Meningeal Spaces

Of the three meningeal "spaces" commonly mentioned in relation to the cranial meninges, only one exists as a space in the absence of pathology:

- The **dura–cranial interface** (extradural or epidural "space") is not a natural space between the cranium and the external periosteal layer of the dura because the dura is attached to the bones. It becomes an **extradural space** only pathologically—for example, when blood from torn meningeal vessels pushes the periosteum away from the cranium (Fig. 7.28C). The potential or pathological cranial epidural space is not continuous with the **spinal epidural space** (a natural space occupied by epidural fat and a venous plexus) because the former is external to the periosteum lining the cranium, and the latter is internal to the periosteum covering the vertebrae.
- The *dura–arachnoid interface* or junction ("subdural space") is likewise not a natural space between the dura and arachnoid. A space may develop in the dural border cell layer as the result of trauma, such as a hard blow to the head (Haines, 1993, 2006).
- The *subarachnoid space*, between the arachnoid and pia, is a real space that contains CSF, trabecular cells, arteries, and veins.

Although it is commonly stated that the brain "floats" in CSF, the brain is suspended in the CSF-filled subarachnoid space by the arachnoid trabeculae.

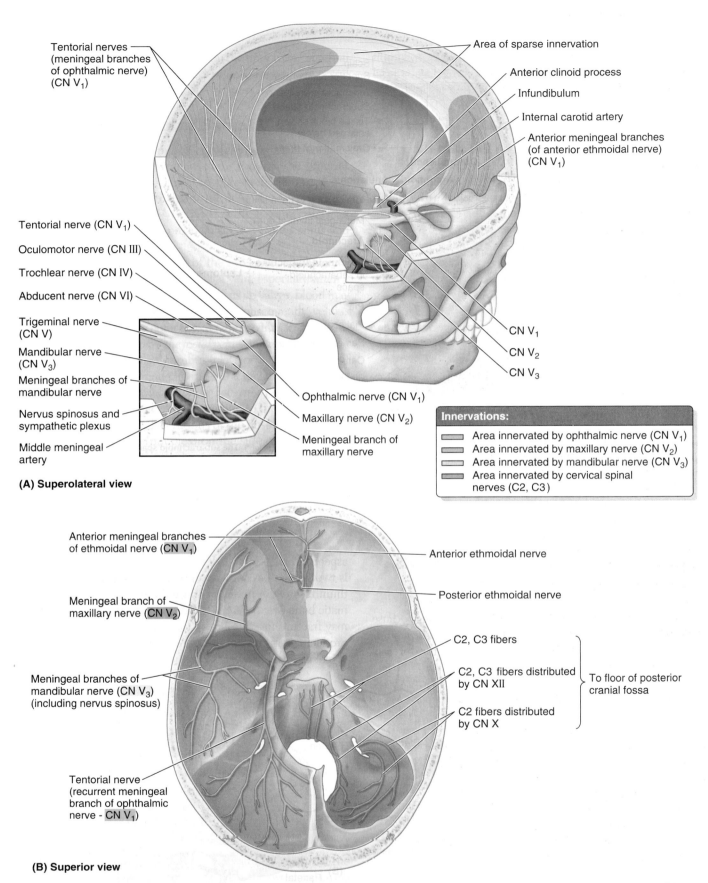

Tentorial nerves (meningeal branches of ophthalmic nerve) (CN V₁)

Area of sparse innervation

Anterior clinoid process

Infundibulum

Internal carotid artery

Anterior meningeal branches (of anterior ethmoidal nerve) (CN V₁)

Tentorial nerve (CN V₁)

Oculomotor nerve (CN III)

Trochlear nerve (CN IV)

Abducent nerve (CN VI)

Trigeminal nerve (CN V)

Mandibular nerve (CN V₃)

Meningeal branches of mandibular nerve

Nervus spinosus and sympathetic plexus

Middle meningeal artery

Ophthalmic nerve (CN V₁)

Maxillary nerve (CN V₂)

Meningeal branch of maxillary nerve

CN V₁

CN V₂

CN V₃

(A) Superolateral view

Innervations:
- Area innervated by ophthalmic nerve (CN V₁)
- Area innervated by maxillary nerve (CN V₂)
- Area innervated by mandibular nerve (CN V₃)
- Area innervated by cervical spinal nerves (C2, C3)

Anterior meningeal branches of ethmoidal nerve (CN V₁)

Anterior ethmoidal nerve

Meningeal branch of maxillary nerve (CN V₂)

Posterior ethmoidal nerve

C2, C3 fibers

C2, C3 fibers distributed by CN XII

Meningeal branches of mandibular nerve (CN V₃) (including nervus spinosus)

C2 fibers distributed by CN X

To floor of posterior cranial fossa

Tentorial nerve (recurrent meningeal branch of ophthalmic nerve - CN V₁)

(B) Superior view

FIGURE 7.34. Innervation of dura mater. A. The right side of the calvaria and brain is removed, and CN V is dissected. The meningeal branches of the maxillary (CN V₂) and mandibular (CN V₃) nerves are distributed to the dura of the lateral part of the anterior and the middle cranial fossae as peri-arterial plexuses that accompany the branches of the middle meningeal artery along with vasomotor sympathetic nerve fibers from the superior cervical ganglion (*inset*). **B.** The internal aspect of the cranial base shows innervation of the dura by branches of the trigeminal and sensory fibers of cervical spinal nerves (C2, C3) passing directly from those nerves or via meningeal branches of the vagus (CN X) and hypoglossal (CN XII) nerves.

Leptomeninx: The arachnoid and pia are continuous parietal and visceral layers, respectively, of the leptomeninx that surround the CSF-filled subarachnoid space. ◆ The arachnoid and pia are connected by fine trabeculae that traverse the subarachnoid space. ◆ The subarachnoid space of the cranial cavity is continuous with that of the vertebral canal. ◆ The arachnoid is normally applied to the internal surface of the dura by CSF pressure. ◆ The pia intimately invests the neural tissue and its surface vasculature, coursing deeply along the vessels as they enter or exit the central nervous system.

Neurovasculature of meninges: The cranial meninges receive blood primarily from the middle meningeal branches of the maxillary arteries. ◆ The dura receives sensory innervation from meningeal branches of all three divisions of the trigeminal nerve and fibers from the C2 spinal ganglion.

BRAIN

Because the brain is usually studied in detail in a separate neuroanatomy course, the brain is covered by only a superficial survey of its gross structure in the typical anatomy course, with attention primarily concerned with the relationship between the brain and its environment—that is, its meningeal coverings, the CSF-filled subarachnoid space, and internal features of its bony encasement (the neurocranium).

Because of their role in the production of CSF (cerebrospinal fluid), the ventricles of the brain and the CSF-producing choroid plexuses found there are also covered. Furthermore, 11 of 12 cranial nerves arise from the brain (see Chapter 9).

Parts of Brain

The **brain** (contained by the neurocranium) is composed of the cerebrum, cerebellum, and brainstem (Fig. 7.36). When the calvaria and dura are removed, **gyri** (folds), **sulci** (grooves), and **fissures** (clefts) of the cerebral cortex are visible through the delicate arachnoid–pia layer. Whereas the gyri and sulci demonstrate much variation, the other features of the brain, including overall brain size, are remarkably consistent from individual to individual.

- The **cerebrum** (L. *brain*) includes the cerebral hemispheres and basal ganglia. The **cerebral hemispheres,** separated by the falx cerebri within the **longitudinal cerebral fissure,** are the dominant features of the brain (Fig. 7.36A-C). Each cerebral hemisphere is divided for descriptive purposes into four lobes, each of which is related to, but the boundaries of which do not correspond to, the overlying bones of the same name. From a superior view, the cerebrum is essentially divided into quarters by the median longitudinal cerebral fissure and the coronal **central sulcus.** The central sulcus separates the **frontal lobes** (anteriorly) from the **parietal lobes** (posteriorly). In a lateral view, these lobes lie superior to the transverse **lateral sulcus** and the temporal lobe inferior to it. The posteriorly placed **occipital lobes** are separated from the parietal and temporal lobes by the plane of the **parieto-occipital sulcus,** visible on the medial surface of the cerebrum in a hemisected brain (Fig. 7.36C).

The anteriormost points of the anteriorly projecting frontal and temporal lobes are the **frontal** and **temporal poles.** The posteriormost point of the posteriorly projecting occipital lobe is the **occipital pole.** The hemispheres occupy the entire supratentorial cranial cavity (Fig. 7.31A & B). The frontal lobes occupy the anterior cranial fossae, the temporal lobes occupy the lateral parts of the middle cranial fossae, and the occipital lobes extend posteriorly over the tentorium cerebelli.

- The **diencephalon** is composed of the epithalamus, dorsal thalamus, and hypothalamus and forms the central core of the brain (Fig. 7.36D).
- The **midbrain,** the rostral part of the brainstem, lies at the junction of the middle and posterior cranial fossae. CN III and IV are associated with the midbrain.
- The **pons** is the part of the brainstem between the midbrain rostrally and the medulla oblongata caudally; it lies in the anterior part of the posterior cranial fossa. CN V is associated with the pons (Fig. 7.36A, C & D).
- The **medulla oblongata** (medulla) is the most caudal subdivision of the brainstem that is continuous with the spinal cord; it lies in the posterior cranial fossa. CN IX, X, and XII are associated with the medulla, whereas CN VI–VIII are associated with the junction of pons and medulla.
- The **cerebellum** is the large brain mass lying posterior to the pons and medulla and inferior to the posterior part of the cerebrum. It lies beneath the tentorium cerebelli in the posterior cranial fossa. It consists of two lateral hemispheres that are united by a narrow middle part, the **vermis.**

Ventricular System of Brain

The ventricular system of the brain consists of two lateral ventricles and the midline 3rd and 4th ventricles connected by the cerebral aqueduct (Figs. 7.37 and 7.38). CSF, largely secreted by the choroid plexuses of the ventricles, fills these brain cavities and the subarachnoid space of the brain and spinal cord.

VENTRICLES OF BRAIN

The **lateral ventricles,** the 1st and 2nd ventricles, are the largest cavities of the ventricular system and occupy large areas of the cerebral hemispheres. Each lateral ventricle

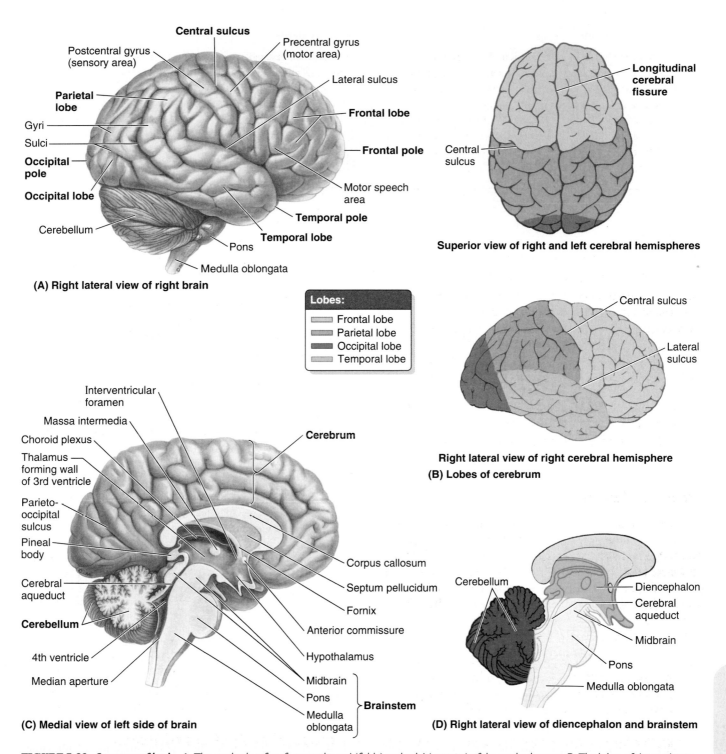

FIGURE 7.36. Structure of brain. A. The cerebral surface features the gyri (folds) and sulci (grooves) of the cerebral cortex. **B.** The lobes of the cerebrum are color coded. Whereas distinct central and lateral sulci demarcate the frontal lobe and anterior boundaries of the parietal and temporal lobes of the cerebrum, the demarcation of the posterior boundaries of the latter and the occipital lobe is less distinct externally. **C.** The medial surface of the cerebrum and deeper parts of the brain (diencephalon and brainstem) are shown after bisection of the brain. The parieto-occipital sulcus demarcating the parietal and occipital lobes is seen on the medial aspect of the cerebrum. **D.** The parts of the brainstem are identified.

opens through an **interventricular foramen** into the 3rd ventricle. The **3rd ventricle,** a slit-like cavity between the right and the left halves of the diencephalon, is continuous postero-inferiorly with the **cerebral aqueduct,** a narrow channel in the midbrain connecting the 3rd and 4th ventricles (Figs. 7.36C and 7.37B).

The pyramid-shaped **4th ventricle** in the posterior part of the pons and medulla extends inferoposteriorly. Inferiorly, it tapers to a narrow channel that continues into the cervical region of the spinal cord as the central canal (Fig. 7.37A). CSF drains into the subarachnoid space from the 4th ventricle through a single **median aperture** and paired **lateral**

Arachnoid granulations

Superior sagittal sinus

Lateral ventricles

Inter-ventricular foramen

3rd ventricle

Communication via lateral apertures

Calvaria

Subarachnoid space containing CSF

Choroid plexus of the lateral ventricle

Cerebral aqueduct

Neurocranium

Straight sinus

4th ventricle

Choroid plexus of the 4th ventricle

Confluence of sinuses

Median aperture

Central canal of spinal cord

(A) Median section with ventricles viewed from the left

Cerebral subarachnoid space

Corpus callosum

3rd ventricle

Optic chiasm

Chiasmatic cistern

Interpeduncular cistern

Pontocerebellar cistern

Spinal subarachnoid space

Septum pellucidum

Choroid plexus of 3rd ventricle

Pineal body

Quadrigeminal cistern

Tentorium cerebelli

Cerebral aqueduct

Choroid plexus of 4th ventricle

Posterior cerebello-medullary cistern

(B) Medial view, right half of hemisected head, sectioned to the right of the superior sagittal and straight sinuses

FIGURE 7.37. Ventricles, subarachnoid spaces, and cisterns. **A.** The ventricular system and circulation of the CSF are shown. The production of CSF is mainly by the choroid plexuses of the lateral, 3rd, and 4th ventricles. The plexuses of the lateral ventricles are the largest and most important. **B.** Subarachnoid cisterns, expanded regions of the subarachnoid space, contain more substantial amounts of CSF.

apertures. These apertures are the only means by which CSF enters the subarachnoid space. If they are blocked, CSF accumulates and the ventricles distend, producing compression of the substance of the cerebral hemispheres.

SUBARACHNOID CISTERNS

Although it is not accurate to say that the brain "floats" in the CSF, the brain actually has minimal attachment to the neurocranium. At certain areas on the base of the brain, the arachnoid and pia are widely separated by subarachnoid cisterns (Fig. 7.37B), which contain CSF, and soft tissue structures

that "anchor" the brain, such as the arachnoid trabeculae, vasculature, and in some cases, cranial nerve roots. The cisterns are usually named according to the structures related to them.

Major intracranial subarachnoid cisterns include the:

• **Cerebellomedullary cistern:** the largest of the subarachnoid cisterns, located between the cerebellum and the medulla; receives CSF from the apertures of the 4th ventricle. It is divided into the **posterior cerebellomedullary cistern** (cisterna magna) and the **lateral cerebellomedullary cistern.**

Frontal lobe cortex
Frontal lobe (white matter)
Anterior horn of lateral ventricle
Head of caudate nucleus
Septum pellucidum
Column of fornix
Thalamus
3rd ventricle
Choroid plexus
Posterior horn of lateral ventricle
Splenium of corpus callosum

FIGURE 7.38. Transverse MRI of brain. CSF surrounding the brain, extending into the sulci and fissures, and occupying the ventricles, appears bright white.

- **Pontocerebellar cistern** (pontine cistern): an extensive space ventral to the pons, continuous inferiorly with the spinal subarachnoid space.
- **Interpeduncular cistern** (basal cistern): located in the interpeduncular fossa between the cerebral peduncles of the midbrain.
- **Chiasmatic cistern** (cistern of optic chiasma): inferior and anterior to the *optic chiasm,* the point of crossing or decussation of optic nerve fibers.
- **Quadrigeminal cistern** (cistern of great cerebral vein): located between the posterior part of the corpus callosum and the superior surface of the cerebellum; contains parts of the great cerebral vein.
- **Cisterna ambiens** (ambient cistern): located on the lateral aspect of the midbrain and continuous posteriorly with the quadrigeminal cistern (not illustrated).

SECRETION OF CEREBROSPINAL FLUID

Cerebrospinal fluid (CSF) is secreted (at the rate of 400–500 mL/day) mainly by choroidal epithelial cells (modified ependymal cells) of the **choroid plexuses** in the lateral, 3rd, and 4th ventricles (Figs. 7.36C, 7.37, and 7.38). The choroid plexuses consist of fringes of vascular pia mater (tela choroidea) covered by cuboidal epithelial cells. They are invaginated into the roofs of the 3rd and 4th ventricles and on the floors of the bodies and inferior horns of the lateral ventricles.

CIRCULATION OF CEREBROSPINAL FLUID

CSF leaves the lateral ventricles through the *interventricular foramina* and enters the 3rd ventricle (Fig. 7.37A). From here, CSF passes through the *cerebral aqueduct* into the 4th ventricle. Some CSF leaves this ventricle through its *median* and *lateral apertures* and enters the *subarachnoid space,* which is continuous around the spinal cord and posterosuperiorly over the cerebellum. However, most CSF flows into the interpeduncular and quadrigeminal cisterns. CSF from the various subarachnoid cisterns flows superiorly through the sulci and fissures on the medial and superolateral surfaces of the cerebral hemispheres. CSF also passes into the extensions of the subarachnoid space around the cranial nerves, the most important of which are the subarachnoid space extensions surrounding the optic nerves (CN II).

ABSORPTION OF CEREBROSPINAL FLUID

The main site of CSF absorption into the venous system is through the **arachnoid granulations** (Figs. 7.35 and 7.37A), especially those that protrude into the superior sagittal sinus and its lateral lacunae (Fig. 7.28D). The subarachnoid space containing CSF extends into the cores of the arachnoid granulations. CSF enters the venous system through two routes: (1) most CSF enters the venous system by transport through the cells of the arachnoid granulations into the dural venous sinuses, and (2) some CSF moves between the cells making up the arachnoid granulations (Corbett et al., 2006).

FUNCTIONS OF CEREBROSPINAL FLUID

Along with the meninges and calvaria, CSF protects the brain by providing a cushion against blows to the head. The CSF in the subarachnoid space provides the buoyancy that prevents the weight of the brain from compressing the cranial nerve roots and blood vessels against the internal surface of the cranium. Because the brain is slightly heavier than the CSF, the gyri on the basal surface of the brain (Fig. 7.42) are in contact with the floor of the cranial cavity when a person is standing erect. In many places at the base of the brain, only the cranial meninges intervene between the brain and cranial bones. In the erect position, the CSF is in the subarachnoid cisterns and sulci on the superior and lateral parts of the brain; therefore, CSF and dura normally separate the superior part of the brain from the calvaria (Fig. 7.37A).

Small, rapidly recurring changes take place in **intracranial pressure** owing to the beating heart; slow recurring changes result from unknown causes. Momentarily large changes in pressure occur during coughing and straining and during changes in position (erect vs. supine). Any change in the volume of the intracranial contents (e.g., a brain tumor, an accumulation of ventricular fluid caused by blockage of the cerebral aqueduct (see Fig. B7.20B), or blood from a ruptured aneurysm) will be reflected by a change in intracranial pressure. This rule is called the **Monro-Kellie doctrine,** which states that the cranial cavity is a closed rigid box and that a change in the quantity of intracranial blood can occur only through the displacement or replacement of CSF.

Arterial Blood Supply to Brain

Although it accounts for only about 2.5% of body weight, the brain receives about one sixth of the cardiac output and one fifth of the oxygen consumed by the body at rest. The *blood supply to the brain* is derived from the internal carotid and vertebral arteries (Fig. 7.39), the terminal branches of which lie in the subarachnoid space. *Venous drainage from the brain* occurs via cerebral and cerebellar veins that drain to the adjacent dural venous sinuses (Fig. 7.29A & B). See also Venous Drainage of Brain on p. 883.

INTERNAL CAROTID ARTERIES

The **internal carotid arteries** arise in the neck from the common carotid arteries (Fig. 7.39). The cervical part of each artery ascends vertically through the neck, without branching, to the cranial base. Each internal carotid artery enters the cranial cavity through the *carotid canal* in the petrous part of the temporal bone. The intracranial course of the internal carotid artery is illustrated and described in Figure 7.40 and demonstrated radiographically in Figure 7.41. In addition to the carotid arteries, the carotid canals contain

venous plexuses and *carotid plexuses of sympathetic nerves* (Fig. 7.40). The internal carotid arteries course anteriorly through the *cavernous sinuses,* with the abducent nerves (CN VI) and in close proximity to the oculomotor (CN III) and trochlear (CN IV) nerves, running in the carotid groove on the side of the body of the sphenoid (Figs. 7.31C and 7.40). The terminal branches of the internal carotid arteries are the **anterior** and **middle cerebral arteries** (Figs. 7.41 and 7.42).

Clinically, the internal carotid arteries and their branches are often referred to as the *anterior circulation of the brain.* The anterior cerebral arteries are connected by the **anterior communicating artery.** Near their termination, the internal carotid arteries are joined to the posterior cerebral arteries by the **posterior communicating arteries,** completing the *cerebral arterial circle* around the *interpeduncular fossa,* the deep depression on the inferior surface of the midbrain between the cerebral peduncles (Figs. 7.42 and 7.43).

VERTEBRAL ARTERIES

The **vertebral arteries** begin in the root of the neck (the prevertebral parts of the vertebral arteries) as the first branches of the first part of the subclavian arteries (Fig. 7.39). The two vertebral arteries are usually unequal in size, the left being larger than the right. The **cervical parts of the vertebral arteries** ascend through the *transverse foramina* of the first six cervical vertebrae. The **atlantic parts of the vertebral arteries** (parts related to the atlas, vertebra C1) perforate the dura and arachnoid and pass through the foramen magnum. The **intracranial parts of the vertebral arteries** unite at the caudal border of the pons to form the *basilar artery* (Figs. 7.29A, 7.39, 7.42 and 7.43C). The vertebrobasilar arterial system and its branches are often referred to clinically as the *posterior circulation of the brain.*

The **basilar artery,** so-named because of its close relationship to the *cranial base,* ascends the *clivus,* the sloping surface from the dorsum sellae to the foramen magnum, through the pontocerebellar cistern to the superior border of the pons. It ends by dividing into the two **posterior cerebral arteries.**

CEREBRAL ARTERIES

In addition to supplying branches to deeper parts of the brain, the cortical branches of each cerebral artery supply a surface and a pole of the cerebrum (Figs. 7.41 and 7.43A & B; Table 7.7). The cortical branches of the:

- **Anterior cerebral artery** supply most of the medial and superior surfaces of the brain and the *frontal pole.*
- **Middle cerebral artery** supply the lateral surface of the brain and the *temporal pole.*
- **Posterior cerebral artery** supply the inferior surface of the brain and the *occipital pole.*

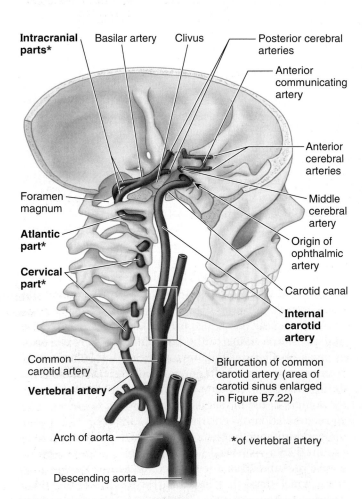

FIGURE 7.39. **Arterial supply to brain.** The bilaterally paired internal carotid and vertebral arteries deliver an abundant supply of oxygen-rich blood.

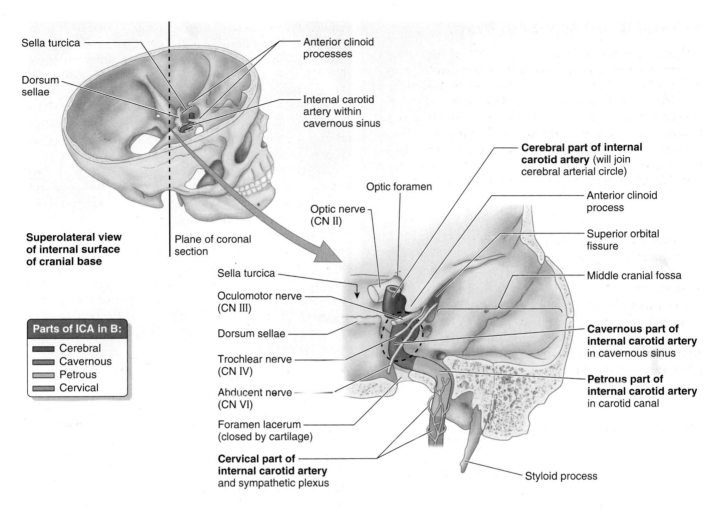

Superolateral view of internal surface of cranial base

Sella turcica

Dorsum sellae

Anterior clinoid processes

Internal carotid artery within cavernous sinus

Plane of coronal section

Parts of ICA in B:

- Cerebral
- Cavernous
- Petrous
- Cervical

Optic foramen

Optic nerve (CN II)

Cerebral part of internal carotid artery (will join cerebral arterial circle)

Anterior clinoid process

Superior orbital fissure

Middle cranial fossa

Sella turcica

Oculomotor nerve (CN III)

Dorsum sellae

Trochlear nerve (CN IV)

Abducent nerve (CN VI)

Foramen lacerum (closed by cartilage)

Cervical part of internal carotid artery and sympathetic plexus

Cavernous part of internal carotid artery in cavernous sinus

Petrous part of internal carotid artery in carotid canal

Styloid process

Posterior view (of right side of anterior portion following bisection in coronal plane)

FIGURE 7.40. Course of internal carotid artery. The orientation drawing (*left*) indicates the plane of the coronal section that intersects the carotid canal (*right*). The cervical part of the internal carotid artery ascends vertically in the neck to the entrance of the carotid canal in the petrous temporal bone. The petrous part of the artery turns horizontally and medially in the carotid canal, toward the apex of the petrous temporal bone. It emerges from the canal superior to the foramen lacerum, closed in life by cartilage, and enters the cranial cavity. The artery runs anteriorly across the cartilage; then the cavernous part of the artery runs along the carotid grooves on the lateral side of the body of the sphenoid, traversing the cavernous sinus. Inferior to the anterior clinoid process, the artery makes a 180° turn, its cerebral part heading posteriorly to join the cerebral arterial circle (Figs. 7.42 and 7.43C).

CEREBRAL ARTERIAL CIRCLE

The **cerebral arterial circle** (of Willis) is a roughly pentagon-shaped circle of vessels on the ventral surface of the brain. It is an important anastomosis at the base of the brain between four arteries (two vertebral and two internal carotid arteries) that supply the brain (Figs. 7.42 and 7.43C; Table 7.7). The arterial circle is formed sequentially in an anterior to posterior direction by the:

- Anterior communicating artery.
- Anterior cerebral arteries.
- Internal carotid arteries.
- Posterior communicating arteries.
- Posterior cerebral arteries.

The various components of the cerebral arterial circle give numerous small branches to the brain.

Venous Drainage of Brain

The thin-walled, valveless veins draining the brain pierce the arachnoid and meningeal layers of dura to end in the nearest dural venous sinuses (Figs. 7.28A and 7.29–7.32), which ultimately drain for the most part into the IJVs. The **superior cerebral veins** on the superolateral surface of the brain drain into the superior sagittal sinus; **inferior** and **superficial middle cerebral veins** from the inferior, postero-inferior, and deep aspects of the cerebral hemispheres drain into the straight, transverse, and superior petrosal sinuses. The **great cerebral vein** (of Galen) is a single, midline vein formed inside the brain by the union of two internal cerebral veins; it ends by merging with the inferior sagittal sinus to form the straight sinus (Fig. 7.29). The cerebellum is drained by **superior** and **inferior cerebellar veins,** draining the respective aspect of the cerebellum into the transverse and sigmoid sinuses (Fig. 7.32).

(A) Anteroposterior view   **(B) Lateral view**

FIGURE 7.41. Carotid arteriograms. A and B. Radiopaque dye injected into the carotid arterial system demonstrates unilateral distribution to the brain from the internal carotid artery. *A,* anterior cerebral artery and its branches; *I,* the four parts of the internal carotid artery; *M,* middle cerebral artery and its branches; *O,* ophthalmic artery. (Courtesy of Dr. D. Armstrong, Associate Professor of Medical Imaging, University of Toronto, Ontario, Canada.)

Olfactory bulb and tract

Corpus callosum

Optic nerve (CN II)

Internal carotid artery

Temporal lobe

Posterior cerebral artery

Superior cerebellar artery

Abducent nerve (CN VI)

Facial nerve (CN VII)

Vestibulocochlear nerve
(CN VIII)

Glossopharyngeal nerve
(CN IX)

Vagus nerve (CN X)

Spinal accessory nerve (CN XI)

Hypoglossal nerve (CN XII)

Frontal lobe

Anterior cerebral artery

Anterior communicating artery

Anterior cerebral artery

Middle cerebral artery

Posterior communicating artery

Oculomotor nerve (CN III)

Trochlear nerve (CN IV)

Trigeminal nerve (CN V)

Basilar artery

Labyrinthine artery

Anterior inferior ⎤ Cerebellar
Posterior inferior ⎦ arteries

Vertebral artery

Anterior spinal artery

Inferior view

FIGURE 7.42. Base of brain with cerebral arterial circle. The internal carotid and basilar arteries converge, divide, and anastomose to form the cerebral arterial circle (of Willis). The left temporal pole is removed to show the middle cerebral artery in the lateral sulcus of the brain. The frontal lobes are separated to expose the anterior cerebral arteries.

FIGURE 7.43. Arterial blood supply of cerebrum.

TABLE 7.7. ARTERIAL BLOOD SUPPLY OF CEREBRAL HEMISPHERES

Artery	Origin	Distribution
Internal carotid:	Common carotid artery at superior border of thyroid cartilage	Gives branches to walls of cavernous sinus, pituitary gland, and trigeminal ganglion; provides primary supply to brain
Anterior cerebral	Internal carotid artery	Cerebral hemispheres, except for occipital lobes
Anterior communicating	Anterior cerebral artery	Cerebral arterial circle (of Willis)
Middle cerebral	Continuation of internal carotid artery distal to anterior cerebral artery	Most of lateral surface of cerebral hemispheres
Vertebral:	Subclavian artery	Cranial meninges and cerebellum
Basilar	Formed by union of vertebral arteries	Brainstem, cerebellum, and cerebrum
Posterior cerebral	Terminal branch of basilar artery	Inferior aspect of cerebral hemisphere and occipital lobe
Posterior communicating	Posterior cerebral artery	Optic tract, cerebral peduncle, internal capsule, and thalamus

BRAIN

Cerebral Injuries

 Cerebral concussion is an abrupt, brief loss of consciousness immediately after a severe head injury. Consciousness may be lost for only a few seconds, as occurs in most knockdowns during boxing. With a more severe injury, such as that resulting from an automobile accident, consciousness may be lost for hours and even days. If a person recovers consciousness within 6 hr, the long-term outcome is excellent (Rowland, 2010). If the coma lasts longer than 6 hr, brain tissue injury usually occurs.

Professional boxers are especially at risk for *chronic traumatic encephalopathy,* or *"punchdrunk syndrome,"* a brain injury characterized by weakness in the lower limbs, unsteady gait, slowness of muscular movements, tremors of the hands, hesitancy of speech, and slow cerebration (use of one's brain). Brain injuries result from acceleration and deceleration of the head that shears or stretches axons (*diffuse axonal injury*). The sudden stopping of the moving head results in the brain hitting the suddenly stationary cranium. Sometimes concussion occurs without loss of consciousness. The absence of loss of consciousness does not mean that the concussion is any less serious. Over 90% of head injuries are referred to as minor traumatic brain injuries.

Cerebral contusion results from brain trauma in which the pia is stripped from the injured surface of the brain and may be torn, allowing blood to enter the subarachnoid space. The bruising results either from the sudden impact of the still-moving brain against the suddenly stationary cranium, or from the suddenly moving cranium against the still-stationary brain. Cerebral contusion may result in an extended loss of consciousness, but if there is no diffuse axonal injury, brain swelling, or secondary hemorrhage, recovery from a contusion may be excellent (Rowland, 2010).

Cerebral lacerations are often associated with depressed cranial fractures (Fig. B7.4, p. 838) or gunshot wounds. Lacerations result in rupture of blood vessels and bleeding into the brain and subarachnoid space, causing increased intracranial pressure and cerebral compression.

Cerebral compression may be produced by:

- Intracranial collections of blood.
- Obstruction of CSF circulation or absorption.
- Intracranial tumors or abscesses.
- Brain swelling caused by *brain edema,* an increase in brain volume resulting from an increase in water and sodium content (Fishman, 2010a).

Cisternal Puncture

CSF may be obtained from the posterior cerebellomedullary cistern through a *cisternal puncture* for diagnostic or therapeutic purposes. The cerebellomedullary cistern is the site of choice in infants and young children; the lumbar cistern is used most frequently in adults (see Chapter 4, Fig. B4.18). The needle is carefully inserted through the posterior atlanto-occipital membrane into the cistern. The subarachnoid space or the ventricular system may also be entered for measuring or monitoring CSF pressure, injecting antibiotics, or administering contrast media for medical imaging.

Hydrocephalus

Overproduction of CSF, obstruction of CSF flow, or interference with CSF absorption results in excess fluid in the cerebral ventricles and enlargement of the head, a condition called *obstructive hydrocephalus* (Fig. B7.20A). The excess CSF dilates the ventricles, thins the cerebral cortex, and separates the bones of the calvaria in infants. Although an obstruction can occur any place, the blockage usually occurs in the cerebral aqueduct (Fig. B7.20B) or an interventricular foramen. *Aqueductal stenosis* (narrow aqueduct) may be caused by a nearby tumor in the midbrain or by cellular debris following intraventricular hemorrhage or bacterial and fungal infections of the central nervous system (Corbett et al., 2006).

Blockage of CSF circulation results in dilation of the ventricles superior to the point of obstruction and increased pressure on the cerebral hemispheres. This condition squeezes the brain between the ventricular fluid and the calvarial bones. In infants, the internal pressure results in expansion of the brain and calvaria because the sutures and fontanelles are still open. It is possible to produce an artificial

(A)

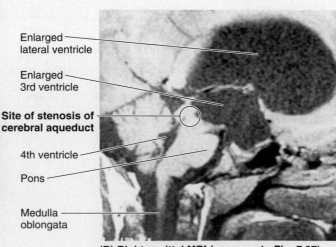

Enlarged lateral ventricle

Enlarged 3rd ventricle

Site of stenosis of cerebral aqueduct

4th ventricle

Pons

Medulla oblongata

(B) Right sagittal MRI (compare to Fig. 7.37)

FIGURE B7.20. Hydrocephalus (A) and aqueductal stenosis (B).

drainage system to bypass the blockage and allow CSF to escape, thereby lessening damage to the brain.

In *communicating hydrocephalus,* the flow of CSF through the ventricles and into the subarachnoid space is not impaired; however, movement of CSF from this space into the venous system is partly or completely blocked. The blockage may be caused by the congenital absence of arachnoid granulations, or the granulations may be blocked by red blood cells as the result of a subarachnoid hemorrhage (Corbett et al., 2006).

Leakage of Cerebrospinal Fluid

Fractures in the floor of the middle cranial fossa may result in CSF leakage from the external acoustic meatus (*CSF otorrhea*) if the meninges superior to the middle ear are torn and the tympanic membrane is ruptured. Fractures in the floor of the anterior cranial fossa may involve the cribriform plate of the ethmoid (see Fig. 7.12A), resulting in CSF leakage through the nose (*CSF rhinorrhea*). CSF can be distinguished from mucus by testing its glucose level; the glucose level of the CSF reflects that of the blood. CSF otorrhea and rhinorrhea may be the primary indications of a cranial base fracture and increased risk of meningitis because an infection could spread to the meninges from the ear or nose (Rowland, 2010).

Anastomoses of Cerebral Arteries and Cerebral Embolism

Branches of the three cerebral arteries anastomose with each other on the surface of the brain; however, if a cerebral artery is obstructed by a *cerebral embolism* (e.g., a blood clot), these microscopic anastomoses are not capable of providing enough blood for the area of cerebral cortex concerned. Consequently, *cerebral ischemia* and *infarction* occur and an area of necrosis results. Large cerebral emboli occluding major cerebral vessels may cause severe neurologic problems and death.

Variations of Cerebral Arterial Circle

Variations in the size of the vessels forming the cerebral arterial circle are common. The posterior communicating arteries are absent in some individuals; in others there may be two anterior communicating arteries. In approximately 1 in 3 persons, one posterior cerebral artery is a major branch of the internal carotid artery. One of the anterior cerebral arteries is often small in the proximal part of its course; the anterior communicating artery is larger than usual in these individuals. These variations may become clinically significant if emboli or arterial disease occur.

Strokes

An *ischemic stroke* denotes the sudden development of focal neurological deficits that are usually related to *impaired cerebral blood flow.* An ischemic stroke is generally caused by an embolism in a major cerebral artery. Strokes are the most common neurologic disorders affecting adults in the United States (Elkind, 2010); they are more often disabling than fatal. The cardinal feature of a stroke is the sudden onset of neurological symptoms.

The cerebral arterial circle is an important means of collateral circulation in the event of gradual obstruction of one of the major arteries forming the circle. Sudden occlusion, even if only partial, results in neurological deficits. In elderly persons, the anastomoses of the arterial circle are often inadequate when a large artery (e.g., the internal carotid) is occluded, even if the occlusion is gradual (in which case function is impaired at least to some degree). The most common causes of strokes are *spontaneous cerebrovascular accidents,* such as cerebral thrombosis, cerebral hemorrhage, cerebral embolism, and subarachnoid hemorrhage (Rowland, 2010).

Hemorrhagic stroke follows the rupture of an artery or a *saccular aneurysm,* a sac-like dilation on a weak part of the arterial wall (Fig. B7.21A). The most common type of saccular aneurysm is a *berry aneurysm,* occurring in the vessels

(A)

Weak part of arterial wall

Berry aneurysm (BA)

Posterior cerebral artery

Basilar artery

(B) BA

(C) BA

FIGURE B7.21.

of or near the cerebral arterial circle and the medium arteries at the base of the brain (Fig. B7.21B). Aneurysms also occur at the bifurcation of the basilar artery into the posterior cerebral arteries.

In time, especially in individuals with *hypertension* (high blood pressure), the weak part of the wall of the aneurysm expands and may rupture (Fig. B7.21C), allowing blood to enter the subarachnoid space. Sudden *rupture of an aneurysm* usually produces a severe, almost unbearable headache and a stiff neck. These symptoms result from gross bleeding into the subarachnoid space.

Brain Infarction

An *atheromatous plaque* at a bend of an artery (e.g., at the bifurcation of a common carotid artery) results in progressive narrowing (*stenosis*) of the artery, producing increasingly severe neurologic deficits (Fig. B7.22). An *embolus* separates from the plaque and is carried in the blood until it lodges in an artery, usually an intracranial branch that is too small to allow its passage. This event usually results in *acute cortical infarction,* a sudden insufficiency of arterial blood to the brain (e.g., of the left parietal lobes). An interruption of blood supply for 30 sec alters a person's brain metabolism. After 1–2 min, neural function may be lost; after 5 min, lack of oxygen (*anoxia*) can result in cerebral infarction. Quickly restoring oxygen to the blood supply may reverse the brain damage (Elkind, 2010).

FIGURE B7.22.

Transient Ischemic Attacks

Transient ischemic attacks (TIAs) refer to neurologic symptoms resulting from *ischemia.* Most TIAs last only a few minutes, but some persist for up to an hour. With major *carotid* or *vertebrobasilar stenosis,* the TIA tends to last longer and causes distal closure of intracranial vessels. The symptoms of TIA may be ambiguous: staggering, dizziness, light-headedness, fainting, and *paresthesias.* Persons with TIAs are at increased risk for myocardial infarction and ischemic stroke (Brust, 2010).

The Bottom Line

BRAIN

Parts of brain: The two hemispheres of the cerebral cortex, separated by the falx cerebri, are the dominant features of the human brain. ♦ Although the pattern of gyri and sulci are highly variable, other features of the brain, including overall brain size, are remarkably consistent from individual to individual. ♦ Each cerebral hemisphere is divided for descriptive purposes into four lobes that are related to, but the boundaries of which do not correspond to, the overlying bones of the same name. ♦ The diencephalon forms the central core of the brain, with the midbrain, pons, and medulla oblongata making the brainstem; the medulla is continuous with the spinal cord. ♦ The cerebellum is the subtentorial brain mass occupying the posterior cranial fossa.

Ventricles of brain: Each cerebral hemisphere includes a lateral ventricle in its core; otherwise, the ventricular system of the brain is an unpaired, median formation that communicates with the subarachnoid space surrounding the brain and spinal cord. ♦ Choroid plexuses secrete CSF into the ventricles, which flows out of them into the subarachnoid space. ♦ CSF is absorbed into the venous system, normally at the same rate at which it is produced, by the arachnoid granulations related to the superior sagittal sinus.

Arterial supply and venous drainage of brain: A continuous supply of oxygen and nutrients is essential for brain function. ♦ The brain receives a dual blood supply from the cerebral branches of the bilaterally paired internal carotid and vertebral arteries. ♦ Anastomoses between these arteries form the cerebral arterial circle. ♦ Anastomoses also occur between the branches of the three cerebral arteries on the surface of the brain. ♦ In adults, if one of the four arteries delivering blood to the brain is blocked, the remaining three are not usually capable of providing adequate collateral circulation; consequently, impaired cerebral blood flow (ischemia) and an ischemic stroke result. ♦ Venous drainage from the brain occurs via the dural venous sinuses and internal jugular veins.

EYE, ORBIT, ORBITAL REGION, AND EYEBALL

The **eye** is the organ of vision and consists of the eyeball and the optic nerve. The *orbit* contains the eyeball and its *accessory visual structures* (L., adnexa oculi). The **orbital region** is the area of the face overlying the orbit and eyeball and includes the upper and lower eyelids and lacrimal apparatus.

Orbits

The **orbits** are bilateral bony cavities in the facial skeleton that resemble hollow, quadrangular pyramids with their bases directed anterolaterally and their apices, posteromedially

(Fig. 7.44A). The medial walls of the two orbits, separated by the ethmoidal sinuses and the upper parts of the nasal cavity, are nearly parallel, whereas their lateral walls are approximately at a right (90°) angle.

Consequently, the axes of the orbits (*orbital axes*) diverge at approximately 45°. The *optical axes* (axes of gaze, the direction or line of sight) for the two eyeballs, are parallel, however, and in the anatomical position run directly anteriorly ("looking straight ahead"), the eyeballs being in the *primary position*. The orbits and orbital region anterior to them contain and protect the **eyeballs** and **accessory visual structures** (Fig. 7.45), which include the:

- *Eyelids*, which bound the orbits anteriorly, controlling exposure of the anterior eyeball.

FIGURE 7.44. Orbits and placement of eyeballs within them. A. Note the orbits' disposition relative to each other and to the optical axes (line of gaze). The orbits are separated by ethmoidal cells and the upper nasal cavity and septum. **B.** The bony walls of the orbit are shown. This anterolateral view allows a view of the orbit and apex, which lie in the sagittal plane and are not well seen in an anterior view.

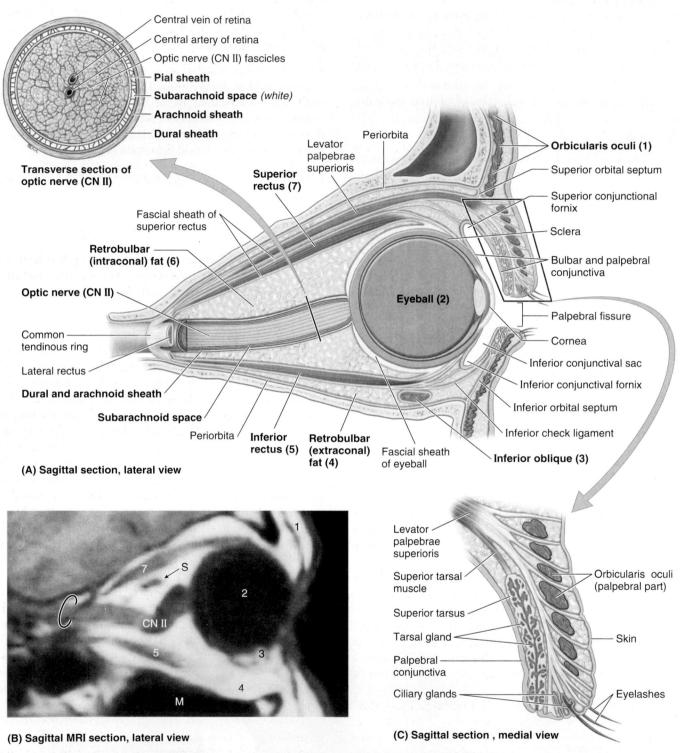

Central vein of retina
Central artery of retina
Optic nerve (CN II) fascicles
Pial sheath
Subarachnoid space *(white)*
Arachnoid sheath
Dural sheath

Transverse section of optic nerve (CN II)

Periorbita

Levator palpebrae superioris

Superior rectus (7)

Orbicularis oculi (1)

Superior orbital septum

Superior conjunctional fornix

Sclera

Fascial sheath of superior rectus

Retrobulbar (intraconal) fat (6)

Optic nerve (CN II)

Eyeball (2)

Bulbar and palpebral conjunctiva

Common tendinous ring

Lateral rectus

Dural and arachnoid sheath

Subarachnoid space

Periorbita

Inferior rectus (5)

Retrobulbar (extraconal) fat (4)

Fascial sheath of eyeball

Inferior oblique (3)

Palpebral fissure

Cornea

Inferior conjunctival sac

Inferior conjunctival fornix

Inferior orbital septum

Inferior check ligament

(A) Sagittal section, lateral view

(B) Sagittal MRI section, lateral view

Levator palpebrae superioris

Superior tarsal muscle

Superior tarsus

Tarsal gland

Palpebral conjunctiva

Ciliary glands

Orbicularis oculi (palpebral part)

Skin

Eyelashes

(C) Sagittal section, medial view

FIGURE 7.45. Orbit, eyeball, and eyelids. A. Sagittal section of orbit demonstrating the contents of the orbit. *Inset,* cross-section of optic nerve (CN II). The subarachnoid space around the optic nerve is continuous with the space between the arachnoid and the pia covering the brain. The numbers refer to structures labeled in part **B. B.** MRI study providing a sagittal section similar to A. *M,* maxillary sinus; *S,* superior ophthalmic vein; *arc,* optic canal. **C.** Detail of the superior eyelid. The tarsus forms the skeleton of the eyelid and contains tarsal glands. (Part **B** courtesy of Dr. W. Kucharczyk, Professor and Neuroradiologist Senior Scientist, Department of Medical Imaging, University Health Network, Toronto, Ontario, Canada.)

- *Extra-ocular muscles,* which position the eyeballs and raise the superior eyelids.
- *Nerves and vessels* in transit to the eyeballs and muscles.
- *Orbital fascia* surrounding the eyeballs and muscles.
- *Mucous membrane (conjunctiva)* lining the eyelids and anterior aspect of the eyeballs, and most of the *lacrimal apparatus,* which lubricates it.

All space within the orbits not occupied by these structures is filled with **orbital fat;** thus, it forms a matrix in which the structures of the orbit are embedded.

The quadrangular pyramidal **orbit** has a base, four walls, and an apex (Fig. 7.44B):

- The **base of the orbit** is outlined by the **orbital margin,** which surrounds the **orbital opening.** The bone forming the orbital margin is reinforced to afford protection to the orbital contents and provides attachment for the *orbital septum,* a fibrous membrane that extends into the eyelids.
- The **superior wall** (roof) is approximately horizontal and is formed mainly by the *orbital part of the frontal bone,* which separates the orbital cavity from the anterior cranial fossa. Near the apex of the orbit, the superior wall is formed by the *lesser wing of the sphenoid.* Anterolaterally, a shallow depression in the orbital part of the frontal bone, called the **fossa for lacrimal gland** (lacrimal fossa), accommodates the lacrimal gland.
- The **medial walls** of the contralateral orbits are essentially parallel and are formed primarily by the **orbital plate of ethmoid bone,** along with contributions from the *frontal process of the maxilla, lacrimal,* and *sphenoid bones.* Anteriorly, the medial wall is indented by the **lacrimal groove** and **fossa for lacrimal sac;** the *trochlea* (pulley) for the tendon of one of the extra-ocular muscles is located superiorly. Much of the bone forming the medial wall is paper thin; the ethmoid bone is highly pneumatized with ethmoidal cells, often visible through the bone of a dried cranium.
- The **inferior wall** (orbital floor) is formed mainly by the *maxilla* and partly by the zygomatic and palatine bones. The thin inferior wall is shared by the orbit and maxillary sinus. It slants inferiorly from the apex to the inferior orbital margin. The inferior wall is demarcated from the lateral wall of the orbit by the **inferior orbital fissure,** a gap between the orbital surfaces of the maxilla and the sphenoid.
- The **lateral wall** is formed by the **frontal process of the zygomatic bone** and the *greater wing of the sphenoid.* This is the strongest and thickest wall, which is important because it is most exposed and vulnerable to direct trauma. Its posterior part separates the orbit from the temporal and middle cranial fossae. The lateral walls of the contralateral orbits are nearly perpendicular to each other.
- The **apex of the orbit** is at the **optic canal** in the *lesser wing of the sphenoid* just medial to the *superior orbital fissure.*

The widest part of the orbit corresponds to the equator of the eyeball (Fig. 7.45A), an imaginary line encircling the eyeball equidistant from its anterior and posterior poles. The bones forming the orbit are lined with **periorbita,** the periosteum of the orbit. The periorbita is continuous:

- At the optic canal and superior orbital fissure with the periosteal layer of the dura mater.
- Over the orbital margins and through the inferior orbital fissure with the periosteum covering the external surface of the cranium (pericranium).
- With the orbital septa at the orbital margins.
- With the fascial sheaths of the extra-ocular muscles.
- With the orbital fascia that forms the *fascial sheath of the eyeball.*

Eyelids and Lacrimal Apparatus

The eyelids and lacrimal fluid, secreted by the lacrimal glands, protect the cornea and eyeballs from injury and irritation (e.g., by dust and small particles).

EYELIDS

The **eyelids** are moveable folds that cover the eyeball anteriorly when closed, thereby protecting it from injury and excessive light. They also keep the cornea moist by spreading the lacrimal fluid. The eyelids are covered externally by thin skin and internally by transparent mucous membrane, the **palpebral conjunctiva** (Fig. 7.45A & C). This part of the conjunctiva is reflected onto the eyeball, where it is continuous with the **bulbar conjunctiva.** This part of the conjunctiva is thin and transparent and attaches loosely to the anterior surface of the eyeball. The bulbar conjunctiva, loose and wrinkled over the sclera (where it contains small, visible blood vessels), is adherent to the periphery of the cornea (Fig. 7.46B). The lines of reflection of the palpebral conjunctiva onto the eyeball form deep recesses, the **superior** and **inferior conjunctival fornices** (Figs. 7.45A and 7.46).

The **conjunctival sac** is the space bound by the palpebral and bulbar conjunctivae; it is a closed space when the eyelids are closed, but opens via an anterior aperture, the *palpebral fissure* (L. *rima palpebrae,* the gap between the eyelids), when the eye is open (eyelids are parted) (Fig. 7.45A). The conjunctival sac is a specialized form of mucosal "bursa" that enables the eyelids to move freely over the surface of the eyeball as they open and close.

The superior (upper) and inferior (lower) eyelids are strengthened by dense bands of connective tissue, the **superior** and **inferior tarsi** (singular = **tarsus**), which form the "skeleton" of the eyelids (Figs. 7.45C and 7.47A). Fibers of the palpebral portion of the *orbicularis oculi* (the sphincter of the palpebral fissure) are in the connective tissue superficial to the tarsi and deep to the skin of the eyelids (Fig. 7.45C). Embedded in the tarsi are **tarsal glands** that produce a lipid secretion that lubricates the edges of the eyelids and prevents them from sticking together when they close. The lipid attaches firmly to the pigment layer of the retina, but can easily be stripped from the sclera. The choroid is continuous anteriorly with the ciliary body.

The **ciliary body,** is a ring-like thickening of the layer posterior to the corneoscleral junction, which is muscular as well as vascular (Figs. 7.49B and 7.50). It connects the choroid with the circumference of the iris. The ciliary body provides attachment for the lens. The contraction and relaxation of the circularly arranged smooth muscle of the ciliary body controls the thickness, and therefore the focus, of the lens. Folds on the internal surface of the ciliary body, the **ciliary processes,** secrete *aqueous humor.* Aqueous humor fills the **anterior segment of the eyeball,** the interior of the eyeball anterior to the lens, suspensory ligament, and ciliary body. (Fig. 7.50B).

The **iris,** which literally lies on the anterior surface of the lens, is a thin contractile diaphragm with a central aperture, the **pupil,** for transmitting light (Figs. 7.49B, 7.50, and 7.51A). When a person is awake, the size of the pupil varies continually to regulate the amount of light entering the eye

(Fig. 7.51B). Two involuntary muscles control the size of the pupil: the parasympathetically stimulated, circularly arranged **sphincter pupillae** decreases its diameter (constrict or contracts the pupil, *pupillary miosis*), and the sympathetically stimulated, radially arranged **dilator pupillae** increases its diameter (dilates the pupil). The nature of the pupillary responses is paradoxical: sympathetic responses usually occur immediately, yet it may take up to 20 min for the pupil to dilate in response to low lighting, as in a darkened theater. Parasympathetic responses are typically slower than sympathetic responses, yet parasympathetically stimulated papillary constriction is normally instantaneous. Abnormal sustained pupillary dilation (*mydriasis*) may occur in certain diseases or as a result of trauma or the use of certain drugs.

INNER LAYER OF EYEBALL

The inner layer of the eyeball is the **retina** (Fig. 7.49C and 7.50). It is the sensory neural layer of the eyeball. Grossly,

Trabecula at iridocorneal angle
Anterior chamber
Dilator pupillae
Iris
Lens
Sphincter pupillae

(A) Superior view

Cornea
Scleral venous sinus (canal of Schlemm)
Sclera
Ciliary body
Ciliary process
Posterior chamber
Zonular fibers

In dim light: (dilated pupil)

In bright light: (constricted pupil)

(B) Anterior view

Dilator pupillae
Postsynaptic sympathetic nerve fiber
Radially-arranged smooth muscle fibers of dilator pupillae
Circularly-arranged smooth muscle fibers of sphincter pupillae
Pupil
Ciliary ganglion
Postsynaptic parasympathetic nerve fiber
Sphincter pupillae

FIGURE 7.51. Structure and function of the iris. A. Iris dissected *in situ.* The iris separates the anterior and posterior chambers of the anterior segment of the eyeball as it bounds the pupil. B. Dilation and constriction of the pupil. In dim light, sympathetic fibers stimulate dilation of the pupil. In bright light, parasympathetic fibers stimulate constricting the pupil.

the retina consists of two functional parts with distinct locations: an optic part and a non-visual retina. The **optic part of the retina** is sensitive to visual light rays and has two layers: a neural layer and pigmented layer. The **neural layer** is light receptive. The **pigmented layer** consists of a single layer of cells that reinforces the light-absorbing property of the choroid in reducing the scattering of light in the eyeball. The **non-visual retina** is an anterior continuation of the pigmented layer and a layer of supporting cells. The non-visual retina extends over the ciliary body (**ciliary part of retina**) and the posterior surface of the iris (**iridial part of retina**), to the pupillary margin.

Clinically, the internal aspect of the posterior part of the eyeball, where light entering the eyeball is focused, is referred to as the **fundus of the eyeball** (ocular fundus). The retina of the fundus includes a distinctive circular area called the **optic disc** (optic papilla), where the sensory fibers and vessels conveyed by the optic nerve (CN II) enter the eyeball (Figs. 7.49C, 7.50A and 7.52). Because it contains no photoreceptors, the optic disc is insensitive to light. Consequently, this part of the retina is commonly called the *blind spot.*

Just lateral to the optic disc is the **macula of the retina** or macula lutea (L. yellow spot). The yellow color of the macula is apparent only when the retina is examined with red-free light. The macula is a small oval area of the retina with special photoreceptor cones that is specialized for acuity of vision. It is not normally observed with an *ophthalmoscope* (a device for viewing the interior of the eyeball through the pupil). At the center of the macula, a depression, the **fovea centralis** (L., central

pit), is the area of most acute vision. The fovea is approximately 1.5 mm in diameter; its center, the **foveola,** does not have the capillary network visible elsewhere deep to the retina.

The optic part of the retina terminates anteriorly along the **ora serrata** (L. serrated edge), the irregular posterior border of the ciliary body (Figs. 7.49C and 7.50A). Except for the cones and rods of the neural layer, the retina is supplied by the **central artery of the retina,** a branch of the ophthalmic artery. The cones and rods of the outer neural layer receive nutrients from the *capillary lamina of the choroid,* or choriocapillaris (discussed in "Vasculature of Orbit" on p. 905). It has the finest vessels of the inner surface of the choroid, against which the retina is pressed. A corresponding system of retinal veins unites to form the **central vein of the retina.**

REFRACTIVE MEDIA AND COMPARTMENTS OF EYEBALL

On their way to the retina, lightwaves pass through the refractive media of the eyeball: cornea, aqueous humor, lens, and vitreous humor (Fig. 7.50A). The *cornea* is the primary refractory medium of the eyeball—that is, it bends light to the greatest degree, focusing an inverted image on the light-sensitive retina of the *fundus of the eyeball.*

The **aqueous humor** (often shortened clinically to "aqueous") occupies the *anterior segment of the eyeball* (Figs. 7.50B and 7.51A). The anterior segment is subdivided by the iris and pupil. The **anterior chamber of the eye** is the space between the cornea anteriorly and the iris/pupil posteriorly. The **posterior chamber of the eye** is between the iris/pupil anteriorly and the lens and ciliary body posteriorly. Aqueous humor is produced in the posterior chamber by the *ciliary processes* of the ciliary body. This clear watery solution provides nutrients for the avascular cornea and lens. After passing through the pupil into the anterior chamber, the aqueous humor drains through a trabecular meshwork at the **iridocorneal angle** into the **scleral venous sinus** (L. *sinus venosus sclerae,* canal of Schlemm) (Fig. 7.51A). The humor is removed by the **limbal plexus,** a network of scleral veins close to the limbus, which drain in turn into both tributaries of the *vorticose* and *anterior ciliary veins* (Fig. 7.50B). Intra-ocular pressure (IOP) is a balance between production and outflow of aqueous humor.

The **lens** is posterior to the iris and anterior to the vitreous humor of the *vitreous body* (Figs. 7.50 and 7.51A). It is a transparent, biconvex structure enclosed in a capsule. The highly elastic **capsule of the lens** is anchored by **zonular fibers** (collectively constituting the **suspensory ligament of the lens**) to the encircling ciliary processes. Although most refraction is produced by the cornea, the convexity of the lens, particularly its anterior surface, constantly varies to fine-tune the focus of near or distant objects on the retina (Fig. 7.53). The isolated unattached lens assumes a nearly spherical shape. In other words, in the absence of external attachment and stretching, it becomes nearly round.

Branches of retinal vessels
(arterioles and venules)

Macula of retina

Optic disc

Ophthalmoscopic view

FIGURE 7.52. Fundus of right eyeball. Retinal venules (wider) and retinal arterioles (narrower) radiate from the center of the oval optic disc. The dark area lateral to the disc is the macula. Branches of retinal vessels extend toward this area, but do not reach its center, the fovea centralis—the area of most acute vision.

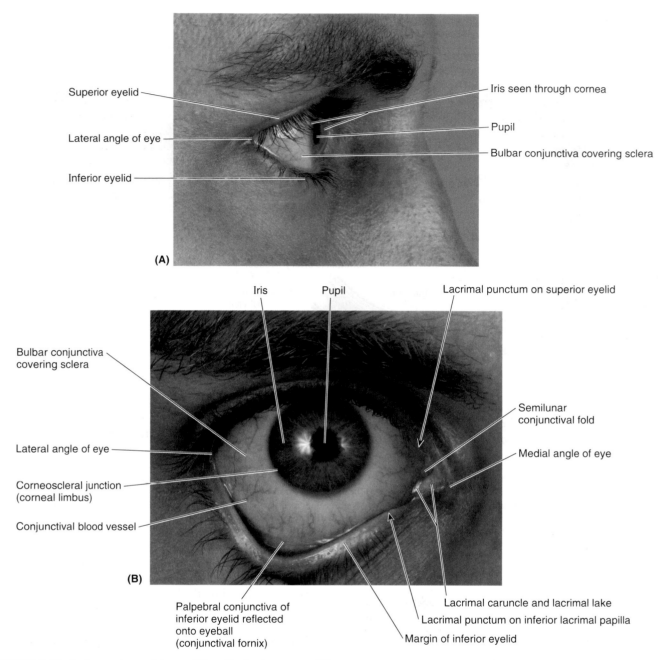

FIGURE 7.64. Surface anatomy of the eye (A) and lacrimal apparatus (B).

The anterior transparent part of the eye is the *cornea*, which is continuous with the sclera at its margins. In a lateral view (Fig. 7.64A), most of the visible part of the eyeball protrudes slightly through the *palpebral fissure*. It is apparent that the cornea has a greater curvature (convexity) than that of the rest of the eyeball (the part covered by sclera); thus a shallow angle occurs at the *corneoscleral junction*, the *corneal limbus* (Fig. 7.64B). The prominence of the cornea also makes movements of the eyeball apparent when the eyelids are closed.

The dark circular opening through which light enters the eyeball, the *pupil*, is surrounded by the *iris* (plural = irides), a circular pigmented diaphragm. The relative size of the pupil and iris varies with the brightness of the entering light; however, the size of the contralateral pupils and irides should be uniform.

Normally, when the eyes are open and the gaze is directed anteriorly, the superior part of the cornea and iris are covered by the edge of the *superior eyelid*, and the inferior part of the cornea and iris are fully exposed above the *inferior eyelid*, usually exposing a narrow rim of sclera. Even slight variations in the position of the eyeballs are noticeable, causing a change in facial expression to a surprised look when the superior eyelid is elevated (as occurs in *exophthalmos*, or protrusion of the eyeballs, caused by hyperthyroidism), or a sleepy appearance (as occurs when the superior eyelid droops, *ptosis*, owing to an absence of sympathetic innervation in Horner syndrome).

The *bulbar conjunctiva* is reflected from the sclera onto the deep surface of the eyelid. The *palpebral conjunctiva* is normally red and vascular and, with experience, can provide some assessment of hemoglobin levels. It is commonly examined in cases of suspected *anemia,* a blood condition commonly manifested by pallor (paleness) of the mucous membranes. When the superior eyelid is everted, the size and extent of the enclosed *superior tarsus* can be appreciated, and commonly the *tarsal glands* can be distinguished through the palpebral conjunctiva as slightly yellow vertical stripes. Under close examination, the openings of these glands (approximately 20 per eyelid) can be seen on the margins of the eyelids, posterior to the two to three rows of emerging cilia or *eyelashes.* As the bulbar conjunctiva is continuous with the anterior epithelium

of the cornea and the palpebral conjunctiva, it forms the *conjunctival sac.* The palpebral fissure is the "mouth," or anterior aperture, of the conjunctival sac.

In the *medial angle of the eye,* a reddish shallow reservoir of tears, the *lacrimal lake,* can be observed. Within the lake is the *lacrimal caruncle,* a small mound of moist modified skin. Lateral to the caruncle is a *semilunar conjunctival fold,* which slightly overlaps the eyeball. The semilunar fold is a rudiment of the nictitating membrane of birds and reptiles. When the edges of the eyelids are everted, a small pit, the *lacrimal punctum,* is visible at its medial end on the summit of a small elevation, the *lacrimal papilla.*

ORBITAL REGION, ORBIT, AND EYEBALL

Fractures of Orbit

The orbital margin is strong to protect the orbital content. However, when the blows are powerful enough and the impact is directly on the bony rim, the resulting fractures usually occur at the three sutures between the bones forming the orbital margin. Because of the thinness of the medial and inferior walls of the orbit, a blow to the eye may fracture the orbital walls while the margin remains intact (Fig. B7.23). Indirect traumatic injury that displaces the orbital walls is called a "blowout" fracture. Fractures of the medial wall may involve the ethmoidal and sphenoidal sinuses, whereas fractures of the inferior wall (orbital floor) may involve the maxillary sinus.

Although the superior wall is stronger than the medial and inferior walls, it is thin enough to be translucent and may be readily penetrated. Thus a sharp object may pass through it and enter the frontal lobe of the brain.

Orbital fractures often result in intra-orbital bleeding, which exerts pressure on the eyeball, causing *exophthalmos* (protrusion of the eyeball). Any trauma to the eye may affect adjacent

structures—for example, bleeding into the maxillary sinus, displacement of maxillary teeth, and fracture of nasal bones resulting in hemorrhage, airway obstruction, and infection that could spread to the cavernous sinus through the ophthalmic vein.

Orbital Tumors

Because of the closeness of the optic nerve to the sphenoidal and posterior ethmoidal sinuses, a malignant tumor in these sinuses may erode the thin bony walls of the orbit and compress the optic nerve and orbital contents. Tumors in the orbit produce *exophthalmos.* The easiest entrance to the orbital cavity for a tumor in the middle cranial fossa is through the superior orbital fissure; tumors in the temporal or infratemporal fossa gain access to this cavity through the inferior orbital fissure. Although the lateral wall of the orbit is nearly as long as the medial wall because it extends laterally and anteriorly, it does not reach as far anteriorly as the medial wall does, which occupies essentially a sagittal plane (Fig. 7.44A). Nearly 2.5 cm of the eyeball is exposed when the pupil is turned medially as far as possible. This is why the lateral side affords a good approach for operations on the eyeball.

Injury to Nerves Supplying Eyelids

Because it supplies the levator palpebrae superioris, a lesion of the oculomotor nerve causes paralysis of the muscle, and the superior eyelid droops (*ptosis*). Damage to the facial nerve involves paralysis of the orbicularis oculi, preventing the eyelids from closing fully. Normal rapid protective blinking of the eye is also lost.

The loss of tonus of the muscle in the inferior eyelid causes the lid to fall away (evert) from the surface of the eyeball, leading to drying of the cornea. This leaves the eyeball unprotected from dust and small particles. Thus, irritation of the unprotected eyeball results in excessive but inefficient lacrimation (tear formation). *Excessive lacrimal fluid* also forms when the lacrimal drainage apparatus is obstructed, thereby preventing the fluid from reaching the inferior part of the eyeball. People often dab their eyes constantly to wipe the tears, resulting in further irritation.

Blowout fracture of orbit

FIGURE B7.23.

The gliding movements of protrusion and retrusion (translation) occur between the temporal bone and the articular disc (superior cavity) (Fig. 7.71); the hinge movements of depression and elevation and the rotational or pivoting movements occur in the inferior compartment. A thickened part of the joint capsule forms the intrinsic **lateral ligament of the TMJ** (Figs. 7.69E and 7.70A), which strengthens the joint laterally and, with the **postglenoid tubercle** (Fig. 7.69A), acts to prevent posterior dislocation of the joint.

Two extrinsic ligaments and the lateral ligament connect the mandible to the cranium. The **stylomandibular ligament,** which is actually a thickening of the fibrous capsule of the parotid gland, runs from the styloid process to the angle of the mandible (Fig. 7.69E & F). It does not contribute significantly to the strength of the joint. The **sphenomandibular ligament** runs from the spine of the sphenoid to the lingula of the mandible (Figs. 7.69F and 7.70C). It is the primary passive support of the mandible, although the tonus of the muscles of mastication usually bears the mandible's weight. However, the sphenomandibular ligaments serve as a "swinging hinge" for the mandible, serving both as a fulcrum and as a check ligament for the movements of the mandible at the TMJs.

The movements of the mandible at the TMJs are shown in Figure 7.71, and the muscles (or forces) producing the movements are summarized in Table 7.10. When the mouth is closed and at rest, the heads of the mandible are held in the retracted position in the mandibular fossae, and the chin is elevated by the tonus of the retractors and elevators of the mandible (Figs. 7.69A & C, 7.70B & C, and 7.71A). When sleeping in the supine or sitting position (head upright), as one enters a state of deep sleep, the tonic contraction relaxes and gravity causes depression of the mandible (the mouth falls open).

FIGURE 7.71. Movements of mandible consequent to movement at TMJs.

TABLE 7.10. MOVEMENTS OF TEMPOROMANDIBULAR JOINT

Movements of Mandible	Muscle(s)
Elevation (close mouth)	Temporalis, masseter, and medial pterygoid
Depression (open mouth)	Lateral pterygoid, suprahyoid, and infrahyoid muscles[a]
Protrusion (protrude chin)	Lateral pterygoid, masseter, and medial pterygoid[b]
Retrusion (retrude chin)	Temporalis (posterior oblique and near horizontal fibers) and masseter
Lateral movements (grinding and chewing)	Temporalis of same side, pterygoids of opposite side, and masseter

[a] The prime mover is normally gravity; these muscles are mainly active against resistance.

[b] The lateral pterygoid is the prime mover here, with minor secondary roles played by the masseter and medial pterygoid.

To enable more than a small amount of depression of the mandible—that is, to open the mouth wider than just to separate the upper and lower teeth—the head of the mandible and articular disc must move anteriorly on the articular surface until the head lies inferior to the articular tubercle (a movement referred to as "translation" by dentists) (Fig. 7.71B). If this occurs without depression, the chin protrudes. Most often, the mandible is depressed (the mouth is opened) as the head of the mandible and articular disc glide toward the articular tubercle, with full depression possible only when the heads and discs are fully protracted (Figs. 7.69B & D and 7.71C). If protraction of head and disc occurs unilaterally, the contralateral head rotates (pivots) on the inferior surface of the articular disc in the retracted position, permitting simple side-to-side chewing or grinding movements over a small range (Fig. 7.71D & E). During protrusion and retrusion of the mandible, the head and articular disc slide anteriorly and posteriorly on the articular surface of the temporal bone, with both sides moving together (Fig. 7.71A & B).

MUSCLES OF MASTICATION

TMJ movements are produced chiefly by the **muscles of mastication.** These four muscles (**temporal, masseter, and medial** and **lateral pterygoid muscles**) develop from the mesoderm of the embryonic first pharyngeal arch; consequently, they are all innervated by the nerve of that arch, the (*motor root of the*) *mandibular nerve* (CN V$_3$). The muscles of mastication are shown in isolation in Figure 7.72 and in situ in Figures 7.68 and 7.74; their attachments, details concerning their innervation, and their main actions are described in Table 7.11. In addition to the movements listed, studies indicate that the superior head of the lateral pterygoid muscle is active during the retraction movement produced by the posterior fibers of the temporalis. Traction is applied to the articular disc so that it is not pushed posteriorly ahead of the retracting mandible.

Generally, depression of the mandible is produced by gravity. The *suprahyoid* and *infrahyoid muscles* are strap-like muscles on each side of the neck (Fig. 7.72E; Table 7.11). They are primarily used to raise and depress the hyoid bone and larynx, respectively—for example, during swallowing (see Chapter 8). Indirectly they can also help depress the mandible, especially when opening the mouth suddenly, against resistance, or when inverted (e.g., standing on one's head). The platysma can be similarly used.

NEUROVASCULATURE OF INFRATEMPORAL FOSSA

The **maxillary artery** is the larger of the two terminal branches of the external carotid artery. It arises posterior to the neck of the mandible and is divided into three parts based on its relation to the lateral pterygoid muscle. The three parts of the maxillary artery and their branches are illustrated in isolation in Figure 7.73, and their courses and distributions

are listed in Table 7.12. Relationships of the maxillary artery and many of its branches are shown in Figure 7.74.

The **pterygoid venous plexus** is located partly between the temporalis and pterygoid muscles (Fig. 7.25). It is the venous equivalent of most of the maxillary artery—that is, most of the veins that accompany the branches of the maxillary artery drain into this plexus. The plexus anastomoses anteriorly with the facial vein via the deep facial vein and superiorly with the cavernous sinus via emissary veins. The extensive nature and volume of the pterygoid venous plexus is difficult to appreciate in the cadaver, in which it is usually drained of blood.

The **mandibular nerve** arises from the trigeminal ganglion in the middle cranial fossa. It immediately receives the motor root of the trigeminal nerve and descends through the foramen ovale into the infratemporal fossa (Fig. 7.75). The branches of CN V$_3$ are the auriculotemporal, inferior alveolar, lingual, and buccal nerves. Branches of CN V$_3$ also supply the four muscles of mastication but not the buccinator, which is supplied by the facial nerve.

The **auriculotemporal nerve** encircles the middle meningeal artery and divides into numerous branches, the largest of which passes posteriorly, medial to the neck of the mandible, and supplies sensory fibers to the auricle and temporal region. The auriculotemporal nerve also sends articular (sensory) fibers to the TMJ (Fig. 7.69E). It conveys postsynaptic parasympathetic secretomotor fibers from the *otic ganglion* to the parotid gland.

The **inferior alveolar nerve** enters the mandibular foramen and passes through the mandibular canal, forming the *inferior dental plexus,* which sends branches to all mandibular teeth on its side. Another branch of the plexus, the *mental nerve,* passes through the mental foramen and supplies the skin and mucous membrane of the lower lip, the skin of the chin, and the vestibular gingiva of the mandibular incisor teeth.

The **lingual nerve** lies anterior to the inferior alveolar nerve (Fig. 7.74). It is sensory to the anterior two thirds of the tongue, the floor of the mouth, and the lingual gingivae. It enters the mouth between the medial pterygoid muscle and the ramus of the mandible and passes anteriorly under cover of the oral mucosa, medial and inferior to the 3rd molar tooth. The **chorda tympani nerve,** a branch of CN VII carrying taste fibers from the anterior two thirds of the tongue, joins the lingual nerve in the infratemporal fossa (Fig. 7.74B). The chorda tympani also carries secretomotor fibers for the submandibular and sublingual salivary glands.

The **otic ganglion** (parasympathetic) is located in the infratemporal fossa, just inferior to the foramen ovale, medial to CN V$_3$ and posterior to the medial pterygoid muscle (Fig. 7.75). Presynaptic parasympathetic fibers, derived mainly from the glossopharyngeal nerve, synapse in the otic ganglion (Fig. 7.66). Postsynaptic parasympathetic fibers, which are secretory to the parotid gland, pass from the otic ganglion to this gland through the auriculotemporal nerve.

or **permanent** (secondary), the type of tooth, and its proximity to the midline or front of the mouth (e.g., medial and lateral incisors; the 1st molar is anterior to the 2nd).

Children have 20 deciduous teeth; adults normally have 32 permanent teeth (Fig. 7.80A & C). The usual ages of the eruption ("cutting") of these teeth are demonstrated in Figure 7.81 and listed in Table 7.13. Before eruption, the developing teeth reside in the alveolar arches as **tooth buds** (Fig. 7.80B).

The types of teeth are identified by their characteristics: **incisors,** thin cutting edges; **canines,** single prominent cones; **premolars** (bicuspids), two cusps; and **molars,** three or more cusps (Fig. 7.80A & C). The **vestibular surface** (labial or buccal) of each tooth is directed outwardly, and the **lingual surface** is directed inwardly (Fig. 7.79B). As used

in clinical (dental) practice, the **mesial surface** of a tooth is directed toward the median plane of the facial part of the cranium. The **distal surface** is directed away from this plane; both mesial and distal surfaces are *contact surfaces*—that is, surfaces that contact adjacent teeth. The masticatory surface is the **occlusal surface.**

PARTS AND STRUCTURE OF TEETH

A tooth has a crown, neck, and root (Fig. 7.82). The **crown** projects from the gingiva. The **neck** is between the crown and root. The **root** is fixed in the tooth socket by the *periodontium* (connective tissue surrounding roots); the number of roots varies. Most of the tooth is composed of **dentine** (L. *dentinium*), which is covered by **enamel** over the crown

(A) Right anterolateral view

(B) Left anterolateral view

(C) Panoramic view

FIGURE 7.80. Secondary dentition. A. The teeth are shown in occlusion. There is a supernumerary midline tooth (mesiodens) in this specimen (*).
B. Maxillary and mandibular jaws of a child acquiring secondary dentition are shown. The alveolar processes are carved to reveal the roots of the teeth and tooth buds. **C.** A pantomographic radiograph of an adult mandible and maxilla is shown. The left lower 3rd molar is not present. *I,* incisor; *C,* canine; *PM,* premolar; *M1, M2,* and *M3,* 1st, 2nd, and 3rd molars. (Part **C** courtesy of M. J. Pharoah, Associate Professor of Dental Radiology, Faculty of Dentistry, University of Toronto, Toronto, Ontario, Canada.)

TABLE 7.13A. DECIDUOUS TEETH

Deciduous Teeth	Central Incisor	Lateral Incisor	Canine	1st Molar	2nd Molar
Eruption (months)[a]	6–8	8–10	16–20	12–16	20–24
Shedding (years)	6–7	7–8	10–12	9–11	10–12

[a] In some normal infants, the first teeth (medial incisors) may not erupt until 12–13 months of age.

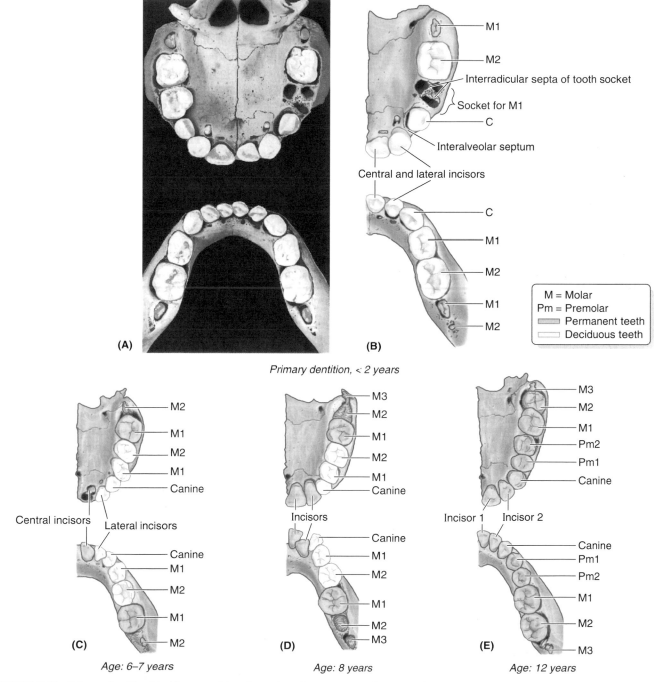

FIGURE 7.81. Primary dentition (deciduous teeth) and eruption of permanent teeth.

TABLE 7.13B. PERMANENT TEETH

Permanent Teeth	Central Incisor	Lateral Incisor	Canine	1st Premolar	2nd Premolar	1st Molar	2nd Molar	3rd Molar
Eruption (years)	7–8	8–9	10–12	10–11	11–12	6–7	12	13–25

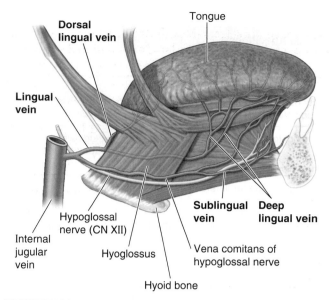

FIGURE 7.93. **Venous drainage of tongue.**

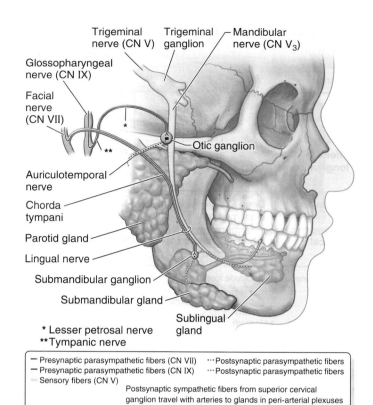

* Lesser petrosal nerve
**Tympanic nerve

— Presynaptic parasympathetic fibers (CN VII)	···Postsynaptic parasympathetic fibers
— Presynaptic parasympathetic fibers (CN IX)	···Postsynaptic parasympathetic fibers
═ Sensory fibers (CN V)	

Postsynaptic sympathetic fibers from superior cervical ganglion travel with arteries to glands in peri-arterial plexuses

FIGURE 7.95. **Innervation of salivary glands.**

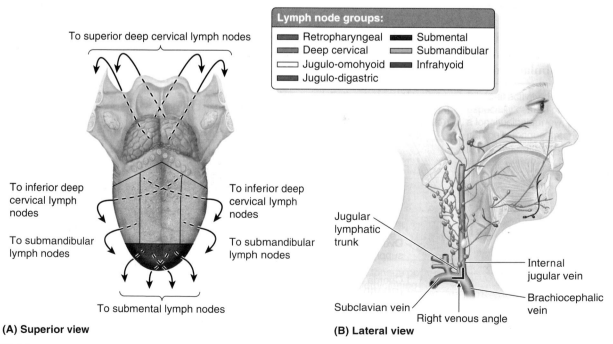

(A) Superior view

(B) Lateral view

FIGURE 7.94. **Lymphatic drainage of tongue. A.** The dorsum of the tongue is shown. **B.** Lymph drains to the submental, submandibular, and superior and inferior deep cervical lymph nodes, including the jugulodigastric and jugulo-omohyoid nodes. Extensive communications occur across the midline of the tongue.

viscid fluid, **saliva,** secreted by these glands and the mucous glands of the oral cavity:

- Keeps the mucous membrane of the mouth moist.
- Lubricates the food during mastication.
- Begins the digestion of starches.
- Serves as an intrinsic "mouthwash."
- Plays significant roles in the prevention of tooth decay and in the ability to taste.

In addition to the main salivary glands, small **accessory salivary glands** are scattered over the palate, lips, cheeks, tonsils, and tongue. The *parotid glands,* the largest of the three paired salivary glands, were discussed earlier in this chapter (p. 914). The parotid glands are located lateral and posterior to the rami of the mandible and masseter muscles, within unyielding fibrous sheaths. The parotid glands drain anteriorly via single ducts that enter the oral vestibule opposite the second maxillary molar teeth (see Fig. 7.65).

SUBMANDIBULAR GLANDS

The **submandibular glands** lie along the body of the mandible, partly superior and partly inferior to the posterior half of the mandible, and partly superficial and partly deep to the mylohyoid muscle (Fig. 7.96). The **submandibular duct,** approximately 5 cm long, arises from the portion of the gland that lies between the mylohyoid and hyoglossus muscles. Passing from lateral to medial, the *lingual nerve* loops under the duct that runs anteriorly, opening by one to three orifices on a small sublingual papilla beside the base of the lingual frenulum (Fig. 7.96B). The orifices of the submandibular

ducts are visible, and saliva can often be seen trickling from them (or spraying from them during yawning). The **arterial supply of the submandibular glands** is from the **submental arteries** (Fig. 7.92). The **veins** accompany the arteries. The **lymphatic vessels** of the glands end in the *deep cervical lymph nodes,* particularly the *jugulo-omohyoid node* (Fig. 7.94B).

The submandibular glands are supplied by presynaptic parasympathetic secretomotor fibers conveyed from the facial nerve to the lingual nerve by the chorda tympani nerve, which synapse with postsynaptic neurons in the submandibular ganglion (Fig. 7.95). The latter fibers accompany arteries to reach the gland, along with vasoconstrictive postsynaptic sympathetic fibers from the superior cervical ganglion.

SUBLINGUAL GLANDS

The **sublingual glands** are the smallest and most deeply situated of the salivary glands (Fig. 7.96). Each almond-shaped gland lies in the floor of the mouth between the mandible and the genioglossus muscle. The glands from each side unite to form a horseshoe-shaped mass around the connective tissue core of the lingual frenulum. Numerous small **sublingual ducts** open into the floor of the mouth along the sublingual folds. The **arterial supply of the sublingual glands** is from the *sublingual* and *submental arteries,* branches of the lingual and facial arteries, respectively (Fig. 7.92). The **nerves of the glands** accompany those of the submandibular gland. Presynaptic parasympathetic secretomotor fibers are conveyed by the facial, chorda tympani, and lingual nerves to synapse in the submandibular ganglion (Fig. 7.95).

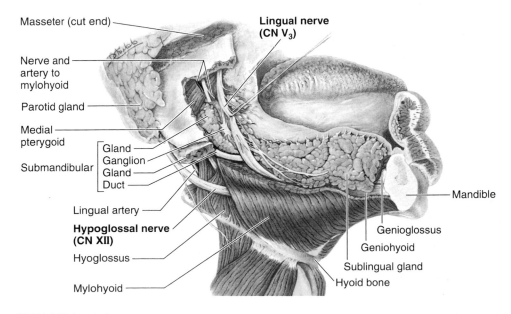

(A) Right lateral view

FIGURE 7.96. Parotid, submandibular, and sublingual salivary glands. A. The body and parts of the ramus of the mandible have been removed. The parotid gland contacts the deep part of the submandibular gland posteriorly. Fine ducts passing from the superior border of the sublingual gland open on the sublingual fold.

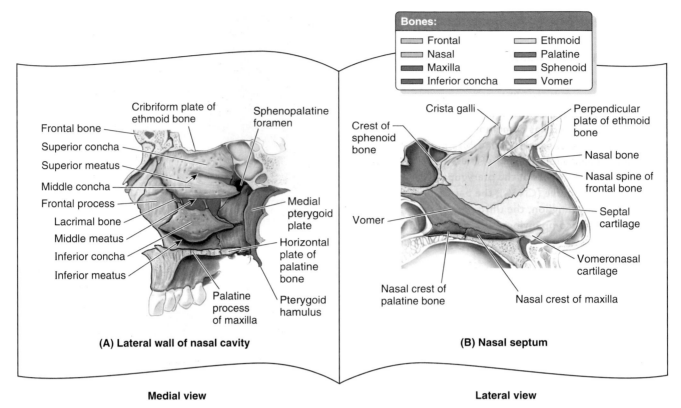

Bones:

☐ Frontal   ☐ Ethmoid
☐ Nasal   ☐ Palatine
☐ Maxilla   ☐ Sphenoid
☐ Inferior concha   ☐ Vomer

(A) Lateral wall of nasal cavity

Frontal bone
Superior concha
Superior meatus
Middle concha
Frontal process
Lacrimal bone
Middle meatus
Inferior concha
Inferior meatus
Cribriform plate of ethmoid bone
Sphenopalatine foramen
Medial pterygoid plate
Horizontal plate of palatine bone
Pterygoid hamulus
Palatine process of maxilla

Medial view

(B) Nasal septum

Crista galli
Crest of sphenoid bone
Vomer
Perpendicular plate of ethmoid bone
Nasal bone
Nasal spine of frontal bone
Septal cartilage
Vomeronasal cartilage
Nasal crest of palatine bone
Nasal crest of maxilla

Lateral view

FIGURE 7.102. Lateral and medial (septal) walls of right side of nasal cavity. The walls are separated and shown as adjacent pages of a book. The medial view shows the right lateral wall of the nasal cavity, and the lateral view shows the nasal septum. The nasal septum has a hard (bony) part located deeply (posteriorly) where it is protected and a soft or mobile part located superficially (anteriorly) mostly in the more vulnerable external nose.

flat bone, forms the postero-inferior part of the nasal septum, with some contribution from the nasal crests of the maxillary and palatine bones. The **septal cartilage** has a tongue-and-groove articulation with the edges of the bony septum.

Nasal Cavities

The term *nasal cavity* refers to either the entire cavity or to the right or left half, depending on the context. The nasal cavity is entered anteriorly through the *nares* (nostrils). It opens posteriorly into the *nasopharynx* through the *choanae* (Fig. 7.9). Mucosa lines the nasal cavity, except for the *nasal vestibule*, which is lined with skin (Fig. 7.103A).

The **nasal mucosa** is firmly bound to the periosteum and perichondrium of the supporting bones and cartilages of the nose. The mucosa is continuous with the lining of all the chambers with which the nasal cavities communicate: the nasopharynx posteriorly, the paranasal sinuses superiorly and laterally, and the lacrimal sac and conjunctiva superiorly. The inferior two thirds of the nasal mucosa is the respiratory area, and the superior one third is the olfactory area (Fig. 7.106B). Air passing over the **respiratory area** is warmed and moistened before it passes through the rest of the upper respiratory tract to the lungs. The **olfactory area** contains the peripheral organ of smell; sniffing draws air to the area.

BOUNDARIES OF NASAL CAVITIES

The nasal cavities have a roof, floor, and medial and lateral walls.

- The *roof of the nasal cavities* is curved and narrow, except at its posterior end, where the hollow *body of the sphenoid* forms the roof. It is divided into three parts (frontonasal, ethmoidal, and sphenoidal) named from the bones forming each part (Fig. 7.102).
- The *floor of the nasal cavities* is wider than the roof and is formed by the *palatine processes of the maxilla* and the *horizontal plates of the palatine bone*.
- The *medial wall of the nasal cavities* is formed by the nasal septum.
- The *lateral walls of the nasal cavities* are irregular owing to three bony plates, the *nasal conchae*, which project inferiorly, somewhat like louvers (Figs. 7.102A, 7.103, and 7.108).

FEATURES OF NASAL CAVITIES

The **nasal conchae** (superior, middle, and inferior) curve inferomedially, hanging like louvers or short curtains from the lateral wall. The conchae (L. shells) or turbinates of many mammals (especially running mammals and those existing in extreme environments) are highly convoluted, scroll-like structures that offer a vast surface area for heat exchange. In both

Frontal sinus

Sphenoidal sinus

Superior concha
Ethmoidal crest
of maxilla
Middle concha
Inferior concha
Atrium
Limen

Nasal vestibule

Vibrissae
(nasal hairs)

(A) Medial view

Nasopharynx

Spheno-ethmoidal recess
Superior nasal meatus
Middle nasal meatus

Pharyngeal opening of pharyngotympanic tube

Inferior nasal meatus

Medial surface of
cerebral hemisphere

Corpus callosum

Third ventricle

Midbrain

Pons

Fourth ventricle

Medulla oblongata

Atlas (C1 vertebra)

Posterior cerebellomedullary
cistern (cisterna magna)

C1

Axis (C2 vertebra)

Spinal cord

Frontal sinus

Rod passed from frontal
sinus through frontonasal
duct, and into ethmoidal
infundibulum
of middle meatus

Ethmoidal bulla

Nasal mucosa

Semilunar hiatus

(B) Medial view

Middle ethmoidal cells
Posterior ethmoidal cells

Form ethmoidal sinuses

Rod passed from sphenoidal
sinus to spheno-ethmoidal recess

Sphenoidal
sinus

Nasopharynx

Pharyngeal
opening of
pharyngotympanic
tube

Orifice of nasolacrimal duct

Rod passed from semilunar hiatus,
through maxillary orifice, into maxillary sinus,
and forced through wall of inferior meatus

FIGURE 7.103. Lateral wall of nasal cavity of right half of head. A. The inferior and middle conchae, curving medially and inferiorly from the lateral wall, divide the wall into three nearly equal parts and cover the inferior and middle meatus, respectively. The superior concha is small and anterior to the sphenoidal sinus and the middle concha has an angled inferior border and ends inferior to the sphenoidal sinus. The inferior concha has a slightly curved inferior border and ends inferior to the middle concha approximately 1 cm anterior to the orifice of the pharyngotympanic tube (approximately the width of the medial pterygoid plate). **B.** This dissection of the lateral wall of the nasal cavity shows the communications through the lateral wall of the nasal cavity. Parts of the superior, middle, and inferior conchae are cut away. The sphenoidal sinus occupies the body of the sphenoid bone; its orifice, superior to the middle of its anterior wall, opens into the spheno-ethmoidal recess. The orifices of posterior, middle, and anterior ethmoidal cells open into the superior meatus, middle meatus, and semilunar hiatus, respectively.

humans with simple plate-like nasal conchae and animals with complex turbinates, a recess or **nasal meatus** (singular and plural; passage(s) in the nasal cavity) underlies each of the bony formations. The nasal cavity is thus divided into five passages: a posterosuperiorly placed *spheno-ethmoidal recess*, three laterally located *nasal meatus* (superior, middle, and inferior), and a medially placed *common nasal meatus* into which the four lateral passages open. The **inferior concha** is the longest and broadest of the conchae and is formed by an independent bone (of the same name, inferior concha) covered by a mucous membrane that contains large vascular spaces that can enlarge to control the caliber of the nasal cavity. The **middle** and **superior conchae** are medial processes of the ethmoid bone.

When infected or irritated, the mucosa covering the conchae may swell rapidly, blocking the nasal passage(s) on that side.

The **spheno-ethmoidal recess,** lying superoposterior to the superior concha, receives the opening of the *sphenoidal sinus,* an air-filled cavity in the body of the sphenoid. The **superior nasal meatus** is a narrow passage between the superior and the middle nasal conchae into which the posterior ethmoidal sinuses open by one or more orifices (Fig. 7.103A). The **middle nasal meatus** is longer and deeper than the superior one. The anterosuperior part of this passage leads into a funnel-shaped opening, the **ethmoidal infundibulum,** through which it communicates with the frontal sinus (Fig. 7.104). The passage that leads inferiorly

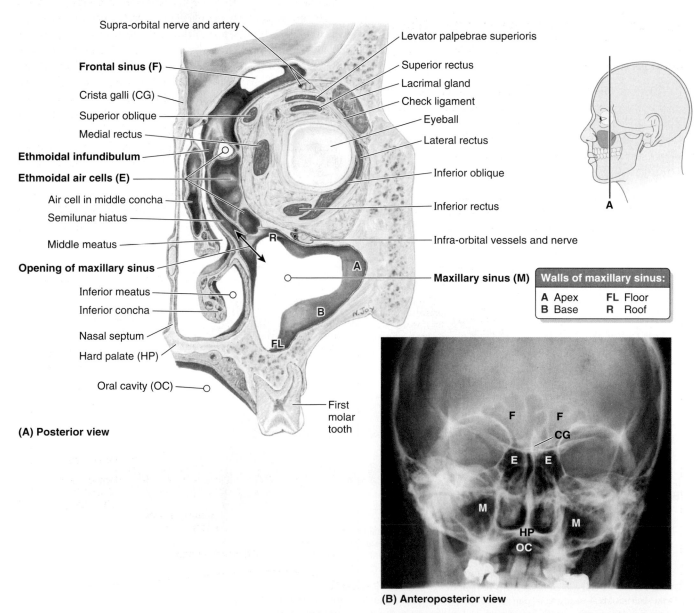

FIGURE 7.104. Coronal section of right half of head. A. The orientation drawing illustrates the plane of the section. Observe the relationship of the orbit, nasal cavity, and paranasal sinuses. The orbital contents, including the four recti and the fascia uniting them, form a circle (a cone when viewed in three dimensions) around the posterior part (fundus) of the eyeball. **B.** Radiograph of cranium demonstrating nasal cavity and paranasal sinuses. Letters refer to structures labeled in part **A.**

from each frontal sinus to the infundibulum is the *fronto-nasal duct* (Fig. 7.103B). The **semilunar hiatus** (L. *hiatus semilunaris*) is a semicircular groove into which the frontal sinus opens. The **ethmoidal bulla** (L. bubble), a rounded elevation located superior to the semilunar hiatus, is visible when the middle concha is removed. The bulla is formed by middle ethmoidal cells that form the *ethmoidal sinuses.*

The **inferior nasal meatus** is a horizontal passage infero-lateral to the inferior nasal concha. The *nasolacrimal duct,* which drains tears from the lacrimal sac, opens into the anterior part of this meatus (see Fig. 7.46A, p. 892). The **common nasal meatus** is the medial part of the nasal cavity between the conchae and the nasal septum, into which the lateral recesses and meatus open.

Vasculature and Innervation of Nose

The *arterial supply of the medial and lateral walls of the nasal cavity* (Fig. 7.105) is from five sources:

1. *Anterior ethmoidal artery* (from the ophthalmic artery).
2. *Posterior ethmoidal artery* (from the ophthalmic artery).
3. *Sphenopalatine artery* (from the maxillary artery).
4. *Greater palatine artery* (from the maxillary artery).
5. *Septal branch of the superior labial artery* (from the facial artery).

The first three arteries divide into lateral and medial (septal) branches. The greater palatine artery reaches the septum via the incisive canal through the anterior hard palate. The

anterior part of the nasal septum is the site of an anastomotic arterial plexus involving all five arteries supplying the septum (*Kiesselbach area*). The external nose also receives blood from first and fifth arteries listed, plus nasal branches of the infraorbital artery and the lateral nasal branches of the facial artery.

A rich **submucosal venous plexus,** deep to the nasal mucosa, provides *venous drainage of the nose via* the spheno-palatine, facial, and ophthalmic veins. The plexus is an important part of the body's thermoregulatory system, exchanging heat and warming air before it enters the lungs. Venous blood from the external nose drains mostly into the facial vein via the angular and lateral nasal veins (see Fig. 7.25). However, recall that it lies within the "danger area" of the face because of communications with the *cavernous (dural venous) sinus* (see the blue box "Thrombophlebitis of Facial Vein," p. 875).

Regarding its *nerve supply of the nose,* the nasal mucosa can be divided into postero-inferior and anterosuperior portions by an oblique line passing approximately through the anterior nasal spine and the spheno-ethmoidal recess (Fig. 7.106). The nerve supply of the postero-inferior portion of the nasal mucosa is chiefly from the maxillary nerve, by way of the *nasopalatine nerve* to the nasal septum, and posterior superior lateral nasal and inferior lateral nasal branches of the *greater palatine nerve* to the lateral wall. The nerve supply of the anterosuperior portion is from the ophthalmic nerve (CN V₁) by way of the **anterior** and **posterior ethmoidal nerves,** branches of the nasociliary nerve. Most of the external nose (dorsum and apex) is also supplied by CN V₁ (via the infratrochlear nerve and the external nasal branch of the

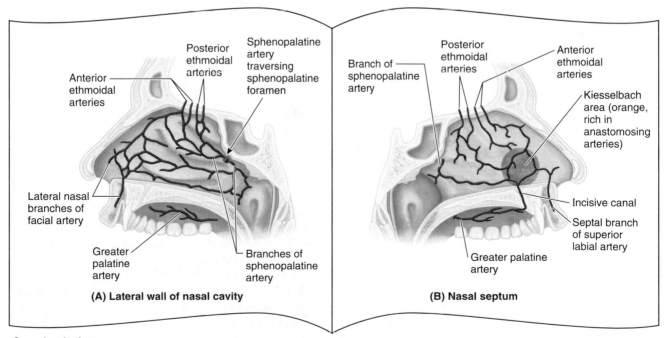

Open-book view

FIGURE 7.105. Arterial supply of nasal cavity. An open-book view of the lateral and medial walls of the right side of the nasal cavity is shown. The left "page" shows the lateral wall of the nasal cavity. The sphenopalatine artery (a branch of the maxillary) and the anterior ethmoidal artery (a branch of the ophthalmic) are the most important arteries to the nasal cavity. The right "page" shows the nasal septum. An anastomosis of four to five named arteries supplying the septum occurs in the antero-inferior portion of the nasal septum (Kiesselbach area, *orange*), an area commonly involved in chronic epistaxis (nosebleeds).

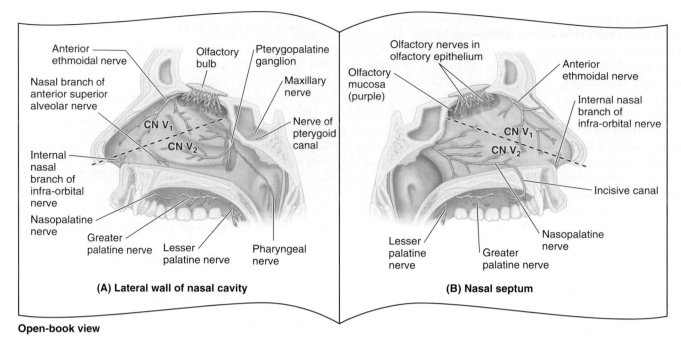

FIGURE 7.106. Innervation of nasal cavity. An open-book view of the lateral and medial (septal) walls of the right side of the nasal cavity is shown. A *dashed line* extrapolated approximately from the spheno-ethmoidal recess to the apex of the nose demarcates the territories of the ophthalmic (CN V_1) and maxillary (CN V_2) nerves for supplying general sensation to both the lateral wall and the nasal septum. The olfactory nerve (CN I) is distributed to the olfactory mucosa superior to the level of the superior concha on both the lateral wall and the nasal septum.

anterior ethmoidal nerve), but the alae of the nose are supplied by the nasal branches of the infra-orbital nerve (CN V_2). The **olfactory nerves,** concerned with smell, arise from cells in the **olfactory epithelium** in the superior part of the lateral and septal walls of the nasal cavity. The central processes of these cells (forming the olfactory nerve) pass through the *cribriform plate* and end in the **olfactory bulb,** the rostral expansion of the **olfactory tract** (Fig. 7.102A).

Paranasal Sinuses

The **paranasal sinuses** are air-filled extensions of the respiratory part of the nasal cavity into the following cranial bones: frontal, ethmoid, sphenoid, and maxilla. They are named according to the bones in which they are located. The sinuses continue to invade the surrounding bone, and marked extensions are common in the crania of older individuals.

FRONTAL SINUSES

The **right** and **left frontal sinuses** are between the outer and inner tables of the frontal bone, posterior to the superciliary arches and the root of the nose (Figs. 7.103, 7.104, and 7.107). Frontal sinuses are usually detectable in children by 7 years of age. The right and left sinuses each drain through a **frontonasal duct** into the *ethmoidal infundibulum,* which opens into the *semilunar hiatus* of the middle nasal meatus. The frontal sinuses are innervated by branches of the *supra-orbital nerves* (CN V_1).

The right and left frontal sinuses are rarely of equal size, and the septum between them is not usually situated entirely

in the median plane. The frontal sinuses vary in size from approximately 5 mm to large spaces extending laterally into the greater wings of the sphenoid. Often a frontal sinus has two parts: a vertical part in the squamous part of the frontal bone, and a horizontal part in the orbital part of the frontal bone. One or both parts may be large or small. When the supra-orbital part is large, its roof forms the floor of the anterior cranial fossa and its floor forms the roof of the orbit.

ETHMOIDAL CELLS

The **ethmoidal cells** (**sinuses**) are small invaginations of the mucous membrane of the middle and superior nasal meatus into the ethmoid bone between the nasal cavity and the orbit (Figs. 7.104, 7.107, and 7.108). The ethmoidal cells usually are not visible in plain radiographs before 2 years of age but are recognizable in CT scans. The **anterior ethmoidal cells** drain directly or indirectly into the middle nasal meatus through the ethmoidal infundibulum. The **middle ethmoidal cells** open directly into the middle meatus and are sometimes called "bullar cells" because they form the *ethmoidal bulla,* a swelling on the superior border of the semilunar hiatus (Fig. 7.103B). The **posterior ethmoidal cells** open directly into the superior meatus. The ethmoidal cells are supplied by the anterior and posterior ethmoidal branches of the *nasociliary nerves* (CN V_1) (Figs. 7.19 and 7.106).

SPHENOIDAL SINUSES

The **sphenoidal sinuses** are located in the body of the sphenoid, but they may extend into the wings of this bone

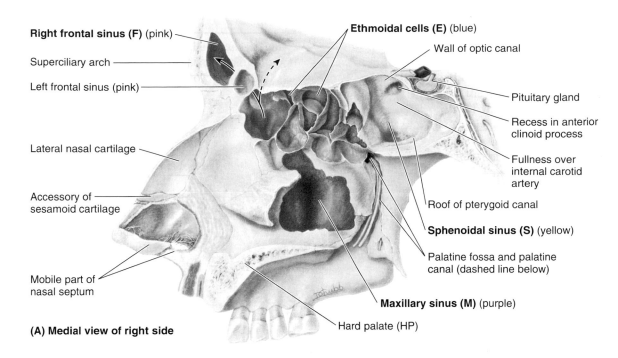

Right frontal sinus (F) (pink)

Superciliary arch

Left frontal sinus (pink)

Lateral nasal cartilage

Accessory of sesamoid cartilage

Mobile part of nasal septum

(A) Medial view of right side

Ethmoidal cells (E) (blue)

Wall of optic canal

Pituitary gland

Recess in anterior clinoid process

Fullness over internal carotid artery

Roof of pterygoid canal

Sphenoidal sinus (S) (yellow)

Palatine fossa and palatine canal (dashed line below)

Maxillary sinus (M) (purple)

Hard palate (HP)

(B) Left lateral radiograph   P Pharynx

FIGURE 7.107. **Paranasal sinuses I. A.** The paranasal sinuses of the right side have been opened from a nasal approach and color coded. An anterior ethmoidal cell (*pink*) is invading the diploë of the frontal bone to become a frontal sinus. An offshoot (*broken arrow*) invades the orbital plate of the frontal bone. The sphenoidal sinus in this specimen is extensive, extending (1) posteriorly, inferior to the pituitary gland, to the clivus; (2) laterally, inferior to the optic nerve (CN II), into the anterior clinoid process; and (3) inferior to the pterygoid process but leaving the pterygoid canal and rising as a ridge on the floor of the sinus. The maxillary sinus is pyramidal. **B.** Radiograph of cranium demonstrating air densities (dark areas) associated with paranasal sinuses, nasal cavity, oral cavity, and pharynx. The letters are defined in part **A.**

(Figs. 7.103 and 7.107). They are unevenly divided and separated by a bony septum. Because of this extensive pneumatization (formation of air cells), the body of the sphenoid is fragile. Only thin plates of bone separate the sinuses from several important structures: the optic nerves and optic chiasm, the pituitary gland, the internal carotid arteries, and the cavernous sinuses. The sphenoidal sinuses are derived from a posterior ethmoidal cell that begins to invade the sphenoid at approximately 2 years of age. In some people, several posterior ethmoidal cells invade the sphenoid, giving rise to multiple sphenoidal sinuses that open separately into the *sphenoethmoidal recess* (Fig. 7.103A). The posterior ethmoidal arteries and the posterior ethmoidal nerves that accompany the arteries supply the sphenoidal sinuses (Fig. 7.105).

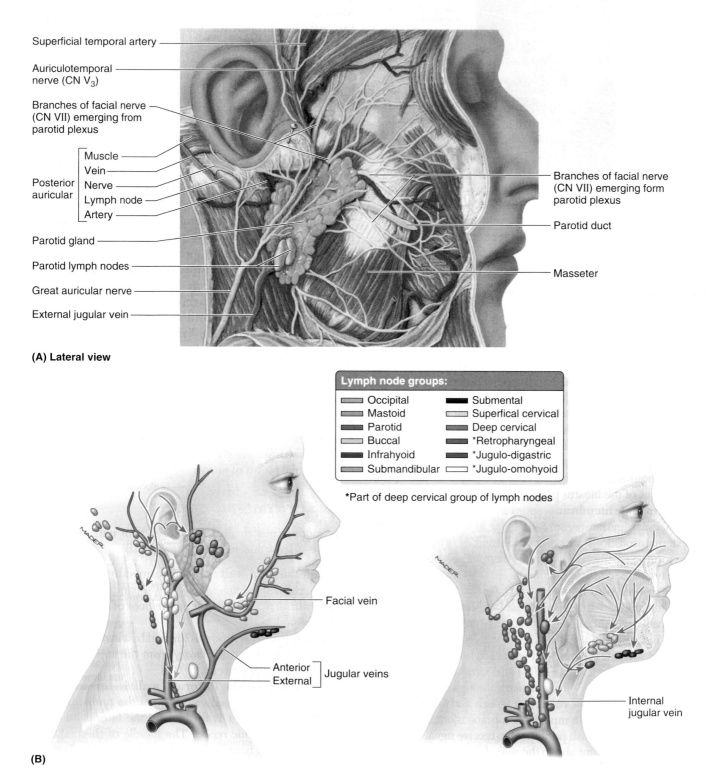

Superficial temporal artery

Auriculotemporal nerve (CN V₃)

Branches of facial nerve (CN VII) emerging from parotid plexus

Posterior auricular
Muscle
Vein
Nerve
Lymph node
Artery

Parotid gland

Parotid lymph nodes

Great auricular nerve

External jugular vein

Branches of facial nerve (CN VII) emerging form parotid plexus

Parotid duct

Masseter

(A) Lateral view

Lymph node groups:

Occipital   Submental
Mastoid   Superfical cervical
Parotid   Deep cervical
Buccal   *Retropharyngeal
Infrahyoid   *Jugulo-digastric
Submandibular   *Jugulo-omohyoid

*Part of deep cervical group of lymph nodes

Facial vein

Anterior
External Jugular veins

Internal jugular vein

(B)

FIGURE 7.111.   Dissection of face and lymphatic drainage of head. A. The posterior auricular and superficial temporal arteries and veins and the great auricular and auriculotemporal nerves provide the circulation and innervation of the external ear. **B.** Lymphatic drainage is to the parotid lymph nodes and the mastoid and superficial cervical lymph nodes, all which drain to the deep cervical nodes.

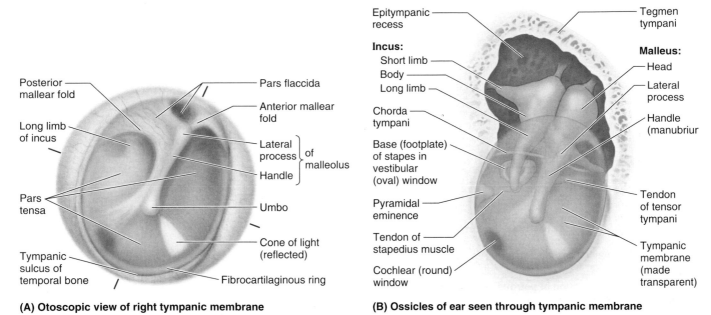

(A) Otoscopic view of right tympanic membrane

(B) Ossicles of ear seen through tympanic membrane

FIGURE 7.112. Tympanic membrane and lateral approach to tympanic cavity. A. An otoscopic view of the right tympanic membrane is demonstrated. The *cone of light* is a reflection of the light of the otoscope. **B.** The tympanic membrane has been rendered semitransparent and the lateral wall of the epitympanic recess has been removed to demonstrate the ossicles of the middle ear in situ.

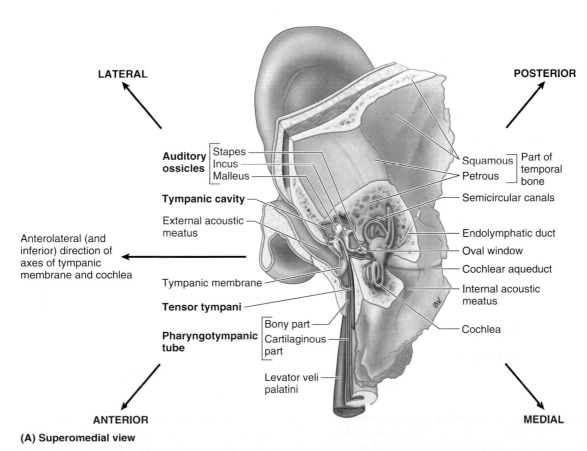

(A) Superomedial view

FIGURE 7.113. General scheme and orientation of components of ear. A. The ear is shown in situ. The external acoustic meatus runs lateral to medial; the axis of the tympanic membrane and the axis about which the cochlea winds runs inferiorly and anteriorly as it proceeds laterally. The long axes of the bony and membranous labyrinths and of the pharyngotympanic tube and parallel tensor tympani and levator palatini muscles lie perpendicular to those of the tympanic membrane and cochlea (i.e., they run inferiorly and anteriorly as they proceed medially).

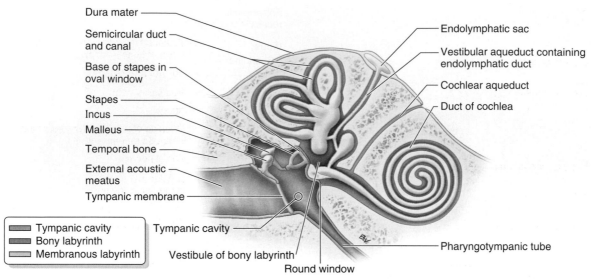

Dura mater

Semicircular duct and canal

Base of stapes in oval window

Stapes

Incus

Malleus

Temporal bone

External acoustic meatus

Tympanic membrane

Endolymphatic sac

Vestibular aqueduct containing endolymphatic duct

Cochlear aqueduct

Duct of cochlea

Tympanic cavity
Bony labyrinth
Membranous labyrinth

Tympanic cavity

Vestibule of bony labyrinth

Round window

Pharyngotympanic tube

(B) Oblique section of petrous temporal bone

FIGURE 7.113. *(Continued)* **B.** The middle and internal parts of the ear are shown. The middle ear lies between the tympanic membrane and the internal ear. Three auditory ossicles stretch from the lateral to the medial wall of the tympanic cavity. The pharyngotympanic tube is a communication between the anterior wall of the tympanic cavity and the lateral wall of the nasopharynx. The internal ear is composed of a closed system of membranous tubes and bulbs, the membranous labyrinth, which is filled with a fluid called endolymph (*orange*) and bathed in surrounding fluid called perilymph (*purple*).

5. The **mastoid wall** (**posterior wall**) features an opening in its superior part, the **aditus** (L. access) **to the mastoid antrum,** connecting the tympanic cavity to the mastoid cells; the canal for the facial nerve descends between the posterior wall and the antrum, medial to the aditus.
6. The anterior **carotid wall** separates the tympanic cavity from the carotid canal; superiorly, it has the **opening of the pharyngotympanic tube** and the **canal for the tensor tympani.**

The **mastoid antrum** is a cavity in the mastoid process of the temporal bone (Fig. 7.114A). The antrum (L. from G., cave), like the tympanic cavity, is separated from the middle cranial fossa by a thin plate of the temporal bone, called the **tegmen tympani.** This structure forms the *tegmental wall* (roof) for the ear cavities and is also part of the floor of the lateral part of the middle cranial fossa. The mastoid antrum is the common cavity into which the mastoid cells open. The antrum and mastoid cells are lined by mucous membrane that is continuous with the lining of the middle ear. Antero-inferiorly, the antrum is related to the canal for the facial nerve.

PHARYNGOTYMPANIC TUBE

The **pharyngotympanic tube** (auditory tube) connects the tympanic cavity to the nasopharynx, where it opens posterior to the inferior nasal meatus (Fig. 7.113). The posterolateral third of the tube is bony, and the remainder is cartilaginous. The pharyngotympanic tube is lined by mucous membrane that is continuous posteriorly with that of the tympanic cavity and anteriorly with that of the nasopharynx.

The *function of the pharyngotympanic tube* is to equalize pressure in the middle ear with the atmospheric pressure, thereby allowing free movement of the tympanic membrane.

By allowing air to enter and leave the tympanic cavity, this tube balances the pressure on both sides of the membrane. Because the walls of the cartilaginous part of the tube are normally in apposition, the tube must be actively opened. The tube is opened by the expanding girth of the belly of the *levator veli palatini* as it contracts longitudinally, pushing against one wall while the *tensor veli palatini* pulls on the other. Because these are muscles of the soft palate, equalizing pressure ("popping the eardrums") is commonly associated with activities such as yawning and swallowing.

The *arteries of the pharyngotympanic tube* are derived from the *ascending pharyngeal artery,* a branch of the external carotid artery, and the *middle meningeal artery* and *artery of the pterygoid canal,* branches of the maxillary artery (Fig. 7.115; Table 7.12).

The *veins of the pharyngotympanic tube* drain into the pterygoid venous plexus. **Lymphatic drainage** of the tube is to the *deep cervical lymph nodes* (Fig. 7.111B).

The **nerves of the pharyngotympanic tube** arise from the *tympanic plexus* (Fig. 7.114B), which is formed by fibers of the glossopharyngeal nerve (CN IX). Anteriorly, the tube also receives fibers from the *pterygopalatine ganglion* (Fig. 7.106A).

AUDITORY OSSICLES

The **auditory ossicles** form a mobile *chain of small bones* across the tympanic cavity from the tympanic membrane to the **oval window** (L. *fenestra vestibuli*), an oval opening on the labyrinthine wall of the tympanic cavity leading to the *vestibule of the bony labyrinth* (Figs. 7.113B and 7.116A). These ossicles are the first bones to be fully ossified during development and are essentially mature at birth. The bone from which they are formed is exceptionally dense (hard).

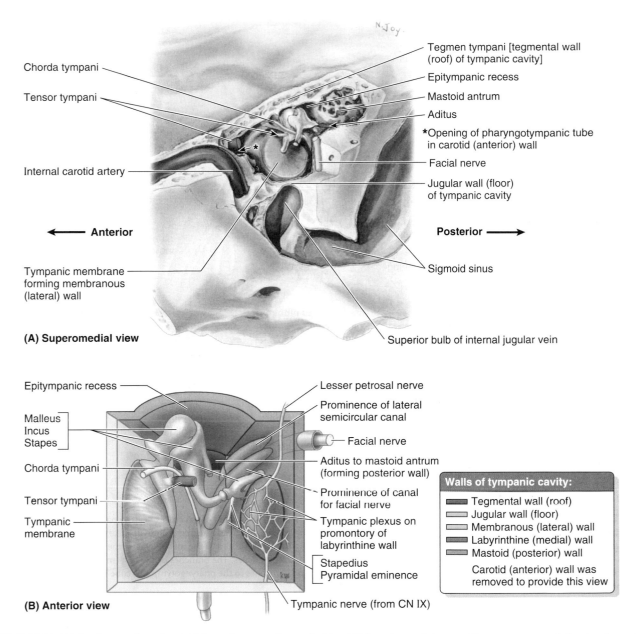

N.Joy.

(A) Superomedial view

Chorda tympani

Tensor tympani

Internal carotid artery

◄───── **Anterior**

Tympanic membrane forming membranous (lateral) wall

Tegmen tympani [tegmental wall (roof) of tympanic cavity]

Epitympanic recess

Mastoid antrum

Aditus

*Opening of pharyngotympanic tube in carotid (anterior) wall

Facial nerve

Jugular wall (floor) of tympanic cavity

Posterior ─────►

Sigmoid sinus

Superior bulb of internal jugular vein

(B) Anterior view

Epitympanic recess

Malleus
Incus
Stapes

Chorda tympani

Tensor tympani

Tympanic membrane

Lesser petrosal nerve

Prominence of lateral semicircular canal

Facial nerve

Aditus to mastoid antrum (forming posterior wall)

Prominence of canal for facial nerve

Tympanic plexus on promontory of labyrinthine wall

Stapedius
Pyramidal eminence

Tympanic nerve (from CN IX)

Walls of tympanic cavity:

- Tegmental wall (roof)
- Jugular wall (floor)
- Membranous (lateral) wall
- Labyrinthine (medial) wall
- Mastoid (posterior) wall

Carotid (anterior) wall was removed to provide this view

FIGURE 7.114. Walls of tympanic cavity. A. This specimen was dissected with a drill from the medial aspect. The tegmen tympani, forming the roof of the tympanic cavity and the mastoid antrum, is fairly thick in this specimen; usually it is extremely thin. The internal carotid artery is the main relation of the anterior wall, the internal jugular vein is the main relation of the floor, and the facial nerve (CN VII) is a main feature of the posterior wall. The chorda tympani passes between the malleus and the incus. **B.** In this view of the middle ear, the carotid (anterior) wall of the tympanic cavity has been removed. The tympanic membrane forms most of the membranous (lateral) wall; superior to it is the epitympanic recess, in which are housed the larger parts of the malleus and incus. Branches of the tympanic plexus provide innervation to the mucosa of the middle ear and adjacent pharyngotympanic tube; but one branch, the lesser petrosal nerve, is conveying presynaptic parasympathetic fibers to the otic ganglion for secretomotor innervation of the parotid gland.

The ossicles are covered with the mucous membrane lining the tympanic cavity; but unlike other bones, they lack a surrounding layer of osteogenic periosteum.

Malleus. The **malleus** (L. a hammer) attaches to the tympanic membrane. The rounded superior **head of the malleus** lies in the epitympanic recess (Fig. 7.116B). The **neck of the malleus** lies against the flaccid part of the tympanic membrane, and the **handle of the malleus** is embedded in the tympanic membrane, with its tip at the umbo; thus the

malleus moves with the membrane. The head of the malleus articulates with the incus; the tendon of the tensor tympani inserts into its handle near the neck. The *chorda tympani* crosses the medial surface of the neck of the malleus. The malleus functions as a lever, with the longer of its two processes and its handle attached to the tympanic membrane.

Incus. The **incus** (L. an anvil) is located between the malleus and the stapes and articulates with them. It has a body and two limbs. Its large **body** lies in the epitympanic recess (Fig. 7.116A),

(A) Superior view of internal surface of cranial base

(B) Anterolateral view of left otic capsule

(C) Anterolateral view of left membranous labyrinth (through transparent otic capsule)

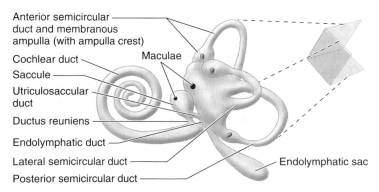

(D) Anterolateral view of left membranous labyrinth

FIGURE 7.117. **Bony and membranous labyrinths of internal ear. A.** This view of the interior of the base of the cranium shows the temporal bone and the location of the bony labyrinth. **B.** The walls of the bony labyrinth have been carved out of the petrous temporal bone. **C.** A similar view of the bony labyrinth occupied by perilymph and the membranous labyrinth is shown. **D.** The membranous labyrinth, shown after removal from the bony labyrinth, is a closed system of ducts and chambers filled with endolymph and bathed by perilymph. It has three parts: the cochlear duct, which occupies the cochlea; the saccule and utricle, which occupy the vestibule; and the three semicircular ducts, which occupy the semicircular canals. The utricle communicates with the saccule through the utriculosaccular duct. The lateral semicircular duct lies in the horizontal plane and is more horizontal than it appears in this drawing.

be isolated (carved) from it using a dental drill. The otic capsule is often erroneously illustrated and identified as being the bony labyrinth. However, *the bony labyrinth is the fluid-filled space,* which is surrounded by the otic capsule, and is most accurately represented by a cast of the otic capsule after removal of the surrounding bone.

Cochlea. The **cochlea** is the shell-shaped part of the bony labyrinth that contains the **cochlear duct** (Fig. 7.117C), the part of the internal ear concerned with hearing. The **spiral canal of the cochlea** begins at the vestibule and makes 2.5 turns around a bony core, the **modiolus** (Fig. 7.118), the cone-shaped core of spongy bone about which the spiral canal of the cochlea turns. The modiolus contains canals for blood vessels and for distribution of the branches of the cochlear nerve. The apex of the cone-shaped modiolus, like the axis of the tympanic membrane, is directed laterally, anteriorly, and inferiorly. The large basal turn of the cochlea produces the *promontory of the labyrinthine wall* of the tympanic cavity (Fig. 7.114B). At the basal turn, the bony labyrinth communicates with the subarachnoid space superior to the jugular foramen through the **cochlear aqueduct** (Fig. 7.113B). It also features the **round window** (L. *fenestra cochleae*), closed by the **secondary tympanic membrane** (Fig. 7.117B & C).

Vestibule of Bony Labyrinth. The **vestibule of the bony labyrinth** is a small oval chamber (approximately 5 mm long) that contains the **utricle** and **saccule** (Fig. 7.117C) and parts of the balancing apparatus (vestibular labyrinth). The vestibule features the *oval window* on its lateral wall, occupied by the base of the stapes. The vestibule is continuous with the bony cochlea anteriorly, the semicircular canals posteriorly, and the posterior cranial fossa by the **vestibular aqueduct** (Fig. 7.113B). The aqueduct extends to the posterior surface of the petrous part of the temporal bone, where it opens posterolateral to the *internal acoustic meatus* (Fig. 7.117A). The vestibular aqueduct transmits the **endolymphatic duct** (Figs. 7.113B and 7.117D) and two small blood vessels.

Semicircular Canals. The **semicircular canals** (**anterior, posterior**, and **lateral**) communicate with the vestibule of the bony labyrinth (Fig. 7.117B). The canals lie posterosuperior to the vestibule into which they open; they are set at right angles to each other. The canals occupy three planes in space. Each semicircular canal forms approximately two thirds of a circle, and is approximately 1.5 mm in diameter, except at one end where there is a swelling, the **bony ampulla.** The canals have only five openings into the vestibule because the anterior and posterior canals have one limb common to both. Lodged within the canals are the *semicircular ducts* (Fig. 7.117C & D).

MEMBRANOUS LABYRINTH

The **membranous labyrinth** consists of a series of communicating sacs and ducts that are suspended in the bony labyrinth (Fig. 7.117C). The labyrinth contains **endolymph,** a watery fluid similar in composition to intracellular fluid, thus differing in composition from the surrounding **perilymph** (which is like extracellular fluid) that fills the remainder of the bony labyrinth. The membranous labyrinth—composed of two divisions, the *vestibular labyrinth* and the *cochlear labyrinth*—consists of more parts than does the bony labyrinth:

- **Vestibular labyrinth:** utricle and saccule, two small communicating sacs in the vestibule of the bony labyrinth.
- Three semicircular ducts in the semicircular canals.
- **Cochlear labyrinth:** cochlear duct in the cochlea.

The **spiral ligament,** a spiral thickening of the periosteal lining of the cochlear canal, secures the *cochlear duct* to the spiral canal of the cochlea (Fig. 7.118). The remainder of the membranous labyrinth is suspended by delicate filaments that traverse the perilymph.

The **semicircular ducts** open into the **utricle** through five openings, reflective of the way the surrounding semicircular canals open into the vestibule. The utricle communicates with the saccule through the **utriculosaccular duct,** from which the *endolymphatic duct* arises (Fig. 7.117D). The **saccule** is continuous with the cochlear duct through the **ductus reuniens,** a uniting duct. The utricle and saccule have specialized areas of sensory epithelium called **maculae.** The **macula of the utricle** (L. *macula utriculi*) is in the floor of the utricle, parallel with the base of the cranium, whereas the **macula of the saccule** (L. *macula sacculi*) is vertically placed on the medial wall of the saccule. The **hair cells in the maculae** are innervated by fibers of the vestibular division of the **vestibulocochlear nerve.** The primary sensory neurons are in the **vestibular ganglia** (Fig. 7.119), which are in the internal acoustic meatus.

The *endolymphatic duct* traverses the *vestibular aqueduct* (Fig. 7.113B) and emerges through the bone of the posterior cranial fossa, where it expands into a blind pouch called the **endolymphatic sac** (Figs. 7.113B, 7.117C and 7.119). The endolymphatic sac is located under the dura mater on the posterior surface of the petrous part of the temporal bone. The sac is a storage reservoir for excess endolymph, formed by the blood capillaries in the membranous labyrinth.

Semicircular Ducts. Each semicircular duct has an **ampulla** at one end containing a sensory area, the **ampullary crest** (L. *crista ampullari*) (Fig. 7.119). The crests are sensors for recording movements of the endolymph in the ampulla resulting from rotation of the head in the plane of the duct. The **hair cells of the crests**, like those of the maculae, stimulate primary sensory neurons, whose cell bodies are in the vestibular ganglia.

Cochlear Duct. The **cochlear duct** is a spiral tube, closed at one end and triangular in cross section. The duct is firmly suspended across the cochlear canal between the *spiral ligament* on the external wall of the cochlear canal (Fig. 7.118) and the **osseous spiral lamina** of the modiolus. Spanning the spiral canal in this manner, the endolymph-filled cochlear duct divides the perilymph-filled spiral canal into two channels that are continuous at the apex of the cochlea at the **helicotrema**, a semilunar communication at the apex of the cochlea.

OVERVIEW

The **neck** is the transitional area between the base of the cranium superiorly and the clavicles inferiorly. The neck joins the head to the trunk and limbs, serving as a major conduit for structures passing between them. In addition, several important organs with unique functions are located here: the larynx and the thyroid and parathyroid glands, for example.

The neck is relatively slender to allow the flexibility necessary to position the head to maximize the efficiency of its sensory organs (mainly the eyeballs but also the ears, mouth, and nose). Thus, many important structures are crowded together in the neck, such as muscles, glands, arteries, veins, nerves, lymphatics, trachea, esophagus, and vertebrae. Consequently, the neck is a well-known region of vulnerability. Further, several vital structures, including the trachea, esophagus, and thyroid gland, lack the bony protection afforded other parts of the systems to which these structures belong.

The main arterial blood flow to the head and neck (the *carotid arteries*) and the principal venous drainage (the *jugular veins*) lie anterolaterally in the neck (Fig. 8.1). Carotid/jugular blood vessels are the major structures commonly injured in penetrating wounds of the neck. The *brachial plexuses of nerves* originate in the neck and pass inferolaterally to enter the axillae and continue into and supply the upper limbs.

In the middle of the anterior aspect of the neck is the *thyroid cartilage,* the largest of the cartilages of the larynx, and the trachea. Lymph from structures in the head and neck drains into cervical lymph nodes.

BONES OF NECK

The skeleton of the neck is formed by the cervical vertebrae, hyoid bone, manubrium of the sternum, and clavicles (Figs. 8.2 and 8.3). These bones are parts of the axial skeleton except the clavicles, which are part of the appendicular skeleton.

Cervical Vertebrae

Seven *cervical vertebrae* form the cervical region of the vertebral column, which encloses the spinal cord and meninges. The stacked, centrally placed vertebral bodies support the head, and the intervertebral (IV) articulations—especially the craniovertebral joints at its superior end—provide the flexibility necessary to allow positioning of the head.

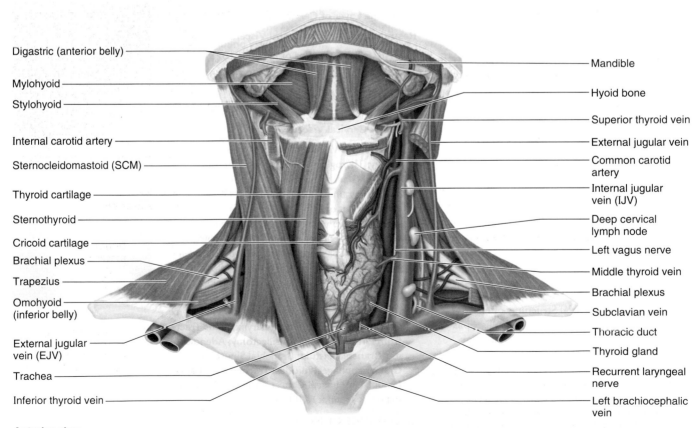

Digastric (anterior belly)
Mylohyoid
Stylohyoid
Internal carotid artery
Sternocleidomastoid (SCM)
Thyroid cartilage
Sternothyroid
Cricoid cartilage
Brachial plexus
Trapezius
Omohyoid (inferior belly)
External jugular vein (EJV)
Trachea
Inferior thyroid vein

Mandible
Hyoid bone
Superior thyroid vein
External jugular vein
Common carotid artery
Internal jugular vein (IJV)
Deep cervical lymph node
Left vagus nerve
Middle thyroid vein
Brachial plexus
Subclavian vein
Thoracic duct
Thyroid gland
Recurrent laryngeal nerve
Left brachiocephalic vein

Anterior view

FIGURE 8.1. Dissection of anterior neck. The fascia has been removed and the muscles on the left side have been reflected to show the hyoid bone, thyroid gland, and structures related to the carotid sheath: carotid artery, internal jugular vein (IJV), vagus nerve (CN X), and deep cervical lymph nodes.

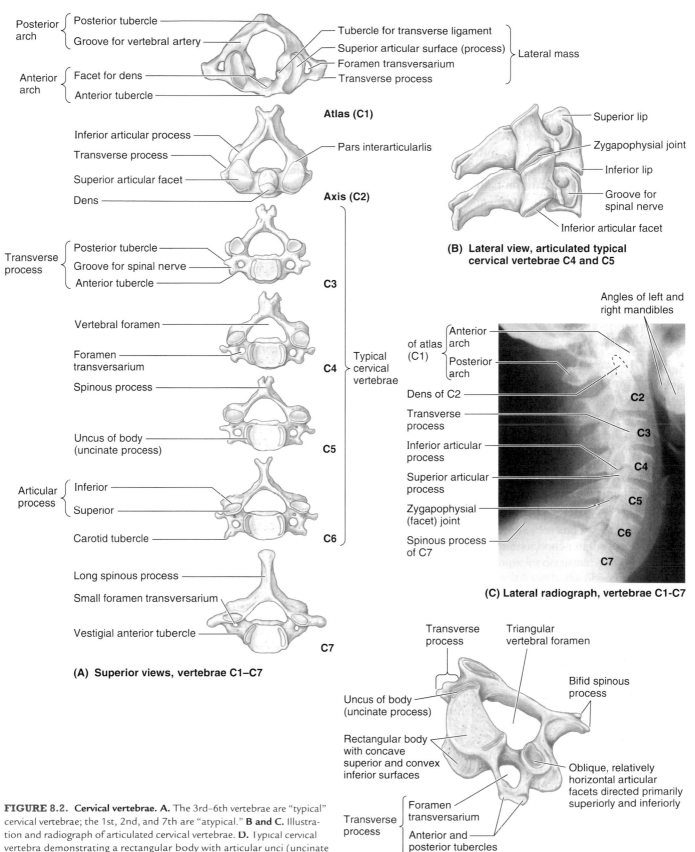

Posterior arch
- Posterior tubercle
- Groove for vertebral artery

Anterior arch
- Facet for dens
- Anterior tubercle

Tubercle for transverse ligament
Superior articular surface (process)
Foramen transversarium
Transverse process
Lateral mass

Atlas (C1)

Inferior articular process
Transverse process
Superior articular facet
Dens
Pars interarticularlis

Axis (C2)

Transverse process
- Posterior tubercle
- Groove for spinal nerve
- Anterior tubercle

C3

Vertebral foramen
Foramen transversarium
Spinous process

C4

Uncus of body (uncinate process)

C5

Typical cervical vertebrae

Articular process
- Inferior
- Superior
Carotid tubercle

C6

Long spinous process
Small foramen transversarium
Vestigial anterior tubercle

C7

(A) Superior views, vertebrae C1–C7

Superior lip
Zygapophysial joint
Inferior lip
Groove for spinal nerve
Inferior articular facet

(B) Lateral view, articulated typical cervical vertebrae C4 and C5

Angles of left and right mandibles

of atlas (C1)
- Anterior arch
- Posterior arch

Dens of C2
Transverse process
Inferior articular process
Superior articular process
Zygapophysial (facet) joint
Spinous process of C7

C2
C3
C4
C5
C6
C7

(C) Lateral radiograph, vertebrae C1-C7

Transverse process
Triangular vertebral foramen
Bifid spinous process

Uncus of body (uncinate process)
Rectangular body with concave superior and convex inferior surfaces

Oblique, relatively horizontal articular facets directed primarily superiorly and inferiorly

Transverse process
- Foramen transversarium
- Anterior and posterior tubercles

(D) Superior oblique view of typical cervical vertebra

FIGURE 8.2. Cervical vertebrae. A. The 3rd–6th vertebrae are "typical" cervical vertebrae; the 1st, 2nd, and 7th are "atypical." **B and C.** Illustration and radiograph of articulated cervical vertebrae. **D.** Typical cervical vertebra demonstrating a rectangular body with articular unci (uncinate processes) on its lateral aspects, a triangular vertebral foramen, a bifid spinous process, and foramina transversaria.

the subclavian artery, and part of the occipital artery. The *thyrocervical trunk*, a branch of the subclavian artery (Figs. 8.9–8.11) most commonly gives rise to a suprascapular artery and a cervicodorsal trunk from its lateral aspect; its terminal branches are the ascending cervical and inferior thyroid artery (discussed on p. 995).

The **suprascapular artery** passes inferolaterally across the anterior scalene muscle and phrenic nerve (Fig. 8.10). It then crosses the third part of the subclavian artery and the cords of the brachial plexus. It then passes posterior to the clavicle to supply muscles on the posterior aspect of the scapula. Alternately, the suprascapular artery may arise directly from the third part of the subclavian artery.

Also arising laterally, the **cervicodorsal trunk** (Weiglein et al., 2005), sometimes known as the transverse cervical artery, further bifurcates into the *superficial cervical artery* (superficial branch of transverse cervical artery) and the *dorsal scapular artery* (deep branch of transverse cervical artery). These branches run superficially and laterally across the phrenic nerve and anterior scalene muscle, 2–3 cm superior to the clavicle. They then cross or pass through the *trunks of the brachial plexus*, supplying branches to

their *vasa nervorum* (blood vessels of nerves). The **superficial cervical artery** passes deep (anterior) to the trapezius accompanying the spinal accessory nerve (CN XI). The **dorsal scapular artery** may arise independently, directly from the third (or, less often, the second) part of the subclavian artery. When it is a branch of the subclavian, the dorsal scapular artery passes laterally through the trunks of the brachial plexus, anterior to the middle scalene. Regardless of its origin, its distal portion runs deep to the levator scapulae and rhomboid muscles, supplying both and participating in the arterial anastomoses around the scapula (Chapter 6). The *occipital artery,* a branch of the external carotid artery, enters the lateral cervical region at its apex and ascends over the head to supply the posterior half of the scalp (Fig. 8.9).

The **subclavian artery** supplies blood to the upper limb. The third part begins approximately a finger's breadth superior to the clavicle, opposite the lateral border of the anterior scalene muscle. It is hidden in the inferior part of the lateral cervical region, posterosuperior to the subclavian vein. The third part of the artery is the longest and most superficial part. It lies on the 1st rib, and its pulsations can be felt by applying deep pressure in the omoclavicular triangle. The artery is in

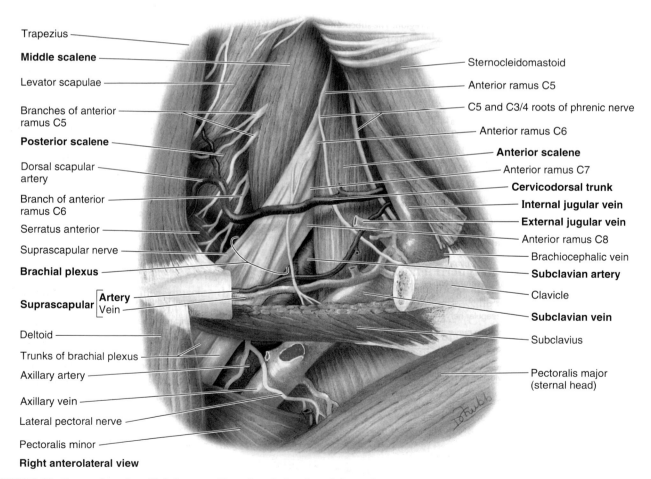

Right anterolateral view

FIGURE 8.10. Deeper dissection of inferior part of lateral cervical region. All fascia, the omohyoid muscle, and the clavicular head of the pectoralis major have been removed to reveal the subclavian vein and third part of the subclavian artery. The internal jugular vein, deep to the SCM, is not in the lateral cervical region but is close to it. The brachial plexus of nerves and subclavian vessels pass to the upper limb, the name of the vessels changing to *axillary* inferior to the clavicle at the lateral border of the 1st rib.

Ascending cervical
Inferior thyroid
Common carotid artery
Vertebral
Cervicodorsal trunk
(transverse
cervical a.)
Thyrocervical trunk
Suprascapular
Costocervical trunk
Subclavian
Internal thoracic
Axillary artery
Brachiocephalic trunk
1st rib

Lateral view of right side

FIGURE 8.11. Subclavian artery: its parts and branches. There are three parts of the subclavian artery: medial (*1*), posterior (*2*), and lateral (*3*) to the anterior scalene muscle. The cervicodorsal trunk (transverse cervical artery) and suprascapular artery occasionally arise directly (or via a common trunk) from the second or third parts of the subclavian artery instead of directly from the thyrocervical trunk via a common trunk, as shown here, or independently.

contact with the 1st rib as it passes posterior to the anterior scalene muscle; consequently, compression of the subclavian artery against this rib can control bleeding in the upper limb. The inferior trunk of the brachial plexus lies directly posterior to the third part of the artery. The branches that occasionally arise from the third part (suprascapular artery, dorsal scapular artery) are aberrant forms of more typical patterns

in which they arise elsewhere (from the thyrocervical trunk via a cervicodorsal trunk in particular).

VEINS IN LATERAL CERVICAL REGION

The **external jugular vein (EJV)** begins near the angle of the mandible (just inferior to the auricle) by the union of the posterior division of the *retromandibular vein* with the *posterior auricular vein* (Fig. 8.12). The EJV crosses the SCM obliquely, deep to the platysma, and enters the antero-inferior part of the lateral cervical region (Fig. 8.8). It then pierces the investing layer of deep cervical fascia, which forms the roof of this region, at the posterior border of the SCM. The EJV descends to the inferior part of the lateral cervical region and terminates in the subclavian vein (Figs. 8.10 and 8.12). It drains most of the scalp and side of the face.

The **subclavian vein,** the major venous channel draining the upper limb, curves through the inferior part of the lateral cervical region. It passes anterior to the anterior scalene muscle and phrenic nerve and unites at the medial border of the muscle with the IJV to form the **brachiocephalic vein,** posterior to the medial end of the clavicle. Just superior to the clavicle, the EJV receives the *cervicodorsal, suprascapular,* and *anterior jugular veins.*

NERVES OF LATERAL CERVICAL REGION

The **spinal accessory nerve (CN XI)** passes deep to the SCM, supplying it before entering the lateral cervical region at or inferior to the junction of the superior and middle thirds of the posterior border of the SCM (Figs. 8.8 and 8.9). The nerve passes postero-inferiorly, within or deep to the investing layer of deep cervical fascia, running on the levator scapulae from which it is separated by the prevertebral layer of fascia. CN XI then disappears deep to the anterior border of

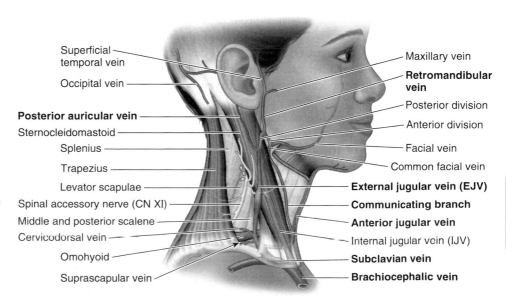

FIGURE 8.12. Superficial veins of neck. The superficial temporal and maxillary veins merge, forming the retromandibular vein, the posterior division of which unites with the posterior auricular vein to form the EJV. The facial vein receives the anterior division of the retromandibular vein before emptying into the internal jugular vein, deep to the SCM. The anterior jugular veins may lie superficial or deep to the investing layer of the deep cervical fascia.

Superficial temporal vein
Occipital vein
Posterior auricular vein
Sternocleidomastoid
Splenius
Trapezius
Levator scapulae
Spinal accessory nerve (CN XI)
Middle and posterior scalene
Cervicodorsal vein
Omohyoid
Suprascapular vein

Maxillary vein
Retromandibular vein
Posterior division
Anterior division
Facial vein
Common facial vein
External jugular vein (EJV)
Communicating branch
Anterior jugular vein
Internal jugular vein (IJV)
Subclavian vein
Brachiocephalic vein

Lateral view

(A)

Platysma

(B)

Key for (B):

A Sternocleidomastoid region
B Lateral cervical region
C Anterior cervical region
D Posterior cervical region
E Suboccipital region
1 Lesser supraclavicular fossa
2 Occipital triangle
3 Omoclavicular triangle
4 Submental triangle
5 Submandibular triangle
6 Carotid triangle
7 Muscular triangle
X Carotid bifurcation
(take pulse inferior to this point)

(C)

SCM
X

Approximated course of spinal accessory nerve (CN XI)

Laryngeal prominence

T
X

Greater supraclavicular fossa

T

Clavicle

Jugular notch

(D)

Angle of mandible

External jugular vein

Laryngeal prominence

SCM

T

CI

S

Key for (C) & (D):

T Trapezius (ant. border)
SCM Sternocleidomastoid
CI Clavicular head
S Sternal head

Jugular notch

Lesser ⎫
Greater ⎭ Supraclavicular fossae

(E)

SCM

Subclavian artery

(F)

FIGURE 8.22. Surface anatomy of neck. A. Contraction of the platysma. **B.** The regions (A–E) and triangles (2–7) of the neck. **C.** The course of the spinal accessory nerve (CN XI). **D.** The landmarks of the anterolateral neck. **E.** Checking the subclavian artery pulse. **F.** Palpation of the submandibular lymph.

if distended by asking the person to take a deep breath and hold it, expiring against resistance (*Valsalva maneuver*) or by using gentle pressure on the inferior part of the vein. These actions impede venous return to the right side of the heart. The EJV is less obvious in children and middle-aged women because their subcutaneous tissues tend to be thicker than those in men.

The great auricular nerve parallels the EJV, approximately a finger's breadth posterior to the vein. Deep to the superior half of the SCM is the cervical plexus, and deep to the inferior half of the SCM are the IJV, common carotid artery, and vagus nerve in the carotid sheath (Fig. 8.21).

The *trapezius*, which defines the *posterior cervical region*, can be observed and palpated by asking the person to shrug the shoulders against resistance (Fig. 8.22B–D). Superiorly, inferior to its attachment to the *external occipital protuberance*, the muscle overlies the *suboccipital region* (see Fig. 4.37).

The inferior belly of the *omohyoid muscle* can just barely be seen and palpated as it passes superomedially across the inferior part of the *lateral cervical region*. Easiest to observe in thin people, the omohyoid muscle can often be seen contracting when they are speaking.

Just inferior to the inferior belly of the omohyoid is the *greater supraclavicular fossa*, the depression overlying the *omoclavicular triangle* (Fig. 8.22C & D). The third part of the subclavian artery passes through this triangle before coursing posterior to the clavicle and across the 1st rib. The greater supraclavicular fossa is clinically important because **subclavian arterial pulsations** can be palpated here in most people. The course of the *subclavian artery* in the neck is represented by a curved line from the *sternoclavicular (SC) joint* to the midpoint of the clavicle. To feel subclavian pulsations, press inferoposteriorly (down and back) immediately posterior to the junction of the medial and middle thirds of the clavicle (Fig. 8.22E). This is the pressure point for the subclavian artery; firmer pressure, compressing the artery against the 1st rib, can occlude the artery when hemorrhage is occurring distally in the upper limb.

The chief contents of the larger *occipital triangle*, superior to the omohyoid muscle, are the spinal accessory nerve (CN XI); cutaneous branches of cervical nerves C2, C3, and C4; and cervical lymph nodes. Because of the vulnerability and frequency of iatrogenic injury of the spinal accessory nerve, it is important to be able to estimate the location of CN XI in the lateral cervical region. Its course can be approximated by a line that intersects the junction of the superior and middle thirds of the posterior border of the SCM and the junction of the middle and lower thirds of the anterior border of the trapezius (Fig. 8.22C).

The cervical viscera and carotid arteries and their branches are approached surgically through the *anterior cervical region*, between the anterior border of the SCM and the midline (Fig. 8.22B). Of the four smaller triangles into which this region is subdivided, the submandibular and carotid triangles are especially important clinically.

The *submandibular gland* nearly fills the *submandibular triangle*. It is palpable as a soft mass inferior to the body of the mandible, especially when the apex of the tongue is forced against the maxillary incisor teeth. The *submandibular lymph nodes* lie superficial to the gland (Fig. 8.14A). These nodes receive lymph from the face inferior to the eye and from the mouth. If enlarged, these nodes can be palpated by moving the fingertips from the angle of the mandible along its inferior border (Figs. 8.22D and F). If continued until the fingers meet under the chin, enlarged *submental lymph nodes* can be palpated in the *submental triangle* (Fig. 8.22B).

The carotid arterial system is located in the *carotid triangle*. This area is important for surgical approaches to the carotid sheath containing the common carotid artery, IJV, and vagus nerve (Figs. 8.15 and 8.21). The carotid triangle also contains the hypoglossal nerve (CN XII) and cervical sympathetic trunk. The *carotid sheath* can be marked out by a line joining the SC joint to a point midway between the mastoid process and the angle of the mandible. The **carotid pulse** can be palpated by placing the index and 3rd fingers on the thyroid cartilage and pointing them posterolaterally between the trachea and SCM. The pulse is palpable just medial to the SCM. The palpation is performed low in the neck to avoid pressure on the *carotid sinus*, which could cause a reflex drop in blood pressure and heart rate (Figs. 8.17 and 8.22B).

SUPERFICIAL STRUCTURES OF NECK: CERVICAL REGIONS

Congenital Torticollis

Torticollis (L. *tortus*, twisted + L. *collum*, neck) is a contraction or shortening of the cervical muscles that produces twisting of the neck and slanting of the head. The most common type of torticollis (wry neck) results from a *fibrous tissue tumor* (L. *fibromatosis colli*) that develops in the SCM before or shortly after birth. The lesion, like a normal unilateral SCM contraction, causes the head to tilt toward, and the face to turn away from, the affected side (Fig. B8.1). When torticollis occurs prenatally, the abnormal position of the infant's head usually necessitates a breech delivery.

Occasionally, the SCM is injured when an infant's head is pulled too much during a difficult birth, tearing its fibers (*muscular torticollis*) (Kliegman et al., 2011). A *hematoma* (localized mass of extravasated blood) occurs that may develop into a fibrotic mass that entraps a branch of the spinal accessory nerve (CN XI) and thus denervates part of the SCM. The stiffness and twisting of the neck results from fibrosis and shortening of the SCM. Surgical release of the SCM from its inferior attachments to the manubrium and

The Bottom Line

DEEP STRUCTURES OF NECK

Prevertebral muscles: The prevertebral muscles, deep to the prevertebral layer of deep cervical fascia, are divided into anterior and lateral vertebral muscles by the neurovascular plane of the cervical and brachial plexuses and subclavian artery. ♦ The anterior vertebral muscles flex the head and neck; however, this movement is normally produced by gravity in conjunction with eccentric contraction of the extensors of the neck. ♦ Thus, the anterior vertebral muscles are called into action mainly when this movement is performed against resistance, probably initiating the movement while the strength of the movement is produced by the SCM. ♦ The lateral vertebral muscles laterally flex the neck, participate in rotation of the neck, and fix or elevate the superiormost ribs during forced inspiration.

Root of the neck: The branches of the arch of the aorta bifurcate and/or traverse the root of the neck, with the branches of the subclavian artery arising here also. ♦ The internal jugular and subclavian veins converge at the root of the neck to form the brachiocephalic veins. ♦ The major lymphatic trunks (right lymphatic duct and thoracic duct) enter the venous angles formed by the convergence of these veins. ♦ The phrenic and vagus nerves enter the thorax by passing anterior to the subclavian arteries and posterior to the brachiocephalic veins. ♦ The sympathetic trunks and recurrent laryngeal nerves traverse the root of the neck posterior to the arteries, as do the visceral structures (trachea and esophagus). ♦ The cervical portion of the sympathetic trunks include three cervical sympathetic ganglia (inferior, middle, and superior), in which presynaptic fibers from the superior thoracic spinal cord synapse with postsynaptic neurons. ♦ These neurons send fibers to the cervical spinal nerves, via gray rami communicantes; to the head and viscera of the neck, via cephalic arterial branches and peri-arterial plexuses; and to the thoracic viscera, via cardiac (cardiopulmonary splanchnic) nerves.

VISCERA OF NECK

The cervical viscera are disposed in three layers, named for their primary function (Fig. 8.26). Superficial to deep, they are the:

1. *Endocrine layer:* the thyroid and parathyroid glands.
2. *Respiratory layer:* the larynx and trachea.
3. *Alimentary layer:* the pharynx and esophagus.

Endocrine Layer of Cervical Viscera

The viscera of the **endocrine layer** are part of the body's endocrine system of ductless, hormone-secreting glands. The *thyroid gland* is the body's largest endocrine gland. It produces *thyroid hormone,* which controls the rate of metabolism, and *calcitonin,* a hormone controlling calcium metabolism. The thyroid gland affects all areas of the body except itself and the spleen, testes, and uterus. The hormone produced by the *parathyroid glands, parathormone* (PTH), controls the metabolism of phosphorus and calcium in the blood. The parathyroid glands target the skeleton, kidneys, and intestine.

THYROID GLAND

The **thyroid gland** lies deep to the sternothyroid and sternohyoid muscles, located anteriorly in the neck at the level of the C5–T1 vertebrae (Fig. 8.26). It consists primarily of right and left **lobes,** anterolateral to the larynx and trachea. A relatively thin **isthmus** unites the lobes over the trachea, usually anterior to the second and third tracheal rings. The thyroid gland is surrounded by a thin **fibrous capsule,** which sends septa deeply into the gland. Dense connective tissue attaches the capsule to the cricoid cartilage and superior tracheal rings. External to the capsule is a loose sheath formed by the visceral portion of the pretracheal layer of deep cervical fascia.

Arteries of Thyroid Gland. The highly vascular thyroid gland is supplied by the superior and inferior *thyroid arteries* (Figs. 8.26B and 8.27). These vessels lie between the fibrous capsule and the loose fascial sheath. Usually the first branches of the external carotid arteries, the **superior thyroid arteries,** descend to the superior poles of the gland, pierce the pretracheal layer of deep cervical fascia, and divide into anterior and posterior branches supplying mainly the anterosuperior aspect of the gland.

The **inferior thyroid arteries,** the largest branches of the thyrocervical trunks arising from the subclavian arteries, run superomedially posterior to the carotid sheaths to reach the posterior aspect of the *thyroid gland.* They divide into several branches that pierce the pretracheal layer of the deep cervical fascia and supply the posteroinferior aspect, including the **inferior poles of the gland.** The right and left superior and inferior thyroid arteries anastomose extensively within the gland, ensuring its supply while providing potential collateral circulation between the subclavian and external carotid arteries.

In approximately 10% of people, a small, unpaired **thyroid ima artery** (L. *arteria thyroidea ima*) arises from the brachiocephalic trunk (see the blue box "Thyroid Ima Artery" on p. 1040); however, it may arise from the arch of the aorta or from the right common carotid, subclavian, or internal thoracic arteries. When present, this small artery ascends on the anterior surface of the trachea, supplying small branches to it. The artery then continues to the isthmus of the thyroid gland, where it divides and supplies it.

(A) Anterior view

Sternohyoid muscle (turned up)

Thyroid cartilage

Sternothyroid muscle

Cricoid cartilage

Thyroid gland (right lobe)

Larynx

Isthmus

Inferior poles

Trachea

Esophagus

(B) Posterior view

Internal carotid artery

External carotid artery

Common carotid artery

Superior thyroid artery

Superior pole

Left parathyroid glands

Inferior thyroid artery

Thyrocervical trunk

Right parathyroid glands

Recurrent laryngeal nerves

(C) Transverse section at level indicated in part A

Inferior view

Thyroid gland

Trachea

Fibrous capsule of thyroid gland

Inferior thyroid artery

C7 vertebra

Esophagus

Sternohyoid

Sternothyroid

Sternocleidomastoid

Pretracheal layer of deep cervical fascia (muscular and visceral layers)

Carotid sheath

Omohyoid

Prevertebral layer of deep cervical fascia

Anterior scalene

Middle scalene

Layers of cervical viscera
- Endocrine layer
- Respiratory layer
- Alimentary layer

(D) Transverse CT scan through lobes of thyroid gland   Inferior views   **(E) Transverse MRI study through thyroid isthmus**

1 Esophagus
2 Trachea
3 Lobes of thyroid gland
4 Thyroid isthmus
5 SCM
6 Sternohyoid muscle
7 Common carotid artery
8 IJV
9 Vertebral artery
10 Vertebral body
11 Spinal cord (surrounded by cerebrospinal fluid in subarachnoid space)
12 Deep muscles of back
13 Retropharyngeal space

FIGURE 8.26. Relationships of thyroid gland. A. The sternothyroid muscles have been cut to expose the lobes of the normal thyroid gland. The isthmus lies anterior to the second and third tracheal rings. **B.** The parathyroid glands are usually embedded in the fibrous capsule on the posterior surface of the thyroid gland. **C–E.** The functional layers of the cervical viscera are indicated. The levels of the imaging studies are close to that shown in part **C.** (Part **D** courtesy of Dr. M. Keller, Medical Imaging, University of Toronto, Toronto, Ontario, Canada. Part **E** Courtesy of Dr. W. Kucharczyk, Professor and Neuroradiologist Senior Scientist, Department of Medical Resonance Imaging, University Health Network, Toronto, Ontario, Canada.)

Tongue
Mandible
Epiglottic vallecula

Epiglottis (E)
Laryngeal vestibule (V)
Ary-epiglottic fold
Vestibular fold
Thyroid cartilage
Saccule
Piriform fossa (recess – P)
Laryngeal ventricle
Middle part of laryngeal cavity
Vocal ligaments (opposed)
Conus elasticus
Infra-glottic cavity (IC)
Cricoid cartilage (C)
Trachea (T)

(A) Posterior view of coronally-sectioned larynx

(B) Coronal MRI study (Plane indicated in Fig. 8.41A & B)

Key for (A):

1 Ary-epiglottic muscle
2 Lateral crico-arytenoid
3 Thyro-arytenoid
4 Vocalis
5 Cricothyroid

Epiglottic tubercle
Epiglottis
Greater horn of hyoid bone
Laryngeal ventricle
Vestibular fold
Ary-epiglottic fold
Vocal fold (cord)
Piriform recess of laryngopharynx
Cuneiform tubercle
Rima glottidis
Corniculate tubercle

(C) Posterosuperior view, looking antero-inferiorly through laryngeal vestibule and rima glottidis

1 Esophagus
2 Thyroid cartilage
3 Lamina of cricoid cartilage
4 Sternothyroid and sternohyoid muscles
5 Common carotid artery
6 IJV
7 Anterior root of spinal nerve
8 SCM
9 Inferior pharyngeal constrictor
10 Vertebral body
11 Spinal cord
12 Vertebral artery

(D) Transverse MRI study of layrnx transecting thyroid cartilage

(E) Transverse MRI study of larynx transecting cricoid cartilage

FIGURE 8.35. Folds and compartments of larynx. A. This coronal section shows the compartments of the larynx: the vestibule, middle compartment with left and right ventricles, and the infraglottic cavity. **B.** This MRI study shows the epiglottic valleculae of the oropharynx, piriform fossae of the laryngopharynx, and vestibular and vocal folds of the larynx. **C.** The rima glottidis (the space between the vocal folds) is visible through the laryngeal inlet and vestibule. The laryngeal inlet is bounded (1) anteriorly by the free curved edge of the epiglottis; (2) posteriorly by the arytenoid cartilages, the corniculate cartilages that cap them, and the interarytenoid fold that unites them; and (3) on each side by the ary-epiglottic fold that contains the superior end of the cuneiform cartilage. **D and E.** The planes of these transverse studies, oriented in the same direction as part **C,** pass superior (**D**) and inferior (**E**) to the rima glottidis. (MRI studies courtesy of Dr. W. Kucharczyk, University Health Network, Toronto, Ontario, Canada.)

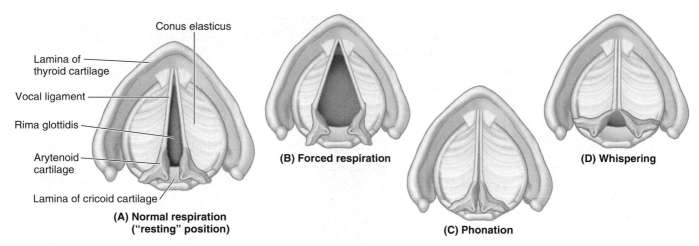

FIGURE 8.36. Variations in shape of rima glottidis. A. The shape of the rima glottidis, the aperture between the vocal folds, varies according to the position of the vocal folds. During normal respiration, the laryngeal muscles are relaxed and the rima glottidis assumes a narrow, slit-like position. **B.** During a deep inhalation, the vocal ligaments are abducted by contraction of the posterior crico-arytenoid muscles, opening the rima glottidis widely into an inverted kite shape. **C.** During phonation, the arytenoid muscles adduct the arytenoid cartilages at the same time that the lateral crico-arytenoid muscles moderately adduct. Air forced between the adducted vocal ligaments produces tone. Stronger contraction of the same muscles seals the rima glottidis (Valsalva maneuver). **D.** During whispering, the vocal ligaments are strongly adducted by the lateral crico-arytenoid muscles, but the relaxed arytenoid muscles allow air to pass between the arytenoid cartilages (intercartilaginous part of rima glottidis), which is modified into toneless speech. No tone is produced.

voice. The lower range of pitch of the voice of postpubertal males results from the greater length of the vocal folds.

The *vestibular folds,* extending between the thyroid and the arytenoid cartilages (Figs. 8.34 and 8.35), play little or no part in voice production; they are protective in function. They consist of two thick folds of mucous membrane enclosing the *vestibular ligaments.* The space between these ligaments is the **rima vestibuli.** The lateral recesses between the vocal and the vestibular folds are the *laryngeal ventricles.*

Laryngeal Muscles. The laryngeal muscles are divided into extrinsic and intrinsic groups.

- **Extrinsic laryngeal muscles** move *the larynx as a whole* (Fig. 8.18; Table 8.3). The *infrahyoid muscles* are depressors of the hyoid and larynx, whereas the *suprahyoid muscles* (and the *stylopharyngeus,* a pharyngeal muscle discussed later in this chapter) are elevators of the hyoid and larynx.
- **Intrinsic laryngeal muscles** move *the laryngeal components,* altering the length and tension of the vocal folds and the size and shape of the rima glottidis (Fig. 8.36). All but one of the intrinsic muscles of the larynx are supplied by the *recurrent laryngeal nerve* (Figs. 8.37, 8.39, and 8.40), a branch of CN X. The cricothyroid is supplied by the external laryngeal nerve, one of the two terminal branches of the *superior laryngeal nerve.*

The actions of the intrinsic laryngeal muscles are easiest to understand when they are considered as functional groups: adductors and abductors, sphincters, and tensors and relaxers. The intrinsic muscles are illustrated in situ in Figures 8.35D & E and 8.38; their attachments, innervation, and main actions are summarized in Table 8.5.

- *Adductors and abductors:* These muscles move the vocal folds to open and close the rima glottidis. The principal adductors are the **lateral crico-arytenoid muscles,**

which pull the muscular processes anteriorly, rotating the arytenoid cartilages so that their vocal processes swing medially. When this action is combined with that of the **transverse** and **oblique arytenoid muscles,** which pull the arytenoid cartilages together, air pushed through the rima glottidis causes vibrations of the vocal ligaments

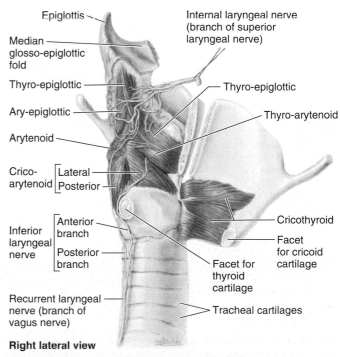

FIGURE 8.37. Muscles and nerves of larynx and cricothyroid joint. The thyroid cartilage is sawn through to the right of the median plane. The cricothyroid joint is disarticulated, and the right lamina of the thyroid cartilage is turned anteriorly (like opening a book), stripping the cricothyroid muscles off the arch of the cricoid cartilage.

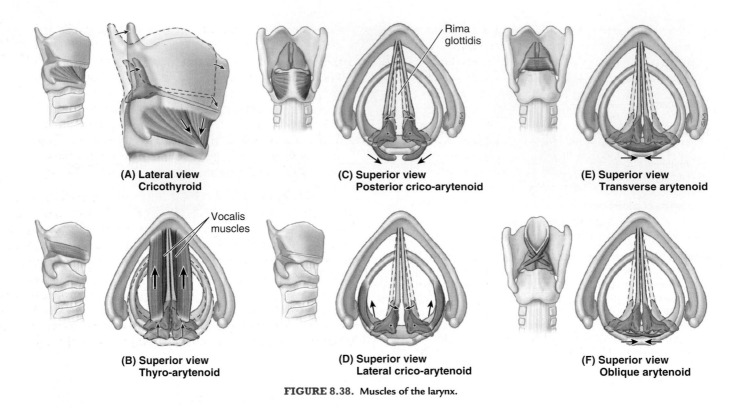

(A) Lateral view
Cricothyroid

(C) Superior view
Posterior crico-arytenoid

Rima
glottidis

(E) Superior view
Transverse arytenoid

Vocalis
muscles

(B) Superior view
Thyro-arytenoid

(D) Superior view
Lateral crico-arytenoid

(F) Superior view
Oblique arytenoid

FIGURE 8.38. Muscles of the larynx.

TABLE 8.5. MUSCLES OF LARYNX

Muscle	Origin	Insertion	Innervation	Main Action(s)
Cricothyroid	Anterolateral part of cricoid cartilage	Inferior margin and inferior horn of thyroid cartilage	External laryngeal nerve (from CN X)	Stretches and tenses vocal ligament
Thyro-arytenoid[a]	Lower half of posterior aspect of angle of thyroid laminae and cricothyroid ligament	Anterolateral arytenoid surface	Inferior laryngeal nerve (terminal part of recurrent laryngeal nerve, from CN X – see Fig. 8.37)	Relaxes vocal ligament
Posterior crico-arytenoid	Posterior surface of lamina of cricoid cartilage	Vocal process of arytenoid cartilage		Abducts vocal folds
Lateral crico-arytenoid	Arch of cricoid cartilage			Adducts vocal folds (inter-ligamentous portion)
Transverse and oblique arytenoids[b]	One arytenoid cartilage	Contralateral arytenoid cartilage		Adduct arytenoid cartilages (adducting intercartilaginous portion of vocal folds, closing posterior rima glottidis)
Vocalis[c]	Lateral surface of vocal process of arytenoid cartilage	Ipsilateral vocal ligament		Relaxes posterior vocal ligament while maintaining (or increasing) tension of anterior part

[a]Superior fibers of the thyro-arytenoid muscles pass into the ary-epiglottic fold, and some of them reach the epiglottic cartilage. These fibers constitute the thyro-epiglottic muscle, which widens the laryngeal inlet.

[b]Some fibers of the oblique arytenoid muscles continue as ary-epiglottic muscles (Fig. 8.39).

[c]This slender muscle slip lies medial to and is composed of fibers finer than those of the thyro-arytenoid muscle.

(phonation). When the vocal ligaments are adducted, but the transverse arytenoid muscles do not act, the arytenoid cartilages remain apart and air may bypass the ligaments. This is the position of whispering when the breath is modified into voice in the absence of tone. The sole abductors are the **posterior crico-arytenoid muscles,** which pull the muscular processes posteriorly, rotating the vocal processes laterally and thus widening the rima glottidis.

- *Sphincters:* The combined actions of most of the muscles of the laryngeal inlet result in a sphincteric action that closes the laryngeal inlet as a protective mechanism during swallowing. Contraction of the *lateral crico-arytenoids, transverse* and *oblique arytenoids,* and *ary-epiglottic muscles* brings the ary-epiglottic folds together and pulls the arytenoid cartilages toward the epiglottis. This action occurs reflexively in response to the presence of liquid or particles approaching or within the laryngeal vestibule. It is perhaps our strongest reflex, diminishing only after loss of consciousness, as in drowning.
- *Tensors:* The principal tensors are the **cricothyroid muscles,** which tilt or pull the prominence or angle of the

thyroid cartilage anteriorly and inferiorly toward the arch of the cricoid cartilage. This increases the distance between the thyroid prominence and the arytenoid cartilages. Because the anterior ends of the vocal ligaments attach to the posterior aspect of the prominence, the vocal ligaments elongate and tighten, raising the pitch of the voice.

- *Relaxers:* The principal muscles in this group are the **thyro-arytenoid muscles,** which pull the arytenoid cartilages anteriorly, toward the thyroid angle (prominence), thereby relaxing the vocal ligaments to lower the pitch of the voice.

The **vocalis muscles** lie medial to the thyro-arytenoid muscles and lateral to the vocal ligaments within the vocal folds. The vocalis muscles produce minute adjustments of the vocal ligaments, selectively tensing and relaxing the anterior and posterior parts, respectively, of the vocal folds during animated speech and singing.

Arteries of Larynx. The laryngeal arteries, branches of the superior and inferior thyroid arteries, supply the larynx (Fig. 8.39). The **superior laryngeal artery** accompanies the internal branch of the superior laryngeal nerve through

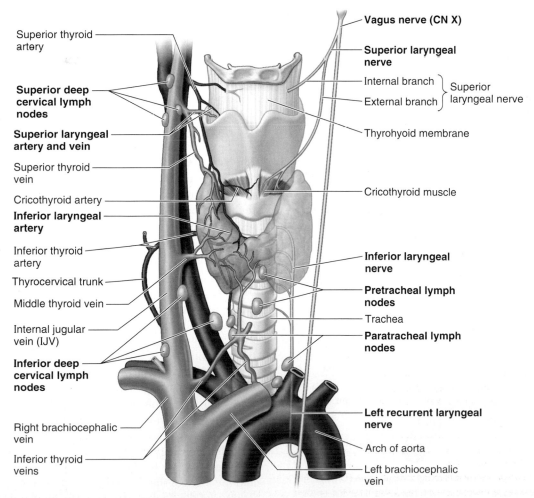

FIGURE 8.39. Vessels, nerves, and lymph nodes of larynx. The superior and inferior thyroid arteries give rise to the superior and inferior laryngeal arteries, respectively; they anastomose with each other. The laryngeal nerves are derived from the vagus (CN X) through the internal and external branches of the superior laryngeal nerve and the inferior laryngeal nerve from the recurrent laryngeal nerve. The left recurrent laryngeal nerve passes inferior to the arch of the aorta.

the thyrohyoid membrane and branches to supply the internal surface of the larynx. The **cricothyroid artery,** a small branch of the superior thyroid artery, supplies the cricothyroid muscle. The **inferior laryngeal artery,** a branch of the inferior thyroid artery, accompanies the *inferior laryngeal nerve* (terminal part of the recurrent laryngeal nerve) and supplies the mucous membrane and muscles in the inferior part of the larynx.

Veins of Larynx. The laryngeal veins accompany the laryngeal arteries. The **superior laryngeal vein** usually joins the superior thyroid vein and through it drains into the IJV (Fig. 8.39). The **inferior laryngeal vein** joins the inferior thyroid vein or the venous plexus of veins on the anterior aspect of the trachea, which empties into the left brachiocephalic vein.

Lymphatics of Larynx. The laryngeal lymphatic vessels superior to the vocal folds accompany the superior laryngeal artery through the thyrohyoid membrane and drain into the **superior deep cervical lymph nodes.** The lymphatic vessels inferior to the vocal folds drain into the *pretracheal* or *paratracheal lymph nodes,* which drain into the **inferior deep cervical lymph nodes** (Fig. 8.39).

Nerves of Larynx. The nerves of the larynx are the superior and inferior laryngeal branches of the vagus nerves (CN X). The **superior laryngeal nerve** arises from the **inferior vagal ganglion** at the superior end of the carotid triangle (Fig. 8.40). The nerve divides into two terminal branches

within the carotid sheath: the internal laryngeal nerve (sensory and autonomic) and the external laryngeal nerve (motor).

The **internal laryngeal nerve,** the larger of the terminal branches of the superior laryngeal nerve, pierces the thyrohyoid membrane with the superior laryngeal artery, supplying sensory fibers to the laryngeal mucous membrane of the laryngeal vestibule and middle laryngeal cavity, including the superior surface of the vocal folds. The **external laryngeal nerve,** the smaller terminal branch of the superior laryngeal nerve, descends posterior to the sternothyroid muscle in company with the superior thyroid artery. At first, the external laryngeal nerve lies on the inferior pharyngeal constrictor; it then pierces the muscle, contributing to its innervation (with the pharyngeal plexus), and continues to supply the cricothyroid muscle.

The **inferior laryngeal nerve,** the continuation of the recurrent laryngeal nerve (a branch of the vagus nerve), enters the larynx by passing deep to the inferior border of the inferior pharyngeal constrictor and medial to the lamina of the thyroid cartilage (Figs. 8.37, 8.39, and 8.40). It divides into anterior and posterior branches, which accompany the inferior laryngeal artery into the larynx. The anterior branch supplies the lateral crico-arytenoid, thyro-arytenoid, vocalis, ary-epiglottic, and thyro-epiglottic muscles. The posterior branch supplies the posterior crico-arytenoid and transverse and oblique arytenoid muscles. Because it supplies all the intrinsic muscles except the cricothyroid, the inferior laryngeal nerve is the primary motor nerve of the larynx. However, it also provides sensory fibers to the mucosa of the infraglottic cavity.

TRACHEA

The **trachea,** extending from the larynx into the thorax, terminates inferiorly as it divides into right and left main bronchi. It transports air to and from the lungs, and its epithelium propels debris-laden mucus toward the pharynx for expulsion from the mouth. The trachea is a fibrocartilaginous tube, supported by incomplete cartilaginous **tracheal cartilages** (rings), that occupies a median position in the neck (Fig. 8.37). The tracheal cartilages keep the trachea patent; they are deficient posteriorly where the trachea is adjacent to the esophagus. The posterior gaps in the tracheal rings are spanned by the involuntary **trachealis muscle,** smooth muscle connecting the ends of the rings (Fig. 8.41). Hence the posterior wall of the trachea is flat.

In adults, the trachea is approximately 2.5 cm in diameter, whereas in infants it has the diameter of a pencil. The trachea extends from the inferior end of the larynx at the level of the C6 vertebra. It ends at the level of the sternal angle or the T4–T5 IV disc, where it divides into the right and left main bronchi (see Chapter 1, p. 114).

Lateral to the trachea are the common carotid arteries and the lobes of the thyroid gland (Fig. 8.39). Inferior to the isthmus of the thyroid gland are the jugular venous arch and the inferior thyroid veins (Fig. 8.16). The brachiocephalic trunk is related to the right side of the trachea in the root of

Inferior vagal ganglion
Superior laryngeal nerve
Superior thyroid artery
Common carotid artery
Vagus nerve (CN X)
Inferior laryngeal nerve
Subclavian artery
Brachiocephalic trunk

Pharyngeal branch
Internal laryngeal nerve
Thyrohyoid
External laryngeal nerve
Cricothyroid
Trachea
Right recurrent laryngeal nerve
Right lateral view

FIGURE 8.40. Laryngeal branches of right vagus nerve (CN X). The nerves of the larynx are the internal and external branches of the superior laryngeal nerve and the inferior laryngeal nerve from the recurrent laryngeal nerve. The right recurrent laryngeal nerve passes inferior to the right subclavian artery.

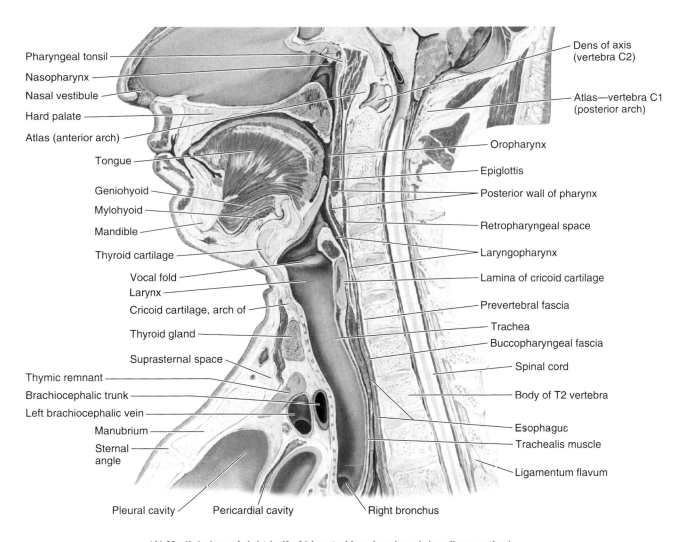

Pharyngeal tonsil
Nasopharynx
Nasal vestibule
Hard palate
Atlas (anterior arch)
Tongue
Geniohyoid
Mylohyoid
Mandible
Thyroid cartilage
Vocal fold
Larynx
Cricoid cartilage, arch of
Thyroid gland
Suprasternal space
Thymic remnant
Brachiocephalic trunk
Left brachiocephalic vein
Manubrium
Sternal angle
Pleural cavity
Pericardial cavity

Dens of axis (vertebra C2)
Atlas—vertebra C1 (posterior arch)
Oropharynx
Epiglottis
Posterior wall of pharynx
Retropharyngeal space
Laryngopharynx
Lamina of cricoid cartilage
Prevertebral fascia
Trachea
Buccopharyngeal fascia
Spinal cord
Body of T2 vertebra
Esophagus
Trachealis muscle
Ligamentum flavum
Right bronchus

(A) Medial view of right half of bisected head and neck (median section)

Plane of coronal MRI study in Fig 8.35B
Tongue
Oropharynx
Genioglossus
Geniohyoid
Hyoid bone
Thyroid cartilage
Vestibular fold
Ventricle
Vocal fold
Trachea
Tracheal ring

Epiglottic vallecula
Epiglottis
Cricoid cartilage
Esophagus

(B) Parasagittal MRI study of pharynx, larynx and trachea

FIGURE 8.41. Median sections of head and neck. A. The pharynx extends from the cranial base to the level of the cricoid cartilage (body of C6 vertebra or the C6–C7 IV disc, as shown here), where it is continuous with the esophagus. **B.** This sagittal section does not demonstrate the continuities of the upper respiratory tract because the soft palate is elevated, closing off the nasopharynx, and the plane of section passes through the vestibular and vocal folds to the side of the rima glottidis. (Part **B** Courtesy of Dr. W. Kucharczyk, University Health Network, Toronto, Ontario, Canada.)

The abundant lymphoid tissue in the pharynx forms an incomplete *tonsillar ring* around the superior part of the pharynx (discussed later in this chapter, p. 1038). The lymphoid tissue is aggregated in certain regions to form masses called *tonsils.* The **pharyngeal tonsil** (commonly called the adenoid when enlarged) is in the mucous membrane of the roof and posterior wall of the nasopharynx (Figs. 8.41A and 8.43). Extending inferiorly from the medial end of the pharyngotympanic tube is a vertical fold of mucous membrane, the **salpingopharyngeal fold** (Figs. 8.42 and 8.43B). It covers the salpingopharyngeus muscle, which opens the pharyngeal orifice of the pharyngotympanic tube during swallowing. The collection of lymphoid tissue in the submucosa of the pharynx near the nasopharyngeal opening, or orifice of the pharyngotympanic tube, is the **tubal tonsils** (Fig. 8.43B). Posterior to the **torus of the pharyngotympanic tube** and the salpingopharyngeal fold is a slit-like lateral projection of the pharynx, the **pharyngeal recess,** which extends laterally and posteriorly.

The **oropharynx** has a digestive function. It is bounded by the soft palate superiorly, the base of the tongue inferiorly, and the palatoglossal and palatopharyngeal arches laterally

(Figs. 8.43 and 8.44A). It extends from the soft palate to the superior border of the epiglottis.

Deglutition (swallowing) is the complex process that transfers a food bolus from the mouth through the pharynx and esophagus into the stomach. Solid food is masticated (chewed) and mixed with saliva to form a soft bolus (mass) that is easier to swallow. Deglutition occurs in three stages:

- **Stage 1:** voluntary; the bolus is compressed against the palate and pushed from the mouth into the oropharynx, mainly by movements of the muscles of the tongue and soft palate (Fig. 8.45A & B).
- **Stage 2:** involuntary and rapid; the soft palate is elevated, sealing off the nasopharynx from the oropharynx and laryngopharynx (Fig. 8.45C). The pharynx widens and shortens to receive the bolus of food as the suprahyoid muscles and longitudinal pharyngeal muscles contract, elevating the larynx.
- **Stage 3:** involuntary; sequential contraction of all three pharyngeal constrictor muscles creates a peristaltic ridge that forces the food bolus inferiorly into the esophagus (Fig. 8.45B-D).

(A) Anterior view through widely opened mouth

Soft palate — Uvula — Posterior wall of oropharynx — *Fold overlying pterygomandibular raphe — Palatopharyngeal arch — Palatoglossal arch (dotted lines) — Palatine tonsils (circled) — Dorsum of tongue

(B) Lateral view

Palatoglossus — Tonsillar branch of facial artery — Styloglossus — Tonsillar bed — Submandibular gland — Glossopharyngeal nerve (CN IX) — Hyoglossus — Stylohyoid ligament — Middle pharyngeal constrictor — Pharyngeal recess — Superior pharyngeal constrictor — Palatopharyngeus — Prevertebral fascia — Retropharyngeal space — **External palatine vein** — Buccopharyngeal fascia — Stylopharyngeus

FIGURE 8.44. Oral cavity and tonsillar bed. A. The oral cavity and palatine tonsils in a young child, with the mouth wide open and the tongue protruding as far as possible. The uvula is a muscular projection from the posterior edge of the soft palate. **B.** In this deep dissection of the tonsillar bed, the palatine tonsil has been removed. The tongue is pulled anteriorly, and the inferior (lingual) attachment of the superior pharyngeal constrictor muscle is cut away.

Deglutition (swallowing)

FIGURE 8.45. Deglutition. A. The bolus of food is squeezed to the back of the mouth by pushing the tongue against the palate. **B.** The nasopharynx is sealed off and the larynx is elevated, enlarging the pharynx to receive food. **C.** The pharyngeal sphincters contract sequentially, creating a "peristaltic ridge," squeezing food into the esophagus. The epiglottis deflects the bolus from but does not close the inlet to the larynx and trachea. **D.** The bolus of food moves down the esophagus by peristaltic contractions.

The **palatine tonsils** are collections of lymphoid tissue on each side of the oropharynx in the interval between the palatine arches (Figs. 8.43 and 8.44A). The tonsil does not fill the **tonsillar sinus** (fossa) between the palatoglossal and palatopharyngeal arches in adults. The submucosal **tonsillar bed,** in which the palatine tonsil lies, is between these arches (Fig. 8.44B). The tonsillar bed is formed by the

superior pharyngeal constrictor and the thin, fibrous sheet of **pharyngobasilar fascia** (Fig. 8.46A & B). This fascia blends with the periosteum of the cranial base and defines the limits of the pharyngeal wall in its superior part.

The **laryngopharynx** lies posterior to the larynx (Figs. 8.41A and 8.43), extending from the superior border of the epiglottis and the pharyngo-epiglottic folds to the inferior

(A) Posterior view

FIGURE 8.46. Pharynx and cranial nerves. A. This dissection shows the posterior aspect of the pharynx and associated structures. The buccopharyngeal fascia has been removed. Of the three pharyngeal constrictor muscles, the inferior muscle overlaps the middle one and the middle one overlaps the superior one. All three muscles form a common median pharyngeal raphe posteriorly.

the cervicodorsal trunk. The main group of deep cervical lymph nodes forms a chain along the IJV, mostly under cover of the SCM. Other deep cervical nodes include the prelaryngeal, pretracheal, paratracheal, and retropharyngeal nodes. Efferent lymphatic vessels from the deep cervical nodes join to form the **jugular lymphatic trunks,** which usually join the thoracic duct on the left side and enter the junction of the internal jugular and subclavian veins (right venous angle) directly or via a short right lymphatic duct on the right.

The **thoracic duct** passes superiorly through the superior thoracic aperture along the left border of the esophagus. It arches laterally in the root of the neck, posterior to the carotid sheath and anterior to the sympathetic trunk and vertebral and subclavian arteries (Fig. 8.51B). The thoracic duct enters the left brachiocephalic vein at the junction of the subclavian and IJVs (*left venous angle*). When the right jugular, subclavian, and bronchomediastinal lymphatic trunks unite to form a *right lymphatic duct*, it enters the right venous angle as the thoracic duct does on the left (Fig. 8.51A). Often, however, these lymphatic trunks enter the venous system independently in the region of the right venous angle.

LYMPHATICS IN NECK
Radical Neck Dissections

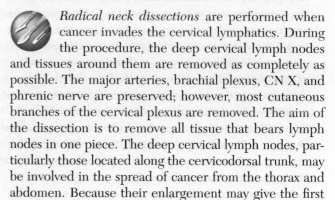 *Radical neck dissections* are performed when cancer invades the cervical lymphatics. During the procedure, the deep cervical lymph nodes and tissues around them are removed as completely as possible. The major arteries, brachial plexus, CN X, and phrenic nerve are preserved; however, most cutaneous branches of the cervical plexus are removed. The aim of the dissection is to remove all tissue that bears lymph nodes in one piece. The deep cervical lymph nodes, particularly those located along the cervicodorsal trunk, may be involved in the spread of cancer from the thorax and abdomen. Because their enlargement may give the first clue to cancer in these regions, they are often referred to as the *cervical sentinel lymph nodes.*

thePoint. **Board-review questions, case studies, and additional resources are available at thePoint.lww.com.**

Summary of Cranial Nerves

FIGURE 9.8. **Distribution of oculomotor (CN III), trochlear (CN IV), and abducent (CN VI) nerves.** CN IV supplies the superior oblique, CN VI supplies the lateral rectus, and CN III supplies five striated extra-ocular muscles (levator palpebrae superioris, superior rectus, medial rectus, inferior rectus, and inferior oblique) and two intra-ocular muscles (ciliary muscle and sphincter pupillae muscle—not shown; see Chapter 7, p. 896).

The oculomotor nerve (CN III) provides the following (Fig. 9.8):

- Motor to the striated muscle of four of the six extra-ocular muscles (*superior, medial,* and *inferior recti* and *inferior oblique*) and superior eyelid (L. *levator palpebrae superioris*); hence the nerve's name.
- Parasympathetic through the ciliary ganglion to the smooth muscle of the sphincter pupillae, which causes constriction of the pupil and ciliary muscle, which produces accommodation (allowing the lens to become more rounded) for near vision.

CN III is the chief motor nerve to the ocular and extra-ocular muscles. It emerges from the midbrain, pierces the dura mater lateral to the sellar diaphragm roofing over the hypophysis, and then runs through the roof and lateral wall of the *cavernous sinus.* CN III leaves the cranial cavity and enters the orbit through the *superior orbital fissure.* Within this fissure, CN III divides into a **superior division** (which supplies the superior rectus and levator palpebrae superioris) and an **inferior division** (which supplies the inferior and medial rectus and inferior oblique). The inferior division also carries presynaptic parasympathetic (visceral efferent) fibers to the *ciliary ganglion,* where they synapse (Fig. 9.4; Table 9.3). Postsynaptic fibers from this ganglion pass to the eyeball in the *short ciliary nerves* to innervate the ciliary body and sphincter pupillae (see Chapter 7, p. 896).

The Bottom Line

OCULOMOTOR NERVE

♦ The oculomotor nerves (CN III) send somatic motor fibers to all extra-ocular muscles, except the superior oblique and lateral rectus. ♦ These nerves also send presynaptic parasympathetic fibers to the ciliary ganglion for innervation of the ciliary body and sphincter pupillae. ♦ These nerves originate from the brainstem, emerging medial to the cerebral peduncles, and run in the lateral wall of the cavernous sinus. ♦ These nerves enter the orbit through the superior orbital fissures and divide into superior and inferior branches.

TROCHLEAR NERVE (CN IV)

Functions: Somatic motor (general somatic efferent) to one extra-ocular muscle (superior oblique).

Nucleus: The **nucleus of the trochlear nerve** is located in the midbrain, immediately caudal to the oculomotor nucleus (Fig. 9.5).

The **trochlear nerve** (CN IV) is the smallest cranial nerve. It emerges from the posterior (dorsal) surface of the midbrain (the only cranial nerve to do so), passing anteriorly around the brainstem. It has the longest *intracranial (subarachnoid) course* of the cranial nerves. The trochlear nerve pierces the dura mater at the margin of the tentorium cerebelli, and passes anteriorly in the lateral wall of the cavernous sinus (Fig. 9.8). CN IV then continues through the superior orbital fissure into the orbit, where it supplies the superior oblique—the only extra-ocular muscle that uses a pulley, or trochlea, to redirect its line of action (hence the nerve's name).

The Bottom Line

TROCHLEAR NERVE

♦ The trochlear nerves (CN IV) supply somatic motor fibers to the superior oblique muscles, which abduct, depress, and medially rotate the pupil. ♦ The trochlear nerves emerge from the posterior aspect of the brainstem. ♦ The nerves run a long intracranial course, passing around the brainstem to enter the dura mater in the free edge of the tentorium cerebelli close to the posterior clinoid process. ♦ The nerves then run in the lateral wall of the cavernous sinus, entering the orbit via the superior orbital fissures.

TRIGEMINAL NERVE (CN V)

Functions: Somatic (general) sensory and somatic (branchial) motor to derivatives of the 1st pharyngeal arch.

Nuclei: There are four trigeminal nuclei (Fig. 9.5)—one motor (**motor nucleus of trigeminal nerve**), and three sensory (**mesencephalic, principal sensory and spinal nuclei of trigeminal nerve**).

The **trigeminal nerve** (CN V) is the largest cranial nerve (if the atypical optic nerve is excluded). It emerges from the lateral aspect of the pons by a large sensory root and a small motor root (Fig. 9.3). The roots of CN V are comparable to the posterior and anterior roots of spinal nerves. CN V is the principal somatic (general) sensory nerve for the head (face, teeth, mouth, nasal cavity, and dura mater of the cranial cavity). The large **sensory root of CN V** is composed mainly of the central processes of the pseudounipolar neurons that make up the sensory **trigeminal ganglion** (Fig. 9.9). The ganglion is flattened and crescent shaped (hence its unofficial name, semilunar ganglion), and is housed within a dural recess (**trigeminal cave**) lateral to the cavernous sinus.

The peripheral processes of the ganglionic neurons form three nerves or divisions: *ophthalmic nerve (CN V₁), maxillary nerve (CN V₂),* and sensory component of the *mandibular nerve (CN V₃).* Maps of the zones of cutaneous innervation by the three divisions resemble the dermatome maps for cutaneous innervation by spinal nerves (Fig. 9.9A). Unlike spinal nerve dermatomes, however, there is little overlap in innervation by the divisions; lesions of a single nerve result in clearly demarcated areas of numbness.

The fibers of the **motor root of CN V** pass inferior to the trigeminal ganglion along the floor of the trigeminal cave, bypassing the ganglion (just as the anterior roots of spinal nerves bypass the spinal sensory ganglia). They are distributed exclusively via the mandibular nerve (CN V₃), blending with the sensory fibers as the nerve traverses the foramen ovale in the cranium. Branches pass to the muscles of mastication, mylohyoid, anterior belly of the digastric, tensor veli palatini, and tensor tympani, which are derived from the 1st pharyngeal arch.

Although CN V conveys no presynaptic parasympathetic fibers from the CNS, all four parasympathetic ganglia are associated with the divisions of CN V. Postsynaptic parasympathetic fibers from the ganglia join branches of CN V and are carried to their destinations along with the CN V sensory and motor fibers (Fig. 9.9; Table 9.3).

Ophthalmic Nerve (CN V₁)

In contrast to the other two CN V divisions, CN V₁ is not a branchial nerve (i.e., it does not supply pharyngeal arch derivatives). It serves structures derived from the paraxial mesoderm of the embryonic frontonasal process. The ophthalmic nerve's association with the other CN V divisions is a secondary occurrence. The somatic (general) sensory fibers of CN V₁ are distributed to skin and mucous membranes and conjunctiva of the front of the head and nose (Fig. 9.9).

Testing CN V₁: The integrity of this division is tested by checking the corneal reflex—touching the cornea, which is also supplied by CN V₁, with a wisp of cotton will evoke a reflexive blink if the nerve is functional (Table 9.4).

Maxillary Nerve (CN V₂)

CN V₂ innervates derivatives of the maxillary prominence of the 1st pharyngeal arch. Exiting the cranial cavity via the foramen rotundum, its somatic (general) sensory fibers are generally distributed to skin and mucous membranes associated with the upper jaw. The pterygopalatine (parasympathetic) ganglion is associated with this division of CN V, involved in innervating the lacrimal gland and glands of the nose and palate.

Mandibular Nerve (CN V₃)

CN V₃ innervates derivatives of the mandibular prominence of the 1st pharyngeal arch. CN V₃ is the only division of CN V to convey somatic (branchial) motor fibers, distributed to the striated muscle derived from mandibular prominence mesoderm, primarily the muscles of mastication. Two parasympathetic ganglia, the otic and submandibular, are associated with this division of CN V; both are concerned with the innervation of salivary glands.

Tables 9.1 and 9.2 provide a general summary of CN V. Table 9.4 summarizes the branches of the three divisions.

(A) Parasympathetic (visceral motor) to lacrimal gland

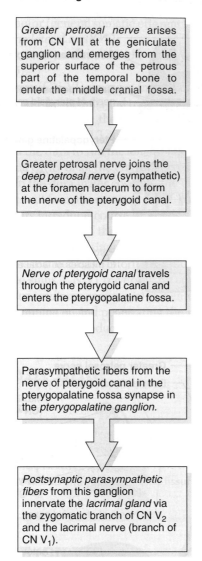

Greater petrosal nerve arises from CN VII at the geniculate ganglion and emerges from the superior surface of the petrous part of the temporal bone to enter the middle cranial fossa.

Greater petrosal nerve joins the *deep petrosal nerve* (sympathetic) at the foramen lacerum to form the nerve of the pterygoid canal.

Nerve of pterygoid canal travels through the pterygoid canal and enters the pterygopalatine fossa.

Parasympathetic fibers from the nerve of pterygoid canal in the pterygopalatine fossa synapse in the *pterygopalatine ganglion*.

Postsynaptic parasympathetic fibers from this ganglion innervate the *lacrimal gland* via the zygomatic branch of CN V_2 and the lacrimal nerve (branch of CN V_1).

(B) Parasympathetic (visceral motor) to submandibular and sublingual glands

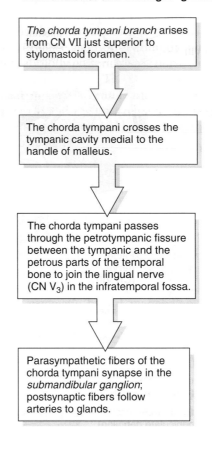

The chorda tympani branch arises from CN VII just superior to stylomastoid foramen.

The chorda tympani crosses the tympanic cavity medial to the handle of malleus.

The chorda tympani passes through the petrotympanic fissure between the tympanic and the petrous parts of the temporal bone to join the lingual nerve (CN V_3) in the infratemporal fossa.

Parasympathetic fibers of the chorda tympani synapse in the *submandibular ganglion*; postsynaptic fibers follow arteries to glands.

FIGURE 9.11. Parasympathetic innervation involving CN VII. A. Innervation of the lacrimal gland. **B.** Innervation of the submandibular and sublingual glands.

The Bottom Line

FACIAL NERVE

♦ The facial nerves (CN VII) supply motor fibers to the stapedius, posterior belly of the digastric, stylohyoid, facial, and scalp muscles. ♦ They also supply presynaptic parasympathetic fibers via the intermediate nerve (smaller root of CN VII) destined for the pterygopalatine and submandibular ganglia via the greater petrosal nerve and chorda tympani, respectively. ♦ CN VII is sensory to some skin of the external acoustic meatus and, via the intermediate nerve, is sensory to taste from the anterior two thirds of the tongue and the soft palate. ♦ CN VII originates from the posterior border of the pons and runs through the internal acoustic meatus and facial canal in the petrous part of the temporal bone. ♦ CN VII exits via the stylomastoid foramen; its main trunk forms the intraparotid nerve plexus.

VESTIBULOCOCHLEAR NERVE (CN VIII)

Functions: Special sensory (special somatic afferent)—that is, special sensations of hearing, equilibrium, and motion (acceleration/deceleration).

Nuclei: Vestibular nuclei are located at the junction of the pons and medulla in the lateral part of the floor of the 4th ventricle; the **cochlear nuclei**, anterior and posterior, are in the medulla (Fig. 9.5).

The **vestibulocochlear nerve** (CN VIII) emerges from the junction of the pons and medulla and enters the *internal acoustic meatus* (Figs. 9.2 and 9.3). Here it separates into the vestibular and cochlear nerves (Fig. 9.12).

- The **vestibular nerve** is composed of the central processes of bipolar neurons in the **vestibular ganglion.**

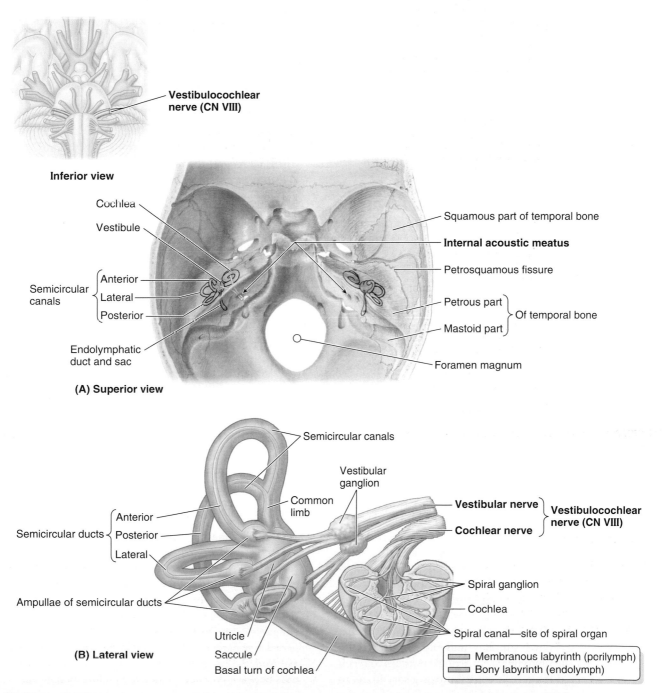

FIGURE 9.12. Vestibulocochlear nerve (CN VIII). A. The internal surface of the cranial base shows the location of the bony labyrinth of the internal ear within the temporal bone. **B.** This view of the bony and membranous labyrinths shows (1) innervation of the cochlea by the cochlear nerve of CN VIII for the sense of hearing and (2) innervation of the vestibular apparatus by the vestibular nerve of CN VIII for equilibrium and motion.

The peripheral processes of the neurons extend to the *maculae of the utricle and saccule* (sensitive to linear acceleration and the pull of gravity relative to the position of the head) and to the cristae of the ampullae of the semicircular ducts (sensitive to rotational acceleration).

- The **cochlear nerve** is composed of the central processes of bipolar neurons in the **spiral ganglion;** the peripheral processes of the neurons extend to the spiral organ for the sense of hearing.

Within the internal acoustic meatus, the two divisions of CN VIII are accompanied by the primary root and intermediate nerve of CN VII and the labyrinthine artery (see Chapter 7).

The Bottom Line

VESTIBULOCOCHLEAR NERVE

♦ The vestibulocochlear nerves (CN VIII) carry fibers concerned with the special senses of hearing, equilibrium, and motion. ♦ The nerves originate from the grooves between the pons and medulla. ♦ They run through the internal acoustic meatus and divide into the cochlear and vestibular nerves. ♦ The cochlear nerve is sensory to the spiral organ (for the sense of hearing). ♦ The vestibular nerve is sensory to the cristae of the ampullae of the semicircular ducts and the maculae of the saccule and utricle (for the sense of equilibration and motion).

GLOSSOPHARYNGEAL NERVE (CN IX)

Functions: *Sensory*—somatic (general) sensory, special sensory (taste), and visceral sensory. *Motor*—somatic (branchial) motor, and visceral (parasympathetic) motor for derivatives of the 3rd pharyngeal arch.

Nuclei: Four nuclei in the medulla send or receive fibers via CN IX: two motor (*nucleus ambiguus* and **inferior salivary nucleus**) and two sensory (*sensory nuclei of the trigeminal nerve* [CN V] and *nuclei of the solitary tract*). Three of these nuclei (in italics) are shared with CN X (Fig. 9.5).

The **glossopharyngeal nerve** (CN IX) emerges from the lateral aspect of the medulla and passes anterolaterally to leave the cranium through the anterior aspect of the *jugular foramen* (Figs. 9.13 and 9.14). At this foramen are the sensory **superior** and **inferior ganglia of CN IX,** which contain the pseudounipolar cell bodies for the afferent components of the nerve. CN IX follows the *stylopharyngeus,* the only muscle the nerve supplies, and passes between the superior and middle pharyngeal constrictor muscles to reach the oropharynx and tongue. It contributes sensory fibers to the *pharyngeal plexus of nerves.* CN IX is afferent from the tongue and pharynx (hence its name) and efferent to the stylopharyngeus and parotid gland.

Somatic (Branchial) Motor

Motor fibers pass to one muscle, the stylopharyngeus, derived from the 3rd pharyngeal arch.

Visceral (Parasympathetic) Motor

Following a circuitous route initially involving the tympanic nerve, presynaptic parasympathetic fibers are provided to the *otic ganglion* for innervation of the parotid gland (Fig. 9.15). The otic ganglion is associated with the mandibular nerve (CN V$_3$), branches of which convey the postsynaptic parasympathetic fibers to the parotid gland.

Somatic (General) Sensory

The general sensory branches of CN IX are as follows (Fig. 9.13):

- The *tympanic nerve.*
- The *carotid sinus nerve* to the carotid sinus, a baro- (presso-) receptor sensitive to changes in blood pressure, and the carotid body, a chemoreceptor sensitive to blood gas (oxygen and carbon dioxide levels).
- The *pharyngeal, tonsillar,* and *lingual nerves* to the mucosa of the oropharynx and isthmus of the fauces (L., throat), including palatine tonsil, soft palate, and posterior third of the tongue. In addition to general sensation (touch, pain, temperature), tactile (actual or threatened) stimuli determined to be unusual or unpleasant here may evoke the gag reflex or even vomiting.

Special Sensory (Taste)

Taste fibers are conveyed from the posterior third of the tongue to the sensory inferior ganglia of CN IX (Fig. 9.14). Details of the distribution of CN IX are outlined in Figure 9.13.

The Bottom Line

GLOSSOPHARYNGEAL NERVE

♦ The glossopharyngeal nerves (CN IX) send somatic motor fibers to the stylopharyngeus and visceral motor (presynaptic parasympathetic) fibers to the otic ganglion for innervation of the parotid gland. ♦ They also send sensory fibers to the posterior third of the tongue (including taste), pharynx, tympanic cavity, pharyngotympanic cavity, carotid body, and carotid sinus. ♦ The nerves originate from the rostral end of the medulla and exit from the cranium via the jugular foramina. ♦ They pass between the superior and the middle pharyngeal constrictors to the tonsillar sinus and enter the posterior third of the tongue.

FIGURE 9.13. Distribution of glossopharyngeal nerve (CN IX). A. CN IX is motor to one striated pharyngeal muscle, the stylopharyngeus. It also carries sensory fibers from the carotid body and carotid sinus, conveying information about blood pressure and gas levels as well as somatic (general) sensation from the internal ear, pharynx, and fauces and taste from the posterior tongue. **B.** The parasympathetic component of CN IX supplies presynaptic secretory fibers to the otic ganglion; postsynaptic fibers pass to the parotid gland via the auriculotemporal nerve (CN V₃).

VAGUS NERVE (CN X)

Functions: *Sensory*—somatic (general) sensory, special sensory (taste), visceral sensory. *Motor*—somatic (branchial) motor and visceral (parasympathetic) motor.

- Somatic (general) sensory from the inferior pharynx, and larynx.
- Visceral sensory from the thoracic and abdominal organs.
- Taste and somatic (general) sensation from the root of the tongue and taste buds on the epiglottis. Branches of the internal laryngeal nerve (a branch of CN X) supply a small area, mostly somatic (general) sensory, but also some special sensation (taste).

- Somatic (branchial) motor to the soft palate; pharynx; intrinsic laryngeal muscles (phonation); and a nominal extrinsic tongue muscle, the palatoglossus, which is actually a palatine muscle based on its derivation and innervation.
- Proprioceptive to the muscles listed above.
- Visceral (parasympathetic) motor to thoracic and abdominal viscera.

Nuclei: *Sensory*—sensory nucleus of the trigeminal nerve (somatic sensory) and nuclei of the solitary tract (taste and visceral sensory). *Motor*—nucleus ambiguus (somatic [branchial] motor) and **dorsal vagal nucleus** (visceral [parasympathetic] motor) (Fig. 9.5).

TABLE 9.5. SUMMARY OF VAGUS NERVE (CN X)

Divisions (Parts)	Branches
Cranial Vagi arise by a series of rootlets from medulla (includes traditional cranial root of CN XI)	Meningeal branch to dura mater (sensory; actually fibers of C2 spinal ganglion neurons that hitch a ride with vagus nerve) Auricular branch
Cervical Exit cranium/enter neck through jugular foramen; right and left vagus nerves enter carotid sheaths and continue to root of neck	Pharyngeal branches to pharyngeal plexus (motor) Cervical cardiac branches (parasympathetic, visceral afferent) Superior laryngeal nerve (mixed) internal (sensory) and external (motor) branches Right recurrent laryngeal nerve (mixed)
Thoracic Vagi enter thorax through superior thoracic aperture; left vagus contributes to anterior esophageal plexus; right vagus to posterior plexus; form anterior and posterior vagal trunks	Left recurrent laryngeal nerve (mixed; all distal branches convey parasympathetic and visceral afferent fibers for reflex stimuli) Thoracic cardiac branches Pulmonary branches Esophageal plexus
Abdominal Anterior and posterior vagal trunks enter abdomen through esophageal hiatus in diaphragm; distribute asymmetrically	Esophageal branches Gastric branches Hepatic branches Celiac branches (from posterior vagal trunk) Pyloric branch (from anterior vagal trunk) Renal branches Intestinal branches (to left colic flexure)

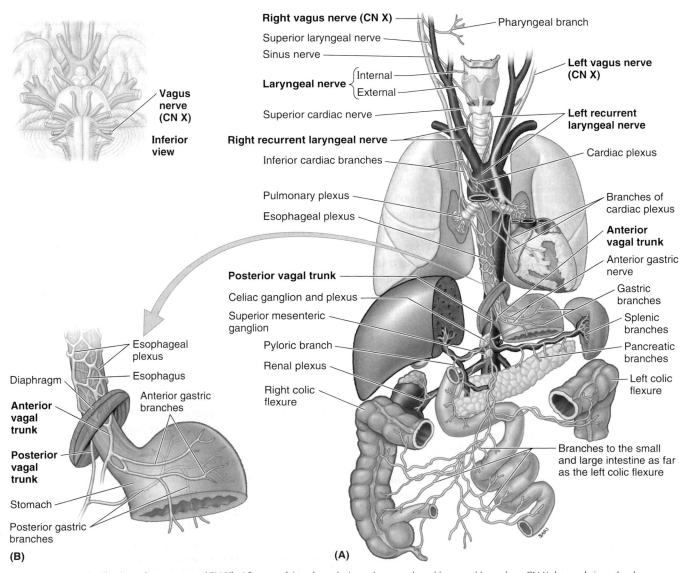

FIGURE 9.16. Distribution of vagus nerve (CN X). After supplying the palatine, pharyngeal, and laryngeal branches, CN X descends into the thorax. The recurrent laryngeal nerves ascend to the larynx, the left from a more inferior (thoracic) level. In the abdomen, the anterior and posterior vagal trunks demonstrate further asymmetry as they supply the terminal esophagus, stomach, and intestinal tract as far distally as the left colic flexure.

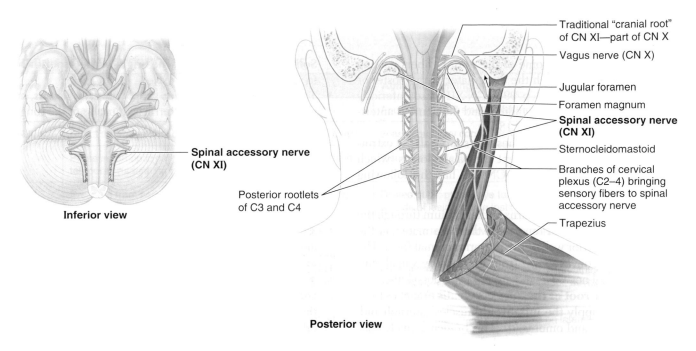

Inferior view

Traditional "cranial root" of CN XI—part of CN X

Vagus nerve (CN X)

Jugular foramen

Foramen magnum

Spinal accessory nerve (CN XI)

Sternocleidomastoid

Branches of cervical plexus (C2–4) bringing sensory fibers to spinal accessory nerve

Trapezius

Spinal accessory nerve (CN XI)

Posterior rootlets of C3 and C4

Posterior view

FIGURE 9.17. Distribution of spinal accessory nerve (CN XI).

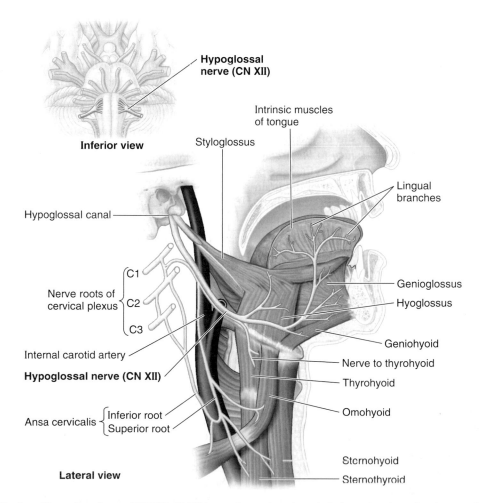

Hypoglossal nerve (CN XII)

Inferior view

Styloglossus

Intrinsic muscles of tongue

Lingual branches

Hypoglossal canal

Nerve roots of cervical plexus — C1, C2, C3

Internal carotid artery

Hypoglossal nerve (CN XII)

Ansa cervicalis — Inferior root / Superior root

Genioglossus

Hyoglossus

Geniohyoid

Nerve to thyrohyoid

Thyrohyoid

Omohyoid

Sternohyoid

Sternothyroid

Lateral view

FIGURE 9.18. **Distribution of hypoglossal nerve (CN XII).** CN XII leaves the cranium through the hypoglossal canal and passes deep to the mandible to enter the tongue, where it supplies all intrinsic and extrinsic lingual muscles, except the palatoglossus. CN XII is joined immediately distal to the hypoglossal canal by a branch conveying fibers from the C1 and C2 loop of the cervical plexus. These fibers hitch a ride with CN XII, leaving it as the superior root of the ansa cervicalis and the nerve to the thyrohyoid muscle. Cervical spinal nerves, not CN XII, supply the infrahyoid muscles.

VESTIBULOCOCHLEAR NERVE

Injuries to Vestibulocochlear Nerve

 Although the vestibular and cochlear nerves are essentially independent, peripheral lesions often produce concurrent clinical effects because of their close relationship. Hence *lesions of CN VIII* may cause *tinnitus* (ringing or buzzing in ears), *vertigo* (dizziness, loss of balance), and impairment or loss of hearing. Central lesions may involve either the cochlear or vestibular divisions of CN VIII.

Deafness

There are two kinds of deafness (hearing loss): *conductive deafness*, involving the external or middle ear (e.g., otitis media, inflammation in the middle ear), and *sensorineural deafness*, which results from disease in the cochlea or in the pathway from the cochlea to the brain.

Acoustic Neuroma

An *acoustic neuroma* (neurofibroma) is a slow-growing benign tumor of the neurolemma (Schwann) cells. The tumor begins in the vestibular nerve while it is in the internal acoustic meatus. The early symptom of an acoustic neuroma is usually loss of hearing. Dysequilibrium (derangement of the sense of equilibrium) and tinnitus occur in approximately 70% of patients (Bruce et al., 2010).

Trauma and Vertigo

People with head trauma often experience headache, dizziness, vertigo, and other features of post-traumatic injury. *Vertigo* is a hallucination of movement involving the person or the environment (Wazen, 2010). It often involves a spinning sensation but may be felt as a swaying back and forth or falling. These symptoms, often accompanied by nausea and vomiting, are usually related to a peripheral vestibular nerve lesion.

GLOSSOPHARYNGEAL NERVE

Lesions of Glossopharyngeal Nerve

Isolated *lesions of CN IX* or its nuclei are uncommon and are not associated with perceptible disability (Brannagan et al., 2010). Taste is absent on the posterior third of the tongue, and the gag reflex is absent on the side of the lesion. Ipsilateral weakness may produce a noticeable change in swallowing.

Injuries of CN IX resulting from infection or tumors are usually accompanied by signs of involvement of adjacent nerves. Because CN IX, CN X, and CN XI pass through the jugular foramen, tumors in this region produce multiple cranial nerve palsies, called the *jugular foramen syndrome*. Pain in the distribution of CN IX may be associated with involvement of the nerve in a tumor in the neck.

Glossopharyngeal Neuralgia

Glossopharyngeal neuralgia (glossopharyngeal tic) is uncommon and its cause is unknown. The sudden intensification of pain is of a burning or stabbing nature. These paroxysms of pain are often initiated by swallowing, protruding the tongue, talking, or touching the palatine tonsil (Brannagan et al., 2010). Pain paroxysms occur during eating when trigger areas are stimulated.

VAGUS NERVE

Isolated *lesions of CN X* are uncommon. Injury to pharyngeal branches of CN X results in *dysphagia* (difficulty in swallowing). Lesions of the superior laryngeal nerve produce anesthesia of the superior part of the larynx and paralysis of the cricothyroid muscle (see Chapter 8). The voice is weak and tires easily. Injury of a recurrent laryngeal nerve may be caused by aneurysms of the arch of the aorta and may occur during neck operations. Injury of the recurrent laryngeal nerve causes hoarseness and *dysphonia* (difficulty in speaking) because of paralysis of the vocal folds (cords). Paralysis of both recurrent laryngeal nerves causes *aphonia* (loss of voice) and *inspiratory stridor* (a harsh, high pitched respiratory sound). Paralysis of recurrent laryngeal nerves usually results from cancer of the larynx and thyroid gland and/or from injury during surgery on the thyroid gland, neck, esophagus, heart, and lungs. Because of its longer course, lesions of the left recurrent laryngeal nerve are more common than those of the right. Proximal lesions of CN X also affect the pharyngeal and superior laryngeal nerves, causing difficulty in swallowing and speaking.

SPINAL ACCESSORY NERVE

 Because of its nearly subcutaneous passage through the posterior cervical region, *iatrogenic* (physician-caused) *injury of CN XI* may occur during surgical procedures such as lymph node biopsy, cannulation of the internal jugular vein, and carotid endarterectomy (see Chapter 8).

HYPOGLOSSAL NERVE

Injury to CN XII paralyzes the ipsilateral half of the tongue. After some time, the tongue atrophies, making it appear shrunken and wrinkled. When the tongue is protruded, its apex deviates toward the paralyzed side because of the unopposed action of the genioglossus muscle on the normal side of the tongue (see Chapter 7).

INTRODUCTION

Bergman RA, Thompson SA, Afifi AK, Saadeh FA: *Compendium of Human Anatomic Variation: Text, Atlas, and World Literature.* Baltimore, Urban & Schwarzenberg, 1988. This useful source has been updated and is available from the Virtual Hospital's Web site *Illustrated Encyclopedia of Human Anatomic Variation* at www.vh.org/Providers/Textbooks/AnatomicVariants/AnatomyHP.html, 2008.

Federative Committee on Anatomical Terminology: *Terminologia Anatomica: International Anatomical Nomenclature.* Stuttgart, Thieme, 1998.

Haines DE (ed): *Fundamental Neuroscience for Basic and Clinical Applications,* 3rd ed. New York, Churchill Livingstone (Elsevier), 2006.

Hutchins JB, Naftel JP, Ard MD: The cell biology of neurons and glia. *In* Haines DE (ed): *Fundamental Neuroscience,* 4th ed. Saunders/Elsevier, 2012.

Keegan JJ, Garrett FD: The segmental distribution of the cutaneous nerves in the limbs of man. *Anat Rec* 102:409, 1948.

Kliegman RM, Stanton BMD, St. Geme J, Schor NF and Behrman RE (eds): *Nelson Textbook of Pediatrics,* 19th ed. Philadelphia, Saunders/Elsevier, 2011.

Kumar V, Abbas AK, Fausto N, Aster J: *Robbins and Cotran Pathologic Basis of Disease,* 8th ed. Philadelphia, Saunders/Elsevier, 2009.

Maklad A, Quinn T, Fritsch B: Intracranial distribution of the sympathetic system in mice: DiI tracing and immunocytochemical labeling. *Anat Rec* 263:99, 2001.

Marieb E and Hoehn K: *Human Anatomy and Physiology,* 9th ed. Menlo Park, CA, Benjamin/Cummings, 2012.

Moore KL, Persaud TVN and Torchia MG: *The Developing Human: Clinically Oriented Embryology,* 9th ed. Philadelphia, Saunders/Elsevier, 2012.

O'Rahilly R: Making planes plain. *Clin Anat* 10:129, 1997.

Ross MH, Pawlina W: *Histology. A Text and Atlas,* 6th ed. Baltimore, Lippincott Williams & Wilkins, 2011.

Salter RB: *Textbook of Disorders and Injuries of the Musculoskeletal System,* 3rd ed. Baltimore, Lippincott Williams & Wilkins, 1998.

Stedman's Medical Dictionary, 28th ed. Baltimore, Lippincott Williams & Wilkins, 2006.

Swartz MH: *Textbook of Physical Diagnosis, History and Examination,* 6th ed. Philadelphia, Saunders/Elsevier, 2009.

Willis MC: *Medical Terminology: The Language of Health Care,* 2nd ed. Baltimore, Lippincott Williams & Wilkins, 2005.

Wilson-Pauwels L, Stewart PA, Akesson E: *Autonomic Nerves: Basic Science, Clinical Aspects, Case Studies.* Hamilton, ON, Decker, 1997.

CHAPTER 1

Bergman RA, Thompson SA, Afifi AK, Saadeh FA: *Compendium of Human Anatomic Variation: Text, Atlas, and World Literature.* Baltimore, Urban & Schwarzenberg, 1988. This useful source has been updated and is available from the Virtual Hospital's Web site Illustrated Encyclopedia of Human Anatomic Variation at www.vh.org/Providers/Textbooks/AnatomicVariants/AnatomyHP.html (accessed May 2004).

Goroll AH and Mulley AG: *Primary Care Medicine: Office Evaluation and Management of the Adult Patient,* 6th ed. Philadelphia: Lippincott Williams & Wilkins, 2009.

Greene MF, Creasy RK, Resnik R, Iams JD, Lockwood CJ and Moore T: *Creasy and Resnik's Maternal-Fetal Medicine,* 6th ed. Philadelphia, Saunders/Elsevier, 2008.

Hardy SGP, Naftel JP: Viscerosensory pathways. *In* Haines DE (ed): *Fundamental Neuroscience for Basic and Clinical Applications,* 3rd ed. New York, Churchill Livingstone (Elsevier), 2006.

Kliegman RM, Stanton BMD, St. Geme J, Schor NF and Behrman RE (eds): *Nelson Textbook of Pediatrics,* 19th ed. Philadelphia, Saunders/Elsevier, 2011.

Kumar V, Abbas AK, Aster JC, Fausto N: *Robbins & Cotran Pathological Basis of Disease,* 8th ed. Philadelphia, Saunders/Elsevier, 2009.

Marx J, Hockberger R, and Walls R: *Rosen's Emergency Medicine: Concepts and Clinical Practice,* 7th ed. St. Louis, Mosby (Elsevier), 2009.

Moore KL, Persaud TVN and Torchia MG: *The Developing Human. Clinically Oriented Embryology,* 9th ed. Philadelphia, Saunders/Elsevier, 2012.

Rowland LP, Pedley TA (ed): *Merritt's Neurology,* 12th ed. Baltimore, Lippincott Williams & Wilkins, 2009.

Shields TW, LoCicero J, Reed CE, and Feins RH: General Thoracic Surgery, Vol. 1. Baltimore, Lippincott Williams & Wilkins, 2009.

Slaby FJ, McCune SK, Summers RW: *Gross Anatomy in the Practice of Medicine.* Philadelphia: Lea & Febiger, 1994.

Standring S (Editor-in-Chief): *Gray's Anatomy: The Anatomical Basis of Medicine and Surgery,* 40th British ed. London, Churchill Livingstone/Elsevier, 2008.

Swartz MH: *Textbook of Physical Diagnosis, History and Examination,* 6th ed. Philadelphia, Saunders/Elsevier, 2009.

Torrent-Guasp F, Buckberg GD, Clemente C, Cox JL, Coghlan HC, Gharib M: The structure and function of the helical heart and its buttress wrapping. I. The normal macroscopic structure of the heart. *Semin Thoracic Cardiovasc Surg* 13:301–319, 2001.

Vilensky JA, Baltes M, Weikel L, Fortin JD, Fourie LJ: Serratus posterior muscles: Anatomy, clinical relevance, and function. *Clin Anat* 14:237–241, 2001.

Wilson-Pauwels L, Stewart PA, Akesson EJ: *Autonomic Nerves—Basic Science, Clinical Aspects, Case Studies.* Hamilton, ON, Canada, Decker, 1997.

CHAPTER 2

Agur AMR, Dalley AF: *Grant's Atlas of Anatomy,* 13th ed. Baltimore, Lippincott Williams & Wilkins, 2013.

Bickley LS, Szilagyi PG: *Bates' Guide to Physical Examination and History Taking,* 10th ed. Baltimore, Lippincott Williams & Wilkins, 2009.

Cantlie J: On a new arrangement of the right and left lobes of the liver. *J Anat Physiol (Lond)* 32:iv, 1898.

Cheng YF, Huang TL, Chen CL, et al.: Variations of the middle and inferior right hepatic vein: Application in hepatectomy. *J Clin Ultrasound* 25:175, 1997.

Ellis H and Mahadevan: *Clinical Anatomy,* 12th ed. Blackwell Scientific, London 2010.

Fruchaud H: Anatomie chirurgicales des hernies de l'aine. Paris, Doin, 1956. [Cited in Skandalakis LJ, Gadacz TR, Mansberger AR Jr, Mitchell WE Jr, Colborn GL, Skandalakis JE: *Modern Hernia Repair: The Embryological and Anatomical Basis of Surgery.* New York, Parthenon, 1996.]

Kliegman RM, Stanton BMD, St. Geme J, Schor NF and Behrman RE (eds): *Nelson Textbook of Pediatrics,* 19th ed. Philadelphia, Saunders, 2011.

Kumar V, Abbas AK, Fausto N: *Robbins & Cotran Pathological Basis of Disease,* 8th ed. Philadelphia, Saunders/Elsevier, 2009.

Magee DF, Dalley AF: *Digestion and the Structure and Function of the Gut* [Karger Continuing Education Series, Vol. 8]. Basel, Karger, 1986.